July 27. 04

Encyclopedic Reference of Molecular Pharmacology

Springer
Berlin
Heidelberg
New York
Hong Kong
London
Milan
Paris
Tokyo

STEFAN OFFERMANNS • WALTER ROSENTHAL (EDS.)

Encyclopedic Reference of
Molecular Pharmacology

With 302 Figures and 136 Tables

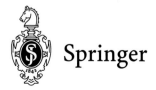

Springer

PROFESSOR DR. STEFAN OFFERMANNS
Pharmakologisches Institut
Universität Heidelberg
Im Neuenheimer Feld 366
69120 Heidelberg
Germany

PROFESSOR DR. WALTER ROSENTHAL
Institut für Pharmakologie,
Freie Universität Berlin,
Thielallee 67-73
D-14195 Berlin,
Germany

ISBN 3-540-42843-7   Springer-Verlag Berlin Heidelberg New York

Library of Congress Cataloging-in-Publication Data

Encyclopedic reference of molecular pharmacology / Stefan Offermanns, Walter Rosenthal, eds.
p. cm.
ISBN 3-540-42843-7 (alk. paper)
1. Molecular pharmacology—Encyclopedias. I. Offermanns, Stefan. II. Rosenthal, Walter.

RM301.65.E53 2003
615'.7'03—dc21
2003041536

Springer-Verlag Berlin Heidelberg New York
a member of BertelsmannSpringer Science+Business Media GmbH

http://www.springer.de

© Springer-Verlag Berlin Heidelberg 2004
Printed in Germany

Production Editor and Typesetting: Frank Krabbes, Heidelberg
Cover design: Erich Kirchner, Heidelberg

Printed on acid-free paper   14/3109 - 5 4 3 2 1 0

We dedicate the *Encyclopedic Reference of Molecular Pharmacology* to Günter Schultz, who has made outstanding contributions to the fields of cellular signal transduction and molecular pharmacology.

Preface

The era of pharmacology, as the science concerned with the understanding of drug action, only began about 150 years ago when Rudolf Buchheim established the first pharmacological laboratory in Dorpat (today Tartu, Estonia). Since then, pharmacology has always been a lively discipline with "open borders", reaching out not only to other life sciences such as physiology, biochemistry, cell biology and clinical medicine, but also to chemistry and physics. In a rather successful initial phase, pharmacologists have devoted their time to describing drug actions either on single organ level or on an entire organism. Over the last few decades, however, research has focused on the molecular mechanisms by which drugs exert their effects. Here, cultured cells or even cell-free systems have served as model systems. As a consequence, our knowledge of the molecular basis of drug actions has increased enormously. The aim of the first *Encyclopedic Reference of Molecular Pharmacology* is to cover this rapidly developing field.

The reductionist approach described above has made it increasingly important to relate the molecular processes underlying drug actions to the drug effect on the level of an organ or whole organism. Only this integrated view will allow the full understanding and prediction of drug actions enabling a rational approach to drug development. On the molecular or even atomic level, new disciplines such as bioinformatics and structural biology have evolved. They have gained major importance within the entire field but are particularly relevant for the rational development and design of new drugs. Finally, the availability of the complete genome sequence of an increasing number of species provides a basis for systematic, genome-wide pharmacological research aimed at the identification of new drug targets and individualised drug treatment (pharmacogenomics and pharmacogenetics). All these aspects are considered in the *Encyclopedic Reference of Molecular Pharmacology*.

The main goal of the *Encyclopedic Reference of Molecular Pharmacology* is to provide up-to-date information on the molecular mechanisms of drug action. Leading experts in the field have provided 159 essays, the core structure of this publication. Most essays describe groups of drugs and drug targets, whereby the emphasis is not just on already exploited drug targets but on potential drug targets as well. Several essays deal with the more general principles of pharmacology, such as drug tolerance, drug addiction or drug metabolism. Others portray important cellular processes or pathological situations and describe how they can be influenced by drugs. The essays are complemented by more than 1600 keywords; essays and keywords are linked to each other. By looking up the keywords or related essays highlighted in each essay the reader can obtain further information related to the respective subject. The alphabetical order of entries makes the encyclopedia very easy to use and help the reader to search successfully. Additionally, all authors are listed alphabetically, together with their essay title, to allow a search by author name.

Apart from very few exceptions, the entries in the main body of the *Encyclopedic Reference of Molecular Pharmacology* do not contain drug names in their titles. Instead, drugs that are commonly used all over the world are listed in the appendix. Also included in the appendix are four extensive sections that contain tables listing proteins such as receptors, transporters or ion channels which are of particular interest as drug targets or modulators of drug action.

The *Encyclopedic Reference of Molecular Pharmacology* provides valuable information for readers with different expectations and backgrounds (from scientists, students and lecturers to informed lay-people) and fills a gap between pharmacology textbooks and specialized review series.

All contributing authors as well as the editors have taken great care to provide up-to-date information. However, inconsistencies or errors may remain, for which we assume full responsibility. We welcome comments, suggestions or corrections and look forward to a stimulating dialog with the readers of the *Encyclopedic Reference of Molecular Pharmacology* whether their comments concern the content of an individual entry or the entire concept.

We are indebted to our colleagues for their excellent contributions. It has been a great experience, both personally and scientifically, to interact with and learn from the 200 plus contributing authors. We would also like to thank Ms. Hana Deuchert and Ms. Katharina Schmalfeld for their excellent and invaluable secretarial assistance during all stages of this project. Within the Springer-Verlag, we are grateful to Dr. Thomas Mager for suggesting the project and also to Frank Krabbes for his technical expertise. Finally, we would like to express our gratitude to Dr. Claudia Lange for successfully managing the project and for her encouraging support. It has been a pleasure to work with her.

Heidelberg / Berlin, June 2003

STEFAN OFFERMANNS and WALTER ROSENTHAL

List of Contributors

ABELL, AMY
National Jewish Center, Immunology & Research Medicine, 1400 Jackson St., Denver, CO 80304, USA
amy.abell@uchsc.edu

ADCOCK, IAN M.
Imperial College London, School of Medicine, National Heart & Lung Institute, Thoracic Medicine, Dovehouse Street, London SW3 6LY, UK
ian.adcock@ic.ac.uk

AGHAJANIAN, GEORGE K.
Yale University School of Medicine, Interdepartmental Neuroscience Program, Section of Neurobiology, Departments of Psychiatry and Pharmacology, 333 Cedar Street, New Haven, CT 06510, USA
george.aghajanian@yale.edu

AKTORIES, KLAUS
Albert-Ludwigs-Universität Freiburg, Institut für Pharmakologie und Toxikologie, Hermann-Herder-Str. 5, 79104 Freiburg, Germany
klaus.aktories@pharmakol.uni-freiburg.de

ANGHELESCU, ION
Freie Universität Berlin, Psychiatrische Klinik und Poliklinik, Universitätsklinikum Benjamin Franklin, Eschenallee 3, 14050 Berlin, Germany
ion.anghelescu@medizin.fu-berlin.de

AUGUSTIN, HELLMUT
Tumor Biology Center Freiburg , Dept. of Vascular Biology and Angiogenesis Research, Breisacher Str. 117, 79106 Freiburg, Germany
augustin@angiogenese.de

BACK, EVELYN
Universität Hohenheim, Institut für Biologische Chemie und Ernährungswissenschaft, Fruwirtstraße12, 70593 Stuttgart, Germany
evelyn_back@uni-hohenheim.de

BADER, MICHAEL
Max-Delbrück-Centrum für Molekulare Medizin (MDC), Robert-Rössle-Str. 10, 13092 Berlin, Germany
mbader@mdc-berlin.de

BAILEY, CLIFFORD J.
Aston University, School of Life and Health Sciences, Birmingham B4 7ET, UK
c.j.bailey@aston.ac.uk

BAKER, JILLIAN G.
Institute of Cell Signalling, Queen's Medical Centre, Medical School, C Floor, Nottingham NG9 4AW, UK,
jillian.baker@nottingham.ac.uk

BANKAITIS-DAVIS, DANUTE
Source Precision Medicine, Medical and Pharmaceutical Services, 2425 N. 55th Street, Suite 111, Boulder, CO 80301, USA

BARKER, ERIC
Purdue University, Department Medicinal Chemistry and Molecular Pharmacology, Robert E. Heine Pharmacy Building, West Lafayette, IN 47907, USA
ericb@pharmacy.purdue.edu

BARTHEL, ANDREAS
Heinrich-Heine-Universität, Klinik für Endokrinologie, Moorenstr. 5, 40225 Düsseldorf, Germany
Andreas.Barthel@uni-duesseldorf.de

BASTIANS, HOLGER
Institut für Molekularbiologie und Tumorforschung (IMT), Emil-Mannkopff-Str. 2, 35033 Marburg, Germany
bastians@imt.uni-marburg.de

BEAVO, JOSEPH A.
University Washington, Department Pharmacology, Box 357280, Seattle, WA 98195-7280, USA
beavo@u.washington.edu

BECK, HEINZ
Universitätskliniken Bonn, Klinik für Epileptologie , Labor für Experimentelle Epileptologie, Sigmund-Freud-Str. 25, 53105 Bonn, Germany
Heinz.Beck@ukb.uni-bonn.de

BECKER, WALTER
RWTH Aachen, Medizinische Fakultät, Institut für Pharmakologie und Toxikologie, Wendlingweg 2, 52057 Aachen, Germany
walter.becker@post.rwth-aachen.de

BECKER, CORD-MICHAEL
Universität Erlangen-Nürnberg, Emil-Fischer-Zentrum, Institut
für Biochemie, Fahrstr. 17, 91054 Erlangen, Germany
cmb@biochem.uni-erlangen.de

BEHRENS, JÜRGEN
Friedrich-Alexander-Universität Erlangen-Nürnberg, Lehrstuhl
für Experimentelle Medizin II, Nikolaus-Fiebiger-Zentrum,
Glueckstrasse 6, 91054 Erlangen, Germany
jbehrens@molmed.uni-erlangen.de

BERGER, MARTIN R
Deutsches Krebsforschungszentrum (DKFZ), D 0301 AG
Toxkologie, Im Neuenheimer Feld 280, 69120 Heidelberg,
Germany
m.berger@dkfz.de

BEVILACQUA, MICHAEL
Source Precision Medicine, Medical and Pharmaceutical Services,
2425 N. 55th Street, Suite 111, Boulder, CO 80301, USA
mbevilac@sourcemedicine.com

BIEL, MARTIN
LMU München, Zentrum für Pharmaforschung, Department
Pharmazie, Box 3686, Butenandtstr. 7, 81377 München, Germany
martin.biel@cup.uni-muenchen.de

BIESALSKI, HANS K.
Universität Hohenheim, Institut für Biologische Chemie und
Ernährungswissenschaft, Fruwirtstraße12, 70593 Stuttgart,
Germany
biesal@uni-hohenheim.de

BLAUKAT, ANDREE
Merck KgaA, Oncology Research Darmstadt, Global Preclinical
R&D, Frankfurter Str. 250, 64293 Darmstadt, Germany
Andree.Blaukat@meck.de

BÖHM, MICHAEL
Medizinische Klinik und Poliklinik III, Abteilung Kardiologie
und Angiologie, 66421 Homburg/Saar, Germany
boehm@med-in.uni-saarland.de

BORKHARDT, ARNDT
University of Gießen, Department of Pediatric Haematology &
Oncology, Children's University Hospital, Feulgenstr. 12, 35392
Gießen, Germany
arndt.borkhardt@paediat.med.uni-giessen.de

BOTTING, REGINA M.
St. Bartholomew's and Royal London School of Medicine and
Dentistry, William Harvey Research Institute, Charterhouse
Square, London EC1 M6BQ, UK
r.m.botting@qmul.ac.uk

BOTTING, JACK
St. Bartholomew's and Royal London School of Medicine and
Dentistry, William Harvey Research Institute, Charterhouse
Square, London EC1 M6BQ, UK

BRÄU, MICHAEL
Justus-Liebig-Universität Gießen, Abteilung Anaesthesiologie und
operative Intensivmedizin, Universitätsklinikum Gießen, Rudolf-
Buchheim-Str. 7, 35392 Gießen, Germany
meb@anaesthesiologie.de

BREYER, MATTHEW D.
Vanderbilt University, School of Medicine, Division of
Nephrology, S3223 MCN, 1161 21st Avenue South, Nashville, TN
37232-2372, USA, matthew.breyer@vanderbilt.edu

BREYER, RICHARD M.
Vanderbilt University, School of Medicine, Division of
Nephrology, S3223 MCN, 1161 21st Avenue South, Nashville, TN
37232-2372, USA
rich.breyer@mcmail.vanderbilt.edu

BROCKMÖLLER, JÜRGEN
Universität Göttingen, Zentrum Pharmakologie und Toxikologie,
Robert-Koch-Str. 40, 37075 Göttingen, Germany
jurgen.brockmoller@med.uni-goettingen.de

BUNZ, FRED
The John Hopkins School of Medicine, Radiation Biology
Program, The John Hopkins Oncology Center, 1650 Orleans
Street, Room 1-146, Baltimore, MD 21231, USA
bunzfre@mail.jhmi.edu

BURNSTOCK, GEOFFREY
Autonomic Neuroscience Institute, Royal Free and University
College Medical School, Rowland Hill Street, London NW3 2PF,
UK, UK
g.burnstock@ucl.ac.uk

CAMERON, ROSS
University of Toronto and The Toronto Hospital, Department of
Pathology, Toronto, Ontario M5G 2C4, Canada
ross.cameron@uhn.on.ca

CASEY, PATRICK
Duke University Medical Center, Department of Molecular
Cancer Biology, C133 LSRCResearch Drive, Durham, NC 27710-
3813, USA
Casey006@mc.duke.edu

CHERONIS, JOHN C.
Source Precision Medicine, Medical and Pharmaceutical Services,
2425 N. 55th Street, Suite 111, Boulder, CO 80301, USA
jcheroni@SourceMedicine.com

CUEVAS, BRUCE
National Jewish Center, Immunology & Research Medicine, 1400
Jackson St., Denver, CO 80304, USA
bruce.cuevas@uchsc.edu

DHEIN, STEFAN
Universität Leipzig, Herzzentrum Leipzig, Klinik für
Herzchirurgie, Strümpell Str.39, 04289 Leipzig, Germany
dhes@medizin.uni-leipzig.de

DOHMEN, JÜRGEN
Universität Köln, Institut für Genetik, Zülpicherstr. 47, 50674
Köln, Germany
j.dohmen@uni-koeln.de

DRAGUHN, ANDREAS
Universität Heidelberg, Institut für Physiologie und
Pathophysiologie, Im Neuenheimer Feld 326, 69115Heidelberg,
Germany
andreas.draguhn@urz.uni-heidelberg.de

EDWARDS, ROBERT
University of San Francisco, Department of Physiology, Box 0444,
room S-762, 513 Parnassus Ave., San Francisco, CA 94143-0444,
USA
edwards@itsa.ucsf.edu

EICHELBAUM, MICHEL F.
Dr. Margarete Fischer-Bosch-Institut für Klinische
Pharmakologie, Auerbachstr. 112, 70376 Stuttgart, Germany
michel.eichelbaum@ikp-stuttgart.de

EXTON, JOHN H.
Vanderbilt University, Howard Hughes Medical Institute,
831 Light Hall, Nashville, TN 37232-0295, USA
john.exton@mcmail.vanderbilt.edu

FALCIANI, FRANCESCO
University of Birmingham, School of Bioscience, Edgbaston,
Birmingham B15 2TT, UK
F.Falciani@bham.ac.uk

FEUERSTEIN, THOMAS
Neurologische Universitätsklinik, Sektion Klinische
Neuropharmakologie, Neurozentrum, Breisacher Str. 64,
79106 Freiburg, Germany
feuer@ukl.uni-freiburg.de

FINSTERBACH, THOMAS
Stanford University Medical School, 161 Beckman Center,
279 Campus Drive, Stanford 94305-5428, USA
tfinster@cmgm.stanford.edu

FLOCKERZI, VEIT
Universität des Saarlandes, Institut für Pharmakologie und
Toxikologie, 66421 Homburg, Germany
veit.flockerzi@uniklinik-saarland.de

FOOTE, MARYANN
Amgen Inc., 1840 DeHavilland Drive, Thousand Oaks,
CA 91230-1799, USA
mfoote@amgen.com

FÖRSTERMANN, ULRICH
Universität Mainz, Pharmakologisches Institut,
Obere Zahlbacher Str. 67, 55101 Mainz, Germany
Ulrich.Forstermann@Uni-Mainz.de

FRANK, JÜRGEN
Universität Hohenheim, Institut für Biologische Chemie und
Ernährungswissenschaft, Fruwirtstraße12, 70593 Stuttgart,
Germany
frank140@uni-hohenheim.de

FUCHS, ELKE
Interdisziplinäres Zentrum für Neurowissenschaften (IZN),
Abteilung Klinische Neurobiologie, Im Neuenheimer Feld 364,
69120 Heidelberg, Germany
E.Fuchs@urz.uni-heidelberg.de

GEISSLINGER, GERD
Universitätsklinikum Frankfurt, Zentrum der Pharmakologie,
Institut für Klinische Pharmakologie, Theodor-Stern-Kai 7,
60590 Frankfurt/Main, Germany
Geisslinger@em.uni-frankfurt.de

GELDART, TOM
Southampton General Hospital, Cancer Sciences Division, CRC
Wessex Medical Oncology Unit, Southampton, UK
trg@soton.ac.uk

GHUYSEN, JEAN MARIE
Institut de Chimie, bâtiment B6, Université de Liège au Sart
Tilman, 4000 Liège, Belgium, Belgium
jmghuysen@ulg.ac.be

GLICK, JENNIFER L.
University Washington, Department Pharmacology, Box 357280,
Seattle, WA 98195-7280, USA
jbelyea@u.washington.edu

GREINACHER, ANDREAS
Ernst-Moritz-Arndt-Universität Greifswald, Institut für
Immunologie und Transfusionsmedizin, Abteilung
Transfusionsmedizin, Klinikum Sauerbruchstraße,
Diagnostikzentrum, 17487 Greifswald, Germany
greinach@mail.uni-greifswald.de

GRÜNDEMANN, DIRK
Medizinische Einrichtungen der Universität Köln, Department of
Pharmacology, Gleueler Str. 24, 50931 Köln, Germany
dirk.gruendemann@uni-koeln.de

GUDERMANN, THOMAS
Philipps-Universität Marburg, Institut für Pharmakologie und
Toxikologie, Fachbereich Humanmedizin, Karl-von-Frisch-Str. 1,
35033 Marburg, Germany
guderman@mailer.uni-marburg.de

HALL, JULIE M.
National Institute of Environmental Health Sciences, Receptor
Biology Section, Laboratory of Reproductive and Developmental
Toxicology, Box 12233, MD B3-02, Research Triangle Park, NC
27709, USA
hall8@niehs.nih.gov

HEIN, LUTZ
Universität Würzburg, Institut für Pharmakologie und
Toxikologie, Versbacherstr. 9, 97078 Würzburg, Germany
hein@toxi.uni-wuerzburg.de

HEINEMANN, UWE
Humboldt-Universität zu Berlin, Johannes-Müller-Institut für
Physiologie, Universitätsklinikum Charité, Campus Charite Mitte,
Tucholskystr. 2, 10117 Berlin, Germany
uwe.heinemann@charite.de

HERMOSILLA, RICARDO
Forschungsinstitut für Molekulare Pharmakologie (FMP)Campus
Berlin-Buch, Robert-Rössle-Str. 10, 13125 Berlin, Germany
hermosilla@fmp-berlin.de

HERWALD, HEIKO
Lund University, H66, Section for Molecular Pathogenesis,
Tornavägen 10, 22184 Lund, Sweden
Heiko.Herwald@medkem.lu.se

HEUSER, ISABELLA
Freie Universität Berlin, Psychiatrische Klinik und Poliklinik,
Universitätsklinikum Benjamin Franklin, Eschenallee 3, 14050
Berlin, Germany
isabella.heuser@medizin.fu-berlin.de

HILL, STEPHEN J.
Institute of Cell Signalling, Queen's Medical Centre, Medical
School, C Floor, Nottingham NG9 4AW, UK
Stephen.Hill@nottingham.ac.uk

HOFMANN, FRANZ
TU München, Institut für Pharmakologie und Toxikologie,
Biedersteiner Str.29, 80802 München, Germany
Pharma@ipt.med.tu-muenchen.de

HÖLLT, VOLKER
Otto-von-Guericke-Universität, Institut für Pharmakologie und
Toxikologie, Leipziger Str. 44, 39120 Magdeburg, Germany
volker.hoellt@medizin.uni-magdeburg.de

HOLSBOER, FLORIAN
Max-Planck-Institut für Psychiatrie, Kraepelinstr. 2-10, 80804
München, Germany
holsboer@mpipsykl.mpg.de

HOLTMANN, HELMUT
Medizinische Hochschule Hannover, Institut für Pharmakologie,
Carl-Neuberg-Str. 1, 30625 Hannover, Germany
Holtmann.Helmut@MH-Hannover.de

HORUK, RICHARD
Berlex BioSciences, Department of Immunology, 15049 San Pablo
Ave., Richmond, 94806, USA
Horuk@pacbell.net

HOYER, DANIEL
Novartis Pharma AG, 360 / 604, 4002 Basel, Switzerland
daniel1.hoyer@pharma.novartis.com

HUCHO, FERDINAND
Freie Universität Berlin, Institut für Biochemie, Thielallee 63,
14195 Berlin, Germany
hucho@chemie.fu-berlin.de

HUPPERTZ, CHRISTINE
Novartis Pharma AG, Cardiovascular and Metabolic Diseases
Research, 4002 Basel, Switzerland
christine.huppertz@pharma.novartis.com

HUWILER, ANDREA
Klinikum der J.W.Goethe-Universität Frankfurt/Main, Institut für
Allgemeine Pharmakologie und Toxikologie, Theodor-Stern-Kai
7, 60590 Frankfurt/Main, Germany
huwiler@em.uni-frankfurt.de

IMOTO, KEIJI
National Institute for Physiological Sciences, Department of
Information Physiology, Myodaiji, Okazaki 444-8585, Japan
keiji@nips.ac.jp

ITO, KIYOMI
Kitasato University, School of Pharmaceutical Sciences, 5-9-1
Shirokane, Minato-ku, Tokyo 108-8641, Japan
itok@pharm.kitasato-u.ac.jp

JAHN, REINHARD
Max-Planck-Institut für biophysikalische Chemie, Abteilung
Neurobiologie, Am Fassberg 11, 37077 Göttingen, Germany
rjahn@gwdg.de

JENTSCH, THOMAS J.
Universität Hamburg, Institut für Molekulare Neurobiologie
Hamburg, Martinistrasse 85, 20246 Hamburg, Germany
jentsch@plexus.uke.uni-hamburg.de

JOHNSON, ROGER A.
State University of New York, Department of Physiology and
Biophysics, SUNY/Health Sciences Center, Stony Brook, NY 11794-
8661, USA
rjohnson@ms.cc.sunysb.edu

JOHNSON, GARY L.
National Jewish Center, Immunology & Research Medicine, 1400
Jackson St., Denver, CO 80304, USA
Gary.Johnson@uchsc.edu

JOHNSTONE, RICKY W.
The Peter MacCallum Cancer Institute, Trescowthick Research
Laboratories, St Andrews Place, East Melbourne, Victoria 3002,
Australia
r.johnstone@pmci.unimelb.edu.au

JOOST, HANS-GEORG
RWTH Aachen, Medizinische Fakultät, Institut für
Pharmakologie und Toxikologie, Wendlingweg 2, 52057 Aachen,
Germany
joost@mail.dife.de

KAEVER, VOLKHARD
Medizinische Hochschule Hannover, Institut für Pharmakologie,
Carl-Neuberg-Str. 1, 30625 Hannover, Germany
Kaever.Volkhard@MH-Hannover.de

KAPUR, SHITIJ
The Centre for Addiction and Mental Health (CAMH), Clarke
Division, Schizophrenia Program, 250 College St., Toronto,
Ontario M5T 1R8, Canada
skapur@camhpet.on.ca

KENAKIN, TERRY P.
GlaxoSmithKline Research and Development, Receptor
Biochemistry, 5 Moore Drive, P.O.Box 13398, Research Triangle
Park, NC 27709, USA
tpk1348@GlaxoWellcome.com

KOBILKA, BRIAN K.
Stanford University Medical School, B-157, Howard Huges
Medical Institute, Beckman Center, Stanford 94305-5428, USA
kobilka@cmgm.stanford.edu

KOCHUPURAKKAL, BOSE
The Weizmann Institute of Science, Dept. Biological Regulation,
POB 26, Rehovot 76100, Israel
Bose.Kochupurakkal@weizmann.ac.il

KOESLING, DORIS
Ruhr-Universität Bochum, Pharmacology and Toxicology,
Medizinische Fakultät MA N1/39, 44780 Bochum, Germany
koesling@iname.com

KORACH, KENNETH S
National Institute of Environmental Health Sciences, Receptor
Biology Section, Laboratory of Reproductive and Developmental
Toxicology, Box 12233, MD B3-02, Research Triangle Park, NC
27709, USA
korach@niehs.nih.gov

KRACHT, MICHAEL
Medizinische Hochschule Hannover, Institut für Pharmakologie,
Carl-Neuberg-Str. 1, 30625 Hannover, Germany
Kracht.Michael@MH-Hannover.de

KRAUSE, GERD
Forschungsinstitut für Molekulare Pharmakologie (FMP),
Campus Berlin-Buch, Robert-Rössle-Str. 10, 13125 Berlin, Germany
gkrause@fmp-berlin.de

KRAUSE, EBERHARD
Forschungsinstitut für Molekulare Pharmakologie (FMP),
Campus Berlin-Buch, Robert-Rössle-Str. 10, 13125 Berlin, Germany
ekrause@fmp-berlin.de

KRÄUSSLICH, HANS-GEORG
Universität Heidelberg, Hygiene-Institut, Abteilung Virologie, Im
Neuenheimer Feld 324, 69120 Heidelberg, Germany
Hans-Georg_Kraeusslich@med.uni-heidelberg.de

KREUTZ, REINHOLD
Freie Universität Berlin, Institut für Klinische Pharmakologie,
Universitätsklinikum Benjamin Franklin, Hindenburgdamm 30,
12200 Berlin, Germany
kreutz@medizin.fu-berlin.de

KRIEGLSTEIN, KERSTIN
Medizinische Fakultät der Universität Göttingen, Zentrum 1
Anatomie, Abteilung Neuroanatomie, Kreuzbergring 36, 37075
Göttingen, Germany
kkriegl@gwdg.de

KUNER, ROHINI
Universität Heidelberg, Pharmakologisches Institut, Im
Neunheimer Feld 366, 69120 Heidelberg, Germany
rohini.kuner@urz.uni-heidelberg.de

KUREBAYASHI, NAGOMI
Juntendo University, School of Medicine, Department of
Pharmacology, 2 - 1 - 1 Hongo, Bunkyo-ku, Tokyo 113-8421, Japan
nagomik@med.juntendo.ac.jp

LANG, THORSTEN
Max-Planck-Institut für biophysikalische Chemie, Abteilung
Neurobiologie, Am Fassberg 11, 37077 Göttingen, Germany
tlang@mpibpc.gwdg.de

LANZER, MICHAEL
Universität Heidelberg, Hygiene-Institut, Abteilung Parasitologie,
69120 Heidelberg, Germany
michael_lanzer@med.uni-heidelberg.de

LARSEN, MOGENS LYTGEN
Aarhus University Hospital, Department of Cardiology, Aarhus,
Denmark
mogenslytkenlarsen@dadlnet.dk

LATCHMAN, DAVID S.
Institute of Child Health, 30 Guilford Street, London WC1N 1EH,
UK
d.latchman@ich.ucl.ac.uk

LEFF, ALAN R.
University of Chicago, Deptartment Of Medicine, MC6076,
Section of Pulmonary and Critical Care Medicine, 5841 South
Maryland Avenue, Chicago, IL 60637, USA
aleff@medicine.bsd.uchicago.edu

LINGE, JENS P.
Institut Pasteur, Unité de Bioinformatigue Structurale, 25-28 rue
du Docteur Roux, 75015 Paris, France
linge@pasteur.fr

LIOUMI, MARIA
Lorantis Ltd., 307 Cambridge Science Park, Cambridge CB4 0WG,
UK
maria.lioumi@lorantis.com

LOHSE, MARTIN
Universität Würzburg, Institut für Pharmakologie und
Toxikologie, Versbacherstr. 9, 97078 Würzburg, Germany
lohse@toxi.uni-wuerzburg.de

LONG, KATHERINE
Copenhagen University, RNA Regulation Centre, Institute of
Molecular Biology, Solvgade 83, 1307 Copenhagen, Denmark
long@mermaid.molbio.ku.dk

LOPATIN, ANATOLI
University of Michigan, Department of Physiology, 7812 Med. Sci.
II, Ann Arbor, MI 48109, USA
alopatin@umich.edu

LÖTSCH, JÖRN
Universitätsklinikum Frankfurt, Zentrum der Pharmakologie,
Institut für Klinische Pharmakologie, Theodor-Stern-Kai 7, 60590
Frankfurt/Main, Germany
j.loetsch@em.uni-frankfurt-de

MACFARLANE, SCOTT
University of Strathclyde, Strathclyde Institute for Biomedical
Sciences, Department of Physiology and Pharmacology, 27 Taylor
St., Glasgow G4ONR, UK
scott.macfarlane@strath.ac.uk

MAMO, DAVID C.
The Centre for Addiction and Mental Health (CAMH), Clarke
Division,, Schizophrenia Program, 250 College St., Toronto,
Ontario M5T 1R8, Canada
dmamo@camhpet.on.ca

MÄNNISTÖ, PEKKA T.
University of Kuopio, Department of Pharmacology and
Toxicology, P.O. Box 162, 70 211 Kuopio, Finnland
Pekka.Mannisto@uku.fi

MARTIN, MICHAEL U.
Medizinische Hochschule Hannover, Institut für Pharmakologie,
Carl-Neuberg-Str. 1, 30625 Hannover, Germany
Martin.Michael@MH-Hannover.de

MEYER, DIETER. K.
Albert-Ludwigs-Universität, Institut für Experimentelle und
Klinische Pharmakologie und Toxikologie , Abteilung 1, Stefan-
Meier-Strasse 19, 79104 Freiburg, Germany
dieter.meyer@pharmakol-uni-freiburg.de

MEYER, AXEL
Interdisziplinäres Zentrum für Neurowissenschaften (IZN),
Abteilung Klinische Neurobiologie, Im Neuenheimer Feld 364,
69120 Heidelberg, Germany
axel.meyer@urz.uni-heidelberg.de

MEYER, THOMAS
Forschungsinstitut für Molekulare Pharmakologie (FMP),
Campus Berlin-Buch, Robert-Rössle-Str. 10, 13125 Berlin, Germany
meyer@fmp-berlin.de

MEYER ZU HERINGDORF, DAGMAR
Universitätsklinikum Essen, Institut für Pharmakologie,
Hufelandstr. 55, 45122 Essen, Germany
meyer-heringdorf@uni-essen.de

MEYERHOF, WOLFGANG
Deutsches Institut für Ernährungsforschung (DIFE), Arthur-
Scheunert-Allee 114-116, 14558 Bergholz-Rehbrücke, Germany
meyerhof@mail.dife.de

Michel, Nico
Deutsches Krebsforschungszentrum (DKFZ), Applied Tumor
Virology Program, Im Neuenheimer Feld 242, 69120 Heidelberg,
Germany
N.Michel@dkfz.de

MICHEL, MARTIN C.
Academisch Medisch Centrum, Afd. Farmacologie, Meibergdreef
15, Amsterdam, 1105 AZ, The Netherlands
m.c.michel@amc.uva.nl

MIEHLE, KONSTANZE
Universität Leipzig, Medizinische Klinik und Poliklinik III,
Philipp-Rosenthal-Str. 27, 04103 Leipzig, Germany
miek@medizin.uni-leipzig.de

MITCHELSON, FREDERICK J.
University of Melbourne, Department of Pharmacology, Victoria
3010, Australia
fjmitc@unimelb.edu.au

MONYER, HANNAH
Interdisziplinäres Zentrum für Neurowissenschaften (IZN),
Abteilung Klinische Neurobiologie, Im Neuenheimer Feld 364,
69120 Heidelberg, Germany
monyer@urz.uni-hd.de

MORSTYN, GEORGE
Amgen Inc., 1840 DeHavilland Drive, Thousand Oaks, CA 91230-
1799, USA
gmorstyn@amgen.com

MOUSA, SHAKER A.
Albany College of Pharmacy &, Head of PRI at Albany, 106 New
Scotland Ave.,, Room 225A, Albany, NY 12208-3492, USA
mousas@acp.edu

MÜLLER, BARBARA
Universität Heidelberg, Hygiene-Institut, Abteilung Virologie, Im
Neuenheimer Feld 324, 69120 Heidelberg, Germany
barbara_mueller@med.uni-heidelberg.de

MÜLLER, ROLF
Institut für Molekularbiologie und Tumorforschung (IMT), Emil-
Mannkopff-Str. 2, 35033 Marburg, Germany
mueller@imt.uni-marburg.de

MÜLLER, MARTIN
Deutsches Krebsforschungszentrum (DKFZ), Applied Tumor
Virology Program, Im Neuenheimer Feld 242, 69120 Heidelberg,
Germany
Martin.Mueller@dkfz.de

MÜLLER, JUDITH
Universitätsklinik Freiburg, Abteilung Frauenheilkunde und
Geburtshilfe I, Universitäts-Frauenklinik, Breisacherstr. 117, 79106
Freiburg, Germany
jmueller@frk.ukl.uni-freiburg.de

MÜLLER-ESTERL, WERNER
Institute for Biochemistry II, University Hospital, Bldg. 75,
Theodor-Stern-Kai 7, 60590 Frankfurt, Germany
wme@biochem2.de

MURAYAMA, TAKASHI
Juntendo University, School of Medicine, Department of
Pharmacology, 2 - 1 - 1 Hongo, Bunkyo-ku, Tokyo 113-8421, Japan
takashim@med.juntendo.ac.jp

NEGULESCU, PAUL A.
Vertex Pharmaceuticals Incorporated, Discovery Biology, 11010
Torreyana Road, San Diego, CA 92121, USA
paul_negulescu@sd.vrtx.com

NICHOLS, COLIN G.
Washington University, Medical School, Department Cellular
Biology, Box 8228, 660 S Euclid Avenue, St. Louis, MO 63110, USA
cnichols@cellbio.wustl.edu

NICKEL, WERNER
Medizinische Klinik und Poliklinik III, Abteilung Kardiologie
und Angiologie, 66421 Homburg/Saar, Germany
wanickl@web.de

NIKKHAH, GUIDO
Neurologische Universitätsklinik, Stereotaktische
Neurochirurgie, Neurozentrum, Breisacher Str. 64, 79106
Freiburg, Germany
nikkhah@nz.ukl.uni-freiburg.de

NILGES, MICHAEL
Institut Pasteur, Unité de Bioinformatigue Structurale,
25-28 rue du Docteur Roux, 75015 Paris, France
nilges@pasteur.fr

NOHR, DONATUS
Universität Hohenheim, Institut für Biologische Chemie und
Ernährungswissenschaft, Fruwirtstraße12, 70593 Stuttgart,
Germany
nohr@uni-hohenheim.de

NÜRNBERG, BERND
Universitätsklinikum Düsseldorf, Institut für Physiologische
Chemie II, Universitätsstraße1, 40225 Düsseldorf, Germany
Bernd.Nuernberg@uni-duesseldorf.de

OAK, JAMES N.
Center for Addiction and Mental Health, Laboratory of Molecular
Neurobiology, 250 College St. W, Toronto, Ontario M5T 1R8,
Canada
james.oak@utoronto.ca

OFFERMANNS, STEFAN
Universität Heidelberg, Pharmakologisches Institut, Im
Neunheimer Feld 366, 69120 Heidelberg, Germany
Stefan.Offermanns@urz.uni-heidelberg.de

OGAWA, YASUO
Juntendo University, School of Medicine, Department of
Pharmacology, 2 - 1 - 1 Hongo, Bunkyo-ku, Tokyo 113-8421, Japan
ysogawa@med.juntendo.ac.jp

OKSCHE, ALEXANDER
Forschungsinstitut für Molekulare Pharmakologie (FMP),
Campus Berlin-Buch, Robert-Rössle-Str. 10, 13125 Berlin, Germany
oksche@fmp-berlin.de

OLIAS, GISELA
Deutsches Institut für Ernährungsforschung (DIFE), Abteilung
Molekulare Genetik, Arthur-Scheunert-Allee 114-116, 14558
Bergholz-Rehbrücke
Olias@ mail.dife.de

OSCHKINAT, HARTMUT
Forschungsinstitut für Molekulare Pharmakologie (FMP),
Campus Berlin-Buch, Robert-Rössle-Straße 10, 13125 Berlin,
Germany
oschkinat@fmp-berlin.de

OSTER, NADJA
Universität Heidelberg, Hygiene-Institut, Abteilung Parasitologie,
Im Neuenheimer Feld 324, 69120 Heidelberg, Germany
Nadja_Oster@med.uni-heidelberg.de

PASCHKE, RALF
Universität Leipzig, Medizinische Klinik und Poliklinik III,
Philipp-Rosenthal-Str. 27, 04103 Leipzig, Germany
pasr@medizin.uni-leipzig.de

PEART, MELISSA
The Peter MacCallum Cancer Institute, Trescowthick Research
Laboratories, St Andrews Place, East Melbourne, Victoria 3002,
Australia
m.peart@pmci.unimelb.edu.au

PETERS, JÖRG
Universität Heidelberg, Pharmakologisches Institut, Im
Neuenheimer Feld 366, 69120 Heidelberg, Germany
joerg.peters@urz.uni-heidelberg.de

PFEIFER, ALEXANDER
LMU München, Molekulare Pharmakologie, Zentrum für
Pharmaforschung, Butenandtstr. 5-13 (Haus C), 81377 München,
Germany
alexander.pfeifer@cup.uni-muenchen.de

PFEILSCHIFTER, JOSEF
Klinikum der J.W.Goethe-Universität Frankfurt/Main, Institut für
Allgemeine Pharmakologie und Toxikologie, Theodor-Stern-Kai
7, 60590 Frankfurt/Main, Germany
Pfeilschifter@em.uni-frankfurt.de

PIN, JEAN-PHILIPPE
Centre National de la Recherche Scientifique, Mechanismes
Moleculaires des Communications Cellulaires, CNRS-UPR9023,
CCIPE, 141 Rue de la Cardonille, 34094 Montpellier, France
pin@montp.inserm.fr

PLEVIN, ROBIN
University of Strathclyde, Strathclyde Institute for Biomedical
Sciences, Department of Physiology and Pharmacology, 27 Taylor
St., Glasgow G4ONR, UK
r.plevin@strath.ac.uk

POLAK, ANNEMARIE
Spitzenrainweg 49, 4147 Aesch, Switzerland
annemarie.polak@bluemail.ch

PONGS, OLAF
Universität Hamburg, Zentrum für Molekulare Neurobiologie,
Martinistrasse 52, 20246 Hamburg, Germany
pointuri@uke.uni-hamburg.de

PÖTZSCH, BERND
Rheinische Friedrich-Wilhelms-Universität, Institut für Exp.
Hämatologie und Transfusionsmedizin der Universität Bonn,
Sigmund-Freud-Str. 25, 53105 Bonn-Venusberg, Germany
bernd.poetzsch@ukb.uni-bonn.de

RADEMANN, JÖRG
Universität Tübingen, Institut für Organische Chemie, Fakultät
Chemie/Pharmazie, Auf der Morgenstelle 18, 72076 Tübingen,
Germany
joerg.rademann@uni-tuebingen.de

REICHARDT, HOLGER M.
Universität Würzburg, Institute of Virology and Immunbiology,
Versbacher Strasse 7, 97078 Würzburg, Germany
holger.reichardt@mail.uni-wuerzburg.de

REIMER, RICHARD
University of San Francisco, Department of Physiology, Box 0444,
room S-762, 513 Parnassus Ave., San Francisco, CA 94143-0444,
USA
rjreimer@stanford.edu

REINHARD, CONSTANZE
Biochemie-Zentrum Heidelberg, Im Neuenheimer Feld 328, 69120
Heidelberg, Germany
reinhard@sunourz.uni-heidelberg.de

REISS, YVONNE
Tumor Biology Center Freiburg , Dept. of Vascular Biology and
Angiogenesis Research, Breisacher Str. 117, 79106 Freiburg,
Germany
reiss@tumorbio.uni-freiburg.de

RESCH, KLAUS
Medizinische Hochschule Hannover, Institut für Pharmakologie,
Carl-Neuberg-Str. 1, 30625 Hannover, Germany
Resch.Klaus@MH-Hannover.de

ROMMELSPACHER, HANS
Freie Universität Berlin, Klinische Neurobiologie, Ulmenallee 32,
14050 Berlin, Germany
hans.rommelspacher@medizin.fu-berlin.de

ROOS, THOMAS C.
Wasserschloß Klinik, Bettenwarfen 2-14, 26427 Neuharlingersiel,
Germany
roos@rehaklinik-neuharlingersiel-klinik.de

ROPER, MICHAEL D.
Source Precision Medicine, Medical and Pharmaceutical Services,
2425 N. 55th Street, Suite 111, Boulder, CO 80301, USA

ROSENTHAL, WALTER
Institut für Pharmakologie, Freie Universität Berlin,
Thielallee 67–73, D-14195 Berlin, Germany,
walter.rosenthal@medizin.fu-berlin.de

ROSSIER, BERNARD C.
Université de Lausanne, Institut de Pharmacologie et de
Toxikologie, Rue de Bugnon 27, 1005 Lausanne, Switzerland
Bernard.Rossier@ipharm.unil.ch

RUDOLPH, UWE
Universität Zürich, Pharmakologisches Institut, Winterthurerstr.
190, 8057 Zürich, Switzerland
rudolph@pharma.unizh.ch

RUEFLI, ASTRID A.
The Peter MacCallum Cancer Institute, Trescowthick Research
Laboratories, St Andrews Place, East Melbourne, Victoria 3002,
Australia
a.ruefli@pmci.unimelb.edu.au

SACHS, GEORGE
University of California at Los Angeles, Center Ulcer Research
VA, Wadsworth Hospital, Membrane Biology Laboratory, 11301
Wilshire Blvd , Bldg 113, Rm 324, Los Angeles, CA 90073, USA
gsachs@ucla.edu

SCHILD, LAURENT
Université de Lausanne, Institut de Pharmacologie et de
Toxikologie, Rue de Bugnon 27, 1005 Lausanne, Switzerland
Laurent.Schild@ipharm.unil.ch

SCHMIDT , ERIK BERG
Hjørring Sygehus, Department of Medicine, 9800 Hjørring,
Denmark
ebs@dadlnet.dk

SCHMIDT, GUDULA
Albert-Ludwigs-Universität Freiburg, Institut für Pharmakologie
und Toxikologie, Hermann-Herder-Str. 5, 79104 Freiburg,
Germany
gudula.schmidt@pharmakol.uni-freiburg.de

SCHNERMANN, JÜRGEN B.
National Institute of Diabetes & Digestive & Kidney Diseases
(NIDDK), MSC 1370, Bldg 10, Rm 4D51, 10 Center Drive,,
Bethseda, MD 29892-1370, USA
jurgens@intra.niddk.nih.gov

SCHÖMIG, EDGAR
Medizinische Einrichtungen der Universität Köln, Department of
Pharmacology, Gleueler Str. 24, 50931 Köln, Germany
edgar.schoemig@medizin.uni-koeln.de

SCHÖNEBERG, TORSTEN
Freie Universität Berlin, Institut für Pharmakologie,
Universitätsklinikum Benjamin Franklin, Thielallee 67-73, 14195
Berlin, Germany
schoberg@zedat.fu-berlin.de

SCHÜLE, ROLAND
Universitätsklinik Freiburg, Abteilung Frauenheilkunde und
Geburtshilfe I, Universitäts-Frauenklinik, Breisacherstr. 117, 79106
Freiburg, Germany
schuele@frk.ukl.uni-freiburg.de

SCHÜLEIN, RALF
Forschungsinstitut für Molekulare Pharmakologie (FMP),
Campus Berlin-Buch, Robert-Rössle-Str. 10, 13125 Berlin, Germany
schuelein@fmp-berlin.de

SCHULTZ, GÜNTER
Freie Universität Berlin, Institut für Pharmakologie, Thielallee
67-73, 14195 Berlin, Germany
gschultz@zedat.fu-berlin.de

SCHÜRMANN, ANNETTE
RWTH Aachen, Institut für Pharmakologie und Toxikologie,
Medizinische Fakultät, Wendlingweg 2, 52057 Aachen, Germany
schuerman@mail.dife.de

SEIBEL, MARKUS J.
University of Sydney, Concord Hospital, Department of
Endocrinology & Metabolism C65, Level 6 - Medical Centre,
Sydney, 2139 NSW, Australia
mjs@anzac.edu.au

SEIFERT, ROLAND
University of Kansas, Department of Pharmacology and
Toxicology, Malott Hall, Room 5064, 12 Wescoe Hall Drive,
Lawrence, KS 66045-7582, USA
rseifert@ku.edu

SEINO, SUSUMU
Chiba University Graduate School of Medicine, Department of
Molecular Medicine, 1-8-1, Inohana, Chuo-ku, Chiba 260, Japan
seino@med.m.chiba-u.ac.jp

SHIEH, CHAR-CHANG
Abbott Laboratories, Department 4PM, Building AP9A 3nd Floor,
100 Abbott Park Road, Abbott Park, IL 60064, USA
char-chang.shieh@abbott.com

SHIN, JAI MOO
University of California at Los Angeles, Center Ulcer Research
VA, Wadsworth Hospital, Membrane Biology Laboratory, 11301
Wilshire Blvd , Bldg 113, Rm 324, Los Angeles, CA 90073, USA
jaishin@ucla.edu

SHTIEGMAN, KEREN
The Weizmann Institute of Science, Dept. Biological Regulation,
POB 26, Rehovot 76100, Israel
Keren.Shtiegman@weizmann.ac.il

SMITH, KELLI E.
Synaptic Pharmaceutical Corporation, 215 College Road,
Paramus, NJ 07652, USA
ksmith@synapticcorp.com

SPANAGEL, RAINER
Klinikum Mannheim, Zentralinstitut für seelische Gesundheit, J
5, 68159 Mannheim, Germany
spanagel@zi-mannheim.de

SPECK, ULRICH
Humboldt-Universität Berlin, Institut für Radiologie,
Universitätsklinikum Charité, Schumannstr. 20/21, 10098 Berlin,
Germany
ulrich.speck@charite.de

STAHLMANN, RALF
Freie Universität Berlin, Institut für Klinische Pharmakologie,
Abteilung Toxikologie, Garystr. 5, 14195 Berlin, Germany
ralf.stahlmann@medizin.fu-berlin.de

STARKE, KLAUS
Universität Freiburg, Pharmakologisches Institut der Universität,
Hermann-Herder-Str. 5, 79104 Freiburg, Germany
Klaus.starke@pharmakol.uni-freiburg.de

STEIN, CHRISTOPH
Freie Universität Berlin, Klinik für Anaesthesiologie und
Operative Intensivmedizin, Hindenburgdamm 30, 12200Berlin,
Germany
christoph.stein@medizin.fu-berlin.de

STEINKÜHLER, CHRISTIAN
Istituto di Ricerche di Biologia Molecolare (IRBM) P. Angeletti,
Via Pontina km 30.600, 00040 Pomezia (Rome), Italy
Christian_Steinkuhler@Merck.com

STRIESSNIG, JÖRG
Universität Innsbruck, Institut für Pharmazie , Department of
Pharmacology and Toxicology, Peter-Mayrstrasse 1, 6020
Innsbruck, Austria
joerg.striessnig@uibk.ac.at

SUGIYAMA, YUICHI
University of Tokyo, Faculty of Pharmaceutical Sciences ,
Department of Pharmaceutics, 7-3-1 Hongo, Bunkio-ku,
Tokyo 108-8641, Japan
sugiyama@mol.f.u-tokyo.ac.jp

SZAMEL, MARTA
Medizinische Hochschule Hannover, Institut für Pharmakologie,
Carl-Neuberg-Str. 1, 30625 Hannover, Germany
Szamel.Marta@MH-Hannover.de

TERRY JR., ALVIN V.
Program in Clinical and Experimental Therapeutics, University
of Georgia College of Pharmacy, CJ-1020, Medical College of
Georgia, Augusta, Georgia 30912-2450, USA
aterry@mail.mcg.edu

TOOMBS, CHRISTOPHER F.
Amgen Inc., Product Development, Mailstop 27-5-A,
1 Amgen Center Drive, Thousand Oaks, CA 91320, USA
ctoombs@amgen.com

TROLLINGER, DAVID B.
Source Precision Medicine, Medical and Pharmaceutical Services,
2425 N. 55th Street, Suite 111, Boulder, CO 80301, USA

TRYON, VICTOR V.
Source Precision Medicine, Medical and Pharmaceutical Services,
2425 N. 55th Street, Suite 111, Boulder, CO 80301, USA
vtryon@sourcemedicine.com

UHLIK, MARK
National Jewish Center, Immunology & Research Medicine,
1400 Jackson St., Denver, CO 80304, USA
mark.uhlik@uchsc.edu

VAN TOL, HUBERT H. M.
Center for Addiction and Mental Health, Laboratory of Molecular
Neurobiology, 250 College St. W., Toronto, Ontario M5T 1R8,
Canada
hubert.van.tol@utoronto.ca

VINKEMEIER, UWE
Forschungsinstitut für Molekulare Pharmakologie (FMP),
Campus Berlin-Buch, Robert-Rössle-Str. 10, 13125 Berlin, Germany
vinkemeier@fmp-berlin.de

WAFFORD, KEITH
Merck, Sharp & Dohme Research Laboratories Terlings Park,
Eastwick Road, Harlow, Essex CM20 2QR, UK
keith_wafford@merck.com

WALKER, MARY W.
Synaptic Pharmaceutical Corporation, 215 College Road,
Paramus, NJ 07652, USA
mwalker@synapticcorp.com

WALLMARK, BJÖRN
Schering AG, Corporate Research, Müllerstraße 178, 13342 Berlin,
Germany
bjoern.wallmark@schering.de

WARKENTIN, THEODORE E.
Hamilton General Hospital, Hamilton Regional Laboratory
Medicine Program, Hamilton Health Sciences, 237 Barton Street
East, Hamilton, Ontario L8L 2X2, Canada
twarken@mcmaster.ca

WAXMAN, DAVID J.
Boston University, Department of Biology, Division of Cell and
Molecular Biology, 5 Cummington St., Boston, MA 02215, USA
djw@bio.bu.edu

WELLING, PETER G.
University of Strathclyde, Department of Pharmaceutical
Sciences, 27 Taylor Street, G4 0NR, Glasgow
peter@pwelling.freeserve.co.uk

WESS, JÜRGEN
National Institutes of Health (NIDDK), Laboratory of Bioorganic
Chemistry, Bldg. 8A , Room B1A-09, Bethseda, MD 20892, USA
jwess@helix.nih.gov

WIEDEMANN, BERND
Universität Bonn, Institut für Mikrobiologie & Biotechnologie,
Abteilung Pharmazeutische Mikrobiologie,
Meckenheimer Allee 168, 53115 Bonn, Germany
B.Wiedemann@uni-bonn.de

WIEGAND, IRITH
Universität Bonn, Institut für Mikrobiologie & Biotechnologie,
Abteilung Pharmazeutische Mikrobiologie,
Meckenheimer Allee 168, 53115 Bonn, Germany
unc30002@uni-bonn.de

WIELAND, FELIX
Biochemie-Zentrum Heidelberg, Im Neuenheimer Feld 328, 69120
Heidelberg, Germany
felix.wieland@urz.uni-heidelberg.de

YARDEN, YOSEF
The Weizmann Institute of Science, Dept. Biological Regulation,
POB 26, Rehovot 76100, Israel
yosef.yarden@weizmann.ac.il

ZANGER, ULRICH M.
Dr. Margarete Fischer-Bosch-Institut für Klinische
Pharmakologie, Auerbachstr. 112, 70376 Stuttgart, Germany
uli.zanger@ikp-stuttgart.de

ZAWATZKY, RAINER
Deutsches Krebsforschungszentrum (DKFZ), (F 0300), Im
Neuenheimer Feld 280, 69120 Heidelberg, Germany
r.zawatzky@dkfz-heidelberg.de

List of Essays

A

ABC Proteins

▶ ATP-binding Cassette Transporter Superfamily
▶ Multidrug Transporter

ABC Transporters

▶ ATP-binding Cassette Transporter Superfamily
▶ Table appendix: Membrane Transport Proteins
▶ Multidrug Transporter

Aβ Amyloid

Aβ amyloid is a 4 kD peptide which is the principle constituent of the Alzheimer amyloid found extracellularly in the brains of Alzheimer patients. Aβ amyloid is cleaved from a larger precursor protein, amyloid precursor protein (APP). APP is a member of a family that includes various proteins. It is present in the dendrites, cell bodies and axons of neurons. Neuronal APP is probably the source of most of the Aβ amyloid deposited in the central nervous system of Alzheimer patients. APP is cleaved by various proteases, α-, β- and γ-secretase. The endopeptidase α-secretase cleaves within the Aβ region of APP, resulting in the secretion of the extracellular domain of APP; hence, the cleavage does not produce the Aβ peptide. In contrast, the β-secretase and γ-secretase cleavages do result in production of the Aβ peptide.

▶ Alzheimer's Disease

ABPs

▶ Actin Binding Proteins

Absence Epilepsy

Absence Epilepsies are a group of epileptic syndromes typically starting in childhood or adolescence and characterised by a sudden lack of attention and mild automatic movements for some seconds to minutes. Absence ▶ epilepsies are generalised, i.e. the whole neocortex shifts into a state of sleep-like oscillations.

▶ Antiepileptic Drugs
▶ Voltage-dependent Ca^{2+} Channels

Absorption

Absorption is defined as the disappearance of a drug from the site of administration and its appearance in the blood ("central compartment") or at its site of action. The main routes of administration are oral or parenteral (injection). After oral administration, a drug has to be taken up (is absorbed) from the gut. Here, the main site of absorption is the small intestine. In this case, only a portion of drug reaches the blood and arrives at its site of action.

▶ Pharmacokinetics

Abstinence Syndrome

The abstinence syndrome (synonym, withdrawal symptom) is observed after withdrawal of a drug to which a person is addicted. For example, the abstinence syndrome after alcohol withdrawal is characterized by tremor, nausea, tachycardia, sweating and sometimes hallucinations.

▶ Drug Addiction
▶ Dependence

Abused Drugs

▶ Drug Addiction
▶ Dependence

ACE Inhibitors

Jörg Peters
Pharmakologisches Institut der Universität
Heidelberg, Heidelberg, Germany
joerg.peters@urz.uni-heidelberg.de

Synonyms

Angiotensin converting enzyme inhibitors

Definition

Angiotensin converting enzyme (ACE) plays a central role in cardiovascular hemostasis. Its major function is the generation of angiotensin (ANG) II from ANG I and the degradation of bradykinin. Both peptides have profound impact on the cardiovascular system and beyond. ACE

inhibitors are used to decrease blood pressure in hypertensive patients, to improve cardiac function and to reduce work load of the heart in patients with cardiac failure.

▶ Blood Pressure Control
▶ Renin-Angiotensin-Aldosteron System

Mechanism of Action

ACE inhibitors inhibit the enzymatic activity of ▶ Angiotensin Converting Enzyme (ACE). This enzyme cleaves a variety of pairs of amino acids from the carboxy-terminal part of several peptide-substrates. The conversion of ANG I to ANG II and the degradation of bradykinin to inactive fragments are considered the most important functions of ACE (1–3). ACE inhibitors are non-peptide analogues of ANG I. They bind tightly to the active sites of ACE, where they complex with a zinc ion and interact with a positively charged group as well as with a hydrophibic pocket. They competitively inhibit ACE with Ki values in the range between 10^{-10} and 10^{-11} (3).

Effects of ACE-inhibitors mediated by the inhibition of ANG II generation:

ANG II is the effector peptide of the renin-angiotensin system (1,2). ANG II is one of the most potent vasoconstrictors, fascilitates norepinephrine release, stimulates aldosterone production and increases renal sodium retention. In addition, ANG II is considered to be a growth factor, stimulating proliferation of various cell types. The actions of ANG II are mediated through two ▶ Angiotensin Receptors, termed AT_1 and AT_2. Most of the cardiovascular functions of ANG II are mediated through the AT_1 receptor.

In some patients with hypertension and in all patients with cardiac failure, the renin-angiotensin system is activated to an undesired degree, burdening the heart. The consequences of diminished ANG II generation by ACE inhibitors are multiple: In patients with hypertension, blood pressure is reduced as a result of (a) decreased peripheral vascular resistance, (b) decreased sympathetic activity, and, (c) reduced sodium and water retention. In patients with cardiac failure, cardiac functions are improved as a result of (a) reduced sodium and water retention (preload and afterload reduction), (b) diminished total peripheral resistance (afterload reduction) and (c) reduced stimulation of the heart by the sympathetic nervous system. A reduction of cardiac hypertrophy appears to be another desired effect of ACE inhibitors. It is mediated at least partially by the reduction of intracardiac ANG II levels. ACE inhibitors furthermore protect the heart from arrhythmia during reperfusion after ischemia, and improve local blood flow and the metabolic state of the heart. These effects are largely mediated by Bradykinin (see below).

In the vasculature, ANG II not only increases contraction of smooth muscle cells, but is also able to induce vascular injury. This can be prevented by blocking ▶ NFκB activation (3) suggesting a link between ANG II and inflammation processes involved in the pathogenesis of arteriosclerosis (see below). Thus, ACE inhibitors not only decrease vascular tone but probably also exert vasoprotective effects.

In the kidney ANG II reduces renal blood flow and constricts preferentially the efferent arteriole of the glomerulus with the result of increased glomerular filtration pressure. ANG II further enhances renal sodium and water reabsorption at the proximal tubulus. ACE inhibitors thus increase renal blood flow and decrease sodium and water retention. Furthermore, ACE inhibitors are nephroprotective, delaying the progression of glomerulosclerosis. This also appears to be a result of reduced ANG II levels and is at least partially independent from pressure reduction. On the other hand, ACE inhibitors decrease glomerular filtration pressure due to the lack of ANG II-mediated constriction of the efferent arterioles. Thus, one important undesired effect of ACE inhibitors is impaired glomerular filtration rate and impaired kidney function.

Another effect of ANG II is the stimulation of ▶ Aldosterone production in the adrenal cortex. ANG II increases the expression of steroidogenic enzymes, such as aldosterone synthase and stimulates the proliferation of the aldosterone producing zona glomerulosa cells. Aldosterone increases sodium and water reabsorbtion at the distal tubuli. More recently it has been recognized that aldosterone is a fibrotic factor in the heart. ACE inhibitors decrease plasma aldosterone levels on a short term scale, thereby not only reducing sodium retention but also preventing aldosterone-induced cardiac fibrotic processes. On a long term scale, however, patients with cardiac failure exhibit high aldosterone levels even when taking ACE inhibitors.

In this context it is important to note that circulating ANG II levels do not remain reduced during long term treatment with ACE inhibitors. This is likely the result of activation of alternative, ACE-independent pathways of ANG II generation. The protective effects of ACE inhibitors on a long term scale, therefore, are not explained by a reduction of circulating ANG II levels. They are either unrelated to inhibition of ANG II generation, or a result of the inhibition of local generation of ANG II. Indeed, due to the ubiquitous presence of ACE in endothelial cells, large amounts of ANG II are generated locally within tissues such as kidney, blood vessels, adrenal gland, heart and brain, and exert local functions without appearing in the circulation (2). Membrane bound endothelial ACE, and consequently local ANG II generation, has been proved to be of greater significance than ANG II generated in plasma by the circulating enzyme. Experimental evidence also indicates that plasma ACE may infact not be relevant to blood pressure control at all.

Effects of ACE inhibitors mediated by the inhibition of Bradykinin degradation:

Kinins are involved in blood pressure control, regulation of local blood flow, vascular permeability, sodium balance, pain, inflammation, platelet aggregation and coagulation. Bradykinin also exerts antiproliferative effects (4). In plasma, bradykinin is generated from high molecular weight (HMW) kininogen, while in tissues lysbradykinin is generated from HMW and low molecular weight (LMW) kininogen. Several effects of bradykinin are explained by the fact that the peptide potently stimulates the NO-pathway and increases prostaglandin synthesis in endothelial cells. In smooth muscle cells and platelets, NO stimulates the soluble guanylate cyclase, which increases cyclic GMP that in turn activates protein kinase G. As a consequence, vascular tone and subsequently systemic blood pressure is decreased, local blood flow is improved and platelet aggregation is prevented.

ACE inhibitors inhibit the degradation of bradykinin and potentiate the effects of bradykinin by about 50–100 fold. The prevention of bradykinin degradation by ACE inhibitors is particularly protective for the heart. Increased bradykinin levels prevent postischemic reperfusion arrhythmia, delays manifestations of cardiac ischemia, prevents platelet aggregation and probably also reduces the degree of arteriosclerosis and the development of cardiac hypertrophy. The role of bradykinin and bradykinin-induced NO release for the improvement of cardiac functions by converting enzyme inhibitors has been demonstrated convincingly with use of a specific bradykinin receptor antagonist and inhibitors of NO-synthase.

In the kidney, bradykinin increases renal blood flow, whereas glomerular filtration rate remains unaffected. Bradykinin stimulates natriuresis and, through stimulation of prostaglandin synthesis, inhibits the actions of antidiuretic hormone (ADH), thereby inhibiting water retention. Bradykinin further improves insulin sensitivity and cellular glucose utilisation of skeletal muscle cells in experimental models. This, however, appears not to be relevant in the clinical context.

Bradykinin exerts its effects via B_1 and B_2 receptors. The inhibition of bradykinin degradation by ACE inhibitors compensatory leads to increased conversion of bradykinin to des Arg-9-bradykinin by kininase I. This peptide still has strong vasodilatatory properties and a high affinity to the B_1 receptor. The clinical relevance of this aspect is not clear. The cardioprotective effects of bradykinin are mediated via B_2 receptors, since they can be blocked by a specific B_2 receptor antagonist (4). On the other hand, kinins increase vascular permeability with the consequence of edema, exhibit chemotactic properties with the risk of local inflammation and they are involved in the manifestation of endotoxic schock. Increased bradykinin levels are thus thought to cause some of the undesired effects observed with ACE inhibitors, such as cough, allergic reactions and anaphylactic responses, for instance angioneurotic edema (5).

Clinical Use (incl. side effects)

ACE inhibitors are approved for the treatment of hypertension and cardiac failure (5). For cardiac failure, many studies have demonstrated increased survival rates independently of the initial degree of failure. They effectively decrease work load of the heart as well as cardiac hypertrophy and relieve the patients symptoms. In contrast to previous assumptions, ACE inhibitors do not inhibit aldosterone production on a long term scale sufficiently. Correspondingly, additional inhibition of aldosterone effects significantly reduces cardiac failure and increases survival even further in patients already receiving diuretics and ACE inhibitors. This can be achieved by coadministration of spironolactone, which inhibits binding of aldosterone to its receptor.

In the treatment of hypertension, ACE inhibitors are as effective as diuretics, β-adrenoceptor antagonists or calcium channel blockers in lowering blood pressure. However, increased survival rates have only been demonstrated for diuretics and β-adrenoceptor antagonists. ACE inhibitors are approved for monotherapy as well as for combinational regimes. ACE inhibitors are the drugs of choice for the treatment of hypertension with renal diseases, particularly diabetic nephropathy, because they prevent the progression of renal failure and improve proteinuria more efficiently than the other drugs.

More than 15 ACE inhibitors are presently available. They belong to three different chemical classes: sulfhydryl compounds such as captopril, carboxyl compounds such as enalapril, and phopshorus compounds such as fosinopril. Sulfhydryl compounds exert more undesired, but also desired effects, since they additionally interact with endogenous SH groups. For instance, these compounds may potentiate NO-actions or act as scavengers for oxygen-derived free radicals. Carboxyl compounds are in general more potent than captopril. Phosporous compounds are usually characterized by the longest duration of action.

Most ACE inhibitors are prodrugs, with the exceptions of captopril, lisinopril and ceranapril. Prodrugs exert improved oral bioavailability, but need to be converted to active compounds in the liver, kidney and/or intestinal tract. In effect, converting enzyme inhibitors have quite different kinetic profiles with regard to half time, onset and duration of action, or tissue penetration.

In general, ACE inhibitors at the doses used to date are safe drugs. In contrast to many antihypertensive drugs, ACE inhibitors do not elicit a reflectory tachycardia and do not influence lipid or glucose metabolism in an undesired manner. Glucose tolerance is even increased. Most undesired effects are class specific and related to the inhibition of ACE. Less dangerous, but often bothersome, are dry cough, related to increased bradykinin levels and loss of taste or impaired taste. The more severe undesired effects are hypotension, hyperkaliemia and renal failure, but those can be easily monitored and appropriately considered. The risk for hypotension increases in combination with diuretics, particularly when ACE inhibitors are initiated in patients who already receive diuretics. The risk of hyperkaliemia increases with coadministration of spironolactone and the risk of renal failure is higher in volume depleted patients or those already exhibiting impaired renal function. Seldom (0.05%) the development of angioneurotic edema occurs (usually) during the first days of treatment and is life threatening. Allergic responses and angioneurotic edema are related to bradykinin. Recently, specific AT_1 receptor antagonists have become available and are used in the management of hypertension and are presently tested for use in cardiac failure. They are believed not to exhibit the bradykinin-related undesired effects. Indeed, undesired effects of AT_1 receptor antagonists are lower than seen with ACE inhibitors. On the other hand, AT_1 receptor antagonists are probably less effective since the patients do not profit from the cardioprotective effects of bradykinin. Studies comparing the effects of ACE inhibitors with AT_1 receptor antagonists are presently underway. ACE inhibitors are contraindicated in pregnancy (risk of abortion, acute renal failure of the newborn) and patients with bilateral stenosis of the renal artery. Special caution should be taken if patients have autoimmunolocial systemic diseases.

References

1. Bader M, Paul M, Fernandesz-Alfonso M, Kaling M, Ganten D (1994). Molecular biology and biochemistry of the renin-angiotensin system Chap. 11, p.214–232; in: Textbook of Hypertension ed: J.D. Swales; Blackwell Scientific Publications. Oxford, London, Edinburgh.
2. Bader M, Peters J, Baltatu O, Müller DN, Luft FC, Ganten D (2001). Tissue renin-angiotensin systems: new insights from experimental animal models in hypertension research. J Mol Med 79:76–102
3. Gohlke P, Unger T (1994). Angiotensin converting enzyme inhibitors Chap 65, p.1115–1127 in: Textbook of Hypertension ed: J.D. Swales; Blackwell Scientific Publications. Oxford, London, Edinburgh.
4. Linz W, Martorana PA, Schölkens B. (1990). Local inhibition of bradykinin degradation in ischemic hearts. J. Cardiovasc Parmacol 15:S99–S109
5. Brogden RN, Todd PA, Sorkin EM (1988) Drugs 36:540–600

Acetylcholine

Acetylcholine is a neurotransmitter in cholinergic nerves which acts on muscarinic or nicotinic cholinoceptors.

► Nicotinic Receptors
► Muscarinic Receptors

Acetylcholinesterase

► Cholinesterase

Acetyltransferase

Acetyltransferase is an enzyme that catalyses the transfer of an acetyl group from one substance to another.

ACPD

ACPD (1-aminocyclopentane-1,3-dicarboxylic acid) is identified as the mGlu selective agonist. Within the 4 stereoisomers, 1S,3R-ACPD activates group-I and group-II mGlu receptors as well as some group-III receptors (mGlu8) at higher concentrations. The 1S,3S-ACPD isomer is one of the first selective group-II mGlu receptor agonists described. These molecules have been widely used to identify the possible physiological functions of mGlu receptors.

▶ Metabotropic Glutamate Receptors

ACTH

▶ Gluco-/Mineralocorticoid Receptors

Actin

▶ Cytoskeleton

Actin Binding Proteins

By binding to F-actin, actin binding proteins (ABPs) stabilize F-actin or regulate its turnover. Known ABPs are proteins such as α-actinin, talin, tensin, filamin, nexilin, fimbrin, and vinculin.

▶ Cytoskeleton

Action Potential

An action potential is a stereotyped (within a given cell) change of the membrane potential from a resting (intracellular negative) value to a depolarized (intracellular positive) value and then back to the resting value. The durations of action potentials range from a couple of milliseconds in nerve cells to hundreds of milliseconds in cardiac cells. Action potentials may be propagated along very elongated cells (e.g. nerves) or from one cell to another *via* electrical gap junctions (e.g. in cardiac tissue).

Activated Partial Thromboplastin Time

Activated partial thromboplastin time (aPTT) is a coagulation assay which measures the time for plasma to clot upon activation by a particulate substance (e.g., kaolin) in the presence of negatively-charged phospholipids.

▶ Anticoagulants

Activation-induced Cell Death

Activation-induced cell death is a specific term used for the apoptosis of T lymphocytes in the periphery. This process is of central importance in the homeostasis of the immune system. For example, an effective response to foreign invaders such as the powerful antigenic stimulus of bacterial super antigens is the extensive proliferation of T lymphocytes with a tremendous expansion of antigen specific T cell clones and efficient immune-mediated clearance of bacteria. This is followed by apoptosis of the majority of these antigen specific T cells, which serve to return the numbers of T cells in the periphery to normal.

Active Site

Catalytic Site

Active Transport

Active transport is permeation of a chemical through biological membranes against the electrochemical gradient. This type of transport requires energy produced by intracellular metabolic processes.

Activins

Activins are growth and differentiation factors belonging to the transforming growth factor-β superfamily. They are dimeric proteins, consisting of two inhibin-β subunits. The structure of activins is highly conserved during vertebrate evolution. Activins signal through type I and type II receptor serine/threonine receptor kinases. Subsequently downstream signals such as Smad proteins are phosphorylated. Activins are present in many tissues of the mammalian organism, where they function as autocrine and/or paracrine regulators of various physiological processes, including reproduction. In the hypothalamus, activins are thought to stimulate the release of gonadotropin-releasing hormone. In the pituitary, activins increase follicle-stimulating hormone secretion and up-regulate gonadotropin-releasing hormon receptor expression. In the ovaries, activins regulate processes such as folliculogenesis, steroid hormone production and oocyte maturation. During pregnancy, activin-A is also involved in the regulation of placental functions.

▶ Receptor Serine/Threonine Receptor Kinase
▶ Transforming Growth Factor-β Superfamily

Acute Phase Reactants

Acute phase reactants (e.g., C-reactive protein) are proteins that increase during inflammation and are deposited in damaged tissues. They were first discovered in the serum, but are now known to be involved in inflammatory processes in the brain (e.g., found in the brain of AD patients and associated with amyloid plaques).

▶ Inflammation

Acyl-CoA

Acyl-CoAs are the activated intermediates of fatty acid metabolism formed by the condensation of fatty acids with Coenzyme A.

Adaptive Immunity

The adaptive or specific arm of the immune system consists of T- and B-lymphocytes and antibodies. T- and B-cells carry antigen receptors that are generated by random genetic rearrangement during the ontogeny of lymphocytes in the bone marrow (B cells) or the thymus (T-cells). The hallmarks of adaptive immunity are the improved and specific defenses by T and B memory cells and antibodies after repeated exposure (immunological memory) to the eliciting antigen.

▶ Immune Defense

Adaptor Proteins

Adaptor proteins are multi-modular proteins containing different protein-protein interaction domains with no intrinsic enzymatic activity. They serve as scaffolds in assembling protein complexes. Their role in fine-tuning signaling networks is becoming more evident.

▶ Growth Factors

Addiction

▶ Drug Addiction
▶ Dependence

Additive Interaction

Additive interaction is interaction in which the combined effect is the sum of the effects of each drug administered separately.

Aδ-fibres

Aδ-fibres are small diameter myelinated afferent fibres. As part of the pain sensory system they are present in nerves that innervate the skin and deep somatic and visceral structures.

▶ Nociception

Adenosine

Adenosine is produced by many tissues, mainly as a by-product of ATP breakdown. It is released from neurons, glia and other cells, possibly through the operation of the membrane transport system. Its rate of production varies with the functional state of the tissue and it may play a role as a autocrine or paracrine mediator (e.g. controlling blood flow). The uptake of adenosine is blocked by dipyridamole, which has vasodilatory effects. The effects of adenosine are mediated by a group of G-protein coupled receptors (the $G_{i/o}$-coupled A_1- and A_3- receptors, and the G_s-coupled A_{2A}-/A_{2B}-receptors). A_1-receptors can mediate vasoconstriction, block of cardiac atrioventricular conduction and reduction of force of contraction, bronchoconstriction, and inhibition of neurotransmitter release. A_2 receptors mediate vasodilatation and are involved in the stimulation of nociceptive afferent neurons. A_3 receptors mediate the release of mediators from mast cells. Methylxanthines (e.g. caffeine) function as antagonists of A_1 and A_2 receptors. Adenosine itself is used to terminate supraventricular tachycardia by intravenous bolus injection.

▶ Purinergic System

Adenosine Receptors

▶ Adenosine
▶ Purinergic System

Adenoviruses

▶ Gene Therapy

Adenylyl Cyclases

ROGER A. JOHNSON
Department of Physiology & Biophysics,
State University of New York, Stony Brook,
New York, USA
rjohnson@ms.cc.sunysb.edu

Synonyms

Adenylyl cyclase (preferred), adenylate cyclase, adenyl cyclase (original), and ATP:pyrophosphate lyase, cyclizing (E.C.4.6.1.1.)

Definition

Adenosine 3':5'-monophosphate (▶ cAMP) modifies cell function and metabolism in virtually all eukaryotic cells through the activation of cAMP-dependent protein kinase, which catalyzes the phosphorylation of numerous proteins or through cAMP-gated ion channels. Cellular levels of cAMP reflect the balance between the actions of adenylyl cyclase and cAMP-phosphodiesterases. Adenylyl cyclases are a family of enzymes that catalyze the formation of cAMP from 5'-ATP. The enzyme occurs throughout the animal kingdom and plays diverse roles in cell regulation.

▶ Guanylyl Cyclases
▶ Phosphodiesterases
▶ Transmembrane Signalling

Basic Characteristics

Mammalian Adenylyl Cyclases

In mammals there are at least ten distinct adenylyl cyclases Isozymes (Fig. 1) and these are central to one of the most important transmembrane signal transduction pathways [1]. All but one of the isozymes are membrane-bound and these are regulated by numerous hormones and neurotransmitters via cell-surface receptors linked via heterotrimeric ($\alpha\beta\gamma$) stimulatory (G_s) and inhibitory (G_i) guanine nucleotide-dependent regulatory proteins (▶ G-proteins) (Fig. 2). $G\alpha_s$ stimulates all of these isozymes except the soluble type X. The isozymes differ more significantly in their responses to G-α_i and to the effects of G-$\beta\gamma$ on $G\alpha_s$-stimulated enzyme. For example, in the pres-

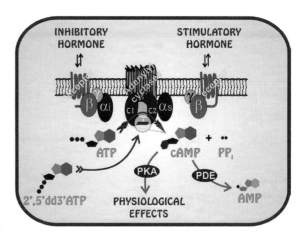

Fig. 2 Membrane localization, topology, and regulation of mammalian adenylyl cyclases.

but significantly stimulates the type II and type IV enzyme, and G-α_i inhibits isozyme types II, III, and V, but is apparently without effect on the other forms (Table 1).

The membrane-bound forms of the mammalian adenylyl cyclases exhibit a putative topology with twelve membrane-spanning regions and two ~40 kD cytosolic domains (C_1 and C_2) (Fig. 2), which share large conserved regions [2]. N-terminal domains are highly variable and likely serve regulatory roles. Differences within other domains of the isozymes are significant and participate in regulation by a variety of agents. The cleft formed by the C1•C2 domains binds substrate and ▶ forskolin (Fig. 3). The active site shares topology and reaction mechanisms with guanylyl cyclases, with which there is considerable homology, and with oligonucleotide polymerases. Each catalyzes a cation-dependent attack of the 3′-OH on the α-phosphate of a nucleoside triphosphate, with pyrophosphate as leaving group. Activation of adenylyl cyclases by α_s•GTP occurs through its interaction with the enzyme's C_2 domain, yielding the active enzyme: GTP•α_s•C [3]. A symmetrical locus on the C_1 domain interacts with α_i. Consequently, agents that affect either the dissociation of either G_i or G_s, or the association of their respective α_s, α_i, or $\beta\gamma$ subunits with adenylyl cyclase could affect rates of cAMP formation in membrane preparations or in intact cells and tissues.

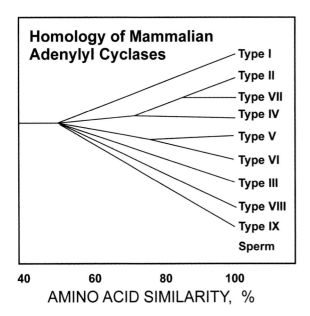

Fig. 1 Adenylyl cyclase isoforms: aminoacid homology. The numbering of adenylyl cyclase isozymes has been in the order of their expression and deduced sequencing. There is substantial homology within the family of membrane-bound forms of the enzyme, yet they are distinctly and selectively regulated by a variety of agents.

Tab. 1 Mammalian adenylyl cyclases and characteristics of their regulation.

Isozyme	Amino Acids	Accession Number[b]	$G\alpha_i$[d,e]	$G\beta\gamma$[f]	Ca^{2+}/ Calmodulin	Protein Kinases	Tissue Distribution[j]
I (bovine)[a]	1134	M25579		↓	EC_{50}~20nM	PKC ↑	brain
II (rat)	1090	M80550	↓	↑	no Δ	PKC[i] ↑↑	brain
III (rat)	1144	M55075	↓	no Δ[g]	↓	PKC ↑	olfactory, brain, adrenal, brown fat
IV (rat)	1064	M80633		↑	no Δ	PKC ↓	ubiquitous
V (rat)	1262	M96159	↓	↓	(no CaM)[h] ↓	PKC ↑	heart, brain
VI (rat)	1180	M96160		↓		PKC ↓ PKA	heart, kidney liver
VII (mouse)	1099	U12919					retina, brain
VIII (rat)	1248(A)	L26986[c]			↑		brain
IX (mouse)	1353	U30602			no Δ		skeletal muscle, heart, brain
X (human)	1610	AF176813	no Δ				testes

Notes:
a) Species designated is that from which the isozyme was originally cloned
b) Structures can be obtained through http://www.ncbi.nlm.nih.gov/
c) Type VIII exhibits three splice variants (A,B,C); accession number is for A.
d) An empty cell implies that no information was available.
e) Arrows indicate increased (up arrow) or decreased (down arrow) adenylyl cyclase activity.
f) Effects of G-$\beta\gamma$ are on G-α_s-stimulated enzyme.
g) No Δ implies that this was tested, but no effect was observed.
h) No CaM: inhibition of adenylyl cyclase was caused by calcium in the absence of calmodulin.
i) Double arrows indicates large effect on activity.
j) Distribution implies evidence of protein expression; this is not a complete listing.

Adenylyl cyclase activity may also be altered by numerous other agents of physiological and biochemical interest. These include agents or enzymes that act on hormone receptors, bacterial toxins that act on G_s and G_i, and agents that act directly on adenylyl cyclase. For example, ► fluoride activates most mammalian adenylyl cyclases indirectly through its effect on Gs. G-α_s is stably activated by poorly hydrolyzable analogs of GTP, e.g. GTPγS or GPP(NH)P, and its activation is hindered by GDPβS. Other important examples include the ADP-ribosyltransferase of *Vibrio cholerae*, which catalyzes the ADP-ribosylation from NAD of G-α_s, leading to stably activated enzyme, and of *Bordetella pertussis*, which ADP-ribosylates G-$\alpha_i\beta\gamma$, which prevents its dissociation and

also leads to elevated adenylyl cyclase activity (cf. G-proteins). These actions contribute to the pathophysiology of these bacteria. Phosphorylation, catalyzed by cAMP-dependent protein kinase (PKA), protein kinase C (PKC), or receptor protein kinases, can elicit altered adenylyl cyclase activity due either to effects directly on the enzyme or indirectly through effects on hormone receptors or G-proteins. By comparison, forskolin [1,3] activates most adenylyl cyclase isozymes by directly binding within the $C_1 \cdot C_2$ cleft. Most isozymes are regulated by Ca^{2+}, either directly through one of the two metal-binding sites (see below), or indirectly through calmodulin [1], which activates a few isozymes, or indirectly through PKC. Although there is substantial homology among the

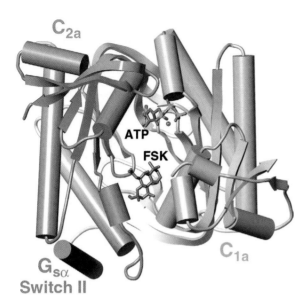

Fig. 3 Crystal structure of adenylyl cyclase. The crystal structure of adenylyl cyclase was first achieved with a $C_2 \cdot C_2$ homodimer and then with the $C_1 \cdot C_2 \cdot \alpha_s$ complex shown here [3]. The Switch II region of $G\alpha_s$ interacts with the C_2 domain to effect activation of adenylyl cyclase. The cleft formed between C_1 and C_2 affords loci for catalysis (ATP) and for activation by forskolin (FSK). The cleft formed by the interaction of the VC_1 and IIC_2 domains of a chimeric adenylyl cyclase contains binding sites for substrate (ATP) and forskolin (FSK). The Switch II domain of $G\alpha_s$ interacts with the C_2 domain of adenylyl cyclase.

membrane-bound forms of the mammalian adenylyl cyclases, the striking differences in the character and extent of regulation by a variety of agents imply that primary and secondary structural characteristics are important determinants in the interactions of the enzyme with cell constituents and hence will regulate enzyme acitivity, the rate of formation of cAMP, and the downstream effects that this will have.

Catalytic Mechanism
Adenylyl cyclases exhibit a reversible bireactant sequential mechanism in which free divalent cations and cation-5'-ATP serve as substrates, and cAMP, metal-PP$_i$, and free divalent cations are products (Fig. 4). For some isozymes, available data suggest that substrate binding and product

release are ordered and for others random. Typically, reaction velocities are considerably greater with Mn^{2+} as the cation than with Mg^{2+}. Maximal velocities observed with various ATP analogs follow the order: 2'-d-5'ATP > ATP > ATPγS > APP(NH)P > APP(CH$_2$)P. Km values for rat brain cyclase are: K_{MnATP}, ~9 μM, $K_{Mn^{2+}}$, ~4 μM, K_{MgATP}, ~60 μM, and $K_{Mg^{2+}}$, ~860 μM. Notably, activation of adenylyl cyclases by hormones or by $G\text{-}\alpha_s$, via the active enzyme configuration $GTP\cdot\alpha_s\cdot C$, causes a reduction in $K_{Mg^{2+}}$ of more than an order of magnitude to ~50 μM, without a change in K_{MgATP}.

Drugs

Activators and Inhibitors
Although agents which indirectly activate or inhibit adenylyl cyclases are common and are even used in the treatment of disease, e.g. blockers of β-adrenergic receptors, hormones, and other drugs targeting G-protein-coupled receptors, drugs acting directly on the enzyme have been less well explored. And for most stimulators and inhibitors that act directly on adenylyl cyclases, isozyme selectivity has not been demonstrated. The main classes of such agents are derivatives of forskolin and of adenine nucleosides. Probably all adenylyl cyclases are inhibited competitively by substrate analogs, which compete with the site and enzyme configuration with which cation-ATP binds (Fig. 4). The best competitive inhibitor is β-L-2',3'-

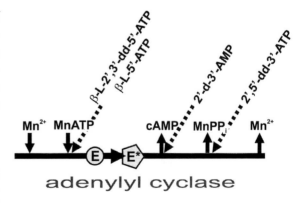

Fig. 4 Reaction sequence for catalysis and inhibition of adenylyl cyclases. E* represents the catalytic transition state.

Tab. 2 Competitive inhibitors of adenylyl cyclase. Assays were performed with detergent-dispersed adenylyl cyclase from rat brain and were conducted with 100 μM MnATP and 5 mM MnCl$_2$ as substrates.

Nucleotide	IC$_{50}$ [μM]
β-L-5'-AMP	200
β-L-2',3'-dd-5'-AMP	62
β-D-5'-AP(CH$_2$)PP	30
β-L-5'-ATP	3.2
β-D-2',3'-dd-5'-ATP	0.76
β-L-2',3'-dd-5'-ATP	0.024

dideoxy-adenosine-5'-triphosphate (β-L-2',3'-dd-5'-ATP; Table 2, Fig. 5) [4], which has been used to identify the ► two metal sites within the catalytic active site [5]. This ligand has also been labeled with ^{32}P in the β-phosphate position and is a useful ligand for reversible, binding displacement assays of adenylyl cyclases [4].

Most membrane-bound forms of the mammalian adenylyl cyclase are inhibited by adenine nucleosides and their 3'-polyphosphates derivatives. These constitute a class of inhibitors historically referred to as P-site ligands. Inhibition by these ligands is conserved with varying sensitivity in all isozymes, save those of bacteria and sperm, and they provide an exquisite means for inhibition of this signal transduction pathway. The most potent of these ligands is 2',5'-dideoxyadenosine-3'-tetraphosphate (2',5'-dd-3'-A4P; Table 3; cf. Fig. 2 for structure of corresponding 3'-triphosphate) [6]. Whereas the most potent ligands in this class contain polyphosphate groups at the 3'-ribosyl position, they are not cell permeable. Membrane permeable ligands include the precursor nucleoside, 2',5'-dd-Ado, and several 9-substituted adenine derivatives, specifically 9-THF-Ade (SQ 22,536), 9-Ara-Ade, 9-Xyl-Ade, and 9-CP-Ade (Table 4). An advantage of 9-CP-Ade, in contrast with the other compounds, is that it is both chemically and metabolically stable. These have been used to lower cellular cAMP levels and to alter function in numerous studies with isolated cells and intact tissues.

To take advantage of the potency of the adenine nucleoside 3'- or 5'-polyphoshate derivatives for studies with intact cells and tissues, it is necessary either to protect the phosphate groups from exonucleotidases or to provide a precursor to these molecules that is cell permeable and is then metabolized into a potent inhibitor by intracellular enzymes. The general term for this type of compound is ► prodrug or pronucleotide. The most interesting members of this class of compound are phorphorylated derivatives of 9-substituted-adenines that are spatially consistent with the phosphate position of 2',5'-dd-3'-AMP and in which the phosphate is protected by any of several protecting ligands. The potency of the best of these compounds is in a range similar to that of 2',5'-dd-3'-ATP. Although the use of these agents to date has been solely with isolated cells, it is likely that they will find applications in other systems as an additional upstream block of the adenylyl cyclase-cAMP-PKA signaling cascade.

Miscellaneous Observations

Since its first description, adenylyl cyclase has been an enzyme family of intense investigation. Consequently, numerous observations have been made of agents that affect its activity, principally in isolated membranes, but also of purified enzyme. Some of these effects are of importance for investigators intending to work with the enzyme. For example, it has been universally observed that the enzyme is protected by thiols, β-mercaptoethanol, 2,3-dimercaptopropanol, and dithiothreitol being the most commonly used.

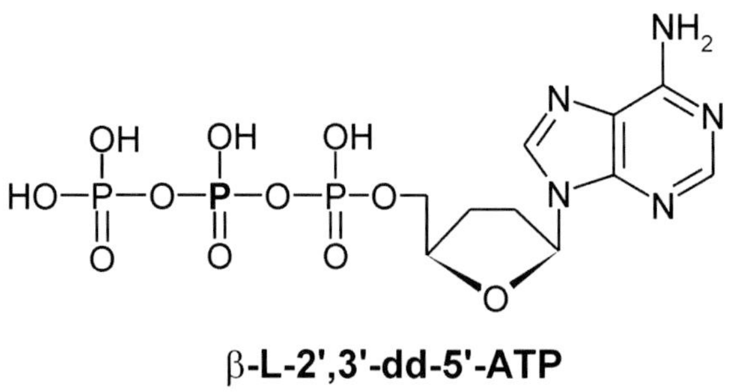

β-L-2',3'-dd-5'-ATP

Fig. 5 A potent, reversibly binding, competitive inhibitor of adenylyl cyclases, labeled with ^{32}P at the β-phosphate.

Tab. 3 **IC$_{50}$ values for inhibition of rat brain adenylyl cyclase by adenosine 3'-phosphates.** Assays were performed with detergent-dispersed adenylyl cyclase from rat brain and were conducted with 100 μM 5'ATP and 5 mM MnCl$_2$ as substrates. Values obtained for 3'-ATP are overestimations due to the formation of 2':3'-cAMP from 3'-ATP that occurs non-enzymatically in the presence of divalent cations.

3'-Phosphate	nucleoside [μM]		
	Ado	2'-d-Ado	2',5'-dd-Ado
none	82	15	2.7
~P	8.9	1.2	0.46
~PP	3.9	0.14	0.10
~PPP	2.0	0.09	0.04
~PPPP	---	0.0105	0.0074

Conversely, adenylyl cyclases are generally susceptible to oxidants, e.g. H$_2$O$_2$, (IC$_{50}$ ~3 μM) and benzoquinone (IC$_{50}$ ~3 μM), and alkylating agents, e.g. N-ethylmaleimide (IC$_{50}$ ~100 μM), *p*-aminophenylarsenoxide (IC$_{50}$ ~40 μM), *p*-aminophenyldichloroarsine (IC$_{50}$ ~80 μM), or *o*-iodosobenzoate (IC$_{50}$ ~10 μM for type I adenylyl cyclase against calmodulin stimulation). Not surprisingly, the crude membrane-bound enzyme is susceptible to thermal inactivation (e.g. 50% inactivation at 35° in 10 min) and the purified enzyme is more labile, but protection is afforded by forskolin, substrate, P-site ligands, Ca^{2+}/calmodulin (e.g. with type I enzyme), and activated G-α_s. Proteases also elevate adenylyl cyclase activity. For example, acrosin, trypsin, and thrombin can cause 5–10 fold activation, and these exhibit some isozyme selectivity (type II > III >> V). The basis for this activation in each case is not known, though serine proteases are known to cleave Gα_i, and this could lead to indirect effects on adenylyl cyclase activity.

All the studies on mammalian adenylyl cyclases notwithstanding, it is unclear if all forms of the enzyme have been identified, whether all modes of regulation have been determined, when during development, cell life cycles, and cell-cell interactions that specific isozymes are expressed, and how these processes are regulated.

Bacterial and Other Adenylyl Cyclases

Adenylyl cyclases are found throughout the animal kingdom and serve a variety of regulatory roles. In some animals, e.g. insects and crustaceans, the enzyme is membrane-bound and is regulated by neurotransmitters and G-proteins in a manner similar to that seen in mammalian systems. Sperm motility, respiration, and fertilization in invertebrates, e.g. sea urchins, all involve changes in adenylyl cyclase activity. Here, too, regulatory mechanisms are similar to those in mammalian systems. In some unicellular organisms, however, adenylyl cyclases have been observed to be soluble whereas in others it is membrane-associated. Structures of enzyme from these latter sources have not been determined, but amino acid sequences have been deduced for some. Available evidence indicates that there is little homology between these adenylyl cyclases and the membrane-bound mammalian form. There are several notable examples. In *Salmonella typhimurium* and *Escherichia coli* regulation of adenylyl cyclase is coordinated with that of carbohydrate permeases by the phosphoenolbpyruvate:sugar phosphotransferase system. This is important for bacterial responses to changes in nutrient levels. The adenylyl cyclase of *Brevibacterium liquifaciens* was the first to be purified and was used to demonstrate the requirement for a α-keto-monocarboxylic acid cofactor and that the catalytic reaction was reversible (reversibility of the reaction was recently shown to occur also for a chimeric mammalian adenylyl cyclase). The adenylyl cyclases of *Bordetella pertussis* and *Bacillus anthracis* are both soluble, Ca^{2+}/calmodulin-dependent but G-protein independent enzymes, which are exported from the respective bacteria. Because these enzymes are then transported into infected cells, adenylyl cyclase actually constitutes a toxic factor in mammals; adenylyl cyclase is the 'edema factor' of *B. anthracis*. It is in *Dictyostelium discoideum* that adenylyl cyclase generates the cAMP that provides the signal for aggregation into a multicellular organism and the development of fruiting bodies. And lastly, in yeast (*Saccharomyces cerevisiae*) the enzyme is membrane bound and is regulated by a G-protein, in this case Ras. As in mammalian systems, it is involved in metabolic control and in mating responses. Given that in many of these other systems additional proteins and cofactors participate in the regulation of adenylyl cyclase activity,

Tab. 4 IC$_{50}$ values for inhibition of rat brain adenylyl cyclase by 9-substituted adenine derivatives. Assays were performed with detergent-dispersed adenylyl cyclase from rat brain and were conducted with 100 μM 5'ATP and 5 mM $MnCl_2$ as substrates.

Adenine Derivative	IC$_{50}$ [μM]
9-CP-Ade	100
9-THF-Ade	20
9-Ara-Ade	30
9-Xyl-Ade	3.2
3'-d-Ado (cordycepin)	13
PMEA	66
PMEApp	0.175
PMEAp(NH)p	0.180

the full elucidation of the roles in which this enzyme activity participates in cell growth, development, and function, is a long way off.

Abbreviations Used Within the Text

Ado, adenosine; 2'-d-Ado, 2'-deoxyadenosine; 3'-d-Ado, 3'-deoxyadenosine; 5'-d-Ado, 5'-deoxyadenosine; 2',5'-dd-Ado, 2',5'-dideoxyadenosine; 2',3'-dd-Ado, 2',3'-dideoxyadenosine; 9-CP-Ade, 9-(cyclopentyl)-adenine; 9-THF-Ade, 9-(tetrahydrofuryl)-adenine (SQ22,536); 9-Ara-Ade, 9-(arabinofuranosyl)-adenine; 9-Xyl-Ade, 9-(xylofuranosyl)-adenine; cAMP, adenosine-3':5'monophosphate; 2'-d-3'-AMP, 2'-deoxyadenosine 3'-monophosphate; 2'-d-3'-ADP, 2'-deoxyadenosine 3'-diphosphate; 2'-d-3'-ATP, 2'-deoxyadenosine 3'-triphosphate; 2',5'-dd-3'-AMP, 2',5'-dideoxyadenosine 3'-monophosphate; 2',5'-dd-3'-ADP, 2',5'-dideoxyadenosine 3'-diphosphate; 2',5'-dd-3'-ATP, 2',5'-dideoxyadenosine 3'-triphosphate; 2',5'-dd-3'-A4P, 2',5'-dideoxyadenosine 3'-tetraphosphate; PMEA, 9-(2-phosphonylmethoxyethyl)-adenine; PMEApp, 9-(2-diphosphorylphosphonylmethoxyethyl)-adenine; PMEAp(NH)p, 9-(2-iminodiphosphorylphosphonylmethoxyethyl)-adenine.

References

1. Sunahara, R.K., Dessauer, C.W., and Gilman, A.G. (1996) Complexity and diversity of mammalian adenylyl cyclases. Ann. Rev. Pharmacol. & Toxicol. 36:461–480
2. Krupinski, J., Coussen, F., Bakalyar, H.A., Tang, W.J., Feinstein, P.G., Orth, K., Slaughter, C., Reed, R.R., and Gilman, A.G. (1989) Adenylyl cyclase amino acid sequence: possible channel- or transporter-like structure. Science 244:1558–1564
3. Tesmer, J.J.G., Sunahara, R.K., Gilman, A.G., and Sprang, S.R. (1997) Crystal structure of the catalytic domains of adenylyl cyclase in a complex with Gsα•GTPγS. Science 278:1907–1916
4. Shoshani, I., Boudou, V., Pierra, C., Gosselin, G., and Johnson, R.A. (1999) Enzymatic synthesis of unlabeled and [β-32P]-labeled ∃-L-2',3'-dideoxyadenosine-5'-triphosphate as a potent inhibitor of adenylyl cyclases and its use as reversible binding ligand. J. Biol. Chem. 274:34735–34741
5. Tesmer, J.J.G., Sunahara, R.K., Johnson, R.A., Gosselin, G., Gilman, A.G., and Sprang, S.R. (1999) Two metal ion catalysis in adenylyl cyclase revealed by its complexes with ATP analogs, Mg^{2+}, Mn^{2+}, and Zn^{2+}. Science 285:756–760
6. Désaubry, L., Shoshani, I., and Johnson, R.A. (1996) Inhibition of adenylyl cyclase by a family of newly synthesized adenine nucleoside 3'-polyphosphates suggests new regulatory pathways. J. Biol. Chem. 271:14028–14034

ADH

Antidiuretic Hormone

▶ Vasopressin/Oxytocin

ADHD

ADHD is ▶ Attention Deficit Hyperactivity Disorder.

▶ Psychostimulants

Adhesion Molecules

Adhesion molecules are transmembrane proteins, which through their extracellular part mediate the interaction of cells with other cells or with extracellular components like the extracellular matrix. On the basis of structural and functional similarities, most adhesion molecules can be grouped into families such as cadherins, integrins, selectins, the immunoglobulin superfamily or the syndecans. While some adhesion molecules are passive in their adhesive function, the adhesiveness of other adhesive molecules can be regulated. Some adhesive proteins are very similar to receptors, in that they not only bind other molecules with high selectivity and affinity, but are also able to transduce the binding into an intracellular signal.

▶ Integrins
▶ Cadherins
▶ Table appendix: Adhesion Molecules
▶ Anti-integrins, therapeutic and diagnostic implications

AdoMet

▶ S-adenosyl -L-methionine

Adrenal Gland

The adrenal gland is a flattened gland situated above each kidney, consisting of a cortex (outer wall) that secretes important steroid hormones and a medulla (inner part) that secretes adrenaline (epinephrine) and noradrenaline (norepinephrine).

▶ Glucocorticoids

Adrenaline

Arenaline (epinephrine) is a catecholamine, which is released as a neurotransmitter from neurons in the central nervous system and as a hormone from chromaffin cells of the adrenal gland. Adrenaline is required for increased metabolic and cardiovascular demand during stress. Its cellular actions are mediated via plasma membrane bound G-protein-coupled receptors.

▶ α-Adrenergic System
▶ β-Adrenergic System

Adrenergic or Noradrenergic Synapses, Receptors and Drugs

Adrenergic or noradrenergic synapses or receptors use either adrenaline or noradrenaline as a chemical transmitter. Drugs stimulating the adrenergic and noradrenergic receptors, respectively. Adrenergic receptors are divided into α and β receptors, both of which are further divided into subtypes like α_{1A}, α_{1B}, α_{2A}, α_{2B}, α_{2C} and β_1, β_2 and β_3 receptors that have different distribution in the body.

▶ α-Adrenergic System
▶ β-Adrenergic System

Adrenoceptor

▶ α-Adrenergic System
▶ β-Adrenergic System

Adrenocorticotropic Hormone

▶ Corticotropin

Adrenomedullin

Human adrenomedullin is a 52-amino acid peptide belonging to the calcitonin/calcitonin gene-related peptide (CGRP)/amylin peptide family. It is synthesized mainly in endothelial cells and elicits vasodilation.

Adverse/Unwanted Reactions

All drugs, in addition to their therapeutic effects, have the potential to do harm, i.e. to cause adverse/unwanted reactions (side effects). These may or may not be related to the principal pharmacological action of the drug. Examples of the second category are toxic effects of metabolites of a drug or immunological reactions.

Affective Disorders

Affective (mood) disorders are characterized by changes in mood. The most common manifestation is depression, arranging from mild to severe forms. Psychotic depression is accompanied by hallucinations and illusions. Mania is less common than depression. In bipolar affective disorder, depression alternates with mania.

▶ Antidepressant Drugs

Affinity

Ligands reside at a point of minimal energy within a binding locus of a protein according to a ratio of the rate the ligand leaves the surface of the protein (k_{off}) and the rate it approaches the protein surface (k_{on}). This ratio is the equilibrium dissociation constant of the ligand-protein complex (denoted $K_{eq} = k_{off}/k_{on}$) and defines the molar concentration of the ligand in the compartment containing the protein that is bound to 50% of the protein at any one instant. The 'affinity' or attraction of the ligand for the protein is the reciprocal of K_{eq}.

▶ Drug-Receptor-Interaction

Agonist

An agonist is a drug or ligand that activates a receptor, by inducing a biological response, when it binds. Between compounds that induce the maximal cellular reaction (full agonists) and antagonists, which do not induce a reaction, there is a spectrum of drugs that induce some but not maximal reaction; they are called partial agonists and have an intrinsic activity, i.e. the ability to induce the cellular reaction, of >0 and <100%.

Between compounds that induce the maximal cellular reaction (full agonists) and antagonists, which do not induce a reaction, there is a spectrum of drugs that induce some but not maximal reaction; they are called partial agonists and have an intrinsic activity, i.e. the ability to induce the cellular reaction, of >0 and <100%.

▶ Drug-Receptor-Interaction
▶ G-protein-coupled Receptors

Agouti-related Protein

The agouti gene encodes a paracrine signaling molecule that antagonizes the effect of melanocyte-stimulating hormone (MSH) at the melanocortin-1 receptor. This effect reduces the synthesis of eumelanin, and is responsible for the agouti hair colour in rodents. Agouti-related protein (AgRP) is similar to the agouti protein (25% identical amino acids), and is an endogenous antagonist of αMSH at the melanocortin-3 and melanocortin-4 receptors. AgRP is a potent orexigen, and down-regulation of AgRP is a major mechanism of the anorexigenic effect of leptin.

AgRP

▶ Agouti-related Protein

Ah Receptor

Members of the CYP1 family and some other drug metabolizing enzymes including *UGT1A6* are collectively induced by polycyclic aromatic hydrocarbons that serve as ligands to a specialized receptor called the Ah (aryl hydrocarbon) receptor which translocates to the nucleus following binding of another protein component called arnt (arnt for Ah receptor nuclear translocator). In the nucleus these two proteins bind DNA and activate transcription.

▶ Arylhydrocarbon Receptor

AIDS

AIDS (acquired immunodeficiency syndrome) is the final stage of disease caused by infection with HIV. In this stage, the virus infection has severely affected the immune system, causing a depletion of CD4+ T-helper cells. AIDS is characterized by the manifestation of typical diseases caused by opportunistic infections (*Pneumocystis carinii* pneumonia, CMV retinitis, candidiasis of the esophagus, cerebral toxoplasmosis), neurological manifestations, cachexia or certain tumors (Kaposi sarcoma of the skin, B cell lymphoma).

▶ Antiviral Drugs

Airway Hyperresponsiveness

Airway hyperresponsiveness is an exaggerated propensity for airways to narrow too easily in response to a wide variety of stimuli. Airway hyperresponsiveness leads to clinical symptoms of wheezing and dyspnea after exposure to allergens, environmental irritants, viral infections, cold air, or exercise.

▶ Glucocorticoids

Airway Surface Liquid

Airway surface liquid (ASL) is the very thin fluid layer (~7 μM) maintained at the apical membrane of airway epithelia. ASL thickness is maintained by a tight control of fluid reabsorption and/or secretion, mediated by sodium and/or chloride channels.

▶ Epithelial Sodium Channel

AKAP

AKAPs are cyclic AMP-dependent protein kinase (PKA)-anchoring proteins, a family of about 30 proteins anchoring PKA at subcellular sites in close vicinity to a certain substrate.

▶ Scaffolding Proteins

Akt

Akt (synonym 'protein kinase B') is a 60 kD serine/threonine protein kinase. Insulin and several growth factors stimulate Akt by a phosphatidylinositol 3'-kinase (PI 3-kinase- dependent phosphorylation of threonine 308 and serine 473 (in the human Akt1-isoform). Akt was initially identified in a T-cell lymphoma as the oncogene product of the transforming AKT8 retrovirus.

▶ Insulin Receptor
▶ Tyrosine Kinases

Alcohol

▶ Ethanol

Alcohol Dehydrogenase

Alcohol dehydrogenase is a cytoplasmic enzyme mainly found in the liver, but also in the stomach. The enzyme accomplishes the first step of ethanol metabolism, oxidation to acetaldehyde, which is further metabolized by ▶ aldehyde dehydrogenase. Quantitatively, the oxidation of ethanol is more or less independent of the blood concentration and constant with time, i.e. it follows zero-order kinetics (▶ pharmacokinetics). On average, a 70-kg person oxidizes about 10 ml of ethanol per hour.

Aldehyde Dehydrogenase

Ethanol is almost entirely metabolized in the liver. The first step, oxidation by alcohol dehydrogenase, yields acetaldehyde, a reactive and toxic compound. Essentially all of the acetaldehyde is converted to acetate by the liver enzyme aldehyde dehydrogenase. Aldehyde dehydrogenase is inhibited by the drug disulfiram. Given alone, disulfiram is a nontoxic substance. However, ethanol consumption in the presence of disulfiram causes an extremely unpleasant reaction characterized by flushing, hyperventilation, vomiting, sweating, tachycardia, hypotension, vertigo and marked distress. The altered response to alcohol is the rational basis for the use of disulfiram in the treatment of chronic alcoholism.

▶ Ethanol

Aldosterone

Aldosterone is a small hydrophobic molecule and belongs to the class of steroid hormones. Aldosterone is the major mineralocorticoid in the body. It binds to the mineralocorticoid receptor. This receptor belongs to the superfamily of steroid hormone receptors, which are located intracellularly and, upon binding of the agonist, translocate into the cell nucleus, where they regulate the transcription of those genes, which contain the appropriate hormone responsive regulatory elements. In the intestine and particularly in the distal tubules of the kidney, aldosterone increases the expression of proteins which modulate the activity of the sodium-potassium ATPase and the amylorid-sensitive sodium channel. As a consequence, sodium reabsorption and, secondarily, potassium excretion increase.

▶ Renin-Angiotensin-Aldosterone System

AlF4⁻

Fluoride forms a tetrahedral ion with aluminum, AlF_4^-, which forms a complex with the GDP $\cdot \alpha\beta\gamma$ form of heterotrimeric G-proteins. In the case of G_s, the complex $AlF_4^- \cdot GDP \cdot \alpha_s\beta\gamma$ behaves much as GTP or the more stable GTP derivatives, GTPγS or GPP(NH)P, and causes the dissociation of G_s and the subsequent activation of adenylyl cyclase through the complex $AlF_4^- \cdot GDP \cdot \alpha_s \cdot C$. AlF_4^- does not activate small, monomeric GTPases.

▶ G-proteins
▶ Adenylyl Cyclases

Alkaloid

Alkaloids are heterocyclic basic compounds and widespread in plants. Many of them have specific targets in organisms. For example, the alkaloids atropine and scopolamine of *Belladonna* are specific antagonists at ▸ muscarinic receptors.

Alkylating Agents

Alkylating agents form covalent bonds with target molecules. They alkylate various nucleophilic moieties such as phosphates. The biological effects of alkylating agents are the consequence of alkylation of DNA. Originally employed as chemical warfare agents, they are now used in the chemotherapy of cancer. Examples are cyclophosphamide and cisplatin.

▸ Antineoplastic Agents

Allele

An allele is one form in which a polymorphism exists. Most genetic polymorphisms are bi-allelic, i.e. they occur in two forms. Other types of genetic polymorphisms such as the VNTR polymorphisms are multi-allelic.

▸ Pharmacogenetics

Allergen

An allergen is usually an inert substance (eg pollen, house dust mite faeces) that can trigger the generation of an inappropriate antigenic response in some individuals. Subsequent exposure of a sensitized individual to the allergen is therefore able to cross-link IgE antibodies on the surface of mast cells and trigger an immune response and histamine release.

▸ Allergy
▸ Histaminergic System

Allergy

KLAUS RESCH, MICHAEL U. MARTIN
Institute of Pharmacology, Hannover Medical School, Hannover, Germany
Resch.Klaus@MH-Hannover.de,
Martin.Michael@MH-Hannover.de

Synonyms

Hypersensitivity

Definition

The term allergy describes inappropriate immune responses to foreign substances after repeated exposure giving rise to irritant or harmful, and eventually fatal reactions. Its incidence depends on two factors: the occurence and nature of an agent eliciting immune reactions (allergen) and the reactivity of the immune system (▸ immune defense). In highly industrialized countries allergies may affect more than 30% of the population caused by poorly understood environmental influences. In addition, a genetically determined predisposition exists to develop an allergy.

▸ Humanized Monoclonal Antibodies
▸ Immune Defense
▸ Immunosuppressive Agents
▸ Inflammation

Basic Mechanisms

Currently allergic reactions are classified into four types on the basis of different reaction patterns. Whereas types I-III are dependent on antibodies, the type IV reaction is mediated by cellular immune reactions.

Type I reaction, anaphylactic reaction
This type of allergic reaction is by far the most common one, and may be responsible for more than 80% of all allergies. Often it is used synonymously with allergy.

In some individuals, exposure to an antigen - then termed allergen - leads to the increased production of specific IgE, a subclass of antibodies

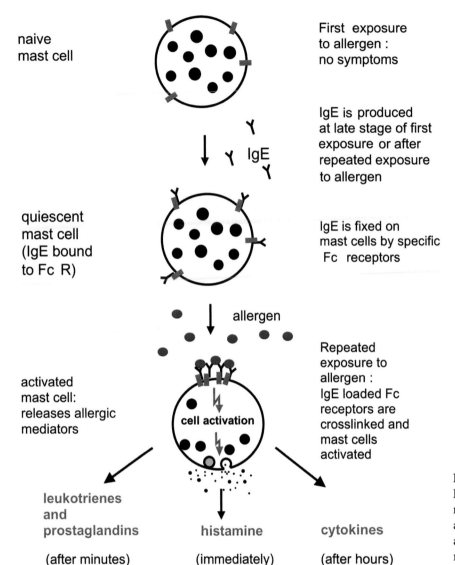

naive
mast cell

First exposure
to allergen :
no symptoms

IgE is produced
at late stage of first
exposure or after
repeated exposure
to allergen

IgE

quiescent
mast cell
(IgE bound
to Fc R)

IgE is fixed on
mast cells by specific
Fc receptors

allergen

activated
mast cell:
releases allergic
mediators

cell activation

Repeated
exposure to
allergen :
IgE loaded Fc
receptors are
crosslinked and
mast cells
activated

leukotrienes
and
prostaglandins

(after minutes)

histamine

(immediately)

cytokines

(after hours)

Fig. 1 Type I Anaphylactic Reaction: IgE-bearing mast cells are activated by allergens to release mediators of acute allergic reactions.

that physiologically is only synthesized in minute quantities. For this bias of the humoral immune response against an allergen, a subgroup of helper T lymphocytes, Th2-cells, plays a key regulatory role by providing the master cytokine interleukin-4 (▶ Immune Defense, ▶ Cytokines). IgE binds with high affinity to receptors (Fcε-receptors) that are present on basophilic granulocytes and most prominently on the closely related mast cells. These cells thus acquire a "borrowed" (as it is, of course, synthesized by B-lymphocytes) allergen specific receptor, which can persist on these cells for long periods, at least several months, perhaps years. If that happens, an individual is "allergic",

i.e. sensitized to an allergen without exhibiting any clinical symptoms and without knowing it. Upon re-exposure to this specific allergen, the mast cells (and the other IgE bearing cells) can immediately recognize the allergen with its IgE antibodies. This results in the crosslinking of the Fcε receptors that in turn triggers activation of the mast cells (or basophils). The consequence is rapid degranulation of preformed vesicles and release of a plethora of mediators into their surrounding (see Fig. 1), the most prominent mediator is histamine which is preformed and stored in vesicles and acts immediately upon release. Within minutes, further mediators like leukotrienes are syn-

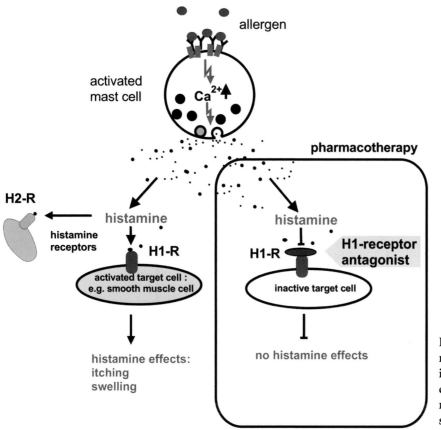

Fig. 2 Histamine H1-receptor antagonists inhibit response of target cells to histamine and relieve hay fever-like symptoms.

thesized. These mediators act in concert on cells in their vicinity which bear the appropriate receptors and thereby cause the clinical symptoms of an immediate allergic reaction. These may be itching (urticaria), local swelling (edema), allergic rhinitis ("hay fever"), constriction of bronchi ("asthma") and, when occurring in a generalized form, "anaphylactic" shock and eventual death. Activated mast cells also start synthesizing protein mediators, termed cytokines, in a process that requires some time (a few hours). These cytokines initiate an acute inflammatory response that in its late phase is characterized by the infiltration of leukocytes and especially eosinophilic granulocytes.

Type II reactions: cytotoxic reaction
As a physiological response to an antigen B lymphocytes initially always secrete antibodies of the IgM class, only in the late stage of the primary response or upon re-exposure to the same antigen, B cells switch immunoglobulin classes and produce either IgG, IgA or IgE (▶ Immune Defense).

In rare situations the antigen, or a metabolite thereof, either alone or bound to a carrier protein, may bind firmly to surfaces of cells. The antigen on the cell surface is now recognized by specific IgG antibodies, and thus the whole cell is labelled as a "foreign" particle that is consequently - but erroneously - destroyed by the complement system or cellular mechanisms. Type II reactions contribute to auto-immune mechanisms (Immunosuppression). They are also responsible for allergic reactions to certain drugs and may induce severe diseases such as drug-induced aplastic anemia or agranulocytosis.

Type III reactions: immune complex reactions
In the case of the type III reaction physiologically produced antibodies, predominantly of the IgG subclasses, bind specifically the soluble antigen and form immune complexes. These immune complexes may bind directly to Fcγ receptors or be coated with complement components and thus be opsonized for uptake by phagocytic cells that nor-

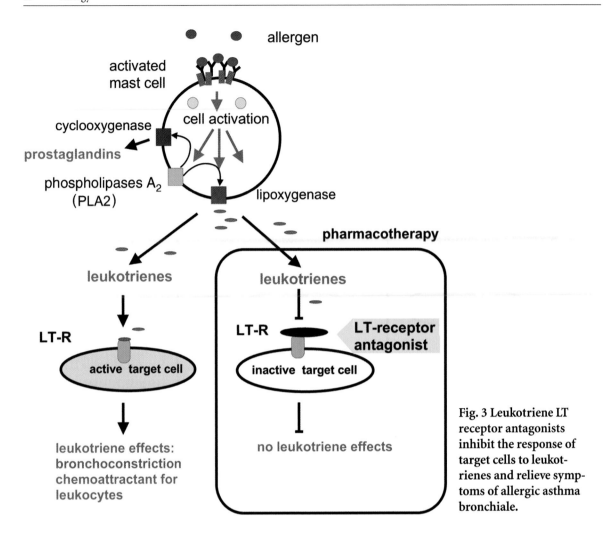

Fig. 3 Leukotriene LT receptor antagonists inhibit the response of target cells to leukotrienes and relieve symptoms of allergic asthma bronchiale.

mally degrade them and thus eliminate them. An "allergic" situation occurs if these immune complexes cannot be ingested appropriately and degraded. Alternatively, and more often, due to a continuous supply of allergen, the phagocytic cell is incapable of coping with the mass of resulting immune complexes. Thus the phagocytic cells respond to the frustraneous or continuous stimulation of Fcγ receptors by secreting a variety of products into their surrounding. These include catabolic enzymes that degrade unspecifically all available biological macromolecules such as proteins, nucleic acids, carbohydrates, or lipids no matter whether these are foreign or belong to the host, resulting in continuous destruction. It should be noted that this mechanism of damage is identical with that occurring in chronic inflammatory diseases (▶ Inflammation) such as in

▶ rheumatoid arthritis or nephritis. Typical allergic type III reactions are pulmonary diseases against inhalative irritants, or ▶ "serum sickness" occurring after administration of high molecular weight proteinacious drugs, originally animal serum applied during passive vaccination, but also murine monoclonal antibodies or other drugs.

Type IV reactions: cellular reactions
At the time when allergic reactions were classified little was known about cellular reactions, thus it appears appropriate today to divide this reaction type in two subgroups.

Type IV a: cellular cytotoxic reactions.
In this type of reaction an antigen elicits the generation of cytotoxic T lymphocytes (▶ Immune Defense). Cytotoxic T lymphocytes (Tc) destroy antigen bearing

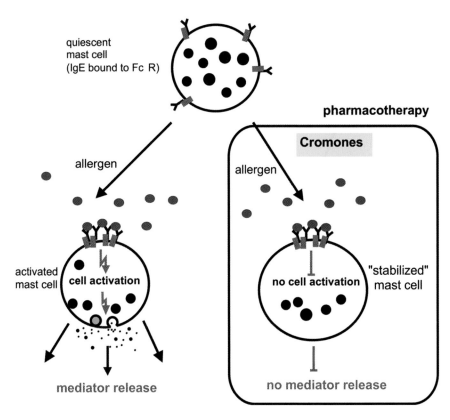

Fig. 4 Cromones "stabilize" mast cells.

cells by inducing apoptosis. This reaction can be viewed as the cellular counterpart to the humoral Type II reactions. They play an important physiological role in the defense of viruses, and can become allergic reactions under the same conditions as described for Type II reactions.

Type IV b reactions: delayed type hypersensitivity reactions (DTH). Antigens commonly induce the activation of T lymphocytes of the T helper type (Th). In the case of Type IV b reactions the predominant responding cell is the Th-1 subtype. By secreting many cytokines, including interferon γ, Th1-lymphocytes recruit and activate granulocytes and monocytic cells to mount an inflammatory response. In that respect the Type IV b reaction can also be viewed as a cellular counterpart of a humoral reaction, specifically of a Type III reaction, being of great importance in chronic inflammatory diseases such as rheumatoid arthritis, and glomerulonephritis, or in autoimmune diseases such as systemic lupus erythematodes. In fact, in these situations both Type III and Type IV b contribute to the chronic inflammatory reaction. With

respect to allergy, Type IV b reactions are relevant for contact ekzema, i.e. the chronic response of skin to many irritants including chromate, nickel, cosmetics, fabrics, etc.

Pharmacological Intervention

General
The ideal and single curative treatment of an allergy is to strictly avoid exposure to the responsible allergen(s). This requires to elucidate the causative agent. A battery of diagnostic methods is available to achieve this including measurement of IgE in blood (RAST), various methods of eliciting allergic reactions in the skin (skin testing), and provocation of clinical symptoms (e.g. in food allergy). Unfortunately, many allergens are difficult to avoid in daily life as they occur ubiquitously or, in the case of occupational exposure, would require a change in profession. Thus, in many cases pharmacological intervention may be necessary to improve the health of the allergic patient.

Type II, III, and IV allergic reactions are variants of physiologic defense mechanisms only rele-

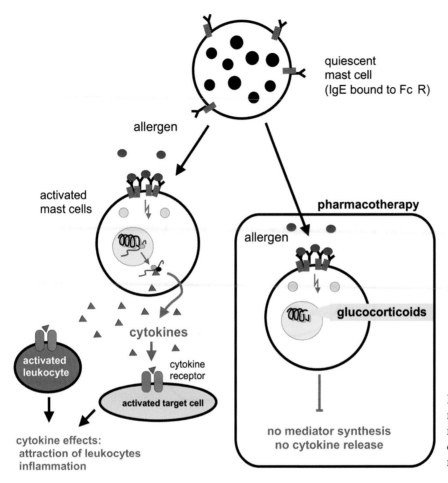

Fig. 5 Glucocorticoids regulate gene expression, resulting in a decrease of cytokine and mediator release.

vant in special situations, which follow a common pathologic pattern. In general, treatment of these forms require anti-inflammatory (▶ Inflammation) or immunosuppressive strategies (Immunosuppression). Therefore, only therapy of Type I reactions will be described here.

Therapy of Type I reactions

(Rush) Immunotherapy (Hyposensitization). The inappropriate production of IgE to an allergen is caused by a Th-2 preponderance upon exposure to the allergen. Immunotherapy aims to influence the undesired Th-2 immune response and shift it to a Th-1 answer. It was found empirically and consists of the application of increasing doses of the allergen within a few days, starting with a very low, clinically inapparent, dose, and ending with a dose close to or above the one which is to be expected

in a natural situation (e.g. after a bee sting). The high dose usually is applied at monthly intervals for up to three years or even longer. An absolute indication for immunotherapy are allergies to bee or wasp poison, which may result in an anaphylatic shock and may be fatal. At least partial relief may be achieved by immunotherapy in patients with allergies against defined pollen, but mostly fails with complex mixtures of allergens such as proteins of pets (epithelia, hair) or proteins in the faeces of mites (house dust allergy). With the availability of modern molecular biology and the achievements of recombinant DNA technology the identification of the responsible structures of allergens and their production in defined quality and quantities may increase the rate of success also with complex allergens or mixture of allergens in future.

Pharmacotherapy

Histamine H1-receptor antagonists. Histamine-H-1-receptor antagonists compete with the binding of histamine to its type 1 receptors which are predominantly located in cells of the vasculature, and thus block its action (Fig. 2). H-1 receptor antagonists are effective when symptoms occur which involve peripheral blood vessels – around which the majority of mast cells are located – such as urticaria, allergic rhinitis ("hay fever") or conjunctivitis. As histamine receptors are also present in the brain, their blockade influences the ability to focus and may result in sleepiness. However, modern second generation H-1 receptor antagonists do not cross the blood-brain barrier and thus do not show this undesired sedative side effect (examples: loratadin, fexofenadin, cetirizin).

Leukotriene antagonists. Leukotrienes are rapidly produced and released during a type I reaction (Fig. 3). They are responsible for a massive bronchoconstriction in allergic bronchial asthma and attract leukocytes, thus being pro-inflammatory. Consequently, antagonists of the LTC receptor have been proven useful in the therapy of ▶ bronchial asthma, often in combination with bronchodilators (example: montelukast).

Cromones. Cromones suppress the release of mediators from mast cells by a mechanism that is not known (Fig. 4). In order to achieve the complete suppressive effect, cromones have to be given prophylactically several days to weeks before exposure to seasonal allergens can be expected, emphasizing the importance of warning systems or calendars (e.g. for pollen) as means for initiating therapy. Cromones also are effective in ongoing allergic responses, but then a few days are required to see benefits for the patient. Cromones are practically insoluble and thus are not absorbed beyond the top layers of tissues. This has the advantage that no systemic side effects occur, on the other hand cromones only act locally and must be applied at the site of action wanted. Cromones have beneficial effects in allergic rhinitis (nose drops or spray), conjunctivitis or bronchial asthma (inhalable preparations) (examples: disodiumcromoglycate or nedocromil).

Glucocorticoids

Topically applied glucocorticoids – "inhalable" glucocorticoids. Glucocorticoids are very effective anti-inflammatory drugs. In Type I allergy they affect several different target cells, the most important being the mast cells and infiltrating T-lymphocytes. In general their action is immunosuppressive (Immunosuppression). On mast cells, glucocorticoids mainly affect the synthesis and release of mediators such as the arachidonic acid metabolites and most prominently the cytokines. The molecular mechanism of glucocorticoid action is complex and can be summarized as a regulatory effect on gene induction and expression (Fig. 5).

Of all glucocorticoids applied to the upper respiratory tract (nose, bronchi) more than 80% may be swallowed and finally absorbed by the gastrointestinal tract. This fraction reaches the circulation after an initial first passage through the liver. "Modern" glucocorticoids for inhalation are chemically modified in a way that they are completely inactviated metabolically by the liver. Thus inhalable glucocorticoids in therapeutic doses are effective in the respiratory tract, but do not give rise to systemic side effects (▶ Glucocorticoids). They play an important role in the long term treatment of ▶ bronchial asthma. They also have beneficial effects in allergic rhinitis ("hay fever"), especially in seasonal forms (example: beclomethason, budesonid).

Glucocorticoid ointments. Glucocorticoid ointments are used to treat allergic skin reactions locally. They should be applied only for limited periods to avoid trophic damage to the skin such as thinning (paper skin).

Systematically applied glucocorticoids. Because of their considerable side effects – which depend on dose and, even more relevant, on the duration of application – systemically applied glucocorticoids are only used in serious allergic diseases. This includes bronchial asthma, autoimmune and chronic inflammatory diseases.

Anaphylactic shock

The most serious acute Type I reaction is the generalized reaction, the anaphylactic shock. Anaphylactic shock results from a generalized release of mediators from mast cells and basophils. The clinical symptoms are manifested predominantly in

- Circulation: Leakage of fluid from the vasculature into the surrounding tissue causes edema, drop in blood pressure and finally hemodynamic shock.
- Heart: Histamine (and also other mediators) induce arrhythmias which can be fatal.
- Respiratory tract: all symptoms associated with allergy can occur, starting from profuse rhinitis to severe asthma and suffocation.
- Gastrointestinal system: cramps and diarrhea.
- Skin: generalized urticaria and erythema.

Treatment

The fate of the patient largely depends on the first 30 minutes of an anaphylactic shock reaction. Thus persons with a known history of hypersensitivity reactions towards bee or wasp poison should always carry an emergency set during the insect season (see below).

1. Intravenous infusion of epinephrin: 0.1 to 0.5 mg epinephrin dissolved in plasma replacement, this can be repeated after 5 minutes.
2. Plasma replacement (any): this should also be used as a continuous access to the intravenous blood.
3. Glucocorticoids: 300 mg to 1 g as bolus
4. H1-histamine receptor antagonist

Emergency set contains:

- a ready to use epinephrine solution in a special syringe allowing sequential application in two doses
- readily resorptive glucocorticoid solution (orally)
- readily resorptive H1 histamine receptor antagonist (**cave:** sedation!!)
- (if available: inhalable epinephrine)

References

1. Allergy and Asthma, supplement to Nature Vol 402, no.6760, 1999.
2. Mygind N, Dahl R, Pedersen S, Thestrup-Pedersen K (1995) Essential Allergy, Blackwell Scientific Publishers, Oxford.
3. Holgate ST, Church MK (1993) Allergy, Gower Medical Publishing, London.

Allodynia

The sensation of pain, following injury or disease, in response to a previously non-noxious stimulus is termed 'allodynia'. Tactile allodynia is caused by recruitment of low-threshold (non-nociceptive) sensory fibers (Aβ) in nociceptive pathways.

▶ Nociception

Alloimmunity

Alloimmunity is the immune response mounted by a host on the basis of differences in major histocompatibility antigens expressed on the surface of a donor cell from the same species as the host.

▶ Immune Defense

Allosteric Modulators

Unlike competitive antagonists that bind to the same domain on the receptor as the agonist, allosteric modulators bind to their own site on the receptor and produce an effect on agonism through a protein conformational change. Allosteric modulators can affect the affinity of the receptor for the agonist or simply the responsiveness of the receptor to the agonist. A hallmark of allosteric interaction is that the effect reaches a maximal asymptote corresponding to saturation of the allosteric sites on the receptor. For example, an allosteric modulator may produce a maximal 10-fold decrease in the affinity of the receptor for the agonist upon saturation of the allosteric sites on the receptor.

Allylamine

▶ Antifungal Drugs

α1-acid Glycoprotein

α1-acid glycoprotein is one of the plasma proteins mainly responsible for the plasma protein binding of drugs. Its level is known to be elevated in some pathological states, such as inflammation.

α-Adrenergic System

Lutz Hein
University of Würzburg, Würzburg, Germany
hein@toxi.uni-wuerzburg.de

Synonyms

α-adrenergic receptors, α-adrenoceptors

Definition

The α-adrenergic system consists of six subtypes of membrane receptors which mediate part of the biological actions of the catecholamines adrenaline and noradrenaline. α-Adrenergic receptors are important regulators of smooth muscle cell contraction (α_1-adrenergic receptors) (1) and pre-synaptic neurotransmitter release (α_2-adrenergic receptors) (2,3). In addition, adrenaline and noradrenaline activate β-adrenergic receptors, which stimulate cardiac contractility and rhythm and inhibit bronchial, vascular and uterine smooth muscle contraction (▶ β-Adrenergic System).

▶ β-Adrenergic System
▶ Catechol-O-Methyltransferase and its Inhibitors
▶ Neurotransmitter Transporters

Basic Characteristics

The adrenergic system is an essential regulator that increases cardiovascular and metabolic capacity during situations of stress, exercise and disease. Nerve cells in the central and peripheral nervous system synthesize and secrete the neurotransmitters noradrenaline and adrenaline. In the peripheral nervous system, ▶ noradrenaline and ▶ adrenaline are released from two different sites: noradrenaline is the principal neurotransmitter of sympathetic neurons that innervate many organs and tissues. In contrast, adrenaline, and to a lesser degree noradrenaline, is produced and secreted from the adrenal gland into the circulation (Fig. 1). Thus, the actions of noradrenaline are mostly restricted to the sites of release from sympathetic nerves, whereas adrenaline acts as a hormone to stimulate many different cells via the blood stream.

Together with dopamine, adrenaline and noradrenaline belong to the endogenous catecholamines that are synthesized from the precursor amino acid tyrosine (Fig. 1). In the first biosynthetic step, tyrosine hydroxylase generates ▶ L-dopa which is further converted to dopamine by the aromatic L-amino acid decarboxylase (▶ Dopa Decarboxylase). Dopamine is transported from the cytosol into synaptic vesicles by a vesicular monoamine transporter. In sympathetic nerves, vesicular dopamine β-hydroxylase generates the neurotransmitter noradrenaline. In chromaffin cells of the adrenal medulla, approximately 80% of the noradrenaline is further converted into adrenaline by the enzyme phenylethanolamine-N-methyltransferase.

Several mechanisms serve to terminate the biological actions of noradrenaline and adrenaline. From the synaptic cleft, most of the released noradrenaline is recycled by re-uptake into the nerve terminals via a specific ▶ noradrenaline transporter. This transporter is selectively blocked by cocaine and tricyclic antidepressants. After re-uptake into the nerve, most of the noradrenaline is transferred into synaptic vesicles and a smaller fraction is destined for degradation by the enzymes ▶ monoamine oxidase (MAO) and ▶ catechol-O-methyltransferase (COMT). COMT plays a major role in the metabolism of circulating catecholamines. MAO and COMT are widely dis-

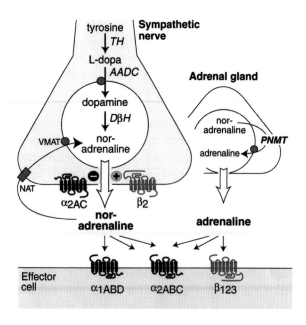

Fig. 1 Synthesis and release of noradrenaline and adrenaline from sympathetic nerve endings (left) and from the adrenal gland (right). Noradrenaline and adrenaline are synthesized from the precursor amino acid tyrosine and are stored at high concentrations in synaptic vesicles. Upon activation of sympathetic nerves or adrenal chromaffin cells, noradrenaline and adrenaline are secreted and can activate adrenergic receptors on surrounding cells (sympathetic nerve), or they enter the blood circulation (adrenaline released from the adrenal gland). Release of noradrenaline from nerve terminals is controlled by presynaptic inhibitory α_2- and activating β_2-adrenergic receptors. Actions of noradrenaline are terminated by uptake into nerve terminals and synaptic vesicles by active transporters (NAT, VMAT) and by uptake into neighboring cells (not shown). Abbreviations: AADC, aromatic L-amino acid decarboxylase; DβH, dopamine β-hydroxylase; NAT, nordadrenaline transporter; PNMT, phenylethanolamine-N-methyltransferase; TH, tyrosine hydroxylase; VMAT, vesicular monoamine transporter.

tributed, and inhibitors of these enzymes are used for the treatment of mental depression (MAO-A inhibitor, moclobemide) or Parkinson's disease (MAO-B inhibitor, selegiline).

The biological actions of adrenaline and noradrenaline are mediated via nine different ▶ G-protein-coupled receptors, which are located in the plasma membrane of neuronal and non-neuronal target cells. These receptors are divided into two different groups, α-adrenergic receptors and β-adrenergic receptors (see β-adrenergic system). The distinction between α- and β-adrenergic receptors was first proposed by Ahlquist in 1948 (4) based on experiments with various catecholamine derivatives to produce excitatory (α) or inhibitory (β) responses in isolated smooth muscle systems. Initially, a further subdivision into presynaptic α_2- and postsynaptic α_1-receptors was proposed. However, this anatomical classification of α-adrenergic receptor subtypes was later abandoned.

At present, six α-adrenergic receptors have been identified by molecular cloning: three α_1-adrenergic receptors (α_{1A}, α_{1B}, α_{1D}) (5) and three α_2-subtypes (α_{2A}, α_{2B}, α_{2C}) (6) (Fig. 2). Due to the lack of sufficiently subtype-selective ligands, the unique physiological properties of these α-receptor subtypes, for the most part, have not been fully elucidated. However, recent studies in mice that carry deletions in the genes encoding for individual α-receptor subtypes have greatly advanced the knowledge about the specific functions of these receptors (3).

α_1-Adrenergic receptors mediate contraction and hypertrophic growth of smooth muscle cells. The three α_1-receptor subtypes share 75% identity in their transmembrane domains, whereas the degree of homology between α_1- and α_2-receptors is significantly smaller (35–40%). Due to discrepancies between the pharmacological subtype classification, mRNA and protein expression data and experiments with cloned α_1-receptor subtypes, some confusion exists in the literature with respect to the assignment of α_1-receptor subtype nomenclature. In the present terminology, α_{1A} (cloned α_{1c}), α_{1B} (cloned α_{1b}) and α_{1D}-receptors (cloned α_{1d}) can be distinguished. All three subtypes seem to be involved in the regulation of vascular tone, with the α_{1A}-receptor maintaining basal vascular tone and the α_{1B}-receptor mediating the constrictory effects of exogenous α_1-agonists. All α_1-receptor subtypes can activate Gq-proteins, resulting in intracellular stimulation of phospholipases C, A_2, and D, mobilization of Ca^{2+} from intracellular stores and activation of mitogen-activated protein kinase and PI3 kinase pathways.

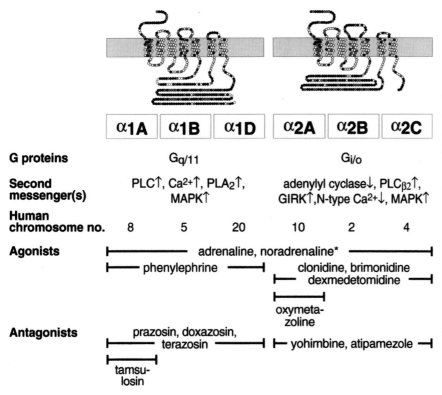

| α1A | α1B | α1D | α2A | α2B | α2C |

G proteins   Gq/11   Gi/o

Second messenger(s)   PLC↑, Ca2+↑, PLA2↑, MAPK↑   adenylyl cyclase↓, PLCβ2↑, GIRK↑, N-type Ca2+↓, MAPK↑

Human chromosome no.   8   5   20   10   2   4

Agonists   —— adrenaline, noradrenaline* ——
⊢—— phenylephrine ——⊣   clonidine, brimonidine
⊢— dexmedetomidine —⊣
⊢———⊣
oxymeta-zoline

Antagonists   prazosin, doxazosin,
⊢—— terazosin ——⊣ ⊢— yohimbine, atipamezole —⊣
⊢——⊣
tamsu-losin

Fig. 2 Subtypes of α-adrenergic receptors, their signaling pathways and agonist and antagonist binding profiles. The proposed topology of α_1- and α_2-adrenergic receptors with 7 transmembrane domains is illustrated. *. Adrenaline and noradrenaline can also activate β-adrenergic receptors (see β-adrenergic system). Abbreviations: PLA$_2$, PLC, phospholipases A, C; GIRK, G-protein-activated inwardly rectifying potassium channel; MAPK, mitogen-activated protein kinase.

Three genes encoding for α_2-adrenergic receptor subtypes have been identified from several species, termed α_{2A}, α_{2B}, and α_{2C}, respectively (Fig. 2). The pharmacological profile of the α_{2A}-subtype differs significantly between species, thus giving rise to the pharmacological subtypes α_{2A} in humans, rabbits and pigs and α_{2D} in rats, mice and guinea pigs (7). Part of the pharmacological difference between α_{2A}- and α_{2D}-receptors can be explained by a Ser-Ala mutation in the fifth transmembrane helix of the α_{2A}-receptor rendering this receptor less sensitive to the antagonists, rauwolscine and yohimbine. α_2-Adrenergic receptors regulate a wide range of signalling pathways via interaction with multiple heterotrimeric G$_i$ proteins (Gα_{i1}, Gα_{i2}, Gα_{i3}) including inhibition of adenylyl cyclase, stimulation of phospholipase D, stimulation of mitogen-activated protein kinases, stimulation of K$^+$ currents and inhibition of Ca^{2+} currents. The three α_2-receptor subtypes have unique patterns of tissue distribution in the central nervous system and in peripheral tissues. The α_{2A}-receptor is expressed widely throughout the central nervous system including the locus coeruleus, brain stem nuclei, cerebral cortex, septum,

hypothalamus and hippocampus. In the periphery, α_{2A}-receptors are expressed in kidney, spleen, thymus, lung and salivary gland. The α_{2B}-receptor primarily shows peripheral expression (kidney, liver, lung and heart) and only low level expression in thalamic nuclei of the central nervous system. The α_{2C}-receptor appears to be expressed primarily in the central nervous system (striatum, olfactory tubercle, hippocampus and cerebral cortex), although very low levels of its mRNA are present in the kidney.

α_{2A}- Receptors and α_{2C}-receptors are located presynaptically in order to inhibit noradrenaline release from sympathetic nerves. Activation of these receptors leads to decreased sympathetic tone, decreased blood pressure and heart rate. Central α_{2A}-receptors mediate sedation and analgesia. α_{2B}-Receptors mediate contraction of vascular smooth muscle, and in the spinal cord they are essential components of the analgesic effect of nitrous oxide. Upon stimulation by agonists, α_1- and α_2-receptor signalling pathways are attenuated by several mechanisms at the receptor and post-receptor levels (see β-adrenergic system).

Drugs

Therapeutically, α_1-receptor-mediated vasoconstriction contributes to the beneficial actions of adrenaline applied as an emergency medicine during hypotensive or anaphylactic shock. Addition of adrenaline or noradrenaline to local anaesthetics prevents diffusion of the local anaesthetic from the site of injection and thereby prolongs its action. α_1-Receptor antagonists including prazosin, doxazosin, terazosin and bunazosin are used to treat patients with hypertension. However, α_1-receptor antagonists are no longer first-line antihypertensive agents since the ALLHAT clinical trial revealed that hypertensive patients taking doxazosin had a higher risk of developing congestive heart failure than patients with diuretic treatment. Tamsulosin is the first α_1-receptor antagonist with selectivity for the α_{1A}-receptor over α_{1B}- and α_{1D}-subtypes. The α_{1A}-selectivity is thought to contribute to the beneficial actions of tamsulosin in the treatment of benign prostate hypertrophy without lowering bood pressure.

At present, no drugs exist that can selectively activate α_2-receptor subtypes. Clonidine stimulates all three α_2-subtypes with similar potency. Clonidine lowers blood pressure in patients with hypertension and it decreases sympathetic overactivity during opioid withdrawal. In intensive and postoperative care, clonidine is a potent sedative and analgesic and can prevent post-operative shivering. Clonidine and its derivative brimonidine lower intraocular pressure of glaucoma patients when applied locally. Moxonidine may have less sedative side effects than clonidine when used as an antihypertensive. It has been suggested that moxonidine activates "imidazoline receptors" instead of α_2-receptors. The α_2-receptor agonists oxymetazoline and xylometazoline are being used as nasal decongestants. At present, α_2-receptor antagonists are not used in human medicine. However, in veterinary practice the α_2-receptor antagonist atipamezole can rapidly reverse anaesthesia mediated by the α_2-agonist medetomidine. In the future, subtype-selective drugs may greatly improve the therapy of diseases involving α_1- or α_2-adrenergic receptor systems.

References

1. Guimaraes S, Moura D (2001) Vascular adrenoceptors: an update. Pharmacol. Rev. 53:319–356
2. Starke K (2001) Presynaptic autoreceptors in the third decade: focus on α_2-adrenoceptors. J. Neurochem. 78:685–693
3. Hein L (2001) Transgenic models of α_2-adrenergic receptor subtype function. Rev. Physiol. Biochem. Pharmacol. 142:162–185
4. Ahlquist, R.P. (1948) A study of the adrenotropic receptors. Am. J. Physiol. 153, 586-600
5. Piascik MT, Perez DM (2001) α_1-Adrenergic receptors: new insights and directions. J. Pharmacol. Exp. Ther. 298:403–410
6. Ruffolo RR, Nichols AJ, Stadel JM, Hieble JP (1993) Pharmacologic and therapeutic applications of α_2-adrenoceptor subtypes. Ann. Rev. Pharmacol. Toxicol. 32:243–279
7. Bylund, D. B., Eikenberg, D. C., Hieble, J. P., Langer, S. Z., Lefkowitz, R. J., Minneman, K. P., Molinoff, P. B., Ruffolo, R. R., Trendelenburg, U. (1994) International Union of Pharmacology nomenclature of adrenoceptors. Pharmacol. Rev. 46, 121-136

α-2 Antiplasmin

α-2 antiplasmin, a naturally occurring inhibitor of fibrinolysis, is a single chain glycoprotein that forms a stable, inactive complex within plasmin and thereby prevents plasmin's activity.

▶ Coagulation/Thrombosis

α-Glucosidase

▶ Oral Antidiabetic Drugs

5α-Reductase

5-α-reductase is an enzyme, which converts testosterone to dihydrotestosterone, which has a greater affinity for androgen receptors. 5-α-reductase is expressed in various peripheral organs. Inhibitors of 5-α-reductase (e.g. finasteride) are used to treat benign prostatic hyperplasia.

▶ Sex Steroid Receptors

α and β tubulin

α and β tubulins associate into heterodimers to form microtubules. Both tubulins have molecular weights of about 50 kD and bind GTP. In higher eukaryotes, there are up to 7 isoforms of α and β tubulin, respectively, which are encoded by different genes.

▶ Cytoskeleton

ALS

▶ Amyotrophic Lateral Sclerosis

Alternative Splicing

Alternative splicing is an important cellular mechanism that leads to temporal and tissue specific expression of unique mRNA products from a single gene. It thereby increases protein diversity by allowing multiple, sometimes functionally distinct, proteins to be encoded by the same gene.

Alzheimer's Disease

Alzheimer's disease is the most common cause of dementia in patients over 60 years of age. It is characterised by loss of recent memory, personality change with perhaps antisocial behaviour, dyslexia, dysgraphia, dysphasia and eventually complete social disintegration. Post mortem examination reveals brain atrophy with reduction in number of cortical neurones. Fibrillary tangles and senile plaques containing amyloid protein are always present in the cortex.

▶ Aβ Amyloid

Ames test

The Ames test measures the reversion from mutant to wild type form (back-mutation) in a culture of *Salmonella*. The test is used to screen large numbers of compounds for their potential mutagenicity.

Amiloride-sensitive Na$^+$ Channel

The amiloride-sensitive Na$^+$ channel (ENaC) is a cell membrane glycoprotein selective for sodium ions, which is composed of three subunits (α, β and γ). Gating of sodium is inhibited by the diuretic amiloride.

▶ Epithelial Na$^+$ Channels

Aminoglycosides

▶ Ribosomal Protein Synthesis Inhibitors

AMP, cyclic

Cyclic AMP (cAMP) is an intracellular (second) messenger generated by adenylyl cyclase from ATP.

▶ Adenylyl Cyclases

AMPA Receptors

AMPAR are L-amino-3-hydroxy-5-methyl-4-isoxazole propionate receptors, a subtype of ionotropic glutamate receptors that are permeable to Na^+, K^+ and sometimes Ca^{2+} ions.

▶ Ionotropic Glutamate Receptors

AMP-activated Protein Kinase

AMP-activated protein kinase (AMPK) is a multi-subunit enzyme, that plays a major role in metabolic regulation of cells. It phosphorylates and inactivates acetyl-CoA carboxylase, a major regulator of lipid biosynthesis. AMPK also induces glucose uptake in skeletal muscles, expression of cAMP-stimulated gluconeogenic genes and expression of muscle hexokinase and glucose transporters (GLUT4). Recently, AMPK has been implicated in the action of biguanides such as metformin, which activates the enzyme.

▶ Biguanides

Amphetamine

Amphetamine and related compounds are indirect acting sympathomimetic agents that are frequently abused due to their stimulant properties on the central nervous system. Amphetamines act by inducing the biogenic amine transporters to reverse or efflux neurotransmitter into the synapse. This drug-induced non-vesicular release of dopamine, norepinephrine and serotonin is thought to be the major action associated with the amphetamines. Clinically, the amphetamines are effective in the treatment of narcolepsy and Attention Deficit Hyperactivity Disorder.

▶ Psychostimulants

AMPK

▶ AMP-activated Protein Kinase

Amyloid Precursor Protein

Amyloid precursor protein (APP) is the precursor of β-amyloid, the main component of senile plaques found in the brain of Alzheimer patients. The production of β-amyloid from APP to the cells from abnormal proteolytic cleavage of the amyloid precursor protein. Enzymes involved in this cleavage may be suitable targets for the therapy of Alzheimer's disease.

▶ Aβ Amyloid

Amyotrophic Lateral Sclerosis

Amyotrophic lateral sclerosis (ALS) is a disease of motor neurons, in which both the upper motor neuron in the cortex and the lower motor neuron in the brain stem and spinal cord degenerate progressively. Neuronal degeneration leads to neurogenic atrophy of muscle and is accompanied by proliferation of astrocytes resulting in scarring of the lateral columns of the spinal cord. Sensory neurons are not affected.

Anabolic Steroids

Anabolic steroids increase muscle mass and strength. They are used by some athletes to enhance performance.

▶ Sex Steroid Receptors

Anaesthesia

▶ General Anaesthetics
▶ Local Anaesthetics

Anaesthetics, general

▶ General Anaesthetics

Anaesthetics, local

▶ Local Anaesthetics

Analeptics

The term analeptics refers to convulsants and respiratory stimulants (i.e. central nervous system stimulants). They comprise a reverse group of agents (for example amphifinazole and doxapram (respiratory stimulants) and strychnine, biculine and picrotoxin). Analeptics are mainly experimental drugs. Only amphifinazole and doxapram are occasionally used for the treatment of acute ventilatory failure.

Analgesia

▶ General Anaesthetics
▶ Analgesics

Analgesics

CHRISTOPH STEIN
Klinik für Anaesthesiologie und Operative Intensivmedizin, Freie Universität Berlin, Berlin, Germany
christoph.stein@medizin.fu-berlin.de

Synonyms

Painkillers; pain medication

Definition

Analgesics interfere with the generation and/or transmission of impulses following noxious stimulation (▶ Nociception) in the nervous system. This can occur at peripheral and/or central levels of the ▶ neuraxis. The therapeutic aim is to diminish the perception of ▶ pain.

▶ Non-steroidal Anti-inflammatory Drugs
▶ Opioid Systems

Mechanism of Action

Analgesics can be roughly discriminated by their mechanisms of action: opioids, non-steroidal anti-inflammatory drugs (NSAIDs), serotoninergic compounds, antiepileptics and antidepressants. Adrenergic agonists, excitatory amino acid (e.g. N-methyl-D-aspartate; NMDA) receptor antagonists, neurokinin receptor antagonists, neurotrophin (e.g. nerve growth factor) antagonists, cannabinoids, and ion channel blockers are currently under intense investigation but are not used routinely yet (1, 7). ▶ Local anaesthetics are used for local and regional anesthetic techniques. Mixed drugs (e.g. tramadol) combine various mechanisms.

Opioids

Opioids act on heptahelical ▶ G-protein-coupled receptors. Three types of opioid receptors (μ, δ, κ) have been cloned. Additional subtypes (e.g. μ_1, μ_2, δ_1, δ_2) have been proposed but are not universally accepted. Opioid receptors are localized and can be activated along all levels of the neuraxis including peripheral and central processes of primary sensory neurons (▶ Nociceptors), spinal cord (interneurons, projection neurons), brainstem, midbrain and cortex (4, 6). All opioid receptors couple to G-proteins (mainly G_i/G_o) and subsequently inhibit adenylyl cyclase, decrease the conductance of voltage-gated Ca^{++} channels and/or open rectifying K^+ channels (6). These effects ultimately result in decreased neuronal activity. The prevention of Ca^{++} influx inhibits the release of excitatory (pronociceptive) neurotransmitters. A prominent example is the suppression of ▶ substance P release from primary sensory neurons both within the spinal cord and from their peripheral terminals within injured tissue (6). At the postsynaptic membrane, opioids produce hyperpolarization by opening K^+ channels, thereby preventing excitation or propagation of action potentials in second order projection neurons. In addition, opioids inhibit sensory neuron-specific tetrodotoxin-resistant Na^+ channels and excitatory postsynaptic currents evoked by ▶ glutamate receptors (e.g. NMDA) in the spinal cord (6). The result is decreased transmission of nociceptive stimuli at all levels of the neuraxis and profoundly reduced perception of pain. The endogenous opioid ligands consist of four peptide families. Three are derived from the known precursors proopiomelanocortin (encoding β-endorphin), proenkephalin (encoding Met-enkephalin and Leu-enkephalin) and prodynorphin (encoding dynorphins). These peptides contain the common Tyr-Gly-Gly-Phe-[Met/Leu] sequence at their amino terminals, known as the opioid motif. β-Endorphin and the enkephalins are potent antinociceptive agents acting at μ and δ receptors. Dynorphins can elicit both pro- and antinociceptive effects via κ-opioid and/or NMDA receptors. A fourth group of tetrapeptides termed endomorphins (with yet unknown precursors) do not contain the pan-opioid motif but they bind to μ-receptors with unprecedented selectivity, resulting in analgesia. Opioid peptides and receptors are expressed throughout the central and peripheral nervous system, in neuroendocrine tissues, and in immune cells (6).

Non-Steroidal Antiinflammatory Drugs (NSAIDs)

NSAIDs inhibit ▶ cyclooxygenases (COX), the enzymes that catalyze the transformation of arachidonic acid (a ubiquitous cell component generated from phospholipids) to prostaglandins and thromboxanes (3). Two isoforms, COX-1 and COX-2, are expressed constitutively in peripheral tissues and in the central nervous system. In response to injury and inflammatory mediators, (e.g. cytokines, growth factors) both isoforms can be upregulated, resulting in increased concentrations of prostaglandins (3). In the periphery, prostaglandins (mainly PGE_2) sensitize nociceptors by phosphorylation of Na^+ channels (7). As a result, nociceptors become more responsive to noxious mechanical (e.g. pressure, hollow organ distension), chemical (e.g. acidosis, ▶ bradykinin, neurotrophins) or thermal stimuli. In the spinal cord PGE_2 blocks glycinergic neuronal inhibition, enhances excitatory amino acid release, and depolarizes ascending neurons. These mechanisms facilitate the generation of impulses within nociceptors and their transmission through the spinal cord to higher brain areas. By blocking one (selective COX-2 inhibitors, coxibs) or both enzymes (nonselective NSAIDs) prostaglandin formation diminishes. Subsequently nociceptors become less responsive to noxious stimuli and spinal neurotransmission is attenuated.

Serotoninergic Drugs

Serotonin (5-hydroxytryptamine; 5-HT) is a monoamine neurotransmitter found in the sympathetic nervous system, in the gastrointestinal tract, and in platelets. It acts on 5-HT receptors expressed at all levels of the neuraxis and on blood vessels. Within the dorsal horn of the spinal cord serotoninergic neurons contribute to endogenous pain inhibition. 5-HT receptors are classified into seven families (5-HT_1–5-HT_7) and at least 14 subtypes. With the exception of 5-HT_3 (a ligand-gated ion channel) all others are G-protein coupled receptors. $5\text{-HT}_{1B/1D}$ agonists (triptans) have been extensively studied and are considered specific for migraine headaches. Migraine is thought to be related to the release of neuropeptides (e.g.

► Calcitonin Gene Related Peptide, ► Substance P) from trigeminal sensory neurons innervating meningeal blood vessels. This leads to vasodilation, an inflammatory reaction, and subsequent pain. Neuronal 5-HT_{1D} receptors localized on trigeminal afferents mediate the triptan-induced inhibition of neurogenic inflammation, with possible additional sites of action for brain penetrating 5-HT_1 agonists in inhibiting nociceptive transmission centrally. In addition, the activation of vascular 5-HT_{1B} receptors constricts meningeal (and coronary) vessels (2). The latter effects have stimulated a search for nonvasoconstrictor approaches such as substance P (neurokinin-1) receptor antagonists, endothelin antagonists and highly selective $5HT_{1D}$ agonists. However, none of them demonstrated clinical antimigraine effects, supporting the view that isolated peripheral trigeminal nerve inhibition is insufficient to relieve acute migraine.

Antiepileptic Drugs

A number of antiepileptics are used in ► neuropathic pain. Different neuropathic pain syndromes have been attributed to certain common mechanisms including ectopic activity in sensitized nociceptors from regenerating nerve sprouts, recruitment of previously "silent" nociceptors, and spontaneous activity in dorsal root ganglion cells. The increase of peripheral neuronal activity is transmitted centrally and results in sensitization of second- and third-order ascending neurons. Among the best studied mechanisms of peripheral and central sensitization are the increased novel expression of Na^+ channels, and increased activity at ► glutamate (NMDA) receptor sites (7). The mechanisms of action of antiepileptics include neuronal membrane stabilization by blockage of pathologically active voltage-sensitive Na^+ channels (carbamazepine, phenytoin, valproate, lamotrigine), blockage of voltage-dependent Ca^{++} channels (gabapentin, lamotrigine), inhibition of presynaptic release of excitatory amino acids (lamotrigine), activation of γ-aminobutyric acid ► (GABA) receptors (valproate, gabapentin), opening of adenosine triphosphate-sensitive K^+channels (K_{ATP}) channels (gabapentin), potential enhancement of GABA turnover/synthesis (gabapentin) and increased nonvesicular GABA release (gabapentin) (5).

Antidepressants

Several antidepressants are used in the treatment of neuropathic pain. They include the classic tricyclic compounds that are divided into nonselective noradrenaline/5-HT reuptake inhibitors (e.g. amitriptyline, imipramine, clomipramine) and preferential noradrenaline reuptake inhibitors (e.g. desipramine, maprotiline), selective 5-HT reuptake inhibitors (e.g. citalopram, paroxetine, fluoxetine) and 5-HT_2 antagonists (nefazodone). The reuptake inhibition leads to a stimulation of endogenous monoaminergic pain inhibition in the spinal cord and brain. In addition, tricyclics have NMDA receptor antagonist, Na^+ channel blocking, and K^+ channel opening effects which can suppress peripheral and central sensitization. Block of cardiac K^+ and Na^+ channels by tricyclics can lead to life-threatening arrhythmias. The selective 5-HT transporter inhibitors lack postsynaptic receptor blocking and membrane stabilization effects (and side effects resulting therefrom) (5).

Clinical Use (incl. side effects)

Analgesics are used in both acute and chronic pain. Whereas acute (e.g. postoperative, posttraumatic) pain is generally amenable to drug therapy, chronic pain is a complex disease in its own right and needs to be differentiated into malignant (cancer-related) and nonmalignant (e.g. musculoskeletal, ► neuropathic, inflammatory) pain. Acute and cancer-related pain are commonly treatable with opioids, NSAIDs and/or local anesthetic blocks. Chronic nonmalignant pain requires a multidisciplinary approach encompassing various pharmacological and non-pharmacological (e.g. psychological, physiotherapeutic) treatment strategies. Various routes of drug administration (e.g. oral, intravenous, subcutaneous, intrathecal, ► epidural, topical, intraarticular, transnasal) are used depending on the clinical circumstances (4). Local anesthetics are used topically and in regional (e.g. epidural) anesthetic techniques for the treatment of acute (e.g. associated with surgery, child birth) and some selected chronic pain syndromes.

Opioids

The commonly available agents (e.g. morphine, codeine, methadone, fentanyl and its derivatives) are μ-agonists. Naloxone is a non-selective antagonist at all three receptors. Partial agonists must occupy a greater fraction of the available pool of functional receptors than full agonists to induce a response (e.g. analgesia) of equivalent magnitude. Mixed agonist/antagonists (e.g. buprenorphine, butorphanol, nalbuphine, pentazocine) may act as agonists at low doses and as antagonists (at the same or a different receptor) at higher doses. Such compounds typically exhibit ceiling effects for analgesia and they may elicit an acute ▶ withdrawal syndrome when administered together with a pure agonist. All three receptors (μ, δ, κ) mediate analgesia but differing side effects. μ-Receptors mediate respiratory depression, sedation, reward/euphoria, nausea, urinary retention, biliary spasm and constipaton. κ-Receptors mediate dysphoric, aversive, sedative and diuretic effects, but do not mediate constipation. δ-Receptors mediate reward/euphoria and, to a lesser degree, respiratory depression and constipation. ▶ Tolerance and physical ▶ dependence occur with prolonged administration of all pure agonists. Thus, the abrupt discontinuation or antagonist administration can result in a withdrawal syndrome. Opioids are effective in the periphery (e.g. topical or intraarticular administration, particularly in inflamed tissue), at the spinal cord (intrathecal or epidural administration), and systemically (e.g. intravenous or oral administration). The clinical choice of a particular compound is mostly based on pharmacokinetic considerations (route of administration, desired onset or duration, lipophilicity) and on side effects associated with the respective route of drug delivery. Dosages can vary widely depending on patient characteristics, type of pain and route of administration. Systemically as well as spinally administered μ-opioids can produce similar side effects, depending on the dosage, with some nuances due to the varying rostral (to the brain) or systemic redistribution of different compounds. For example, lipophilic drugs are preferred for intrathecal application because they are trapped in the spinal cord and less likely to migrate to the brain within the cerebrospinal fluid. Small, systemically inactive doses are used in the periphery and are therefore devoid of side effects (4, 6). Opioids remain the most effective drugs for the treatment of severe acute and cancer-related chronic pain. Detrimental side effects are usually preventable by careful dose titration and close patient monitoring, or they are treated by co-medication (e.g. laxatives) or naloxone. Current research aims at the development of opioids with restricted access to the brain (1, 4, 6).

NSAIDs

Less severe pain states (associated with e.g. arthritis, menstruation, headache, minor surgery, early stages of cancer) are commonly treated with nonselective NSAIDs (e.g. aspirin, acetaminophen, ibuprofen, indomethacin, diclofenac). NSAIDs are mostly used orally. Over-the-counter availability and self medication have led to frequent abuse and toxicity. Side effects have been attributed mostly to COX-1 inhibition leading to a blockade of thromboxane production with subsequent impairment of platelet function (accounting for gastrointestinal and other bleeding disorders), a decrease of tissue-protective prostaglandins (accounting for gastrointestinal ulcers, perforation, gastric outlet obstruction) and a decrease of renal vasodilatory prostaglandins (accounting for nephrotoxicity). The development of selective COX-2 inhibitors (coxibs) was driven by the assumption that COX-2 expression is selectively induced in inflamed tissue and that the constitutive tissue-protective COX-1 would be spared. It has now become clear that COX-2 expression is also constitutive in many tissues (e.g. gastrointestinal epithelium, vascular endothelium, smooth muscle cells, brain, spinal cord) (3). Experimental evidence suggests that COX-2 inhibition may exacerbate late phases of inflammation, impair ulcer healing and decrease formation of prostacyclin (which normally inhibits platelet activation and produces vasodilation). In clinical trials, selective COX-2 inhibitors have been associated with an increased risk of thrombosis, angina pectoris, myocardial infarction, hypertension, stroke, and death from major cardiovascular events (3). Both classes of COX inhibitors can cause rare anaphylactic reactions. Currently, nonselective NSAIDs remain the mainstay in the treatment of arthritis, minor headache, menstrual, minor postsurgical, and dental pain.

Serotoninergic Drugs

Triptans can be applied orally, subcutaneously or transnasally and have been used for over 10 years in the treatment of migraine. All triptans narrow coronary arteries via 5-HT_{1B} receptors by up to 20% at clinical doses and should not be administered to patients with risk factors or manifest coronary, cerebrovascular or peripheral vascular disease. Some triptans have the potential for significant drug-drug interactions (e.g. with monoamine oxidase inhibitors, propranolol, cimetidine, hepatic P450-metabolized medications, p-glycoprotein pump inhibitors). Rational use of triptans should be restricted to patients with disability associated with migraine (2).

Antiepileptic Drugs

Various antiepileptics (carbamazepine, phenytoin, valproate, gabapentin, lamotrigine, pregabalin) have been used for neuropathic pain and more recently also for migraine prophylaxis. They are frequently co-administered with antidepressants. The commonest adverse effects are impaired mental (somnolence, dizziness, cognitive impairment, fatigue) and motor function (ataxia) which may limit clinical use, particularly in elderly patients. Serious side effects have been reported, including hepatotoxicity, thrombocytopenia and life-threatening dermatologic and hematologic reactions. Plasma drug concentrations should be monitored (5).

Antidepressants

Antidepressants are used in neuropathic pain and migraine prophylaxis. Tricyclics require monitoring of plasma drug concentrations to achieve optimal effect and avoid toxicity, unless sufficient pain relief is obtained with a low dose (e.g. up to 75 mg/day of imipramine or amitriptyline). In patients with ischemic heart disease there may be increased mortality from sudden arrythmia, and in patients with recent myocardial infarction, arrythmia or cardiac decompensation tricyclics should not be used at all. Tricyclics also block histamine, cholinergic and α-adrenergic receptor sites. Adverse events include fatigue, nausea, dry mouth, constipation, dizziness, sleep disturbance, blurred vision, irritability/nervousness and sedation (5).

References

1. Brower V (2000) New paths to pain relief. Nature Biotechnol. 18:387–391
2. Ferrari MD, Roon KI, Lipton RB, Goadsby PJ (2001) Oral triptans (serotonin 5-$HT_{1B/1D}$ agonists) in acute migraine treatment: a meta-analysis of 53 trials. Lancet 358:1668–1675
3. FitzGerald GA, Patrono C (2001) The coxibs, selective inhibitors of cyclooxygenase-2. N. Engl. J. Med. 345(6):433–442
4. Kalso E, Smith L, McQuay HJ, Moore A (2002) No pain, no gain: clinical excellence and scientific rigour – lessons learned from IA morphine. Pain 98:269-75.
5. Sindrup SH, Jensen TS (1999) Efficacy of pharmacological treatments of neuropathic pain: an update and effect related to mechanism of drug action. Pain 83:389–400
6. Stein C, Machelska H, Schäfer M (2001) Peripheral analgesic and antiinflammatory effects of opioids. Z. Rheumatol. 60(6):416–424
7. Woolf CJ, Salter MW (2000) Neuronal plasticity: increasing the gain in pain. Science 288:1765–1768

Anandamide

Arachidonylethanolamine (anandamide) is one of the endogenous cannabinoids (endocannabinoids) which derives from N-arachidonylphosphatidylethanolamine (NAPE).

▶ Endocannabinoid System

Anaphylactic Shock

The term anaphylactic shock describes a severe generalized type I allergic reaction associated with cardiovascular shock, airway constriction and heart arrhythmias, which, if left untreated, may cause death.

▶ Allergy

Androgen Receptor

▶ Sex Steroid Receptors

Androgens

Androgens stimulate the development of secondary sexual characteristics. They also increase mass and strength of skeletal muscles (anabolical effect). Substantial androgen deficiency is associated with as decrease of libido. The main naturally occuring androgen is testosterone.

▶ Sex Steroid Receptors

Anemia, macrocytic hyperchromic

Macrocytic or magaloblastic anemia is caused by disturbances of DNA synthesis. It occurs, for example, in both folic acid and vitamin B12 deficiencies. Hematopoesis is slowed down due to reduced DNA synthesis and a reduced number of abnormally large (macrocytic) and hemaglobinrich (hyperchromic) erythrocytes is released.

▶ Vitamin B12

Angel Dust

Phencyclidine

▶ Psychotomimetic Drugs

Angina Pectoris

Angina pectoris is a clinical syndrome caused by transient myocardial ischemia. Typically, patients suffer from a squeezing substernal discomfort (hence the name). The pain may radiate to the left shoulder but also to other regions of the body. In addition, patients may suffer from dyspnoea and tachycardia. The drug of choice for the treatment of angina pectoris is glyceryl trinitrate.

▶ NO-Synthases
▶ Guanylylcyclases
▶ Calcium Channel Blockers

Angioblast

An angioblast is an endothelial cell precursor cell.

▶ Angiogenesis and Vascular Morphogenesis

Angiogenesis and Vascular Morphogenesis

HELLMUT G. AUGUSTIN, YVONNE REISS
Tumor Biology Center Freiburg, Freiburg,
Germany
augustin@angiogenese.de,
reiss@tumorbio.uni-freiburg.de

Definition

▶ Angiogenesis and Vascular Morphogenesis comprise all mechanisms and processes that lead to the development of new blood and lymphatic vessels. These include vasculogenesis, sprouting and non-sprouting angiogenesis (intussusception), vessel assembly and maturation, and vascular remodeling. The formation of new blood vessels takes place primarily during embryonic devel-

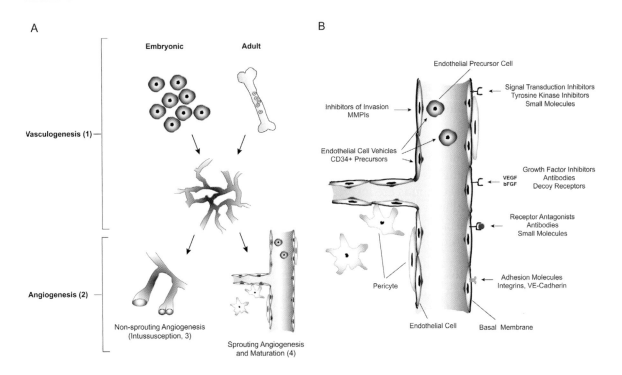

Fig. 1 Molecular mechanisms of vasculogenesis and angiogenesis (Fig. 1A) and the corresponding targets for therapeutic intervention (Fig. 1B). The primary formation of of blood vessels occurs through mechanisms of vasculogenesis (1). Vasculogenesis refers to the formation of a vascular network from precursor cells (angioblasts) as it occurs developmentally by *in situ* differentiation or in the adult by distal recruitment of angioblastic stem cells from the bone marrow. The secondary level of vascular morphogenesis describes the angiogenic formation of blood vessels. Angiogenesis refers to the formation of vessels and vascular networks from preexisting vascular structures (2). This can occur through classical sprouting angiogenesis (3) or through mechanisms of non-sprouting angiogenesis (4). The growing vascular network assembles and matures, eventually allowing directional blood flow. Pharmacological intervention of angiogenesis is based on different strategies interfering directly or indirectly with the endothelium as indicated in Fig. 1B.

opment and is physiologically limited to few organs in the healthy adult, such as the female reproductive system. Pathologic angiogenesis is widespread and is associated with diseases as diverse as tumors, wound healing, inflammatory diseases, skin diseases, eye diseases, and joint diseases.

▶ Growth Factors

Basic Mechanisms

Vasculogenesis and Angiogenesis

The supply of oxygen and nutrients are critical determinants for mammalian cell survival. There-

fore, cells are located within a distance of 100 μm to maximally 150 μm of blood vessels. Multicellular organisms must recruit new blood vessels in order to achieve growth by mechanisms termed vasculogenesis and angiogenesis. The regulation of this process is tightly controlled by a balance of pro- and antiangiogenic molecules, and is degenerated in various diseases, especially cancer. Pharmacological intervention of angiogenesis can be achieved by interfering with the molecular inducers of the angiogenic cascade or with molecular determinants of the immature neovasculature.

The assembly of a primitive vascular plexus during embryonic development occurs from endothelial precursor cells (▶ **Angioblasts**) that differentiate *in situ*. This process is termed vasculogenesis (Fig. 1A). Vasculogenic vessel growth by the distal recruitment of endothelial precursor cells from the bone marrow has also been described in the adult. Yet, the quantitative contribution of vasculogenic vessel growth in the adult has not been defined.

The first primitive vascular plexus expands by angiogenesis, the sprouting of new capillaries from pre-existing vessels, and intussusception, a process in which interstitial tissue columns are inserted into the lumen of pre-existing vessels (also termed non-sprouting angiogenesis; Fig. 1A). Sprouting and non-sprouting angiogenesis contribute to an increasing complexity of the growing vascular network. The network assembles and matures by the recruitment of smooth muscle cells and ► pericytes, eventually allowing directional flow of blood. The morphogenic events leading to a mature vascular network involve several additional steps including vessel assembly, maturation, acquisition of vessel identity and organotypic differentiation. Vascular remodeling describes the adaptational reorganization of an existing, mature vasculature in pathological conditions.

Molecular Regulators of the Angiogenic Cascade

The growth of blood vessels is regulated by a fine tuned balance of angiostimulatory and angioinhibitory molecules. To date, more than 20 stimulators and 20 inhibitors have been identified (Table 1), and the composition of the "angiogenic cocktail" has not been well defined for most situations involving angiogenesis. Of the many angioregulatory molecules, three families of molecules, the VEGFs, the ► angiopoietins, and the Ephrins stand out. They act selectively or preferentially on the vascular system and have thus to be considered as key regulatory molecules of the angiogenic cascade, in contrast to the large list of pleiotrophic growth factors that exert a variety of biological functions in addition to their angiogenesis-inducing capacity.

The best characterized angiogenic growth factor is ► vascular endothelial growth factor (VEGF) which fulfills all criteria to be considered as master switch of the angiogenic cascade. This has been most unambiguously demonstrated in gene targeting experiments in mice which have shown that disruption of just one VEGF allele is not compati-

ble with life and leads to early embryonic lethality. VEGF, now designated VEGF-A, is a member of a still growing family of growth factors comprising VEGF-A, VEGF-B, VEGF-C and VEGF-D. VEGF molecules exert their vascular specificity through the limited expression of their corresponding receptors, VEGF-R1, VEGF-R2, and VEGF-R3 which are almost exclusively expressed by blood and lymphatic endothelial cells. VEGF-A is one of the most potent inducers of blood vessel angiogenesis and vascular permeability. It exists in five different splice forms ($VEGF_{121}$, $VEGF_{145}$, $VEGF_{165}$, $VEGF_{189}$, and $VEGF_{206}$) and signals primarily through VEGF-R2. VEGF-R1 appears to act as a co-receptor with an approximately 20 fold higher affinity to VEGF than VEGF-R2. The signaling functions of VEGF-R1 have not yet been determined. Correspondingly, VEGF-B has been identified as a VEGF-R1 specific growth factor whose function has not fully been defined. VEGF-C and VEGF-D bind to both VEGF-R2 and VEGF-R3. VEGF-R2 activation drives blood vessel angiogenesis, whereas VEGF-R3 signaling has been shown to be critically involved in controlling lymphatic vessel growth.

► Placenta growth factor (PlGF) is a VEGF-related molecule (PlGF-1 and PlGF-2) that exclusively binds to VEGF-R1. PlGF is dispensable for embryonic and reproductive angiogenesis but plays important roles in pathologic angiogenesis as it relates to tumor growth or cardiac ischemia.

Despite its requisite role in angiogenesis, VEGF must act in concert with other growth factors. The angiopoietins (Ang-1 and Ang-2) were discovered as ligands for the endothelial cell receptor tyrosine kinase Tie-2. Gene ablation experiments in mice suggested a role of the Ang/Tie-2 system in vessel remodeling and stabilization of the growing neovasculature. There are now four members of the angiopoietin (Ang) family, although Ang-3 and Ang-4 may represent widely diverged counterparts of the same gene locus in mouse and man. All known angiopoietins bind to Tie-2, and no ligands have yet been identified for the second Tie receptor, Tie-1. Ang-1 acts as an agonistic Tie-2 ligand and is involved in regulating vessel maturation and remodeling by acting as a survival factor for endothelial cells and controlling the association with mural cells (pericytes and smooth muscle cells). Low level constitutive Tie-2 phosphor-

Tab. 1 Positive and negative endogenous regulators of angiogenesis.

Stimulators	Inhibitors
Peptide growth factors VEGF-A, -B, -C, -D PlGF Ang-1 FGF-1, -2 PDGF-BB TGF-α HGF IGF-1	*Proteolytic peptides* Angiostatin (plasminogen fragment) Endostatin (collagen XVIII fragment) Vasostatin (calreticulin fragment) Tumstatin (collagen IV fragment) Antithrombin III fragment *Inhibitors of enzymatic activity* TIMP-1, -2, -3, -4 PAI-1, -2
Multifunctional cytokines/immune mediators TNF-α (low dose) MCP-1	*Multifunctional cytokines/immune mediators* TNF-α (high dose)
CXC-chemokines IL-8	*CXC-chemokines* PF-4 IP-10 Gro-β
Enzymes PD-ECGF, thymidine phosphorylase Angiogenin (ribonuclease A homolog)	
	Extracellular matrix molecules Thrombospondin
Hormones Estrogens Prostaglandin-E$_1$, -E$_2$ Follistatin Proliferin	*Hormones/metabolites* 2-ME Proliferin-related protein
Oligosaccharides Hyalorunan oligosaccharides Gangliosides	*Oligosaccharides* Hyaluronan, HMW species
Hematopoietic growth factors Erythropoietin G-CSF GM-CSF	

Abbreviations: VEGF, vascular endothelial growth factor; -A, -B, -C, -D; PlGF, placenta growth factor; Ang, angiopoietin; FGF, fibroblast growth factor; PDGF, platelet-derived growth factor; TGF, transforming growth factor; HGF, hepatocyte growth factor; IGF, insulin-like growth factor; TNF, tumor necrosis factor; MCP, monocyte chemoattractant protein; IL, interleukin; PD-ECGF, platelet-derived endothelial cell growth factor; G-CSF, granulocyte-colony stimulating factor; GM-CSF, granulocyte-macrophage colony stimulating factor; TIMP, tissue metalloproteinase inhibitor; PAI, plasminogen activator inhibitor; PF, platelet factor; IP-10, interferon-γ-inducible protein-10; 2-ME, 2-Methoxyestradiol; HMW, high molecular weight

ylation appears to be involved in maintaining the quiescent phenotype of the resting vasculature. In turn, Ang-2 functions are more complex. Ang-2 acts as a functional antagonist of Ang-1 by binding to Tie-2 without exerting signal transducing functions. Intriguingly, Ang-2 is almost exclusively produced by endothelial cells and acts as an auto-crine regulator of vessel stabilization and destabi-lization. As such, Ang-2 may facilitate angiogen-esis in the presence of angiogenic activity (e.g. VEGF stimulation) or induce vessel regression in the absence of angiogenic activity (e.g. during regression of the cyclic ovarian corpus luteum).

The Eph receptor tyrosine kinases comprise the largest known family of tyrosine kinase recep-tors and interact in a specific, yet somewhat pro-miscuous manner with their corresponding Ephrin ligands. Although initially characterized as regulators of axonal outgrowth in the nervous sys-tem, recent gene inactivation experiments in mice have revealed key roles for ephrin-B2 and its Eph-B2, Eph-B3, and Eph-B4 receptors during vascular development (▶ ephrin-B Molecules). Mouse embryos lacking ephrin-B2 or Eph-B4 (or the combination of Eph-B2 and Eph-B3) suffer dra-matic defects in early angiogenic remodeling that are similar to those seen in mice lacking Ang-1 or Tie-2. Moreover, ephrin-B2 and Eph-B4 display remarkable asymmetric arterio-venous expres-sion patterns, with ephrin-B2 selectively marking arterial vessels and Eph-B4 preferentially being expressed by venous endothelial cells. This asym-metric expression pattern suggests a critical role of ephrin-B2 and Eph-B4 in establishing arterial versus venous identity of the growing vasculature.

Angiogenic activation induces a complex gene expression program in endothelial cells enabling the cells to execute the complex molecular tasks required to grow new blood vessels. The invasive ingrowth of angiogenic endothelial cells involves a distinct set of adhesion molecules including the integrin heterodimers $\alpha_v\beta_3$ and $\alpha_v\beta_5$ as well as the homotypic endothelial cell-specific adhesion mol-ecule VE-cadherin. Likewise, sprouting endothe-lial cells display a shift of their proteolytic balance towards a proinvasive phenotype, involving the plasminogen activator (tPA and uPA) and plas-minogen activator inhibitor system (PAI). Ang-iogenic endothelial cells deposit their own extra-cellular matrix, rearrange their cytoskeleton, and turn on their proliferative machinery. All of these molecular systems are extensively being explored to therapeutically interfere with the angiogenic process.

Angiogenesis in Pathological Conditions

Abnormal vessel growth is involved in numerous pathological conditions. Pioneering work more than 30 years ago has shown that the growth of solid tumors is critically dependent on the supply with new blood vessels. While some of this supply may be provided by mechanisms of vessel coop-tion, the process whereby a growing tumor is preying on the pre-existent vasculature, the pri-mary mechanism of tumor vascularization appears to be the angiogenic growth of blood ves-sels from the tumor neighboring blood vessels. Tumor cells release pro-angiogenic growth factors, such as VEGF, which diffuse into nearby tissues where they bind and activate receptors on endothelial cells of pre-existing blood vessels. Secretion of proteolytic enzymes, such as matrix metalloproteinases (MMPs), results in the degra-dation of basement membrane and extracellular matrix components, allowing endothelial cells to invade and proliferate, and form new lumen-con-taining vessels. Tumor angiogenesis involves the specific molecular regulators of the angiogenic cascade that control developmental or reproduc-tive angiogenesis. However, tumor angiogenesis also involves additional mechanisms that include the pleiotrophic angiogenic growth factors, for example as a consequence of the inflammatory response usually associated with tumor growth.

Besides tumor angiogenesis, an increasing list of diseases is now recognized to critically depend on either increased or reduced angiogenesis. For example, increased angiogenesis occurs during diabetic retinopathy, macula degeneration, arthritic joint diseases, and hyperproliferative skin diseases. In turn, reduced angiogenesis may have a negative impact on wound healing and the regen-erative processes associated with ischemic dis-eases as they occur in the heart or during periph-eral limb ischemia.

Pharmacological Intervention

Both, angioinhibitory as well as angiostimulatory therapies are presently being explored extensively for a number of indications. Angioinhibitory ther-apies are being developed most intensely to thera-peutically interfere with tumor angiogenesis and tumor growth (Fig. 1B). Other major antiang-iogenic therapies that are currently in clinical development target retinal diseases (diabetic retinopathy, macula degeneration), joint diseases (arthritis), as well as hyperproliferative skin diseases (psoriasis). In turn, angiostimulatory therapies are being developed to stimulate wound healing angiogenesis, peripheral limb ischemia, and arteriogenic growth of collaterals during cardiac ischemia.

Antiangiogenic Tumor Targeting

Antiangiogenic tumor targeting is conceptually a particularly attractive therapeutic target for a number of reasons: (1) As an oncofetal mechanism that is mostly downregulated in the healthy adult, targeting of angiogenesis should lead to minimal side effects even after prolonged treatment, (2) tumor-associated angiogenesis is a physiological host mechanism and its pharmacological inhibition should, consequently, not lead to the development of resistance, (3) each tumor capillary potentially supplies hundreds of tumor cells and the targeting of the tumor vasculature should, thus, lead to a potentiation of the antitumorigenic effect, and (4) in contrast to the interstitial location of tumor cells, direct contact of the vasculature to the circulation allows efficient access of therapeutic agents.

A number of approaches have been taken to inhibit tumor angiogenesis and other diseases involving angiogenesis (Table 2). Pharmacological inhibition of angiogenesis is aimed at interfering with the angiogenic cascade or the immature neovasculature. Pharmacological agents may be synthetic or semi-synthetic substances, endogenous inhibitors of angiogenesis, or biological antagonists of the angiogenic cascade. In contrast, vascular targeting is aimed at utilizing specific molecular determinants of the neovasculature for the delivery of a biological, chemical, or physical activity that will then locally act angiocidal or tumoricidal. A comprehensive website summarizing the status of tumor antiangiogenic compounds in various stages of clinical trial is maintained by the National Cancer Institute at: www.cancer.gov/clinicaltrials/developments/anti-angio-table. Following is a survey of the most important substances currently in clinical development.

Specific Synthetic and Biological Antagonists of the Angiogenic Cascade

Specific inhibition of any of the key regulators of the angiogenic cascade is one of the most specific and selective ways to interfere with angiogenesis. A number of experimental strategies have been taken to interfere with the interaction of VEGF with its receptors. These include antisense and antibody approaches to inhibit VEGF, the development of small molecular weight antagonists to the VEGF receptors, as well as the use of soluble VEGF receptors. Difficulties with some of the first generation-specific inhibitors of angiogenesis in clinical trials, including the discontinuation of the phase III clinical trial involving a humanized neutralizing antibody to VEGF (Avastin), has severely set back the field of antiangiogenesis research. Yet, a number of new generation small molecular weight VEGF receptor antagonists are rapidly proceeding in various stages of clinical trials (e.g., SU11248 [Pharmacia], ZD6474 [AstraZeneca], PTK787/ZK222584 [Novartis/Schering]).

Inhibitors of the angiopoietin/Tie-2 and Ephrin/Eph systems are in preclinical development that parallels the biological target validation of these molecules. As vascular assembly, maturation, and homeostasis regulating molecules, therapeutic interference with these molecular systems may hold promise for a number of vascular indications.

Interference with specific cell-cell and cell-matrix adhesion mechanisms is another rapidly advancing approach to therapeutically interfere with angiogenesis. Antagonistic antibodies to the integrin heterodimer $\alpha_v\beta_3$ have shown to be effective in interfering with the interaction of angiogenic endothelial cells with their extracellular matrix, causing the cells to detach and die by apoptosis. Likewise, VE-cadherin acts as a homotypic cell-cell adhesion molecule and can be used to target the angiogenic vasculature.

The growing list of endogenous inhibitors of angiogenesis holds great promise for therapeutic applications. Substances most advanced in clinical development include Interleukin-12, Endostatin, Thrombospondin, and Tumstatin. As endogenous substances, these molecules have a long half-life in the plasma and are, thus, particularly attractive for long-term treatments. Thrombospondin has been most extensively studied as an endogenous

Tab. 2   Antiangiogenic therapeutic strategies.

Substance	Mechanism / Approach
Biological antagonists	
VEGF inhibitors	Humanized neutralizing antibodies, antisense oligonucleotides
VEGF receptor blockers	Small receptor tyrosine kinase antagonists
Soluble receptors	Inhibition with soluble VEGF-R1 or soluble Tie-2
$\alpha_v\beta_3$ integrin antagonists	Induce angiogenic endothelial cell apoptosis
Endogenous inhibitors	
Angiostatin	Plasminogen fragment (antiangiogenic mechanism unknown)
Endostatin	Collagen XVIII fragment (antiangiogenic mechanism unknown)
Vasostatin	Calreticulin fragment
Tumstatin	Collagen IV fragment
IL-12	Induces IP-10
Interferon-α	Decreases FGF production
Platelet factor-4	Inhibits endothelial cell proliferation
Thrombospondin	Antiangiogenic mechanism unknown
Synthetic / semisynthetic inhibitors	
Carboxyamidotriazole	Calcium channel blocker
CM101	Analog of group β streptococcus toxin, binds to tumor endothelium, induces inflammation
Marimastat	Metalloproteinase inhibitor, inhibits endothelial cell invasion
Pentosan polysulfate	Inhibits heparin binding growth factors
TNP470	Analog of fumagillin, inhibits cell migration and proliferation
Thalidomide	Polycyclic teratogen, antiangiogenic mechanism unknown
Vascular targeting	
Regional TNF-α therapy	Isolated limb perfusion to target in transit metastases
Antibody targeting	Use of mono-and bispecific antibodies to target components of angiogenic blood vessels (e.g. VEGF receptors, endoglin, L19 antigen) to deliver specific angio- and/or tumoricidal activity
Vascular gene therapy	Transfer of dominant-negative receptors or suicide genes under the control of angiogenic endothelial cell specific promoters

inhibitor of angiogenesis and work is underway to exploit Thrombospondin to locally inhibit skin angiogenesis, e.g. during psoriasis. A better understanding of the molecular mechanisms through which these molecules act may greatly advance the field and may lead to the rational design of synthetic small molecular mimetics of endogenous inhibitors of angiogenesis.

Non-specific Synthetic and Biological Angiogenesis Inhibitors

Systematic screening experiments have identified more than 100 synthetic compounds with potent antiangiogenic activity. The mode of action for most of these molecules is not well understood, but approximately 40 compounds are well advanced in clinical trials. The first substances to have entered clinical trials was the fumagillin-derivative AGM 1470. Fumagillin is an antibiotic that was identified as an endothelial cell migration and proliferation inhibiting substance. The mechanism of action of AGM 1470 is poorly understood, but it was shown that it binds and inhibits the metalloprotease methionine aminopeptidase (MetAp-2). Other antibiotics with antiangiogenic activity are minocycline and herbimycin A. Carboxyamidotriazole (CAI) inhibits the calcium influx into cells and suppresses the proliferation of endothelial cells. It inhibits angiogenesis and metastasis, but it is not an endothelial cell-specific substance. Similarly, the metalloproteinase inhibitors (MMPIs) Marimastat (BB2516) and Batimastat (BB94) are not vascular-specific substances, but are both antiangiogenic and anti-tumorigenic by inhibiting invasion of endothelial cells as well as tumor cells. The poor performance of some MMPIs in clinical trials has led to the development of novel metalloproteinase inhibitors such as BMS-275291, Col-3, and Neovastat. Thalidomide appears to be a promising antitumorigenic and antiangiogenic substance: Originally developed as a hypnosedative drug in the late 1950s and subsequently withdrawn from the market as a consequence of its teratogenic effects, it has been selectively reintroduced in the last few years for use in various disorders thought to act on an autoimmune or inflammatory basis. The mechanism of thalidomide's antiangiogenic activity is not known but it probably impedes cell migration by downregulating β-integrins. Pentosan polysul-

fate (xylanopolyhydrogensulfate) is a semi-synthetic sulfated heparinoid polysaccharide. It has been used as an anticoagulant for many years. It exerts antiangiogenic activity by interfering with the binding of angiogenic growth factors to the cell surface. Another substance that has entered clinical trials is the analog of a group B streptococcal toxin (GBS toxin) that has been designated CM101. The polysaccharide CM101 binds preferentially to a subset of tumor endothelial cells and induces a massive local inflammatory reaction that in turn acts tumoricidal.

Vascular Targeting

The goal of vascular targeting is to utilize specific molecular determinants of angiogenic endothelium to deliver substances or activities that destroy the vasculature. Following this concept, targeting human tissue factor to endothelial cells using a bispecific antibody to an angiogenic endothelial cell marker on the tumor vasculature leads to localized thrombosis. In consequence, the tumor regresses as a result of the massive infarction. Vascular targeting has also been employed in advanced extremity soft tissue sarcomas through regional high dose TNF-α therapy. In these experiments, an isolated limb perfusion system was used to preferentially target TNF-α to tumor-associated endothelial cells causing a rapid destruction of the sarcoma-associated microvasculature. Similarly, genetic targeting experiments are underway to direct suicide genes, such as herpes simplex virus thymidine kinase (HSV-TK) to proliferating endothelial cells by employing endothelial cell specific promoters. Lastly, the single chain antibody L19, binding a fibronectin variant that is selectively expressed in the tumor subendothelial basement membrane, is extensively being explored as target for vascular targeting strategies.

Proangiogenic Therapies

Antiangiogenesis research has driven the field. Yet, there are a number of indications which may benefit from an induction of angiogenesis, including wound healing, cardiac ischemia, and peripheral limb ischemia. Various approaches have been taken to therapeutically deliver angiogenic cytokines such as VEGF and FGF-2. These include the local administration of recombinant proteins and gene therapeutic delivery of angiogenic cytokines. Individual cytokine therapy may have limitations as it may induce a neovascular response but may not be able to induce the growth of a patent neovascular network that is stable for prolonged periods of time. This notion has led to alternative strategies aimed at inducing the complex endogenous angiogenic program and not just a single cytokine. For example, experiments are underway to locally induce hypoxia-inducible factor-1 (HIF-1), a key regulator of the hypoxia response program that is able to control the complex endogenous program of angiogenesis induction.

Clinical Implementation of Angiomanipulatory Therapies

It is difficult to foresee which of the more than 50 compounds presently pursued in clinical trials will eventually enter the clinic. The original intense enthusiasm in the field has been dampened by sobering results in some clinical trials including discontinuation of some phase III clinical trials. Furthermore, too many compounds have too rapidly entered clinical trials before completing a stringent preclinical evaluation.

Despite this cautionary note, some angiomanipulatory therapies are already in clinical use. The most widespread – and likewise most ignored – established antiangiogenic therapy is the chemotherapeutic and radiotherapeutic treatment of tumors. Chemo- and radiotherapy targets proliferating cells. Endothelial cell proliferation is a key step of the angiogenic cascade and antiproliferative therapies do not just target the proliferative tumor cell compartment but also the proliferative endothelial cell compartment. Likewise, the vascular endothelium with its proximity to the iron containing blood compartment is a preferential target of radiotherapeutic intervention. These observations have long been recognized. Yet, it is not clear to this date to what extent the targeting of the proliferating endothelial cell pool contributes to the therapeutic efficacy of established chemotherapies and radiotherapies. Low dose continuous chemotherapy (metronomic therapy) has been proposed as a strategy to redirect standard chemotherapy protocols to preferentially target the angiogenic endothelial cell compartment in tumors.

Some of the advanced antiangiogenic compounds will be approved for clinical use in the next few years. It is now widely recognized that these compounds may not be very effective in monotherapies. The challenge of antiangiogenic tumor therapies, thus, lies in the establishment of the most rational and effective combination therapies between antiangiogenesis and other established therapeutic modalities (chemotherapy, radiotherapy).

In contrast to antiangiogenic therapies, the first proangiogenic therapies have already been approved for clinical use. Direct laser-assisted myocardial revascularization (DMR) is an approved technique in the US, Europe, and parts of Asia to create numerous myocardial channels. This results in the induction of a massive inflammatory reaction which in turn induces angiogenesis. The other FDA-approved proangiogenic therapy is the use of recombinant human platelet-derived growth factor (Regranex) for use in the treatment of diabetic neuropathic foot ulcers.

References

1. Jain RK, Carmeliet P (2001) Vessels of death or life. Sci Am 285:38–45
2. Yancopoulos GD, Davis S, Gale NW, Rudge JS, Wiegand SJ, Holash J (2000) Vascular-specific growth factors and blood vessel formation. Nature 407:242–248
3. Jussila L, Alitalo K (2002) Vascular growth factors and lymphangiogenesis. Physiol Rev 82:673–700
4. Scappaticci FA (2002) Mechanisms and future directions for angiogenesis-based cancer therapies. J Clin Oncol 20:3906–3927

Angiogenic Switch

The angiogenic shift is a shift in the balance of proangiogenic to antiangiogenic activity which is considered to be a critical rate limiting step during tumor progression in the transition of a tumor from an avascular to a vascular state.

▶ Angiogenesis and Vascular Morphogenesis

Angiopoietins

Angiopoietins are growth factor ligands of the receptor tyrosine kinase Tie-2 which are critical regulators of vascular assembly and differentiation.

▶ Angiogenesis and Vascular Morphogenesis

Angiotensin

▶ Renin-Angiotensin-Aldosterone System

Angiotensin Converting Enzyme

Angiotensin converting enzyme (ACE) is identical to kininase II. It is an essential component of both the renin-angiotensin system and the kallikrein-kinin system. Three different foms of ACE are known. It exists as a membrane bound protein with a molecular weight of 150-180 kD, anchored to the cytoplasmatic membrane of endothelial cells and as a circulating protein of similar size. The enzyme consists of two highly homologous lobes with an active site in each lobe. Interestingly, although still of uncertain consequence, the active sites exhibit different catalytic profiles and different affinities for ACE inhibitors. A third, smaller form of ACE (90 kD) with only one active site is expressed in mature germ cells.

The substrate specificity of ACE is low. ACE cleaves a variety of pairs of amino acids from the carboxy-terminal part of several peptide substrates. The conversion of ANG I to ANG II and the degradation of bradykinin to inactive fragments are considered the most important functions of ACE. Both peptides have profound impact on the cardiovascular system and beyond. ACE is thus an important target for ACE inhibitors. These compounds are frequently and efficiently used in the treatment of hypertension and cardiac failure.

▶ ACE Inhibitors
▶ Renin-Angiotensin-Aldosterone System
▶ Antihypertensive Drugs

Angiotensin Receptors

Angiotensin receptors mediate the effects of angiotensin (ANG) II, the effector peptide of the renin-angiotensin system. Two receptors termed AT1 and AT2 have been characterised in detail. Both receptors belong to the superfamily of G-protein coupled receptors. Most of the cardiovascular functions of ANG II are mediated through the AT_1 receptor. This receptor is usually $G_{q/11}$- coupled and its activation leads to intracellular calcium surges and protein kinase C activation. Downstream of the G protein activation, small GTP-binding proteins such as RAS and RHOA and tyrosine kinase cascades are activated. These include members of the MAP-Kinase and JAK/STAT pathways. Finally transcription factors, such as AP-1, NF-kappa-Band the STATs(signal transducer and activators of transcription) are activated, which initiates the expression of growth related genes and/or is involved in inflammatory processes. This explains the effects of ANG II on growth, proliferation and its assumed role in inflammation. The functions of the AT_2 receptor are still a matter of debate. The AT_2 receptor is probably involved in differentiation processes, inhibits proliferation and induces apoptosis and thus may partially counteract some effects of AT_1 receptor activation. It is expressed during embryonic development in a tightly controled manner. In adults it is expressed in adrenal gland and ovary and its expression is induced during inflammatory processes and tissue damage. At present, there are no drugs available, which specifically inhibit or stimulate the AT_2 receptor.

▶ Renin-Angiotensin-Aldosterone System

Angiotensinogen

▶ Renin-Angiotensin-Aldosterone System

Anion Exchange Resin

Anion exchange resins are basic polymers with a high affinity for anions. Because different anions compete for binding to them, they can be used to sequester anions. Clinically used anion exchange resins such as cholestyramine are used to sequester bile acids in the intestine, thereby preventing their reabsorption. As a consequence, the absorption of exogenous cholesterol is decreased. The accompanying increase in low density lipoprotein (LDL)-receptors leads to the removal of LDL from the blood and, thereby, to a reduction of LDL cholesterol. This effect underlies the use of cholestyramine in the treatment of hyperlipidaemia.

▶ HMG-CoA-reductase-inhibitors

Antacids

Antacids are neutralizing agents. Examples are magnesium hydroxide, magnesium trisylicate and aluminium hydroxide. Prior to the introduction of histamine-H_2 receptor antagonists (histaminergic system) and proton pump inhibitors, they were the standard drugs for the treatment of duodenal/peptic ulcers. Today their clinical use is limited to the treatment of dyspepsia and the symptomatic relieve for patients with peptic ulcers.

Antagonist

An antagonist is a drug or ligand that binds to a receptor without activating it. Thus an antagonist can block the ability of an agonist to induce a biological signal through its receptor.

▶ Drug Receptor Interaction
▶ G-protein-coupled Receptors

Anthelminthic Drugs

Anthelminthic drugs are used for the treatment of worm infections. They represent a small but diverse group of drugs with regard to both their chemical structure and their mechanism of action. Like antimicrobial agents they are effective against certain types of worm and ineffective against others. The benzimidazoles (mebendazole, thiabendazole and albendazole) are broad-spectrum agents and the main group of anthelminthics used in the clinic. They induce multiple biochemical changes. However, their main mechanism of action appears to be inhibition of microtubule formation by binding to free parasitic β-tubulin. The spectrum of worms includes nematodes (e.g. the common round worm and the worm causing trichiniasis, *Trichinella spiralis*) and some cestodes. The drug of choice for the treatment of river blindness (caused by *Onchocerca volvulus*) is ivermectin. Trematodes (e.g. *Schistosoma* species causing bilharzia) are sensitive to praziquantel.

Anthracyclines

Anthracyclines are cytotoxic antibiotics isolated from *Streptomyces peucetius* or synthetic derivates of these antibiotics. Chemically, they consist of a tetracyclin ring to which an amino sugar, daunosamine, is attached by glycosidic linkage. Examples are doxorubicin, daunorubicin, epirubicin and idarubicin. They intercalate with DNA or RNA and thereby inhibit their synthesis. In addition, they cause single- and double-strand breaks in DNA, probably by inhibition of the enzyme topoisomerase II.

Clinically, they are used in various types of cancer with the individual compound exhibiting a specific spectrum. For example, doxorubicin is used for the treatment of malignant lymphoma but also for the treatment of solid tumors, particularly breast cancer. In addition to the typical unwanted effects of cytotoxic drugs (e.g. bone marrow depression), this group of drugs causes cardiac damage (cardiotoxic effect).

▶ Antineoplastic Agents

Antiarrhythmic Drugs

STEFAN DHEIN
Universität Leipzig, Herzzentrum Leipzig,
Klinik für Herzchirurgie, Leipzig, Germany
dhes@medizin.uni-leipzig.de

Synonyms

Antiarrhythmics

Definition

Antiarrhythmic drugs are substances that block cardiac ionic channels, thereby altering the cardiac action potential. This results in changes of the spread of activation or the pattern of repolariza-

tion. Thereby, these drugs suppress cardiac arrhythmia.

These drugs can be classified according to Vaughan-Williams (Table 1): (a) sodium channel blockers; slowing the spread of activation (▶ Class I Antiarrhythmic Drugs) with prolongation of the action potential (class IA), with shortening of the action potential (class IB) or without effect on action potential duration (class IC), (b) β-adrenoceptor antagonists; slowing sinus rhythm and atrioventricular conduction (▶ Class II Antiarrhythmic Drugs), (c) potassium channel blockers; prolonging the action potential (▶ Class III Antiarrhythmic Drugs), (d) calcium channel blockers; mainly slowing atrioventricular conduction (▶ Class IV Antiarrhythmic Drugs), and (not included in this classification) (e) digitalis glycosides, (f) adenosine and (g) atropine.

▶ K$^+$ Channels
▶ Voltage-dependent Na$^+$ Channels

Mechanism of Action

Basic Considerations
Normal rhythmic activity is the result of the activity of the sinus node generating action potentials that are conducted via the atria to the atrioventricular node, which delays further conduction to the His-Tawara-Purkinje system. From the

Tab. 1 Classification of antiarrhythmic drugs according to Vaughan-Williams (6).

Class	Effects	Drugs
I	Block of sodium channel	
I a	With prolongation of action potential	Quinidine, Procainamide, Disopyramide, Ajmaline, Prajmaline
I b	With shortening of action potential	Lidocaine, Mexiletine, Tocainide, Phenytoin, Aprindine
I c	With only little effect on action potential duration	Lorcainide, Flecainide, Propafenone
II	β-adrenoceptor antagonists	Propranolol, Metoprolol and others
III	Block of repolarizing potassium channels, prolongation of action potential	Amiodarone, Dronedarone, Sotalol, Dofetilide, Ibutilide
IV	Block of calcium channels	Verapamil, Diltiazem

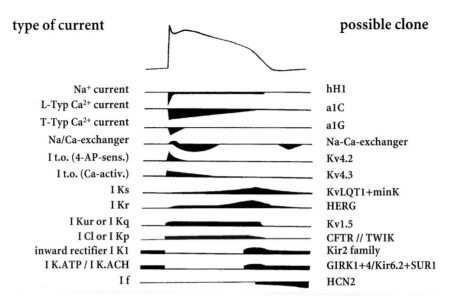

Fig. 1 Transmembrane ionic currents of the cardiac action potential. In the middle of the figure a typical cardiac action potential is shown as can be obtained from the ventricular myocardium (upper trace). Below, the contribution of the various transmembrane currents is indicated. Currents below the zeroline are inward, currents above the zero line are outward fluxes. In the left column the name of the current is given and in the right column the possible clone; redrawn and modified after (5).

Purkinje fibers, action potentials propagate to the ventricular myocardium. Arrhythmia means a disturbance of the normal rhythm either resulting in a faster rhythm (tachycardia, still rhythmic) or faster arrhythmia (tachyarrhythmia) or slowed rhythm (bradycardia, bradyarrhythmia).

Arrhythmia is either the result of impaired conduction or enhanced electrical activity. However, in all arrhythmias, conduction and intercellular communication are important since arrhythmia only occurs if the altered electrical activity in one region is transduced to the whole organ.

Antiarrhythmic drugs can either influence electrical activity of the single cell or can interfere with the spread of activation.

In the following, the cardiac action potential is explained (see Fig. 1): An action potential is initiated by depolarization of the plasmamembrane due to the pacemaker current (I_f) (carried by Na^+) [in sinus nodal cells] or to depolarization of the neighboring cell. Depolarization opens the fast Na^+ channel resulting in a fast depolarization (phase 0 of the action potential). These channels then inactivate and can only be activated if the

membrane is hyperpolarized again. This fast upstroke is followed by a short incomplete repolarization (activation of the transient outward rectifier $I_{t.o.}$ carried by K^+, phase 1). Next, the action potential remains quiet constant for about 50–350 ms (plateau phase, phase 2), which is the result of inward Ca^{++} current (via L-type Ca^{++} channels) and simultaneous activation of the repolarizing potassium current, the delayed rectifier I_K (which has three components: rapid, $I._{K.r}$, ultrarapid, $I_{K.ur}$, slow component: $I_{K.s}$). This is followed by complete ▶ repolarization of the membrane to -80 mV via activation of the delayed rectifier (phase 3), while the Ca^{++} channels close during this phase. During an action potential it is not possible to elicit a second action potential since the fast Na^+ channel is inactivated. This period is called refractory period.

Not all cells in the heart express the fast sodium channel. Thus, sinus nodal and atrioventricular nodal cells lack the fast Na^+ channel and instead generate their action potentials via opening of Ca^{++} channels. This is the basis for their sensitivity to Ca^{++} antagonists.

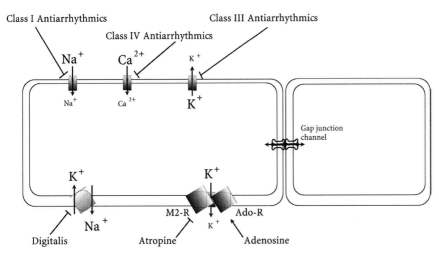

Fig. 2 Targets of the various antiarrhythmic drugs. The K^+ channel, regulated by acetylcholine (via M_2 receptors) or adenosine (via A_1 receptors), plays a role only in supraventricular tissues. The action potential which is generated in one cell propagates to the neighboring cell via the gap junction channel.

Action potential propagation along the fiber is mainly dependent on the Na^+ channel availability, which is a function of the resting membrane potential. Propagation from cell to cell is possible via intercellular gap junction channels. These channels can be regulated by a number of stimuli. Thus, low pH, high $[Ca^{++}]_i$ or low $[ATP]_i$ result in a closure of these channels leading to conduction disturbances and arrhythmias in myocardial infarction.

There are several basic mechanisms of arrhythmia:

a) a single cell or group of cells capable of a pacemaker potential may generate extrastimuli (enhanced automaticity).

b) a cell may generate oscillating afterpotentials which reach the threshold for activation of the Na^+ channel (triggered activity).

c) a cell generates late afterdepolarizations (typically induced by catecholamines or digitalis) following a complete repolarization that may elicit an action potential.

d) a cell may produce early afterdepolarizations that are depolarization during incomplete repolarization. This is possible if the action potential is considerably prolonged.

e) Furthermore, under certain conditions (e.g. local unidirectional block) it is possible that the activation wavefront is delayed and encounters areas already repolarized. This may result in a circulating wavefront (= reentrant circuit ▶ reentrant arrhythmia), from which centrifu-

gal activation waves originate and elicit life threatening ventricular fibrillation.

f) a block of propagation may occur in the specific conduction system leading to bradyarrhythmia (sinuatrial block, atrioventricular block, bundle block).

Antiarrhythmic treatment is based upon modulation of the ionic currents mentioned above. A principal problem with this therapy is that the electrophysiology of all cells is targeted and not specifically the arrhythmogenic focus. As a consequence, all antiarrhythmics acting at transmembrane ionic channels possess a risk for elicitation of arrhythmia (= proarrhythmic risk).

Molecular Mechanism of Action

Class I, III and IV antiarrhythmics bind to and block transmembrane ionic channels (Fig. 2). Class I antiarrhythmics block the fast Na^+ channel. This channel switches from a resting state to an open state, and then time- and voltage-dependently inactivates (inactivated state) (Fig. 3). The block of this channel by an antiarrhythmic drug is a ▶ state-dependent block: a class I compound like lidocaine enters the channel in its open state and binds to the inactivated state, altering the kinetics of recovery from inactivation. If the channel switches to its resting state the affinity for lidocaine is less and the drug dissociates from the channel. This is the basis for the use dependence of block: the kinetics of dissociation determines the interval after which a subsequent action

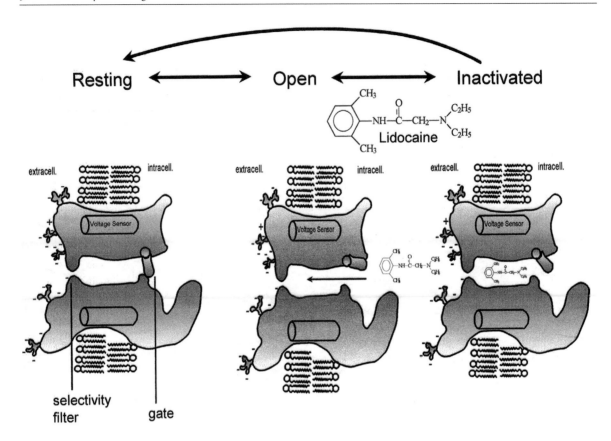

Fig. 3 Binding of class I antiarrhythmic drugs to the cardiac sodium channel. Summary of the modulated receptor hypothesis as an explanation of state-dependent block of Na^+ channels by local anaesthetics such as lidocaine. The Na^+ channel switches between resting, open and inactivated state. On the extracellular side a selectivity filter controls the ions passing through the channel. On the intracellular side the inactivation gate can close the channel. A class I antiarrhythmic drug (lidocaine) enters the channel during its open state and binds with its lipophilic moiety to the inactivated state, the hydrophilic part of the molecule extending into the water-filled channel pore blocking it.

potential is not influenced. That means that an action potential early after the foregoing action potential will be suppressed while another after a long interval will not be altered.

Drugs with fast dissociation will only suppress high frequency arrhythmia (high use-dependence). Drugs with a long dissociation time constant will suppress action potentials at normal frequency as well. Class IB drugs exhibit the shortest time constant (0.2–0.4 s; highest use-dependence), while class IC drugs have the longest dissociation time constant (2–250 s; no use-dependence). Class IA antiarrhythmics show an intermediate dissociation time constant (5–50 s).

Class I drugs (Na^+ channel blockers) suppress action potential amplitude, reduce depolarization velocity and propagation velocity, prolong total refractory period and reduce automaticity. These drugs have no or little influence on slow Ca^{++} carried action potentials (AV- or sinus nodal cells). All these drugs exert negative inotropic effects and a strong proarrhythmic effect especially in patients with structural heart disease and, thus, cannot be used in patients after myocardial infarction.

Class IA possess a marked proarrhythmic risk for the induction of ▶ torsade de pointes arrhythmia (life-threatening polymorphic ventricular tachycardia observed with most action potential prolonging drugs).

Quinidine, the classical class IA drug, binds to the open state of the Na^+ channel, and prolongs the action potential by block of the delayed rectifier. In higher concentrations, L-type Ca^{++} channels are inhibited. Quinidine exerts antimuscarinic effects, thereby accelerating AV nodal conduction and antagonising α-adrenergic effects. Typial untoward effects include vomiting, diarrhoea, allergies, immunological effects and hepatitis.

Ajmaline (intravenously only) and its orally applicable prodrug prajmaline are classified as class IA drugs, but due to their long dissociation time constant can also be considered as class IC compounds.

Further class IA drugs include the open state blockers procainamide and disopyramide with electrophysiological effects similar to those of quinidine; procainamide lacks the antimuscarinic and antiadrenergic effects. Characteristic side effects of procainamide are hypotension and immunological disorders.

Class IB drugs like lidocaine, phenytoin or mexiletine preferentially bind to the inactivated state. Lidocaine, a local anaesthetic, can be used intravenously for antiarrhythmic treatment. It is one of the classical drugs used in emergency medicine for the treatment of ventricular fibrillation. The side effects of lidocaine are typical for local anaethetics including dizziness, tremor, nystagmus, seizures or nausea.

The antiepileptic drug phenytoinis, an orally available class IB antiarrhythmic, is mainly effective in digitalis-induced arrhythmias. This drug exhibits nonlinear pharmacokinetics and a number of side effects including neuropathy, gingival hyperplasia, hepatitis, immunological disorders and suppression of white blood cells.

Class IC antiarrhythmic drugs such as flecainide or propafenone block the Na^+ channel (open state; propafenone: open and inactivated state) with a very long dissociation time constant so that they alter normal action potential propagation. Flecainide increased mortality of patients recovering from myocardial infarction due to its proarrhythmic effects (CAST study). Action potential is shortened in Purkinje fibers but prolonged in the ventricules.

Propafenone possesses antagonistic effects due to its similarity to propranolol β-adrenoceptor. In high concentrations it blocks calcium channels and, thus, exerts prominent negative inotropic effects. Its adverse effects include proarrhythmic effects, worsening of heart failure and (due to β-adrenoceptor blockade) bradycardia and bronchospasm.

Class II drugs are classical β-adrenoceptor antagonists such as propranolol, atenolol, metoprolol or the short-acting substance esmolol. These drugs reduce sinus rates, exert negative inotropic effects and slow atrioventricular conduction. Automaticity, membrane responsiveness and effective refractory period of Purkinje fibers are also reduced. The typical extracardiac side effects are due to β-adrenoceptor blockade in other organs and include bronchospasm, hypoglycemia, increase in peripheral vascular resistance, depressions, nausea and impotence.

Class III antiarrhythmic drugs block the repolarizing K^+ channel thereby prolonging the action potential duration and lengthen the refractory period. The classical class III antiarrhythmic compounds like sotalol block the rapid component of the delayed rectifier, I_{Kr}. However, at higher heart rates the repolarization is mainly carried by the slow component I_{Ks} and, thus, the action potential prolonging effect of these agents is progressively reduced with increasing heart rate (inverse use-dependence). Class III antiarrhythmics can induce early afterdepolarizations and torsade de pointes.

d,l-sotalol is a racemate of l-sotalol, a β-adrenoceptor antagonist, and d-sotalol, an inhibitor of both I_{Kr} and I_{Ks}. This substance exhibits a strong inverse use-dependence. Regarding the beneficial antiarrythmic effects, studies with only l-sotalol showed that the racemate is superior. However, due to β-adrenoceptor blockade d,l-sotalol can induce bronchoconstriction, increase in peripheral vascular resistance, negative inotropy, depressions, hypoglycemia and bronchospasm. A serious side effect is the induction of torsade de pointes arrhythmia (ca. 3%).

Amiodarone blocks several ionic channels; besides predominant blockade of I_{Kr} and I_{Ks}, I_f, I_{Na}, $I_{Ca.L}$, $I_{Ca.T}$ are inhibited. Moreover, amiodarone acts as an antagonist at both α- and β-adrenoceptors. Inverse use-dependence is less than with sotalol. The action potential prolonging effect is slowly developing (steady state after 2–5 months). Side effects include defects of vision, corneal depositions, neurological disorders, pigmentation, photosensibilization, torsade de pointes arrhythmia and AV-block. Moreover, alterations of thyroid function and lung fibrosis are observed.

Since alterations of thyroid function by amiodarone are related to the iodine substitution of the drug, the iodine-free derivative dronedarone has been developed with similar electrophysiological effects as amiodarone.

Newly developed class III drugs comprise dofetilide, a specific I_{Kr} blocker, and ibutilide, which blocks I_{Kr} and activates the slow I_{Na}. Both drugs lack hemodynamic side effects. These drugs are scheduled for the treatment of atrial fibrillation and atrial flutter. As with class III drugs, they can induce torsade de pointes arrhythmia.

Class IV antiarrhythmic drugs (Ca^{++} entry blockers) inhibit L-type Ca^{++} channel. For antiarrhythmic purposes, only those Ca^{++} channel antagonists are used with higher affinity to the heart (i.e. verapamil, diltiazem) than to the vasculature (as nifedipine). These drugs have the strongest electrophysiological effects on sinus and atrioventricular node. They reduce sinus rate, slow atrioventricular conduction, prolong refractory period of the AV node and exert a strong negative inopropic effect.

Verapamil is a phenylalkylamine blocking L-type Ca^{++} channels in a use-dependent manner. The drug binds to the inactivated state of the channel. Diltiazem is a benzothiazepine derivative with a profile of action most similar to that of verapamil.

Other Antiarrhythmic Compounds

Digitalis glycosides exert parasympathomimetic effects leading to slowing of sinus rate and predominantly to prolongation of atrioventricular conduction time. This latter action is used for the control of the ventricular response frequency in the treatment of atrial fibrillation with digitalis.

Adenosine activates the atrial A_1-adenosine receptor, which opens the $I_{K.ACh}$ channel leading to hyperpolarization, slowing of spontaneous depolarization, reduces sinus rate and atrioventricular conduction. The drug has to be administered intravenously. Due to its extremely short half-life time (0.6–1.5 s) the effects are only tran-

sient. As a vasorelaxant it may produce pronounced hypotension.

The anti-muscarinic drug atropine can also be used for antiarrhythmic treatment. Muscarinic receptors (M_2 subtype) are mainly present in supraventricular tissue and in the AV node. They inhibit adenylcyclase via G_i proteins and thereby reduce intracellular cAMP. On the other hand, activation of the M_2 receptor leads to opening of hyperpolarizing $I_{K.ACh}$ and inhibits the pacemaker current I_f probably via the $\beta\gamma$-subunit of the G_i protein associated with this receptor. The results are hyperpolarization and slower spontaneous depolarization. Muscarinic receptor antagonists like atropine lead to increased heart rate and accelerated atrioventricular conduction.

Intravenous administration of magnesium sulfate (1–5 g) is used for the termination of torsade de pointes arrhythmia. The underlying electrophysiological mechanism is not well understood. It includes changes of the current-voltage relationship of I_{K1} and Ca^{++} channel blockade.

Clinical Uses

Clinical uses of antiarrhythmics have been restricted after CAST due to their proarrhythmic risk, and preference is given to electrophysiological methods.

Supraventricular bradycardia is treated by implantation of a pacemaker device or has been treated pharmacologically with atropine. Supraventricular paroxysmal tachycardia is treated with ajmaline or prajmaline. Supraventricular tachyarrhythmias typically can be terminated using adenosine.

The risk of atrial flutter is a 2:1 transmission to the ventricles generating a high ventricular rate. The therapeutic goal is to reduce transmission to 3:1 or 4:1 by administration of either β-adrenoceptor antagonists, Ca^{++} channel blockers or amiodarone.

The most common arrhythmia in humans is atrial fibrillation. Because of the lack of rhythmic atrial activation, irregular ventricular rhythms and thromboembolism result. There are two possible therapeutic goals: control of heart rate or return to sinus rhythm. For frequency control, β-adrenoceptor antagonists, Ca^{++} channel blockers and digitalis can be used. For conversion to sinus rhythm, electrophysiological ablation is the therapy of choice. Alternatively, a pharmacological attempt with class IA drugs or class IC drugs can be made. Thereafter, relapse to atrial fibrillation has to be prevented by amiodarone or β-adrenoceptor antagonists.

Atrioventricular block in general is treated by implantation of an electrical pacemaker. A pharmacological alternative (although no longer used today) was atropine.

Ventricular extrasystoles are treated only if they may degenerate into life-threatening arrhythmia. In milder forms the proarrhythmic risk of the drugs overshadows their benefits. In such cases β-adrenoceptor antagonists may be attempted. For the treatment of ventricular extrasystoles, such as series or runs of extrasystoles, amiodarone or sotalol are used. In the absence of structural heart disease, class I antiarrhythmic drugs can be considered an alternative. However, they may not be administered during the post-infarction period.

Ventricular fibrillation should be terminated by electrical defibrillation. Alternatively, lidocaine can be injected intravenously. In cases with lower frequency, ventricular tachyarrhythmia class I drugs such as ajmaline, flecainide or propafenone are more effective. For prophylaxis treatment, amiodarone or sotalol may be helpful or the implantation of a cardioverter-defibrillator system.

Torsade de pointes arrhythmia can be terminated by intravenous (not oral) administration of large doses of magnesium.

References

1. The Cardiac Arrhythmia Suppression Trial Investigators (1991) Mortality and morbidity in patients receiving encainide, flecainide or placebo. New Engl J Med 324:781
2. Dhein S (1998) Gap junctional channels in the cardiovascular system: pharmacological and physiological modulation. Trends Pharmacol Sci 19:229–241
3. Hille B (1992) Ionic channels of excitable membranes. Sunderland: Sinauer Assoc. pp.1–423
4. Hondeghem LM, Katzung BG (1984) Antiarrhythmic agents: the modulated receptor mechanism of action of sodium and calcium channel-blocking drugs. Annu Rev Pharmacol Toxicol 24:387–423
5. Rosen DM (1996) Antiarrhythmic drugs. In: Hardman JG, Limbird LE (Eds): Goodman & Gilman's The pharmacological basis of therapeutics. New York: McGraw-Hill pp.839–874
6. Vaughan-Williams EM (1994) A classification of antiarrhythmic actions reassessed after a decade of new drugs. J Clin Pharmacol 24:129
7. Zipes DP, Jalife J (1995) Cardiac electrophysiology. From cell to beside. Philadelphia: Saunders Inc.

Antibiotics

Originally, the term antibiotics referred to substances produced by microorganisms that suppressed the growth of other organisms. Today, the term antibiotics often includes synthetic antimicrobial agents.

▶ Microbial Resistance to Drugs
▶ β-lactam Antibiotics
▶ Ribosomal Protein Synthesis Inhibitors

Antibodies

Antibodies are involved in the humoral immune response. They recognize foreign substances (antigens) and trigger immune responses by the host. For the former, they possess interaction sites for a specific antigen. These interaction sites (Fab portions) are highly variable between antibodies produced by different clones of B cells. For the latter, they possess a constant region (Fc portion). Engineered antibodies are increasingly used for the treatment of human diseases.

▶ Immune Defense
▶ Humanized Monoclonal Antibodies

Anticoagulants

THEODORE E. WARKENTIN
Hamilton Regional Laboratory Medicine
Program, Hamilton Health Sciences, and
Department of Pathology and Molecular
Medicine, McMaster University, USA
twarken@mcmaster.ca

Synonyms

Oral anticoagulants, usually coumarin derivatives (e.g., warfarin, phenprocoumon); heparin, either unfractionated heparin (UFH) or low-molecular weight heparin (LMWH); danaparoid (heparinoid); fondaparinux (indirect factor Xa-inhibiting pentasaccharide); drotrecogin α (recombinant human activated protein C [APC]); direct thrombin inhibitors (DTIs), including hirudin derivatives (e.g., lepirudin, desirudin, bivalirudin) and small molecule active site inhibitors (e.g., argatroban, ximelagatran)

Definition

Anticoagulants inhibit ▶ coagulation by preventing ▶ thrombin generation and, ultimately, fibrin formation (1). They represent one of the two major classes of antithrombotic drugs, the other being antiplatelet agents. Anticoagulants are widely used to treat and prevent thrombosis involving arteries, veins and intra-cardiac chambers.

In general, arterial thrombi are platelet-rich ("white clots") and form at ruptured atherosclerotic plaques, leading to intraluminal occlusion of arteries that can result in end-organ injury (e.g., myocardial infarction, stroke). In contrast, venous thrombi consist mainly of fibrin and red blood cells ("red clots"), and usually form in low-flow veins of the limbs, producing deep vein thrombosis (DVT); the major threat to life results when lower extremity (and, occasionally, upper extremity) venous thrombi embolize via the right heart chambers into the pulmonary arteries, i.e., pulmonary embolism (PE).

▶ Antiplatelet Drugs
▶ Coagulation/Thrombosis
▶ Fibrinolytics

Mechanism of Action

Overview of Coagulation

Fig. 1 shows a simplified scheme of the coagulation cascade. Coagulation is usually triggered physiologically when ▶ tissue factor (TF), usually found in extravascular sites, binds to circulating factor VII(a) following vessel injury. TF/VII(a) complexes activate factor X, generating factor Xa. Factor Xa, together with a cofactor (factor Va), forms "prothrombinase" on phospholipid surfaces on activated platelets. Prothrombinase generates the key procoagulant enzyme, thrombin (factor IIa), from prothrombin (factor II). Various positive feedback loops help to convert a small procoagulant stimulus into a thrombin burst. For example, TF/VII(a) complexes also activate factor IX to IXa, which acts with a cofactor (VIIIa) to form the "tenase" complex that activates factor X to Xa. Other positive feedback loops initiated by thrombin include activation of factors V to Va, VIII to VIIIa and XI to XIa (not shown in Fig. 1).

Coagulation is regulated by three major inhibitory systems. (1) Antithrombin (AT, formerly, antithrombin III) inhibits circulating thrombin, Xa, IXa, XIa and TF/VII(a). However, AT does not inhibit thrombin bound to fibrin ("clot-bound thrombin") or surface-bound Xa. (2) The protein C natural anticoagulant pathway is triggered when thrombin binds to a receptor (thrombomodulin, TM) on endothelial cell surfaces: TM-bound thrombin activates protein C to activated protein C (APC), which together with a cofactor (protein S) degrades factors Va and VIIIa, thus down-regulating thrombin generation in the TM-rich microcirculation (3). Tissue factor pathway inhibitor (TFPI) binds to, and inhibits, factor Xa; subsequently, TFPI/Xa complexes inhibit VII(a) within VII(a)/TF.

The most commonly used anticoagulants – coumarins and heparins – inhibit various steps involving "propagation" of the coagulation cascade. Several newer agents inhibit thrombin directly. Drugs that inhibit initiation of coagulation are under investigation.

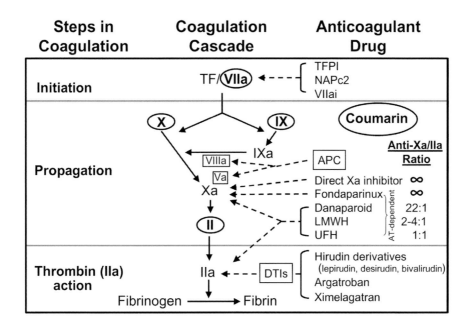

Fig. 1 Effects of Anticoagulants on the Coagulation Cascade. Coumarin agents alter the synthesis of four procoagulant zymogens (VII, X, IX, II), shown within circles. The other anticoagulants affect various coagulation factors (dotted arrows). Abbr.: APC, activated protein C; AT, antithrombin; DTIs, direct thrombin inhibitors; LMWH, low-molecular-weight heparin; NAPc2, nematode anticoagulant protein; TF, tissue factor, TFPI, tissue factor pathway inhibitor; UFH, unfractionated heparin; VIIai, active site-blocked VIIa. (Modified from 1, with permission from Chest).

Oral Anticoagulants (Coumarins)

Most oral anticoagulants are coumarin derivatives that act via ▶ vitamin K antagonism (2; Fig. 2). Vitamin K is required for post-translational modification of certain glutamate (glu) residues in four procoagulant factors (II, VII, IX, X). Addition of a carboxyl group (COO-) to each glu residue (to form γ-carboxyglutamate, or gla, residues) causes these vitamin K-dependent factors to become functional ▶ zymogens (proenzymes), as they now can bind to phospholipid surfaces via Ca2+-recognizing gla regions. Protein C and protein S are vitamin K-dependent anticoagulant factors.

The two most widely used coumarins are warfarin (US, Canada and UK) and phenprocoumon (continental Europe). The long half-life (60 h) of prothrombin means that coumarin cannot achieve therapeutic anticoagulation for at least 5 days following initiation. Thus, for patients with acute thrombosis, oral anticoagulants are usually started only when the patient is receiving a rapidly-active agent, usually UFH or LMWH.

Disadvantages of oral anticoagulants include a narrow therapeutic index (bleeding risk) and their highly variable dose-response relation (ongoing need for monitoring).

Maintenance doses vary widely among patients (e.g., from 1 to 20 mg/d for warfarin), and are influenced by diet (variable vitamin K intake) and medications that affect coumarin metabolism (decreased drug clearance: e.g., cotrimoxazole, amiodarone, erythromycin; increased clearance: e.g., barbiturates, carbamazepine, rifampin). Thus, regular monitoring is needed even during long-term maintenance therapy. This is performed using the ▶ prothrombin time (PT), which is usually expressed as the ▶ international normalized ratio (INR).

AT-Dependent Anticoagulants: Heparins, Danaparoid and Fondaparinux

Heparin is a highly sulfated ▶ glycosaminoglycan (3). Usually obtained from pig intestine or beef lung, UFH contains polymer varying from 3000–

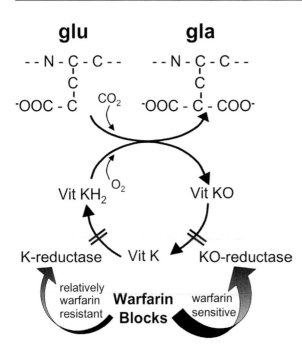

Fig. 2 Coumarin (Warfarin) and the Vitamin K Cycle.
Abbr.: glu, glutamate; gla, γ-carboxy-glutamate.
(Modified from 2, with permission from Chest.).

30,000 D (mean, 15,000 D; range, 10–90 monosaccharide units). Chemical or enzymatic methods can be used to make LMWH preparations that vary from 1000–10,000 D (mean, 4500 D; range, 3–30 monosaccharide units). A specific five saccharide sequence ("AT-binding pentasaccharide") present within up to one-third of UFH chains binds to AT, greatly increasing the efficiency of AT to inactivate thrombin, Xa, IXa, XIa, and TF/VII(a). AT is most efficient at inactivating thrombin and Xa, as shown by higher second order rate constants (8900 and 2500 $M^{-1}s^{-1}$, respectively compared with values of 300—450 for VII(a)/TF, IXa and XIa, respectively). Catalysis by UFH increases AT-mediated inhibition 1,000-fold.

Besides containing the specific AT-binding pentasaccharide sequence, heparin molecules must be at least 18 monosaccharide units long to bind to both AT and thrombin; in contrast, AT bound to any pentasaccharide-containing heparin — even with a chain length <18 monosaccharide units — will inhibit factor Xa. Thus, whereas UFH catalyzes inhibition of thrombin and Xa equally well, LMWH preferentially inhibits factor Xa (usual anti-Xa/anti-IIa ratio, 2–4:1) (Fig. 3). LMWH preparations (e.g., ardeparin [Normiflo], dalteparin [Fragmin], enoxaparin [Lovenox], reviparin [Clivarin], tinzaparin [Innohep]) differ in both jurisdictional availability and composition, and cannot be assumed to be interchangeable.

The ▶ activated partial thromboplastin time (aPTT) is usually used to monitor the anticoagulant effect of UFH, with the target aPTT level corresponding to an anti-factor Xa level of 0.35–0.70 U/mL (i.e., a ratio of patient/control aPTT of 1.5–2.5 for many aPTT reagents). However, prolongation of the aPTT is not sufficiently great to permit monitoring of LMWH therapy by this test. Nevertheless, since the shorter LMWH polymers have less non-specific binding to plasma proteins, LMWH anticoagulation is quite predictable. Thus, weight-adjusted LMWH dosing without monitoring is standard practice. Particularly during inflammation (high levels of UFH-binding proteins), high doses of UFH may be needed to prolong the aPTT and anti-factor Xa levels into the therapeutic range (heparin "resistance"). Anticoagulant monitoring of LMWH using anti-factor Xa levels may be needed in renal failure as LMWH accumulates.

Danaparoid (Orgaran; mean MW, 6000 D) is a mixture of non-heparin glycosaminoglycans derived from pig gut (dermatan sulfate, heparan sulfate, chondroitin sulfate). The anti-Xa/anti-IIa ratio (22:1) is even greater than seen with LMWH. The anti-IIa effect may be mediated in part by dermatan sulfate, which catalyzes thrombin inhibition by heparin cofactor II.

Fondaparinux, the factor Xa-binding pentasaccharide (Arixtra, MW 1728 D), is prepared synthetically, unlike UFH, LMWH and danaparoid, which are obtained from animal sources. Despite only inactivating free factor Xa, clinical trials indicate that fondaparinux is an effective antithrombotic agent (4).

In addition to the AT-dependent agents discussed above, various direct Xa inhibitors (e.g., tick anticoagulant peptide, antistatin, DX-9065a) are undergoing clinical testing. Unlike fondaparinux, these drugs also inhibit surface-bound Xa within prothrombinase.

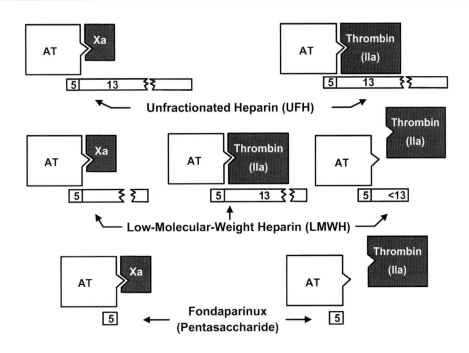

Fig. 3 Relative effects of UFH, LMWH, and fondaparinux on AT-mediated inhibition of factor Xa and thrombin (IIa). Whereas UFH catalyzes inhibition of Xa and thrombin equally well, only LMWH chains of 18 saccharide units or longer catalyze thrombin inhibition; thus, the anti-Xa/anti-IIa ratio of LMWH preparations ranges from 2:1 to 4:1. In contrast, fondaparinux exclusively inhibits Xa. (Modified from 3, with permission from Chest.)

Activated Protein C (APC)

Protein C is a vitamin K-dependent natural anticoagulant activated by thrombin to form APC in the presence of the endothelial receptor, TM. APC proteolyzes factors Va and VIIIa, thus down-regulating thrombin generation. APC may also have anti-inflammatory properties, as recombinant human APC (drotrecogin α, Xigris) reduces mortality in ▶ septicemia. Nonactivated protein C concentrates, prepared from pooled plasma, are also available for use in patients with congenital or acquired protein C deficiency.

Direct Thrombin Inhibitors (DTIs)

There are two major classes of DTIs: hirudin derivatives and small molecule active site inhibitors. Hirudin is a 65-amino acid polypeptide produced by the medicinal leech, which binds irreversibly and with high affinity to both the active site and exosite I (fibrinogen binding site) regions of thrombin, resulting in stable non-covalent hirudin-thrombin complexes (dissociation constant, ~10^{-14} M). Hirudin binds to both circulating and clot-bound thrombin. Lepirudin (Refludan, MW ~7000 D) and desirudin (Revasc) closely resemble hirudin. In contrast, bivalirudin (Angiomax, MW ~2180 D) is a 20-amino acid oligopeptide consisting of the active site and exosite I regions of hirudin connected by a short "spacer". All three agents are obtained by recombinant technology.

Two small molecule DTIs are argatroban (Novastan, MW 527 D) and the oral thrombin inhibitor, ximelagatran (Exanta, MW 474 D) (Ximelagatran is an inactive pro-drug: after absorption, it is metabolized to the active DTI, melagatran [MW 430 D]). In general, DTIs are monitored using the ▶ aPTT, although the high predictability of blood levels with oral administration of ximelagatran offers the possibility (now under investigation) that blood monitoring may not be necessary with this agent.

Factor VII(a)/Tissue Factor Pathway Inhibitors

Recombinant TFPI (tifacogin) directly inhibits VII(a)/TF complexes. Unlike recombinant APC, TFPI did not reduce mortality in clinical trials of septicemia. Recombinant nematode anticoagulant protein (NAPc2) is a small hookworm protein that binds to a non-catalytic site on both X and Xa, thus inhibiting VII(a)/TF. The half-life of NAPc2 is long (48 h), resembling that of factor X. Active site-blocked VIIa (factor VIIai) achieves an anticoagulant effect by competing with VII(a) for binding to TF.

Clinical Use (incl. side effects)

Both UFH and LMWH are used when rapid anticoagulation is needed, such as acute venous thromboembolism (DVT and/or PE), acute coronary insufficiency (acute myocardial infarction or unstable angina) or for ▸ percutaneous coronary intervention (PCI). UFH is also used for intraoperative anticoagulation during cardiac surgery employing cardiopulmonary bypass (CPB) as well as during vascular surgery. ▸ Protamine sulfate is used to reverse UFH anticoagulation after heart surgery.

Treatment of DVT or PE consists of therapeutic-dose heparin, given as intravenous UFH or subcutaneous LMWH with overlapping oral anticoagulation. Until the early 1990s, UFH was usually given alone for five days, followed by at least five days of UFH/coumarin overlap, then several months of coumarin anticoagulation. Now, coumarin is often started within 24 h of initiating UFH or LMWH. Duration of coumarin typically ranges from as low as 6 to 8 weeks (small calf-vein DVT in a transient prothrombotic situation, such as post-surgery) to indefinite (multiple prior DVTs complicating a chronic hypercoagulability state). Often, treatment of DVT or PE employing LMWH followed by oral anticoagulants occurs exclusively in an outpatient setting.

Prevention of DVT and PE (antithrombotic prophylaxis) is another common indication for UFH, LMWH or coumarin, especially following surgery or immobilizing trauma. Fondaparinux recently received approval for prevention of DVT and PE after hip and knee surgery.

Coumarin is also widely used for long-term anticoagulation in chronic atrial fibrillation (particularly to avoid cardioembolic strokes), to prevent DVT or PE in patients with chronic hypercoagulability (e.g., congenital AT or protein C deficiency) or to prevent atherothrombosis in patients with atherosclerosis. LMWH therapy is often appropriate for patients with cancer-associated hypercoagulability or to prevent or treat thrombosis during pregnancy.

Danaparoid, lepirudin and argatroban are important options for rapid anticoagulation when UFH or LMWH are contraindicated (e.g., heparin-induced thrombocytopenia). Desirudin is approved in some jurisdictions for antithrombotic prophylaxis after hip replacement surgery. Bivalirudin is an alternative to heparin for anticoagulation during ▸ PCI. Ximelagatran is being evaluated for chronic anticoagulation (potential coumarin replacement). Recombinant TFPI (tifacogin), NAPc2 and VIIai are under clinical study.

Side Effects

Bleeding is the most common adverse effect of anticoagulants (1-3) and is often associated with overdosing. When bleeding occurs during anticoagulation within the target therapeutic range, factors such as recent surgery or gastrointestinal lesions often coexist. For bleeding caused by coumarin overdosing, vitamin K will reverse anticoagulation beginning at least 4 h after administration. More urgent reversal can be achieved by coagulation factor replacement using plasma or prothrombin complex concentrates. Rapid reversal of UFH is achieved by ▸ protamine sulfate (1 mg protamine for 100 U heparin). However, only about 60% of the anticoagulant effect of LMWH is neutralized by protamine. Specific antidotes are not available for danaparoid, fondaparinux, DTIs or inhibitors of the VII(a)/TF pathway. Thus, careful patient selection and anticoagulant monitoring are usually needed to reduce bleeding risk with these newer agents.

Unusual adverse effects sometimes occur with coumarin or heparin (2,5). For example, coumarin-induced skin necrosis is a rare complication of oral anticoagulants characterized by (sub)dermal microvascular thrombosis that usually begins 3 to 6 days after commencing coumarin. Typically, central tissue sites such as the breast, abdomen and thigh are affected. Congenital abnormalities of the protein C natural anticoagulant pathway are implicated in some patients. A related syndrome of microvascular thrombosis can lead to limb gangrene in some patients treated with oral anticoagulants during ▶ thrombocytopenia and hypercoagulability. This syndrome of coumarin-induced venous limb gangrene has been linked to severe protein C depletion during use of warfarin to treat DVT complicated by metastatic cancer or heparin-induced thrombocytopenia.

As many as 3 to 5% of postoperative patients who receive UFH for two weeks develop heparin-induced thrombocytopenia (HIT). This hypercoagulable state is caused by IgG antibodies that recognize complexes between heparin and platelet factor 4 (a platelet α-granule protein). Paradoxically, patients with HIT remain at high risk for thrombosis, even when heparin is discontinued or heparin is replaced with coumarin. To avoid coumarin-induced venous gangrene, alternative anticoagulants such as danaparoid, lepirudin or argatroban should be given, and coumarin delayed until substantial resolution of thrombocytopenia has occurred. Long-term UFH treatment can cause ▶ osteoporosis, likely because heparin both decreases bone formation by osteoblasts and increases bone resorption by osteoclasts. Both HIT and osteoporosis are less likely to occur with LMWH.

Coumarins are generally contraindicated for use during pregnancy, particularly the first trimester. This is because γ-carboxyglutamate (gla)-containing proteins are found in bone. Thus, pharmacologic vitamin K antagonism can cause embryopathy (chondrodysplasia punctata). LMWH is an attractive option for many pregnant women who require anticoagulation.

References

1. Weitz JI, Hirsh J (2001) New anticoagulant drugs. Chest 119 (Suppl.):95S–107S
2. Hirsh J, Dalen JE, Anderson DR et al., (2001) Oral anticoagulants: mechanism of action, clinical effectiveness, and optimal therapeutic range. Chest 119 (Suppl.):8S–21S
3. Hirsh J, Warkentin TE, Shaughnessy SG et al. (2001) Heparin and low-molecular-weight heparin: mechanisms of action, pharmacokinetics, dosing, monitoring, efficacy, and safety. Chest 119 (Suppl.):64S–94S
4. Turpie AG, Gallus AS, Hoek JA (2001) A synthetic pentasaccharide for the prevention of deep-vein thrombosis after total hip replacement. N Engl J Med 344:619–625
5. Warkentin TE, Kelton JG (2001) Temporal aspects of heparin-induced thrombocytopenia. N Engl J Med 344:1286–1292

Anticonvulsants

▶ Anti-epileptic Drugs

Antidepressant Drugs

FLORIAN HOLSBOER
Max Planck Institute of Psychiatry, Munich, Germany
holsboer@mpipsykl.mpg.de

Synonyms

Antidepressants; mood elevators.

Definition

Antidepressants are small heterocyclic molecules that after oral administration enter the circulation and pass the blood brain barrier to bind at numerous sites in the brain. They are used for treatment of depression, panic disorders, social phobia, obsessive compulsive disorder and other affective illnesses.

▶ Antipsychotic Drugs
▶ Neurotransmitter Transporters
▶ Serotoninergic System

Mechanisms of Action

Most currently available antidepressants enhance neurotransmission of ▶ biogenic amines, mainly ▶ norepinephrine and ▶ serotonin. Once released

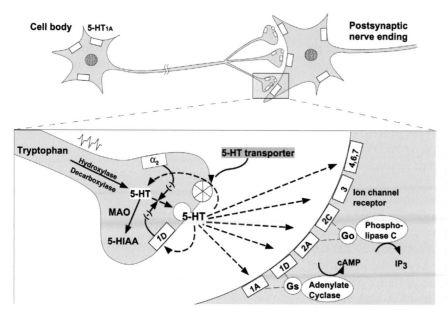

Fig. 1 Schematic illustration of serotonergic neurotransmission. Through blockade of the serotonin transporter at presynaptic terminals, the cell membrane receptor-mediated signalling pathways, principally through adenylate cyclase or phospholipase C, are enhanced.

from specialized vesicles at the presynaptic nerve terminal ▶ neurotransmitters enter the synaptic cleft and bind to respective receptors at the postsynaptic cell membrane, thus modulating the associated signalling cascades (Fig. 1). Additionally they bind to presynaptically localized receptors that regulate the amount of transmitter released. The cell membrane of presynaptic nerve terminals also contains ▶ reuptake transporters that clear the synaptic cleft from biogenic amines. Once reshuffled into the presynaptic compartment the neurotransmitter is degraded by ▶ monoamine oxidase (MAO). These two molecular processes, reuptake through specific transporters and enzymatic degradation by MAO, are targeted by antidepressant drugs. For example, the ▶ selective serotonin reuptake inhibitors (SSRI) which became the mainstay for the vast majority of depressed patients treated prevent clearance of serotonin from the synaptic cleft by blocking the presynaptic transporter and thus amplify receptor mediated events postsynaptically (▶ serotoninergic system). Analogous effects are those by norepinephrine reuptake inhibitors, while MAO-inhibitors act by reducing norepinephrine or serotonin degradation and thus increase the releasable amount of neurotransmitter from the respective vesicles. Antidepressants do not exert prompt effects as it takes weeks or months until clinical amelioration

occurs. The exact mode of action by which antidepressants work is still not resolved but there is consensus that their primary action, i.e. binding to cell membrane receptors, triggers a manifold of events which we are only beginning to decipher.

One such hypotheses submits that most antidepressants enhance the expression of ▶ cyclo-AMP response element binding protein (CREB) which is a transcription factor that after phosphorylation binds to cyclo-AMP response elements (CRE) localized in the promoter region of many genes including that coding for ▶ brain derived neurotrophic factor (BDNF) (1). The latter neurotrophin was found to be decreased in the hippocampus of chronically stressed rats, serving as animal model of depression. When treated with antidepressants, BDNF expression increases, possibly through enhanced phospho-CREB driven transactivation of the BDNF gene. This hypothesis is in keeping with the frequently observed reduction of depressed patients hippocampus volume (estimated by magnetic resonance imaging), a limbic brain structure pertinent for cognitive function, and expressing BDNF at high levels. Some preliminary studies support that antidepressants increase adult neurogenesis in this brain area, a phenomenon also associated with increased levels of phospho-CREB. The hypothesis that phospho-CREB is involved in adult neurogenesis is also strengthened by experiments with transgenic mice overexpressing a dominant negative isoform of CREB where the Ser[133] is mutated preventing phosphorylation-induced transactivation of CREB. Overexpression of mutant CREB prevented decreased neurogenesis in adult hippocampus. While many pieces of this hypothesis are in line with an antidepressant-induced enhancement of neurogenesis, evidence is lacking that this effect is the same through which antidepressants regulate emotional states. Morphological studies on brains of depressives failed to detect evidence for neuronal deterioration in the hippocampus. Also the increase of BDNF gene transcriptionas induced by antidepressants is possibly an unspecific response to a xenobiotic molecule. Whether increased transcription of BDNF conveys antidepressant effects is yet not proven, as mouse mutants where BDNF production is lowered by heterozygous gene deletion failed to show behavioral abnormalities. Also, data on drug-induced changes in BDNF peptide concentrations are not giving a clear picture.

Another hypothesis derives from the clinical observation that impaired stress hormone regulation is a cardinal symptom among patients with an acute major depressive episode (2). If stress hormones (primarily cortisol secreted by adrenocortical glands and corticotropin released from the pituitary) are monitored longitudinally in these patients, those who respond to drug treatment show a swift neuroendocrine normalization while those where stress hormone regulation continues to be altered have a much worse outcome, i.e. they fail to respond or they relapse. Studies using transgenic mice with glucocorticoid receptor impairment show some behavioral and functional features reminiscent of depression. Some of these abnormalities disappear under antidepressants, which is in line with a drug-induced improvement of corticosteroid receptor function. When ligand-activated, these gluco- and mineralocorticosteroid receptors form homo- and heterodimers that interact with ▶ corticotropin releasing hormone (CRH) in many ways. This is of relevance in this context because clinical and basic studies have shown that overexpression of CRH in many brain areas is causally related to development and course of depression. The effect of antidepressants has therefore consequences upon CRH secretion and it is believed that these antidepressants may work through this corticosteroid receptor driven signalling pathway, suppressing the depressogenic and anxiogenic effects of CRH acting through CRH type 1 receptors (CRHR1). Thus, the antidepressant-induced behavioral and neuroendocrine changes in patients together with their observed molecular actions upon stress hormone signalling pathways have triggered the search for new pharmacological approaches to understand how antidepressants might work and ultimately to discover better drugs (3).

In the absence of a robust pathogenetic model for depression, hypotheses-driven research has limitations that hopefully can be overcome by unbiased approaches. The availability of cDNA microarrays allowing one to study a huge amount of genes which are simultaneously regulated in the brains of mice under long-term treatment with antidepressants will shift the emphasis from the "usual suspects" (such as serotonin and its receptors) to yet unheard candidate genes (4).

Clinical Use

Antidepressants were serendipitously discovered in the 1950s and the first generation of these drugs was constituted by tricyclic molecules. The refinement among the second and third generation of these drugs resulted in molecules that have less side effects, are better tolerated and consequently enjoy much better acceptance. In fact, the percentage of Americans treated for depression tripled nationwide. Simultaneously patient visits to doctors for depression fell by a third through the last 5 years. Such figures do not yet apply for Europe, where alternative treatments, especially herbals (St. Johns Wort is the best selling antidepressant in Germany), continue to play a predominant role. Given the personal and socioeconomic burden of depression the undertreatment of this disabling clinical condition seems neither ethical nor prudent.

While antidepressants have proven to be effective drugs, several drawbacks and caveats need to be resolved. This can be most likely achieved by enforced ▶ pharmacogenetic approaches in combination with refined clinical research: Matching patients to the antidepressant that is most likely to be effective and less likely to harm through adversive reactions is the main goal of all modern therapies. Patient characteristics including sex, age, anxiety level, premedication and family history (genetic load) do not predict better or worse response to a particular antidepressant drug or drug class (e.g. an SSRI). However, the fact that all drugs are equally effective between comparison groups does not mean that they are equally effective for individual patients. It is now hoped that combination of clinical data, including functional assessments, e.g. neuroendocrine, neuroimaging, neuropsychology together with information from genotyping, i.e. identification of a collection of single nucleotide polymorphisms (SNPs) will ultimately lead to choosing a first line antidepressant based upon individual data. Indeed small studies surmized that a serotonin transporter polymorphism may explain some of the variability in response to SSRIs.

In practice, a genotype guided medication selection is yet not in reach, but several minor innovations emerging from hypothesis driven research are. The current antidepressive pipeline contains two promising candidates: ▶ Substance P, a peptide from the tachykinin family, which binds preferentially at the NK_1-receptor, was suspected to play a role in causality of depression. Several clinical studies testing NK_1-receptor antagonists showed promising results and a number of pharmaceutical companies are developing drugs antagonizing NK- receptors. Another neuropeptide is CRH that seems to be causally related to symptoms of depression through activation of CRHR1, which led to the development of CRHR1 antagonists as potential antidepressants. A first clinical study supported such a possibility.

Another new development of immediate clinical usefulness is the analysis of genetic variability in the cytochrome P450 enzyme system in patients, which may elucidate clinically relevant changes in drug metabolisation and adverse reactions. For example, if a patient receives an SSRI such as Prozac, which blocks the P4502D6 enzyme, and an antiarrhytmic, which is metabolised by the same enzyme, a fatal increase of the cardiotropic drug may occur. Other possible candidates involved in pharmacokinetics are P-glycoproteins, which are important regulators of a drug's blood-brain barrier passage. It was recently shown that antidepressants are substrates of P-glycoprotein, which, if overexpressed, can extrude the antidepressant out of the brain cells into the circulation thus preventing central effects that may lead to therapy resistance (5).

References

1. Duman RS, Nakagawa S, Malberg J (2001) Regulation of adult neurogenesis by antidepressant treatment. Neuropsychopharmacology 25:836–844
2. Holsboer F (2000) The corticosteroid receptor hypothesis of depression. Neuropsychopharmacology 23:477–501
3. Holsboer F (2001) Antidepressant drug discovery in the postgenomic era. World J. Biol. Psychiatry 2:165–177
4. Landgrebe J, Welzl G, Metz T, van Gaalen MM, Ropers H, Wurst W, Holsboer F (2002) Molecular characterisation of antidepressant effects in the mouse brain using gene expression profiling. J. Psychiatr. Res. 36:119-29.
5. Uhr M, Steckler T, Yassouridis A, Holsboer F (2000) Penetration of amitriptyline, but not fluoxetine, into brain is enhanced in mice with blood-brain barrier deficiency due to mdr1a P-glycoprotein gene disruption. Neuropsychopharmacology 22:380–387

Antidiabetic Drugs

Antidiabetic drugs is the general term for drugs that lower blood glucose concentrations and are used in the treatment of diabetes mellitus. Antidiabetic drugs are typically categorized as either *oral* (sulphonylureas, prandial insulin releasers, metformin, thiazolidinediones, alpha-glucosidase inhibitors) which are used to treat most type 2 (non-insulin-dependent) diabetic patients, or *insulin* (given parenterally) which is used to treat all type 1 and some type 2 diabetic patients.

▶ Oral Antidiabetic Drugs
▶ Insulin
▶ Diabetes Mellitus

Antidiarrhoeal Agents

Antidiarrhoeal drugs are used for the symptomatic treatment of diarrhoea (the frequent passage of liquid faeces). Commonly used antidiarrhoeal drugs are opioids including codeine, diphenoxylate and loperamide. They reduce the motility of the intestine. Other antidiarrhoeal agents (chalk, charcoal, methyl cellulose) probably act by adsorbing toxins or microorganisms causing diarrhoea. Bismuth subsalicylate is used for the treatment of traveller's diarrhoea. It mainly reduces fluid secretion in the bowel.

Antidiuretic Hormone

▶ Vasopressin

Antidysrhythmic Drugs

▶ Antiarrhythmic Drugs

Anti-emetic Drugs

▶ Emesis

Antiepileptic Drugs

UWE HEINEMANN, ANDREAS DRAGUHN[#], HEINZ BECK[*]
Johannes-Müller-Institut für Physiologie, Universitätsklinikum Charité, Humboldt-Universität zu Berlin; [#]Institut für Physiologie und Pathophysiologie, Universität Heidelberg; [*]Labor für Experimentelle Epileptologie, Klinik für Epileptologie, Universitätskliniken Bonn, Germany
Uwe.heinemann@charite.de,
andreas.draguhn@urz.uni-heidelberg.de,
Heinz.Beck@ukb.uni-bonn.de

Definition

▶ Epilepsy is a chronic neurological disorder that affects about 0.6–0.8% of the general population worldwide. The clinical hallmark of epilepsy is recurrent ▶ seizures, which disrupt normal brain function. A large number of different types of epilepsies and epileptic syndromes have been distinguished. Many specific syndromes start in infancy and are accompanied by further developmental, neuropsychological and metabolic alterations, mostly of unknown origin. Generally, epilepsies with a focal origin (focal epilepsies) are discriminated from epilepsies with a generalized beginning (primary generalized epilepsies).

At the cellular level, focal and general convulsions correspond to synchronized high-frequency ▶ discharges of large groups of neurons, which disrupt normal information processing. Depending on the areas of the CNS recruited into the abnormal discharge, clincal symptoms observed during focal seizures may vary considerably. Thus, discharges within limited areas of the motor cortex may lead only to mild motor seizures, while seizure activity in the ▶ temporal lobe may cause complex semiologies that include behavioral automatisms and loss of conciousness. Focal seizures without loss of conciousness are termed simple partial seizures, whereas focal seizures with loss of conciousness are named complex partial seizures. In some epilepsies, initially focal seizures spread to involve most of the cerebral cortex (secondary generalized seizures).

Primary generalized seizures are also heterogeneous with respect to their clinical features. Such seizures can impose as ▶ absence epilepsy, which is characterized by a brief interruption of conciousness due to highly synchronized neuronal activity involving thalamocortical networks without increases in neuronal firing rate. On the other hand, ▶ tonic-clonic convulsions with loss of consciousness are often also primarily generalized.

▶ GABAergic System
▶ Ionotropic Glutamate Receptors
▶ Voltage-dependent Ca^{2+} Channels
▶ Voltage-gated K^+ Channels

Basic Mechanisms

Both focal and generalized epilepsies are heterogeneous with respect to their etiology and the principles of therapy.

Basic Mechanisms Underlying Focal Epilepsies

A large group of focal epilepsies arises as a consequence of developmental lesions, CNS tumors, trauma or inflammatory processes, which may be located in neocortical areas as well as the mesial temporal lobe. In a second group of patients, no such causal factor can be identified. Very frequently, such epilepsies arise from a focus within the ▶ hippocampus, which shows characteristic neuropathological and molecular changes. Only few focal epilepsies seem to be due to a mutation in ▶ ion channel genes. In contrast, a large number of generalized epilepsies is thought to have a genetic basis, and the chromosomal localization or the gene mutation has been identified in some of these disorders.

Many patients with focal epilepsies respond well to antiepileptic drugs, but a sizeable portion continues to have seizures even in the presence of optimal therapeutic drug concentrations. For unknown reasons, patients with an epileptic focus residing in the temporal lobe (Temporal Lobe Epilepsy, TLE) often develop pharmaco-resistant epilepsy. Therefore, considerable attention has been focused on unravelling the cellular changes underlying hyperexcitability in this form of epilepsy. Identifying such changes is of obvious importance in determining promising novel therapeutic strategies.

In focal epilepsies a number of functional and morphological changes are observed which may act in concert to support enhanced excitability. Such changes have been intensively investigated in order to develop targets for drug design.

▶ Altered density of voltage-dependent ion currents in neurons: Such changes may considerably affect the firing properties of neurons. They may also affect how neurons integrate a given synaptic input.

▶ Altered synaptic properties: Numerous changes in the properties of inhibitory (GABAergic) and excitatory (glutamatergic) synapses have been reported. While the simple adage of an imbalance between inhibitory and excitatory neurotransmission in epilepsy is not generally applicable, some forms of inhibition are lost or impaired in epilepsy. Likewise, an increased function of glutamate receptors has been demonstrated in some brain areas.

▶ Formation of novel aberrant synapses, axonal sprouting: In addition to altered properties of inhibitory and excitatory synapses, numerous synapses are newly formed in chronically epileptic tissue. In some regions, as in the dentate gyrus, the subiculum and area CA1 of the hippocampus, excitatory neurons form recurrent synapses terminating within the same region. This, and other forms of recurrent sprouting are thought to constitute a positive feedback pathway facilitating seizure generation in this area. Very little is known about the elementary properties of newly formed synapses.

▶ Altered properties of glial cells: Glial cells are centrally involved in regulating the size of the extracellular space and the composition of the extracellular milieu, amongst other important tasks. In particular, glial cells normally take up K^+ released by neurons during repetitive neuronal activity. Preventing excessive increases in the extracellular K^+ concentration is important because they may enhance excitability of surrounding neurons. In chronic epilepsy, one of the numerous changes occurring in glial cells is the loss of the capacity to take up K^+.

Clearly, the largest difficulty in chronic focal epilepsy is to identify amongst the numerous changes that might plausibly affect excitability those that are most important in mediating hyperexcitability. Because of the lack of molecular targets with a proven causal role in mediating seizures, design of anticonvulsant drugs has been driven mainly by considering which drugs potently limit excitability in normal brain tissue or normal animals. It must be also stressed that, in focal epilepsies, our knowledge extends mainly to the cellular changes that underlie hyperexcitability in the chronic stage of the disease. The factors governing the development of the epileptic condition in humans are much less clear, and the design of substances aimed at inhibiting the progression of epilepsy is in its first stages.

Primary Generalized Epilepsies

Primary generalized epilepsies are a heterogeneous group of diseases. Some of the generalized epilepsies are hereditary, and several genetic mutations of ion channels or membrane receptors linked to this disorder have been identified. In others, the pathogenesis is less clear. Absence epilepsies present with a characteristic 3/s discharge in the electroencephalogram, and the mechanism for similar aberrant discharges have been well studied in animal models. It is thought that thalamic projection neurons that have the capacity to generate burst discharges mediated by low-threshold Ca^{2+} channels provide a phasic excitation of interneurons. These interneurons in turn inhibit thalamic projection neurons via GABAreceptors, resulting in a pronounced hyperpolarization. This hyperpolarization removes inactivation of low-threshold Ca^{2+} channels, subsequently enabling these neurons to generate a new, Ca^{2+} channel-dependent burst discharge. Thus, rhythmogenesis seems to rely on the interplay between low-threshold Ca^{2+} channel-dependent bursting and GABA-mediated inhibition. Accordingly, absence epilepsies respond well to substances blocking low-threshold Ca^{2+} channels (ethosuximide, trimethadione), as well as to some GABAantagonists (which are still in an experimental stage for this indication).

Substances Acting on Voltage-Dependent Ion Channels

With few exceptions, information on the anticonvulsant pharmacology of specific ion channel subunits analyzed in expression systems is scarce. Hitherto, a first understanding of the mechanism of action of most antiepileptic drugs has evolved from analyses of somatic ion channel pharmacology either in isolated neurons from human or rodent neurons, or cell culture models.

Voltage-Dependent Na⁺ Channels. A large number of anticonvulsant drugs commonly in use for focal epilepsies act on fast voltage-dependent Na^+ channels at clinically relevant concentrations (carbamazepine, phenytoin, lamotrigine). Most of these anticonvulsant drugs display three distinct effects on Na^+ channels:

- A shift of the voltage-dependence of inactivation to a hyperpolarizing direction, resulting in a lower fraction of channels available for activation at action potential threshold.
- A reduction of the peak Na^+ channel conductance.
- A pronounced slowing of Na^+ channel recovery from the inactivated state.

The latter effect results in a prolongation of the time required after an action potential for inactivated Na^+ channels to become available again. This prolongation would be expected to inhibit repetitive firing only if the time between action potentials is not long enough to permit recovery of Na^+ channels, i.e. at high discharge frequencies. Indeed, phenytoin, carbamazepine and lamotrigine have been shown to preferentially inhibit high frequency but not low frequency firing (see Fig. 1). It has to be noted that this mechanism is most probably invoked not only at somatodendritic Na^+ channels, but also at presynaptic Na^+ channels. In the latter case, application of one of the antiepileptic drugs mentioned above would be expected to preferentially inhibit transmitter release induced by high frequency presynaptic action potentials.

In addition to inhibiting fast voltage-dependent Na^+ currents, many anticonvulsants also suppress persistent Na^+ currents, in some cases even more efficiently. This mechanism may also be important in the anticonvulsant action of these substances because persistent Na^+ currents are thought to give rise to high frequency burst discharges in some neurons.

Voltage-Dependent Ca²⁺ Channels. A number of anticonvulsant drugs also display effects on Ca^{2+} channels. In most cases, effects on Ca^{2+} channels

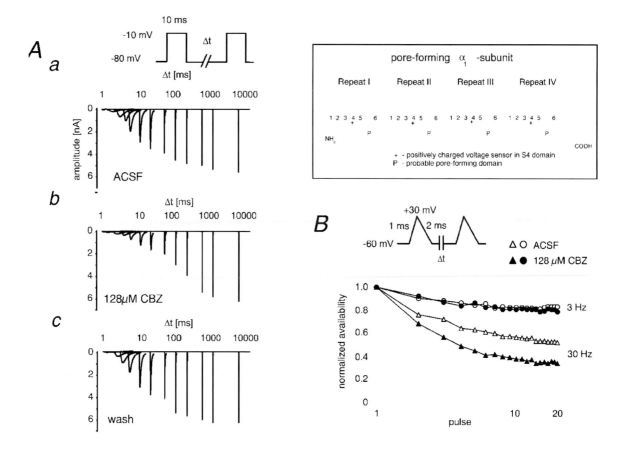

Fig. 1 Effects of carbamazepine on voltage-dependent Na⁺ channels. A: Fast recovery from inactivation can be analyzed in double pulse experiments using the whole-cell patch clamp technique. Recordings shown are from rat hippocampal dentate granule neurons. Inactivation is induced with a conditioning pulse (10 ms, -10 mV), after which recovery of Na⁺ channels from inactivation is monitored by a test pulse applied at various intervals following the conditioning pulse (inset, Fig. 1A). Representative traces after various recovery intervals are displayed on an exponential time scale. Application of 128 μM CBZ causes a marked slowing of the time course of recovery. **B: Use-dependent block of Na⁺ channels by CBZ.** Trains of mock action potentials were applied as voltage commands at different frequencies. Application of CBZ reduces Na⁺ channel availability preferentially during high-frequency stimulation. Inset: General molecular structure of pore-forming α subunits of voltage-dependent Na⁺ channels.

with a depolarized threshold of activation are small at clinically relevant concentrations. In the case of gabapentin, binding to a Ca²⁺ channel accessory subunit has been demonstrated, but whether this binding affects channel function is unknown. In contrast, Ca²⁺ channels with a hyperpolarized threshold of activation (low-threshold channels) are sensitive to a number of drugs (i.e. ethosuximide, trimethadione through its metabolite dimethadione, phenytoin, lamotrigine). As stated above, the activity of ethosuximide and trimethadione against absence epilepsy is thought to be due to their inhibition of low-threshold Ca²⁺ channels. The differing anticonvulsant profile of lamotrigine and phenytoin may be due to the fact that the three pore-forming subunits underlying low-threshold Ca²⁺ channels are differentially sensitive to anticonvulsant drugs.

Tab. 1 **Summary of the known spectrum of actions of a selection of antiepileptic drugs.** This synopsis refers only to actions demonstrated within or close to therapeutic concentrations of drugs. Abbreviations: (+) to (+++) weak to strong efficacy, (-) no efficacy, (?) not investigated. HVA: high threshold Ca^{2+} channels, T: T-type Ca^{2+} channels, L: L-type Ca^{2+} channels, I_{NaP}: persistent sodium current, DR: delayed rectifier K^+ channels, KCNQ: KCNQ subtypes of K^+ channels.

	Voltage-dependent Ion channels			Neurotransmitter Receptors			NT release	Other mechanisms
	Na^+	Ca^{2+}	K^+	GABA	NMDA	AMPA		
Phenytoin	+++	++ (T)	+ (DR)	?	?	?	++	Calmodulin and cyclic nucleotide-dependent second messenger systems
Carbamazepine	+++	-	?	-	+	?	?	Adenosine receptors
Lamotrigine	+++	++	-	-	-	-	?	
Valproic acid	+++	+	+	?	?	?	++	Increase in brain GABA, decrease in brain aspartate
Ethosuximide	+ ($I_{Na,p}$)	+++ (T)	+	?	?	?	-	Inhibition of Na^+/K^+ ATPase
Trimethadione	?	+++ (T,L)	?	?	?	?	?	
Phenobarbital	-	+	?	+++	?	?	++	
Diazepam	+	-	-	+++	-	-	-	
Felbamate	++	?	?	?	+++	?	?	
Gabapentin	-	+ (HVA)	+	-	-	-	+	Increased GABA synthesis, GDH, GAD, GABA-aminotransferase
Vigabatrin	?	?	?	?	?	?	+++	GABA-transaminase inhibition
Tiagabine	?	?	?	?	?	?	+++	
Losigamone	?	++	?	++	?	?	?	
Ramecemide	?	?	?	?	?	?	?	
Topiramate	++	?	?	++	-	?	?	
Levetiracetam	-	- (T), + (HVA)	?	?	?	?	?	GABA-T, GAD
Retigabine	?	?	+++ (KCNQ)	?	?	?	?	

Voltage-Dependent K^+ Channels. Up-modulation of voltage-dependent K^+ channels may be a plausible mechanism to reduce cellular excitability and action potential-dependent neurotransmitter release. However, the number of novel antiepileptic drugs developed that target potassium channels is small. Interestingly, it has recently been discovered that a mutation resulting in a moderate loss of function of KCNQ2/3 K^+ channels causes a focal form of epilepsy. The novel anticonvulsant

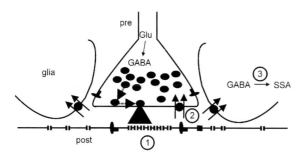

Fig. 2 The GABAergic synapse as a target of anticonvulsent drugs. GABA is synthesized from glutamate in the presynaptic terminal and is packed into small synaptic vesicles. After release, GABA actavates postsynaptic ion channels (GABA$_A$R, marked "1") which mediate the cloride influx and thereby the inhibition of the postsynaptic cell. From the synaptic cleft, GABA is removed into the presynaptic terminal and into a adjacent glia cells by GABA-uptake ("2"). A fraction of the transmitter is degraded into succinyl-semialdehyde by GABA-transaminase ("3"), which is present in glia cells as well as in neurons. Pre- and postsynaptic metabotrophic GABA$_B$R are indicated by elipsoid bodies in the cell membrane but are no major target for anticonvulsants presently in use. GABAergic drugs against epilepsy act as positive modulators of the GABA$_A$R ("1"), blockers of GABA-uptake ("2") or inhibitors of GABA degradation ("3").

retigabine, which enhances the activity of this very channel type, displays a high clinical efficacy in these patients.

Substances Acting on Neurotransmitter Receptors
A large fraction of anticonvulsants are based on the attempt to boost inhibitory synaptic transmission in order to restore the balance between inhibition and excitation in epileptic tissue. The first drug using this mechanism of action was phenobarbitone, which was introduced into clinical practice in 1912. Today, there are at least three different targets of anticonvulsant drugs at the synaptic level, all centered on the main inhibitory transmitter GABA (γ-aminobutyric acid).

GABAergic Synapses. Based on the key elements in synaptic inhibitory transmission, three classes of drugs can be distinguished:

▶ GABA receptor modulators. These substances yield a potentiation of synaptic responses to GABA by changing the affinity of the GABA receptor (benzodiazepines) or enhancing the open probability of this ligand-gated ion channel (barbiturates). Benzodiazepines are especially useful against status epilepticus but are also used as an adjunctive therapy in partial and generalised seizures. Clinically used substances are clobazepam, clonazepam, clorazepate, diazepam, lorazepam, midazolam and nitrazepam. Barbiturates (esp. phenobarbitone) are used in tonic-clonic and partial seizures, in status epilepticus and in neonatal seizures. Chronic treatment with benzodiazepines and barbiturates is complicated due to the sedative side effects and, most importantly, development of tolerance.

▶ GABA-uptake blockers. Block of GABA-uptake prolongs the presence of the transmitter in the synaptic cleft and thereby strengthens the postsynaptic effects of synaptically released GABA. Tiagabine, a derivative of nipecotic acid, is in clinical use as an add-on therapy against simple and complex partial seizures. Like all substances that generally increase GABAergic transmission, tiagabine has sedative side effects.

▶ Blockers of GABA catabolism. Blocking the GABA-degrading enzyme GABA-transaminase increases the concentration of GABA in synaptic terminals and enhances or stabilises the inhibitory transmission. A "new" anticonvulsant designed for this purpose is γ-vinyl-GABA (Vigabatrin), but it should be noted that valproate has the same effect. Vigabatrin is used as an adjunctive therapy in partial and secondary generalized seizures. It is very efficient against infantile spasms and is being used in Lennox-Gastout (together with sodium valproate and benzodiazepines). Side effects of vigabatrin include neuropsychiatric (especially mood) disturbances as well as retinopathic changes. Novel experimental approaches are aimed at increasing GABA synthesis, rather than blocking its degradation, by potentiating the action of the GABA-synthesizing enzyme glutamate decarboxylase.

One of the oldest antiepileptic drugs, bromide, has been reported to boost inhibition by an unknown mechanism. Bromide is still in use in certain cases of tonic-clonic seizures and in pediatric patients with recurrent febrile convulsions and others. The mechanism of action may include a potentiation of GABAergic synaptic transmission, although the precise target is not known.

Excitatory Amino Acid Antagonists. The complementary approach to boosting inhibition, i.e. antagonising the effects of the excitatory neurotransmitter ► glutamate (► GABAergic System), has been less fruitful so far. Antagonists of the NMDA-subtype of glutamate receptors show anticonvulsant activity in animal experiments but have not been introduced into clinical use due to severe neuropsychological side effects. An exception may be felbamate, which seems to exert at least part of its effect by a block on NMDA receptors. Antagonists of two other glutamate receptor subclasses (AMPA- and Kainate-receptors) are under development. Topiramate, a new anticonvulsant drug, partially blocks kainate-receptors and thus may provide the first example of an AED with effects against excitatory neurotransmission.

Substances with Unknown or Mixed Mechanism of Action

It should be pointed out that most anticonvulsants have more than one effect on neuronal excitability or synaptic transmission. A prominent example is valproic acid, which affects GABAergic transmission (probably by enhancing cellular GABA-content), glutamatergic synaptic transmission by reducing sythesis of excitatory amino acids as well as voltage-dependent ion channels (see Table 1).

Drugs with unknown mechanism of action are gabapentin, bromides (but see above effects on GABAergic transmission) and adrenocorticotropic hormone (ACTH), which is used in infantile spasms.

References

1. Antiepileptic Drugs. Editors René H. Levy, Richard H. Mattson, Brian S. Meldrum, Fritz E. Dreifuss, J. Kiffin Penry. Raven Press, New York.
2. Bialer M, Johannessen SI, Kupferberg HJ, Levy RH, Loiseau P, Perucca E (2001) Progress report on new antiepileptic drugs: a summary of the Fifth Eilat Conference (EILAT V). Epilepsy Res. 43(1):11–58

Antiestrogen

Antiestrogens are estrogen/estrogen receptor antagonists.

► Sex Steroid Receptor
► Selective Sex Steroid Receptor Modulators

Antifibrinolytic Drugs

► Fibrinolytics

Antifungal Drugs

ANNEMARIE POLAK
Aesch, Switzerland
annemarie.polak@bluemail.ch

Synonyms

Antimycotic drugs, antimycotics, fungicides

Definition

► Fungi cause diseases in plants, animals and humans. Antifungal drugs (fungicides) are therefore used in agriculture, animal and human medicine. In this paragraph, only antifungal drugs used for human chemotherapy are described.

Antifungal drugs inhibit the growth of fungi in tissue (► fungistatic activity) by a number of different mechanisms; some of the agents even kill the fungal cell (► fungicidal effect). Antifungal drugs are used for the treatment of established fungal diseases; however, in immunosuppressed patients at high risk they are also used as prevention or empiric therapy.

Antifungal drugs are classified according to their mode of action and/or their chemical class. Four chemical classes have mainly contributed to the actual armentory of antifungal drugs: The broadest class is the one of ► azoles, (imidazoles and triazoles) followed by ▶ polyenes; ▶ allylamines and ▶ morpholines. Some individual compounds are used in dermatology.

Mechanism of Action

The difficulty of killing the eukaryotic fungal cell without damaging the host is perhaps more akin to the problems of cancer chemotherapy than those of antibacterial treatment. Biochemical studies have identified a number of potential targets for antifungal chemotherapy, including cell wall synthesis, membrane sterol biosynthesis, nucleic acid synthesis, metabolic inhibition and macronuclear biosynthesis. The cell wall synthesis is the only fungal-specific target, since the fungal cell wall has an unique molecular structure; all other pathways (enzymatic steps) in the fungal cell are closely related to the ones used in human cells.

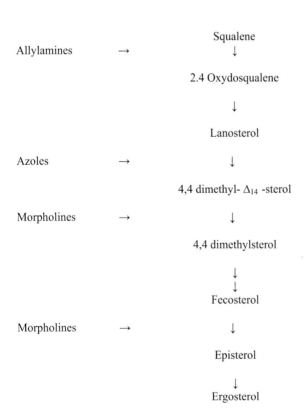

Fig. 1 Antifungal Drugs

Sterol Biosynthesis Inhibitors

Most antifungals on the market (▶ Azoles, ▶ Allylamines, ▶ Morpholines, Tolnaftate, Tolciclate) interfere with the various enzymatic steps involved in the cascade of ergosterol synthesis from squalene to ergosterol; this pathway being the Achille's heel of the fungal cell. Ergosterol is the essential component of the fungal membrane and exerts two functions: it is the bulk membrane component and it regulates cell growth and proliferation. All sterol biosynthesis inhibitors induce depletion of the essential ergosterol and accumulation of a wrong sterol moiety, consequently disturbing the function of the cell membrane. The morphological changes seen in all cells treated with a sterol biosynthesis inhibitor are similar, all including thickening of the cell wall by chitin deposits.

The imidazoles and triazole (▶ Azoles) (for example, ketoconazole, itraconazole, fluconazole, voriconazole) interfere with cytochrome P_{450}-dependent lanosterol C_{14} demethylase, leading to depletion of ergosterol and accumulation of lanosterol in the membrane. At the molecular level, one of the nitrogen atoms of the azole ring binds to the haeme moiety of cytochrome P_{450}. Only compounds with higher specific binding to the fungal cytochrome than to the human one can be used as systemic antifungal drugs. Compared with the imidazoles, the triazoles have a much higher affinity for fungal cytochrome than for human cytochrome P_{450} enzyme steps. In addition to the main interactions with the P_{450} cytochrome, azoles may inhibit cytochrome C oxidase and peroxidative enzymes, they may also interfere with phospholipids. The fact that miconazole and itraconazole are fungicidal is thought to be the result of a direct membrane interaction, leading to the loss of cytoplasmic constituents.

Allylamines. Allylamines (terbinafine, naftifine) interfere with the ergosterol pathway at the level of squalene epoxidase leading to the depletion of ergosterol and the accumulation of squalene. Again, only compounds with a higher specificity for the fungal enzyme than for the human enzyme can be used for systemic use. A clear correlation exists between growth inhibition and degrees of

A

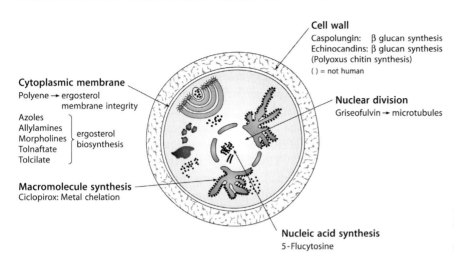

Cell wall
Caspolungin: β glucan synthesis
Echinocandins: β glucan synthesis
(Polyoxus chitin synthesis)
( ) = not human

Cytoplasmic membrane
Polyene → ergosterol
        membrane integrity

Nuclear division
Griseofulvin → microtubules

Azoles
Allylamines
Morpholines   ergosterol
Tolnaftate   biosynthesis
Tolcilate

Macromolecule synthesis
Ciclopirox: Metal chelation

Nucleic acid synthesis
5-Flucytosine

Fig. 2 Antifungal Drugs – Targets of antifungal activity.

sterol biosynthesis inhibition; the fungicidal effect is more correlated to the intracellular accumulation of squalene.

Morpholines. Morpholines (amorolfine) interfere at two levels of the ergosterol pathway, the Δ_{14}-reductase and the Δ_7- Δ_8-isomerase leading to depletion of ergosterol and accumulation of an unplanar sterol ignosterol. With the inhibition of two steps in the same pathway, a natural synergistic effect is built into the molecule so that the risk of appearance of resistant mutants is low and efficacy high.

Drugs Binding Directly to Ergosterol (amphotericin B, nystatin, candicidin)

The current model for the mechanism of the ▶ polyene Amphotericin B (Amph B), is based on the formation of a 1:1 Amph B/Ergosterol aggregate, which associates into a transmembrane channel with a large –OH lined aqueous pore down the middle. The result of the interaction between Amph B and the sterols is the disturbance of the ergosterol function leading to increased permeability, disruption of the proton gradient and leakage of potassium. The fungicidal effect, however, has been linked to irreversible inhibition of the membrane ATPase.

5-Fluorocytosine (5FC). 5-Fluorocytosine (5FC), a mock pyrimidine, is the only antifungal drug that acts as true antimetabolite. 5FC is taken up into the fungal cell, deaminated to 5-fluorouracil (5FU) which is the active principle responsible for the killing of the fungal cell. Fungi lacking the cytosine deaminase are resistant to 5FC. Intracellularly, 5FU acts along two different pathways: it is incorporated as 5-flurouridine monophophate into the RNA and it inhibits after conversion to 5-fluoro-deoxyuridine monophosphate the thymidylate synthetase leading to inhibition of DNA synthesis. 5FU itself cannot be used for antifungal therapy due to its toxicity for mammalian cells.

Glucan Synthase Inhibitors

Echinocandins (i.e. caspofungin), semisynthetic lipopeptides, inhibits the synthesis of β-(1,3)-D-glucan, an integral component of the fungal cell wall not present in mammalian cells.

Griseofulvin. Griseofulvin is the first antimycotic drug detected that is only active against ▶ dermatophytes. Its activity manifests as nuclear and mitotic abnormalities followed by distortions in the hyphal morphology.

Hydroxypyridones (Ciclopirox, rilopirox). The primary mode of action of this class of antimycotics is interference with uptake and accumulation of products required for cell membrane synthesis. In higher concentrations it causes a disturbance of the cellular permeability. Some investigations show an interaction with Fe(III)- ions; the compounds acting as chelators. Very high concentrations interfere with the function of fungal mitochondria.

Clinical Use (incl. side effects)

Fungal diseases divide themselves into three classes: superficial (topical, local) mycoses (▶ dermatomycoses and gynaecological infections) subcutaneous and organ mycoses. This division is important not especially for microbiological reasons, but in the view of the different problems arising during treatment. Superficial mycoses are not life threatening, but they are irritating. Subcutaneous mycoses are also not life threatening but are associated with a high morbidity, and deep mycoses, especially in immunosuppressed patients, are life threatening showing a high mortality rate in patients if untreated. The treatment schedules (dose, duration of treatment, galenical formulation) are strongly dependent on the localisation of the fungal disease, on the pathogenicity of the fungi and on the conditions of the host. Additionally, the diagnosis of the disease is not always guaranteed, therefore, a clear-cut, simple description of clinical usage for antifungal drugs is not possible.

Due to the divergence of fungal diseases there is neither single best treatment nor a superior drug for all diseases. However, a superior drug does exist for dermatomycoses caused by dermatophytes, namely the allylamine terbinafine (TER). For the treatment of deep mycoses in immunosuppressed patients the most efficacious drug is the polyene Amph B.

The therapy of ▶ dermatomycoses and acute vaginal infections is unproblematic. A large choice of various drugs (all chemical classes and compounds discussed above) in different galenical formulations (crèmes, tinctures, sprays, ovula, powder, shampoo, nail lacquer and tablets) exists. All drugs topically applied – used in various treatment schedules – show high efficacy and a low incidence of adverse reactions. For the treatment of onychomycoses without matrix involvement two nail lacquers (a morpholine and hydroxypyron) are on the market showing high efficacy with low (<1%) adverse reactions after topical therapy for several months. A combination therapy with a topical and a systemically applied antifungal drug is the most efficacious and the most economic therapy for onychomycosis with matrix involvement. Systemic therapy is indicated if the dermatomycosis is widespread. The highest cure rate is achieved with TER. TER is well tolerated in adults and children. In ca 5% of the patients, mild and reversible side effects have been observed: gastrointestinal, skin, central nervous system, respiratory events and loss of taste. For acute vaginal candidosis the treatment of choice with the highest compliance and best efficacy is one daily dose of fluconazole.

Three fungal infections – Madura feet (mycetoma), chromomycosis and ▶ sporotrichosis – fall into the category of subcutaneous mycoses, their distribution is mainly in tropical and subtropical areas. The ideal treatment for madura feet caused by fungi is not yet established; the azoles are of some benefit, however, neither the optimal drug, dose, nor the treatment schedules are known. Chromomycosis responds well to itraconazole (ITRA) monotherapy or the combination of 5FC plus ITRA. ITRA has been set up as standard therapy for cutaneous and lymphatic sporotrichosis.

Systemic Mycoses

Systemic mycoses are caused either by true pathogenic fungi (endemic in distinct areas of USA/South America) or by opportunistic fungi that induce severe infections in immunosuppressed patients. The arsenal for the treatment of deep organ mycoses is relatively small: Amph B, 5FC, azoles (fluconazole (FLU), ITRA, voriconazole (NDA filing)) and CAS.

The polyene Amph B (intravenous formulation) has the broadest spectrum, is fungicidal and shows its superiority in immunosuppressed patients. Its only drawback is its infusion-related toxicity and its negative influence on renal function. Acute reactions to Amph B – usually fever chills, rigor and nausea – can be ameliorated by concomitant administration of meperidine, acetomiophen or hydrocortisone. Additionally, there is the possibility of tailoring time and duration of infusion. Prevention of the chronic tubular injury is feasible by salt loading. Encapsulation of Amph B into liposomes or complexing of the drug with other lipid carriers brings a major reduction of nephrotoxicity. Three lipid-associated forms are now available (Ambisome, Amph B lipid complex and Amph B colloidal dispension). Due to its toxic side effects Amph B is not widely used for prevention; it is, however, often used as empiric therapy with high success rates.

Due to the rapid appearance of resistance, 5FC is only used as a combination partner for the intensive therapy of established severe fungal infections caused by *Candida spp, Cryptococcus neoformans* and *Aspergillus sp*. Anorexia, nausea, vomiting, diarrhoea and or abdominal pain occur in 6% of the patients. Of greater concern is the potential for bone marrow depression (seen in 5% of the patients, all with elevated 5FC levels).

Azoles. Generally the azoles are well tolerated in children and adults; mild side effects like nausea and vomiting are seen in <5% of the patients treated with FLU.

Attention has to be given to the problem of interaction between azoles and other drugs; these are based on two mechanisms:
- inhibition of absorption of the azoles leading to lower bioavailability or
- interference with the activity of hepatic microsomal enzymes, which alters the metabolism and plasma levels of azole, the interacting drug or both. This latter induces often increased toxicity of the concomitant drug.

With FLU, only few drug interactions are seen, namely with rifampicin (reduction of FLU), phenytoin, cyclosporin, tolbutamide and warfarin (increasing levels of concomitant drug). The interactions with ITRA are more significant than with FLU: H2 antagonists and all drugs increasing intragastric pH decrease the absorption of ITRA. Interactions due to hepatic enzymes are seen with rifampicin (reducing the levels of ITRA to undedectable levels), phenytoin, isoniazid, carbamazepin, phenobarbital, midazolam, triazolam, digoxin, lovastatin terfenadine, warfarin and cyclosporin. The list of interacting drugs is still increasing.

Oral FLU is well established as first line therapy for oropharyngeal candidosis and *Candida* oesophagitis and for maintenance therapy in AIDS patients with meningeal cryptococcosis. FLU (oral or intravenous) is also efficacious in candidemia without neutropenia. It shows efficacy in prevention (attention: *Aspergillus sp*. are not in the spectrum) and empiric therapy. ITRA, being fungicidal against *Aspergillus sp*., shows promising

results in aspergillosis, especially under intravenous therapy, and is used as maintenance therapy in AIDS patients with histoplasmosis. ITRA is the first line therapy for histoplasmosis and blastomycosis in HIV-negative patients. A combination of ITRA plus 5FC may be the optimal therapy of phaeohyphomycoses.

The glucan synthase inhibitor caspofungin (intravenous formulation) is new on the market for the treatment of invasive aspergillosis in patients whose disease is refractory to, or who are intolerant of, other therapies. During the clinical trials fever, infused vein complications nausea, vomiting and in combination with cyclosporin mild transient hepatic side effects were observed. Interaction with tacrolismius and with potential inducer or mixed inducer/inhibitors of drug clearance was also seen.

References

1. AHFS First New Drug overview. Caspofungin.
2. De Carli L, Larizza L. (1988) Griseofulvin: Mutat Res 195:91–126
3. Gupta AK, Einarson TR, Summerbell R.C, Shear NH (1998) Drug 55:645–74
4. Hoeprich PD (1995) Antifungals.
5. Korting HC, Grundmann-Kollmann M (1997) The hydroxypyridones. Mycoses 40:243–247
6. Polak A (1997) Prog. Drug Res. 44:221–297

Antigen

An antigen is a molecule recognised by specific receptors on cells of the immune system such as B lymphocytes.

▶ Immune Defense
▶ Humanized Monoclonal Antibodies

Antigen-presenting Cells

Antigen-presenting cells (APCs) are cells of the immune system that are able to process and present foreign antigens to effector cells (e.g. cyto-toxic T-cells or T-helper cells). The antigen is presented in the context of an MHC-I or MHC-II molecule on APCs in the presence of so-called co-stimulatory molecules to activate the effector cells.

▶ Immune Defense

Antigen Presentation

Antigen presentation is the key mechanism allowing T lymphocytes to survey whether intracellular pathogens exist in the cells of the body. As T lymphocytes can only recognize antigen in the form of peptides presented on specific molecules termed major histocompatibility complex (MHC), antigen-presenting cells instruct T cell reaction and thus the development of adaptive immunity. Professional antigen presenting cells (MHC class II positive) are dendritic cells, monocytes/macrophages and B lymphocytes.

▶ Immune Defense

Antigen Receptors

Each T- and B-lymphocyte carries on its surface one type of receptor which recognizes one specific antigen. T cells carry the heterodimeric T cell antigen receptor consisting of an alpha and beta chain. This receptor recognizes a peptide presented by a MHC (major histocompatibility complex) molecule. B-cells express an immunoglobulin on their surface which can recognize epitopes on antigens of different sizes and qualities without the need for presentation. Both forms of antigen receptors are created by random genetic rearrangement during the ontogeny of each individual lymphocyte. Both types of antigen receptors require additional transmembrane molecules for signal transduction.

▶ Immune Defense

Anti-gout Drugs

ROLAND SEIFERT
The University of Kansas, Lawrence, KS, USA
rseifert@ku.edu

Synonyms

Drugs for the treatment/management of ▶ gout and/or ▶ hyperuricemia

Definition

Pathophysiology and clinical manifestations of gout

▶ Uric acid is the end product of purine catabolism in man. Purines originate from food and the degradation of nucleic acids and nucleotides. ▶ Xanthine oxidase (XOD) is the key enzyme in purine degradation. XOD converts hypoxanthine to xanthine, and xanthine to uric acid, respectively (Fig. 1). Uric acid is filtered in the glomerulus of the kidney, is almost completely absorbed in the proximal tubules and secreted more distally (Fig. 2). At physiological pH (~7.4), uric acid exists predominantly in its ionic form (urate). At lower pH, the fraction of uric acid molecules (protonized form) increases. This is important because uric acid possesses a lower solubility than urate. Thus, a decrease in pH, as it occurs in inflamed tissue and in the tubules, facilitates the formation of uric acid crystals, which are the initial cause of gout. In most mammals, the enzyme uricase converts uric acid to the more soluble allantoin, but humans do not express uricase. Of importance for therapeutic intervention is the fact that xanthine and hypoxanthine are more soluble than uric acid. Specifically, by preventing uric acid formation through XOD inhibition, the excretion of xanthine and hypoxanthine increases, and the risk of uric acid crystal formation decreases. An increase of the serum uric acid concentration above 416 µmol/L is referred to as hyperuricemia and is associated with an increased risk of uric acid crystal formation and acute attacks of gouty arthritis. With a serum uric acid level of 535 µmol/L, the annual incidence of gouty arthritis is 4.9–5.7%.

Hyperuricemia can have genetic causes or acquired causes. A defect of hypoxanthine-gua-

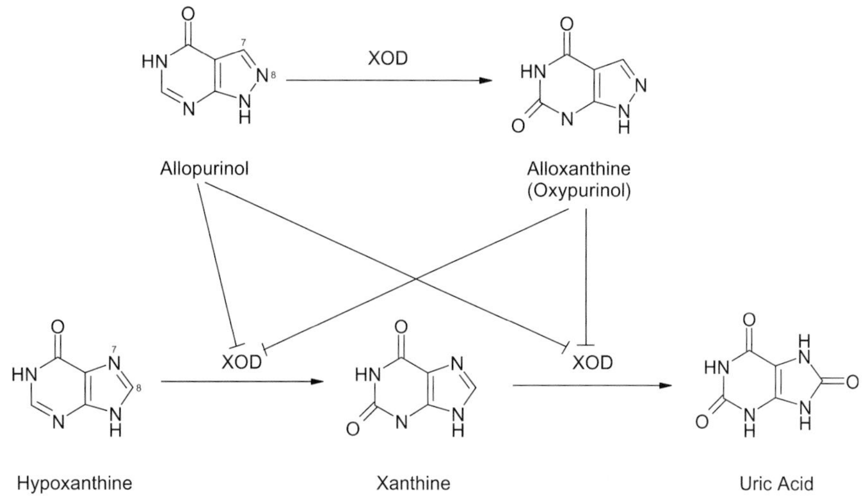

Fig. 1 Xanthine oxidase-catalyzed reactions. Xanthine oxidase converts hypoxanthine to xanthine and xanthine to uric acid, respectively. Hypoxanthine and xanthine are more soluble than uric acid. Xanthine oxidase also converts the uricostatic drug allopurinol to alloxanthine. Allopurinol and hypoxanthine are isomers that differ from each other in the substitution of positions 7 and 8 of the purine ring system. Although allopurinol is converted to alloxanthine by xanthine oxidase, allopurinol is also a xanthine oxidase inhibitor. Specifically, at low concentrations, allopurinol acts as a competitive inhibitor, and at high concentrations it acts as a non-competitive inhibitor. Alloxanthine is a non-competitive xanthine oxidase inhibitor. XOD, xanthine oxidase.

nine phosphoribosyl transferase is the cause of Lesch-Nyhan syndrome, resulting in increased uric acid production. Among the genetically caused defects, impaired renal uric acid secretion is a very common cause of gout. Myeloproliferative diseases, a purine-rich diet (*e.g.*, meat, beer, beans, peas, oatmeal, spinach), obesity and alcoholism are common causes of acquired hyperuricemia and result from increased uric acid production. Renal diseases and the application of certain drugs such as the tuberculostatic drug pyrazinamide, thiazide diuretics, loop diuretics, acetylsalicylic acid at doses of up to 1–2 g/day, and the immunosuppressant cyclosporin A are acquired causes of impaired uric acid secretion.

Gout is the consequence of hyperuricemia and is caused by uric acid deposits in joints, tendons, bursae, kidney and urinary tract. In the USA, the prevalence of gout is ~1% for all ages and both sexes. The prevalence of gout is higher in men than in women and exceeds 5% in men ≥65 years. These epidemiologic data are important for drug therapy since older patients are more sensitive to side effects of anti-gout drugs than younger

patients. In the initial stage, gout is characterized by asymptomatic hyperuricemia. In the second stage, the disease manifests itself by acute gouty arthritis. The third (intercritical) stage is asymptomatic, and the fourth stage is characterized by progressive uric acid deposits in joints, tendons, bursae, kidney and urinary tract (tophus formation). Uric acid deposits result in the deformation and loss of function of joints and recurrent episodes of urate lithiasis. Uric acid deposits in the kidney and urate lithiasis can ultimately result in renal failure.

Fig. 3 illustrates important pathophysiologic events leading to acute gouty arthritis. Once the concentration of uric acid exceeds its solubility, uric acid crystals form in the synovial fluid of joints. Subsequently, the uric acid crystals are phagocytosed by synoviocytes that form the inner cell layer of joints. Next, synoviocytes release numerous mediators of inflammation including leukotriene B_4 (LTB_4), prostaglandin E_2 (PGE_2), platelet-activating factor (PAF), histamine, interleukins (ILs) 1, 6 and 8 and tumor necrosis factor-α that in conjunction with products of the comple-

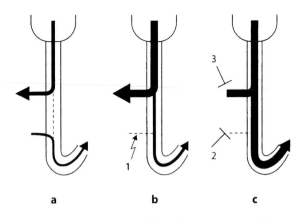

Fig. 2 Reabsorption and secretion of uric acid in the proximal renal tubulus. a, Normal situation. Uric acid is completely reabsorbed in the proximal segment of the renal tubulus and secreted more distally. **b, Situation in untreated hyperuricemia.** In most genetically caused cases of gout, uric acid secretion is defective (1). **c, Situation in hyperuricemia under treatment with uricosouric drugs. 2,** Inhibition of uric acid secretion by uricosuric drugs at low doses. **3,** Inhibition of uric acid secretion and reabsorption by uricosuric drugs in therapeutic doses. The inhibition of uric acid secretion with low doses of uricosuric drugs can further increase blood levels of uric acid and induce attacks of acute gouty arthritis.

ment cascade (C5a and C3a) and kinins (bradykinin) induce an inflammatory response. Moreover, LTB_4, PAF, C5a and IL-8 attract polymorphonuclear leukocytes (neutrohpils). Neutrophils migrate into affected joints along a concentration gradient of these inflammatory mediators (chemotaxis). Accordingly, LTB_4, PAF, C5a and IL-8 are also referred to as chemoattractants. Once present in joints, neutrophils phagocytose uric acid crystals. Uric acid crystals and chemoattractants trigger the release of cytotoxic lysosomal enzymes, NADPH oxidase-catalyzed formation of reactive oxygen species, LTB_4 formation and the release of other pro-inflammatory molecules from neutrophils. The latter molecules attract additional neutrophils and mononuclear phagocytes. Moreover, neutrophils generate lactate that decreases the pH within the joint and further accelerates uric acid crystal formation. Oxygen radicals and lysosomal enzymes cause damage to tissues. Thus, the

presence of uric acid crystals in joints triggers a vicious cycle, resulting in an extremely painful inflammation. A typical localization of acute gouty arthritis is the first metatarsal joint of the foot (podagra). The diagnosis of acute gouty arthritis is confirmed by the detection of urate crystals in the joint or tophus.

▶ Inflammation

Anti-gout drugs
Fig. 4 shows the structures of commonly employed anti-gout drugs. The treatment of acute gouty arthritis aims at rapidly reducing the pain and inflammatory reaction. This aim can be achieved by treatment with colchicine. In addition, ▶ non-steroidal anti-inflammatory drugs (NSAIDs), ▶ glucocorticoids and adrenocorticotropic hormone (ACTH) can be used to treat acute gouty arthritis. However, since NSAIDs and glucocorticoids are used in numerous other commonly occurring inflammatory conditions, they are not *per se* considered specific anti-gout drugs. Glucocorticoids can be given systemically (orally, intramuscularly or intravenously) or locally into afflicted joints. The long-term goals of gout treatment are the prevention of acute gouty arthritis, the prevention of urate lithiasis and renal failure and the resorption of existing uric acid deposits in the joints and urinary tract. The long-term therapy aims at reducing the serum concentration of uric acid below 357 µmol/L. Therapy with the ▶ uricostatic drug allopurinol and the ▶ uricosuric drugs benzbromarone, sulfinpyrazone or probenecid can accomplish the long-term goals. These drugs are well tolerated in most patients. Uricostatic and uricosuric drugs can be combined. Additionally, low doses of colchicine can be used to prevent the occurrence of acute gouty arthritis. However, as is unfortunately often the case with classic diseases, there are only few well conducted clinical studies assessing the clinical efficacy and safety of anti-gout drugs.

Mechanism of Action

Colchicine
Colchicine is an alkaloid from the autumn crocus *Colchicum autumnale*. Colchicine binds to the cytoskeletal protein ▶ tubulin and, thereby, pre-

vents microtubule formation. As a result, colchicine inhibits neutrophil chemotaxis and the influx of these cells into areas containing uric acid crystals (Fig. 3). Colchicine also inhibits neutrophil phagocytosis. As a result, colchicine interrupts the vicious cycle of inflammation in gouty arthritis. However, because of its mechanism of action, colchicine is most effective only when given in the early stages of gouty arthritis, i.e. within 24 hours. Otherwise, the inflammatory reaction may be too advanced. Specifically, colchicine is effective in > 90% of patients when given within the first few hours after the start of the attack, but after 24 hours, the responsiveness decreases to 75%. Given the very significant side effects of colchicine, it is absolutely crucial to initiate colchicine therapy as early as possible.

Allopurinol

Allopurinol is an analog of hypoxanthine and is converted to alloxanthine by XOD. Both allopurinol and hypoxanthine inhibit XOD (Fig. 1). Alloxanthine is a non-competitive inhibitor of XOD as is allopurinol at high concentrations. At low concentrations, allopurinol is a competitive inhibitor of XOD. As a result of XOD inhibition, the formation of the poorly soluble uric acid is reduced, whereas the formation of the more soluble metabolites hypoxanthine and xanthine is increased. Because of the good solubility of hypoxanthine and xanthine, formation of hypoxanthine/xanthine crystals is a rare complication of allopurinol treatment. Another consequence of XOD inhibition is the accumulation of the precursor of xanthine, inosine. Inosine inhibits the key enzyme of *de novo* purine synthesis, phosphoribosyl-pyrophosphate amidotransferase. The allopurinol metabolite allopurinol ribonucleotide also inhibits phosphoribosyl-pyrophosphate amidotransferase. Inhibition of purine biosynthesis contributes to the anti-hyperuricemic effects of allopurinol.

Uricosuric drugs

Depending on the dose applied, uricosuric drugs inhibit tubular reabsorption and tubular secretion of uric acid in the kidney differentially (Fig. 2). At low (subtherapeutic) doses, uricosuric drugs inhibit uric acid secretion without inhibiting reabsorption. Therefore, low doses of uricosuric drugs

can actually increase serum levels of uric acid and trigger acute attacks of gouty arthritis. At higher, i.e. therapeutic doses, uricosuric drugs inhibit both tubular secretion and tubular reabsorption. Since inhibition of tubular reabsorption is quantitatively more important than inhibition of tubular secretion, the net effect is an increased renal elimination of uric acid. In order to avoid formation of uric acid crystals in the kidney and urinary tract, it is important that the pH of the urine is kept > 6.0. This goal can be achieved by the oral administration of potassium sodium hydrogen citrate, sodium bicarbonate or acetazolamide. In addition, it is mandatory that the patient drinks at least 3L per day to avoid formation of uric acid crystals.

New strategies

Based on the pathophysiological events in gouty arthritis shown in Fig. 3, new therapeutic strategies for the treatment of gout may be developed. Specifically, complement components, bradykinin, LTB_4, PGE_2, PAF, histamine, interleukins and other cytokines exert their biological effects through specific receptors. Thus, antagonists for specific receptors and/or antibodies against specific signaling molecules or receptors may alleviate the clinical symptoms. However, the clinical efficacy of such drugs depends on the relative contribution of the respective mediator of inflammation in the pathogenesis of gouty arthritis, which has yet to be assessed. NSAIDs that selectively inhibit cyclooxygenase 2 (COX-2) are assumed to specifically inhibit prostanoid formation in inflamed areas but not in other locations such as the gastric mucosa. Accordingly, COX-2 inhibitors have less gastrointestinal side effects than the classic NSAIDs with no or little selectivity for COX-2 relative to COX-1. However, COX-2 inhibitors may have other side effects, and COX-1 inhibition may be of some relevance for the therapeutic efficacy of NSAIDs.

Clinical Use (incl. side effects)

Colchicine

Daily doses of 3–8 mg (6–8 times 0.5–1.0 mg) are used for the treatment of acute gouty arthritis. For prophylaxis, daily doses of 0.5–1.5 mg are used, but the use of colchicine for prophylaxis is controver-

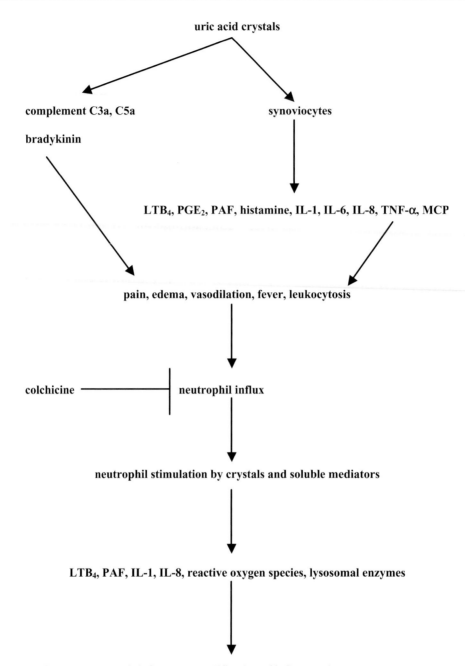

◄ **Fig. 3 Important pathophysiologic events in acute gouty arthritis.** Uric acid crystals activate the complement cascade, the formation of kinins and the release of various mediators of inflammation from synoviocytes that phagocytose uric acid crystals. The combined action of the released mediators induces a strong inflammatory reaction that is further enhanced by neutrophils. Neutrophils migrate along a concentration gradient to loci in which C5a, LTB_4, PAF and IL-8 are produced (chemotaxis). Accordingly, C5a, LTB_4, PAF and IL-8 are also referred to as chemoattractants. Neutrophils phagocytose uric acid crystals. Upon exposure to uric acid crystals and chemoattractants, neutrophils release various mediators of inflammation, reactive oxygen species and lysosomal enzymes. The concerted effects of all theses compounds amplify the inflammatory reaction even further. Colchicine interrupts the vicious cycle of inflammation predominantly by inhibiting neutrophil chemotaxis. IL-1, interleukin 1; IL-6, interleukin 6; IL-8, interleukin 8; LTB_4, leukotriene B_4; MCP, monocyte chemoattractant protein; PAF, platelet-activating factor; PGE_2, prostaglandin E_2; TNF-α, tumor necrosis factor-α.

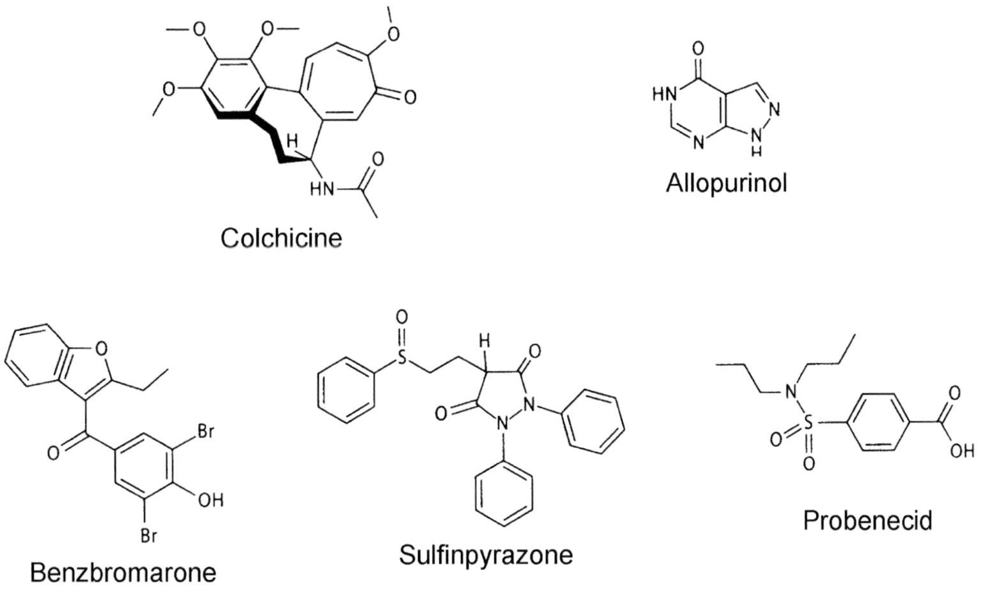

Colchicine

Allopurinol

Benzbromarone

Sulfinpyrazone

Probenecid

Fig. 4 Structures of commonly used anti-gout drugs. Colchicine is an alkaloid from the autumn crocus *Colchicum autumnale* and inhibits tubulin polymerization. Allopurinol is an isomer of xanthine and inhibits uric acid formation (uricostatic drug). Benzbromarone, sufinpyrazone and probenecid are uricosuric drugs and inhibit uric acid reabsorption in the proximal tubulus of the kidney.

sial. The side effects of colchicine are very significant. About 80% of the patients experience gastrointestinal problems including nausea, vomiting and diarrhea. The anti-mitotic effects of colchicine can result in thrombocytopenia, agranulocytosis, hair loss and azoospermia. In the central nervous system, confusion, ascending paralysis, respiratory failure and seizures have been reported. These side effects can be explained by the fact that intact microtubules are essential for proper transport functions in neuronal axons. Moreover, colchicine can cause myopathy. Because of the significant side effects, many physicians prefer to treat acute gouty arthritis with NSAIDs or glucocorticoids. Although colchicine is a classic anti-gout drug, colchicine can also be used to treat other inflammatory diseases including amyloidosis, Dupuytren's contracture, Behcet's syndrome, vasculitis, various forms of hepatic cirrhosis, pulmonary fibrosis, pericarditis and various inflammatory diseases of the skin. Colchicine is extensively metabolized through the hepatic cytochrome CYP 3A4. Accordingly, inhibitors of CYP 3A4 such as diltiazem, gestodene, grapefuit juice, ketoconazole and macrolide antibiotics prolong and enhance the pharmacological (and toxic) effects of colchicine. Drugs that are inactivated via CYP 3A4 such as steroid hormones, lidocaine, midazolam, quinidine, terfenadine, nifedipine and verapamil can also prolong colchicine action. Because of its anti-mitotic effects, colchicine should not be used in pregnant women.

Allopurinol

The daily dose of allopurinol is 300–600 mg. In combination with benzbromarone, the daily allopurinol dose is reduced to 100 mg. In general, allopurinol is well tolerated. The incidence of side effects is 2–3%. Exanthems, pruritus, gastrointestinal problems and dry mouth have been observed. In rare cases, hair loss, fever, leukopenia, toxic epidermolysis (Lyell syndrome) and hepatic dysfunction have been reported. Allopurinol inhibits the metabolic inactivation of the cytostatic drugs azathioprine and 6-mercaptopurine. Accordingly, the administered doses of azathioprine and 6-mercaptopurine must be reduced if allopurinol is given simultaneously.

Uricosuric drugs

Benzbromarone. The daily dose of benzbromarone is 50–200 mg. In combination with allopurinol, the benzbromarone dose is reduced to 20 mg. Benzbromarone is well tolerated. Rare side effects are headaches, gastrointestinal problems and exanthems.

Probenecid. The daily dose of probenecid is 0.5–3.0 g. Probenecid is well tolerated, and there are few serious side effects. In less than 10% of the treated patients, gastrointestinal disturbances, hypersensitivity and skin reactions occur.

Sulfinpyrazone. The daily dose of sulfinpyrazone is 200–400 mg. The side effects of sulfinpyrazone are comparable with those of probenecid. A potential therapeutic advantage of sulfinpyrazone in patients with coronary heart disease and thromboembolic diseases is its inhibitory effect on platelet aggregation.

References

1. Star VL, Hochberg MC (1993) Prevention and management of gout. Drugs 45:212–222
2. Terkeltaub RA (1993) Gout and mechanisms of crystal-induced inflammation. Curr Opin Rheumatol 5:510–516
3. Emmerson BT (1996) The management of gout. New Engl J Med 334:445–451
4. Schlesinger N, Schuhmacher HR Jr (2001) Gout: can management be improved? Curr Opin Rheumatol 13:240–244
5. Lange U, Schumann C, Schmidt KL (2001) Current aspects of colchicine therapy. Classical indications and new therapeutic uses. Eur J Med Res 6:150–160

Antihistamines

The term antihistamines describes drugs which bind to the H_1-histamine receptor and antagonize (block) the histamine effect in Type I allergic responses.

▶ Histaminergic System
▶ Allergy

Antihyperglycaemic

▶ Antidiabetic Drugs

Antihypertensive Drugs

REINHOLD KREUTZ
Freie Universität Berlin, Berlin, Germany
kreutz@medizin.fu-berlin.de

Synonyms

Antihypertensives; blood pressure lowering drugs

Definition

Reducing blood pressure by pharmacological means reduces cardiovascular morbidity and mortality rates. Benefits include protection from stroke, coronary events, heart failure, progression of renal disease, progression to more severe hypertension, and, most importantly mortality from all causes. Owing to the complexity of the pathogenesis of hypertension, antihypertensive drugs are directed against a variety of pharmacological targets in various cell types in different organs involved in blood pressure control.

▶ ACE Inhibitors
▶ Blood Pressure Control
▶ Ca^{2+} Channel Blockers
▶ Diuretics
▶ Renin-Angiotensin-Aldosterone System

Mechanism of Action

The fundamental mechanisms involved in blood pressure control have been outlined in chapter 'Blood pressure control'. In addition to direct neuronal modulation of arterial pressure two neurohumoral systems, i.e. the sympathetic nervous system and the renin-angiotensin-aldosterone system (RAS) play a pivotal role in blood pressure control. Both systems are always either directly or indirectly affected by treatment with any antihypertensive drug. Antihypertensives agents can be categorized into seven different drug classes (Fig. 1) (1). Centrally-acting antihypertensive drugs can be classified according to their relative affinities to α_2- and imidazoline (I_1) receptors. Clonidine is considered as a mixed α_2- and I_1-agonist, whereas moxinidine acts as a relative selecitve I_1-agonist. Methyldopa is a selective α_2-agonist. Administration of clonidine results in decreased cardiac output, a preservation of baroreflexes with a relative reduction in tendency of heart rate to rise, and little change in peripheral resistance. Methyldopa decreases sympathetic outflow predominantly to the α_1-receptors of the arterioles, thereby reducing peripheral resistance with little (but some) effect on the heart. The baroreceptor arc is impaired because of the effect on arterioles (2). Direct vasodilators such as minoxidil and hydralazine work by opening potassium channels in vascular smooth muscle cells in arterioles, which leads to K^+ efflux and hyperpolarization. Since the heart is not directly affected, direct vasodilators lead when used alone to reflex increases in heart rate and force of contraction; a significant neurohumoral activation of both the sympathetic nervous system and RAS occurs. Because of the activation of counter-regulatory systems, the simultaneous use of β-blockers and diuretics is generally required (3). Selective α_1 blockers inhibit the action of norepinephrine (noradrenaline) at arteriolar receptors, thereby leading also to activation of counter-regulatory systems (4). Calcium channel blockers act primarily as inhibitors of vasoconstriction by blocking L-type calcium channels in vascular smooth muscle cells. However, there are two different main classes (dihydropyridines and non-dihydropyridines), which work on different sites within the L-channel and hence produce different effects in the kidney, heart and vasculature. The non-dihydropyridines verapamil and diltiazem blunt increases in heart rate in response to exercise and have both negative inotropic and negative chronotropic (verapamil>diltiazem) effects; most dihydropyridines do not have major cardiodepressant effects because the long-acting agents slightly increase sympathetic nervous system tone, while this negative effect is even more pronounced with short-acting agents. In general, dihydropyridines lead to increases in heart rate and do not blunt the increase in heart rate response to exercise. Calcium channel blockers have a slight (transient) natriuretic effect (5). The competitive inhibition of β-blockers on β-receptors results in numerous effects on functions that regulate blood pressure, including a reduction in cardiac output, a decrease in renin release, perhaps a decrease in both central sympathetic nervous outflow and peripheral resistance. The view that the primary effect is a reduction in cardiac output as a result from the blockade of cardiac β$_1$-receptors with a subsequent reduction of heart rate and myocardial contractility has been questioned. Indeed, it seems that although cardiac output usually falls acutely and remains lower chronically, peripheral resistance on the other hand rises acutely but falls towards, if not to, normal with time. Thus, the hemodynamic hallmark of chronic established hypertension, that is an increased peripheral resistance, is also normalized by β-blockers. All currently available β-blockers antagonize cardiac β$_1$-receptors competitively, but they vary in their degree of β$_2$-receptor blockade in extra cardiac tissues. However, there seems to be little difference in antihypertensive efficacy among those that are more or less cardio- or β1-selective. Although the presence of intrinsic sympathomimetic activity (ISA) in some compounds such as pindolol and acebutolol could in theory translate into some beneficial effects, there is little convincing evidence that partial agonism confers significant clinical benefits. The newer compounds carvedilol and nebivolol produce additional vasodilator features that are attributable either to the additional blockade of α-receptors (carvedilol) or endothelial nitric oxide release (nevibolol) (6). The mode of action of diuretics depends on their major site of action within the nephron (Fig. 1). These differences determine their relative efficacy as expressed in the maximal percentage of filtered sodium excreted. Sixty percent of the filtered sodium is reabsorbed in the proximal tubule of the nephron. Thirty percent is reabsorbed in the thick ascending limb of Henle by ▶ Na$^+$/K$^+$/2Cl$^-$ cotransport, which is inhibited by loop diuretics. Seven percent is reclaimed by Na$^+$/Cl$^-$ cotransport in the distal convoluted tubule, which is inhibited by thiazide diuretics. The last 2% is reabsorbed via the ▶ epithelial sodium channel (ENaC) in the cortical collecting duct, which is

a target either directly (amiloride, triamterene) or indirectly via the mineralocorticoid receptor (spironolactone) for potassium-sparing agents (Fig. 1).

Agents acting in the proximal tubule are seldom used to treat hypertension. Treatment is usually initiated with a thiazide-type diuretic. Chlorthalidone and indapamide are structurally different from thiazides but are functionally related. If renal function is severely impaired (i.e. serum creatinine above 2.5 mg/dl), a loop diuretic is needed. A potassium-sparing agent may be given with the diuretic to reduce the likelihood of hypokalemia. By themselves, potassium-sparing agents are relatively weak antihypertensives (7). In general, there are four ways to reduce the activity of the RAS. The first way is the use of β-blockers to reduce renin release from the juxtaglomerular (JG). The second way, the direct inhibition of the activity of renin, although being actively investigated has not been successful in the clinical arena thus far. The third way is to inhibit the activity of the ▶ angiotensin converting enzyme (ACE), which converts the inactive decapeptide angiotensin I to the potent octapeptide angiotensin II (Ang II), by agents referred to as ACE inhibitors. Thus, these agents inhibit the biosynthesis of Ang II and thereby decrease the availability of Ang II at both angiotensin type 1 (AT$_1$) and angiotensin type 2 (AT$_2$) receptors. The fourth way is to use a competitive and selective antagonist at the AT$_1$ receptor (i.e. AT$_1$ antagonists) and thereby to inhibit the classical effects mediated by Ang II such as vasoconstriction and aldosterone release. ACE inhibitors exhibit additional effects that are independent from RAS such as on kinins, since ACE is also a kininase. Although the clinical relevance is not fully understood, blood pressure effects mediated via inhibition of breakdown of bradykinin may contribute to the vasodilatory effects of ACE inhibitors. Some of the latter effects could be mediated via kinin stimulation of prostaglandin production. In addition to these effects on vascular tone, multiple other effects may contribute to the antihypertensive effects of ACE inhibitors. The blunting of the expected increase in sympathetic nervous activity typically seen after vasodilation is potentially of greater importance for the documented clinical benefits of ACE inhibitors. As a result, heart rate is not increased as is seen with direct vasodilators, α-blockers and less pronounced with dihydropyrid-

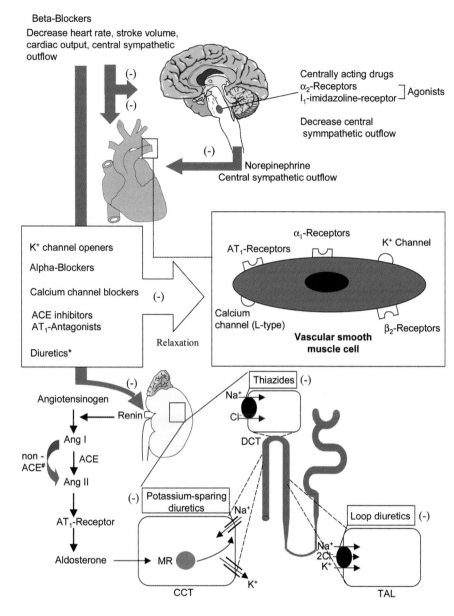

Beta-Blockers
Decrease heart rate, stroke volume, cardiac output, central sympathetic outflow

Centrally acting drugs
α_2-Receptors
I_1-imidazoline-receptor — Agonists

Decrease central symmpathetic outflow

Norepinephrine
Central sympathetic outflow

K⁺ channel openers
Alpha-Blockers
Calcium channel blockers
ACE inhibitors
AT_1-Antagonists
Diuretics*

Relaxation

α_1-Receptors
AT_1-Receptors
K⁺ Channel
Calcium channel (L-type)
β_2-Receptors
Vascular smooth muscle cell

Angiotensinogen
Renin
Ang I
non-ACE#   ACE
Ang II
AT_1-Receptor
Aldosterone → MR
CCT
K⁺

Thiazides (-)
Na⁺
Cl⁻
DCT

Potassium-sparing diuretics
Na⁺

Loop diuretics (-)
Na⁺
2Cl⁻
K⁺
TAL

Fig. 1 Site of action of different classes of antihypertensive drugs.
Antihypertensive drugs are directed against a variety of pharmacological targets in various cell types in different organs involved in blood pressure control. The most important targets in the brain, heart, vasculature (vascular smooth muscle cells), and the kidney (nephron) are shown. *Some diuretics produce some direct vasodilation; # non-ACE, conversion of angiotensin I (Ang I) to angiotensin II (Ang II) may occur independent from ACE due to the activity of other enzymes in different tissues such as chymase in the heart; DCT, distal convoluted tubule (DCT); CCT, cortical collecting duct; TAL, thick ascending limb of the loop of Henle; (-), indicates inhibition. Modified according to reference 3.

ine calcium channel blockers. The presence of the complete RAS within various tissues including the vasculature, kidney, heart and brain has been demonstrated and the activation of the RAS at the tissue level seems to play – beyond its role on blood pressure regulation – an important role for the manifestation and progression of hypertensive target organ damage in these organs. Our understanding of the molecular mechanisms by which Ang II contributes to both structural and functional changes, e.g. due to its growth factor capacity, at the tissue level continues to expand. Consequently, the inhibition of

tissue ACE may play an important role for the prevention and regression of hypertensive target organ damage that has been documented for these agents in experimental and clinical studies.

The major obvious difference between AT_1 antagonists and ACE inhibitors is the absence of an increase in kinins that may be responsible for some of the beneficial effects of ACE inhibitors and probably their side effects. Direct comparison between the two types of drugs show little differences in antihypertensive efficacy but cough, a common side effect seen with ACE inhibitors, is

Tab. 1 Common side effects of antihypertensive drugs.

Class of Drug		Side Effects
ACE inhibitors		cough, hyperkalemia, skin reactions
AT$_1$-antagonists		hyperkalemia (less frequent compared with ACE inhibitors)
Calcium channel blockers	Dihydropyridine	pedal edema, headache
	Non-Diyhdropyridine	constipation (verapamil); headache (diltiazem)
Diuretics		frequent urination, hyperuricemia, hyperglycemia, hyperlipidemia
Centrally acting drugs	α2-receptor agonists	sedation, dry mouth, rebound hypertension
	Imidazoline-receptor agonists	
Central neuronal blockers (reserpine)		depression, sedation, nasal congestion
α-blockers		orthostatic hypotension, rapid drop of blood pressure after first dose, pedal edema, dizziness
β-blockers		fatigue, hyperglycemia, bronchospasm
Potassium channel openers		hypertrichosis (minoxidil); lupus-like reactions and pedal edema (hydralazine)

Modified according to reference 3

not provoked by AT$_1$ antagonists, although angioedema and ageusia have also been reported for these newer agents.

Clinical Use (incl. side effects)

Recent consensus committees, including the Sixth Report of the Joint National Committee on Prevention, Detection, Evaluation, and Treatment of High Blood Pressure (JNC VI) and the World Health Organisation-International Society of Hypertension (WHO-ISH) Guidelines Subcommittee, have modified traditional treatment recommendations in several important ways.

Criteria for initiation of drug treatment now take into consideration total cardiovascular risk rather than blood pressure alone, such that treatment is now recommended for persons whose blood pressure is in the normal range but still bear a heavy burden of cardiovascular risk factors. Thus, the role of simultaneous reduction of multiple cardiovascular risk factors in improving prognosis in hypertensive patients is stressed. In addi-

tion, more aggressive blood pressure goals are recommended for hypertensive patients with comorbid conditions such as diabetes mellitus or renal insufficiency.

Finally, drug treatment in the elderly is of great importance and warrants special attention with regard to safety and tolerability, since systolic blood pressure is recognized as an important target for treatment, particularly in older persons. The benefits of antihypertensive treatment in the elderly and in patients with isolated systolic hypertension are greater than in younger persons.

As a consequence for drug treatment, an increasing number of patients will be treated with antihypertensive compounds and the importance of tailoring the choice of antihypertensive drug treatment to the patients individual profile of concomitant cardiovascular risk factors/comorbid conditions has to be emphasized. Moreover, it is reasonable to individualize antihypertensive treatment on the basis of each patient's personal needs with respect to tolerability, convenience and quality of life. Initiation of treatment with a drug that is expected to be well tolerated and therefore likely to be effective in lowering blood pressure over time is prudent (common side effects are listed in Table 1). Long-acting agents are preferable because adherence to therapy and consistency of blood pressure control are superior when the drug is taken once a day. Low-dose, fixed-dose combination therapy can be used in place of monotherapy as initial treatment or as an alternative to adding a second agent of a different therapeutic class to unsuccessful monotherapy. The advantage of this approach is that low doses of drugs that act by different mechanisms may have additive or synergistic effects on blood pressure with minimal dose-dependent adverse effects. Giving the patient a single tablet provides an additional benefit. A case in point represents the well-established combination of an ACE inhibitor or AT1-antagonist with low-dose hydrochlorothiazide, which does not produce more side effects than placebo.

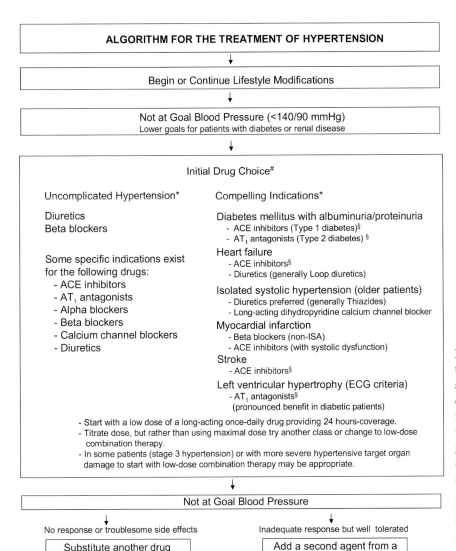

Fig. 2 Algorithm for the treatment of hypertension. # Unless contraindicated; * based on randomized controlled trials; § Evidence suggests that the beneficial effects of ACE inhibitors can be duplicated with AT_1 antagonists (and probably *vice versa*). Thus, ACE inhibitors could be substituted by AT_1 antagonists in the case of troublesome side effects, such as cough under treatment with ACE inhibitors. Modified according to reference 5.

Many of the concepts of antihypertensive treatment put forward are adopted from the algorithms recommended by the JNC VI (Fig. 2). Treatment should always include lifestyle modifications. For the minority of hypertensive patients without comorbid conditions, target organ damage, or concomitant cardiovascular disease, the JNC VI recommends starting drug therapy with a diuretic (i.e. thiazides) or β-blocker because these agents had been proven to lower morbidity and mortality compared with placebo in randomized controlled trials. Secondly, they are less costly than newer classes of drugs. Therefore, the era of placebo-controlled trials is past and any new agents can only be compared against the gold standard of diuretics and β-blockers. Overall, these early trials with diuretics and β-blockers established a greater reduction of risk related to stroke (–40%) than the risk related to coronary heart disease (–14%). While diuretics are more effective in preventing stroke than β-blockers the opposite holds true for cardiac risk. A reduction in cardiovascular risk has also been documented for the ACE-inhibitor captopril and in elderly patients with isolated systolic hypertension for the dihydropyridine calcium channel blocker (nitrendipine). However, outcome trials comparing two anti-hypertensives require large groups of patients, because the risk in patients with mild-to-moderate essential hypertension is low, and intervention trials are usually limited to duration of 5 years. Therefore, differences between drug classes have been documented when patients with higher absolute cardiovascular risk and/or comorbid conditions were studied. Compelling indications that have been established in randomized controlled trials are summarized in Fig. 2.

References

1. Brunner HR, Gavras H (2000) Angiotensin blockade for hypertension: a promise fulfilled. Commentary. Lancet 359:990–992
2. Carretero OA, Oparil S (2000) Essential Hypertension. Part II: Treatment. Circulation 101:329–335
3. Tarif N, Bakris GL (2000) Pharmacologic treatment of essential hypertension. In: Johnson RJ, Feehally J (eds) Comprehensive clinical nephrology. Mosby, London, p37.1–37.11
4. Kaplan NM (1998) Clinical hypertension, 7th edition.Williams & Wilkins, Baltimore.
5. Joint National Committee on Prevention, Detection, Evaluation, and Treatment of High Blood Pressure (1997). The Sixth Report of the Joint National Committee on Prevention, Detection, Evaluation, and Treatment of High Blood Pressure (JNC VI). Arch Int Med 157:2413–2446

Anti-inflammatory Drugs

► Glucocorticoids
► Non-steroidal Anti-inflammatory Drugs

Anti-integrins, therapeutic and diagnostic implications

SHAKER A. MOUSA
Albany College of Pharmacy, Albany, USA
mousas@acp.edu

Definition

Integrins are a widely expressed family of cell adhesion receptors via which cells attach to extracellular matrices either to each other or to different cells. All integrins are composed of αβ heterodimeric units, expressed on a wide variety of cells, and most cells express several integrins. The interaction of integrins with the cytoskeleton and extracellualr matrix appears to require the presence of both subunits. The binding of integrins to their ligands is cation-dependent. Integrins appear to recognize specific amino acid sequences in their ligands. The best studied is the RGD sequence found within a number of ► matrix proteins including fibrinogen, vitronectin, fibronectin, thrombospondin, osteopontin and VWF. However, other integrins bind to ligands via non-RGD binding domain such as the α4β1 integrin receptors that bind and recognize the LDV sequence within the CS-1 region of fibronectin. There are at least 8 known β subunits and 14 α subunits (1, 2, 3,

4). Although the association of the different β and α subunits could in theory result in more than 100 integrins, the actual diversity is restricted.

▶ Angiogenesis and Vascular Morphogenesis
▶ Antiplatelet Drugs

Basic Characteristics

Integrin adhesion receptors contain an extracellular face that engages adhesive ligands and a cytoplasmic face that engages with intracellular proteins. The interactions between the cell adhesion molecules and extracellular matrix proteins are critical for cell adhesion and for anchorage-dependent signaling reactions in normal and pathological states. For example, platelet activation induces a confirmational change in integrin αIIb/β3, thereby converting it into a high affinity fibrinogen receptor. Fibrinogen binding then triggers a cascade of protein tyrosine kinases, phosphatases and recruitment of numerous other signaling molecules into F-actin-rich cytoskeletal assemblies in proximity to the cytoplasmic tails of αIIb and β3 (5). These dynamics appear to influence platelet functions by coordinating signals emanating from integrins and G protein-linked receptors (5). Studies of integrin mutations confirm that the cytoplasmic tails of αIIb/β3 are involved in integrin signaling presumably through direct interactions with cytoskeletal and signaling molecules (5). Blockade of fibrinogen binding to the extracellular face of αIIb/β3 has been shown to be an effective way to prevent arterial ▶ thrombosis after coronary angioplasty in myocardial infarction and unstable angina patients (6).

Pathophysiology and Therapeutic Potential
The role of integrins has been found in various pathological processes, including ▶ angiogenesis, thrombosis, apoptosis, cell migration and proliferation. These processes lead to both acute and chronic diseases such as ocular diseases, metastasis, unstable angina, myocardial infarction, stroke, ▶ osteoporosis, and a wide range of inflammatory diseases, vascular remodeling and neurodegenerative disorders. A breakthrough in this field is evident from the role of the platelet αIIbβ3 integrin in the prevention, treatment and diagnosis of various thromboembolic disorders. Additionally, significant progress in the development of leukocyte α4β1 antagonists for various inflammatory indications and αv integrin antagonists for angiogenesis and vascular-related disorders has been achieved.

β1 Integrins

α4β1 Integrin. The largest numbers of integrins are members of the β1 integrins, also known as the very late antigen (VLA) subfamily because of its late appearance after activation. There are at least seven receptors characterized from this subfamily, each with different ligand specificity. Among the most studied include the α4β1 and α5β1 receptors. The leukocyte integrin α4β1 is a cell adhesion receptor that is predominantly expressed on lymphocytes, monocytes and eosinophils (7).

Potent and Selective Small Molecule Antagonists of α4β1 Integrins. The α4β1 integrins are heterodimeric cell surface molecules central to leukocyte-cell and leukocyte-matrix adhesive interactions. The integrin α4β1, expressed on all leukocytes except neutrophil, interacts with the immunoglobin superfamily member VCAM-1 and with an alternately spliced form of fibronectin. Additionally, the integrin α4β7 is also restricted to leukocytes and can bind not only to VCAM1 and fibronectin, but also to MAdCAM the mucosal addressin or homing receptor, which contains Ig-like domains related to VCAM-1 (8). *In vivo* studies with α4β1 monoclonal antibodies in several species demonstrate that the interactions between these integrins and their ligands play a key role in immune and ▶ inflammatory disorders (9) and selected ones are in clinical trials.

α5β1 Integrin in Angiogenesis. In contrast to collagen, expression of the extracellular matrix protein fibronectin in provisional vascular matrices precedes permanent collagen expression and provides signals to vascular cells and fibroblasts during blood clotting and wound healing, atherosclerosis and hypertension (10). Fibronectin expression is also upregulated on blood vessels in granulation tissues during wound healing. These observations suggest a possible role for this isoform of fibronectin in angiogenesis. Evidence was recently provided that both fibronectin and its receptor integrin α5β1 directly regulate angiogenesis (11). Thus, integrin antagonist for α5β1 integrin might be a useful target for the inhibition of angiogenesis associated with human tumor growth; neovascular related ocular and inflammatory diseases.

α5β1 Integrin and Bacterial Invasion. Recent studies suggested a key role for α5β1 integrin in certain bacterial invasion of human host cells leading to antibiotic resistance (12).

β3 Integrins

Intravenous and Oral Platelet αIIb/β3 Receptor Antagonists: Potential Clinical Utilities. There is an urgent need for more efficacious antithrombic drugs superior to aspirin or ticlopidine for the prevention and treatment of various cardiovascular and cerebrovascular thromboembolic disorders. The realization that the platelet integrin αIIbβ3 is the final common pathway for platelet aggregation regardless of the mechanism of action prompted the development of several small molecule αIIb/β3 receptor antagonists for intravenous and/or oral antithrombotic utilities. Platelet αIIb/β3 receptor blockade represents a very promising therapeutic and diagnostic strategy of thromboembolic disorders. Clinical experiences (efficacy/safety) gained with injectable αIIbβ3 antagonists (Abciximab, Eptifibatide, Aggrastat) elucidate the safety and efficacy of this mechanism in combination with other antiplatelet and anticoagulant therapies.

Orally Active GPIIb/IIIa Antagonists. A high level of platelet antagonism has been required when GPIIb/IIIa antagonists have been employed for acute therapy of coronary arterial diseases using intravenous GPIIb/IIIa antagonists with heparin and aspirin. Interaction with aspirin and other antiplatelet and anticoagulant drugs lead to shifts in the dose-response curves for both efficacy and unwanted side effects, such as increased bleeding time. More recently, all oral GPIIb/IIIa antagonists with or without aspirin but not with anticoagulant were withdrawn because of a disappointing outcome (no clinical benefit or increased thrombotic events). This raises a lot of serious questions with regard to the potential of oral GPIIb/IIIa antagonists as compared to the well-

documented success of intravenous GPIIb/IIIa antagonists (6,13).

GPIIb/IIIa Integrin Receptor Antagonists in the Rapid Diagnosis of Thromboembolic Events. The role of the platelet integrin GPIIb/IIIa receptor and its potential utility as a radio-diagnostic agent in the rapid detection of thromboembolic events has been demonstrated (14). This approach may be useful for the non-invasive diagnosis of various thromboembolic disorders.

Integrin αvβ3 Antagonists Promote Tumor Regression by Inducing Apoptosis of Angiogenic Blood Vessels. Antagonists of integrin αvβ3 inhibit the growth of new blood vessels into tumors cultured on the chick chorioallantoic membrane without affecting adjacent blood vessels, and also induce tumor regression (15). Antagonists of αvβ3 also inhibit angiogenesis in various ocular models of retinal neovascularization (16,17).

Integrin αvβ3 in Restenosis. The calcification of atherosclerotic plaques may be induced by osteopontin expression, since osteopontin is a protein with a well-characterized role in bone formation and calcification. Vascular smooth muscle cell migration on osteopontin is dependent on the integrin αvβ3 and antagonists of αvβ3 prevent both smooth muscle cell migration and restenosis in some animal model (18).

Integrin αvβ3 Antagonists Versus Anti- αvβ3 and αvβ5. Since the recognition of at least two αv integrin pathways for cytokine-mediated angiogenesis, αvβ3 and αvβ5 antagonists may be more effective in certain indications as compared to a specific anti- αvβ3. However, further work is needed to document this notion.

Potential Role of αvβ3 Antagonists in Osteoporosis. RGD analogs have been shown to inhibit the attachment of osteoclasts to bone matrix and to reduce bone resorptive activity *in vitro*. The cell surface integrin, αvβ3, appears to play a role in this process. RGD analogs may represent a new approach to modulating osteoclast-mediated bone resorption and may be useful in the treatment of osteoporosis (19).

Integrins αvβ3 Ligands. Therapeutics: A number of potent small molecule antagonists for αvβ3 integrin are under preclinical investigations for various angiogenesis or vascular-mediated disorders (20).

Site directed delivery: This approach of conjugating αvβ3 integrin ligand with a chemotherapeutic agent for optimal efficacy and safety in cancer is under investigation. Earlier work demonstrated the validity of this concept (21).

Diagnostics: Imaging metastatic cancer using technetium-99m labeled RGD-containing synthetic peptide has been demonstrated. Additionally, detection of tumor angiogenesis *in vivo* by αvβ3-targeted magnetic resonance imaging (MRI) was demonstrated (22,23,24).

References

1. Ruoslahti E and Pierschbacher M. (1986) Arg-Gly-Asp: A versatile cell recognition sequence. Cell 44:517–518

2. Hynes R O. (1992) Integrins: versatility, modulation and signaling in cell adhesion. Cell 69:11–25

3. Cox D, Aoki T, Seki J, Motoyama Y, Yoshida K. (1994) The pharmacology of the integrins. Med Res Rev 14(2):195–228

4. Albelda SM and Buck CA. (1990) Integrins and other cell adhesion molecules. FASEB J 4:2868–2880

5. Pelletier A J, Bodary S C, and A D Levinson. (1992) Signal transduction by the platelet integrin αIIbβ3: induction of calcium oscillations required for protein-tyrosine phosphorylation and ligand-induced spreading of stably transfected cells. Mol Biol Cell 3:989–998

6. Mousa SA. (1999) Antiplatelet therapies: From Aspirin to GPIIb/IIIa receptor antagonists and beyond. Drug Discovery Today 4(12):552–561

7. Hamann A, Andrew DP, Jablonski-Westrich D, Holzmann B, Butcher EC. (1994) Role of α4-integrins in lymphocyte homing to mucosal tissues in vivo. J. Immunol. 152:3282–3293

8. Berlin C, Berg EL, Briskin MJ, Andrew DP, et al. (1994) α4β7 integrin mediates lymphocyte binding to the mucosal vascular addressin MAdCAM-1. Cell 74:185–195

9. Lin K-C, Castro AC. (1998) Very late antigen 4 (VLA4) antagonists as anti-inflammatory agents. Current Opinion in Chemical Biology 2:453–457

10. Magnusson, M.K. and Mosher, D.F. (1998) Fibronectin: Structure, assembly, and cardiovascular implications. Arterioscler. Thromb. Vasc. Biol. 18:1363–1370

11. Kim S, Mousa S, Varner J. (2000) Requirement of integrin α5β1 and its ligand fibronectin in angiogenesis. American J. Pathology 156:1345–1362

12. Cue D, Southern S, Southern P, Prabhakar J, Lorelli W, Smallhear J, Mousa S, Cleary P (2000) A nonpeptide integrin antagonist can inhibit epithelial cell ingestion of streptococcus pyogenes by blocking α5β1-fibronectin-M1 protein complexes. Proc. Nat. Acad. Sci. 97(6):2858–2863

13. Quinn M, Fitzgerald DJ. (1998) Long-term administration of glycoprotein IIb/IIIa antagonists. Am Heart J 135(5 Pt 2 Su):S113–118

14. Mousa SA, Bozarth JM, Edwards S, Carroll T, Barrett J. (1998) Novel technetium 99m-labeled GPIIb/IIIa receptor antagonists as potential imaging agents for venous and arterial thrombosis. Coronary Artery Disease 9:131–141

15. Brooks P C., Stromblad S , Klemke R , et al. (1995) Anti-integrin αvβ3 blocks human breast cancer growth and angiogenesis in human skin. J Clin Invest 96:1815–1822

16. Friedlander M, Brooks P C, Shaffer R , et al. (1995) Definition of two angiogenic pathways by distinct αv integrins. Science 27:1500–1502

17. Luna J, Tobe T, Mousa S, et al. (1996) Antagonists of integrin αvβ3 inhibit retinal neovascularization in a murine model. Lab Invest. 75:563–573

18. Srivatsa SS, Tsao P, Holmes DR, Schwartz RS, Mousa SA. (1997) Selective αvβ3 integrin blockade limits neointima hyperplasia and lumen stenosis in stented porcine coronary artery injury in Pig. Cardiovascular Res. 36:408–428

19. Horton MA, Taylor ML, Arnett TR, Helfrich MH. (1991) Arg-Gly-Asp (RGD) peptides and the anti-vitronectin receptor antibody 23C6 inhibit dentine resorption and cell spreading by osteoclasts. Exp Cell Res 195:368–375

20. Mousa SA, Lorelli W, Mohamed S, Batt DG, Jadhav PK, Reilly TM. (1999) αvβ3 integrin binding affinity and specificity of SM256 in various species. J. Cardiovascular Pharmacology 33:641–646

21. Arap W, Pasqualini, Ruoslahti E. (1998) Cancer treatment by targeted drug delivery to tumor vasculature in a mouse model. Science 279:377–380

22. Sipkins DA, Cheresh DA, Kazemi MR, Nevin LM, Bednarski MD, King CP. (1998) Detection of tumor

angiogenesis in vivo by avb3-targeted magnetic resonance imaging. Nature Medicine 4(5):623–626
23. Sivolapenko GB, Skarlos D, Pectasides D, et al. (1998) Imaging of metastatic melanoma utilizing a technetium-99m labeled RGD-containing synthetic peptide. Eur J Nucl Med 25(10):1383–1389
24. Haubner R, Wester HJ, Reuning U, et al. (1999) Radiolabeled α(v)β3 integrin antagonists: a new class of tracer for tumor targeting. J Nucl Med 40(6):1061–1071

Antimalarial Drugs

▶ Antiprotozoal Drugs

Antimetabolite

Antimetabolites are compounds that inhibit the utilization of an essential nutrient. When used as anticancer agents, they are often analogs of nucleotide precursors.

▶ Antineoplastic Agents

Antimicrobial Agents

Antimicrobial drugs are used for the treatment of diseases caused by microorganisms (bacterial or viral infections).

▶ β-Lactam Antibiotics
▶ Ribosomal Protein Synthesis Inhibitors
▶ Quinolons
▶ Antiviral Drugs
▶ Microbial Resistance to Drugs

Antimode

The antimode is the cut-off value separating different functionally defined groups in a bi-modal or multi-modal frequency distribution.

▶ Pharmacogenetics

Antineoplastic Agents

MARTIN R. BERGER
Deutsches Krebsforschungszentrum (DKFZ),
Heidelberg, Germany
m.berger@dkfz.de

Synonyms

Anticancer drugs, cytostatic drugs, cytotoxic drugs, anti-tumor drugs

Definition

Cancer or neoplastic disease is a genomic disorder of the body's own cells which start to proliferate in an uncontrolled fashion that is ultimately detrimental to the individual. Antineoplastic agents are used in conjunction with surgery and radiotherapy to restrain that growth with curative or palliative intention. The domain of antineoplastic chemotherapy is cancer that is disseminated and therefore not amenable to local treatment modalities such as surgery and radiotherapy.

▶ Cancer, molecular mechanisms of therapy

Mechanism of Action

Development and Characteristics of Cancer Cells
The genesis of cancer cells can be modeled by the formula:
Cancer = f{Exposure, Genetic disposition, Age}
'*Exposure*' denotes the impact of exogenous factors that can be of chemical (chemical carcinogens), physical (UV or γ-irradiation) or of biological (viruses, bacteria) origin. '*Genetic disposition*'

indicates the germline transmission of genes associated with cancer development, and '*Age*' points to the fact that certain cellular injuries that cause mutations and lead to cancer development are not reversible but accumulate with time. Thus, a cancer cell is characterized by genetic abnormalities such as chromosomal alterations as well as activation of cellular ▶ proto-oncogenes to oncogenes and inactivation of ▶ tumor suppressor genes. As result of these changes they show autonomous proliferation, dedifferentiation, loss of function, invasiveness and metastasis formation. Furthermore, drug resistance (primary or acquired in response to treatment with antineoplastic drugs) is a common phenomenon.

Growth of Cancer Cells

Proliferation of cancer cells is not restricted by ▶ contact inhibition as for normal cells but rather by the supply of growth factors and nutrients. Once a cell has become malignant and its descendants have the necessary blood supply, the initial growth rate is exponential and follows approximately the pattern shown in Fig. 1. The subsequent loss of logarithmic growth is related to insufficient supply of nutrients, which drives cancer cells to either die or exit the cell cycle. As a result, larger tumors contain only a certain ratio of dividing cells which is termed growth fraction. The resultant steady state growth is depicted by the so-called Gompertz function (Fig. 2).

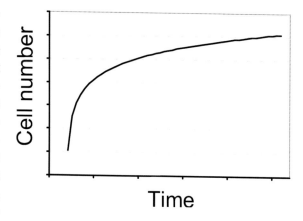

Fig. 2 Growth curve of tumor cells according to Gompertz.

Anticancer drugs can be grouped into several classes according to their mechanism of action and origin. These are (1) alkylating agents and related compounds which act by forming covalent bonds with cellular macromolecules such as DNA, (2) anti-metabolites which block metabolic pathways that are vital for cell survival or proliferation, (3) cytotoxic antibiotics of microbial origin and (4) plant derivatives which both interfere with mammalian cell division, (5) hormonal agents which suppress hormone secretion, block hormone synthesis or antagonize hormone action, (6) biological response modifiers which enhance the host's response to cancer cells, (7) antibodies which recognize antigens specific for cancer cells, and (8) miscellaneous agents which do not fit into the classes described above.

General effects include cytostatic or cytotoxic effects, the latter being related to killing a constant fraction of cells. The mode of action of antineoplastic agents is not causal because it does not reverse the basal changes that have led to the development of cancer cells but symptomatic since it aims at their destruction. However, cytotoxicity is generally not restricted towards cancer cells but affects all (quickly) dividing cells, especially those from bone marrow, gastrointestinal tract, hair follicles, gonads and growing tissues in children (lack of selectivity).

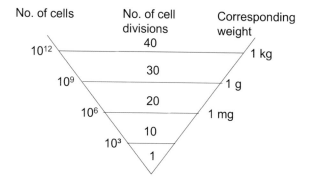

Fig. 1 Relationship of cell number, number of cell divisions, and corresponding weight.

The limited efficacy of anticancer drugs can be explained by the compartment model of dividing (growth fraction, compartment A) and non dividing (compartment B) cells. The majority of antineoplastic drugs acts upon cycling cells and will hit, therefore, compartment A only.

Alkylating Agents and Related Compounds

Alkylating agents are activated spontaneously or enzymatically to give rise to an electrophilic species that can form covalent bonds with nucleophilic cellular constituents. Reaction of monofunctional alkylating agents with DNA bases leads to induction of single strand breaks, that of bifunctional alkylating agents to ▶ crosslink formation between bases of the same strand of DNA (intrastrand crosslink) or two complementary strands (interstrand crosslink). Replicating cells are more susceptible to these drugs since parts of the DNA are unpaired and not protected by proteins. Therefore, although alkylating agents are not cell cycle specific, cells are most susceptible to alkylation in late G1 and S phases of the cell cycle resulting in block at G2 and subsequent apoptotic cell death.

Cells that survive these damages may undergo mutations that results in cancer development. This is reason for the carcinogenicitiy of alkylating agents.

The most important subgroup is that of nitrogen mustard derivatives. Nitrogen mustard was developed in relation to sulphur mustard, the 'mustard gas' used during World War I that was found to suppress ▶ leukopoiesis. Nitrogen mustard was the first drug to induce a remission in a lymphoma patient at the end of World War II, but has been abandoned since then. The highly reactive R-N-bis-(2-choroethyl) group, however, is part of many drugs in current use, such as cyclophosphamide, melphalan and chlorambucil. The activity of cyclophosphamide is dependent on P450 mixed function oxidases-mediated activation into active and/or toxic metabolites. One of the toxic metabolites is acrolein, which causes hemorrhagic cystitis if not prevented by the antidote mesna. Mesna is a sulphydryl donor and interacts specifically with acrolein to form a non-toxic compound.

Other subgroups of alkylating agents are the nitrosoureas (examples: carmustine, BCNU; lomustine, CCNU) and the triazenes (example:

dacarbazine, DTIC). Platinum derivatives (cisplatin, carboplatin, oxaliplatin) have an action that is analogous to that of alkylating agents (formation of crosslinks) and therefore are appended to this class.

Alkylating agents are used for treating solid tumors as well as leukemias and lymphomas. Their broad spectrum of activity is reason for their inclusion in many past and current chemotherapy schedules. Platinum derivatives are especially useful in treating testicular and ovarian cancers. All alkylating agents depress bone marrow function and cause gastrointestinal side effects. With prolonged use, depression of gametogenesis occurs leading to sterility and an increased risk of leukemias as well as other malignancies.

Anti-metabolites

Anti-metabolites interfere with normal metabolic pathways. They can be grouped into folate antagonists and analogues of purine or pyrimidine bases. Their action is limited to the S- phase of the cell cycle and they therefore target a smaller fraction of cells as compared with alkylating agents. The main folate antagonist is methotrexate. In structure, folates are based on three elements: a heterobicyclic pteridine, p-aminobenzoic acid and glutamic acid. The latter moiety is polyglutamated within cells, which causes a prolonged intracellular half-life and, as compared with monoglutamate, an increased affinity to dihydrofolate reductase, the target enzyme of antifolates. This enzyme catalyses the reduction of dihydrofolate to tetrahydrofolate, and its inhibition interferes with the transfer of mono-carbon units that are needed for purine- and thymidylate synthesis and thus blocks the synthesis of DNA, RNA, and protein. Methotrexate has a higher affinity for dihydrofolate reductase than the normal substrate (dihydrofolate) and inhibits thymidylate synthesis at a ten-fold lower concentration (1 nM) than purine synthesis. Methotrexate is toxic to normal tissues (especially the bone marrow) and causes hepatotoxicity following chronic therapy. Acute toxicity following iatrogenic error or high dose therapy can be rescued by using folinic acid, a form of tetrahydrofolate, as antidote.

Purine- and pyrimidine analogs are characterized by modifications of the normal base or sugar moieties. The uridine analog 5-fluorouracil is converted intracellularly into fluorouridine-mono-phosphate (FUMP) and fluorodeoxyuridine-monophosphate (FdUMP). Further phosphoryla-tion leads to the respective triphosphates FUTP and FdUTP. FdUMP inhibits the enzyme thymidi-late synthase and thus blocks the generation of thymidine, whereas FUTP and FdUTP are incor-porated into RNA and DNA, respectively. Gemcit-abine is a cytosine analog in which the pentose moiety contains two fluorine atoms at position 2 of the sugar ring. This drug is converted into the respective diphosphate, which inhibits ribonucle-otide reductase, and the triphosphate, which after incorporation into DNA causes masked termina-tion of DNA chain elongation since the altered base sequence cannot be efficiently repaired. Cyto-sine arabinoside is a cytosine analog with a 'wrong' pentose that after phosphorylation to the respective triphosphate inhibits DNA polymerase. The purine analogs mercaptopurine and fludarab-ine are converted into fraudulent nucleotides and inhibit DNA polymerase. The main unwanted effects are gastrointestinal epithelial cell damage and myelotoxicity.

Cytotoxic Antibiotics

Cytotoxic antibiotics affect normal nucleic acid function by intercalating between DNA bases, which blocks reading of the DNA template and also stimulates ▶ topoisomerase II dependent DNA-double strand breaks. In addition, metabo-lism of the drugs gives rise to free radicals that cause cytotoxicity by affecting two main targets: They damage DNA and injure membranes by direct interaction or via oxidative damage. Cyto-toxic antibiotics are poorly absorbed from the gut and therefore are given intravenously. They have long half-lives (1–2 days), and are eliminated by metabolism.

Anthracyclins (e.g. doxorubicin, epirubicin, and idarubicin) are the most important subgroup. They consist of a four-ringed planar quinone structure attached to an amino sugar group. In addition to the general unwanted effects, anthra-cyclins can cause cumulative, dose-related cardio-toxicity leading to heart failure and hair loss. Epi-rubicin is less cardiotoxic than doxorubicin.

Mitoxantrone has a three-ringed planar qui-none structure with amino-containing side chains and exerts dose-related cardiotoxicity and bone

marrow depression. Mitomycin C is a non-planar tricyclic quinone that is activated to give an alkylating metabolite. Bleomycins are metal-chelating glycopeptides that degrade DNA causing chain fragmentation and release of free bases. This subgroup causes little myelosuppression but pul-monary fibrosis, mucocutaneous reactions and hyperpyrexia. Actinomycin D (dactinomycin) is a chromopeptide that intercalates in the minor groove of DNA between adjacent guanosine/cyto-sine pairs and interferes with RNA polymerase, thus preventing transcription. Unwanted effects include nausea, vomiting and myelosuppression.

In general, the mechanisms of action are not cell cycle specific, although some members of the class show greatest activity at certain phases of the cell cycle, such as S-phase (anthracyclins, mitox-antrone), G1- and early S-phases (mitomycin C) and G2- and M-phases (bleomycins).

Plant Derivatives

Plant derivatives comprise several subgroups with diverse mechanisms of action.

Some are mitosis inhibitors that affect microtu-bule function and hence the formation of the mitotic spindle, others are topoisomerase I and II inhibitors.

Vinca alkaloids (vincristine, vinblastine, vindesine) are derived from the periwinkle plant (*Vinca rosea*); they bind to tubulin and inhibit its polymerisation into microtubules and spindle for-mation, thus producing metaphase arrest. They are cell cycle specific and interfere also with other cellular activities that involve microtubules, such as leukocyte phagocytosis, chemotaxis and axonal transport in neurons. Vincristine is mainly neuro-toxic and mildly hematotoxic, vinblastine is mye-losuppressive with very low neurotoxicity whereas vindesine has both moderate myelotoxicity and neurotoxicity.

Taxanes (paclitaxel, docetaxel) are derivatives of yew tree bark (*Taxus brevifolia*); they stabilize microtubules in the polymerized state leading to non-functional microtubular bundles in the cell. Inhibition occurs during G2- and M phases. Tax-anes are also radiosensitizers. Unwanted effects include bone marrow suppression and cumulative neurotoxicity.

Epipodophyllotoxins (etoposide, teniposide) are derived from mandrake root (*Podophyllum peltatum*); they inhibit topoisomerase II thus causing double-strand breaks. Cells in S- and G2-phases are most sensitive. Unwanted effects include nausea and vomiting, myelosuppression and hair loss.

Camptothecins (irinotecan, topotecan) are derived from the bark of the Chinese tree Xi Shu (*Camptotheca accuminata*); they inhibit topoisomerase I thus effecting double-strand breaks. Unwanted effects include diarrhea and reversible bone marrow depression.

Hormonal Agents

Tumors derived from hormone sensitive tissues can remain hormone dependent and are then amenable to therapeutic approaches with hormonal agents. These include hormones with opposing (apoptotic) action, hormone antagonists, and agents that inhibit hormone synthesis.

Glucocorticoids have inhibitory (apoptotic) effects on lymphocyte proliferation and are used to treat leukemias and lymphomas. Estrogens (fosfestrol) are used to block the effect of androgens in prostate cancer. Progestogens (megestrol, medroxyprogesteroneacetate) have been useful for treating endometrial carcinoma, renal tumors, and breast cancer.

Gonadotropin releasing hormone analogs (goserelin, buserelin, leuprorelin, triptorelin) inhibit gonadotropin release and thus lower testosterone or estrogen levels. They are used to treat breast cancer and prostate cancer.

Hormone antagonists (tamoxifen and toremifen bind to the estradiol receptor, flutamide binds to the androgen receptor) are used for treating breast and prostate cancer.

Aromatase inhibitors (aminogluthetimide, formestane, trilostane) block the formation of estrogens from precursor steroids and thus lower estrogen levels. They have been used for treating breast cancer.

Side effects are less prominent in type and extent as compared with cytostatics and include typical hormonal or lack of hormone-like effects.

Biological Response Modifiers

Agents that enhance the host's response against neoplasias or force them to differentiate are termed biological response modifiers. Examples include interleukin 2, which is used to treat renal cell carcinoma, interferon α, which is active against hematologic neoplasias, and tretinoin, which is a powerful inducer of differentiation in certain leukemia cells by acting on retinoid receptors. Side effects include influenza like symptoms, changes in blood pressure and edema.

Antibodies

Recombinant ▶ humanized monoclonal antibodies have been used recently to target antigens that are preferentially located on cancer cells. Examples include trastuzumab and rituximab, which are used to treat HER2 positive breast cancer and B-cell type lymphomas, respectively. Unwanted side effects include anaphylactic reactions.

Miscellaneous Agents

Antineoplastic agents that cannot be grouped under subheadings 1–7 include miltefosine, which is an alkylphosphocholine that is used to treat skin metastasis of breast cancer, and crispantase, which breaks down asparagine to aspartic acid and ammonia. It is active against tumor cells that lack the enzyme asparaginase, such as acute lymphoblastic leukemia cells. Side effects include irritation of the skin in the case of miltefosine and anaphylactic reactions in the case of crispantase.

Clinical Use

Cancer treatment is a multimodality treatment, i.e. surgery is combined with radiotherapy and antineoplastic chemotherapy. The latter treatment mode is used mainly for cancers that have disseminated. Different forms of cancer differ in their sensitivity to chemotherapy with antineoplastic agents. The most responsive include lymphomas, leukemias, choriocarcinoma and testicular carcinoma, while solid tumors such as colorectal, pancreatic and squamous cell bronchial carcinomas generally show a poor response. The clinical use of antineoplastic agents is characterized by the following principles.

1. The therapeutic ratio of antineoplastic agents, which is defined by the dose necessary to cause a significant anti-cancer effect divided by the dose effecting significant side effects, is generally low (near to one).
2. The intention to treat a cancer patient can vary between curative and palliative, pending on the

prognosis. Antineoplastic therapy with curative intention is based on high dosages and takes into account severe side effects that have to be tolerated by patients in order to receive the optimal treatment. Palliative therapy with cytotoxic agents aims at maximum life quality for a patient who cannot be cured. This includes palliation of symptoms like pain, fractures, and compression of vital tissues that are caused by cancer growth, but tries to accomplish this aim with dosages of cytostatics that bring about as few side effects as possible.

3. Generally, combination therapy with antineoplastic agents is superior to monotherapy. The reason is that several different mechanisms of action can be combined, thus lowering the risk of rapid induction of resistance, and the dosages of the single agents can be reduced. This, in turn, decreases the incidence in side effects caused by the single agents and, in addition, the side effects will not sum up if the respective toxicity profiles differ from each other.

4. To be successful antineoplastic therapy often has to be applied for considerable periods of time. The initial therapy period is being termed 'induction therapy' which is then followed by a 'maintenance therapy' and possibly a 're-induction therapy'.

5. The therapeutic success is measured by its effect on tumor size and can be described as tumor remission (complete or partial), stable disease, or progression of the tumor. Also, the impact of a therapy is related to time and can be measured as disease-free interval, time to progress, or overall survival time.

6. Patients receiving cytotoxic chemotherapy very often need concomitant administrating of antiemetic therapy. Such protocols start well in advance of administering the cytotoxic agent, and last for a reasonable time with regard to pharmacokinetics of the antineoplastic agent. In addition, side effects of antineoplastic therapy are made better tolerable by supportive care.

7. Few side effects can be alleviated by the use of antidotes. An example is the prevention of hemorrhagic cystitis caused by cyclophosphamide by the concomitant infusion of mesna.

References

1. DeVita VT, Hellman S, Rosenberg SA (2001) Cancer, Principles & Practice of Oncology, Lippincott Williams & Wilkins, Philadelphia
2. Forth, Henschler, Rummel (2001) Allgemeine und spezielle Pharmakologie und Toxikologie, Urban & Fischer, München

Anti Obesity Drugs

CHRISTINE HUPPERTZ
Cardiovascular and Metabolic Diseases, Novartis Pharma AG, Basel, Switzerland
christine.huppertz@pharma.novartis.com

Synonyms

None (appetite suppressants are only a subgroup of anti obesity drugs)

Definition

Obesity is defined as excess adiposity (fat mass) for a given body size. The definition is based on an approximation of body fat - the body mass index (BMI), measured as body weight in kilograms divided by the squared height in metres (kg/m²). A BMI of 30 or more is a commonly-used criterion for defining obesity in both sexes, individuals with a BMI between 25 and 30 are considered overweight. Obesity develops when energy intake exceeds expenditure over a prolonged period of time. The prevalence of obesity in industrialised countries is approximately 20–25% of the adult population. It is frequently associated with other diseases such as arterial hypertension (high blood pressure) and type 2 diabetes (▶ Diabesity), which makes it a major health issue. For a drug to have a significant impact on body weight it must ultimately either reduce energy intake, increase energy expenditure, or both. Anti-obesity drugs should be taken in conjunction with a low calorie diet and exercise and may be part of a sequential or combined treatment to circumvent or reduce compensatory mechanisms. Anti obesity drugs should induce weight loss as reduced fat mass, and should help to maintain the reduced weight, thereby reducing the risk of obesity-associated co-morbidities.

▶ Appetite Control
▶ Diabetes Mellitus

Mechanism of Action

When energy intake chronically exceeds expenditure, even a slight daily energy gain results in obesity. Excess energy is stored in the high caloric form of triglycerides. Environmental factors, such as the general availability of high calorie food or the limited need for physical exercise, and genetic factors that evolved to increase energy efficiency (▶ Thrifty Gene Hypothesis) contribute to the development of obesity.

Energy balance is regulated through a complex feedback loop between peripheral fat depots and the brain in which the hormone ▶ leptin plays an essential role (Fig. 1) (1,2). Leptin is produced by white adipose tissue (WAT) in proportion to adipocyte size and number and is secreted into the blood. It crosses the blood brain barrier via a saturable transport system and reaches its receptors in the ▶ hypothalamus, the brain region that is critical for regulation of energy homeostasis. Stimulation of leptin receptors initiates a signaling cascade that ultimately affects energy homeostasis by affecting feeding behaviour, neuroendocrine and reproductive functions. Feeding behaviour, i.e. meal size and frequency, is in addition regulated by a short-term feedback loop in which afferent signals originating in the oral cavity and the gastrointestinal (GI) tract during and after a meal are transmitted to a region in the hindbrain. This brain region communicates with higher brain areas such as the hypothalamus and the cerebral cortex where the various signals are integrated. Body weight is thus regulated in a complex manner involving feeding behaviour, control mechanisms of digestion, absorption, energy metabolism, expenditure and storage.

Reduction of Energy Intake: Appetite Suppression
There is a complex network of various neuropeptides, monoamines and their respective receptors in the hypothalamus to control food intake and metabolism.

The hypothalamic neuropeptides affecting food intake include α-melanocyte stimulating hormone (α-MSH), a melanocortin produced by cleavage of pro-opiomelanocortin (POMC), which exerts anorectic (food intake-reducing) effects via stimulation of the melanocortin 4 receptor (MC4R), a G protein-coupled receptor that is expressed in various brain regions including the hypothalamus. Agouti-related protein (AGRP) antagonises the effects of α-MSH at MC4R, thus having orexigenic effects. The importance of melanocortinergic pathways in the regulation of body weight has been demonstrated by genetic studies in obese mice and obese humans. Neuropeptide Y (NPY) is assumed to mediate its strong orexigenic effects through the G protein-coupled receptors Y1R, Y5R and possibly additional subtypes. The neuropeptides mentioned above are expressed in so-called first-order neurons, as they are regulated directly by leptin. Elevated leptin levels reflecting increased energy stores stimulate the expression of the anorexigens POMC/ α-MSH and cocaine- and amphetamine-regulated transcript (CART), which are co-expressed in one population of hypothalamic neurons, and decrease the expression of the orexigens NPY and AGRP, which are co-expressed in a distinct neuron population. These peptides are thereby regulated by leptin in a concerted manner to maintain a steady body weight. It is generally agreed that neuropeptides further downstream from leptin include galanin, melanin concentrating hormone (MCH) and the orexins (also termed hypocretins), which all exert orexigenic effects. New genes and new findings with known peptides or hormones such as ghrelin and insulin are constantly being added to the list of anorectic or orexigenic pathways. Their importance is as yet unclear, but they could change the current view of the complex pathways involved in energy homeostasis.

The neural circuits regulating feeding may also be influenced directly by a sensor of metabolic fuels in the brain. This hypothesis was recently raised again, based on the findings suggesting that inhibitors of fatty acid synthase inhibited food intake through actions in the brain, presumably via increased levels of the substrate of fatty acid synthase, malonyl CoA.

A

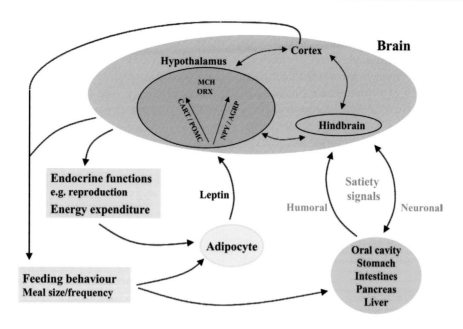

Fig. 1 Regulation of feeding behaviour and fat stores by central and peripheral pathways. Leptin is secreted by adipocytes and circulates to the brain, where it binds to its receptors in the hypothalamus. Here a cascade is initiated that ultimately regulates food intake, various endocrine systems, and (at least in rodents) energy expenditure. Elevated leptin levels reflecting increased energy stores downregulate the expression of the orexigenic peptides neuropeptide Y (NPY) and agouti-related protein (AGRP), which are co-localized in a population of neurons, and stimulate the expression of the anorexigenic peptides pro-opiomelanocortin (POMC) and cocaine- and amphetamine-regulated transcript (CART), which are co-localized in a different neuron population. These neurons project further to other brain centres which ultimately communicate with the cerebral cortex, where feeding behaviour is finally coordinated. The level of food intake will in turn affect fat depots, thus completing the feedback loop between the CNS and the periphery. Feeding behaviour, defined by frequency and size of meals, is in addition regulated in a short-term loop. During and after a meal, various signals are generated in the periphery including taste signals from the oral cavity, gastric distension and humoral signals (e.g. cholecystokinin) from secretory cells of the gastrointestinal (GI) tract. These afferent signals are transmitted mainly by the vagus nerve to the hindbrain. This brain region communicates with higher brain areas such as the hypothalamus and the cerebral cortex. MCH, melanin concentrating hormone, ORX orexins.

In response to a meal, peripheral signals are generated in the GI tract to serve as satiety factor. The onset of satiety is a response to neural and humoral factors, such as gut distension and release of the gut peptide cholecystokinin (CCK). In addition, some peptides can modulate nutrient absorption and passage through the GI tract, including regulation of the autonomic nervous system. Glucagon-like peptide 1 (GLP-1), which is processed from proglucagon in the pancreas, intestinal cells and in the CNS, presumably regulates feeding by both delaying gastric emptying and suppressing food intake. A recent paper describes anorectic effects of a related peptide, GLP-2.

Reduction of Energy Intake: Inhibition of Absorption

Inhibition of the absorption of fat represents the most efficient approach for reduction of caloric intake. In the intestine, triglycerides are split into free fatty acids (FFAs) and monoglycerides by lipases, the targets for orlistat (see below). After hydrolysis, FFAs cross the membranes of the epithelial cells lining the intestinal wall. Once inside the epithelial cell, FFAs are donated to acyl-CoA synthetase in the endoplasmic reticulum by fatty acid-binding proteins (FABPs). Acyl-CoA is then transferred to 2-monoacylglycerol to resynthesize triglycerides. Acyl CoA:diacylglycerol acyltransferase (DGAT) is a key enzyme responsible for the final step in the glycerol phosphate pathway of triglyceride synthesis. The absorption of dietary fat involves several steps catalysed by proteins that might represent promising drug targets.

Increase of Energy Expenditure

Energy expenditure includes three main components: a) basal metabolism, i.e. the constant intracellular processes necessary to sustain life, b) physical activity and c) adaptive thermogenesis, i.e. energy dissipated in the form of heat in response to environmental changes, such as exposure to cold and alterations in diet (3). The stimulation of thermogenesis has raised much interest as a possible mechanism to treat obesity, especially once the mitochondrial uncoupling proteins (UCPs) were identified (4). UCP1 is selectively expressed in brown adipose tissue (BAT), which is the major site of thermogenesis in rodents. Activation of the sympathetic nervous system in response to cold stress or high fat diet activates β3-adrenoreceptors of the BAT, resulting in increased cAMP levels and stimulation of protein kinase A (PKA). PKA phosphorylates and activates hormone-sensitive lipase, thereby promoting the release of free fatty acids. These serve both as fuel for mitochondrial respiration and as activators of UCP1. UCP1 dissipates the transmembrane proton gradient coupled to the oxidation of metabolites, releasing energy as heat. In addition, there is a chronic response, i.e. UCP1 is transcriptionally upregulated, and mitochondrial biogenesis is stimulated through mechanisms involving a transcriptional coactivator of the nuclear peroxisome proliferator-activated receptor-γ (PPARγ), with the acronym PGC-1 (PPARγ coactivator-1). In adult humans, BAT is present in only very small amounts, the major thermogenic tissue being skeletal muscle. Since UCP3 is expressed almost exclusively in skeletal muscle in higher mammals, the selective stimulation of UCP3 may be a challenging target for obesity treatment.

Modulation of Fat Storage

Processes involved in the storage of fat, including adipocyte differentiation, angiogenesis or apopto-

sis, could also be targeted as a way to reduce fat mass. Adipocyte differentiation includes various steps, i.e. initial commitment of mesenchymal stem cells to preadipocytes, the proliferation of preadipocytes, a step in which HMGI-C (high-mobility group (HMG) I-type protein) appears to play a critical role, and the final differentiation program. The transcription factor and nuclear hormone receptor PPARγ can control adipocyte differentiation and cross-regulation between and PPARγ and C/EBPα- (CAAT/enhancing binding proteins) is required to maintain the differentiated state of the adipocyte. Once the mature adipocyte has been formed, the amount of stored lipid can be modulated through lipogenesis or lipolysis, where perilipin seems to come into play. However, all these potential approaches to reduce the ability to synthesize or store fat will be safe only if associated with an increase in fat oxidation and/or with a reduction of fat absorption. Otherwise, the inability to deliver excess calories to adipose tissue could have serious secondary consequences as lipids accumulate in the blood or various organs.

A safer anti-obesity approach could be the stimulation of BAT (rich in mitochondria and UCP-1, highly developed in rodents for thermogenesis) formation in man, involving either *de novo* recruitment from preadipocytes or interconversion of white adipose tissue, which is the major site for triglyceride storage.

Clinical Use (incl. side effects)

Obesity treatment aims at a sustained loss of 5–10% of body weight, which has been shown to reduce the risk of obesity-associated co-morbidities such as hypertension and diabetes. Since body fat is likely to be regulated homeostatically, a change in either intake or expenditure alone will face resistance as compensatory adjustments are made. It is possible that combined drug therapy will solve this problem.

At present, only sibutramine, an appetite suppressant, and orlistat, an inhibitor of fat absorption, are approved anti-obesity drugs for long-term (12 months) treatment. All other drugs for obesity treatment are approved for short-term use only and are either catecholaminergic or serotonergic CNS-active (activating the sympathetic nervous system) anorectic agents (e.g. phentermine).

Sibutramine

Sibutramine, a CNS active appetite suppressant, exerts its effects by acting as a norephinephrine, serotonin and dopamine reuptake inhibitor. It is taken in combination with a reduced-calorie diet. Sibutramine is contra-indicated in patients with poorly controlled hypertension and patients with a history of cardiovascular heart disease.

Orlistat

Orlistat is taken with meals since the mechanism of action is to reduce the absorption of fatty acids by inhibition of triglyceride hydrolysis through its action as a gastric and pancreatic lipase inhibitor. Orlistat represents an overall safe treatment for obesity, given that the drug is minimally absorbed. Side effects of orlistat include malabsorption of fat-soluble vitamins and steatorrhea (fatty stools).

Comment on the First Leptin Trials

Leptin has proved to be an efficient treatment for the rare form of obesity associated with leptin deficiency. By contrast, the results of the first clinical trial with human leptin in obese patients (without leptin deficiency) were less promising. This may be explained by the hypothesis that the leptin system evolved as a mechanism to protect against starvation and that the hormone plays its physiological role only at low plasma concentrations. Therefore only little can be gained from increasing leptin levels above normal. Furthermore, the fact that obese patients still overeat despite high plasma leptin concentrations suggests that they are resistant to leptin.

References

1. Chiesi M, Huppertz C, Hofbauer KG (2001) Pharmacotherapy of obesity: targets and perspectives. Trends Pharmacol Sci 22(5):247–254
2. Spiegelman BM, Flier JS (2001) Obesity and the regulation of energy balance. Cell 104:531–543
3. Lowell BB, Spiegelman BM (2000) Towards a molecular understanding of adaptive thermogenesis. Nature 404:652–660
4. Crowley V, Vidal-Puig AJ (2001) Mitochondrial uncoupling proteins (UCPs) and obesity. Nutr Metab Cardiovasc Dis 11(1):70–75

Antiparasitic Drugs

Antiparasitic drugs are used for the treatment of parasitic infections caused by pathogenic protozoa or helminths (worms).
Antihelmintic Drugs

▶ Antiprotozoal Drugs

Anti-parkinson Drugs

T.J. FEUERSTEIN, G. NIKKHAH
Neurozentrum, Freiburg, Germany
feuer@ukl.uni-freiburg.de;
nikkhah@nz.ukl.uni-freiburg.de

Synonyms

Antiparkinsonian drugs

Definition

Parkinsonism is a clinical syndrome comprising ▶ bradykinesia, muscular ▶ rigidity, ▶ resting tremor and impairment of postural balance. The pathological hallmark of Parkinson's disease is a loss of more than 60–70% of pigmented dopaminergic neurons of the substantia nigra pars compacta with the appearance of intracellular inclusions known as ▶ Lewy bodies. Without treatment, idiopathic Parkinson's disease progresses over 5 to 10 years to a rigid, akinetic state leading to complications of immobility, e.g. pneumonia and pulmonary embolism. The distinction between Parkinson's disease and other causes of parkinsonism is important because parkinsonism arising from other causes is usually more refractory to treatment with antiparkinsonian drugs.

▶ Dopamine System

Mechanisms of Action

Pathophysiology

The primary deficit in Parkinson's disease is a loss of dopaminergic neurons in the substantia nigra pars compacta and a corresponding loss of dopaminergic innervation of the caudate nucleus and the putamen (forming the striatum). This suggests that replacement of dopamine could restore function. Physiologically, dopamine is synthesized from tyrosine in terminals of nigrostriatal neurons by the sequential action of the enzymes tyrosine hydroxylase, yielding the intermediary L-dihydroxyphenylalanin (L-DOPA), and aromatic L-amino acid decarboxylase (the corresponding prodrug L-DOPA is the most effective agent in the treatment of Parkinson's disease, see below.). The subsequent uptake and storage of synthesized dopamine in vesicles is blocked by reserpine, an earlier antipsychotic drug and admixture to anti-hypertensive medicines, which is known to induce parkinsonism. Release of dopamine is triggered by depolarization leading to entry of Ca^{2+} and ▶ exocytosis. The (pre- and) postsynaptic actions of dopamine are mediated by two types of dopamine receptors, both of which are seven-transmembrane-region receptors. The D_1-receptor-family (consisting of D_1 and D_5 receptors) stimulates the synthesis of intracellular cAMP and phosphatidyl inositol hydrolysis, the D_2-receptor-family (D_2, D_3 and D_4 receptors) inhibits cAMP synthesis and modulates K^+ and Ca^{2+} channels. D_1 and D_2 proteins are abundant in the striatum; striatal D_3 expression is rather low. Most ▶ antipsychotics block D_2 receptors and may lead to the adverse event of parkinsonism.

The following model of basal ganglia function accounts for the Parkinson syndrome as a result of diminished dopaminergic neurotransmission in the striatum (Fig.). The basal ganglia modulate the flow of information from the neocortex to the motoneurons in the spinal cord. The striatum receives excitatory glutamatergic input from the neocortex (red solid arrows). The majority of striatal neurons are projection neurons to other basal ganglia nuclei (blue GABAergic neurons) and a small subgroup are interneurons that interconnect neurons within the striatum (yellow cholinergic neurons). Nigrostriatal dopaminergic neurons (green) innervate GABAergic neurons (blue, 2, 3) and cholinergic interneurons (yellow, 1). The outflow of the striatum proceeds as the direct and the indirect pathway. The direct pathway projects directly to the output stages of the basal ganglia, the substantia nigra pars reticulata and the globus pallidus medialis, which contain GABAergic neurons (blue). These in turn relay to the thalamus, which provides excitatory input to the neocortex (red broken arrows). Since two inhibitory GABAergic neurons are arranged successively, the stimulation of the direct pathway at the level of the striatum (by glutamatergic corticostriatal afferents or via 2) results in an increased excitatory outflow from the thalamus to the neocortex. The opposite effect, i.e. a decreased excitatory outflow from the thalamus, is the result when the stimulation of the first chain link of the direct pathway, GABAergic neurons in the striatum, is abolished.

This is the case when the excitatory D_1 receptors on these striatal GABAergic projection neurons are no longer activated since the transmitter dopamine is reduced (green broken arrows at 2). The indirect pathway is composed of striatal GABAergic neurons (blue) that project to the globus pallidus lateralis (to blue GABAergic neurons). This inhibitory structure in turn innervates glutamatergic neurons of the subthalamic nucleus (red) to diminish the excitation of subthalamic neurons. The subthalamic nucleus provides excitatory glutamatergic outflow to the output stage, i.e., to GABAergic neurons (blue) of the substantia nigra pars reticulata and the globus pallidus medialis. Thus, the net effect of stimulating the indirect pathway at the level of the striatum is to reduce the excitatory outflow from the thalamus to the neocortex. Striatal neurons forming the indirect pathway express inhibitory D_2 receptors (3 in the Fig.), counteracting the excitation through glutamatergic corticostriatal afferents. Thus, dopamine released in the striatum reduces the activity of the indirect pathway through D_2 receptors, but increases the activity of the direct pathway through D_1 receptors. A reduced dopaminergic neurotransmission in the striatum (depicted as green broken line) ultimately reduces the thalamic excitation of the motor cortex.

What is the reason for the rather selective degeneration of nigrostriatal dopaminergic neurons in Parkinson's disease? Apart from their oxidative metabolism leading to the production of reactive compounds as in every cell (hydrogen peroxide, superoxide anion radical), dopaminergic neurons seem to be additionally compromised by an extra accumulation of hydrogen peroxide due to the metabolic conversion of dopamine to 3,4-dihydroxyphenylacetaldehyde (DOPAL) plus hydrogen peroxide by the enzyme monoamine oxidase (MAO) (4). In the presence of ferrous iron hydrogen peroxide undergoes spontaneous conversion (Fenton reaction), forming a hydroxyl free radical, one of the most risky species of all reactive compounds. Levels of iron are high in the substantia nigra; whether the excess iron exists in a form capable of participation in redox chemistry, however, is unclear. In addition, the increase in iron occurs only in the advanced stages of Parkinson's disease suggesting that this increase may be a secondary, rather than a primary initiating event (2). Despite this objection, hydroxyl free radicals are generated from hydrogen peroxide without the catalytic help of ferrous iron in the presence of DOPAL: Thus, the one MAO product, DOPAL, is a cofactor in the generation of the hydroxyl radical from the other MAO product, hydrogen peroxide, which is also produced enzymatically by superoxide dismutase from the superoxide anion radical. Since MAO is located on the outer mitochondrial membrane adjacent to the free radical sensitive permeability transition pore, its products including the hydroxyl free radical may function as cell death messengers leading to ▶ apoptosis. Apart from this local mechanism, reactive oxygen species can lead to DNA damage, peroxydation of membrane lipids, and neuronal death. Because parkinsonian brains are free of pathological sign of necrosis, apoptosis is the likely or predominant mechanism for death of nigrostriatal dopamine neurons.

Neuromelanin, a dark coloured pigment and product of the oxidative metabolism of dopamine, is found in the cytoplasm of dopaminergic neurons of the human substantia nigra pars compacta (for review see 6,7). Neuromelanin deposits increase with age, matching the age distribution of Parkinson's disease. Neuromelanin functions as a redox polymer and may promote the formation of reactive oxygen free radicals, especially in the presence of iron that accumulates in neuromelanin. However, as stated above, iron accumulation occurs mainly in later stages of the disease. In the

absence of significant quantities of iron, neuromelanin can act as an antioxidant in that it can interact with and inactivate free radicals. Thus, it is unclear at present whether neuromelanin has a more protective or more destructive impact on dopaminergic neurons of the substantia nigra compacta.

A genetic defect of complex I of the mitochondrial respiratory chain has been demonstrated specifically for the substantia nigra in Parkinson's disease. This finding matches the observation that the neurotoxin 1-methyl-4-phenyl-1,2,3,6-tetrahydropyridine (MPTP), which causes a Parkinson-like syndrome in humans, acts via inhibition of complex I by its neurotoxic metabolite 1-methyl-4-phenylpyridine (MPP$^+$), thus destroying dopaminergic neurons in the substantia nigra. Despite this obvious specificity, the question arises whether dopaminergic neurons are more vulnerable to this mitochondrial deficit *per se* compared with other neurons and whether there is differential vulnerability to complex I inhibition within the dopaminergic midbrain population. In addition, which are the death transducers of mitochondrial dysfunction? Apart from increased accumulation of reactive oxygen species and their functional consequences (see above) due to defective mitochondria, dopaminergic neurons express alternative types of ▶ K_{ATP} channels in the plasma membrane. The channels mediate their differential response to mitochondrial complex I inhibition; that is opening of K_{ATP} channels due to a diminished ATP/ADP ratio. Thus, a subpopulation of dopaminergic neurons might tonically hyperpolarize and reduce their physiological spontaneous activity as a neuroprotective response whereas other dopaminergic neurons, expressing other types of K_{ATP} channels, may not survive.

Symptomatic Drug Therapy and Curative Treatments of the Future

While advances in the symptomatic drug therapy (summarized in the next paragraph) have certainly improved the lives of many Parkinson patients, the goal of current research is to develop treatments that can prevent, retard or reverse the death of dopaminergic neurons in the substantia nigra pars compacta (and of other neurons involved in the pathogenesis of Parkinson's disease

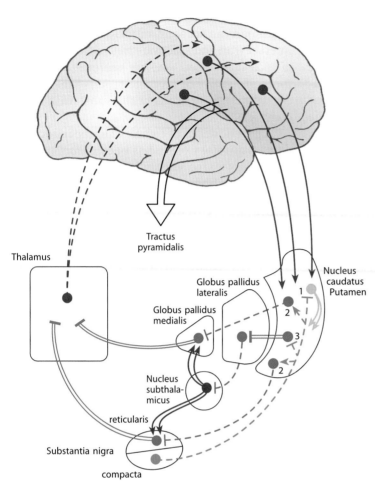

Fig. 1 **Extrapyramidal wiring diagram of the basal ganglia in Parkinson's disease.** Arrow heads: activation; arrow beams: inhibition; solid lines: normal neurotransmission; double lines: increased neurotransmission; broken lines, diminished neurotransmission; red: glutamate excitatory; blue: GABA inhibitory; green: dopamine excitatory (D_1 receptors, 2) and inhibitory (D_2 receptors, 1, 3); yellow: acetylcholine. (from Feuerstein TJ. Antiparkinsonmittel, Pharmakotherapie des Morbus Parkinson. In: 7).

not mentioned in this essay; see 3 for further details).

In view of the pathophysiological aspects of dopaminergic cell death as discussed above, the following future therapies seem conceivable:

Pharmacological reduction of oxidative stress or prevention of iron load seems feasible, despite disappointing results of clinical trials with the free radical scavenger tocopherol and the MAO inhibitor selegiline (see below).

Antiapoptotic strategies, e.g. caspase inhibitors, may develop into more causal drug therapies of the future. Also neural growth factors are an important area for drug development.

The above mentioned role of K_{ATP} channels of nigral dopaminergic neurons supports the idea of K_{ATP} channel activation as a novel neuroprotective strategy in the early stages of Parkinson's disease.

Clinical Use (incl. side effects)

The therapeutic and adverse effects of L-DOPA result from its intracerebral decarboxylation to dopamine. Oral L-DOPA is rapidly absorbed by the intestinal active transport system for aromatic amino acids, where dietary amino acids may act as competitors. The same is true at the corresponding aromatic amino acid carrier of the blood-brain-barrier. L-DOPA is usually coadministered with a peripherally acting inhibitor of aromatic L-amino acid decarboxylase (benserazide, carbidopa) that prevents (dopamine-induced) nausea and vomiting, cardiac arhythmias and orthostatic hypotension, and increases the fraction of L-DOPA that remains unmetabolized and available to cross the blood-brain-barrier. Entacapone is a selective inhibitor of catechol-O-methyltransferase whose activity is primarily in the peripheral nervous system. Entacapone further increases the fraction of L-DOPA crossing the blood-brain-barrier and thus prolongs its action and reduces fluctuations in response. In early Parkinson's disease, when some buffering capacity of remaining striatal dopaminergic nerve terminals is still present, the degree of motor improvement due to L-DOPA is highest (7). With time, however, the patient's motor state may fluctuate dramatically with each drug dose. Increasing the frequency of administration can improve this situation, while increasing the L-DOPA dose may induce dyskinesias, i.e. excessive and abnormal involuntary movements (1). In view of the above mentioned dopamine autotoxicity, might L-DOPA accelerate the disease progression? Although no convincing evidence for such an effect has yet been obtained, a pragmatic therapeutic approach may be appropriate, i.e. to use L-DOPA only when required by a functional impairment of the patient not otherwise treatable.

Alternatives to L-DOPA are direct agonists of striatal dopamine receptors (e.g. pergolide, cabergoline) that are not metabolized in a manner that leads to increased free radical formation. Their use may reduce endogenous release of dopamine and the need for exogenous L-DOPA, possibly with the consequence of a delay in the progression of the disease. At present, however, there are no clinical data to support a neuroprotective effect of dopamine receptor agonists. In contrast to the prodrug L-DOPA, these agonists do not depend on the functional capacities of nigrostriatal nerve terminals, which may be advantageous in late stage Parkinson's disease where L-DOPA-induced fluctuations are frequent. In addition, clinically used dopamine agonists have durations of action substantially longer than L-DOPA. However, despite these pharmacokinetic advantages, the clinical efficacy of the currently available agonists that preferentially activate dopamine D_2 receptors is less than that of L-DOPA. Due to their peripheral activity, dopamine receptor agonists may cause orthostatic hypotension and nausea. Typical central adverse events in elderly patients are hallucinosis or confusion, similar to that observed with L-DOPA.

The mode of action of selegiline, which slightly improves parkinsonian symptoms, is unclear. At clinically used doses it inhibits the MAO-B isoenzyme whereas MAO-A prevails in dopaminergic terminals. Selegiline is metabolized to (-)-desmethyldeprenyl, which seems to be the active principle in its antiapoptotic effects in animal models, and further to (-)-amphetamine and (-)-methamphetamine, which antagonize its rescuing effects. The (-)-amphetamines release biogenic amines including dopamine from their storage sites in nerve terminals, although with less potency than their (+)-enantiomers. This may partly explain the symptomatic relief seen with selegiline. Developmental drugs, structurally related to selegiline which exhibit virtually no MAO-B or MAO-A inhibiting properties and which are not further metabolized to amphetamines, show neurorescuing properties that are qualitatively similar, but about 100-fold more potent compared to those of selegiline. Glyceraldehyde-3-phosphate dehydrogenase, a glycolytic enzyme with multiple other functions including an involvement in apoptosis, seems to be the molecular target for these neuroprotective selegiline-related drugs of the future.

Antagonists of muscarinic acetylcholine receptors were widely used since 1860 for the treatment of Parkinson's disease before the discovery of L-DOPA. They block receptors that mediate the response to striatal cholinergic interneurons. The antiparkinsonian effects of drugs like benzatropine, trihexyphenidyl and biperiden are moderate; the resting tremor may sometimes respond in a favorable manner. The adverse effects, e.g. constipation, urinary retention and mental confusion, may be troublesome, especially in the elderly.

Low affinity use-dependent NMDA receptor antagonists meet the criteria for safe administration into patients. Drugs like amantadine and memantine have modest effects on Parkinson's disease and are used as initial therapy or as adjunct to L-DOPA. Their adverse effects include dizziness, lethargy and sleep disturbance.

References

1. Bezard E, Brotchie JM, Gross CE (2001) Pathophysiology of Levodopa-induced dyskinesias: potential for new therapies. Nat Rev Neurosci 2:577–588
2. Double KL, Gerlach M, Youdim MB, Riederer P (2000) Impaired iron homeostasis in Parkinson's disease. J Neural Transm Suppl 60:37–58

3. Dunnett SB, Björklund (1999) Prospects for new restorative and neuroprotective treatments in Parkinson's disease. Nature 24;399:32–39

4. Foley P, Riederer P (1999) Pathogenesis and preclinical course of Parkinson's disease. J Neural Transm Suppl 56:31–74

5. Forth W, Henschler D, Rummel W, Förstermann U, Starke K, eds. Allgemeine und spezielle Pharmakologie und Toxikologie. Urban & Fischer, pp 327-333, 2001

6. Lang AE, Lozano AM (1998a) Pakinson's disease. First of two parts. New Eng J Med 339:1044–1053

7. Lang AE, Lozano AM (1998b) Parkinson's disease. Second of two parts. New Engl J Med 339:1130–1143

Antiplatelet Drugs

STEFAN OFFERMANNS
Pharmakologisches Institut, Universität Heidelberg, Heidelberg, Germany
Stefan.Offermanns@urz.uni-heidelberg.de

Synonyms

Platelet inhibitors, platelet aggregation inhibitors

Definition

Platelets play a central role in ▶ primary hemostasis. They are also important in pathological processes leading to ▶ thrombosis. Antiplatelet drugs are primarily directed against platelets and inhibit platelet activation by a number of different mechanisms. They are used for the prevention and treatment of thrombotic processes, especially in the arterial vascular system.

▶ Anticoagulants
▶ Anti-integrins, therapeutic and diagnostic implications
▶ Coagulation/Thrombosis

Mechanism of action

Antiplatelet therapy is an important means in the prevention and treatment of thromboembolic artery occlusions in cardiovascular diseases. Platelets are discoid cell fragments, derived from megakaryocytes in the bone marrow, that circulate freely in the blood. Under normal conditions they neither adhere to each other nor to other cellular surfaces. However, when blood vessels are damaged at their luminal side, platelets adhere to the exposed subendothelium. This adhesion is mediated by ▶ collagen and ▶ von Willebrand factor (vWf) both of which are exposed at or have been deposited at the subendothelial surface. Adherent platelets release various factors (see below) that activate other nearby platelets resulting in the recruitment of more platelets at the site of vascular injury.

Initially, activated platelets change their shape, an event immediately followed by the secretion of platelet granule contents (including ADP, ▶ fibrinogen and serotonin) as well as by platelet aggregation. Aggregation of platelets is mediated

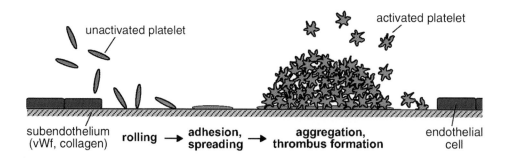

Fig. 1 Platelet adhesion, activation, aggregation and thrombus formation on subendothelial surface at an injured blood vessel. VWf, von Willebrand factor deposited at subendothelial surface.

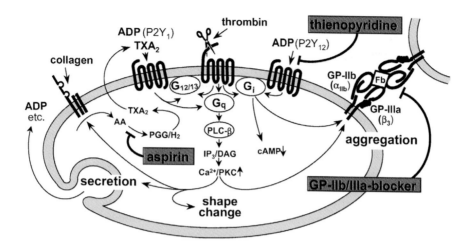

Fig. 2 Mechanisms of platelet activation, together with sites of drug action. Most platelet activators function directly or indirectly through G-protein coupled receptors and induce several intracellular signalling pathways that eventually lead to secretion of granule contents, change of shape, and inside-out activation of GP-IIb/IIIa (integrin $\alpha_{IIb}\beta_3$). Activation of GP-IIb/IIIa allows fibrinogen (Fb) or vWf to cross bridge adjacent platelets. The main pathway that leads to platelet activation involves the G_q/phospholipase C-β (PLC-β)-mediated formation of inositol 1,4,5 trisphosphate (IP_3) and diacyl glycerol (DAG). This in turn results in the release of Ca^{2+} from intracellular stores and the activation of protein kinase C (PKC) isoforms. Aspirin blocks the conversion of arachidonic acid (AA) to prostaglandin G_2 and H_2 (PGG/H_2) by irreversibly inhibiting cyclo-oxygenase-1. Active metabolites of thienopyridines block ADP(P_2Y_{12})-receptors on platelets and GPIIb/IIIa-blockers interfere with fibrinogen- and vWf-mediated platelet aggregation. TXA_2 stands for thromboxane A_2.

by fibrinogen or vWf. They connect platelets by bridging complexes of glycoprotein IIb/IIIa (▶ integrin $\alpha_{IIb}\beta_3$) on adjacent platelets, forming a platelet aggregate. Each platelet contains about 50,000 to 80,000 glycoprotein IIb/IIIa (GP-IIb/IIIa) molecules on its surface. In order to bind fibrinogen and ▶ vWf, GP-IIb/IIIa has to be converted from a low affinity/avidity state to a high affinity/avidity state by a process described as inside-out signalling that is initiated during platelet activation (Fig. 1). The rapid formation of a 'platelet plug' at sites of vascular injury is the main mechanism of primary hemostasis. This is followed by a strengthening of the primary thrombus due to the formation of fibrin fibrils by the coagulation cascade. Platelets also play an important role in pathological conditions since they can become activated on ruptured atherosclerotic plaques or in regions of disturbed blood flow. This in turn leads to thromboembolic complications that underlie common diseases such as myocardial infarction or thrombotic stroke.

Among the main stimuli able to induce full platelet activation, including shape change, secretion and aggregation, are collagen, thrombin, ADP and thromboxane A_2 (TXA_2). Collagen acts primarily through integrin $\alpha_2\beta_1$ and glycoprotein VI, whereas thrombin, ADP and thromboxane A_2 (TXA_2) function through heptahelical, ▶ G-protein-coupled receptors (Fig. 2).

TXA_2 is produced by activated platelets by the sequential conversion of arachidonic acid by phospholipase A_2, ▶ cyclooxygenase-1 (COX-1) and thromboxane synthase. Similar to ADP, TXA_2 acts as a positive feedback mediator. In vascular endothelial cells, COX-1 is involved in the generation of prostacyclin, which inhibits platelet activation and leads to vasodilation. Low doses of acetylsalicylic acid (aspirin) have an antiplatelet effect by inhibiting the TXA_2 production by irreversibly acetylating COX-1 at serine-530 close to the active site of the enzyme. This results in impaired platelet function for the rest of its lifespan (7–10 days). Anucleated platelets, in contrast to nucleated cells, are unable to *de novo* synthesize COX-1. The aspirin doses required for this antiplatelet effect are therefore considerably lower than those necessary to achieve inhibition of prostacyclin formation in endothelial cells or analgetic and antipyretic effects. Following oral administration of aspirin, platelets are exposed to a relatively high concentration of aspirin in the portal blood. This may further contribute to the relatively high sensitivity of platelets toward the action of aspirin. Most other tissues are partly protected by presystemic metabolisation of aspirin to salicylate through esterases in the liver. Since platelets are the major source of TXA_2 production and action, inhibitors of thromboxane synthase and TXA_2 receptor (TP) antagonists are being developed. TXA_2 synthesis inhibitors may have some disadvantages as they lead to the accumulation of cyclic endoperoxides (e.g. PGH_2) that are themselves agonists at the TXA_2 receptor.

The proteolytic enzyme thrombin is known to play a crucial role in the overall thrombotic event leading to both, arterial and venous thrombosis by transforming fibrinogen into fibrin and by serving as a direct platelet activator. Thrombin exerts its effects on platelets via G-protein-coupled protease-activated receptors (PAR-1 and PAR-4 in human platelets). Thrombin-dependent receptor activation is achieved by cleaving an N-terminal extracellular peptide. Exposure of the newly generated N-terminal region functions as a tethered ligand for the receptor. Substances that directly bind to thrombin have been developed. The 65 amino acid long protein hirudin, originally isolated from the medical leech, *Hirudo medicinalis*, as well as related analogues have been recombinantly produced. They bind with the stoichiometry of 1:1 to thrombin and prevent its proteolytic action on fibrinogen as well as its binding to and the activation of PAR.

ADP is released from activated platelets by the secretion of dense granules and acts through at least three receptors. These are the ionotropic purinoceptor $2X_1$ ($P2X_1$) and two G-protein coupled receptors, the G_q-coupled purinoceptor $2Y_1$ ($P2Y_1$) and the G_i-coupled $P2Y_{12}$ receptor. The latter has also been termed $P2T_{AC}$ or $P2_{cyc}$ and is targeted by a group of antiplatelet agents - the thienopyridines - such as ticlopidine and clopidogrel. To become activated, ticlopidine and clopidogrel require biotransformation by the hepatic CYP-1A enzyme into an active metabolite. The active metabolite irreversibly modifies the $P2Y_{12}$ receptor.

Most antiplatelet drugs only partially inhibit platelet activation. In contrast, blockers of GP-IIb/IIIa interfere at the end of the pathway common to platelet aggregation. They prevent fibrinogen and vWf from binding to activated GP-IIb/IIIa and can therefore completely inhibit platelet aggregation. The first GP-IIb/IIIa antagonist developed was a hybrid human/murine monoclonal antibody. Its Fab fragment, termed abciximab, is clinically used and functions in a noncompetitive manner. An alternative approach to block GP-IIb/IIIa involves the use of peptides that mimic short protein sequences of fibrinogen or vWf. Several peptides (e.g. the cyclic heptapeptide eptifibatide) or non-peptidic, low molecular weight compounds (e.g. tirofiban, lamifiban) have been developed and function as competitive antagonists. Prodrugs of peptidomimetic compounds (e.g. xemilofiban, orbofiban, lefradafiban or sibrafiban) that are transformed into active metabolites in the body can be administered orally.

Clinical use

Due to the pivotal role of platelets in thrombus formation, especially in the arterial system, inhibition of platelet function has become a central pharmacological approach. This is done to prevent and treat thromboembolic diseases such as coronary heart disease, peripheral and cerebrovascular disease and is also used during as well as after invasive coronary interventions.

Aspirin leads to maximal antithrombotic effects at doses much lower than required for other actions of the drug. Clinical trials have demonstrated that aspirin is maximally effective as an antithrombotic drug at daily doses of 75–320 mg. Higher doses have no advantage but increase the frequency of side effects, especially bleeding and upper gastrointestinal symptoms. Despite the development of various other compounds, aspirin has remained the gold standard for antiplatelet drugs due to its relative safety and extremely low cost. Several studies have demonstrated a beneficial role for aspirin as an adjunctive therapy in unstable angina and acute myocardial infarction.

Mortality and disease progression were significantly reduced by low dose aspirin treatment. Patients with a history of arterial thromboembolism including myocardial infarction, stroke, transient ischemic attack or unstable angina were shown to benefit from low dose aspirin treatment in several trials. The overall rate of mortality, as well as the occurrence of further vascular events appeared to be reduced in these patients. The results of these studies led to the recommendation to use aspirin for secondary prevention of arterial thromboembolism. However, aspirin is not generally recommended for primary prevention of arterial thromboembolism. A possible beneficial effect, such as a decreased risk of non fatal myocardial infarction, may outweigh the risk of hemorrhagic complications only in a population already at high risk of cardiovascular diseases but not in a population of average health. Aspirin may also be beneficial as a prophylactic agent to reduce the risk of deep venous thrombosis and pulmonary embolism. However, the effectiveness compared to existing therapies remains to be determined; ▶ anticoagulants are still the mainstay of treatment in these conditions.

Thienopyridines are principally suited to treat conditions that respond to aspirin. Ticlopidin, but not clopidogrel, can lead to fatal neutropenia. Gastrointestinal problems and skin rashes can occur with both drugs but are more frequently seen when ticlopidine is used. In various trials, clopidogrel has been shown to be safe and similarly effective as aspirin. In patients at high risk from cerebrovascular events, thienopyridines seem to be somewhat more effective than aspirin in preventing serious vascular complications. Thienopyridines may be used instead of aspirin when the latter is not tolerated. However, aspirin still remains the first choice in most cases due to its low cost, relative safety and well documented efficacy. Studies are under way to test whether aspirin, given together with clopidogrel has advantages under certain clinical conditions.

Currently GP-IIb/IIIa antagonists are mainly used in controlled trials. So far, their use is restricted to interventional cardiology such as percutaneous transluminal revascularization with balloon angioplasty or intracoronary stenting, to acute coronary syndromes like unstable angina and to acute myocardial infarction. The main complications are bleeding and thrombocytopenia. The bleeding risk appears to increase further with concommittant therapy with heparin at standard doses. Currently, a number of available GP-IIb/IIIa antagonists that are to be administered orally, are under investigation to treat acute coronary syndromes. Although to date treatment with GP-IIb/IIIa antagonists is still in the phase of clinical trials, the trials appear to have a promising outcome. However, the use of GP-IIb/IIIa antagonists for standard clinical applications still awaits further verification. It is also not clear whether GP-IIb/IIIa antagonists will prove useful for vascular pathologies other than coronary artery disease such as cerebrovascular and peripheral artery disease.

References

1. George JN (2000) Platelets. Lancet 355:1531-1539
2. Awtry EH, Loscalzo J (2000) Aspirin. Circulation 101:1206–1218
3. Bennet JS (2001) Novel platelet inhibitors. Annu. Rev. Med. 52:161–184
4. Antiplatetelet Trialists' Collaboration (2002) Collaborative meta-analysis of randomised trials of antiplatelet therapy for prevention of death, myocardial infarction, and stroke in high risk patients. BMJ 324:71-86
5. Bhatt DL, Topol EJ (2003) Scientific and Therapeutic Advances in Antiplatelet Therapy. Nat. Rev. Drug Discov. 2:15-28

Antiprogestins

Antiprogestins are progesterone antgonists such as mifepristone (RU 38486), ORG 31710, ZK 137 316, ZK 230 211, ZK98299 (Onapristone).

▶ Sex Steroid Receptor

Antiprotozoal Drugs

Nadja Oster, Michael Lanzer
Hygiene-Institut, Universität Heidelberg,
Germany
Michael_Lanzer@med.uni-heidelberg.de;
Nadja_Oster@med.uni-heidelberg.de

Synonyms

Protocidal drugs, antiprotozoan chemotherapeutics

Definition

Protozoa are unicellular eukaryotes and a subregnum of the animal kingdom. Some protozoa exhibit a parasitic life style (Parasite) and are pathogenic to man and/or animals. Examples of important infectious diseases of man with protozoan etiology are malaria (*Plasmodium spp.*), toxoplasmosis (*Toxoplasma gondii*), African sleeping sickness (*Trypanosoma brucei gambiense and rhodesiense*), Chagas' disease (*Trypanosoma cruzi*), visceral and cutaneous Leishmaniasis (*Leishmania spp.*), amoebic dysentery and liver abscess (*Entamoeba histolytica*), lamblic diarrhoea (*Giardia lamblia*) and vaginitis (*Trichomonas vaginalis*). Antiprotozoal drugs are substances used in the treatment of diseases caused by protozoa.

Mechanism of Action

In the following chapter, the most important antiprotozoal drugs including their modes of action will be discussed (Tab. 1).

Antimalarial drugs

The 4-aminoquinoline chloroquine (Fig. 1) was once the first line drug in the global campaigns against ▶ malaria. Indiscriminate use and low compliance have resulted in the generation of chloroquine resistant malarial parasites, which today are widespread and compromise the application of chloroquine in many places of the world. Chloroquine targets the intraerythrocytic stages of malarial parasites (protozoa of the genus *Plasmodium* (Fig. 2)). Its mode of action is intricately linked with plasmodial heme metabolism (Fig. 3). During development within erythrocytes, *Plasmodia* feed on the host cell's hemoglobin, which is digested within an acidic food vacuole. Heme released during this process is highly cytotoxic and destabilizes membranes by facilitating ion exchange. Malarial parasites have developed three independent pathways to detoxify heme: 1) crystallization to insoluble and inert ▶ hemozoin; 2) peroxidative degradation; and 3) glutathione-dependent degradation. Chloroquine, which accumulates in the food vacuole, prevents heme detoxification by forming a stable complex with heme. The heme-chloroquine complexes have an enhanced affinity for membranes than does heme alone, thus potentiating the cytotoxic activity of heme. The build up of toxic membrane-associated heme-chloroquine molecules eventually destroys the integrity of the parasite's membranes (Fig. 3).

The arylaminoalcohol quinine was the first antimalarial known in the Western world. It was originally produced from the bark of the chinchona tree and sold as a powdery substance, which became known as Jesuits' powder. Several potent antimalarials are derived from quinine, including mefloquine, halofantrine and quinidine, the dextrarotatory diastereoisomer of quinine. All arylaminoalcohols seem to affect heme detoxification or cause other changes in the parasite's food vacuole, although their precise mode of action is still pending.

Artemisinin is another antimalarial drug that apparently interferes with heme detoxification. The prevailing hypothesis on artemisinin's mode of action is that reductive cleavage of its peroxide bridge, possibly by intracellular transition metal ions, such as Fe^{2+} (present in heme), generates radicals, which, in turn, would alkylate or hydroxylate biomolecules leading to the death of the parasite. Artemisinin is derived from the Chinese plant qinghaosu (*Artemisia annua*) and its derivatives, artesunate and artemether, are used in clinical practice.

Primaquine, an 8-aminoquinoline, is used in the treatment of malaria caused by *P. vivax* and *P. ovale*. These two malarial parasites produce dormant stages (hypnozoites) in the liver, which may cause relapses of the disease. Primaquine targets

Tab. 1 Protozoal diseases, etiologic agents and antiprotozoal drugs.

Disease	Etiologic Agent	Drugs
Malaria		Chloroquine, mefloquine, quinine/quinidine, halofantrine, artemisinin derivates, atovaquone/proguanil, primaquine, pyrimethamine/sulfadoxine
- tropical malaria	*Plasmodium falciparum*	
- tertian malaria	*Plasmodium vivax and ovale*	
- quartan malaria	*Plasmodium malariae*	
Visceral leishmaniasis (Kala-Azar), cutaneous leishmaniasis, mucocutaneous leishmaniasis	*Leishmania spp.*	Antimonial preparations (sodium stibogluconate), amphotericin B, liposomal amphotericin B, pentamidine
African sleeping sickness	*Trypanosoma brucei gambiense*	Suramine, pentamidine, eflornithine, melarsoprol
	Trypanosoma brucei rhodesiense	Suramine, melarsoprol
Chagas' Disease	*Trypanosoma cruzi*	Nifurtimox, benznidazole
Toxoplasmosis	*Toxoplasma gondii*	pyrimethamine/ sulfadiazine (+ folinic acid substitution)
Giardiasis (acute diarrhoea, chronic diarrhoea and malabsorption)	*Giardia lamblia*	Metronidazole
Intestinal amoebiasis (dysentery), amoebic liver abscess	*Entamoeba histolytica*	Metronidazole or chloroquine against invasive stages; diloxanid furoate for eradication of cysts
Diarrhoea in immunocompromised hosts and travellers	*Cyclospora cayetenensis*	Cotrimoxazole
Diarrhoea in immunocompromised hosts	*Cryptosporidium parvum*	
	Isospora belli	Cotrimoxazole, pyrimethamine/sulfadoxine
	Microspora	Albendazole
Vaginal infections and prostatitis	*Trichomonas vaginalis*	Metronidazole

these hypnozoites, although its mode of action remains obscure.

Pyrimethamine, cycloguanil and sulfadoxine (sulfadiazine) are folate antagonists that interfere with the folic acid biosynthesis pathway in malarial parasites and other protozoa, including *Toxoplasma gondii* (Fig. 4). Folate is an essential precursor of the pyrimidine dTTP and the amino acids serine and methionine. Both protozoa and mammalian cells require folate for DNA and protein synthesis. However, protozoa can either synthesize dihydrofolate *de novo* or salvage folate precursors, whereas mammalian cells have no *de novo* dihydrofolate synthesis and must rely on dietary sources. By acting as an analogue of p-aminobenzoic acid, sulfadoxine (sulfadiazine) inhibits the dihydropteroate synthase (DHPS), which now fails to convert dihydropteroate to hydroxymethyldihy-

Antimalarial drugs :

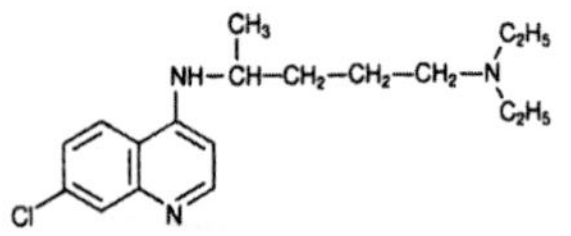

Chloroquine

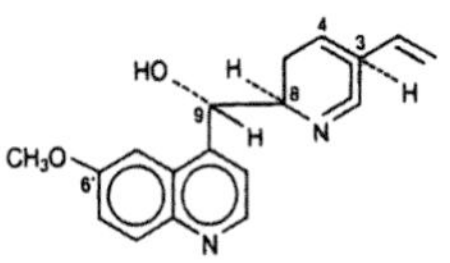

Quinine

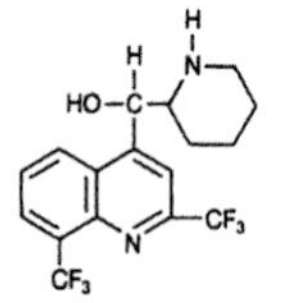

Mefloquine

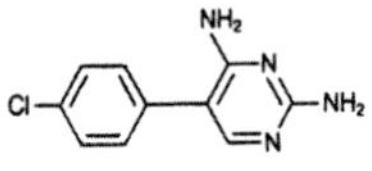

Pyrimethamine

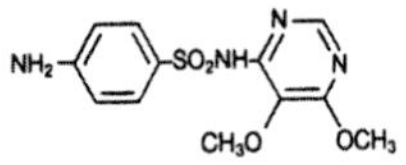

Sulfadoxine

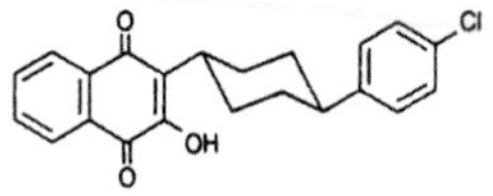

Atovaquone

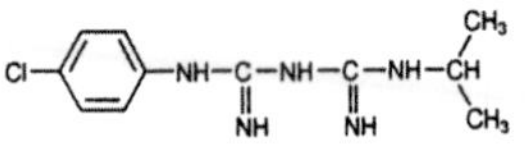

Proguanil

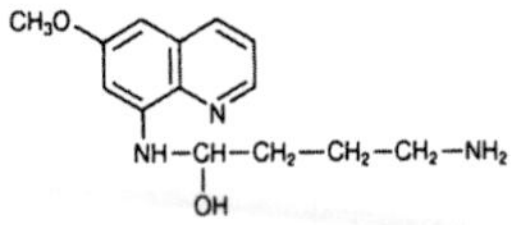

Primaquine

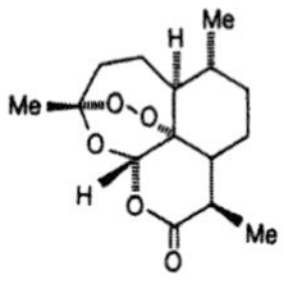

Artemisinin

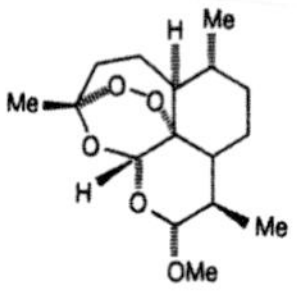

Artemether

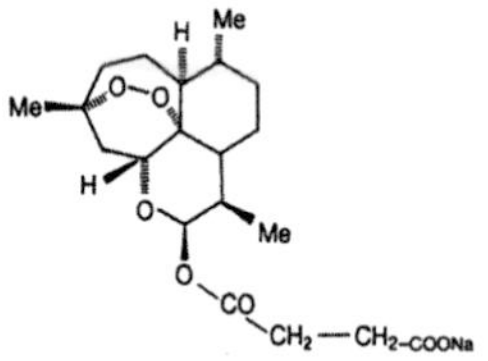

Artesunate

Antitrypanosomal drugs :

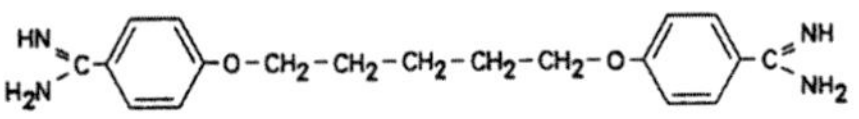

Pentamidine

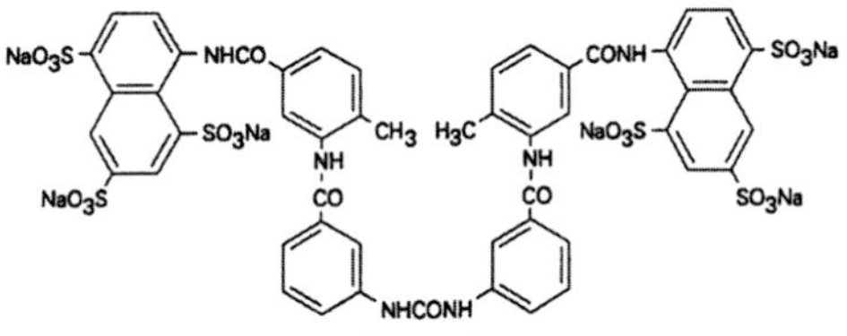

Suramin

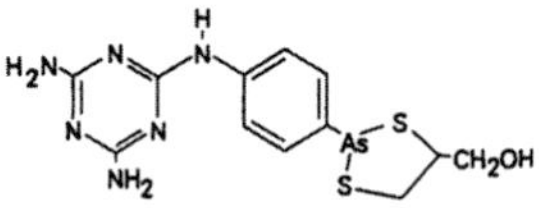

Melarsoprol

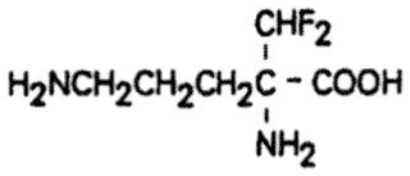

Eflornithine

Drug against anaerobic protozoa :

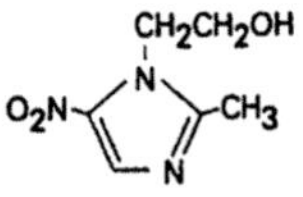

Metronidazole

Fig. 1 Chemical structures of antiprotozoal drugs.

dropterin, resulting in a lack of dihydrofolate in the parasite. This mechanism does not affect the mammalian cells.

Pyrimethamine and cycloguanil, the active metabolite of proguanil, act further downstream in the folic acid pathway by inhibiting the dihydrofolate reductase/thymidylate synthase enzyme complex. In mammalian cells dihydrofolate reductase (DHFR) and thymidylate-synthase (TS) are two independent enzymes. The protozoan DHFR/TS enzyme complex has a higher affinity for pyrimethamine and cycloguanil than does human DHFR, which explains their high antiprotozoal activity. To avoid deficiency of folic acid in patients treated with folate antagonists, folinic acid should be given during therapy.

Atovaquone, a hydroxynaphthoquinone, selectively inhibits the respiratory chain of protozoan mitochondria at the cytochrome bc1 complex (complex III) by mimicking the natural substrate, ubiquinone. Inibition of cytochrome bc1 disrupts the mitochondrial electron transfer chain and leads to a breakdown of the mitochondrial membrane potential. As resistance to atovaquone occurs rapidly in the field it is combined with proguanil.

Proguanil appears to have a dual activity: Part of it is metabolized to cycloguanil, which subsequently inhibits the protozoan dihydrofolate reductase/thymidylate synthase (see above). In addition, the native form, proguanil itself, exerts a potent antimalarial activity, especially in combination with other antimalarial drugs. The target of proguanil is separate from DHFR/TS.

Antitrypanosomal Drugs

Eflornithine (difluoromethylornithine, DFMO) is used in the treatment of African sleeping sickness caused by *Trypanosoma brucei gambiense*. It inhibits the ornithine decarboxylase of the polyamine pathway in both the trypanosome and the mammalian cell by acting as an irreversible competitor of the natural substrate, ornithine. Inhibition of ornithine decarboxylase results in depletion of the products of polyamine synthesis, putrescine, spermidine and spermine, which are essential for biosynthesis of nucleic acids and proteins. The assumed reason why eflornithine harms the parasite but not mammalian cells is that rates of production of ornithine decarboxylase in the

parasite are much lower than in the mammalian cells. Enzyme inhibition is compensated by immediately replenishing ornithine decarboxylase in the latter but not in the parasite. Eflornithine is only effective against *T. brucei gambiense*.

Melarsoprol, an arsenic compound, is the most efficient drug against intracerebral parasites in both *T. brucei gambiense* and *T. brucei rhodesiense* infection. Melarsoprol accumulates via an amino-purine transporter in trypanosomes, but the precise mechanism of action is still a matter of debate. Due to its high toxicity, use of melarsoprol should be restricted to cerebral stage trypanosomiasis only.

The antitrypanosomal mechanisms of suramine and pentamidine are not yet understood. It has been shown that both drugs inhibit a number of trypanosomal enzymes but the importance of these effects on the therapeutic efficacy needs to be further investigated. Suramine and pentamidine both can only be used in the treatment of blood stage trypanosomiasis because they cross the blood-brain barrier poorly.

Drugs Against Anaerobic Protozoa

Metronidazole is effective in the treatment of infections caused by *Giardia lamblia*, *Entamoeba histolytica* and ▶ *Trichomonas vaginalis*. The drug becomes active in its reduced state. Reduction of metronidazole to hydroxymetronidazole only occurs under strongly reducing conditions. In some anaerobic protozoa and bacteria such conditions are achieved when ferrodoxin is reduced by the fermentation enzyme pyruvate:ferrodoxin oxidoreductase (POR). Ferrodoxin can then transfer one electron to metronidazole to form hydroxymetronidazole. POR does not occur in mammalian cells. The corresponding enzyme to POR in mammalian cells is pyruvate decarboxylase, which is not able to establish a reducing potential high enough for metronidazole reduction. Therefore conversion of metronidazole to hydroxymetronidazole does not occur in mammalian cells and, hence, the drug cannot harm them. In protozoa or bacteria, hydroxymetronidazole affects the DNA by complex formation and strand cleavage, causing death of the cells.

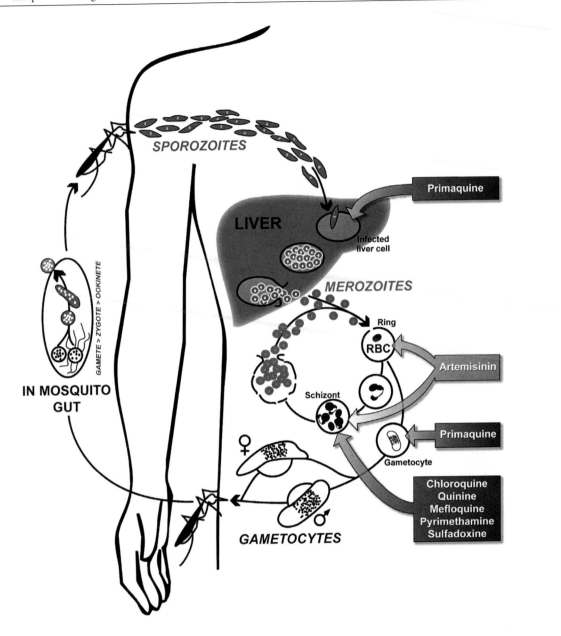

Fig. 2 Life cycle of malarial parasites and developmental activity of various antimalarial drugs. Malarial parasites, protozoa of the genus *Plasmodium,* are transmitted to humans by the bite of infected *Anopheles*mosquitoes. The transmitted stages, termed sporozoites, invade liver cells where they replicate to form merozoites. Upon rupture of the infected hepatocyte, merozoite are released into the blood stream where they infect erythrocytes. Within the erythrocyte, the parasite develops from a ring stage to a trophozoit, and then to schizont. When the infected erythrocyte finally ruptures, merozoites are released, which again invade erythrocytes. Some intraerythocytic ring stages develop to sexual stages (gametocytes). These can be ingested by feeding *Anophelines* and are then able to complete the life cycle in the mosquito by developing to gametes, zygotes, ookinets and finally sporozoites. Primaquine is the only drug effective against liver forms of all *Plasmodia* including dormant stages of *P. vivax* and *P. ovale.* Additionally, it acts against gametocytes. Artemisinin destroys intraerythrocytic ring stage parasites and schizonts. The so-called schizonticidal drugs, chloroquine, quinine, mefloquine, pyrimethamine and sulfadoxine, act against intraerythrocytic schizonts.

Clinical Use (incl. side effects)

Due to its low toxicity and low price, chloroquine was the drug of choice for the treatment of uncomplicated malaria. Today, chloroquine frequently fails in the treatment of malaria because of widespread resistance. Chloroquine is still used in prophylaxis of malaria, usually in combination with proguanil. Other medical applications include extraintestinal infections with *Entamoeba histolytica* and treatment of rheumatic diseases. The dosage independent side effects of chloroquine comprise itching rash, gastrointestinal discomfort and neurotoxicity. Retinopathy appears life dosage dependent after 5–6 years of prophylaxis with chloroquine.

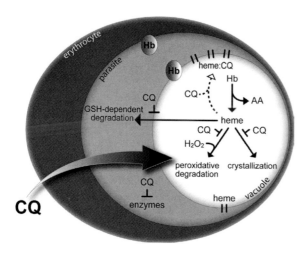

Fig. 3 Model of chloroquine's interactions with *P. falciparum*. Chloroquine's mode of action is associated with heme detoxification. Heme is released from hemoglobin (Hb), which is ingested by the parasite and degraded to amino acids (AA) in the parasite's acidic food vacuole. Chloroquine (CQ) inhibits heme crystallization as well as heme degradation mediated by glutathione (GSH) or hydrogen peroxide (H_2O_2). Chloroquine also inhibits enzymes that require heme as a prosthetic group. Chloroquine forms a complex with heme and enhances the association of heme with membranes, resulting in membrane perforation. The host erythrocyte, the parasite, acidic vesicles and the parasite's food vacuole are shown in different shades of gray.

Quinine is the drug of choice for the treatment of complicated malaria. Side effects can be tinnitus, vomiting, dysphoria, prolongation of QT interval and black water fever. Malaria-induced hypotension and hypoglycaemia can exacerbate under treatment with quinine. Intoxication can lead to deafness and blindness. Quinidine has higher cardiotoxic properties than quinine does.

Mefloquine is used for the treatment of uncomplicated malaria and for malaria prophylaxis in areas with high prevalence of chloroquine resistance. Mefloquine is hardly used for malaria control in endemic areas due to its high costs. The principal side effects of mefloquine are vomiting and neuropsychiatric disorders.

Halofantrine is no longer recommended for the treatment of malaria because of its cardiotoxicity (prolongation of QT-interval).

Artemisinin is used for the treatment of uncomplicated malaria in areas with high multidrug resistance. Due to its short half-life time it cannot be used for prophylaxis of malaria. Side effects are rare and of limited importance, such as gastrointestinal discomfort, headache and dizziness.

Pyrimethamine/sulfadiazine is used for the treatment and prophylaxis of toxoplasmosis in immunocompromised patients, and for the treatment of pregnant women with acute toxoplasmosis and children with congenital toxoplasmosis. Pyrimethamine/sulfadoxine is effective in the treatment and prophylaxis of *P. falciparum* malaria. Unfortunately, widespread use and the simple resistance mechanism (resistance is conferred by single point mutations within the corresponding enzymes) have resulted in the emergence and spread of resistant malarial parasites. Side effects induced by pyrimethamine comprise severe cutaneous eruptions and agranulocytosis. Megaloblastic anemia can occur when folinic acid is not supplemented. As pyrimethamine is suspected to be teratogenic it should not be given during the first trimenon. In case of acute toxoplasmosis in the first 15 weeks of pregnancy, spiramycin should be administered instead. Towards the end of pregnancy sulfadoxine/ sulfadiazine are suspected to cause kernicterus in the newborn and should therefore be omitted. Other side effects of sulfadoxine resemble those of other sulfonamides and include severe cutaneous reactions, liver failure and haematological reactions.

Atovaquone/proguanil is used in combination for the treatment and prophylaxis of malaria in areas with multi-drug resistance pattern. Atovaquone alone is used for the treatment and prophylaxis of *Pneumocystis carinii* infection and *Toxoplasma gondii* in immunocompromised patients. The problem of single application of atovaquone is its high potential to induce resistance, and by this recrudescence of the disease. Principal side effects of atovaquone are gastrointestinal discomfort and headache. Proguanil is known to cause ulcerations of the oral mucosa. Melarsoprol is used for the treatment of cerebral African trypanosomiasis, irrespective of the etiologic agent. Melarsoprol is the most efficacious substance to eliminate intracerebral parasites. The administration has to be considered carefully because severe and fatal side effects are common, and the use of melarsoprol for the treatment of sleeping sickness is only justified by the usually fatal outcome of the disease in its late stage. The principal side effect is reactive encephalopathy along with altered mental state, loss of consciousness and seizures. Other side effects are peripheral polyneuropathy, tremor, febrile reactions and skin complications especially if the drug has not been administered strictly intravenously.

Eflornithine is used in late stage trypanosomiasis with *T. brucei gambiense*. The side effects are less severe than those of melarsoprol. Reversible leucopenia and anemia resulting from bone marrow suppression and watery diarrhoea are the most common adverse effects. Convulsions are seen rarely and if, as a single event.

Pentamidine is used in the treatment of early stage African sleeping sickness caused by *Typanosoma brucei gambiense* and of leishmaniasis as well as for the treatment and prophylaxis of *Pneumocystis carinii* pneumonia in HIV-infected patients. Activity against intracerebral trypanosomes is poor. The most important side effect of pentamidine is acute anaphylactoid reaction along with a decrease of blood pressure, dizziness, loss of consciousness, dyspnoea, tachycardia and vomiting.

Suramine is used only in the treatment of early stage trypanosomiasis as the compound poorly crosses the blood-brain barrier. It is effective

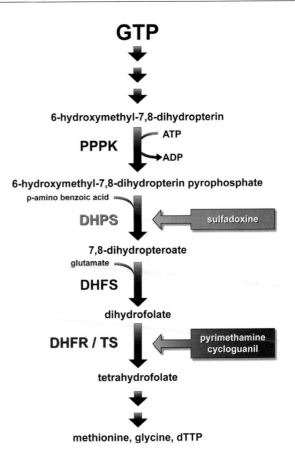

Fig. 4 Mode of action of folate antagonists in protozoa. Protozoa are capable of *de novo* synthesis of dihydrofolate, a precursor of thymidine, serine and methionine; 6-hydroxymethyl-7,8-dihydropterin pyrophosphate pyrophosphokinase (PPPK) and dihydropteroate synthase (DHPS) form one enzyme complex with two distinct active sites. The PPPK transforms GTP to 6-hydroxymethyl-7,8-dihydropterin and then to 6-hydroxymethyl-7,8-dihydropterin pyrophosphate. The product is linked to p-aminobenzoic acid (PABA) by dihydropteroate synthetase (DHPS), forming 7,8-dihydropteroate. Sulfadoxine exerts its activity by acting as a substrate analogue of PABA in this reaction. Glutamate is added to 7,8-dihydropterate by dihydrofolate synthase (DHFS) resulting in dihydrofolate. Dihydrofolate reductase (DHFR) and thymidylate synthase (TS) form a single enzyme complex with two enzymatically active sites. The catalytic site responsible for DHFR activity converts dihydrofolate into tetrahydrofolate. Pyrimethamine and cycloguanil exert their antimalarial activity by inhibiting the protozoal DHFR. The site of DHFR/TS responsible for TS activity converts tetrahydrofolate into deoxythymidintriphosphate (dTTP).

against *T. brucei rhodesiense* as well as *T. brucei gambiense*. Side effects of suramine are hypersensitivity reaction (especially in concomitant onchocerciasis), fever, arthritis, urticaria, proteinuria, polyneuropathy and stomatitis.

Metronidazole is used for the treatment of infections caused by *Trichomonas vaginalis, Giardia lamblia, Entamoeba histolytica* and anaerobic bacteria and for the treatment of Crohn's disease. Adverse effects are generally mild including gastrointestinal discomfort, alcohol intolerance, headache and dizziness. Long-term use of metronidazole can lead to neurotoxic sequelae such as peripheral neuropathy and seizures.

References

1. Folley M, Tilley L (1998) Quinoline antimalarials: Mechanisms of action and resistance and prospects for new agents. Phamacol Ther 79(1):55–87
2. Samuelson J (1999) Why metronidazole is active against both bacteria and parasites. Antimicrob Agents Chemother 43(7):1533–1541
3. Sanchez C, Lanzer M (2000) Changing ideas on chloroquine in *Plasmodium falciparum*. Curr Op Infect Dis 13:653–658
4. Srivastata IK, Vaidya AB (1997) Atovaquone, a broad spectrum antiparasitic drug, collapses mitochondrial membrane potential in a malarial parasite. J Biol Chem 272(7):3961–3966
5. Wang CC (1995) Molecular mechanisms and therapeutic approaches to the treatment of African trypanosomiasis. Annul Rev Pharmacology Toxically 35:93–127

Antipsychotic Drugs

DAVID C. MAMO, SHITIJ KAPUR
PET Centre - Schizophrenia Division, Centre for Addiction and Mental Health, Toronto, Canada
dmamo@camhpet.on.ca, skapur@camhpet.on.ca

Synonyms

Typical antipsychotic drugs: neuroleptic drugs, conventional antipsychotic drugs, older antipsychotic drugs; Atypical antipsychotic drugs: novel antipsychotic drugs, serotonin/dopamine antagonists, $5HT_{2A}/D_2$ antagonists

Definition

Antipsychotic drugs are effective in alleviating psychotic manifestations of a number of neurodegenerative and psychiatric disorders, especially ▸ schizophrenia. They are generally divided in two main groups based on their propensity to cause motor side effects and sustained elevation of plasma ▸ prolactin levels at clinically effective doses. Older or "typical" antipsychotic drugs (e.g. chlorpromazine and haloperidol) are associated with a high incidence of motor adverse effects and usually cause hyperprolactinemia. Newer antipsychotic drugs (clozapine, risperidone, olanzapine, quetiapine and ziprasidone) are called "atypical" antipsychotic drugs because they cause significantly lower motor side effects and usually avoid hyperprolactinemia.

▸ Antidepressant Drugs
▸ Dopamine System
▸ Serotoninergic System

Mechanism of Action

The serendipitous discovery of the antipsychotic effect of chlorpromazine in 1952 brought renewed hope in the treatment of psychotic disorders. The observation of chlorpromazine's antagonism of dopamine receptors heralded the introduction of multiple antipsychotic drugs based on their common ability to cause catalepsy in laboratory animals leading to the dopamine hypothesis of schizophrenia. Central to the dopamine hypothesis is that all known antipsychotic medications, including atypical antipsychotic medications, bind to dopamine-D_2 receptors (D_2-receptors). ▸ Positron emission tomograpghy (PET) studies have shown a direct relationship between central D_2-c receptor occupancy and clinical effects of antipsychotic medications, with clinical response occurring only when at least 60% of central D_2-receptors are occupied while ▸ extrapyramidal side effects (EPS) occur at D_2-receptor occupancy above 80% (1). Antipsychotic doses resulting in D_2-receptor occupancy higher than 80% result in more adverse effects with no additional clinical benefit, consistent with earlier observations that increasing the antipsychotic medication beyond this 'neuroleptic threshold' resulted in no additional benefit other than possibly decreasing clinical measures of hostility.

The introduction of clozapine presented a major challenge to the dopamine hypothesis. Not only does it show a modest clinical superiority over older antipsychotic agents (i.e. it is effective in some patients who do not respond to older antipsychotic drugs) but it does so without causing EPS or hyperprolactinemia. Pharmacologically, clozapine has been shown to have a low affinity for dopamine D_2-receptors (resulting in 20–70% occupancy) and a high affinity for serotonin ($5HT_2$) receptors (>80% occupancy). This gave rise to the hypothesis that its atypical nature was related to its high $5HT_2$-receptor (specifically $5HT_{2A}$-receptor) affinity relative to its low D_2-receptor affinity (2). However, some authors now challenge the role of $5HT_{2A}$ antagonism in the uniqueness of clozapine (1). A number of trials using drugs known to be antagonists of the $5HT_{2A}$-receptor (but not of dopamine receptors) have failed to show clozapine-like efficacy. Similarly, the $5HT_{2A}$-receptors are saturated by clozapine at sub-therapeutic doses, indicating that $5HT_{2A}$-receptor antagonism is not sufficient to effect an antipsychotic response. There are some case reports suggesting that augmentation of older antipsychotic medications with specific $5HT_2$-receptor antagonists may potentiate the antipsychotic efficacy, but this remains to be tested in controlled clinical trials. In summary, it has been suggested that clozapine's low EPS and avoidance of hyperprolactinemia is attributable to $5HT_2$ antagonism, but some degree of D_2-receptor antagonism may still be necessary for an antipsychotic response.

The $5HT_2/D_2$ hypothesis was influential in the introduction of four new antipsychotic medications (risperidone, olanzapine, quetiapine and ziprasidone), all having in common a high ratio of $5HT_2/D_2$ receptor affinity and lower incidence of both EPS and hyperprolactinemia (2). However, at least in the case of risperidone and olanzapine (and possibly also ziprasidone) this 'atypical' nature appears to be lost in a dose-dependent manner resulting in the appearance of EPS and sustained hyperprolactinemia at higher doses.

Indeed, the relationship between dopamine D_2-receptor occupancy and clinical effects (response and EPS) for risperidone and olanzapine in human subjects studied with PET is very similar to that found with older antipsychotic drugs (i.e. a threshold >60% D_2-receptor occupancy for clinical response and >80% D_2-receptor occupancy for EPS). On the other hand, clozapine and quetiapine are clinically effective at lower D_2-receptor occupancy without showing sustained hyperprolactinemia. Some studies evaluating the ratio of D_2-receptor occupancy in extrastriatal regions relative to the striatum suggested that atypical antipsychotic medications preferentially bind to extrastriatal (i.e. limbic) D_2-receptors when compared to typical antipsychotic drugs. However, data from a study using kinetic analysis (a technique that avoids a number of the limitations of ratio studies) in non-human primates is not consistent with this hypothesis.

Recent studies suggest that the apparent low striatal D_2-receptor occupancy may be a result of quetiapine and clozapine's loose binding to D_2-receptors (i.e. high k_{off} resulting in low ▸ affinity for D_2-receptor) (1). Hence endogenous dopamine and low concentrations of radioligands (used in these experiments) may displace an appreciable amount of bound drug resulting in underestimation of D_2-receptor occupancy. In one study, patients treated with quetiapine at doses ranging from 300–600mg/day showed normal prolactin levels and less than 20% D_2-receptor occupancy 12 hours after their last dose. However, transiently elevated prolactin levels and appreciable (64%) dopamine D_2-receptor binding were noted two hours after drug administration. Similarly clozapine (350mg/day) resulted in 71% D_2-receptor occupancy 1–2 hours after administration, declining to 55% and 26% after 12 and 24 hours, respectively. While these findings await replication they raise the possibility that different pharmacodynamic properties of dopamine receptor antagonists may be sufficient to explain their varying degrees of 'atypicality' (3). The transient dopamine receptor occupancy may also account for clozapine's clinical superiority, since it has been shown that repeated transient dopamine receptor antagonism results in sensitization of the dopamine system, while continuous receptor antagonism results in tolerance and up-regulation of the system.

While all antipsychotic medications have a robust acute effect on delusions, auditory hallucinations and disorganized behaviour (also known as 'positive symptoms'), and maintenance treatment has been shown to decrease both relapse and hospitalization rates, their effect on negative symptoms (apathy, avolition, alogia and affective flattening) and related cognitive disturbance (e.g. attentional problems and disrupted working memory) is at best marginal. Newer antipsychotic medications, especially clozapine, have been shown to have some effect on negative symptoms and selected cognitive measures when compared to older antipsychotics such as haloperidol, but this topic remains controversial due to the difficulty in distinguishing primary negative symptoms from secondary (i.e. adverse) effects of the (older) medications (3). *In vivo* measurements of extracellular dopamine levels using microdialysis in rodents and primates have shown that while both acute administration of clozapine and haloperidol result in an increase in dopamine levels in the striatum, clozapine results in higher dopamine levels in the prefrontal cortex compared with haloperidol. With chronic administration of clozapine in rodents, the increased dopamine release is maintained only in the prefrontal cortex but not in the striatum. It has been postulated that this modulation of prefrontal dopaminergic transmission may be involved in its effects on cognitive and negative symptoms, which are known to be associated with decreased prefrontal activity in functional neuroimaging studies (4).

It is thought that the mesolimbic dopaminergic projections from ventral tegmental area (VTA) are involved in the clinical response to antipsychotic drugs, and that in contrast to older antipsychotic drugs, newer antipsychotic drugs may act preferentially on these neurons. Acute administration of haloperidol in anaesthetized rodents has been shown to increase firing rate of neurons in the substantia nigra (SN) as well as the VTA. On the other hand daily administration for three weeks leads to a decline in the activity in these dopaminergic neurons below that at baseline, an electrophysiological phenomenon known as 'depolarization block'. All antipsychotic medications have the ability to cause a depolarization block in the VTA, and their ability to cause depo-

larization block in the SN is related to their propensity to cause EPS in human subjects. Clozapine causes a depolarization block in the VTA but not in the SN, consistent with involvement of the mesolimbic system in its antipsychotic effect (5).

In summary, the mechanism of action of antipsychotic drugs appears to be intricately linked with the normalization of a disrupted state of dopaminergic transmission. Remission of positive symptoms and the emergence of extrapyramidal side effects are associated with specific levels of striatal dopamine D_2-receptor occupancy. An increased ratio of $5HT_2/D_2$-receptor antagonism and/or altered pharmacodynamic properties of atypical antipsychotic drugs resulting in loose binding to D_2-receptors may be involved in the decreased incidence of motor side effects with some newer antipsychotic drugs, while antipsychotic action may involve activity of these drugs on the mesolimbic ascending dopaminergic neurons. Preferential activity and modulation of prefrontal dopaminergic activity by atypical antipsychotic drugs may be related to their effects on cognitive and negative symptoms of schizophrenia.

Clinical Use (incl. side effects)

Antipsychotic medications are indicated in the treatment of acute and chronic psychotic disorders. These include schizophrenia, schizoaffective disorder and manic states occurring as part of a bipolar disorder or schizoaffective disorder. The co-adminstration of antipsychotic medication with antidepressants has been shown to increase the remission rate of severe depressive episodes that are accompanied by psychotic symptoms. Antipsychotic medications are frequently used in the management of agitation associated with delirium, dementia and toxic effects of both prescribed medications (e.g. L-dopa used in Parkinson's disease) and illicit drugs (e.g. cocaine, amphetamines and PCP). They are also indicated in the management of tics that result from Gilles de la Tourette's syndrome, and widely used to control the motor and behavioural manifestations of Huntington's disease.

The choice of antipsychotic medications is largely dependent on considerations related to their individual side effect profile. Older antispychotic medications are generally divided into high, moderate and low potency drugs, potency being related to their propensity for causing EPS. ▶ Tardive dykinesia is the most common and potentially most disabling long-term side effect. The neuroleptic malignant syndrome is the most severe neurological side effect and consists of hyperthermia, autonomic instability and muscle stiffness that may result in dehydration, renal failure and death. Early diagnosis and management has resulted in decreased mortality from this condition. In addition to neurological side effects, other systems may also be affected by typical antipsychotic medications. In contrast to the neurological side effects, the incidence of these side effects are generally inversely proportional to the potency of the drug used. These include autonomic effects (e.g. tachicardia, dry mouth, urinary retention, constipation), hematologic effects (e.g. neutropenia and, rarely, agranulocytois), neurological (sedation, seizures), endocrine (e.g. weight gain, galactorrhoea, obesity, hypercholsterolemia and hypergylcemia) and dermatological effects (e.g. photosensitivity).

The atypical antipsychotic drugs were introduced with the goal of minimizing neurological adverse effects associated with older antipsychotic medications. However, these medications are not free of serious adverse effects including dose-related parkinsonism (risperidone and olanzapine), dose-related risk of seizures (clozapine), endocrinological manifestations (including diabetes, weight gain and hypercholesterolemia) and haematological abnormalities (neutropenia and agranulocytosis with clozapine). Nonetheless, while older antipsychotic medications remain the most widely used antipsychotic medications globally, the use of newer antipsychotic medications has largely dominated the market in Western Europe and North America. The principle clinical advantage that has led to this shift in prescribing practice is undoubtedly the decreased incidence of neurological side effects, which are associated with significant morbidity and poor outcome largely secondary to non-compliance. Indeed, they are generally recommended as first line agents in the treatment of psychotic disorders, with typical antipsychotic drugs reserved for patients having previously been successfully maintained on these medications or requiring parenteral antipsychotic drugs (e.g. short-acting intramuscular neurolep-

tics for agitation, and long-acting "depot neuroleptics" for patients who are non-compliant with oral medication). While atypical antipsychotic medications are more acceptable to patients, their impact on the long-term outcome of schizophrenia remains to be established. Moreover, continued vigilance for their potentially significant long-term side effects including obesity, hypercholesterolemia and impaired glucose tolerance is warranted.

All antipsychotic medications are effective in alleviating positive and negative symptoms of schizophrenia, while atypical antipsychotic agents have been associated with some superior efficacy in reduction of negative symptoms. Following an adequate trial of antipsychotic treatment (8–12 weeks of treatment with adequately dosed antipsychotic drug) in acute schizophrenia, 60% of patients show significant improvement or remission compared with 20% of patients treated with placebo. Of the 40% who do not respond, approximately half respond to subsequent trials with other antipsychotic medications. The acute phase of the illness is treated with an oral antipsychotic medication titrated to the appropriate clinically effective dose. This may be supplemented by short-acting intramuscular antipsychotic agents in patients in whom rapid sedation is clinically indicated (e.g. severe agitation). Patients failing to respond to an adequate trial of an antipsychotic medication should be switched to another antipsychotic drug from a different pharmacological class. Patients who fail to respond or show only partial response to two adequate trials of antipsychotic drugs (including at least one atypical antipsychotic drug) or experience severe neurological side effects (e.g. tardive dyskinesia) should be considered for a trial of clozapine (6). Significant inter-individual variability in dose requirements is commonly seen, and this may be influenced by sex, age and concomitant medications. Increasing the dose beyond that which causes extrapyramidal side effects results in no additional clinical advantage. Regular monitoring for extrapyramidal side effects is warranted especially during the first three months of treatment, followed by screening for EPS and tardive dyskinesia every six months or following any medication or dose changes. Patients are maintained on the clinically effective dose for the next three to six months. Following the resolution of the acute phase, the dose may be decreased to address any adverse effects having significant functional or emotional impact on the patient's well-being.

The duration of treatment is generally considered to be indefinite in patients diagnosed with schizophrenia, though selected patients recovering from a first psychotic episode may be considered for gradual taper of medication after at least one-year of treatment and with close psychiatric follow up. Patients with a history of multiple psychotic episodes should be stable for at least five years before considering a trial off medication. When considering discontinuation of antipsychotic treatment, an individualized approach is recommended with careful consideration of certain aspects of the disease course (e.g. severe occupational impairment when acutely ill, history of suicidal attempts and violence). Symptom-targeting strategies and drug holidays have been tried in the past, but for most patients this is no longer recommended since it is associated with very high relapse rates. Finally, with the resolution of the acute phase of the psychotic episode, psychosocial, occupational and cognitive difficulties need to be addressed, since they usually persist with significant impact on the patients' functional status.

In summary, antipsychotic drugs have a significant impact on the acute resolution and the maintenance of remission of symptoms of schizophrenia, enabling focus on rehabilitation efforts directed at residual cognitive, social and occupational disabilities. The advent of atypical antipsychotic drugs brought lesser motor side effects and renewed hope to patients and families affected by this devastating illness. It is hoped that a better understanding of pharmacological mechanisms underlying the clinical superiority of drugs like clozapine will lead to the development of new treatment strategies with better efficacy and improved side effect profile.

References

1. Kapur S, Seeman P. (2001) Does fast dissociation from the dopamine D2 receptor explain the action of atypical antipsychotics? A new hypothesis. Am J Psychiatry 158:360–369

2. Meltzer HY. (1999) The role of serotonin in antipsychotic drug action. Neuropsychopharmacology 21:106S–115S

3. Kapur S, Remington G. (2001) Atypical antipsychotics: new directions and challenges in the treatment of schizophrenia. Annu Rev Med 52:503–517

4. Youngren KD, Inglis FM, Pivirotto PJ, Jedema HP, Bradberry CW, Goldman-Rakic PS, Roth RH, Moghaddam B. (1999) Clozapine preferentially increases dopamine release in the rhesus monkey prefrontal cortex compared with the caudate nucleus. Neuropsychopharmacology 20:403–12

5. Grace AA, Bunney BS, Moore H, and Todd CL. (1997) Dopamine-cell depolarization block as a model for the therapeutic actions of antipsychotic drugs. TINS 20:31–37

6. Canadian Clinical Practice Guidelines for the Treatment of Schizophrenia. (1998) Can J Psychiatry 1–CPG

Antipyretic Agents

Antipyretic agents are used for the treatment of fever. The most commonly used antipyretics are acetylsalicylic acid and paracetamol (synonym acetaminophen).

▶ Non-steroidal Anti-inflammatory Drugs

Antiretroviral Agents

▶ Antiviral Drugs

Antirheumatoid Drugs

Antirheumatoid drugs are employed in the treatment of rheumatoid disease (rheumatoid arthritis). The characteristic feature of this autoimmune disease is a persistent inflammation of peripheral joints. The inflammatory process leads to joint damage and subsequently to marked functional impairment. Inflammatory cytokines play a major role in the pathogenesi of the disease. Drugs used in the therapy of rheumatoid arthritis are ▶ nonsteroidal anti-inflammatory drugs, ▶ glucocorticoids, ▶ immunosuppressive agents and disease-motifying antirheumatoid drugs (DMARDs). DMARDs are not analgesic, but they suppress the inflammatory process. DMARDs include drugs with cytotoxic and immunosuppressant activity (azathioprine, cyclosporin, methotrexate), gold compounds (auranofin and sodium aurothiomalate), anti-malarial drugs (chloroquine and hydroxychloroquine) and sulphasalazine. The last is also used for the treatment of chronic inflammatory bowel disease.

▶ NSAID
▶ Glucocorticoids
▶ Immunosuppressive Agents
▶ Inflammation

Antisense Oligonucleotides and RNA Interference

ARNDT BORKHARDT
Universität Gießen, Children's University Hospital, Gießen, Germany
arndt.borkhardt@paediat.med.uni-giessen.de

Synonyms

Antisense DNA; reverse complementary oligonucleotides.

Definition

Antisense therapy means the selective, sequence-specific inhibition of gene expression by single-stranded DNA oligonucleotides. In contrast, ▶ RNA interference (RNAi) is triggered by double-stranded RNA (dsRNA) and causes sequence-specific mRNA degradation of single-stranded target RNAs in response to dsRNA. The mediators of mRNA degradation are small interfering RNA duplexes (▶ siRNAs), which are produced from long dsRNA by enzymatic cleavage in the cell. siR-

NAs are approximately 21-nucleotide length and have a base-paired structure with 2-nucleotide 3'-overhangs. Beyond their value for target validation, antisense molecules and siRNAs also hold great potential as gene-specific therapeutic and more than thirty synthetic oligonucleotides have entered clinical trials for treatment of viral diseases, cancer and inflammatory diseases.

▶ Gene Therapy
▶ Genetic Vaccination

Description

Antisense Oligonucleotides (ASON) are sequences of usually 17–30 bases of single-stranded DNA that hybridize to specific genes or their mRNA products by ▶ Watson-Crick base-pairing and disrupt their function. In most cases ASON bind to the expressed mRNA of their target gene, although in rarer cases the ASON also prevent normal gene transcription by directly forming triplex-helix structures with target DNA. The short length of a typical ASON facilitates cell internalization and increases hybridization efficiency by reducing base-mismatch errors. Once hybridization has occurred the ASON-mRNA complex becomes a substrate for intracellular ▶ RNAses (e.g. RNAse-H) that catalyzes mRNA degradation and allows ASON to recycle for another base-pairing with the next target mRNA molecule. The net result of this process is a sustained decrease of target mRNA translation and a lower intracellular level of the corresponding protein (Fig. 1).

The therapeutic utility of systemically administered ASON had been limited by their short plasma half-life (sometimes even less than 3 minutes). This is due to their sensitivity of nuclease digestion. When ASON are chemically modified, e.g. by replacing the oxygen in the phosphodiester bond with sulfur (phosphorothiorate), they have a increased stability in biological fluids while their antisense effect is maintained.

Another problem with employment of ASON in a larger clinical setting is their poor uptake and inappropriate intracellular compartmentalization, e.g. sequestration in endosomal or lysosomal complexes. In addition, there is a need for a very careful selection of the ASON-mRNA pair sequences that would most efficiently hybridize.

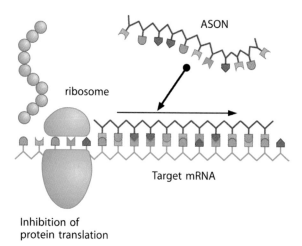

ASON

ribosome

Target mRNA

Inhibition of
protein translation

Fig. 1 Schematic representation of the action of antisense oligonucleotides: they bind to their respective target mRNA preventing protein translation.

To date, several computer programs are used to predict the secondary and tertiary structures of the target mRNA and, in turn, which of the mRNA sequences are most accessible to the ASON. However, even with these sophisticated techniques, the choice of base-pairing partners still usually includes a component of empiricism. Despite the principal limitations, it has become clear that ASON can penetrate into cells and mediate their specific inhibitory effect of the protein synthesis in various circumstances.

The basic concept of the use of ASON can be modified in several ways: 1. Antisense RNA, that is expressed intracellularly following transfection with antisense genes. 2. ► Ribozymes that are small RNA molecules with endoribonuclease activity, exhibiting catalytic sequence-specific cleavage of the target. The ribozymes were widely modified and can be further subdivided according to their structural features in group I ribozymes, hammerhead ribozymes, hairpin ribozymes, ribonucelase P (RNase P), and hepatitis delta virus ribozymes.

Examples of applied ASON therapeutics

The number of ongoing clinical trials represents a growing interest in antisense technology.

1. ASON to inhibit angioplasty re-stenosis. Patients suffering from coronary stenosis can be successfully treated by percutaneous transluminal coronary angioplasty (PTCA). However, in up to 50% of the patients re-stenoses occur necessitating a repeated PTCA: ASON emerged as a potentially useful strategy to prevent such re-stenoses in animal models and the first clinical trials are currently in progress.

2. ASON against HIV infection. Once HIV has infected the cell, the genomic RNA of the retrovirus is used to code for a double-stranded cDNA intermediate. This cDNA is integrated into the genome of the host cell by the viral integrase. RNA identical to the genomic RNA of the virus will be transcribed from the DNA of this provirus by the infected cell. In experimental systems, ASON were used to target various parts of the viral life cycle, e.g. genomic RNA reverse transcription, viral mRNA transcription, and viral translation. In this regard, GEM 91, a 25-mer ASON against the HIV-1 gag gene, has been extensively studied.

3. ASON for targeting the bcl-2 proto-oncogene in human cancers. The bcl-2 protein is a major apoptosis inhibitor originally identified by its involvement of a chromosomal translocation t(14;18) found in follicular Non-Hodgkin Lymphoma. Beside lymphomas, bcl-2 is upregulated in several other tumours, e.g. leukemia, breast cancer, melanoma, prostate cancer, small and non-small lung carcinoma. In most of these studies, a 18-mer phosphothiorate ASON targeting the first six codons of bcl-2 (ISIS G3139) was used. The bcl-2 antisense therapy was feasible and showed potential antitumor activity. However, the mean inhibition of bcl-2 expression was only moderate and the clinical significance of this small decline was uncertain. Beside bcl-2, a large variety of other ► oncogenes have been targeted in cancer cell models. Table 1 gives an overview of such attempts.

4. Formivirsen to treat cytomegalovirus-induced retinitis in HIV-infected patients. The first antisense drug approved by the US Food and Drugs Administration (FDA) was formivirsen (ISIS 2922) that targets the CMVIE2 protein. Formivirsen was approved for the treatment of cytomegalovirus-induced retinitis in patients with AIDS. One or both eyes can be affected and it is not unusual for patients to suffer from severe vis-

ual impairment or even blindness as a result of untreated infections. But the conventional treatment of CMV-retinitis also remains problematic, in particular for patients who cannot take, do not respond or become resistant to standard therapy by gancyclovir, foscarnet and cidofovir. The main drawback of formivirsen is its need for local administration by intravitreal injection. Of note, the inhibitory effect of formivirsen for cytomegalovirus replication *in vitro* is about 30 times higher than for gancyclovir, the conventional treatment of choice for CMV infection. Table 2 summarizes current ASON-mediated therapies against viral infections.

Non-sequence specific activities of ASON

A rather unexpected stimulation of lymphocyte proliferation by ASON was frequently observed. Of note, the phosphorothiorate backbone of a given ASON has immunstimulatory properties itself which are independent of its DNA sequence. In contrast, the stimulatory effect of unmodified oligonucleotides are dependent on a simple unmethylated ▶ CpG dinucleotide motif. The increasing number of ▶ CpG motifs generally increases the level of activation of B-lymphocytes. In addition, ASON may have effects of cytokine or immunoglobulin secretion, or may alter the DNA binding activity of transcription factors. These non-antisense immune-enhancing (or sometimes immune-suppressing) effects are generally recognised as a undesirable side-effect. However, they may have therapeutic utility of their own, even though the mechanisms are not yet fully understood.

In general, systemic treatment with ASON is well-tolerated and side-effects are dose-dependent. Among these, thrombocytopenia, hypotension, fever, increasing liver enzymes, and complement activation were most frequently seen (1).

RNA interference and the mechanism of siRNA-mediated gene silencing

Description: Introduction of double-stranded RNA (dsRNA) into cells leads to the sequence-specific destruction of endogenous RNA that match the dsRNA. The remarkable potency of the RNAi reaction enables a complete "knock-down" of a specific protein. The key enzyme required for processing of long dsRNAs to siRNA duplexes is

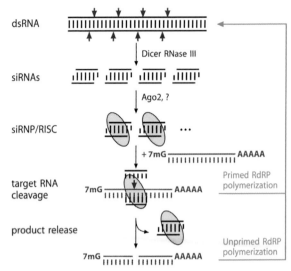

Fig. 2 A model for RNA interference: dsRNA is processed to 21– to 23–nt siRNA duplexes by Dicer RNase III and possibly other dsRNA-binding factors. The siRNA duplexes are incorporated into the RISC endonuclease (RNAi-inducing silencing complex), which targets homologous mRNAs for degradation. Ago2 and yet to be characterised proteins are believed to be required for RISC formation. The RISC complex mediates sequence-specific target RNA degradation. In plants and nematodes, it is thought that targeted RNAs may also function as templates for double-strand RNA synthesis giving rise to transitive RNAi. Two possibilities have been suggested, siRNA-primed dsRNA synthesis or unprimed synthesis from aberrant RNA, which could represent the cleaved target RNA. In mammals or in fruit fly, however, RdRP (RNA dependent RNA polymerase) genes have yet not been identified and the major mechanism of siRNA action is believed to be endonucleolytic target RNA cleavage guided by siRNA-protein complexes (RISC).

the RNase III enzyme ▶ Dicer. The silencing effect is long lasting, typically several days, and extraordinarily specific, because one nucleotide mismatch between target and the central region of the siRNA is frequently sufficient to prevent silencing. A schematic illustration of the mechanism of RNAi is shown in Fig. 2. siRNAs can be rapidly chemically synthesized and are now broadly available. More recently, it has also become possible to express siRNAs from short inverted repeat genes in order to silence genes expressed in somatic

A

Tab. 1 Malignant disorders as potential targets for ribozyme gene therapy.

Target gene	Gene product	Ribozyme-induced change of function
bcr-abl	Tyrosine kinase	Inhibition of cell proliferation and colony formation.
PML/RAR α	Transcriptional regulator	Inhibition of cell prolifeation; induction of apoptosis; increase in sensitivity against ATRA.
AML1/MTG8	Transcription factor	Inhibition of cell proliferation; induction of apoptosis
N-*ras*, H-*ras*, K-*ras*	Signal transduction pathway	Inhibition of cell proliferation and colony formation; change in morphology, enhanced melanin synthesis; decrease of *in vivo* tumorigenicity.
EGFR	Receptor tyrosine kinase	Inhibition of cell proliferation and colony formation; decrease of *in vivo* tumorigenicity.
c-*erbB-2* (HER2/neu)	Receptor tyrosine kinase	Inhibition of cell proliferation; decrease of *in vivo* tumorigenicity.
c-*erbB-4*	Receptor tyrosine kinase	Inhibition of mitogenesis and colony formation; decrease of *in vivo* tumorigenicity.
Estrogen receptor	Transcriptional regulator	Inhibition of cell-cycle progression.
Androgen receptor	Transcriptional regulator	Inhibition of androgen receptor transcriptional activity.
c-*fms*	Growth factor receptor	Inhibition of cell proliferation.
RET	Receptor tyrosine kinase	Inhibition of colony formation.
mdr-1	Drug-efflux pump	Reduction in resistance to chemotherapeutic drugs.
c-*fos*	Transcirptional regulator	Change in morphology; reduction in resistance to chemotherapeutic drugs.
CD44	Cell adhesion molecule	n.d.
VLA-6	Adhesion receptor	Decrease of *in vitro* invasion and *in vivo* metastatic ability
MMP-9	Matric metalloproteinase	Decrease of *in vivo* metastatic ability
CAPL (S100A4)	Calcium-binding protein	Decrease of *in vitro* invasion; reduction in expression of MMP-2, MT1-MMP, and TIMP-1; decrease of *in vivo* metastatic ability
Pleiotrophin	Growth factor	Inhibition of colony formation; decrease of *in vivo* tumor growth, tumor angiogenesis, and metastatic ability
VEGF-R1/VEGF-R2	Growth factor	n.d.
VEGF	Growth factor	n.d.

Tab. 1 Malignant disorders as potential targets for ribozyme gene therapy. (Continued)

Target gene	Gene product	Ribozyme-induced change of function
bFGF-BP	bFGF-binding protein	Reduction of release of biologically active bFGF; decrease of *in vivo* tumor growth and tumor angiogenesis
Telomerase	Ribonucleoprotein	Suppression of telomerase activity; inhibition of cell proliferation; change in morphology; induction of apoptosis
bcl-2	Anti-apoptotic protein	Induction of apoptosis
PKC-α	Anti-apoptotic protein	Induction of apoptosis

Tab. 2 Viral disorders with malignant complications as potential targets for ribozyme gene therapies.

Virus	Malignant complication	Target gene for ribozymes	Ribozyme-induced change of function
Human papilloma virus (HPV)	Cervical cancer, oral cancer	E6, E7	Inhibition of cell proliferation and colony formation
Epstein-Barr virus (EBV)	Burkitt's lymphoma, nasopharyngeal carcinoma, lymphoproliferative disorders in immuno-suppressed patients (AIDS, transplant recipients)	EBNA-1	Inhibition of cell proliferation
Hepatitis B virus (HBV)	Hepatocellular carcinoma	Progenomic RNA	Inhibition of viral gene expression
Hepatitis C virus (HCV)	Hepatocellular carcinoma	5' untranslated/cor region	Inhibition of viral gene expression

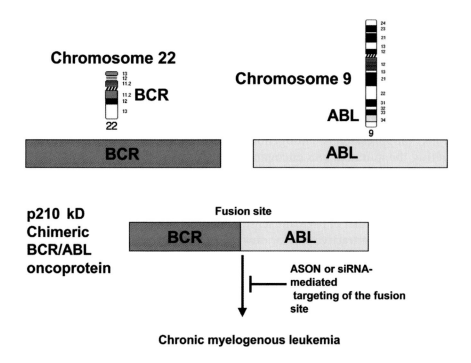

Fig. 3 The translocation between chromosomes 9 and 22 is the classical prototype of chromsomal translocations in human leukaemias. The translocation fuses two unrelated genes, BCR from chromosome 22 and ABL from chromosome 9, to an oncogenic hybrid gene. The resulting BCR/ABL protein has, as compared to the normal ABL protein, an increased kinase activity leading to pathologic phosphorylation of several downstream targets. This results in oncogenic growth and inhibition of apoptosis. The fusion site is tumour cell-specific and can be targeted either by ASON or siRNA mediated approaches.

cells. The RNAs were expressed under the control of a compact ▶ RNA polymerase III promoter, which normally drives the expression of human H1 RNA, the RNA subunit of RNase P enzyme. The short hairpin loop constructs gave rise to siRNAs, presumably because Dicer RNase III recognizes these hairpin RNAs and excises siRNAs. Transfection of plasmids encoding siRNAs therefore represents an alternative to direct siRNA transfection and may facilitate certain applications of gene targeting. A prerequisite for the application of siRNAs for validation and therapeutic applications is the need for a functional RNAi machinery within the targeted cells or tissue to bind to siRNAs and mediate mRNA degradation.

siRNAs are highly sequence-specific reagents and discriminate between single mismatched target RNA sequences and open new avenues for gene therapy. mRNAs coding for mutated proteins, which give rise to dominant genetic disorders and

neoplastic growth, may be down-regulated by specific siRNAs.

With respect to targeting viral gene products expressed in virus-infected cells, it should be considered that infectious mammalian viruses may express inhibitors of RNAi similar to plant viruses. siRNAs were successfully used for the silencing of genes expressed from respiratory syncytial virus (RSV), a negative strand RNA virus causing childhood respiratory diseases. Especially in leukemias and lymphomas the oncogene activation frequently occurs through reciprocal ▶ chromosomal translocations. These translocations split genes on both partner chromosomes leading to juxtaposition of part of each gene in the joint segments and the creation of a composite gene. Silencing of these tumour-specific chimeric mRNAs by siRNAs or ASON may become fusion gene-specific tumour therapy (Fig. 3). The extraordinary sequence specificity of the RNAi mechanism may also allow the targeting of individual polymorphic alleles expressed in loss-of-heterozygosity tumour cells as well as point-mutated transcripts of ▶ transforming oncogenes such as RAS. The great potential of RNAi-mediated tumour therapy was recently demonstated by Brummelkamp *et al.* who used a retroviral version of their plasmid vector system "pSUPER" (suppression of endogenous RNA) for targeting the mutated RAS oncogene. They strongly inhibited the expression of mutated K-ras^{V12} while leaving other ras isoforms unaffected. This extraordinary sequence specificity of RNAi which clearly exceeds that of DNA antisense approaches, makes it a very attractive tool for cancer therapy. Brummelkamp *et al.* demonstrated the power of RNAi-mediated gene therapy not only in cell culture but, encouragingly, in an animal model as well (2). The latter finding, together with recent reports about the successful application of RNAi in mice predicts further studies in which transgenic or knock-in mice carrying such oncogenic alleles will by treated by RNA-based therapeutics.

With respect to future medical applications, siRNAs were recently directed against a pathological transcript associated with the spinobulbular muscular atrophy (SBMA) in tissue culture. Together with the Huntington's disease, SBMA belongs to a growing group of neurodegenerative disorders caused by the expansion of trinucleotide repeats. Targeting the CAG expanded mRNA transcript by dsRNA may be an attractive alternative to commonly used therapeutic strategies that, beyond symptomatic treatment, mainly focus on the inhibition of the toxic effects of the polyglutaminated protein. Caplen*et al.* successfully targeted pathologic RNA of the androgene receptor in human kidney 293T cells that was introduced by transfection of a plasmid encoding the expanded CAG construct. Therapeutically most important, the authors achieved a rescue of the polyglutamine-induced cytotoxicity in cells treated with dsRNA molecules (3). Even if this study did not knock down an endogenous disease-related transcript the approach underlines the remarkable broad potency and sequence-specificity of RNAi-mediated gene therapy. Whether the RNAi pathway is functionally active in various neuronal cells irrespective of their state of differentiation remains to be shown.

In sum, RNAi clearly has the potential to change the nucleic-based therapies for cancer, infectious diseases and many other diseases (4). However, the universality of this approach, the types of genes that can be silenced using this strategies in human cells, remain unknown to date.

References

1. Tamm, I., Dorken, B., and Hartmann, G. (2001) Antisense therapy in oncology: new hope for an old idea? Lancet 358:489–497.
2. Brummelkamp, T. R., Bernards, R., and Agami, R. (2002) Stable suppression of tumorigenicity by virus-mediated RNA interference. Cancer Cell 2:243–247.
3. Caplen, N. J., Taylor, J. P., Statham, V. S., Tanaka, F., Fire, A., and Morgan, R. A. (2002) Rescue of polyglutamine-mediated cytotoxicity by double-stranded RNA- mediated RNA interference. Human Molecular Genetics 11:175–184.
4. Paddison, P. J., and Hannon, G. J. (2002) RNA interference: the new somatic cell genetics? Cancer Cell 2:17–23.

Antithyroid Drugs

K. MIEHLE, R. PASCHKE
III. Medical Department, University of Leipzig, Leipzig, Germany
pasr@medizin.uni-leipzig.de

Synonyms

Thionamides

Definition

Antithyroid drugs block thyroid hormone production in the thyroid gland and are therefore used for the treatment of hyperthyroidism. Substances described here belong to the thionamide group. Other drugs utilized to treat hyperthyroidism are β-blocking agents, and seldom lithium.

Thionamides are heterocyclic compounds that contain a thiourylene group. Thiouracil was the first widely used antithyroid drug. Further studies

Tab. 1 Different treatment strategies depending on the cause of hyperthyroidism.

	Graves' Disease	Thyroid Autonomy toxic nodule toxic multinodular goiter
Etiology	- organ specific autoimmune disease - TSH receptor antibody production	constitutively activating somatic mutation in TSH receptor or in Gs α
Remission after Antithyroid Drug Treatment	in 40-50% of patients 1 year after treatment withdrawal	no remission
Antithyroid Drug Treatment	1 year	until euthyroid
Treatment with Radioiodine or Surgery	if relapse after 1 year of antithyroid drug treatment	after euthyroidism is achieved

led to the introduction of substances with fewer side effects. Three drugs of this type are currently in use: methimazole, carbimazole and propylthiouracil (1). Thiouracil and propylthiouracil belong to the subgroup of pyrimidines, whereas methimazole and carbimazole belong to the thioglyoxalines. The goitrogenic properties of several substances were first recognized in the 1940s when thyroid enlargement was noticed in rats that had been given sulfaguanine to study the antibiotic effects of sulfaguanidine on the intestinal flora (1,2). Others noted the development of goiters in rats fed with phenylthiocarbamide. Later it was concluded that the effect of thiourea and the sulfonamides was due to the inhibition of thyroid hormone synthesis. It was first suggested that the entire thiourylene grouping (NH.CS.NH) would be necessary for antithyroid activity. Further studies revealed that only the thiocarbamide group (S=C-N) is essential for antithyroid activity (2).

Mechanism of Action

Synthesis of thyroid hormones occurs in several steps. At first, inorganic iodide is actively concentrated by thyroid follicular cells by the sodium iodide symporter. After oxidation to iodine (= iodination) it is bound to tyrosine residues thus forming monoiodothyronine (MIT) or diiodothyronine (DIT). MIT and DIT are coupled to form ▶ triiodothyronine (T_3) or ▶ thyroxine (T_4). Both iodination and coupling occur at the apical membrane of the thyroid follicular cell and within the ▶ thyroglobuline (Tg) molecule, and are catalyzed by the enzyme ▶ thyroid peroxidase (TPO). TPO is a hemoprotein enzyme with binding sites for both iodine and tyrosine. In model systems, TPO has no catalytic activity in the absence of H_2O_2. Therefore, it is assumed that H_2O_2 production is important also for thyroid hormone formation *in vivo*. TPO degrades H_2O_2 in a catalase-like reaction releasing O_2. Several iodination intermediates were postulated for this reaction, for instance TPO–bound iodinium (I^+) and TPO–bound hypoiodite (I^-). T3 and T4 are stored in the follicular lumen bound to thyroglobuline. The re-entry of Tg into the thyroid follicular cell involves a macropinocytosis process. Thyroid hormones are released after proteolysis of Tg. Type I and type II 5′ deiodinase generate the active hormone T_3 by reductive deiodination of the phenolic ring of T4 (6).

Antithyroid drugs inhibit the thyroid peroxidase-mediated iodination and coupling. Inactivation of TPO by antithyroid drugs involves a reaction between the drugs and the oxidized heme group produced by the interaction between TPO and H_2O_2. Results of several studies suggested that antithyroid drugs bind to the enzyme either at the same site as iodide or at a nearby site, and that the binding interferes with the binding of iodide (2,6). The type of inhibition depends on the extent of TPO inactivation and drug oxidation. These rates depend mainly on the iodine to drug concentration ratio. At a high iodine to drug ratio the inhibition of iodination is reversible and TPO is only

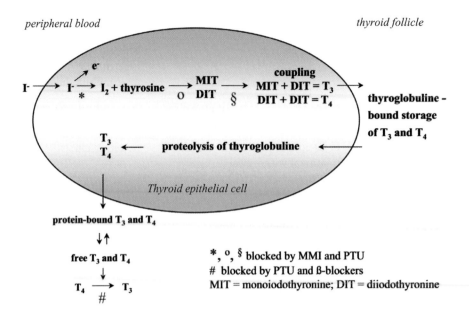

Fig. 1 Synthesis and secretion of thyroid hormones and mechanisms of action of antithyroid drugs. Iodine is actively concentrated by the thyroid gland (sodium iodide transporter). After oxidation it is bound to thyrosine residues thus forming monoiodothyronine (MIT) or diiodothyronine (DIT). MIT and DIT are coupled to triiodothyronine (T_3) or thyroxine (T_4) and are stored in thyroid follicles bound to thyroglobuline. Thyroid hormones are released by proteolysis. In the peripheral blood, T_4 is converted to T_3. Antithyroid drugs act by inhibiting the thyroid peroxidase-mediated formation of T_3 and T_4 (§) and compete with iodothyronine residues for oxidized iodine (o). Moreover, they inhibit iodine oxidation (*). PTU, but not MMI, inhibits the monodeiodination (#) of thyroxine to triiodothyronine.

partially inactivated. Under these conditions, extensive drug oxidation occurs. When the iodine to drug ratio is low, iodination is irreversibly inhibited. This is associated with rapid and complete inactivation of TPO (2,6).

PTU, but not MMI, has an additional peripheral effect. It inhibits the monodeiodination of thyroxine to triiodothyronine by blocking the enzyme 5′ monodeiodinase (1). In humans the potency of MMI is at least 10 times higher than that of PTU, whereas in rats PTU is more potent than MMI. The higher potency of MMI in humans is probably due to differences in uptake into the thyroid gland and subsequent metabolism, because *in vitro* inhibition of thyroid peroxidase by MMI is not significantly more potent than by PTU (1, 6). Whether antithyroid drugs have additional immunosuppressive actions in Graves' disease is a matter of discussion (1, 6).

Pharmacokinetics

Absorption of MMI from the gastrointestinal tract occurs rapidly and almost completely. Peak serum concentrations increase linearly with dose and are in the range of 300 ng/ml 1 to 2 h after oral ingestion of 15 mg MMI (1). *In vitro* carbimazole is an effective inhibitor of iodination without prior hydrolysis to MMI. In contrast, carbimazole itself is inactive *in vivo*. During absorption and in serum it is almost completely converted to methimazole (2). 10 mg carbimazole is equivalent to 6.7 mg MMI (6). MMI is virtually not protein bound. The total volume distribution is about 40 liters. The serum half life is 4–6 h and remains unchanged in hyperthyroid patients. Patients with hepatic disease have prolonged plasma disappearance, whereas in kidney disease the metabolism is unchanged. Because of its lipophilic character the transplacental passage and excretion in breast milk is high (1,2). Little MMI is excreted in urine. Little is known about the products of metabolism of MMI and their way of excretion (1).

PTU is also well absorbed from the gastrointestinal tract. Peak serum concentrations are in the range of 3 µg/ml after an oral dose of 150 mg, and is reached 1 hour after drug ingestion. 80–90% of PTU is protein bound. The total volume distribution is around 30 l for PTU. The serum half life of PTU is 75 min. It is not altered in patients with thyrotoxicosis, renal disease and, in contrast to MMI, in liver disease. PTU is mostly excreted in the urine after hepatic conjugation with glucuronide (1,2). Biotransformation of PTU primarily occurs at the S group. It results in substantial loss of antiperoxidase activity. The metabolites, 6-n-propyluracil, S-methyl-PTU, PTU disulfide and PTU glucuronide, are only weakly active or completely inactive as thyroid peroxidase inhibitors. Because of its high protein binding and ionization at a physiologic pH, PTU is excreted in breast milk to a lesser degree than MMI (1).

Both drugs, MMI and PTU, are actively concentrated by the thyroid gland. Intrathyroidal concentrations of MMI are in the range of 5×10^5 M. There is no difference in intrathyroidal concentrations of MMI 3–6 h and 17–20 h after ingestion of 10 mg of carbimazole. Little is known about intrathyroidal concentrations of PTU. Eight hours after a single dose of 10 mg of MMI or 100 mg of PTU inhibition of intrathyroidal organification of iodide is about 90% and 60% respectively (2). This may be one reason for the longer effect of MMI compared with PTU. MMI can be administered once daily, whereas PTU should be applied 3 times a day.

Metabolism of the drugs by TPO is largely iodine dependent. Under conditions of reversible inhibition of iodination, the drugs are rapidly metabolized to higher oxidation products such as sulfonate and sulfate, with disulfide as an intermediate. If there is irreversible inhibition of iodination (higher drug to iodide ratio), some of the drug is oxidized only to the disulfide stage, but the TPO is simultaneously inactivated and no iodination is observed (2,6).

Clinical Use (incl. side effects)

Clinical Use

In patients with a first episode of ▶ Graves' disease, thionamides are used for long-term treatment to achieve remission of the organ-specific autoimmune disease. The standard therapy in Europe is a 1–1.5 year course of antithyroid drug treatment. In contrast, ▶ radioiodine is the preferred initial treatment in North America (4, 6). The relapse rate following antithyroid drug treatment is approximately 50% within 1 to 2 years. Most relapses occur within the first 12 months (4, 6). After an unsuccessful course of antithyroid drug treatment there is little chance that a second course will result in permanent remission (4, 6). Therefore a definite treatment, i. e. surgery or radioiodine, should be performed. Various parameters have been tested for their ability to predict the outcome of the individual patient after withdrawal of antithyroid drug therapy, but until now, the studies have failed to identify reliable markers with predictive statistical significance for the individual patient (4, 6). In ▶ thyroid autonomy that is mainly caused by somatic ▶ TSH receptor or Gsα mutations (5) a spontaneous remission (e. g. by nodule apoplexia) is very uncommon. Therefore, antithyroid drug treatment is only used to render patients euthyroid before ablative treatment.

Initial daily doses of 10–40 mg and 100–600 mg are recommended in clinical practice for MMI and PTU, respectively (1). Several studies have shown that treatment of hyperthyroidism with single daily doses of 10–40 mg of MMI is effective in the induction of euthyroidism in 80–90% of patients within 6 weeks (6). Intrathyroidal drug accumulation is one cause for the efficiency of a single daily dose regimen. Moreover, a once daily dose yields better patients' compliance. Single daily doses of PTU have been shown to be less effective in achieving euthyroidism than administration of 3 divided doses a day. If a once daily dose regimen is considered for the treatment of hyperthyroidism, MMI is preferred to PTU (1, 6).

The response to thionamides depends on the dose and the environmental iodine intake. It occurs faster in subjects living in countries with moderately low iodine intake than in areas with iodine sufficiency (1, 6). Drug doses should be gradually decreased to the minimal maintenance dose as the serum thyroid hormone levels fall. The aim is to restore the euthyroid state within 1 to 2 months. The "block-and-replace regimen" with the simultaneous administration of an antithyroid drug and L-thyroxine is used in case of poor patients compliance or if follow-up is difficult (4).

Side Effects

Antithyroid drugs have several side effects. The most frequent side effects are maculopapular rashes, pruritus, urticaria, fever, arthralgia and swelling of the joints. They occur in 1–5% of patients (1, 6). Loss of scalp hair, gastrointestinal problems, elevations of bone isoenzyme of alkaline phosphatase and abnormalities of taste and smell are less common. The incidence of all these untoward reactions is similar with MMI and PTU (1,2). PTU may cause slight transient increases of serum aminotransferase and γ-glutamyl transpeptidase concentrations. The side effects usually appear within the first weeks or months after starting treatment and mostly resolve despite continued therapy. They occur more frequently with higher drug doses (1,2, 6). If they are severe enough to alter treatment, it is possible to change from MMI to PTU or vice versa, although there is an estimated cross sensitivity of about 50% (6). Most of the minor side effects are considered to be allergic reactions. Serious side effects such as bone marrow-depression, vasculitis, systemic lupus-like syndrome, cholestatic jaundice, hepatitis, hypoglycemia due to antiinsulin antibodies and hypoprothrombinemia are rare. They occur in approximately 0.2–0.5% of patients (1). Depression of the bone marrow mostly appears as agranulocytosis, but also aplastic anemia and thrombocytopenia can be found. Symptoms of agranulocytosis like sore throat, fever and stomatitis are rare. Because of the sudden onset of agranulocytosis it can often not be detected in time by the routine leucocyte cell count which should be performed repeatedly during the first 3 months of treatment (1, 6). Agranulocytosis is an absolute contraindication to further antithyroid drug treatment. Therefore, patients should be advised to stop taking the drug immediately if sore throat, pharyngitis or fever occur, and immediately seek medical attention and an urgent blood cell count. Most patients recover from agranulocytosis after discontinuation of antithyroid drugs. But deaths have been reported in 20% of patients despite treatment with intravenous broad spectrum antibiotics. Granulocyte colony-stimulating factor has been administered, but did not yield a better outcome in the treatment of antithyroid drug-induced agranulocytosis compared with antibiotic therapy only. The risk of agranulocytosis is greater in patients given larger doses and in older patients (1,2, 6). Vasculitis and lupus-like syndrome occur much more frequently with PTU than with MMI; their cause is not known. Treatment consists of discontinuation of the drug and the use of high doses of glucocorticoids. Major side effects usually occur within the first 3 months after the start of antithyroid drug treatment but can also appear during prolonged treatment and after reinstitution of the drug (1,2, 6).

References

1. Cooper DS (2000) Treatment of thyrotoxicosis. In: Braverman LE, Utiger RD (eds) Werner and Ingbar: The Thyroid. Lippincott Williams & Wilkins, Philadelphia, p 691–715
2. Marchant B, Lees J, Alexander WD (1978) Antithyroid drugs. Pharmacology & Therapeutics. Part B: General & Systematic Pharmacology 3:305–348
3. Weetman A (2000) Graves' disease. New England Journal of Medicine.343:1236–1248
4. Paschke R, Ludgate M (1997) The thyrotropin receptor in thyroid diseases. New England Journal of Medicine.337:1675–1681
5. Taurog A (2000) Thyroid hormone synthesis: Thyroid iodine metabolism. In: Braverman LE, Utiger RD (eds) Werner and Ingbar: The Thyroid. Lippincott Williams & Wilkins, Philadelphia, p 61–85
6. Miehle K, Paschke R (2003) Therapy of hyperthyroidism. Experimental and Clinical Endocrinology and Diabetes. In press

Antitrypanosomal Drugs

Despite the enthusiasm shown by Robert Koch and Paul Ehrlich in African sleeping sickness, progress in the control of this disease achieved since the 19th century is sobering. Only four substances have been introduced, in total, in the therapy of African sleeping sickness, although the incidence of this disease has increased tremendously during the past decades with an estimated 50 million people at risk of infection and approximately 20 000 new cases reported each year. Suramin, the oldest of the antitrypanosomal drugs, was discovered by Paul Ehrlich and introduced in 1922. It was followed by pentamidine in 1937. Both drugs are only effective against early stages of the disease. The first and only drug effective against cerebral stages of African trypanosomiasis, of both *T. brucei gambiense* and *T. brucei rhodesiense* type, is melarsoprol, which has been in use for more than 50 years. It is still the drug of choice in most endemic areas despite its marked tendency to induce reactive encephalitis. Since then, drug and vaccine development in this field has declined to near zero. The only new antitrypanosomal substance so far has been eflornithine (difluoromethylornithine), which was introduced in 1990. It was originally developed for cancer therapy and proved later to be effective against intracerebral *T. b. gambiense*.

Nowadays, treatment of African sleeping sickness with the prevailing drugs faces three major problems: 1) severe side effects, especially of melarsoprol; 2) wide spread drug resistance;and 3) lack of interest in drug development and production due to a low return of investment. To make matters worse, in recent years the producers of melarsoprol as well as eflornithine have tried to stop the production of these drugs entirely. A vaccine against trypanosomiasis is also not in sight, and efforts are complicated by the parasite's ability to constantly change the antigenic properties of its surface coat, a phenomenon called antigenic variation.

▶ Antiprotozoal Drugs

Antituberculosis Drugs

Antituberculosis drugs or antimycobacterial agents are specifically used for the treatment of tuberculosis (*Mycobacterium tuberculosis* infections). First-line drugs in tuberculosis therapy are isoniazid, rifampicin, ethambutol, pyrazinamide and streptomycin (▶ Ribosomal Protein Synthesis Inhibitors). In order to minimize the development of drug resistance, a compound drug therapy is employed. In a first phase of two months, a combination of three drugs is employed. In a second phase of about four months, a combination of two drugs is used. A major problem is the increasing resistance of *Mycobacterium tuberculosis* strains against the first-line drugs. Infections caused by resistant strains are treated with combinations of second-line agents (e.g. capreomycin and cycloserine).

Antitussives

Antitussives are used for the symptomatic treatment of cough. Usually, cough is a protective reflex for the removal of secretions and particulate matter from the respiratory tract. Only inappropriate cough, caused, e.g. by respiratory tract infections or tumors, requires treatment. The opioid codeine (methylmorphine; opioid system) depresses the "cough center" in the brainstem and is a highly effective antitussive. Other centrally acting antitussives are dextromethorphan and noscapine.

Antiviral Drugs

HANS-GEORG KRÄUSSLICH, BARBARA MÜLLER
Abteilung Virologie, Universitätsklinikum
Heidelberg, Heidelberg, Germany
Hans-Georg_Kraeusslich@med.uni-heidelberg.de,
barbara_mueller@med.uni-heidelberg.de

Synonyms

Antivirals, virostatics

Definition

Viruses are small infectious agents composed of a nucleic acid genome (DNA or RNA) encased by structural proteins and in some cases a lipid ▶ envelope. They are the causative agents of a number of human infectious diseases, the most important for public health today being ▶ AIDS, ▶ hepatitis, ▶ influenza and measles. In addition, certain viruses contribute to the development of cancer. Antiviral drugs inhibit viral replication by specifically targeting viral enzymes or functions and are used to treat specific virus-associated diseases.

▶ Interferons
▶ Viral Proteases

Mechanism of Action

Basic Principles

Viruses are obligatory intracellular parasites that can only replicate within an appropriate host cell. They rely on host cell-derived factors and mechanisms and encode only few enzymes and other proteins of their own. Consequently, interfering with virus replication without inflicting damage to the host requires highly specific approaches and there is no general mechanism of action for virostatics. In contrast to antibacterial agents, where fundamental differences between prokaryotic and human cells (e.g. bacterial cell wall synthesis) can be exploited to inhibit a broad range of bacteria without significant toxicity to the patient, antiviral drugs are mostly highly selective for a specific virus or a limited number of related viruses. Furthermore, many human virus infections are acute and are rapidly controlled by the immune system. In these cases, the highest ▶ viremia - i.e. the time when the patient would benefit the most from causative antiviral treatment - usually preceeds the clinical manifestation of symptoms and the diagnosis by serological methods. For these reasons, the number of currently available antiviral drugs is low compared to chemotherapeutics effective against other classes of infectious agents. Most antivirals have been developed to control chronic or recurrent virus infections, and in many cases antiviral treatment does not result in elimination of the virus but rather reduction of virus replication and alleviation of symptoms. In principle, antivirals can be targeted at any of the viral replication steps outlined in Fig. 1. (a) Binding: Viruses attach to their host cells via binding of a viral surface protein to a receptor molecule on the plasma membrane. This interaction is highly specific and presents a very attractive target for antiviral intervention. The most advanced compounds in this class are the human immunodeficiency virus (HIV) co-receptor antagonists. These substances (peptides or bicyclam derivatives) bind to and block the cellular chemokine receptors CCR5 or CXCR4, respectively, which are required in addition to the CD4 receptor to mediate HIV entry. Some co-receptor antagonists are currently in clinical trials. (b) Entry of the virus into the cell and release of the viral genome (uncoating): Although this process is not characterized in its entirety for most viruses, random screening has identified amantadine/rimantadine, which inhibit this step in **influenza** A replication. In addition, entry inhibitors specific for ▶ HIV or ▶ picornaviruses, respectively, are under development. (c) Replication of the viral genome: Viruses contain either single- or double-stranded DNA or RNA genomes and employ a variety of replication strategies. Thus, there is no general mechanism or replication enzyme common to viruses. However, to accomodate for various replication strategies, many viruses encode their own polymerase(s), the biochemical and structural properties of which differ in some respects from those of the host cell polymerases. This can be exploited to specifically interfere with viral genome replication, and a number of inhibitors targeting viral replicases have been developed as antiviral drugs. (d) Expression of viral genes leads to the production of virus proteins: The basic machineries for transcription of virus genes and translation of mRNA into viral proteins largely rely on cellular factors and are therefore difficult to target. Many viruses encode proteins regulating transcription or mRNA transport and modification (e.g. the HIV Tat and Rev proteins), which are potential candidates for inhibition. However, drugs specifically interfering with viral gene expression have not yet been developed. (e) Virus assembly comprises transport of the virion components to the assembly site, formation of an ordered ▶ capsid structure and in some cases morphological maturation of the particle into a fully infectious state. Capsid stability depends on multiple interactions between viral structural proteins, and interfering with only a few interactions should suffice to disturb the ordered

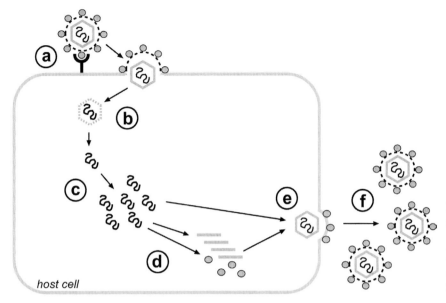

A

Fig. 1 Basic steps of viral replication: (a) binding, (b) entry, (c) genome replication, (d) gene expression, (e) assembly, (f) release.

host cell

capsid architecture essential for infectivity. The subunit interfaces, unlike viral enzymes, do not have correlates in the host cell. This should allow the design of efficient and specific inhibitors, but to date insufficient understanding of the molecular processes involved and the lack of suitable assay systems has prevented the development of assembly inhibitors for antiviral therapy. However, highly effective antiviral drugs targeting the process of virion maturation (▶ protease inhibitors) have been developed against HIV. (f) Virus release from the producing cell is required for virus spread: It can be accomplished by cell lysis, exocytosis or, in the case of many enveloped viruses, by budding from the plasma membrane. Virus budding is a complex process involving a number of host cell derived factors, and drugs targeting the budding process itself have not yet been developed. However, the recently introduced influenza neuraminidase inhibitors are effective by blocking the release and spread of influenza viruses.

Interferon (IFN) differs from *bona fide* antiviral drugs since it is a natural defense protein of the host organism and does not directly interfere with the viral replication steps. Interferons are small glycoproteins inducing immune modulatory and antiviral activities. They are secreted by lymphocytes, leukocytes and fibroblasts in response to foreign nucleic acids (dsRNA). IFNs are classi-

fied into three groups α, β and γ, and the different classes are produced from different cell types. Recombinant IFN-α is used in the treatment of chronic hepatitis B and C.

Mechanisms of Action of Currently Used Antiviral Drugs

The only drugs acting at the initial steps in virus replication currently in use are the adamantane derivatives, amantadine and rimantadine. Amantadine inhibits influenza virus replication and has been in clinical use since the early 1970s, but its mechanism of action was elucidated only 20 years later. It blocks the M2 ion channel in the envelope of influenza A virus, thereby inhibiting virus uncoating. Adamantanes are not efficient against influenza B, which lacks the M2 protein. Drugs inhibiting the binding and entry of HIV are currently under development and their introduction into clinical use can be expected. A promising concept is represented by T-20. This peptide derivative binds to a helix in the envelope protein gp41, which is exposed upon binding of HIV to its host cell. Binding of T-20 blocks a conformational rearrangement of gp41 molecules into a 6-helix bundle that is required to mediate fusion of viral and cellular membranes. Entry inhibitors specific for entero-and rhinoviruses are drugs based on the substance pleconaril. It binds to a hydrophobic pocket on the surface of picornavirus capsids resulting in conformational changes of the ► capsid that interfere with the release of the viral RNA genome into the host cell. Such drugs have been developed but are not yet approved for therapy.

Polymerase inhibitors with different mechanisms of action account for the largest group of currently available antiviral drugs. The most important class are the chain terminating nucleoside analogs (Fig. 2). The prototype of this class is acyclovir (ACV) which is used against herpes simplex (HSV) and ► varicella zoster viruses (VZV). ACV is an acyclic analog of the nucleoside thymidine, with carbon atoms C2 and C3 missing from the deoxyribose ring. Phosphorylation by ► HSV thymidine ► kinase (TK) inside an infected cell yields ACV-monophosphate, which is further converted into ACV-triphosphate by cellular enzymes and then serves as a substrate for the HSV polymerase. ACV incorporation into DNA results in chain termination due to the lack of the 3'OH group required for further elongation. Since both monophosphorylation and incorporation into DNA are preferably carried out by viral enzymes, selectivity on two levels reduces toxicity to uninfected cells. Efficacy of phosphorylation and incorporation into DNA are not correlated: whereas penciclovir (oral prodrug: famciclovir) is a much better substrate for TK than ACV, penciclovir triphosphate is incorporated less efficiently by the viral polymerase than ACV-triphosphate. An optimal inhibitor should be a good substrate for both viral enzymes. Human cytomegalovirus (HCMV) lacks a *tk* gene and is relatively insensitive to ACV, but a protein encoded by gene *UL97* of HCMV is able to phosphorylate the nucleoside analog ganciclovir (GCV). This analog also efficiently interferes with cellular DNA polymerisation, and thus has a higher toxicity than ACV. Resistance against GCV can develop through mutations in either *UL97* (90%) or the viral polymerase gene. The alternative drug cidofovir is a cytosine phosphonate analog, which only depends on cellular enzymes for its conversion into the active form. Thus, its efficacy is not affected by mutations in *UL97*. A direct inhibitor of viral polymerase, which does not require intracellular activation, is foscarnet (phosphonoformic acid). The chain terminating mechanism is shared by another important group of antivirals, the nucl-

eosidic and nucleotidic ► reverse transcriptase (RT) inhibitors (NRTI and N+RTI), which inhibit the RT of HIV. A number of different NRTIs are available in different formulations, e.g. azidothymidine (AZT), ddI, ddC and d4T. All of these are nucleoside analogs, in which the 3'OH group is missing or replaced by another functional group, e.g. an azido group in AZT. NRTI are also applied as prodrugs which have to be phosphorylated by cellular kinases into their active triphosphate form. N+RTIs (Tenofovir, Adefovir) are monophosphorylated derivates. In this case the first - and often rate-limiting step of activtion is circumvented. Hepatitis B virus (HBV) (► Hepatitis), another important human pathogen, also encodes an RT, and several nucleoside/nucleotide analogs originally developed against HIV (e.g. lamivudine, adefovir) are also active against HBV. Lamivudine (3TC) has been tested for the treatment of hepatitis and is considered a promising candidate anti-HBV drug. As obvious from this example, chain terminators are not exclusively selective for the particular viral polymerase targeted, since nucleoside analogs bind to the relatively conserved active site of polymerases. Thus, a certain degree of inhibition of cellular polymerases also has to be taken into account. Furthermore, soon after the introduction of AZT for the treatment of AIDS patients in 1987, it became apparent that although it was possible to lower the viral load by up to 80% through AZT monotherapy, the therapeutic success was limited by the rapid emergence of drug resistant virus. The same unfortunately holds true for other NRTI, and resistance development against nucleoside inhibitors is also observed in the case of HBV and herpesviruses. The search for alternative anti-HIV drugs led to the discovery of another class of polymerase inhibitors, the so-called non-NRTI (NNRTI). NNRTI in clinical use are nevirapine, delavirdine and efavirenz. These polycyclic compounds do not mimic nucleosides, but act as allosteric inhibitors inducing conformational changes that lock the polymerase active site in an inactive conformation. Unlike NRTI, NNRTI are highly specific for the RT of HIV.

Another antiviral nucleoside analog is the guanosine analog ribavirin, which is active against certain RNA viruses (hepatitis C virus, respiratory syncytial virus, lassavirus) and is administered in

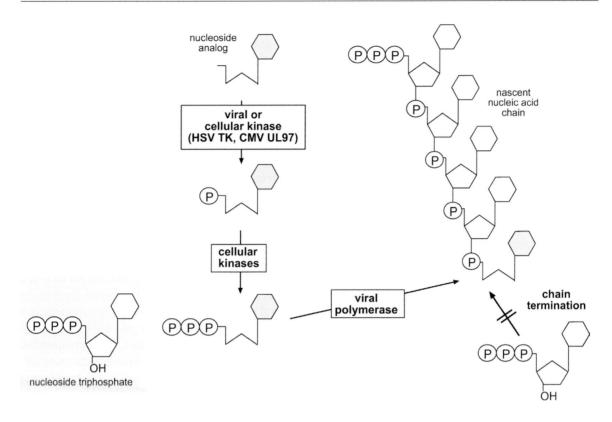

Fig. 2 Mechanism of action of chain terminating nucleoside analogues.

combination with IFN-α for treatment of chronic hepatitis C. Its mechanism of action is not completely elucidated. It is known that ribavirin-monophosphate inhibits cellular inosine mono-phosphate dehydrogenase and this leads to depletion of the cellular GTP pool, which can interfere with viral genome replication or mRNA capping.

Antiretroviral drugs interfering with a later replication step are ► protease (PR) inhibitors affecting HIV infectivity. Like other retroviruses, HI-virions are released from the cell as immature, non-infectious particles, in which the capsid is assembled from the structural polyprotein Gag. Concomitant with release, Gag is cleaved into its functional subdomains by the viral ► PR, leading to a structural rearrangement of the capsid essential for virion infectivity. Thus, PR inhibitors are effective anti-HIV drugs. Retroviral PR are aspartyl proteases, and inhibitors of members of this class (renin, pepsin) had been investigated prior the onset of the AIDS epidemic. These inhibitors

are peptidomimetics resembling substrates in which the scissile peptide bond is replaced by a non-cleavable structural analog of the substrates ► transition state. Further modifications result in optimized selectivity, stability and bioavailability of the compounds. Based on this concept and detailed structural and biochemical information about HIV PR, effective inhibitors were designed, several of which are used for the treatment of AIDS patients (saquinavir, ritonavir, indinavir, nelfinavir, amprenavir, lopinavir; tipranavir and atazanavir are expected to be introduced soon)

The influenza virus inhibitors, zanamivir and oseltamivir, act outside the cell after virus particles have been formed. The drugs have been designed to fit into the active site of the viral envelope enzyme neuraminidase, which is required to cleave sialic acid off the surface of the producing cells. When its activity is blocked, new virus particles stay attached to the cell surface through binding of the virus protein hemagglutinin to sialic acid and are prevented from spreading to other cells.

Clinical Use (incl. side effects)

Only a limited spectrum of viral infections can be currently treated with antiviral drugs; otherwise prevention by vaccination (if possible) and hygiene measures are the only options. Influenza can be treated with amantadine or rimantadine. Both drugs are only effective against influenza A and cause significant side effects including dizziness, lightheadedness, insomnia and nausea. Thus, the newer neuraminidase inhibitors zanamivir (aerosol) and oseltamivir (oral), active against influenza A and B and with lower risk of side effects, may be preferable. Since potential side effects include bronchospasm, these drugs are not recommended for patients with chronic pulmonary disease or asthma. In any case, treatment needs to be started within 36–48 h after the manifestation of the first symptoms and only alleviates the course of disease. Amantadine is also approved for prophylactic treatment of exposed persons with particularly high risk of influenza-associated complications. Infections with the herpesviruses ▶ HSV and ▶ VZV are treated with acyclovir (orally available prodrug: valaciclovir) or famciclovir. Intravenous treatment is indicated for herpes virus encephalitis, neonatal HSV infection, and HSV and VZV reactivation under immunosuppression. Herpes genitalis and herpes zoster are treated orally, and topical acyclovir treatment is used against herpes labialis. Alternative HSV and VZV treatment is possible using idoxuridine or vidarabin. Foscarnet can be used against resistant viruses but has a higher risk of side effects (nephrotoxicity). Indications for the use of ganciclovir are ▶ CMV chorioretinitis in ▶ AIDS patients and CMV colitis. It is also used to prevent interstitial pneumonia in immunosuppressed patients. Ganciclovir is more toxic than acyclovir and causes neutropenia in about 40% of patients. Alternatively, CMV infection can be treated with cidofovir or foscarnet, which are also effective against ganciclovir-resistant CMV but have an even higher toxicity. In pharmacologically immunosuppressed transplant recipients, ganciclovir or acyclovir are administered to prevent CMV or HSV disease, respectively. An anti CMV drug based on a new mechanism of action is Fomivirsen. It is an antisene RNA which inhibits the synthesis of a viral protein and is approved for intra-vitreal treatment of CMV retinitis.

A combination therapy of IFN-α ('pegylated', i.e. coupled to polyethylene glycol, which prevents its rapid clearance from the body) and ribavirin over 24–48 weeks is the most effective way to treat chronic hepatitis C. Therapeutic success depends on virus genotype and viral load, but overall this treatment eliminates the virus in about 60% of patients. A major side effect of this combination therapy is hemolytic anemia, attributed to ribavirin. Patients with chronic hepatitis B, characterized by elevated serum alanine aminotransferase levels and detectable HBe antigen for >6 months, are currently treated with IFN-α alone. Reduction of viral replication and clinical improvement can be accomplished in about 30–40% of treated patients. Fatigue, muscle aches, headache, nausea and diarrhea are common side effects of interferon. The most common serious side effect is depression. The use of antiviral nucleoside analogs against HBV is limited by the frequent development of resistant virus variants.

The broadest spectrum of antiviral drugs is available against HIV. However, monotherapy with any of these drugs leads to rapid treatment failure due to selection and further evolution of resistant viruses. Since acquisition of resistance mutations requires virus replication, an efficient therapy regimen and patient compliance are paramount to minimize resistance development. Currently, AIDS patients in developed countries are treated with a combination therapy known as HAART (highly active antiretroviral therapy) involving at least 3 different anti-HIV drugs from the classes mentioned above (NRTI, NNRTI, PRI). Treatment is currently indicated when the patient shows symptoms of AIDS or has a CD4+ cell count below 350/μl or a plasma viral load above 55,000 genome copies/ml. Treatment decisions in other cases are complex and need to be made on an individual basis. Triple therapy is also recommended as prophylaxis following accidental exposure to the virus. In this case, it is crucial that treatment is started within 1–2 h. The introduction of HAART led to a significant decrease in AIDS morbidity and mortality. However, severe side effects (neutropenia, neurological problems, lipodystrophy) can occur especially under prolonged therapy, and even under HAART, resistant and multi-resistant viruses emerge and are transmitted. Thus, HAART requires selection of a suitable drug combination by a physician experienced in AIDS therapy, constant monitoring of viral load and individual adjustment in case of treatment failure or intolerable side effects. Successful treatment in the case of HIV infection does not mean eradication of the virus and therapy has to be continued over many years, probably life-long. For this reason, future goals do not only include the discovery of new anti-HIV drugs, but also the improvement of existing drugs in terms of galenics, side effects and possible combination formulations that make it easier to follow the therapy scheme. Finally, it should be noted that HAART is not available in developing countries, where most of the millions of HIV-infected people live.

High replication rates, error-prone polymerase as well as replication strategies favouring genetic recombination result in rapid virus evolution. Thus, the emergence of drug resistant variants is a general problem for antiviral therapy. Successful antiviral strategies will probably have to be combination therapies employing different drugs. Experiences indicate that co-treatment with two or even three drugs does not prevent viral resistance development, and broadening of the antiviral arsenal is a key issue. Future additions to this arsenal will result from different approaches: First, availability of alternative and improved drugs based on the same mechanisms of action or on the same principles (e.g. inhibition of viral enzymes by substrate analogs) can be expected. For example, lead compounds that inhibit the third enzyme of HIV, integrase have been defined and may be the basis for new anti-HIV drugs. Second, as the molecular understanding of viral biology increases and suitable assay systems for *in vitro* screening can be established, other steps of viral replication that are currently not accessible (assembly, transcriptional and post-transcriptional regulation or virus release) could become targets of chemotherapeutic intervention. Third, there are attempts to include new and experimental therapeutic approaches, such as the use of antisense RNA, siRNA (small interfering RNA) or gene therapy, into antiviral strategies.

References

1. Fields Virology (2001) 4th ed., Knipe D, Howley PM ed., Lippincott Williams & Wilkins.
2. Principles of Virology (2000) Flint SJ, Enquist LW, Krug RM, Racaniello VR, Skalka AM ed., ASM Press.
3. Antiretroviral therapy (2001) DeClercq EDA ed., ASM Press.

Anxiety

Anxiety is a normal reaction. Pathological anxiety interferes with daily-life activities and may be accompanied by autonomic symptoms (chest pain, dyspnoea and palpitations). Severe forms include phobic anxiety and panic disorder.

▶ Benzodiazepines

Anxiolytics

Anxiolytics are drugs used for the treatment of anxiety disorders. Apart from benzodiazpines, a frequently used anxiolytic is the $5HT_{1A}$ (serotonin) receptor agonist buspiron, which has no sedative, amnestic or muscle-relaxant side effects, but whose action takes about a week to develop. Furthermore, it is less efficaceous than the benzodiazepines. Buspiron's mechanism of action is not fully understood.

▶ Anxiety
▶ Benzodiazepines

APCs

▶ Antigen-presenting Cells
▶ Immune Defense

Apoptosis

ROSS CAMERON
Department of Pathology, University of Toronto
and The Toronto Hospital, Toronto, Canada
ross.cameron@uhn.on.ca

Synonyms

▶ Programmed Cell Death (antonym: ▶ Necrosis)

Definition

Apoptosis is involved in the programmed elimination of cells. This is a mechanism for the elimination of excess or damaged cells. Apoptosis also occurs during embryonic and fetal development. In adult life, apoptosis regulates the size of organs and tissues. In pathological conditions, apoptosis is responsible for the reduction of cells in different types of atrophy and in the regression of hyperplasia. It develops spontaneously in cancer cells and it is increased in both neoplasms and during normal cell proliferation triggered by a variety of agents applied in cancer chemotherapy. Apoptosis is enhanced by cell mediated immune reactions and various toxins that also produce necrosis. Apoptosis develops in four different phases: Firstly, the presence of genes regulates the occurrence of programmed cell death. Secondly, various signals, such as calcium ions, glucocorticoid hormones and sphingomyelin, trigger the genetic program. Initiation of apoptosis can also occur by an unbalanced signalling such as lack of growth factor or by the inhibitory effects of molecules such as toxins or toxicants. Thirdly, the progression of apoptosis leads to the expression of genes manifesting in structural alterations such as cytoskeletal changes, cell shrinkage, nuclear ▶ pyknosis, chromatin changes and ▶ DNA fragmentation. Finally, death and engulfment of the whole cell or cell fragments by phagocytosis (▶ phagocyte) terminates the apoptotic process.

Basic Mechanisms

Apoptosis is a process that is regulated by genetic mechanisms, induced by various signalling factors, mediated through plasma membrane receptors and specific ligands, and proceeds to completion through effector molecules such as caspases. Caspases interact with mitochrondria and leads to expansion of effector molecules and ultimately results in DNA fragmentation and phagocytosis of the apoptotic cells by neighbouring cells and professional phagocytic cells or macrophages.

There are a number of specific evidences that transcription of genes is required for cell death: Firstly in developing Drosophila cells, specific genes are transcriptionally activated 1–2 hours before the cells die. In the developing worm, *C. elegans*, there are a number of genes that are involved and associated with the death of developing cells. These genes are given the name *ced-1*, etc. If mutation in *ced-9* occurs, then programmed cell death of most cells of the worm proceeds and leads to eventual death of the nematode. Several other of the genes of *C. elegans* have been shown to be associated with various aspects of cell death. The cytoskeletal reorganization involved in developmental and program cell death is associated with the activation of the *ced-5* gene. The transcription products of *ced-3* are involved in the activation of apoptosis and are structurally homologous to the mammalian protein ▶ caspase-1.

A number of physiologic and pharmacologic stimuli can induce the process of apoptosis, these include steroids, withdrawal of trophic hormones or other growth factors, anti-cancer drugs such as methotrexate and oxidants or other cytotoxic chemicals. The effect of these stimuli are mediated through cell surface receptors that are specific for the apoptotic process.

One of the important cell surface receptor proteins is the receptor ▶ Fas-L which is found on many cells and is involved in transducing the apoptotic signals into the effector intracellular program. For example, with ▶ activation induced cell death of T-cells, the mature lymphocytes are activated by T-cell-receptor interaction with antigen presenting cells. The activated T-cells express Fas-L that binds to the Fas-expressing activating T-cells to produce apoptosis. The ligation of Fas then triggers a release and activation of various effector molecules called caspases. Specific caspases such as caspase-8 then cleave the molecule ▶ BID, which is a normal inducer of the cell death process once it has become truncated or cleaved.

The cleaved BID molecule is then translocated into mitochondria where it is involved in the permeabilization of inner mitochondrial membranes, rupture of the outer mitochondria membranes and release of cell death factors such as cytochrome C and apoptosis-inducing factor or AIF. The release of cytochrome C stimulates more caspases to be released in a cascade.

The interaction of BID with the mitochondria involves the specific process of ▸ mitochondrial permeability transition pore opening, which is a inner membrane-generated large channel that combines with the outer mitochondrial membrane to make a pore. The opening of this pore leads to free radical generation such as ▸ reactive oxygen species, release of calcium into the cytosol and further caspase activation. The build up of caspases leads to cytoskeletal reorganization and also the stimulation of changes in the nuclear membrane pore complex. There is an increase in endonucleolytic activity that cleaves the DNA into 50–300 kilobase high molecular weight fragments that appear by electron microscopy as chromatin condensation. In addition, there is a further endonuclease activation that leads to proteolysis and this results in smaller 10–40 kilobase fragments of DNA. This leads to an appearance, on examining the DNA fragments, of an oligonucleosome ladder. The specific fragmentation of the DNA lent itself to the development of a method for *in situ* labelling of DNA breaks in nuclei, in tissue sections and cells in culture. This method is called ▸ TUNEL.

Pharmacological Intervention

Many drugs have been found to induce apoptosis in experimental conditions or as side effects. Some of these actions are direct by effecting the death pathway, some drugs interfere with biochemical mechanisms and these effects lead indirectly to apoptosis. For example, azide administration inhibits ATP synthesis, diptheria toxin interferes with protein synthesis, and in both cases subsequently apoptosis is induced. Since a variety of pharmacological agents provoke the same reaction, it may be that the effect of drugs is associated with a non-specific stress response leading to the formation of apoptotic bodies.

▸ Chemotherapy drugs are a major example of pharmacological agents that serve as inducers of the process of apoptosis in a number of tissues and with a number of different cell types. Most prominent of this class of inducers are cytosine arabinoside, doxorubicin, etoposide, methotrexate and Taxol. Several mechanistic steps have been identified by studying the effects of cytosine arabinoside on the process of apoptosis in various cell types. It has been demonstrated that mitogen-activated protein kinase and protein kinase C are critical to the apoptotic effects of cytosine arabinoside in promyelocytic leukemic cells. This effect is mediated through the Fas and Fas ligand system. The chemotherapy drug Taxol shows cytotoxicity to tumour cell lines in the form of apoptosis at low dose concentration and cell death by the mechanism of necrosis at drug concentrations that are much higher *in vitro*. The cytotoxic effect of Taxol has been shown to be mediated by its polymerization of microtubules and blockage of entry into the S phase of the cell cycle in these tumor cell lines.

▸ Glucocorticoids are very active physiologic and pharmacologic agents in the induction of apoptosis of a number of cell types, especially lymphocytes. These effects are mediated through the glucocorticoid receptor, a cell surface receptor on leukocytes, which is a steroid hormone receptor that also mediates cytokine interleukin-5 production by lymphocytes. One major effect of glucocorticoids appears to be cell cycle arrest in the G1 phase. A number of specific pharmacologic agents, including betamethazone, triamcinolone, dexamethazone and clobetasol are inducers of apoptosis by means of transcriptional activation of glucocorticoid receptor.

References

1. Cameron RG, Feuer G (2000) Incidence of Apoptosis and its Pathological and Biochemical Manifestations. In "Cameron RG, Feuer G (eds). Apoptosis and its Modulation by Drugs." Springer, Heidelberg, p1–35
2. Arends MJ, Wyllie AJ (1991) Apoptosis: Mechanisms and Roles in Pathology. International Review of Experimental Pathology 32:223–254
3. Mignotte B, Vayssiere JL (1998) Mitochondria and Apoptosis. EJB 252:1–15

4. Savill J, Fadok V, Henson P, Haslett C (1993) Phagocyte recognition of cells undergoing apoptosis. Immunol Today 14:131–136

5. Cameron R, Feuer G (2001) The Effect of Drugs and
Toxins on the Process of Apoptosis. Drug Metabolism and Drug Interactions. 18:1–32

Appetite Control

WALTER BECKER, #HANS-GEORG JOOST
Institute of Pharmacology und Toxicology,
RWTH Aachen, Aachen, Germany; #German
Institute of Human Nutrition;
Potsdam-Rehbrücke, Germany
walter.becker@post.rwth-aachen.de,
joost@mail.dife.de

Synonyms

Control of food intake, regulation of ingestive
behaviour

Definition

Appetite control is a complex function of the brain
that regulates feeding behaviour. This function
integrates cognitive and emotional factors with a
complex array of signals from the gastrointestinal
tract and from adipose tissue. The feeding behaviour controls and is balanced by acute energy
requirements and the long-term storage of substrate as fat.

▶ Anti Obesity Drugs
▶ Diabetes Mellitus
▶ Neuropeptide Y

Basic Mechanisms

Feeding behaviour is subject to both short-term
regulation during a single meal and long-term regulation related to the maintenance of body weight
and fat content. As a complex function of the
brain, ingestive behaviour is controlled by psychological and cognitive factors such as sociocultural
context (e.g. eating habits), experience (sensory
preferences) or emotional status (mood). Appetite
control also integrates information about the status of peripheral organs, particularly the gastrointestinal tract and adipose tissue (1). Two main
groups of signals can be distinguished: (a) Satiety
signals secreted from gastrointestinal organs, and
(b) adiposity signals that are proportionate to
body fat stores. A key factor of this control system
is that energy intake is primarily controlled by
adjustment of meal size rather than meal onset,
allowing the organism to initiate meals at times
that are convenient and to adapt eating patterns to
individual constraints (food availability) and
activities (circadian rhythm).

Satiety Signals

Satiety-inducing signals are conveyed to the brain
by afferent nerve fibers that are sensitive to
mechanical or chemical stimulation of the stomach and small intestine during food ingestion. In
addition, humoral signals such as
▶ cholecystokinin (CCK) are released upon nutrient stimulation of neuroendocrine cells located in
the gastrointestinal wall. These satiety signals converge in the nucleus tractus solitarii in the brainstem and induce meal termination in the absence
of hypothalamic control, as demonstrated in
decerebrate rats. ▶ CCK is the paradigmatic
humoral satiety signal, and its action has been
studied extensively in multiple species including
human. Exogenous administration of CCK dose-
dependently reduces meal size. This effect is synergistically enhanced by other factors that limit
meal size, such as gastric distension. Specific CCK-
A receptor antagonists stimulate food intake in
rats, indicating that endogenous CCK contributes
to the termination of meals. However, repeated
administration of CCK before each meal does not
reduce caloric intake of free-feeding mice or rats
because the animals compensate the reduced meal
size by increasing the number of meals.

Adiposity Signals

It has long been postulated that appetite and food
intake are controlled by signals that originate from
adipose tissue (lipostat hypothesis, (2)). When
energy uptake is greater than total body energy
expenditure (basal metabolic rate, i.e. thermogenesis plus basal muscle activity), excess substrate is
stored as fat. In the long-term control of feeding
behaviour, enlarging fat depots transmit signals to

the brain that inhibit food intake. Both feeding behaviour and energy expenditure (adaptive thermoregulation) are subject to regulation by the brain, in particular by the hypothalamus.

Insulin as a Satiety/Adiposity Signal. The first hormonal signal found to comply with the characteristics of both a satiety and an adiposity signal was insulin (1). Insulin levels reflect substrate (carbohydrate) intake and stores as they rise with blood glucose levels and fall with starvation. In addition, they may reflect the size of adipose stores, because a fatter person secretes more insulin than a lean individual in response to a given increase of blood glucose. This increased insulin secretion in obesity can be explained by the reduced insulin sensitivity of liver, muscle and adipose tissue. Insulin is known to enter the brain, and direct administration of insulin to the brain reduces food intake. The adipostatic role of insulin is supported by the observation that mutant mice lacking the neuronal insulin receptor (NIRKO mice) develop obesity.

Leptin as an Adiposity Signal. ▶ Leptin is a cytokine produced and secreted by adipose tissue in proportion to the body fat content (3). Mice and humans lacking leptin or its receptor develop a severe hyperphagia and a dramatic degree of obesity that is considerably more pronounced than that of the NIRKO mouse. Thus, leptin is the key adiposity signal in rodents and humans. Leptin secretion appears to reflect the metabolic status of the adipocyte rather than the sheer size of triglyceride deposits, and leptin levels may transiently be dissociated from total body fat. Nonetheless, over the course of a day with unrestricted food supply, plasma leptin levels reliably reflect the amount of total body fat. Local administration of leptin into the brain results in reduced food intake. The vast majority of patients with obesity have elevated serum levels of leptin. Thus, it is believed that the polygenic obesity is due to leptin resistance rather than to inadequate leptin secretion, or to a reduced blood/brain transport of the cytokine.

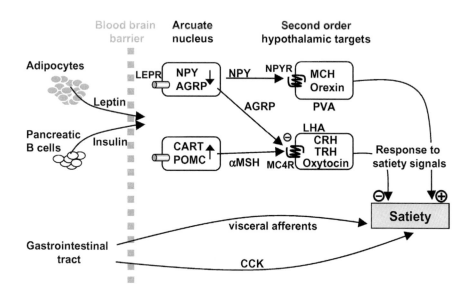

Fig. 1 Diagram of pathways integrating satiety and adiposity signals. Satiety is the net output from brainstem centres that leads to the termination of an individual meal. Satiety is primarily determined by neural and humoral inputs from the gastrointestinal tract (satiety signals). Response to satiety signals is modulated by descending anabolic or catabolic pathways originating in the hypothalamus. Adiposity signals circulate in proportion to total body fat and enter the brain. They stimulate secretion of anorexigenic peptides (αMSH, CART), and inhibit expression of orexigens (NPY, AgRP) in the arcuate nucleus. Secondary target neurons in the paraventricular nucleus (PVN) and the lateral hypothalamic area (LHA) integrate signals from neurons in the arcuate nucleus, and connect them with central autonomic pathways that modulate satiety.

Appetite-Regulating Pathways in the Arcuate Nucleus of the Hypothalamus

Two distinct populations of neurons in the arcuate nucleus have been identified as the most relevant target cells of leptin (Fig. 1 (2,4)). Leptin inhibits expression of the orexigenic peptides NPY (▸ Neuropeptide Y) and AgRP (▸ Agouti-related Protein) in one subset of neurons, and stimulates production of the anorexigenic peptides αMSH (α-melanocyte-stimulating hormone) and ▸ CART (cocaine- and amphetamine-regulated transcript) in the other. Insulin receptors are also highly concentrated in the arcuate nucleus, and insulin appears to elicit similar changes in these neuropeptides as leptin.

The Melanocortin Signalling System. Considerable evidence indicates that the molecules of the melanocortin system are key mediators of the response to leptin. AgRP and αMSH are antagonistic ligands for a common receptor, the melanocortin 4 receptor (MC4R). αMSH is an anorexigenic neuropeptide that activates MC4R and thereby reduces appetite, whereas AgRP is an orexigen that acts as an endogenous antagonist of the receptor and suppresses its activation by αMSH. The critical role of the melanocortin system in appetite regulation is supported by the effects of spontaneous and experimental mutations of AgRP, αMSH, and MC4R in mice. Moreover, patients with complete loss of ▸ proopiomelanocortin (POMC), the precursor molecule of αMSH, develop severe hyperphagia and are overweight, and 4–5% of all cases of severe human obesity appear to be due to mutations in the MC4R gene.

Role of NPY. The second neuropeptide effector of leptin, NPY, has long been known to be a potent orexigen when directly injected into the hypothalamus. Hyperphagia of the leptin-deficient *ob/ob* mice is attenuated by knockout of NPY, supporting the role of NPY as a downstream effector of leptin. However, the neuropeptide is not an indispensable transmitter of adiposity signals, since lean mice which lack NPY show a normal feeding behaviour. The effects of NPY on appetite regulation appears to be mediated by different receptor subtypes (NPY1R, NPY2R and NPY5R).

Second Order Hypothalamic Targets in Adiposity Signalling

The pathways by which the neurons of the arcuate nucleus affect food intake and energy expenditure are not well understood. However, stimulation and lesioning studies have identified the ▸ lateral hypothalamic area (LHA) and the ▸ paraventricular nucleus (PVN) as two areas of the hypothalamus with an important role in energy homeostasis. Lesions of the LHA cause anorexia, whereas ablation of the PVN cause a hyperphagic obesity syndrome. Consistent with these results, LHA neurons express the orexigenic neuropeptides ▸ MCH and ▸ orexin. PVN neurons produce several neuropeptides that are anorexigenic when administered directly into the brain (CRH, TRH, oxytocin), in addition to their better known roles as endocrine regulators. LHA and PVN receive rich inputs from axons of NPY/AgRP- and αMSH/CART-producing neurons in the arcuate nucleus.

Other Hormones, Peptides and Neurotransmitters Involved in Appetite Control

Many other neuropeptides including galanin, ghrelin and ▸ glucagon-like peptide-1 and 2 (GLP-1/GLP-2) have been described to participate in appetite control (Table 1). In addition, the neurotransmitters norepinephrine, dopamine and serotonin are known to be involved in appetite regulation. The role of the monoamines in energy homeostasis is illustrated by effects of drugs (see below). Agonists of α_1 adrenoceptors, 5-HT$_{2C}$ serotonin receptors and dopamine receptors (D1 and/or D2) suppress appetite. However, the relevant neural circuits that use these transmitters are not very well defined. A control system mediating appetite-stimulating effects is the cannabinoid signalling. Recently, endocannabinoids have been added to the list of signals that act downstream of leptin. Leptin reduces levels of the endocannabinoid anandamide in the hypothalamus of normal rats, and mice that lack the cannabinoid receptor 1 (CB1) show reduced food intake under conditions of low leptin levels (after fasting).

Pharmacological Intervention

Appetite-Suppressing Drugs

The increasing prevalence of obesity and its consequences has stimulated the search for appetite-

Tab. 1   Hormones, peptides and neurotransmitters implicated in appetite control.

Molecule	Effect of icv injection on food intake	Effect of gene deletion on food intake	Response to adiposity signals	Receptor	Effect of receptor defect on food intake
Satiety signals					
Cholecystokinin (CCK)	↓		-	CCK-A	↑ (↔[a])
Adiposity signals					
Leptin	↓	↑↑	-	LEPRb	↑↑
Insulin	↓		-	IR	↑[b]
Orexigenic					
Neuropeptide Y (NPY)	↑	↔(↓[c])	↓	NPY2R NPY5R[d]	↑ ↑
Agouti-related peptide (AgRP)	↑		↓	MC4R[d,e]	↑
Melanin-concentrating hormone (MCH)	↑	↓	↓	MCHR1 MCHR2	↑[f]
Orexin A and B (hypocretins)	↑	↔[g]	↓	HCRTR1 HCRTR2	
Galanin	↑	↔		GALR1-3	
Ghrelin	↑		↓	GHSR	
Endocannabinoids	↑			CB1	↔ (↓[h])
Anorexigenic					
α-melanocyte-stimulating hormone (αMSH)	↓	↑[i]	↑	MC4R	↑
Cocaine-and amphetamine regulated transcript (CART)	↓		↑	?	
Corticotropin-releasing hormone (CRH)	↓		↑	CRHR1 CRHR2	↔ (↑[j]) ↔
Urocortin	↓		↑	CRHR1 CRHR2	↔(↑[j]) ↔
Thyreotropin-releasing hormone (TRH)	↓		↑	THRH	
Glucagon-like peptide (GLP-1,2)	↓			GLPR	↔
Serotonin	↓			5-HT$_{1B}$ 5-HT$_{2C}$	↑
Noradrenaline	↓ (↑)			α$_1$,(α$_2$)	

[a] normal basal food intake in knockout mice, but stimulatory response to CCK is abolished
[b] neuron-specific insulin receptor knockout
[c] reduction of hyperphagia was observed in leptin-deficient mice that also lack NPY
[d] other receptor isoforms may also be relevant
[e] AgRP acts antagonistic on MC4 receptors
[f] mice exhibit hyperphagia but are lean due to hyperactivity and altered metabolism
[g] knockout mice exhibit narcolepsy
[h] reduced feeding response to fasting in CB1 knockout mice
[i] αMSH deficiency in patients with mutations in the precursor, proopiomelanocortin (POMC)
[j] normal basal food intake in knockout mice, but inhibitory response to urocortin is attenuated

suppressing drugs as anti-obesity agents (5). Therapy based on nutritional and behavioural counselling produces almost always only a temporary weight loss. The existing drugs that target adrenergic and serotonergic pathways (e.g. metamphetamine, phentermine, fenfluramine, sibutramine) have a negative reputation of toxicity and limited efficacy. The recent insights in appetite control as outlined above have provided new candidate targets for the search of appetite suppressing drugs. Since obesity is usually a chronic disorder that requires life-long therapy, anti-obesity drugs need to meet high safety standards.

β-Phenylethylamine Drugs. The appetite-suppressing effect of β-phenylethylamine drugs is either related to their sympathomimetic effect (metamphetamine, phentermine, diethylpropion), to increased serotonergic transmission (fenfluramine), or both (sibutramine). Compared with metamphetamine, phentermine and diethylpropion appear to have little abuse potential but exhibit the typical side effects of sympathomimetic drugs (insomnia, hypertension). In a 36 week trial, the weight-reducing effect of phentermine persisted for 20 weeks with no further weight reduction thereafter. Use of fenfluramine was terminated after a high incidence of valvular heart disease was reported in patients treated with a combination of phentermine and fenfluramine. The same rationale to combine serotonergic and noradrenergic action underlies the therapy with sibutramine, a serotonin-norepinephrine reuptake inhibitor. Weight reduction by 5–10% was achieved over 24 weeks of treatment with sibutramine in doses from 10–15 mg/d. Weight was regained when the drug was stopped, indicating that a continuous therapy would be necessary to achieve the useful but limited therapeutic effect. This general limitation is likely to apply for any novel drugs that target central noradrenergic and/or serotonergic pathways, e.g. agonists of the $5\text{-}HT_{2C}$ serotonin receptor.

Leptin. Leptin has been shown to markedly reduce appetite and weight in the extremely rare individuals who lack leptin. In contrast, in the first clinical study of patients with polygenic obesity and elevated leptin levels, weight loss was variable and relatively small. This disappointing result may be explained by the leptin resistance consistently observed in obese humans and rodents. However, it cannot be excluded that a small subpopulation of obese patients is susceptible to the cytokine. Major efforts are currently underway to develop new drugs that target hypothalamic pathways downstream of leptin (e.g., NPY receptor antagonists, MC4R agonists, CRH agonists).

Drugs with Appetite-Stimulating Effects

Stimulation of appetite and weight gain has frequently been observed as a side effect of long term therapy with various psychoactive drugs. Prominent examples are the tricyclic (e.g., imipramine) and heterocyclic (e.g., mirtazepine) antidepressants but also selective serotonin reuptake inhibitors (e.g., paroxetine), neuroleptic drugs (e.g., olanzapine) and lithium. Although it is reasonable to assume that these drugs interfere with central serotonergic and/or adrenergic signalling, the exact mechanism of their appetite-stimulating effect and the receptors involved are unknown. Stimulation of appetite by cyproheptadine, an antihistamin/antiserotonin agent, is believed to reflect antagonism of serotonin receptors.

Treatment of Cachexia and Anorexia. In the palliative treatment of cachexia and anorexia in advanced cancer and AIDS patients, modest relief can be achieved with appetite-stimulating drugs. Various pharmacologic strategies have been tested, including corticosteroids, anabolic steroids, megestrol acetate, cyproheptadine and dronabinol (δ-9-tetrahydrocannabinol). The cannabinoid receptor agonist dronabinol is approved in the US for stimulation of appetite in AIDS patients. Megestrol is so far the only agent associated with increased appetite and weight gain in patients with cancer.

References

1. Schwartz MW, Woods SC, Porte D Jr, Seeley RJ, Baskin DG (2000) Central nervous system control of food intake. Nature 404:661–671
2. Spiegelman BM, Flier JS (2001) Obesity and the regulation of energy balance. Cell 104:531–453
3. Friedman JM, Halaas JL (1998) Leptin and the regulation of body weight in mammals. Nature 395:763–770

4. Ahima RS, Osei SY (2001) Molecular regulation of eating behavior: new insights and prospects for therapeutic strategies. Trends Mol Med. 7:205–213
5. Bray GA, Tartaglia LA (2000) Medicinal strategies in the treatment of obesity. Nature 404:672–677

aPTT

▶ Activated Partial Thromboplastin Time
▶ Anticoagulants

Aquaporins

Aquaporins (AQP or water channels) are intrinsic membrane proteins that serve as selective pores through which solute-free water crosses the plasma membrane. There are several types of AQP; more than 10 different mammalian AQP have been identified to date. In mammals they are expressed in several tissues and organs, such as red blood cells, eye, kidney, brain, inner ear, lung, digestive tract, pancreas, liver, glands, testis and sperm. Closely related AQP proteins have been isolated from plants, insects and bacteria.

▶ Vasopressin/Oxytocin

Aquaretic Agents

Aquaretic agents promote the eliminationof water by the kidney without major losses of salts. They are particularly useful in situations where excess of dilutional water needs to be eliminated without affecting the salt metabolism, e.g. congestive heart failure, some stages of hypertension, and some metabolic states.

▶ Vasopressin/Oxytocin

AR

▶ Androgen Receptor

Arachidonic Acid

The 20 carbon fatty acid, 5,8,11,14-eicosatetranoic acid is an important lipid formed from membrane phospholipids by the action of phospholipse A_2 It serves as a precursor for a variety of important mediators like eicosanoids (prostaglandins, leukotrienes and HETEs) or the endogenous cannabinoid receptor ligand, anandamide.

▶ Phospholipases
▶ Cyclooxygenases

Area Postrema

The area postrema is a circumventricular brain region positioned on the dorsal surface of the medulla on the floor of the fourth ventricle. The blood-brain barrier and the cerebrospinal fluid-brain barrier are absent in this region and consequently many substances that do not pass across capillaries in other regions of the brain can do so in the area postrema. The chemoreceptor trigger zone (CTZ), located in the lateral area postrema is sensitive to blood-borne emetogens. Nerves from the CTZ connect with the vomiting centre.

▶ Emesis

Area under the Curve

Area under the Curve (AUC) refers to the area under the curve in a plasma concentration-time curve (▶ Pharmacokinetics). It is directly proportional to the amount of drug which has appeared in the blood ("central compartment"), irrespective of the route of administration and the rate at which the drug enters. The ▶ bioavailability of an orally administered drug can be determined by comparing the AUCs following oral and intravenous administration.

Arginine Vasopressin

▶ Vasopressin/Oxytocin

Aromatase

Aromatase is the enzyme which converts androgens to estrogens. Inhibitors of aromatase are clinically used for the treatment of breast cancer. Examples are the steroidal androstenedione analogs formestane and exemestane and the imidazoles anastrozole, vorozole, and letrozole.

Arousal

Arousal is a state of vigilance regulated by subcortical parts of the nervous system, especially connections between the nuclei of the amygdala, the hypothalamus and the brain stem. These unconscious responses prepare the body for action.

▶ Psychostimulants

Array

An array is the physical substrate to which biological samples are attached to create features (spots). In gene expression, profiling arrays are hybridised with labeled sample and then scanned and analysed to generate data.

▶ Microarray Technology

Arrestins

Arrestins act as adaptor proteins that bind to phosphorylated G-protein-coupled receptors (GPCR) and link the receptors to clathrin-coated pits. β-Arrestins are essential in the internalization of many GPCRs.

▶ β-Adrenergic System
▶ G-protein-coupled Receptors

Arrhythmias

▶ Antiarrhythmic Drugs

Arteriogenesis

Arteriogenesis is the growth of collateral vessels from a pre-existing arteriolar network to bypass an ischemic area (e.g., following cardiac ischemia).

▶ Angiogenesis and Vascular Morphogenesis

Arylhydrocarbon Receptor

The arylhydrocarbon (Ah) receptor belongs to the PAS superfamily of proteins and although distinct in biochemical structure, functions much like the classical nuclear receptors. The Ah receptor binds a variety of small planar xenobiotics including dioxins. The receptor normally resides in the cytoplasm with a dimer of Hsp90, which holds it in a ligand binding form. After ligand binding, the Ah receptor translocates from the cytoplasm into the nucleus and exchanges its chaperone (Hsp90) for the Ah receptor nuclear translocator (ARNT). The Ah receptor-ARNT heterodimer then binds to the dioxin responsive element and activates the transcription of downstream target genes. Among the activated target genes are those encoding enzymes, which metabolize xenobiotics like cytochrome P450, monooxygenase families 1A and 1B (CYP1A and CYP1B), glutathione S-transferase and glucuronyltransferase. Other genes, which are involved in cellular signaling and growth control, such as the c-jun proto-oncogene, cytokines or components of the basic cell-cycle machinery have also been shown to be induced through the Ah receptor.

▶ PAS Domain
▶ Dioxins
▶ Nuclear Receptor Regulation of Drug-metabolizing P450 Enzymes

ASF Family of Transporters

The Amphiphilic Solute Facilitator family of transporters are simple in the sense that no specific source of energy is used for operation (such as hydrolysis of ATP or gradients of inorganic solutes).

▶ Organic Cation Transporters

ASL

▶ Airway Surface Liquid

Asn-linked Glycosylation

Asn-linked glycosylation is the addition of carbohydrate groups to peptides or proteins through specific glycosyltransferases. Glycosyltransferases within the lumen of the endoplasmic reticulum recognize an Asn-X-Ser/Thr motif (X can be any amino acid but not proline) and link carbohydrates *via* a N-acetylglucosamine to the amino group of the asparagine residue.

▶ Intracellular Transport
▶ Protein Trafficking and Quality Control

ASON

ASON stands for antisense oligonucleotides.

▶ Antisense Oligonucleotides and RNA Interference

Aspartyl Proteinases

Aspartyl proteinases are proteinases that utilize the terminal carboxyl moiety of the side chain of aspartic acid to effect peptide bond hydrolysis.

▶ Non-viral Proteases

Aspirin

Aspirin is the brand name of acetylsalicylic acid. It is the most widely used analgesic, antipyretic and anti-inflammatory drug. Its main mode of action is irreversible acetylation of cyclooxygenases.

▶ Cyclooxygenases

Assay

An assay is used to measure the effect of the test compound on the target.

▶ High-throughput Screening

Asthma

▶ Bronchial Asthma

Astrocytes

Astrocytes are a category of glial cells in the vertebrate central nervous system with long radial processes. Astrocytes provide structural support to nerve cells and help to control their chemical and ionic extracellular environment.

Atherogenesis

Atherogenesis is the process that leads to changes in the arterial blood vessels, including deposition of cholesterol (atherosclerosis). It is the pathophysiological process behind the vast majority of heart attacks.

▶ HMG-CoA-reductase-inhibitors

Atherosclerotic Plaques

Atherosclerotic plaques are lesions in the arterial vessels which arise during the process of atherogenesis. Most cases of acute heart attacks are caused by rupture of an atherosclerotic plaque.

▶ HMG-CoA-reductase-inhibitors

Atopy

Atopy is the propensity to develop allergic reactions mediated by immunoglobulin E.

▶ Allergy

ATP

ATP is a purine nucleotide involved in extracellular signalling, as well as acting as an intracellular energy source.

ATP-binding Cassette Transporter Superfamily

ATP-binding cassette (ABC) transporters (proteins) are characterized by having so-called ATP-binding cassette domains. ABC proteins function as pumps, channels, and channel regulators (receptors). They have multiple membrane-spanning segments and nucleotide-binding folds (domains) (NBFs or NBDs) in the cytoplasmic side, which contain highly conserved Walker motifs and an ABC signature sequence. Cystic fibrosis transmembrane conductance regulator, P-glycoprotein,canalicular multispecific organic anion transporter, and sulfonylurea receptor are typical ABC proteins.

▶ Multidrug Transporter
▶ ATP-dependent K$^+$ Channel

ATP-dependent K$^+$ Channel

SUSUMU SEINO
Chiba University Graduate School of Medicine, Chiba, Japan
seino@med.m.chiba-u.ac.jp

Basic Characteristics

The ATP-dependent potassium (K$^+$) channel, also known as the ATP-sensitive K$^+$ channel or ATP-regulated K$^+$ (K$_{ATP}$) channel, was first discovered in cardiac myocytes, and is characterized by channel inhibition when intracellular ATP is increased. K$_{ATP}$ channels were found subsequently in many other tissues including pancreatic β-cells, skeletal muscle, smooth muscle, brain, pituitary, and kidney and in mitochondria. K$_{ATP}$ channels are weakly inwardly rectifying K$^+$-selective channels, and their regulation is essentially voltage-independent (▶ Inward Rectification). Although K$_{ATP}$ channel activity is regulated primarily by intracellular ATP and MgADP, which opens and closes them, respectively, there are also various other intracellular factors involved, including phosphorylation by protein kinase A (PKA) and phosphatidylinositol phosphates. K$_{ATP}$ channels of various composition play distinct and crucial physiological roles in different tissues by linking cell metabolism to membrane potential.

▶ Inward Rectifier K$^+$ Channels
▶ K$^+$ Channels
▶ Oral Antidiabetic Drugs
▶ Voltage-gated K$^+$ Channels

Molecular Structure and Composition of K$_{ATP}$ Channels

K$_{ATP}$ channels comprise two different subunits, an ▶ inwardly rectifying K$^+$ channel subfamily (Kir6.0) member (Kir6.1 or Kir6.2) and a receptor (SUR1 or SUR2) for ▶ sulfonylureas widely used in treatment of type 2 (non-insulin dependent) diabetes mellitus. Kir6.1 and Kir6.2 have two transmembrane domains (TMDs) connected by a pore-forming region (H5 region), which serves as part of the K$^+$-selective filter. However, the glycine (G)-tyrosine (Y)-glycine (G) motif in the H5 region, which is highly conserved among K$^+$ channels, is not present in either Kir6.1 or Kir6.2. The motif in this region of these subunits is glycine (G)-phenylalanine (F) -glycine (G). SUR, a member of the ▶ ATP-binding cassette (ABC) transporter (protein) superfamily, has three TMDs (TMD0, TMD1, and TMD2) consisting of 5, 6, and 6 membrane spanning regions and two nucleotide binding folds (or binding domains), NBF1 and NBF2 (NBD1 andNBD2) in the cytoplasmic side. NBF1 and NBF2 are located in the loop between TMD1 and TMD2 and in the C-terminus, respectively. There are several variants of SUR2 derived from alternative splicing of SUR2 mRNA. SUR2A and SUR2B are major variants that differ in the 42 amino acids of the C-terminus, resulting in SUR2B having a C-terminus similar to that of SUR1. Kir6.1 or Kir6.2 serves as the pore-forming subunit, while the SUR subunit serves as the regulatory subunit. K$_{ATP}$ channels are octameric complexes of Kir6.1 or Kir6.2 and SUR subunits in 4:4 stoichiometry. The various combinations of Kir6.1 or Kir6.2 and SUR subunits constitute K$_{ATP}$ channels with distinct nucleotide and pharmacological properties in different tissues. Kir6.2 and SUR1 subunits constitute the K$_{ATP}$ channel in pancreatic β-cells and ventromedial hypothalamus (VMH). Kir6.2 and SUR2A subunits constitute the K$_{ATP}$ channel in cardiac myocytes and, probably, in skeletal muscle. Kir6.2 and SUR2B subunits constitute the K$_{ATP}$ channel in smooth muscle. Kir6.1 and SUR2B subunits constitute the nucleoside diphosphate-dependent K$^+$ channel in vascular smooth muscle that is somewhat insensitive to ATP, activated by nucleoside diphosphates, and sensitive to the sulfonylurea glibenclamide.

Regulation of K$_{ATP}$ Channels

Nucleotides. Inhibition of K$_{ATP}$ channel activity by ATP is mediated primarily by the Kir6.2 subunit, while stimulation of the activity by MgADP is mediated primarily by the SUR subunit. The N- and C-termini of Kir6.2 interact cooperatively to modulate channel inhibition by ATP. Although four molecules of ATP can bind to each channel molecule, binding of a single ATP molecule to a Kir6.2 molecule is sufficient to induce channel closure. The inhibitory effect of ATP is also modulated by the SUR subunit. SUR has the highly conserved Walker A and B motifs and the SGGQ ABC signature in each NBF. NBF2 of SUR subunits is important in mediation of channel stimulation by MgADP and, presumably, for ATPase activity. Of the SUR subunits, SUR1 has the highest affinity to MgADP at NBF2. Other Mg^{2+}-bound nucleotides, including MgATP, MgGTP, and MgUDP, also have stimulatory effects on the K$_{ATP}$ channel through NBF1 or NBF2.

Phosphatidylinositol Phosphates (PIPs). ▶ Phosphatidylinositol phosphates (PIPs) antagonize ATP inhibition of K$_{ATP}$ channels in pancreatic β-cells,

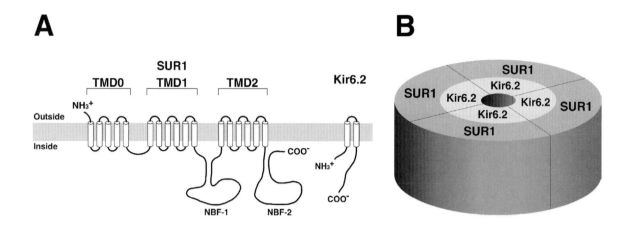

Fig. 1 Model of K$_{ATP}$ channel structure. A, Membrane topology of SUR1 and Kir6.2. SUR has three transmembrane domains, TMD0, TMD1, and TMD3, consisting of five, six, and six transmembrane segments, respectively. The transmembrane segments (M1, M2) and K+ ion pore-forming region (H5) of Kir6.2 are shown. **B**, **Heteromultimeric structure of the K$_{ATP}$ channel.** The K$_{ATP}$ channel is an octameric protein assembled with four Kir6.2 subunits and four SUR1 subunits.

cardiac myocytes and skeletal muscles. Particularly, phosphatidylinositol-4, 5-bisphosphate (PIP$_2$) induces a marked decrease in the ATP-sensitivity of Kir6.2/SUR channels. PIPs bind positive charges in the cytoplasmic region of the Kir6.2 subunit, stabilizing the open state of the channel by antagonizing the inhibitory effect of ATP. PIP$_2$ also inhibits sensitivity to the sulfonylurea tolbutamide. The run-down of K$_{ATP}$ channels seen in isolated patches may result from hydrolysis of PIP$_2$, and the restoration of channel activity by MgATP may involve membrane lipid phosphorylation, that is, the synthesis of PIP$_2$ that may activate K$_{ATP}$ channels.

Phosphorylation. Exogenous PKA catalytic subunits activate native β-cell type K$_{ATP}$ channels. Both the Kir6.2 and SUR1 subunits contain consensus sites for phosphorylation by PKA. Phosphorylation of Kir6.2 stimulates activity of Kir6.2/SUR1 channels while phosphrylation of SUR1 affects basal properties, including burst duration, interburst interval, and open probability, and increases channel expression at the cell surface.

Trafficking to the Plasma Membrane. Unlike other Kir subunits, Kir6.1 and Kir6.2 cannot form functional channels at the cell surface in the absence of

a SUR subunit. This is due to the presence of an endoplasmic reticulum (ER) retention signal (RXR) in the C-terminal region of Kir6.1 and Kir6.2. SUR1 subunit, which also contains an ER retention signal in the cytoplasmic region between TM11 and NBF-1, fails to traffic to the plasma membrane when expressed alone. Kir6.2 subunits and SUR subunits mask each other's ER retention signals, allowing trafficking to the cell surface.

Physiological Functions of K$_{ATP}$ Channels

Role of the K$_{ATP}$ Channel in Insulin Secretion. Insulin secretion is regulated by a variety of factors including nutrients, hormones and neurotransmitters. Among these, glucose is physiologically the most important. Glucose uptake and subsequent metabolism produces ATP. The increased ATP/ADP ratio closes the K$_{ATP}$ channels, which depolarizes the β-cell membrane and opens the voltage-dependent calcium channels (VDCC) to calcium influx. The rise in intracellular calcium concentration in the β-cells triggers insulin granule exocytosis. Sulfonylureas close the K$_{ATP}$ channels directly to stimulate insulin secretion. Studies of Kir6.2 and SUR1 knockout mice demonstrate that the pancreatic β-cell K$_{ATP}$ channel (Kir6.2/

A

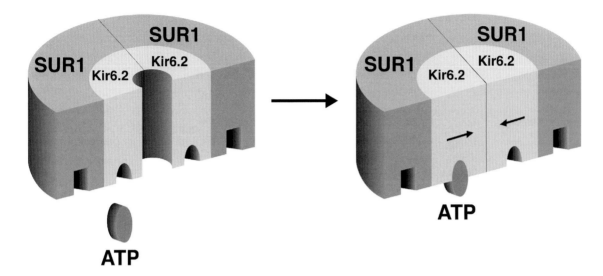

B

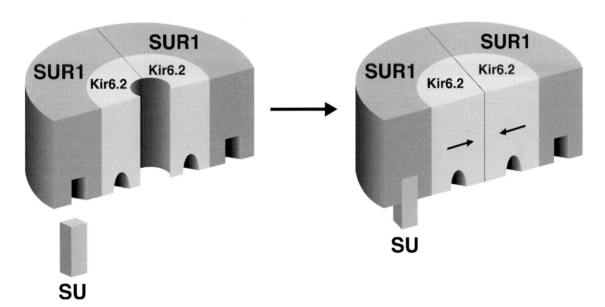

Fig. 2 **Closure of the pancreatic β-cell type K$_{ATP}$ channel by ATP and sulfonylurea. Increased ATP caused by glucose metabolism closes the K$_{ATP}$ channel by binding to the Kir6.2 subunit (A). Sulfonylureas close the channel by binding to the SUR1 subunit (B).** The SUR2 subunit has binding sites for benzamide-derivatives in addition to sulfonylureas (SU). Although there are four binding sites for the ATP molecule and four binding sites for the sulfonylurea molecule in each channel complex, occupation of only one of these sites by ATP or sulfonylurea is sufficient to close the channel.

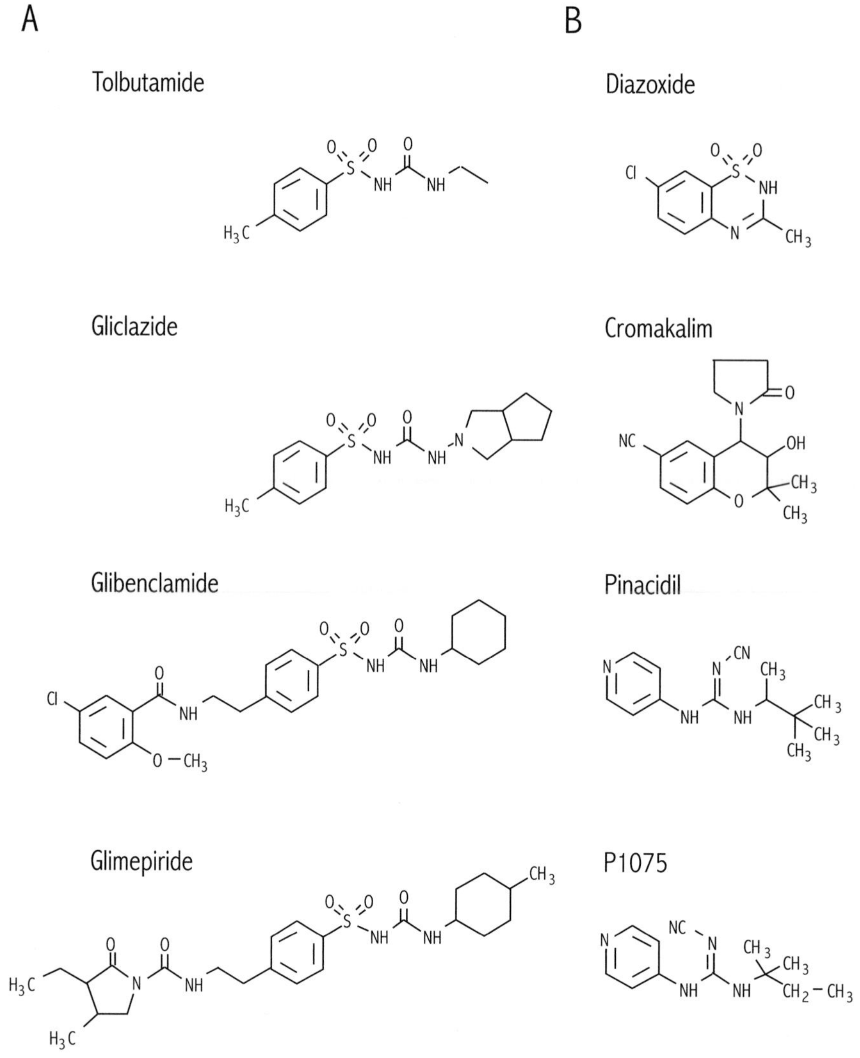

A

Tolbutamide

B

Diazoxide

Gliclazide

Cromakalim

Glibenclamide

Pinacidil

Glimepiride

P1075

Fig. 3 Chemical structure of K$_{ATP}$ channel blockers (A) and openers (B).

SUR1 channel) is critical in the regulation of glucose-induced and sulfonylurea-induced insulin secretion.

Role of the K$_{ATP}$ Channel in Glucagon Secretion. The ventromedial hypothalamus (VMH) possesses the highest density of glucose responsive (GR) neurons, which play a critical role in glucose homeostasis and are involved in glucagon secretion during hypoglycemia. The K$_{ATP}$ channel in the VMH consists of SUR1 and Kir6.2, the same molecular composition as the pancreatic β-cell K$_{ATP}$ channel. A study of Kir6.2 knockout mice demonstrates that the K$_{ATP}$ channels in the VMH function as glucose sensors for glucagon secretion during

hypoglycemia. The VMH K$_{ATP}$ channels have been found to consist of Kir6.2 and SUR1. This raises a clinically important issue, as hypoglycemia occurs during sulfonylurea treatment in some diabetic patients. It is not known currently which of the sulfonylureas inhibit the K$_{ATP}$ channels in the VMH and might impair glucagon secretion during sulfonylurea-induced hypoglycemia.

Role of the K$_{ATP}$ Channel in Cardiac Function. Sarcolemmal K$_{ATP}$ channels consist of Kir6.2 and SUR2A subunits. Pinacidil, a KCO, induces outward current and action potential shortening that is blocked by glibenclamide. The sarcolemmal K$_{ATP}$ channel mediates the depression in cardiac excitability and contractility induced by KCOs. ▶ Ischemic preconditioning (IPC) is a phenomenon in which brief intermittent periods of ischemia paradoxically protect the myocardium against a more prolonged ischemic insult, the result of which is a marked reduction of infarct size. Kir6.2-containing sarcolemmal K$_{ATP}$ channels contribute at least in part to ischemic preconditioning. Mitochondrial K$_{ATP}$ channels, of which the molecular composition has not yet been determined, are also thought to play an important role in ischemic preconditioning.

Role of the K$_{ATP}$ Channels in Generalized Seizure. The substantia nigra pars reticulata (SNr), the area of the highest expression of K$_{ATP}$ channels in the brain, plays a key role in the control of seizures. SNr neuron activity is inactivated during hypoxia by the opening of the post-synaptic K$_{ATP}$ channels. However, the activity of these neurons is enhanced in Kir6.2 knockout mice, indicating the participation of K$_{ATP}$ channels in the suppression of SNr neuronal activity during hypoxia and their involvement in a protective mechanism against generalized seizure.

Drugs

Pharmacology of K$_{ATP}$ Channels

Sulfonylureas. The SUR subunits are the target of the most widely used therapeutic drugs. Sulfonylureas including tolbutamide, gliclazide, glibenclamide (glyburide) and glimepiride are clinically used in the treatment of type 2 diabetes. They bind to SUR1 to close the pancreatic β-cell K$_{ATP}$ (Kir6.2/SUR1) channels to stimulate insulin secretion, but the affinities for SUR1 of the various sulfonylureas differ. Occupation of only one of the four sulfonylurea-binding sites per channel complex (four molecules of Kir6.2 and four molecules of SUR1) is sufficient to induce K$_{ATP}$ channel closure. The affinities of the sulfonylureas were estimated by measurement of competition with radiolabeled glibenclamide. The rank of binding potency to SUR1 parallels the ability of the sulfonylureas to close the K$_{ATP}$ channels and stimulate insulin secretion. Kir6.2/SUR1 (β-cell type K$_{ATP}$ channels), Kir6.2/SUR2A (cardiac and skeletal muscle type K$_{ATP}$ channels), and Kir6.2/SUR2B (smooth

muscle K$_{ATP}$ channel) K$_{ATP}$ channels show different sensitivities to the various sulfonylureas. For example, β-cell type K$_{ATP}$ channels are blocked by tolbutamide and gliclazide bound with high affinity, while cardiac and skeletal muscle type K$_{ATP}$ channels are not. Both Kir6.2/SUR1 channels and Kir6.2/SUR2A channels are blocked by glibenclamide and glimepiride, as are Kir6.2/SUR2B channels. Tolbutamide and gliclazide have a sulfonylurea moiety, but glibenclamide and glimepiride have a benzamide group moiety in addition. SUR1 may possess separate high affinity binding sites for sulfonylureas and for benzamide groups, while SUR2 on the other hand, may have only high affinity binding sites for the benzamide group. Because there are distinct effects of the various sulfonylureas on SUR2A and SUR2B, there may be differing actions of these drugs on the various K$_{ATP}$ channels in native tissues.

Meglitinide-related Compounds. Meglitinide, a benzamide derivative, shares a nonsulfonylurea moiety with glibenclamide. Meglitinide also blocks both Kir6.2/SUR1 channels and Kir6.2/SUR2A channels. Several newly developed non-sulfonylurea hypoglycemic agents such as nateglinide (A-4166), repaglinide and mitiglinide (KAD1229 or S21403) are structurally related to meglitinide. Although the meglinitide-related compounds all inhibit Kir6.2/SUR1 channels to stimulate insulin secretion, they have differing pharmacological effects on Kir6.2/SUR2A and Kir6.2/SUR2B channels. ▶ Meglinitide-related compounds have clinical potentials for the treatment of type 2 diabetes.

K$^+$ Channel Openers (KCOs). The K$_{ATP}$ channels in various tissues exhibit different responses to K$^+$ channel openers (KCOs) including diazoxide, pinacidil, nicorandil, and minoxidil sulfate. Diazoxide is used to inhibit insulin secretion, nicorandil is used for the treatment of angina, and minoxidil sulfate is used to stimulate hair growth in male baldness. All of these KCOs act directly on the SUR subunits. The binding of KCOs to a SUR subunit seems to require ATP hydrolysis in the NBFs. The tissue specific differences in the responses of K$_{ATP}$ channels to KCOs are conferred by the SUR subunit. Diazoxide activates Kir6.2/SUR1 and Kir6.2/SUR2B channels but not Kir6.2/SUR2A channels. Inhibition of the channels by diazoxide is effective only in the presence of Mg-nucleotide. However, Kir6.2/SUR2A channels become as sensitive to diazoxide as Kir6.2/SUR1 channels in the presence of MgADP. The effect of diazoxide may require hydrolysis of ATP by the NBFs of the SUR subunit. Pinacidil strongly activates Kir6.2/SUR2A channels but only slightly activates Kir6.2/SUR1 channels. Nicorandil, an anti-anginal agent, activates Kir6.2/SUR2A, Kir6.2/SUR2B and Kir6.1/SUR2B channels but not Kir6.2/SUR1 channels, suggesting that it acts through SUR2 subunit.

Imidazolines. Many drugs containing an imidazoline moiety such as phentolamine stimulate insulin secretion. Phentolamine acts directly on the Kir6.2 subunit. Although the ATP-molecule contains an imidazoline group, the binding site of phentolamine is not identical to the ATP-binding site.

Persistent Hyperinsulinemic Hypoglycemia of Infancy (PHHI)

▶ PHHI, also referred to as familial hyperinsulinism (HI) and formerly called pancreatic nesidioblastosis, is a rare metabolic disorder occurring in neonates and infants which is characterized by excessive insulin secretion despite severe hypoglycemia. PHHI is an autosomal recessive hereditary disease occurring approximately in 1/50,000 births in Western countries. The disease is characterized by severe hypoglycemia with inappropriate, excessive insulin secretion in neonates and infants. The protein-coding regions of the SUR1 gene and the Kir6.2 gene are composed of 39 exons and a single exon, respectively. Many of the mutations in the SUR1 gene have been identified in PHHI patients, most of which in SUR1 occur in NBF-1 or NBF-2. Mutations of Kir6.2 also have been shown to cause PHHI. The mechanisms by which mutations of SUR1 or Kir6.2 cause K_{ATP} channel dysfunction in PHHI include physical uncoupling of the SUR1 subunits and the Kir6.2 subunits, impaired MgADP activation, impaired trafficking to the plasma membrane, and impaired K^+-ion permeation. The pancreatic β-cells are continuously depolarized as a result so that continuous calcium influx leads to hypoglycemia due to unregulated insulin secretion.

References

1. Noma A (1983) ATP-regulated K^+ channels in cardiac muscle. Nature 305:147–148
2. Inagaki N, Gonoi T, Clement IV JP, Namba N, Inazawa J, Gonzalez G, Aguilar-Bryan L, Seino, S, Bryan J (1995) Reconstitution of IK$_{ATP}$: an inward rectifier subunit plus the sulfonylurea receptor. Science 270:1166–1170
3. Miki T, Nagashima K, Tashiro F, Kotake K, Yoshitomi H, Tamamoto A, Gonoi T, Iwanaga T, Miyazaki J, Seino S (1998) Defective insulin secretion and enhanced insulin action in K_{ATP} channel-deficient mice. Proc. Natl. Acad. Sci. USA. 95:10402–10406
4. Seino, S (1999) ATP-sensitive potassium channels: a model of heteromultimeric potassium channel/receptor assemblies. Annu Rev Physiol 61:337–362
5. Ashcroft F, Gribble, F (2000). New windows on the mechanism of action of K_{ATP} channel openers. TIPS 21:439–445

ATP-powered pump

▶ Table appendix: Membrane Transport Proteins

Atrial Fibrillation

Cardiac arrhythmia with a rapid and irregular activity in different areas within the upper chambers (atria) of the heart is also known as atrial fibrillation.

▶ Antiarrhythmic Drugs

Atrial Natriuretic Peptide

The atrial natriuretic peptide (ANP) belongs to a family of hormones that have structural similarity and some biological actions in common, such as natriuresis and hemoconcentration. It is synthesized and secreted by the cardiac atrium in response to increased atrial pressure. ANP is believed to act physiologically in an opposing manner to arginine vasopressin (AVP).

▶ Guanylyl Cyclases

Attention Deficit Hyperactivity Disorder

Key features of Attention Deficit Hyperactivity Disorder (ADHD) - with a highly differing prevalence of 0.1 to 10% - are distractibility and difficulties in sustaining attention and focusing on a task. These symptoms are associated with impulsiveness, regardless of consequences. Comorbidity is high, boy to girl ratio is 4:1.

▶ Psychostimulants

Atypical Neuroleptic

▶ Antipsychotic Drugs

AUC

AUC is the area under the (drug) concentration time curve.

▶ Area under the Curve

Autacoid

Autacoids are literally 'self-medicating agents' that are liberated from, or produced by, cells in response to a stimulus. They differ from hormones in that they usually act locally after release, rather than reaching their target organ *via* the bloodstream.

▶ Histaminergic System

Autoimmune Disease

Autoimmune disease originates from the development of autoreactive T- and B-lymphocytes. These cells are sensitized and react to ubiquitous or specific antigens of host cells provoking chronic inflammatory reactions. Most autoimmune diseases are characterized by the presence of autoreactive antibodies.

▶ Interferons
▶ Immunosuppressive Agents

Autonomic Nervous System

The autonomic nervous system is that part of the nervous system concerned with autonomic control of visceral and cardiovascular systems.

Autoreceptors

Autoreceptors are presynaptic receptors (Synaptic transmission) activated by the neurotransmitter released from the same neuron. They either stimulate or inhibit subsequent transmitter release. The classical example is the presynaptic α_2 adrenoceptor which is activated by noradrenaline and inhibits its further release.

▶ α-Adrenergic System
▶ Synaptic Transmission
▶ Histaminergic System

Axon

An axon is a long nerve cell process which transmits the action potential and ends as the synapse.

Axonal Membrane

The axonal membrane is a lipid bilayer in the nerve fibre. Ionic channels and other proteins are located in the membrane to achieve electrical activity. Action potentials are generated and conducted along the membrane.

▶ Local Anaesthetics

Azole

▶ Antifungal Drugs

B

BAC

A Bacterial Artificial Chromosome (BAC) is a vector that allows the propagation of larger exogenous DNA fragments, up to several hundred kb. BACs are propagated in recombination-deficient strains of *E. coli*. They are more stable and easier to handle than yeast artificial chromosomes (YACs).

▶ Transgenic Animal Models

Back Propagation

Back propagation is the propagation of action potentials from the soma distally to dendrites. If the dendrites are passive cable transmitting distally evoked postsynaptic potentials to the soma, the dendrites do not have to generate action potentials. Direct patch clamp measurements demonstrated the back propagation of action potentials.

▶ Voltage-dependent Na$^+$ Channels

Bacterial Toxins

GUDULA SCHMIDT, KLAUS AKTORIES
Institut für Experimentelle und Klinische Pharmakologie und Toxikologie, Albert-Ludwigs-Universität Freiburg, Freiburg, Germany
Gudula.Schmidt@pharmakol.uni-freiburg.de;
Klaus.Aktories@pharmakol.uni-freiburg.de

Definition

Bacterial protein toxins are proteins that are released by the pathogen into the environment. Thereafter, they target eukaryotic cells to damage the membrane, to induce pathogenic signalling by acting on membrane receptors or to disturb cell signaling and cell function after entry into the cytosol. The three major aims of bacteria producing toxins are i. to enter the host organism, ii. to inhibit the hosts immune system, and iii. to produce an appropriate host niche for their own development.

Protein toxins acting intracellulary are often composed of two subunits (A/B model). One subunit is catalytic (A-subunit) and the other is responsible for binding and cell entry (B-subunit). Following binding to an extracellular membrane receptor, the toxins are endocytosed. From the endosomes the A-subunit is directly (pH dependent) transferred into the cytosol (e.g., diphtheria toxin and anthrax toxin) or the toxin is transported in a retrograde manner via the Golgi to the ER (e.g., cholera toxin), where translocation into the cytosol occurs.

▶ Cytoskeleton
▶ Exocytosis
▶ Small GTPases

Mechanism of Action

Toxins Modifying Target Proteins

Protein toxins of this type are generally very potent and efficient because they act catalytically. The toxins activate or inactivate eukaryotic key proteins involved in essential cellular functions usually by covalent modification. One subfamily catalyzes the ADP-ribosylation of target proteins. For unknown reasons many toxins of this subfamily modify eukaryotic GTPases. Examples are the di-chain diphtheria toxin from toxigenic *Corynebacterium diphtheriae* and the single-chain *Pseudomonas aeruginosa* exotoxin A, which ADP-ribosylates elongation factor 2 at diphthamide to cause inhibition of protein synthesis. Pertussis toxin from *Bordetella pertussis* and cholera toxin from *Vibrio cholerae* act on heterotrimeric G proteins. Pertussis toxin consists of the catalytic subunit S1 and five binding subunits (S2, S3, 2xS4 and S5) with masses of ~11–26 kD. Cholera toxin consists of a ~28 kD A-subunit and five B-subunits (~12 kD). Whereas pertussis toxin ADP-ribosylates the α-subunits of the Gi subfamily of G proteins (exception Gz) at a cysteine residue, cholera toxin and the related *E. coli* heat labile toxins ADP-ribosylate α-subunits of the Gs subfamily at an arginine residue. Pertussis toxin-induced ADP-ribosylation blocks the interaction of the G protein with heptahelical receptors (GPCR). The ADP-ribosylation of Gs inhibits the intrinsic GTPase activity and persistently activates the G protein. Increase in cellular cAMP, activation of protein kinase A and subsequent disturbance of cellular electrolyte secretion is suggested to be the cause of cholera toxin-induced diarrhea.

Small GTPases of the Rho family are ADP-ribosylated (e.g., at Asn41 of RhoA) and inactivated by C3-like toxins from *C. botulinum, C. limosum* and *S. aureus*. These proteins have a molecular mass of 23–30 kD and consist only of the enzyme domain. Specific inhibition of Rho functions (Rho but not Rac or Cdc42 are targets) is the reason why C3 is widely used as a pharmcological tool.

Another subfamily of ADP-ribosylating toxins modifies G-actin (at Arg177), thereby inhibiting actin polymerization. Members of this family are for example *Clostridium botulinum* C2 toxin and *Clostridium perfringens* iota toxin. These toxins are binary in structure. They consist of an enzyme component and a separate binding component, which is structurally related to the binding component of anthrax toxin.

The above mentioned Rho GTPases are glucosylated by the family of large clostridial cytotoxins. Important members of this toxin family are *Clostridium difficile* toxins A and B, which are implicated in antibiotic-associated diarrhea and pseudomembranous colitis. The large clostridial cytotoxins are single chain toxins with molecular masses of 250–308 kD. The enzyme domain is located at the N-terminus. The toxins are taken up from an acidic endosomal compartment. They glucosylate RhoA at Thr37; also Rac and Cdc42 are substrates. Other members of this toxin family such as *C. sordellii* lethal toxin possess a different substrate specificity and modify Rac but not Rho. In addition, Ras subfamily proteins (e.g., Ras, Ral and Rap) are modified. As for C3, they are widely used as tools to study Rho functions.

Rho GTPases are activated by *E. coli* cytotoxic necrotizing factors 1 and 2 (CNF1, 2) and by the *Bordetella* dermonecrotic toxin (DNT). CNF1 and CNF2 are closely related toxins sharing more than 90% identity in their amino acid sequences. Both toxins are single chain proteins with molecular masses of about 115 kD. The cell-binding domain of CNF1 is located at the N terminus and the catalytic domain at the C terminus of the toxin. DNT is a protein of ~160 kD that shares significant homology with CNF in the catalytic domain.

All these toxins activate the small GTP binding proteins of the Rho family by deamidation (CNFs) and transglutamination (DNT) of a glutamine residue (e.g., Gln63 of RhoA), which is necessary for GTP hydrolysis. Moreover, the inactivation of Rho GTPases by GAP (GTPase-activating protein) is blocked by CNF and DNT. According to the functions of Rho GTPases, the toxins cause formation of stress fibers, filopodia and membrane ruffles, and induce cell flattening and multinucleation The role of CNFs in the pathogenesis of *E. coli* infections is still unclear. CNF and DNT are dermonecrotic after intradermal application.

The anthrax toxin is a tripartite toxin and consists of the binding component PA (protective antigen), the lethal factor (LF), which is a metalloprotease, and the edema factor (EF), which is a calmodulin dependent adenylylcyclase. Both enzyme components are translocated via PA into target cells. PA is activated by furin-induced cleavage and forms heptamers, which are similar to the binding components of C2 toxin and iota toxin. In the low pH compartment of endosomes, the heptamers form pores to allow translocation of LF and EF. LF cleaves the amino-terminus of the MAPK-kinase thereby inhibiting this enzyme. The functional consequence is the blockade of the ras-MAPK signalling pathway that controls cell proliferation. Whether this is the reason for the LT-induced cell death of macrophages is not clear.

Shiga-toxin is produced i. by *Shigella dysenterica*, the cause of bacillary dysentery, ii. by certain *E. coli* strains (EHEC, enterohaemorrhagic *E. coli*; cause of the hemolytic uremic syndrome, HUS) and iii. by various enterobacteriaceae (e.g., *Enterobacter cloacae*). The toxin consists of an A-subunit of ~32 kD and a pentameric B-subunit (7.7 kD each). The toxin enters cells after retrograde transport to the Golgi. In the cytosol, the A-subunit acts as a N-glycosidase to remove one adenine residue in position 4324 of the 28S-rRNA at the ribosome and blocks protein biosynthesis.

Clostridial neurotoxins are mainly bichain toxins having a ~50 kD enzyme component and a ~100 kD binding/ translocation subunit. They are the cause of botulism, a generalized flaccid paralysis of skeletal muscles mainly acquired by food poisoning, and tetanus, which occurs subsequently to wound infection. Botulism is induced by *Clostridium botulinum* neurotoxins types A, B, C1 , D, E, F and G. Tetanus is induced by tetanus toxin from *Clostridium tetani*. The toxins belong to the most potent agents known. About 1 ng of botulinum toxin per kg body mass may be lethal for man or animal. The toxins are zinc-metalloproteases and cleave synaptic peptides involved in transmitter release. Botulinum neurotoxins B, D, F and G and tetanus toxin cleave synaptobrevin; neurotoxins A and E cleave SNAP25, and neurotoxin C cleaves syntaxin. The botulinum neurotoxins induce flaccid muscle paralysis (botulism) because they act presynaptically at the peripheral neuromuscular junction to block acetylcholine release. Tetanus toxin is taken up at the neuromuscular junction but is then transported in a retrograde manner to the spinal cord. Within the spinal cord tetanus toxin migrates to interneurons annd blocks the release of inhibitory transmitters to cause spastic paralysis.

Bacterial Phospholipases

The α-toxin from *Clostridium perfringens* is involved in the pathogenesis of gas gangrene and the sudden death syndrome of young animals. This toxin is a zinc-metalloenzyme with phospholipase activity. Other phospholipase C-toxins are from *Listeria monocytogenes* and from *Mycobacterium tuberculosis*. The phospholipase C-toxin from *Bacillus cereus* is specific for phosphatidylinositol. It cleaves phosphatidylinositol and its glucosyl derivatives. In cell biology, this toxin can be used as a tool to study whether a protein is anchored to GPI. A second phospholipase C-toxin produced by *Bacillus cereus* is specific for sphingomyelin. Cleavage of sphingomyelin generates ceramide, a second messenger involved in processes like apoptosis and differentiation.

Superantigens

Like physiological ligands, bacterial toxins can influence cells by binding to cell surface molecules. Best known are the superantigens produced by *Staphylococcus* strains. Superantigens are bivalent molecules that bind to the major histocompatibility complex (MHC) class II and to the variable regions of the T-cell receptor. This bridging leads to the activation of the T-cell receptor in the absence of an antigenic peptide. This unspecific activation of T-cells is followed by a massive release of cytokines which is thought to play a role in diseases like toxic shock syndrome and some exanthemas.

Pore-forming Toxins

Pore-forming toxins act by punching holes into mammalian cell membranes. Many different types are known. They can be divided into toxins forming small holes and large-pore forming toxins. Pore-forming toxins oligomerize in the plasma membrane of the mammalian cell to build circular structures. These ring-like structures can be composed of a few molecules, generating small pores that allow the exchange of ions and nucleotides (*Aeromonas* aerolysin, *Staphylococcus aureus* α-toxin). Large pores, which allow the passage of peptides or proteins are formed by toxins which insert up to 50 molecules into the plasma membrane generating a pore with up to 35 nm in diameter. Examples for such toxins are *Streptococcus pyrogenes* streptolysin O or *Clostridium tetani* tetanolysin.

Tab. 1 Intracellular acting exotoxins.

Toxin	Protein substrate	Activity	Functional consequences
Diphtheria toxin, *Pseudomonas* Exotoxin A	Elongation factor 2	ADP-ribosylation	Inhibition of protein synthesis (diphtheria, *Pseudomonas* infection)
Cholera toxin, heat labile *E.coli* toxins	G_s-proteins	ADP-ribosylation	Activation of adenylate cyclase (cholera, 'traveller'-diarrhea)
Pertussis toxin	$G_{i,o}$-proteins	ADP-ribosylation	Inhibition of G protein signalling (whooping cough)
C. botulinum C2-toxin and related toxins	Actin	ADP-ribosylation	Inhibition of actin polymerization
C. botulinum C3-toxin and related toxins	Rho proteins	ADP-ribosylation	Inhibition of RhoA, B ,C Destruction of the cytoskeleton
E.coli CNF 1 und 2	Rho proteins	deamidation	Activation of RhoA, Rac, Cdc42
Bordetella DNT	Rho proteins	transglutamination	Activation of RhoA, Rac, Cdc42
C. difficile toxin A and B	Rho proteins	glucosylation	Inactivation of Rho proteins Destruction of the cytoskeleton
Botulinum-Neurotoxins (A-G), Tetanus toxin	Synaptic peptides: a) Synaptobrevin b) Syntaxin c) SNAP25	Zinc dependent endoprotease	Cleavage of synaptic peptides Inhibition of transmitter release (Tetanus, Botulism)
Shiga toxins and related toxins from *E.coli*	No proteins (!) 28S rRNA	N-Glycosidase	Cleavage of 28S rRNA Inhibition of protein synthesis

Injected toxins are directly delivered into the cytosol of eukaryotic target cells by the bacterial Type III secretion Apparatus. The pathogens (e.g., *Pseudomonas aeruginosa*, *Yersinia* and *Salmonella*) produce a set of proteins that are delivered into mammalian cells by this complex type-III secretion machinery dependent on the direct contact between bacterium and host cells. Some of these injected toxins (e.g., Yops in the case of Yersinia) are not covalently modifying mammalian targets but act modulatory on important signal transduction pathways; they act as molecular mimics of cellular proteins. For example, they regulate the activity of small GTP binding proteins as exchange factors to activate the small G-proteins or as activators of GTP-hydrolysis to inhibit them. Notably, *Salmonella* produces two contrary acting molecular mimics. They inject an activator of Rho GTPases (SopE) to induce ruffling and the uptake of the bacteria into the mammalian cell, and they inject an inactivator of Rho GTPases (SptP), probably to switch off the induced cytoskeletal rearrangements.

Clinical Uses

Botulinum neurotoxins are widely used as therapeutic agents to cause reduction or paralysis of skeletal muscle contraction. They are used to treat cervical dystonia, which causes regional involuntary muscle spasms often associated with pain. Moreover, they are used in strabism, blepharospasm, hemifacial spasm and achalasia. Meanwhile, a number of studies indicate efficacy for botulinum toxin for the treatment of tension headache and migraine, but further studies are necessary to demonstrate its short-term and long-term efficacy. Botulinum toxin is also used as a cosmetic agent and the effects occur after injection into the muscle after few days and last for several months. The treatment can be repeated several times without major development of anti-neurotoxin antibodies.

In the case of anti-neurotoxin antibody production, the treatment is continued with a different botulinum neurotoxin.

Some toxins (for example the diphtheria toxin) are used as immunotoxins, fused to antibodies against cell surface molecules, for example to deplete T-cells as targeted therapy for cutaneous T cell lymphoma. Under current investigation is further the use of bacteria with the type-III secretion system (for example salmonella) producing only an injected toxin-antigen fusion protein as live vaccines. The aim is to directly deliver protein fragments into antigen-presenting cells to improve immunisation.

References

1. Aktories, K., G. Schmidt, and I. Just. 2000. Rho GT-Pases as targets of bacterial protein toxins. Biol. Chem. 381:421–426
2. Schiavo, G., van der Goot, F.G. 2001. The bacterial toxin toolkit. Nature Reviews molcellbiol. 2:530–537

Bacteriophage

A bacteriophage (or phage) is a virus, made up of a DNA or RNA core and a protein coat, that may infect bacteria.

▶ Humanized Monoclonal Antibodies

Barbiturates

Barbiturates are salts of barbituric acid. They can be used as hypnotics, sedatives, general anaesthetics and antiepileptics. Similar to benzodiazepines they have modulatory effects on the $GABA_A$ receptor.

▶ GABAergic System

Baroreceptor Reflex

The baroreceptor reflex is a central reflex mechanism, which reduces heart rate following an increase in blood pressure. Each change in blood pressure is sensed by baroreceptors in the carotid arteries, which activate the autonomic nervous system to alter heart rate and thereby readjust blood pressure.

▶ Blood Pressure Control

Bartter's Syndrome

Bartter's syndrome (antenatal Bartter syndrome, hyperprostaglandin E syndrome) is an electrolyte disorder that has now been recognized to be caused by mutations in at least three transport proteins responsible for NaCl absorption in the loop of Henle. Besides mutations in the $Na^+/K^+/$2Cl-cotransporter, Bartter's syndrome can also be caused by mutations in the K channel that is present in the apical membrane of the ascending limb (ROMK or KIR1.1). This K channel is a K-recycling pathway and its operation is a prerequisite for NaCl absorption through NKCC2. Clinically, Bartter syndromes types I and II are indistinguishable. In contrast, a milder form of Bartter's syndrome is caused by mutations in the basolateral chloride channel (ClC-Kb), an exit pathway for cellular Cl.

▶ Diuretics

Basal Activity

Basal activity is the enzymatic or other activity of a protein normally governed by interaction with a ligand or other activator molecule in the absence of that activator.

Basal Ganglia

Basal ganglia are a group of subcortical nuclei which are essential for the coordination of movements (so-called extrapyramidal system). They include the caudate nucleus, putamen, globus pallidus, and lentiform nucleus. Damage of the basal ganglia results in involuntary movements, as are observed in Parkinson's disease and Huntington's chorea.

▶ Anti-parkinson Drugs

Basophils

Basophils constitute a subgroup of circulating blood cells (leucocytes). In many aspects they resemble non-circulating mast cells (Allergy). Upon binding of antibody of the IgE class, basophils release histamine and other proinflammatory agents.

▶ Allergy

bax

bax is a *bcl-2* homolog that forms dimers with *bcl-2* and acts to accelerate apoptosis.

▶ Apoptosis

bcl-2

bcl-2 (B-cell lymphoma-related gene) is major mammalian gene that is known to inhibit apoptosis.

▶ Apoptosis
▶ BID

BDNF

BDNF (brain-derived neurotrophic factor) is a neurotrophin, i.e. a target derived growth factor which is expressed in the brain predominantly in the hippocampus. It acts through its tyrosine kinase receptor, trkB which after ligand activation induces phosphorylation of intracellular signalling proteins on tyrosine residues. BDNF expression is suppressed by stress hormones, and increased by antidepressants through a yet unknown mechanism.

▶ Neurotrophic Factors

Benign Familial Neonatal Convulsions

Benign familial neonatal convulsion is an idiopathic form of epilepsy beginning within the first six months after birth. Seizures include generalized and mixed, starting with tonic posture, ocular symptoms, and apnea, and often progressing to clonic movements and motor automatisms.

▶ Antiepileptic Drugs

Benzoapyrene

One of the most studied of the polyaromatic hydrocarbone (PAH) is benzo(a)pyrene (BaP), which is present in coal tar at coke oven plants. The BaP content of coal tar is between 0.1% and 1% and it contributes to the serious potential health effects on employees exposed to coke oven emissions. The largest sources of BaP are open burning and home heating with wood and coal. The latter alone contributes 40 percent of all the BaP released each year in the USA.
Industries that burn wood, gas, oil or coal contribute most of the rest of airborne B(a)P. Studies on

animals have shown that contact with BaP and PAH can cause skin cancer, but the effects of breathing or ingesting them are not yet well enough studied to draw a conclusion as to other cancers. Animal tests have shown that exposure to BaP may cause reproduction difficulty. The U.S. government considers BaP a human carcinogen.

Benzodiazepines

UWE RUDOLPH

Institute of Pharmacology and Toxicology, University of Zürich, Zürich, Switzerland
rudolph@pharma.unizh.ch

Definition

The term benzodiazepine refers to a chemical structure consisting of a heterocyclic ring system in which the two N atoms are mostly located in postions 1 and 4 (1,4-benzodiazepines), e.g. in diazepam (Fig. 1). Benzodiazepines have found wide therapeutic applications as ▶ anxiolytics, sedatives, hypnotics, anticonvulsants and central muscle relaxants.

▶ GABAergic System

Mechanism of Action

Enhancement of GABA Response

▶ GABA is the major inhibitory neurotransmitter in the mammalian central nervous system. Its fast synaptic actions are mediated by ▶ GABA$_A$Receptors, which are located on postsynaptic membranes. GABA$_A$ receptors have a central pore with selectivity for chloride ions. Upon binding of GABA to GABA$_A$ receptors, negatively-charged chloride ions flow into the postsynaptic neuron, leading - in most cases - to hyperpolarization of the postsynaptic membrane and thus functional inhibition. In addition to a binding site for the physiological neurotransmitter GABA, most GABA$_A$ receptors contain binding sites for ▶ allosteric modulators, e.g. benzodiazepines, ▶ barbiturates and ▶ neurosteroids. Benzodiazepines bind to a common modulatory site that is

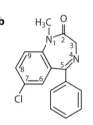

Fig. 1 A) Chemical structure of classical [1,4] benzodiazepines. R1, R2, R2', R3 and R7 denote variable suibstitutents. B) Chemical structure of the prototypical benzodiazepine diazeapm.

therefore called benzodiazepine site. However, the ligands of the benzodiazepine site are not limited to ligands of the benzodiazepine structure. In particular, the imidazopyridine zolpidem, a widely used hypnotic, and zopiclone, a cyclopyrrolone, also bind to the benzodiazpine site. The basic mechanism of action of benzodiazepines and non-benzodiazepines acting via the benzodiazepine site appears to be the same.

The binding of a benzodiazepine to the benzodiazepine site of the GABA$_A$ receptor enhances GABAergic inhibition by increasing the opening frequency of the GABA-gated ion channel. This leads to a shift of the GABA dose-response curve to the left, so that at any given concentration of GABA, the response is increased (Fig. 2). This can also be viewed as an increase in the affinity of GABA for the receptor. The action of benzodiazepines is use-dependent and self-limiting. Use-dependence indicates that benzodiazepines are only active in the presence of GABA. In the absence of GABA, benzodiazepines do not have an effect on their own, i.e., their action is dependent on the precondition that GABA is present and the respective synapse thus in use. Furthermore, benzodiazepines are not able to increase the response to GABA beyond its physiological maximum at

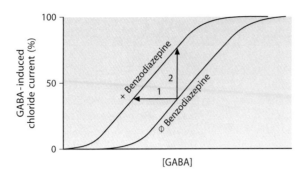

Fig. 2 Schematic representation of the potentiation of the GABA-induced chloride current by benzodiazepines. The GABA dose-response curve is shifted to the left in the presence of benzodiazepines (arrow 1). The chloride current that is induced by a submaximal concentration of GABA is increased (arrow 2). Benzodiazepines are effective only in the presence of GABA (use-dependence) and cannot increase the inhibition by high concentrations of GABA (self-limiting action).

high GABA concentrations, which is referrred to as the self-limiting nature of their action. The magnitude of the effect of benzodiazepines depends on the amount of GABA present in the synapse and thus synaptic activity. The self-limiting feature may help explain why the enhancement of GABA transmission by benzodiazepines is typically safe even at high doses, whereas overdoses with drugs that do not display this self-limiting feature, e.g. barbiturates, are life-threatening.

Subtype-Specificity of BZ Actions

$GABA_A$ receptors that contain the $\alpha 1$, $\alpha 2$, $\alpha 3$ and $\alpha 5$ subunits in combination with β and γ subunits can bind classical benzodiazepines, e.g. diazepam, whereas $GABA_A$ receptors that contain the $\alpha 4$ and $\alpha 6$ subunits do not bind classical benzodiazepines. Essentially all benzodiazepines that are currently in clinical use bind indiscriminately to $GABA_A$ receptors that contain the $\alpha 1$, $\alpha 2$, $\alpha 3$ and $\alpha 5$ subunits. The only clinically used drug that displays a significant subtype selectivity is the imidazopyridine hypnotic, zolpidem. Zolpidem has a high affinity at $GABA_A$ receptors containing the $\alpha 1$ subunit, an intermediate affinity at $GABA_A$ receptors containing the $\alpha 2$ or $\alpha 3$ subunits and no affinity at $GABA_A$ receptors containing the $\alpha 5$ subunit. The

$GABA_A$ receptor subtype-specificity of benzodiazepine actions was assessed in genetically engineered mice. Whereas the diazepam-sensitive $\alpha 1$, $\alpha 2$, $\alpha 3$ and $\alpha 5$ subunits have a histidine residue in a conserved position in the N-terminal extracellular domain (H101 in $\alpha 1$, H101 in $\alpha 2$, H126 in $\alpha 3$, H105 in $\alpha 5$), the diazepam-insensitive $\alpha 4$ and $\alpha 6$ subunits have an arginine residue at the homologous position. By mutating the conserved histidine residue in the $\alpha 1$, $\alpha 3$ and $\alpha 5$ subunits to arginine residues the $GABA_A$ receptors containing the respective subunits were rendered diazepam-insensitive. Using this approach, it was discovered that the sedative and antergrade amnesic action of diazepam, and in part also the anticonvulsant action of diazepam, are mediated by $GABA_A$ receptors containing the $\alpha 1$ subunits, while the anxiolytic action of diazepam is mediated by $GABA_A$ receptors containing the $\alpha 2$ subunit. The central muscle relaxant action of diazepam is mediatedby $GABA_A$ receptors containing the $\alpha 2$, $\alpha 3$ or $\alpha 5$ subunits (1–4). The anxiolytic action of diazepam is observed at much lower doses than the muscle relaxant action. Interestingly, $GABA_A$ receptors containing the $\alpha 3$ subunit were not involved in mediating the anxiolytic-like action of diazepam in ethological tests of anxiety, indicating that this response is not dependent on neurons in the reticular activating system where the $\alpha 3$ subunit is expressed.

	$\alpha 1$	$\alpha 2$	$\alpha 3$	$\alpha 5$
Sedation	+	–	–	–
Anterograde amnesia	+	ND	ND	ND
Anticonvulsant activity	+	–	–	–
Anxiolysis	–	+	–	–
Myorelaxation	–	+	+	+

Fig. 3 Dissection of benzodiazepinepharmacology. The functional roles of $GABA_A$ receptor subtypes mediating particular actions of diazepam are indicated. A "+" sign indicates that the respective response is mediated by the respective receptor subtype, a "-" sign indicates that the respective response is apparently not mediated by the respective receptor subtype. ND = not determined.

These findings demonstrate that subtype-selective drugs are likely to be of benefit, e.g. as anxiolytics without sedative and anterograde amnesic side effects. A remarkable step in this direction was the development of L-838,417, which is a partial agonist at $GABA_A$ receptors containing the $\alpha 2$, $\alpha 3$ and $\alpha 5$ subunits but has no activity at $GABA_A$ receptors containing the $\alpha 1$ subunit. This compound is active as an anxiolytic and anticonvulsant, but apparently does not impair motor performance (4).

Interestingly, while the sedative action of diazepam is mediated by $GABA_A$ receptors containing the $\alpha 1$ subunit, its ▶ REM sleep inhibiting action, its enhancement of sleep continuity and its effect on the ▶ EEG spectra in sleep and waking are mediated by $GABA_A$ receptors that do not contain the $\alpha 1$ subunit, indicating that the hypnotic effect of diazepam and its EEG fingerprint can be dissociated from its sedative action (5).

Agonists and Inverse Agonists

Drugs that bind to the benzodiazepine site of the $GABA_A$ receptor and enhance GABA responses, are termed agonists. Essentially all ligands at the benzodiazepine site that are in clinical use are agonists. In contrast, inverse agonists diminish GABA responses. They are not in clinical use and have effects opposite to those of the agonists, e.g., they are convulsant and anxiogenic.

The Antagonist Flumazenil

Although flumazenil binds with high affinity to the benzdiazepine site of $GABA_A$ receptors, it has practically no action when given alone. However, flumazenil competitively blocks the action of benzodiazepine site agonists. Flumazenil can be used to terminate the action of benzodiazepines, e.g. after a benzodiazepine overdose. It may also serve as a diagnostic tool in this regard.

Pharmacokinetic Considerations

The benzodiazepines currently on the market differ in their pharmacokinetic properties, in particular the duration of action, which guides the use of the drug to be used. The half-life is largely determined by the rate of metabolic degradation of the parent drug. In addition, long-acting metabolites (e.g. desmethyldiazepam) are generated that may contribute to the duration of action. Short-acting drugs might be used for patients with difficulties to fall asleep, with the expectation that there is no hangover effect on the next day. Long-acting drugs may be used if reawakening during the entire night is to be prevented. Short-acting benzodiazepines may have a half-life in the range of 2–6 hours, e.g. midazolam, triazolam and oxazepam, medium-acting benzodiazepines a half-life in the range of 10–12 hours, e.g. lorazepam and lormetazepam, and long-acting benzodiazepines a half-life in the range of 20–50 hours, e.g. diazepam and clobazam.

Clinical Use

Benzodiazepines are amongst the most frequently prescribed drugs; they have well established uses in the treatment of anxiety disorders (anxiolytics) (6) and insomnia, preanaesthetic sedation, suppression of seizures and muscle relaxation.

Benzodiazepines are used as tranquilizers to relieve anxiety states, e.g. in generalized anxiety disorder and panic attacks. The anxiolytic effects are observed at low doses, suggesting that only a small number of $GABA_A$ receptors need to be modulated to obtain the anxiolytic effect. As outlined previously, this action is most likely mediated by $GABA_A$ receptors containing the $\alpha 2$ subunit. In contrast, higher doses of benzodiazepines and thus a higher receptor occupancy is needed for the sedative action of diazepam, which is mediated by $GABA_A$ receptors containing the $\alpha 1$ subunit. When diazepam is used as an anxiolytic, sedative side effects are frequently troublesome. The reduction of the reactivity to external stimuli is the basis for the use of benzodiazepines as hypnotics in the treatment of sleep disorders. The anticonvulsant activity of diazepam can be explained by the GABAergic inhibition of neuronal reponsiveness to excitatory inputs. Benzodiazepines (lorazepam and diazepam) are the drugs of choice in the treatment of status epilecpticus. Their use in the chronic treatment of epilepsy (e.g. clonazepam) is limited by the development of ▶ tolerance.

The definition of desired therapeutic and side effects in the case of the benzodiazepines very much depends on the clinical problem in question. The sedative and hypnotic actions are desired effects in the treatment of insomnia but undesired effects in the treatment of anxiety disorders. Effects that are usually undesired include daytime drowsiness, potentiation of the sedative effects of ethanol and anterograde amnesia. They are mediated via the benzodiazepine site of $GABA_A$ receptors, since they can be antagonized with flumazenil.

Repeated administration may lead to the development of tolerance to certain benzodiazepine effects, in particular to the sedative, anticonvulsant and muscle relaxant effects and to the development of ▸ physical dependence, which can include withdrawal anxiety, insomnia, convulsions and sensory hyperactivity and thus be similar to the symptoms that lead to the treatment. To avoid ▸ withdrawal symptoms, chronic treatment is discontinued by gradually tapering out the dose over a long period of time. The neurobiological nature of the adaptive changes which occur after long-term treatment or withdrawal from long-term treatment are poorly understood. Because of the adaptive changes that occur under chronic treatment, the long-term use of benzodiazepines is generally not recommended. For treament of insomnia, benzodiazepines should not be given for more than e.g. four weeks. For the treatment of anxiety disorders, benzodiazepines should not be used for more than e.g. six months. Because of their potentiation of the sedative action of ethanol, benzodiazepines should not be used in patients with alcohol abuse. Likewise, the potential nontherapeutic use of benzodiazepines for the purpose of euphoria has to be kept in mind, and particular care should be taken when treating patients with a history of drug abuse.

References

1. Rudolph U, Crestani F, Benke D, Brünig I, Benson JA, Fritschy J-M, Martin JR, Bluethmann H, Möhler H. (1999) Benzodiazepine actions mediated by specific γ-aminobutyric acid$_A$ receptor subtypes. Nature 401:796–800
2. Löw K, Crestani F, Keist R, Benke D, Brünig I, Benson JA, Fritschy J-M, Rülicke T, Bluethmann H, Möhler H, Rudolph U (2000) Molecular and neuronal substrate for the selective attenuation of anxiety. Science 290:131–134
3. Crestani F, Keist R, Fritschy J-M, Benke D, Vogt K, Prut L, Blüthmann H, Möhler H, Rudolph U (2002) Trace fear conditioning involves hippocampal α5 $GABA_A$ receptors. Proc Natl Acad Sci USA 13:8980-8985
4. McKernan RM, Rosahl TW, Reynolds DS, Sur C, Wafford KA, Atack JR, Farrar S, Myers J, Cook G, Ferris P, Garrett L, Bristow L, Marshall G, Macaulay A, Brown N, Howell O, Moore KW, Carling RW, Street LJ, Castro JL, Ragan CI, Dawson GR, Whiting PJ (2000) Sedative but not anxiolytic properties of benzodiazepines are mediated by the $GABA_A$ receptor α1 subtype. Nat Neurosci 3:587–592
5. Tobler I, Kopp C, Deboer T, Rudolph U (2001) Diazepam-induced changes in sleep: role of the α1 $GABA_A$ receptor subtype. Proc Natl Acad Sci USA 98:6464–6469
6. Shader RI, Greenblatt DJ (1993) Use of benzodiazepines in anxiety disorders. New Engl J Med 328:1398–1405

Benzothiazepines

Benzothiazepines (e.g. Diltiazem) block dihydropyridine-sensitive HVA calcium channels .

▸ Ca^{2+} Channel Blockers
▸ Voltage-dependent Ca^{2+} Channels

Beri-Beri

Beri-beri or clinically manifest (Vitamin B_1) thiamine deficiency exists as infantile beri-beri or adult beri-beri. Infantile beri-beri occurs in exclusively breastfed infants of thiamine-deficient mothers. Adults can develop different forms of the disease, depending on their constitution, environmental conditions, the relative contribution of other nutrients to the diet and the duration and severity of deficiency. Firstly, there is a so-called dry or atrophic (paralytic or nervous) form, which includes peripheral degenerative polyneuropathy, muscle weakness and paralysis. Secondly, a wet or exudative (cardiac) form exists, in which typical symptoms are lung and peripheral oedema and ascites. Finally, there is a cerebral form, that can occur as Wernicke encephalopathy or Korsakoff psychosis. This last form mostly affects chronic alcoholics with severe thiamine deficiency.

▶ **Vitamin B1 (Thiamin)**
▶ **Vitamines, watersoluble**

β-Adrenergic System

MARTIN J. LOHSE
Universität Würzburg, Würzburg, Germany
lohse@toxi.uni-wuerzburg.de

Synonyms

β-adrenoceptor system

Definition

The β-adrenergic system defines the effects of the ▶ Sympathetic System mediated via β-adrenergic receptors (synonym: β-adrenoceptors). These are G-protein-coupled receptors primarily causing an activation of adenylyl cyclases. They mediate a plethora of cardiovascular, smooth muscle and metabolic effects. β-Adrenergic receptor antagonists are used to treat various cardiovascular diseases, including hypertension, coronary artery disease and myocardial infarction, but also glaucoma and hyperthyroidism. β-Adrenergic receptor agonists are used to treat bronchial asthma and premature labor.

▶ α-Adrenergic System
▶ Antiarrhythmic Drugs
▶ Antihypertensive Drugs
▶ Catechol-O-Methyltransferase and its Inhibitors

Basic Characteristics

The sympathetic nervous system secretes the ▶ Catecholamines noradrenaline (norepinephrine) from nerve endings and adrenaline (epinephrine) from the adrenal medulla. Noradrenaline is stored in the varicosities (≈nerve endings) of the sympathetic nervous system, often together with ATP or neuropeptide Y. Adrenaline is stored in vesicles of the chromaffin cells of the adrenal medulla together with its precursor noradrenaline at a ratio of ≈4:1. Release of noradrenaline and adrenaline is subject to inhibitory control by presynaptic α_{2A}- and α_{2C}-adrenergic receptors, and to – less pronounced – stimulation via presynaptic β_2-adrenergic receptors (see chapter on α-adrenergic system).

Adrenaline and noradrenaline act on a total of nine adrenergic receptor subtypes, three of them belonging to the β-adrenergic receptor subfamily. These are termed β_1, β_2 and β_3. All adrenergic receptors couple to ▶ G-proteins. G_s is the primary G-protein for all three β-adrenergic receptors and mediates activation of ▶ Adenylyl Cyclase, i.e. results in an increase of intracellular cAMP-levels. Activation of ▶ Protein Kinase A (PKA) is the main effector pathway of elevated cAMP, but cAMP can also activate cyclic-nucleotide-dependent ion channels and inhibit the metabolism of cGMP by phosphodiesterases. Additional signaling pathways have been suggested mainly for the β_2-subtype, they include activation of G_i as well as stimulation of ▶ MAP-kinase pathways. G-protein-independent signaling pathways have been suggested by a variety of experiments, but their biochemical or physiological relevance has never been clearly demonstrated.

All adrenergic receptors are heptahelical, i.e. they have seven transmembrane helices that form a ligand-binding pocket. Amino acids essential for ligand binding have been mapped extensively for the β_2-adrenergic receptor; they are located in transmembrane helices 3, 5 and 6. Receptor activation involves an agonist-induced intramolecular conformational change that causes a relative movement of the transmembrane helices 3 and 6. This is thought to lead to a rearrangement of the intracellular parts of the receptor which couple to G-proteins, most notably the part of the third intracellular loop that is adjacent to transmembrane helix 6.

In addition to agonist-induced activity, many receptors, including the β-adrenergic receptors, display spontaneous or constitutive activity. This means, that the unoccupied receptor has some likelihood to adopt an active conformation, couple to G-proteins and generate an intracellular signal. Some compounds classified as antagonists (e.g. propranolol) can suppress constitutive activity and are therefore termed inverse agonists. Constitutive activity is more pronounced for the β_2-than the β_1-subtype, but has not yet been investigated for the β_3-receptor.

The agonist-induced conformational change not only causes receptor activation and generation of an intracellular signal, but also a number of biochemical processes that dampen the signal and cause desensitization of the receptor (Fig. 1). These include (1) phosphorylation of the receptor by members of the G-protein-coupled receptor kinase (GRK) family, followed by binding of the inhibitor proteins β-arrestins which prevents further contact of the receptor with its G-protein, (2) phosphorylation by the second-messenger activated protein kinases protein kinases A and C (PKA and PKC), which directly impairs G-protein-coupling, (3) translocation of the receptors into clathrin-coated pits and internalization into endosomes. Movement of receptors into clathrin-coated pits and binding of β-arrestin may also be required for non-conventional signaling, such as activation of MAP-kinases. Most internalized receptors are recycled back to the cell surface, but some are degraded. The regulatory processes described above are most pronounced for the β_2-subtype, and least for the β_3-subtype; they have also been demonstrated for other G-protein-coupled receptors, e.g. the α_2-adrenergic receptors. In addition to these regulatory processes at the level of the receptor itself, the receptor mRNA-levels can be down-regulated, at least in part by destabilization via mRNA-binding proteins.

β-Adrenergic receptors mediate a plethora of cardiovascular, smooth muscle and metabolic effects. Cardiac β_1-adrenergic receptors increase the frequency, electrical conduction and force of cardiac contractions as well as cardiac relaxation; they represent the strongest stimulus for the heart. At the same time they increase the generation of ectopic impulse generation and thereby the risk of arrhythmias. These effects are mediated by ▶ Protein Kinase A-mediated phosphorylation of calcium channels (resulting in enhanced calcium influx) as well as of phospholamban, a negative regulator of the sarcoplasmic calcium ATPase ▶ SERCA (resulting in enhanced uptake of calcium into the stores of the sarcoplasmic reticulum). A second important localization of β_1-adrenergic receptors are the cells of the juxtaglomerular

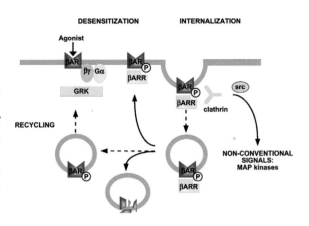

Fig. 1 Desensitization, internalization and recycling of β-adrenergic receptors. Activation of β-adrenergic receptors causes its phosphorylation by members of the G-protein-coupled receptor kinases (GRKs). Cytosolic β-arrestins then bind to the phosphorylated receptors and prevent further interaction with G-proteins. β-Arrestin-bound receptors assemble in clathrin-coated pits, where the complex appears to interact with other proteins, including dynamin and src-kinase. This leads (a) to the activation of non-conventional signaling pathways (raf-kinases, MAP-kinases, JNK-kinases), and (b) to the internalization of the receptors to endosomes. Endosomal receptors become either dephosphorylated and recycle back to the cell surface; some endosomal receptors undergo lysosomal degradation.

apparatus, where they increase the release of renin and thus cause stimulation of the renin-angiotensin-system.

β_2-Adrenergic receptors are located primarily on smooth muscle cells and mediate relaxation. This results in bronchodilatation, relaxation of the uterus and vasodilatation (partially mediated by β_1-adrenergic receptors). Liver β_2-adrenergic receptors trigger a protein kinase cascade that results in inhibition of glycogen synthase and activation of phosphorylase and thereby trigger the mobilization of glucose from glycogen stores.

β_3-Adrenergic receptors stimulate lipase and cause the breakdown of triglycerides to fatty acids in fat cells. It is still not clear to what extent this process is mediated by the β_3- or the β_2-subtype. Together with the mobilization of glucose from the liver, lipolysis provides the energy sources for the sympathetic "fight-or-flight" reaction.

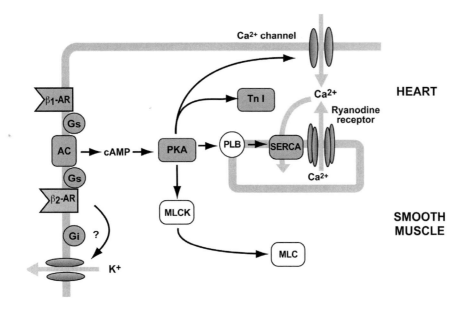

Fig. 2 β-Adrenergic signaling in cardiac muscle (predominantly β₁) and smooth muscle (predominantly β₂)
cells. Proteins that become more active after activation of β-adrenergic receptors are depicted in gray, those
which become less active are depicted in white. Both receptors couple to G_s and lead to activation of adenylyl
cyclases, generation of cyclic AMP and activation or protein kinase A (PKA). In *heart muscle cells*, PKA causes
phosphorylation of L-type calcium channels (increased Ca^{2+}-influx; relevant site of phosphorylation uncertain),
troponin I (TnI; diminishes affinity of troponin C for Ca^{2+} and thus enhances relaxation) and phospholamban
(PLB; leads to less inhibition of the sarcoplasmic Ca^{2+} ATPase, SERCA, which pumps Ca^{2+} into the sarcoplasmic
stores. This in turn enhances relaxation and enhances Ca^{2+}-release during the next beat) All this leads to more
rapid and forceful contraction as well as relaxation. In *smooth muscle cell* the signaling pathways are less clear.
PKA-mediated phosphorylation of myosin light chain kinase (MLCK) causes reduced activity of this kinase,
which in turn leads to decreased phosphorylation of myosin light chains and, hence, reduced contraction. A second postulated mechanism for relaxation is hyperpolarization via activation of K^+-channels; the signaling pathway is unclear and might involve coupling of β₂-receptors to G_i.

Drugs

Agonists as well as antagonists of β-adrenergic
receptors are used for the treatment of a variety of
conditions. β-Adrenergic receptor antagonists
belong to the most frequently used classes of
drugs.

The main use of β-adrenergic receptor agonists (β-sympathomimetic drugs) is the symptomatic treatment of bronchial asthma. Stimulation
of β₂-adrenergic receptors on smooth muscles
produces dilatation of the airways and reduces airway resistance. Although β₂-adrenergic receptor
activation inhibits inflammatory mediator release
from mast cells and other inflammatory cells,
there is no major effect of these drugs on airway
inflammation associated with asthma. β₂-Adren-

ergic receptor agonists are the most effective bronchodilators known. In order to reduce unwanted
systemic effects (most notably tachycardia and
arrhythmia) inhaled β₂-selective compounds are
the drugs of choice; a high first-pass effects helps
to reduce systemic effects of the major fraction of
the inhaled drug that reaches the gastrointestinal
tract. The most frequently used compounds are
fenoterol and salbutamol, which have a rapid
onset and a short duration of action. Newer
lipophilic compounds such a formoterol and salmeterol have a much longer duration of action (up
to 12 h), presumably because they are retained in
the plasma membrane after dissociation from the
receptor, i.e. they remain in the immediate vicinity
and can thus re-associate with the receptor.

β_2-Adrenergic receptor agonists are also used to treat premature labor by causing uterine relaxation. Fenoterol and ritodrine are frequently used. The effectiveness of long-term tocolysis is controversial, since both desensitization of the receptors and the symptomatic nature of this treatment may limit their effects to 1–2 days according to one large study.

Non-selective β-adrenergic receptor agonists, particularly adrenaline (epinephrine), are used in cardiovascular emergency situations, most importantly cardiopulmonary resuscitation and anaphylactic shock. They are given to produce stimulation of cardiac electrical activity via β_1-receptors, inhibition of mast cell mediator release via β_2-receptors, and bronchodilatation via β_2-receptors as well as α_1- and α_2-receptor-mediated vasoconstriction.

Relatively selective stimulation of β_1-adrenergic receptors can be achieved with dobutamine. This is a racemic drug of which both isomers activate the β_1-receptor, and in addition the (–) isomer activates α_1-receptors whereas the (+) isomer activates β_2-receptors; the simultaneous activation of α_1- and β_2-receptors results in no major net effect on peripheral resistance, and thus the overall cardiovascular effects are mediated by β_1-stimulation leading to increases in cardiac contractility and output. Dobutamine is used for the short-term treatment of acute cardiac failure and for diagnostic purposes in stress echocardiography.

Clinically used β-adrenergic receptor antagonists are either β_1-selective (e.g. bisoprolol, metoprolol, atenolol, betaxolol) or non-selective, i.e. with similar affinity for the β_1- and the β_2-subtype (e.g. propranolol, timolol, celiprolol). Many compounds classified as antagonists are in fact inverse agonists, for example metoprolol, bisoprolol, timolol or propranolol; inverse agonism is more pronounced at β_2- than at β_1-receptors because the latter possess a lower constitutive activity.

Some compounds possess a partial agonist activity (PAA, or intrinsic sympathomimetic activity ISA); examples are pindolol or celiprolol. These drugs produce less bradycardia but may be therapeutically less efficient.

Blockade of β-adrenergic receptors is important in the treatment of many cardiovascular diseases. Supraventricular and ventricular tachycardias are treated by reducing pacemaker currents in the SA-node, slowing AV-conduction and decreasing ectopic impulse generation. This is achieved via reductions in pacemaker currents and Ca^{2+}-currents (class II antiarrhythmic drugs).

Blockade of cardiac β_1-adrenergic receptors (preferentially with β_1-selective drugs) reduces cardiac frequency, cardiac output, cardiac O_2-consumption and probably prevents β-adrenergically induced cardiac remodeling. Therefore, they are first-line drugs in the treatment of hypertension, angina, myocardial infarction and cardiac failure. In the latter case, treatment must by initiated with very low doses to prevent acute decompensation.

Non-selective β-adrenergic receptor antagonists (e.g. propranolol) can suppress tachycardia and tremor in patients with hyperthyroidism or tremor caused by stress or nervousness.

β-Adrenergic receptor antagonists can reduce aqueous humor production in the eye and thereby reduce intraocular pressure. This is why they are the most frequently used class of drugs in glaucoma. Timolol is the best-established compound, followed by levobunolol and others. High concentrations of these compounds are applied to the eye, and it is, therefore, not really clear whether the effects are indeed mediated via specific interactions with β-adrenergic receptors.

References

1. Brodde OE (1991) β1- and β2-adrenoceptors in the human heart: properties, function, and alterations in chronic heart failure. Pharmacol. Rev. 43:203–242
2. Danner S, Lohse MJ (1999) Regulation of β-adrenergic receptor responsiveness. Reviews Physiol. Biochem. Pharmacol. 136:183–223
3. Hall RA, Premont RT, Lefkowitz RJ (1999) Heptahelical receptor signaling: beyond the G protein paradigm. J Cell Biol. 145:927–932
4. Lohse MJ, Strasser RH, Helmreich EJM (1993) The β-adrenergic receptors. In: New Comprehensive Biochemistry (Hucho F, ed.), Elsevier, Amsterdam, pp. 137–180

β Barrel

A beta barrel is a three-dimensional protein fold motif in which beta strands connected by loops form a barrel-like structure. This fold motif is found in many proteins of the immunoglobulin family and of the chymotrypsin family of serine proteases.

β-blockers

β-blockers are antagonists of β-adrenergic receptors.

▸ β-adrenergic System

β-cell

▸ Pancreatic β-cell

11β-HSD II

▸ 11β-hydroxysteroid Dehydrogenase Type II
▸ Glucocorticoids
▸ Epithelial Na⁺ Channel

11β-hydroxysteroid Dehydrogenase Type II

11β-hydroxysteroid dehydrogenase type II (11β-HSD II) is a steroid metabolizing enzyme which is specifically expressed in epithelial tissues such as kidney or colon. 11β-HSD II is an NAD^+-dependent enzyme which has a low K_m for physiological glucocorticoids. The reaction in the dehydroge-

nase direction is essentially irreversible. 11β-HSD II converts active glucocorticoids into their inactive ketoform, e.g. cortisol into cortisone. Since aldosterone posseses a cyclic 11,18-hemiacetyl-group, it is not a substrate for 11β-HSD II. Thus, this mechanism ensures protection of mineralocorticoid target tissues from transcriptional activation by glucocorticoids. Mutations in the 11β-HSD II gene are responsible for the syndrome of apparent mineralocorticoid excess.

▸ Glucocorticoids

β-lactam Antibiotics

JEAN-MARIE GHUYSEN
Centre d'Ingenierie des Proteines, University of Liège, Liège, Belgium
jmghuysen@ulg.ac.be

Synonyms

Wall peptidoglycan inhibitors

Definition

▸ β-lactam antibiotics are bicyclic or monocyclic azetidinone ring-containing compounds (Fig. 1). They kill bacteria by preventing the assembly of (4→3) peptidoglycans. These covalently closed net-like polymers form the matrix of the cell wall by which the bacteria can divide and multiply despite their high internal osmotic pressure.

▸ Microbial Resistance to Drugs
▸ Quinolones
▸ Ribosomal Protein Synthesis Inhibitors

Mechanism of Action

▸ Peptidoglycans of the (4→3) and (3→3) types (Fig. 2) are comprised of glycan chains made of alternating β-1,4-linked N-acetylglucosamine and N-acetylmuramic acid residues. The D-lactyl groups on carbon C_3 of the muramic acids are substituted by L-alanyl-γ-D-glutamyl-L-diaminoacyl-D-alanine stem tetrapeptides. In the (4→3) peptidoglycans, peptides borne by adjacent glycan chains are cross-linked through direct linkages or cross bridges (comprised of one or several intervening amino acid residues) that extend from the D-alanine residue at position 4 of a stem peptide to the ω-amino group at position 3 of another stem peptide. Lipid II (Fig. 3) is the immediate biosynthetic precursor. A disaccharide bearing a L-alanyl-γ-D-glutamyl-L-diaminoacyl-D-alanyl-D-alanine stem pentapeptide (the diamino acid residue of which can be either free, i.e. unsubstituted, or substituted by one or several amino acid residues, i.e. branched) is exposed on the outer face of the plasma membrane, linked to a C_{55}-undecaprenyl via a pyrophosphate. From this precursor, the formation of polymeric (4→3) peptidoglycans relies on glycosyl transferases ensuring glycan chain elongation and acyl transferases ensuring peptide cross-linking. Acyl transferases of the SxxK superfamily (▶ SxxK Acyl Transferases) are implicated in cross-linking. With x denoting a variable amino acid residue, they have a specific bar code in the form of three motifs, SxxK, SxN (or analogue) and KTG (or analogue), occurring at equivalent places and roughly with the same spacing along the polypeptide chains. As a result of the polypeptide folding, the motifs are brought close to each other at the immediate boundary of the catalytic centre between an all-α domain and an α/β domain. SxxK acyl transferases identify N-acyl-D-alanyl-D-alanine sequences as carbonyl donors, produce a N-acyl-D-alanyl moiety linked as an ester to the serine residue of the invariant motif SxxK and transfer the peptidyl moiety to an amino group (transpeptidation) or a water molecule (carboxypeptidation). SxxK acyl transferases identify penicillin (used as a generic term for β-lactam antibiotics) as a suicide carbonyl donor. Because the serine-ester linked penicilloyl enzyme that SxxK acyl transferases produce is inert and stable, they are immobilized, at least for a long time, in the form of penicillin-binding proteins, in short PBPs. A constellation of genes code for PBPs of varying amino acid sequences and functionalities. PBPs occur as free-standing polypeptides and as protein fusions. This combinatorial system of structural modules results in a massive increase in diversity.

Lethal Target Proteins

▶ SxxK PBP fusions of classes A and B are the lethal targets of β-lactam antibiotics. The PBP fusions of class A are comprised of an SxxK acyl transferase module of class A, linked to the carboxy end of a glycosyl transferase module having its own five motif-bar code, itself linked to the carboxy end of a membrane anchor. They convert the disaccharide-pentapeptide units borne by lipid II precursor molecules into nascent polymeric (4→3) peptidoglycans. Glycan chain elongation strictly depends on the glutamic acid residue of motif 1 of the glycosyl transferase module. It is aided by the neighbouring aspartic acid residue of motif 1 and the glutamic acid residue of motif 3 of the same module. Peptide cross-linking between elongated glycan chains is then carried out by the associated SxxK acyl transferase module. The PBP fusions of class B are comprised of an SxxK acyl transferase module of class B, linked to the carboxy end of a linker module having its own three-motif bar code, itself linked to a membrane anchor. They are components of morphogenetic apparatus that control wall expansion, ensure cell-shape maintenance and carry out septum formation. Likely, the linker modules ensure that the associated SxxK acyl transferase modules are positioned in an active conformation within the morphogenetic apparatus where they need to be. The essential PBP fusions of classes A and B are large bodies studded with positively and negatively charged magnets. In turn, the electrostatic negative wells that surround the β-lactam antibiotic backbones, e.g. $CON-C-CON-C-COO^-$ in the penams and 3-cephems, $C=N-CO-CON-C-COO^-$ in mecillinam, and $CON-C-CON-SO_3^-$ in aztreonam (Fig. 1) are coplanar but their location, shape and strength vary depending on the bicyclic or monocyclic framework and the nature of the substituents of the azetidinone ring. Binding of β-lactam antibiotics to the SxxK acyl transferase modules of the PBP fusions lead to the formation of Michaelis complexes that are ligand- and enzyme-specific hydrogen bonding networks. *Escherichia coli* is killed in a number of ways; via cell lysis as a result of the selective inactivation of the PBP fusions of class A, Eco1a and Eco1b (they can substitute for each other), by cephaloridine and cefsulodin; via transformation of the cells into round bodies as a result of the selective inactiva-

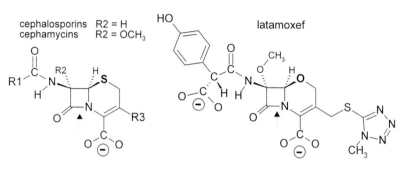

Penams

benzylpenicillin

mecillinam

3-Cephems

cephalosporins R2 = H
cephamycins   R2 = OCH$_3$

Oxacephems

latamoxef

Carbapenems

imipenem
thienamycin

Monobactams

aztreonam

Fig. 1 Bicyclic (penams, 3-cephems, oxacephems and carbapenems) and monocyclic (aztreonam) β-lactam antibiotics. Rupture of the scissile amide bond of the azetidinone ring (arrow) by the SxxK acyl transferases implicated in (4→3) peptidoglycan synthesis results in the formation of long-lived, serine-ester-linked acyl derivatives. The inactivated enzymes behave as penicillin-binding proteins or PBPs.

tion of the cell-cycle PBP fusion of subclass B2, Eco2, by mecillinam and thienamycin; via cell filamentation as a result of the selective inactivation of the cell-cycle PBP fusion of subclass B3, Eco3, by mezlocillin, cefaperazone, cefotaxime, cefuroxime, cephalothin and aztreonam; or via different combinations of these morphological alterations by ampicillin, benzylpenicillin, carbenicillin and cefoxitin.

β-Lactamase-Mediated Resistance

▶ SxxK free-standing PBPs are peptidoglycan-hydrolases of one kind or another. Loss of these auxilliary cell-cycle proteins causes varying morphological aberrations, but is not fatal. Likely, conversion of free-standing PBPs into β-lactam antibiotic-hydrolysing enzymes, with loss of peptidase

activity and conservation of the polypeptide fold, gives rise to the SxxK β-lactamases. On good β-lactam substrates, the β-lactamase catalytic centres can turn over 1000 times or more per second. In some bacteria, β-lactamase synthesis is inducible. The protein BlaR of *Bacillus licheniformis* is a SxxK penicillin sensory-transducer. A SxxK penicillin sensor, related to β-lactamases of class D by statistically significant similarity indexes, is exposed on the outer face of the plasma membrane. It is linked to a four α-helix bundle signal transmitter embedded in the plasma membrane, itself linked to a signal emitter, in the cytosol, that possesses the consensus sequence of a Zn^{2+}-dependent peptidase. As an independent entity, the penicillin sensor is a high affinity PBP. Signal reception by the full size BlaR does not involve

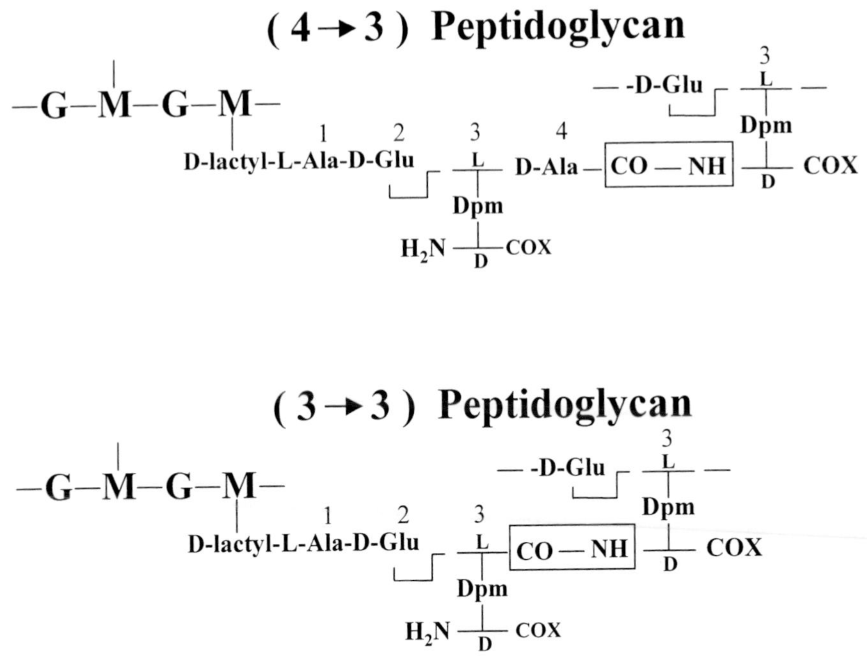

(4 → 3) Peptidoglycan

$$-G-M-G-M-$$

D-lactyl-L-Ala-D-Glu   1   2   3   4   D-Ala — | CO — NH | — COX

— -D-Glu   3 L — Dpm

L — Dpm

H_2N — COX

(3 → 3) Peptidoglycan

$$-G-M-G-M-$$

D-lactyl-L-Ala-D-Glu   1   2   3

— -D-Glu   3 L — Dpm

L — | CO — NH | — COX

Dpm

H_2N — COX

Fig. 2 (4→3) Peptidoglycan (the synthesis of which is susceptible to β-lactam antibiotics) and (3→3) peptidoglycan (the synthesis of which is resistant to antibiotics) in *Escherichia coli* and *Mycobacterium tuberculosis*. G: N-acetylglucosamine. M: N-acetylmuramic acid (*i.e.* N-acetylglucosamine with a D-lactyl substituent on carbon C_3). Dpm: *meso*-diaminopimelic acid. In *E. coli* and *M. tuberculosis*, the stem peptides are unbranched. COX: COOH (in *E. coli*) or $CONH_2$ (in *M. tuberculosis*).

penicilloylation of the serine residue of motif SxxK of the penicillin sensor. Hence, fusion of a free standing PBP to another polypeptide can result in a hybrid that performs gene regulation, unblocking transcription of the β-lactamase-encoding gene.

PBP-mediated resistance

There are at least two modes of intrinsic resistance to β-lactam antibiotics. Determinants conferring a decreased susceptibility to β-lactam antibiotics evolve by the accumulation of point mutations in genes that code for essential PBP fusions of classes A and/or B. The shuffling and capture of DNA sequences from commensal *Streptococci* having a reduced susceptibility to the drug gives rise to *Streptococcus pneumoniae* pathogens in which mosaic genes code for mosaic PBP fusions of classes A and/or B of decreased affinity for the drug. Mosaic and wildtype PBP fusions of a same

class (and same subclass) differ by up to 15% amino acid residues. Mosaic PBPs occur also in *Neisseria meningitidis* and *N. gonorrhoeae* strains. Another mode of intrinsic resistance is the capacity of bacterial pathogens of manufacturing, in addition to a penicillin-susceptible (4→3) peptidoglycan, a penicillin-resistant (3→3) peptidoglycan in which cross-linking involves the diamino acid residues at position 3 of the stem peptides (Fig. 2). The mechanisms of (3→3) peptidoglycan assembly from lipid II precursor molecules, and its diverse growth phase-dependence in different bacterial species remain to be elucidated. *Enterococcus faecium* in the exponential phase of growth, manufactures a (3→3) peptidoglycan in varying proportions of total peptidoglycan and resist β-lactam antibiotics at varying levels. *E. faecium* produces a SxxK protein fusion, Efam5, which is extremely resistant to β-lactam antibiotics although it bears the linker and acyl transferase

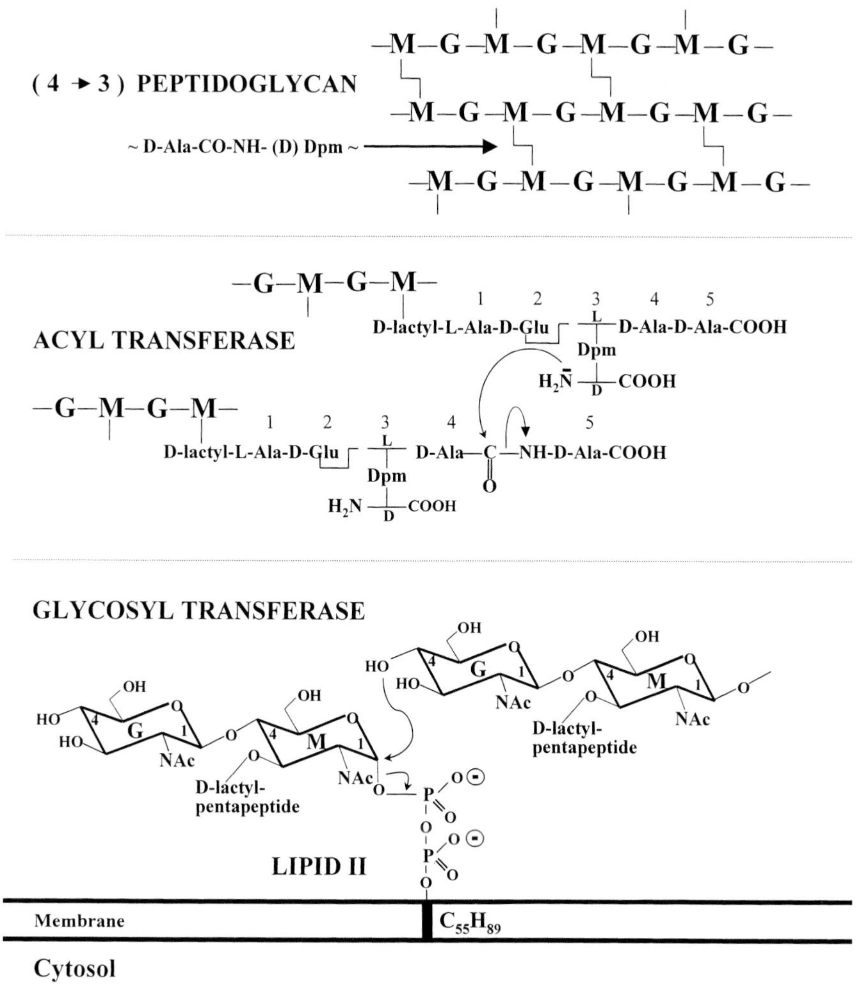

B

Fig. 3 Lipid II precursor (bottom) and polymeric (4→3) peptidoglycan of *Escherichia coli* and *Mycobacterium tuberculosis*. Glycosyl transferase and acyl transferase-catalysed reactions. G: N-acetylglucosamine. M: N-acetylmuramic acid. Dpm: *meso*-diaminopimelic acid. (3→3) Peptidoglycan cross-linking (Fig. 2) may proceed *via* the formation, in a penicillin-resistant manner, of a N-acyl-L-diaminoacyl moiety linked as an ester to the serine residue and the transfer of the peptidyl moiety to the ω-amino group of the diamino acid residue of another peptide.

bar codes of the PBP fusions of class B. Orthologues of Efam5 are produced by other *Enterococci* and *Staphylococcus* strains. *Mycobacterium tuberculosis* and *M. leprae* produce a set of SxxK protein fusions that, in all likelihood, are penicillin-resistant counterparts of the PBP fusions. The walls of mycobacteria grown to stationary phase are mixtures of (4→3) and (3→3) peptidoglycans. Conditions similar to stationary phase may prevail when *M. tuberculosis* and *M. leprae* dwell in host macrophages and Schwann cells, respectively. Making a (3→3) peptidoglycan in a penicillin-resistant manner under these stress conditions, may explain the lack of efficiency of the β-lactam antibiotics as therapeutic agents against tuberculosis and leprosy.

Clinical Use

Because the SxxK PBP fusions are specific to the prokaryotes, the β-lactam antibiotics have a high selective toxicity without marked side effects except for possible allergic reactions. Resistance is a problem of great concern. The use of antibiotics functions to fuel the continuing emergence of novel β-lactamases and intrinsic resistance determinants among bacterial pathogens.

References

1. van Heijenoort J (1996) Murein synthesis. In F.C. Neidhart et al. (ed.) Escherichia coli and Salmonella: Cellular and Molecular Biology. 2nd ed. ASM Press, Washington, DC. pp1025–1035

2. Goffin C, Ghuysen JM (1998) The multimodular penicillin-binding proteins: an enigmatic family of orthologs and paralogs. Microbiol. Mol. Biol. Rev. 62:1079–1093

3. Hardt K et al. (1997) The penicillin sensory-transducer BlaR involved in the inducibility of β-lactamase synthesis in Bacillus licheniformis is embedded in the plasma membrane via a four α-helix bundle. Mol. Microbiol. 23:935–944

4. Lepage S et al. (1997) Dual multimodular class A penicillin-binding proteins in Mycobacterium leprae. J. Bacteriol. 179:4627–4630

β-Lactamases

▶ β-lactam Antibiotics

BH4

▶ (6R)-5,6,7,8-tetrahydro-L-biopterin

BH Domain

BH domains or Bcr (breakpoint cluster region) homology domains are homologus to the GTPase activating protein domain of the Bcr gene product. Although the p85 BH domain specifically interacts with the Rho family proteins Cdc42 and Rac1, no GTPase-activating activity has been attributed to it.

▶ Phospholipid Kinases

Bicuculline

Bicuculline is a competitive antagonist at the $GABA_A$ receptor. It is a plant alkaloid.

▶ $GABA_A$ Receptor

BID

BID is a member of the Bcl-2 gene family, which encode proteins that function either to promote apoptosis or to inhibit apoptosis as in the proteins derived from Bcl-2. These proteins can exist as monomers or they can dimerize. For example, if two promoting Bcl-2 family proteins dimerize then apoptosis will be greatly enhanced. Conversely, if dimerization of an inhibitory and promotor protein occurs, then the effects are cancelled out. The Bcl-2 family of proteins are localized to the outer mitochondrial or outer nuclear membranes.

▶ Apoptosis

Biguanides

▶ Oral Antidiabetic Drugs

Bimodal Distribution

A bimodal distribution is a frequency distribution of a certain phenotype with two peaks separated by an antimode.

▶ Pharmacogenetics

Bioavailability

Bioavailability is the amount of drug in a formulation that is released and becomes available for absorption or the amount of the drug absorbed after oral administration compared to the amount absorbed after intravenous administration (bioavailability = 100%), judged from areas remaining under plasma drug concentration-time curves.

▶ Area under the Curve (AUC)

Biogenic Amines

Acetylcholine, serotonin, norepinephrine, epinephrine, dopamine, and histamine are often collectively referred to as biogenic amines. These agents play key roles in neurotransmission and other signaling functions. They are relatively small in size and contain a protonated amino group or a permanently charged ammonium moiety. ▶ Acetylcholine, ▶ serotonin, norepinephrine (▶ Norepinephrine/Noradrenalin), ▶ epinephrine, ▶ dopamine, and ▶ histamine are often collectively referred to as biogenic amines. These agents play key roles in neurotransmission and other signaling functions. They are relatively small in size and contain a protonated amino group or a permanently charged ammonium moiety. Biogenic amines are synthesized in nerve cells from amino acids. They are released from vesicles localized in presynaptic terminals into the synaptic cleft. Biogenic amines bind to cell membrane located receptors at postsynaptic terminals. The synaptic cleft is cleared of biogenic amines through reuptake transporters located at the presynaptic terminal or by enzymes degradating the amines.

Bioinformatics

MICHAEL NILGES, JENS P. LINGE
Unité de Bio–Informatique Structurale, Institut Pasteur, Paris, France
nilges@pasteur.fr, linge@pasteur.fr

Synonyms

Related: Computational Biology, Computational Molecular Biology, Biocomputing

Definition

Bioinformatics derives knowledge from computer analysis of biological data. These can consist of the information stored in the genetic code, but also experimental results from various sources, patient statistics and scientific literature. Research in bioinformatics includes method development for storage, retrieval and analysis of the data. Bioinformatics is a rapidly developing branch of biology and is highly interdisciplinary, using techniques and concepts from informatics, statistics, mathematics, chemistry, biochemistry, physics and linguistics. It has many practical applications in different areas of biology and medicine.

▶ Molecular Modelling

Description

The history of computing in biology goes back to the 1920s when scientists were already thinking of establishing biological laws solely from data analysis by induction (e.g. A.J. Lotka, Elements of Physical Biology, 1925). However, only the development of powerful computers, and the availability of experimental data that can be readily treated by computation (for example, DNA or amino acid sequences and three–dimensional structures of proteins) launched bioinformatics as an independent field. Today, practical applications of bioinformatics are readily available through the world wide web, and are widely used in biological and medical research. As the field is rapidly evolving, the very definition of bioinformatics is still the matter of debate.

The relationship between computer science and biology is a natural one for several reasons. First, the phenomenal rate of biological data being produced provides challenges; massive amounts of data have to be stored, analysed and made accessible. Second, the nature of the data is often such that a statistical method, and hence computation, is necessary. This applies in particular to the information on the building plans of proteins and of the temporal and spatial organisation of their expression in the cell encoded by the DNA. Third, there is a strong analogy between the DNA sequence and a computer program (it can be shown that the DNA represents a Turing Machine).

Analyses in bioinformatics mainly focus on genome sequences, macromolecular structures, and functional genomics experiments (e.g. expression data, yeast two–hybrid screens). But bioinformatic analysis is also applied to various other data, e.g. taxonomy trees, relationship data from metabolic pathways, the text of scientific papers, and patient statistics. A large range of techniques is used, including primary sequence alignment, protein 3D structure alignment, phylogenetic tree construction, prediction and classification of protein structure, prediction of RNA structure, prediction of protein function, and expression data clustering. Algorithmic development is an important part of bioinformatics, and techniques and algorithms were specifically developed for the analysis of biological data (e.g., the dynamic programming algorithm for sequence alignment).

Bioinformatics has a large impact on biological research. Giant research projects such as the Human Genome Project [4] would be meaningless without the bioinformatics component. The goal of sequencing projects, for example, is not to corroborate or refute a hypothesis, but to provide raw data for later analysis. Once the raw data is available, hypotheses may be formulated and tested in silico. In this manner, computer experiments may answer biological questions which cannot be tackled by traditional approaches. This has led to the founding of dedicated bioinformatics research groups as well as to a different work practice in the average bioscience laboratory where the computer has become an essential research tool.

Three key areas are the organisation of knowledge in databases, sequence analysis and structural bioinformatics.

Organizing Biological Knowledge in Databases

Biological raw data is stored in public ▶ databanks (such as Genbank or EMBL for primary DNA sequences). The data can be submitted and accessed via the world wide web. Protein sequence databanks like trEMBL provide the most likely translation of all coding sequences in the EMBL databank. Sequence data are prominent, but also other data are stored, e. g. yeast two–hybrid screens, expression arrays, systematic gene knockout experiments, and metabolic pathways.

The stored data need to be accessed in a meaningful way, and often contents of several databanks or databases have to be accessed simultaneously and correlated with each other. Special languages have been developed to facilitate this task, such as the Sequence Retrieval System (SRS) and the Entrez system. An unsolved problem is the optimal design of inter–operating database systems. ▶ Databases provide additional functionality such as access to sequence homology searches and links to other databases and analysis results. For example, SWISSPROT [1] contains verified protein sequences and more annotations describing the function of a protein. Protein 3D structures are stored in specific databases (for example, the Protein Data Bank [2], now curated and developed by the Research Collaboratory for Structural Bioinformatics). Organism specific databases have been developed (such as ACEDB, the A C. Elegans DataBase for the *C. elegans* genome, FLYBASE for *D. melanogaster* etc). A major problem are errors in databanks and databases (mostly errors in annotation), in particular since errors propagate easily through links.

Also databases of scientific literature (such as PUBMED, MEDLINE) provide additional functionality, e.g. they can search for similar articles based on word–usage analysis. Text recognition systems are being developed that extract automatically knowledge about protein function from the abstracts of scientific articles, notably on protein–protein interactions.

Analysing Sequence Data

The primary data of sequencing projects are DNA sequences. These become only really valuable through their annotation. Several layers of analysis with bioinformatics tools are necessary to arrive from a raw DNA sequence at an annotated protein sequences:

▶ establish the correct order of sequence contigs to obtain one continuous sequence;

▶ find the tranlation and transcription initiation sites, find promoter sites, define open reading frames (ORF);

▶ find splice sites, introns, exons;

▶ translate the DNA sequence into a protein sequence, searching all six frames;

▶ compare the DNA sequence to known protein sequences in order to verify exons etc with homologuous sequences.

Some completely automated annotation systems have been developed (e.g., GENEQUIZ), which use a multitude of different programs and methods.

The protein sequences are further analysed to predict function. The function can often be inferred if a sequence of a ▶ homologous protein with known function can be found. Homology searches are the predominant bioinformatics application, and very efficient search methods have been developed [3, 4]. The often difficult distinction between orthologous sequences and paralogous sequences facilitates the functional annotation in the comparison of whole genomes. Several methods detect glycolysation, myristylation and other sites, and the prediction of signal peptides in the amino acid sequence give valuable information about the subcellular location of a protein.

The ultimate goal of sequence annotation is to arrive at a complete functional description of all genes of an organism. However, function is an ill-defined concept. Thus, the simplified idea of "one gene – one protein – one structure – one function" cannot take into account proteins that have multiple functions depending on context (e.g., subcellar location and the presence of cofactors). Well-known cases of "moonlighting" proteins are lens crystalline and phosphoglucose isomerase. Currently, work on ontologies is under way to explicitly define a vocabulary that can be applied to all organisms even as knowledge of gene and protein roles in cells is accumulating and changing.

Families of similar sequences contain information on sequence evolution in the form of specific conservation patters at all sequence positions. Multiple sequence alignments are useful for
- building sequence profiles or Hidden Markov Models to perform more sensitive homology searches. A sequence profile contains information about the variability of every sequence position, improving structure prediction methods (secondary structure prediction). Sequence profile searches have become readily available through the introduction of PsiBLAST [3];
- studying evolutionary aspects, by the construction of phylogenetic trees from the pairwise differences between sequences: for example, the classification with 70S, 30S RNAs established the

separate kingdom of archeae;
- determining active site residues, and residues specifc for subfamilies;
- predicting protein–protein interactions;
- analysing single nucleotide polymorphisms to hunt for genetic sources of deseases.

Many complete genomes of microorganisms and a few of eukaryotes are available [5, 6]. By analysis of entire genome sequences a wealth of additional information can be obtained. The complete genomic sequence contains not only all protein sequences but also sequences regulating gene expression. A comparison of the genomes of genetically close organisms reveals genes responsible for specific properties of the organisms (e.g., infectivity). Protein interactions can be predicted from conservation of gene order or operon organisation in different genomes. Also the detection of gene fusion and gene fission (i.e, one protein is split into two in another genome) events helps to deduce protein interactions.

Structural Bioinformatics
This branch of bioinformatics is concerned with computational approaches to predict and analyse the spatial structure of proteins and nucleic acids. Whereas in many cases, the primary sequence uniquely specifies the three–dimensional (3D) structure, the specific rules are not well understood, and the protein folding problem remains largely unsolved. Some aspects of protein structure can already be predicted from amino acid content. Secondary structure can be deduced from the primary sequence with statistics or ▶ neural networks. When using a multiple sequence alignment, secondary structure can be predicted with an accuracy above 70%.

3D models can be obtained most easily if the 3D structure of a homologous protein is known (homology modelling, comparative modelling). A homology model can only be as good as the sequence alignment; whereas protein relationships can be detected at the 20% identity level and below, a correct sequence alignment becomes very difficult, and the homology model will be doubtful. From 40 to 50% identity the models are usually mostly correct; however, it is possible to have 50% identity between two carefully designed protein sequences with different topology (the so-called JANUS protein). Remote relationships that are undetectable by sequence comparisons may be detected by sequence–to–structure fitness (or ▶ threading) approaches; the search sequence is systematically compared to all known protein structures. Ab initio predictions of protein 3D structure remains the major challenge; some progress has been made recently by combining statistical with ▶ force-field based approaches.

Membrane proteins are interesting drug targets. It is estimated that membrane receptors form 50% of all drug targets in pharmacological research. However, membrane proteins are under-represented in the PDB structure database. Since membrane proteins are usually excluded from structural genomics initiatives due to technical problems, the prediction of transmembrane helices and solvent accessibility is very important. Modern methods can predict transmembrane helices with a reliability greater than 70%.

Understanding the 3D structure of a macromolecule is crucial for understanding its function. Many properties of the 3D structure cannot be deduced directly from the primary sequence. Obtaining better understanding of protein function is the driving force behind ▶ structural genomics efforts, which can be thus understood as part of ▶ functional genomics. Similar structure can imply similar function. General structure–to–function relationships can be obtained by statistical approaches, for example, by relating secondary structure to known protein function or surface properties to cell location.

The increased speed of structure determination necessary for the structural genomics projects make an independent validation of the structures (by comparison to expected properties) particularly important. Structure validation helps to correct obvious errors (e.g., in the covalent structure) and leads to a more standardized representation of structural data, e.g., by agreeing on a common atom name nomenclature. The knowledge of the structure quality is a prerequisite for further use of the structure, e.g in molecular modelling or drug design.

In order to make as much data on the structure and its determination available in the databases, approaches for automated data harvesting are being developed. Structure classification schemes, as implemented for example in the SCOP, CATH, and FSSP databases, elucidate the relationship between protein folds and function and shed light on the evolution of protein domains.

Combined analysis of structural and genomic data will certainly get more important in the near future. Protein folds can be analysed for whole genomes. Protein–protein interactions predicted on the sequence level, can be studied in more detail on the structure level. Single nucleotide polymorphisms can be mapped on 3D structures of proteins in order to elucidate specific structural causes of disease.

More detailed aspects of protein function can be obtained by ▶ force–field based approaches. Whereas protein function requires protein dynamics, no experimental technique can observe it directly on an atomic scale, and motions have to be simulated by molecular dynamics (MD) simulations. Free energy differences (for example between binding energies of different protein ligands) can be characterized by MD simulations. Molecular mechanics or molecular dynamics based approaches are also necessary for homology modelling and for structure refinement in X–ray crystallography and NMR structure determination.

Drug design exploits the knowledge of the 3D structure of the binding site (or the structure of the complex with a ligand) to construct potential drugs, for example inhibitors of viral proteins or RNA. In addition to the 3D structure, a force field is necessary to evaluate the interaction between the protein and a ligand (to predict binding energies). In virtual screening, a library of molecules is tested on the computer for their capacities to bind to the macromolecule.

Pharmacological Relevance

Many aspects of bioinformatics are relevant for pharmacology. Drug targets in infectious organisms can be revealed by whole genome comparisons of infectious and non–infectious organisms. The analysis of single nucleotide polymorphisms reveals genes potentially responsible for genetic deseases. Prediction and analysis of protein 3D structure is used to develop drugs and understand drug resistance.

Patient databases with genetic profiles, e.g. for cardiovascular diseases, diabetes, cancer, may play an important role in the future for individual health care by integrating personal genetic profile into diagnosis, despite obvious ethical problems. The goal is to analyse a patient's individual genetic profile and compare it with a collection of reference profiles and other related information. This may improve individual diagnosis, prophylaxis and therapy.

References

1. Bairoch A, Apweiler R (2000) The SWISS–PROT protein sequence database and its supplement TrEMBL in 2000. Nucleic Acids Res. 28:45–48
2. Berman HM, Westbrook J, Feng Z, Gilliland G, Bhat TN, Weissig H, Shindyalov IN, Bourne PE (2000) The Protein Data Bank. Nucleic Acids Res. 28:235–242
3. Altschul SF, Madden TL, Schaffer AA, Zhang J, Zhang Z, Miller W, Lipman DJ (1997) Gapped BLAST and PSI–BLAST: a new generation of protein database search programs. Nucleic Acids Res. 25:3389–3402
4. Pearson WR (2000) Flexible sequence similarity searching with the FASTA3 program package. Methods Mol. Biol. 132:185–219
5. The Genome International Sequencing Consortium (2001) Initial sequencing and analysis of the human genome. Nature 409:860–921
6. JC Venter et al. (2001) The sequence of the human genome. Science 291:1304–1351

Biopterin

▶ (6R)-5,6,7,8-tetrahydro-L-biopterin

Biotin

▶ Vitamins, watersoluble

BiP

BiP is a molecular chaperone (relative molecular mass 78 KD) found in the lumen of the endoplasmic reticulum. BiP is related to the Hsp70 family of heat-shock proteins and was originally described as immunoglobulin heavy chain binding protein.

▶ Protein Trafficking and Quality Control

Bipolar Disorder

Bipolar disorder, or manic depressive illness, is a severe mental illness characterized by recurring episodes of mania and depression.

▶ Antidepressant Drugs
▶ Galanin Receptors

Bisphosphonates

Bisphosphonates are pyrophosphate analogues that accumulate in bone and inhibit osteoclast activity. Nitrogen-containing bisphosphonates such as alendronate, risedronate, ibandronate or zoledronate are distinguished from non-aminobisphosphonates such as clodronate or etidronate. Bisphosphonates are among first-line treatments for benign and malignant bone diseases.

▶ Bone Metabolism

Bisubstrate Analogs

Bisubstrate analogs are compounds that contain features of both substrates for an enzymatic reaction in which two substrates are used.

▶ Lipid Modifications

BK$_{Ca}$ channel

A BK$_{Ca\ channel}$ belongs to the ▶ K$^+$ channels with a large conductance, controlled by the membrane potential and the submembrane Ca^{2+} concentration.

Blastocyst

The blastocyst is an early embryonic stage in mammalian development. Murine blastocysts can be harvested at day 3.5 p.c. Their inner cell mass contains embryonic stem cells. Multiple murine embyonic stem cell lines have been established. Embryonic stem cells carrying genetically engineered mutations are injected into blastocysts, which are subsequently implanted into pseudopregnant foster mothers.

▶ Transgenic Animal Models

Blood-brain Barrier

The blood-brain barrier arises because capillaries in the brain are more impermeable than those in other organs. This appears to be due largely to the presence of tight junctions between endothelial cells, rather than pores, as well as the close association of perivascular extensions of astrocytes with the capillaries. The blood brain-barrier is permeable to water, glucose, sodium chloride and non-ionised lipid-soluble molecules but large molecules such as peptides as well as many polar substances do not readily permeate the barrier.

Blood:Gas Partition Coefficient of Anaesthetics

The term partition coefficient is defined as the ratio of the concentration of an agent in two phases at equilibrium. In the case of inhalation anaesthetics, the blood:gas partition coefficient, i.e. the ratio of the concentration of the anaesthetic in the blood and in the inspired air, determines the rate of induction of and recovery from the anaesthetic state. A low blood:gas partition coefficient implies fast induction and recovery.

▶ General Anaesthetics

Blood Pressure Control

REINHOLD KREUTZ
Freie Universität Berlin, Berlin, Germany
kreutz@medizin.fu-berlin.de

Synonyms

Physiology of blood pressure; control of ▶ hypertension

Definition

The blood pressure represents the tension or pressure of the blood within the arteries that is exerted against the arterial wall *in vivo*. Blood pressure is a quantitative trait that is highly variable. In population studies, blood pressure has a normal distribution that is slightly skewed to the right. The regulation of blood pressure within the intravascular system is a complex interaction of a number of systems and mechanisms. A chronic elevation of blood pressure or hypertension is a substantial health problem affecting 25% of the adult population in industrialised societies. Despite important advances in our understanding of the pathophysiology of hypertension and the availability of effective treatment strategies it still remains a major modifiable risk factor for cardiovascular and renal disease. There is no specific level of blood pressure where clinical complications start to occur; thus the definition of hypertension is arbitrary but needed in clinical practice for patient assessment and treatment.

The relevance of clinical conditions with chronic low blood pressure or hypotension has been questioned, with the exception of a few rare clinical syndromes. Temporary increases or decreases of blood pressure are often seen in clinical medicine in the context of acute illnesses or interventions.

▶ Antihypertensive Drugs
▶ Renin-Angiotensin-Aldosterone System
▶ Smooth Muscle Tone Regulation

Basic Mechanisms

The circulation is divided into several compartments: the high-pressure arterial circuit, which contains 13% of the blood volume, the capillary bed containing 7% of the blood volume, and the low-pressure venous bed, which contains 64% of the blood volume. The pulmonary circulation contains 9% and the heart 7% of the blood volume. Although the venous system stores and propels large volumes of blood and regulates cardiac output by venous return to the heart, in considering blood pressure control attention is focused on the high-pressure arteries. The basic function of the circulation is to provide nutrients to peripheral tissues. Blood vessels in local tissue beds regulate blood flow in relation to local needs. Blood flow (Q) is defined by Ohm's law and varies directly with the change in pressure (P) across a blood vessel and inversely with the resistance R (Q = P/R). It can be seen that pressure varies directly with blood flow and resistance (P = QR). Blood pressure is produced by the contraction of the left ventricle (producing blood flow) and by the resistance of the arteries and arterioles. Systolic pressure, or maximum blood pressure, occurs during left ventricular systole. Diastolic pressure, or minimum blood pressure, occurs during ventricular diastole. The difference between systolic and diastolic pressure is the pulse pressure (▶ Systolic and Diastolic Blood Pressure and Pulse Pressure).

Although blood pressure control follows Ohm's law and seems to be simple, it underlies a complex circuit of inter-related systems. Hence, numerous physiologic systems that have pleiotropic effects and interact in complex fashion have been found to modulate blood pressure. Because of their number and complexity it is beyond the scope of the current account to cover all mechanisms and feedback circuits involved in blood pressure control. Rather, an overview of the clinically most relevant ones is presented. These systems include the heart, the blood vessels, the extracellular volume, the kidneys, the nervous system, a variety of humoral factors, and molecular events at the cellular level. They are intertwined to maintain adequate tissue perfusion and nutrition. Normal blood pressure control can be related to cardiac output and the total peripheral resistance. The stroke volume and the heart rate determine cardiac output. Each cycle of cardiac contraction propels a bolus of about 70 ml blood into the systemic arterial system. As one example of the interaction of these multiple systems, the stroke volume is dependent in part on intravascular volume regulated by the kidneys as well as on myocardial contractility. The latter is, in turn, a complex function involving sympathetic and parasympathetic control of heart rate; intrinsic activity of the cardiac conduction system; complex membrane transport and cellular events requiring influx of calcium, which lead to myocardial fibre shortening and relaxation; and affects the humoral substances (e.g. catecholamines) in stimulation heart rate and myocardial fibre tension.

The regulation of the total peripheral resistance also involves the complex interactions of several mechanisms. These include baroreflexes and sympathetic nervous system activity; response to neurohumoral substances and endothelial factors; myogenic adjustments at the cellular level, some mediated by ion channels and events at the cellular membrane; and intercellular events mediated by receptors and mechanisms for signal transduction. As examples of some of these mechanisms, there are two major neural reflex arcs (Fig. 1). Baroreflexes are derived from high-pressure baroreceptors in the aortic arch and carotid sinus and low-pressure cardiopulmonary baroreceptors in ventricles and atria. These receptors respond to stretch (high pressure) or filling pressures (low pressure) and send tonic inhibitory signals to the brainstem (nucleus tractus solitarius). If blood pressure increases and tonic inhibition increases, inhibition of sympathetic efferent outflow occurs and decreases vascular resistance and heart rate. If blood pressure decreases, however, less tonic inhibition ensues from the baroreflexes and both heart rate and peripheral vascular resistance increase, thereby increasing blood pressure. In addition, the neural control of renal function produces alterations in renal blood flow; glomerular filtration rate (GFR); excretion of sodium, other ions, and water; and release of renin and other vasoactive substances. These, in turn, have effects on the regulation of intravascular volume, vascular resistance and blood pressure. Activation of carotid chemoreceptors is also transmitted to the vasomotor centre and responds not only to arterial pressure but also to oxygen tension and carbon dioxide tension (in opposite directions). A drop in blood pressure, a drop in oxygen tension, or a rise in dioxide tension results in increased sympathetic outflow to the adrenal medulla, heart, and resistance vessels.

Numerous vasoactive substances have major effects on blood vessels, the heart, the kidneys, and the central nervous system (CNS) and often serve to counterbalance one another. As examples of physiologic actions, norepinephrine (noradrenaline), via α-adrenergic mechanisms, is a potent vasoconstrictor, while epinephrine (adrenaline), via α- and β-adrenoceptors, increases primarily heart rate, stroke volume, systolic blood pressure and pulse pressure. The ▶ renin-angiotensin aldosteron system generates angiotensin II (Ang II). Ang II, in turn, constricts vascular smooth muscle, stimulates aldosterone secretion, potentiates sympathetic nervous system activity, leads to salt and water reabsorption in the proximal tubule, stimulates prostaglandin, nitric oxide, and endothelin release, increases thirst, and is a growth factor. Aldosterone activates the epithelial sodium channel (ENaC) in the cortical collecting duct in the kidney, leading to sodium reabsorption and potassium excretion. Prostaglandin E and prostacyclin act to counterbalance vasoconstriction by Ang II and norepinephrine.

Vasopressin (antidiuretic hormone [ADH]) secretion increases in response to decreased blood volume and/or reductions in effective blood volume via a decrease in inhibitory tone from both low-pressure and high-pressure baroreceptors to the hypothalamus. The neuronal pathways that mediate hemodynamic regulation of vasopressin release are completely different from those involved in osmoregulation and unlike the latter, small decreases in blood pressure or blood volume have little effect on vasopressin secretion. A rise in blood pressure causes a decrease in secretion of vasopressin related to increased baroreceptor activity, which inhibits hypothalamic vasopressin-releasing hormones. Vasopressin works by causing water conservation at the distal collecting duct of nephron. This alone, however, is a relatively inefficient mechanism of increasing intravascular volume because conserved water is distributed among total body water and only a small portion is intravascular. In addition, vasopressin is a potent vasoconstrictor and the greater vasopressin secretion observed in response to more sever hypovolemia or hypotension serves as a mechanisms to stave off cardiovascular collapse during periods of large reductions of blood pressure or blood volume. Two important endothelial derived factors have opposite effects on the blood vessels: nitric oxide is a vasodilator whereas the endothelins, particularly endothelin-1, are vasoconstrictors. The kallikrein-kinin system produces vasodilator kinins, which in turn may stimulate prostaglandins and nitric oxide. Natriuretic peptides induce vasodilation, induce natriuresis, and inhibit other vasoconstrictors (renin-angiotensin, sympathetic nervous system and endothelin).

When the temporal sequence of adjustments of blood pressure is analysed it seems, that CNS mechanisms (e.g. baroreflexes) will provide regulation of the circulation within seconds to minutes. Other mechanisms, such as the renin-angiotensin-aldosterone system and fluid shifts, occur over minutes to hours. Only the kidneys seem to have the ability for long-term adjustment in blood pressure, predominantly through regulation of extracellular volume. This theoretical concept has recently been – although indirectly – confirmed by genetic approaches applied to the analysis of rare familial syndromes of high blood pressure, i.e. hypertension, or low blood pressure, i.e. hypotension. In those studies carried out in families with monogenetic forms of the disease several molecular pathways have been successfully delineated. All defects identified so far raise or lower blood pres-

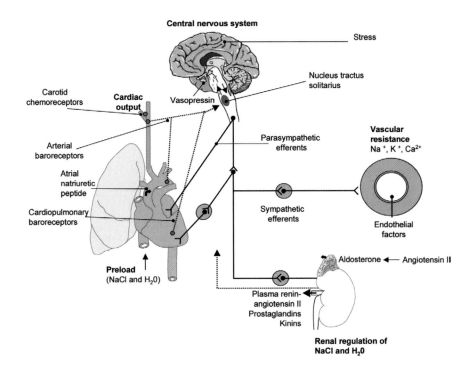

Fig. 1 Basic mechanisms involved blood pressure control. The most important organs involved in blood pressure control are shown (for explanations see text). In these organs a variety of different cell types and molecular events are related to blood pressure control. Physiological effects are initiated by a wide spectrum of vasoactive substances: (1) catecholamines such as norepinephrine and ephineprine bind to different adrenergic receptors (α_1, α_2, β_1, β_2) causing protein phosphorylation and increased intracellular calcium via G-protein-coupled receptors linked to ion channels or second messengers (cyclic nucleotides, phosphoinositide hydrolysis); (2) Ang II as the effector peptide of the RAS binds to angiotensin (AT_1, AT_2 and others)-receptors causing increased intracellular calcium and protein phosphorylation via second messenger, phosphoinositide hydrolysis, and activated protein kinases, and aldosterone secretion. (3) Endothelial derived factors such as nitric oxide (NO) increase levels of cGMP and activation of protein kinases, while endothelins (most importantly endothelin-1 [ET-1]) activate G-proteins, phospholipase C and L-type calcium channels. (4) The effects of atrial natriuretic peptide (ANP) and of brain and C-type natriuretic peptides are mediated via cGMP upon stimulation of three different receptors.

Additional cellular events linked to the activity of blood pressure regulating substances involve membrane sodium transport mechanisms; Na^+/K^+ ATPase; Na^+/Li^+ countertransport; Na^+-H^+ exchange; Na^+-Ca^{2+} exchange; Na^+-K^+2Cl transport; passive Na^+ transport; potassium channels; cell volume and intracellular pH changes; and calcium channels.

sure through a common pathway by increasing or decreasing salt and water reabsorption by the nephron. Thus, these studies point to the kidney as a (the) pivotal organ for chronic (genetic) determination of blood pressure.

Pharmacological Intervention

The morbid consequences of high blood pressure have been documented by epidemiologic studies, which demonstrate a strong positive and continuous correlation between blood pressure and the risk of cardiovascular disease (stroke, myocardial infarction, heart failure), renal disease and mortality. This correlation is more robust with systolic than with diastolic blood pressure. While hypertension was once thought to be 'essential' for perfusion of tissues through sclerotic and narrowed blood vessels and to maintain a normal sodium balance, the pathologic nature of elevated blood pres-

Tab. 1 Definitions and classifications of blood pressure levels.

Category	Systolic [mm Hg]		Diastolic [mm Hg]	Stroke mortality Relative risk
Optimal	< 120	and	< 80	1.00
Normal	< 130	and	< 85	1.73
High normal	130–139	or	85–90	2.14
Hypertension				
Stage 1 (mild)	140–159	or	90–99	3.58
Subgroup: borderline	140–149	or	90–94	
Stage 2 (moderate)	160–179	or	100–109	6.90
Stage 3 (severe)	≥ 180	or	≥ 110	9.66
Isolated systolic hypertension	≥ 140	and	< 90	
Subgroup: borderline	140–149	and	< 90	

The higher category applies, if systolic and diastolic blood pressure values of a patient fall into different categories.

sure has become clear. Essential, primary, or idiopathic hypertension is defined as high blood pressure in which causes such as renovascular disease, renal failure, pheochromocytoma, aldosteronism, or other causes of secondary hypertension or monogenic (mendelian) forms are not present. Essential hypertension accounts for 95% of all cases of hypertension. This condition is a heterogeneous disorder, with different patients having different causal factors that lead to high blood pressure. There are no established clinical or laboratory tests to identify the factors that are responsible for the blood pressure elevation in an individual patient. Consequently, pharmacologic treatment of essential hypertension is largely empiric. Clinical treatment algorithms try to account for co-morbidities and expected or observed side effects of drugs in individual patients. Pharmacologic treatment should always be implemented 'on top' of non-pharmacologic interventions such as control of body weight, alcohol intake, salt intake and modifications of lifestyle as necessary in the individual patient. Randomised trial of pharmacologic treatment of hypertension have documented that blood pressure reduction lowers morbidity and mortality, with dramatic reduction in stroke and smaller reductions in cardiac and renal disease (for details see ▶ Antihypertensive Drugs).

As a result of such studies hypertension has been operationally defined as the blood pressure level above which therapeutic intervention has clinical benefit. As increasingly aggressive intervention has continued to demonstrate benefits, this level has gradually reduced over time and is commonly defined as systolic blood pressure ≥140 mmHg and/or diastolic blood pressure ≥90 mmHg (Table 1). Isolated systolic hypertension is defined as systolic blood pressure ≥140 mmHg and diastolic blood pressure <90 mmHg.

Moreover, in patients with certain co-morbidities, such as diabetes mellitus, left ventricular dysfunction or chronic nephropathy, lower blood pressures levels in the range of 130/80 mmHg (125/75 mmHg for nephropathies with overt proteinuria >1 g per day) are currently established as target blood pressure. Individuals with high normal blood pressure tend to maintain pressure that are above average for the general population and are at greater risk for development of definite hypertension and cardiovascular events than the general population. These observations leave open the question of whether there is an 'optimal' blood pressure in the general population, and whether small reductions in blood pressure across the entire population, rather than larger targeted reductions, would have benefit.

Nonetheless, in patients with established hypertension according to the above criteria, antihypertensive drug treatment is one of the most important means to prevent or reduce overall cardiovascular and renal disease. There is hope that the information gained from the Human Genome Project and from ongoing research aimed at dissecting the genetic basis of hypertension in both human populations and animal models will foster the development of more effective and targeted, i.e. pharmacogenetic, treatments based on the genotype of the individual patient.

References

1. Carretero OA, Oparil S (2000) Essential Hypertension. Part I: Definition and Etiology. Circulation 101:329–335
2. Lifton RP, Gharavi AG, Geller DA (2001) Molecular mechanisms of human hypertension. Cell 104:545–556
3. Lawton WJ, DiBona (2000) Normal blood pressure control and the evaluation of hypertension. In: Johnson RJ, Feehally J (eds) Comprehensive clinical nephrology. Mosby, London, p37.1–37.11
4. Kaplan NM (1998) Clinical hypertension, 7th edition.Williams & Wilkins, Baltimore
5. Joint National Committee on Prevention, Detection, Evaluation, and Treatment of High Blood Pressure (1997). The Sixth Report of the Joint National Committee on Prevention, Detection, Evaluation, and Treatment of High Blood Pressure (JNC VI). Arch Int Med 157:2413–2446

B Lymphocyte

A B lymphocyte is a specific type of white blood cell (leucocyte) derived from bone marrow stem cells. Each B lymphocyte expresses an immunoglobulin (antibody) specific for a particular antigen. Following antigenic stimulation, a B lymphocyte may differentiate and multiply into plasma cells that secrete large quantities of monoclonal antibody.

▶ Immune Defense
▶ Humanized Monoclonal Antibodies

BMPs

▶ Bone Morphogenetic Proteins

Body Mass Index

▶ Anti-obesity Drugs

Bombesin-like Peptides

Bombesin-like peptides are a group of biologically active peptides, which are structurally related, including bombesin (a tetradecapeptide originally derived from amphibians), gastrin-releasing peptide (GRP), neuromedin B (NMB), and GRP_{18-27} (previously named "neuromedin C"). Bombesin and bombesin-like peptides have a wide range of functions. They have been shown to promote cell growth, including that of carcinoma cell lines, they are involved in smooth muscle contraction and in the regulation of the body temperature. Bombesin / bombesin-like peptides also mediate endocrine responses, such as the release of gastrin, cholesystokinin, and pancreatic polypeptide. This group of peptides has been involved in the regulation of various behavioral responses, the regulation of pain and the modulation of feeding behavior. Bombesin / bombesin-like peptides exert their effects through a group of ▶ G-protein coupled receptors, which signal through $G_{q/11}$(BB1, BB2, BB3). While BB1 responds mainly to NMB and bombesin, BB2 responds to GRP and bombesin.

Bone Formation

Bone formation is the building of new bone through osteoblasts. Bone formation, which is part of the bone remodelling process, includes the synthesis of organic matter (mostly collagen type I) and subsequent mineralisation.

▶ Bone Metabolism

Bone Metabolism

MARKUS J. SEIBEL
Department of Endocrinology & Metabolism
C65, Medical Centre/ Concord Hospital,
University of Sydney, Sydney, Australia
mjs@anzac.edu.au

Synonyms

Bone Turnover, Skeletal Turnover, Skeletal Metabolism, Bone Remodelling

Definition

Bone Metabolism comprises the processes of ▶ bone formation and ▶ bone resorption, the key actions by which skeletal mass, structure and quality are accrued and maintained throughout life. In the mature skeleton, anabolic and catabolic actions are mostly balanced (coupling) due to the tight regulation of the activity of bone forming (▶ osteoblast) and bone resorbing (▶ osteoclast) cells through circulating osteotropic hormones and locally active cytokines.

Basic Mechanisms:

Structure of Bone

Most bones of the human skeleton are composed of two structurally distinct types of tissue: compact (dense) and trabecular (cancellous, spongy) bone (1). Both types contain the same elements: *cells* (osteocytes) which are embedded in a *mineralised matrix* and connected by small canals ("*canaliculi*"). In compact bone, which makes up 85% of the skeleton, these components form elongated cylinders of concentric lamellae surrounding a central blood vessel (called osteon or Haversian system). In contrast, cancellous bone forms thin, interconnected spicules. Compact bone constitutes the outer parts of many bones ("com-

pacta"), shows a high degree of mineralisation, a comparatively low number of cells, and provides the framework for the interior cancellous parts of bone. The latter consists of a sponge-like network of small beams (trabeculae) with a larger number of cells distributed over a huge surface. Consequently, the metabolic rate of cancellous bone is much higher than that of compact bone (see below).

Biochemistry of Bone

Bone is composed of approximately 70% mineral (mainly hydroxyapatite $[Ca_{10}(PO_4)_6(OH)_2]$ crystals) and 30% organic matter (i.e. cells, collagen and non-collagenous proteins). Most of the latter is synthesised by local osteoblasts. 90% of the organic extracellular matrix of bone consists of type I collagen, which assembles into fibrils and is then covalently cross-linked to generate tensile strength. Of the non-collagenous proteins, osteocalcin, bone sialoprotein and osteopontin are the most abundant. Most of the non-collagenous proteins play important roles in the organisation of the extracellular matrix (cell-cell and cell-matrix attachment, cell migration, growth, development, fibril formation). Besides these components, several specific enzymes and small peptides are an integral part of the organic matrix and play an important role in skeletal metabolism (see below). The calcium-collagen-cell composite ensures the two main functions of bone: providing a structural framework and a reservoir for mineral ions.

Mechanisms of Bone Remodelling

Bone is a metabolically active tissue that throughout life undergoes constant *remodelling*. The term "*modelling*" is restricted to the period of skeletal growth, when the size and shape of the bone is determined. Skeletal modelling and remodelling are achieved by two counteracting processes: bone formation and bone resorption. While bone formation is achieved through osteoblasts, bone resorption is attributed to osteoclast activity. As bone remodelling is part of the body's mineral (calcium / phosphate) homeostasis and a mechanism for repair and adaptation, all cellular events are regulated by systemic and local modulators: parathyroid hormone (PTH), 1,25-dihydroxyvitamin D_3, sex and other steroid hormones, calci-

Tab. 1 Strategies and compounds that influence bone turnover.

Inhibitors of Osteoclast Activity	Stimulators of Osteoblast Activity
Currently in Use	*Currently in Use*
Bisphosphonates	Fluorides
Calcitonins & synthetic analogues	Parathyroid Hormone
Oestrogens	Calcitriol & analogues
Selective Oestrogen Receptor Modulators (SERMs, e. g. Raloxifene)	Androgens
Testosterone	
Vitamin D	
Vitamin D metabolites & analogues	
Under Development	*Under Development*
Ipriflavone	PTH-rP & analogues
Statins	High dose oestrogens
Calcium receptor modulators	Statins
Osteoprotegerin	Strontium salts
Anti-cytokines (e. g. IL-1, TNFs, IL-1 receptor constructs)	Growth Factors (e. g. GH, IGFs, FGFs)
Proton pump inhibitors	Prostaglandins & PG mimetics
Nitric oxide modulators	Endothelins & analogues
Enzyme inhibitors (e. g. metalloproteinases, cathepsin K)	Amylin & analogues
Adhesion molecule inhibitors	Mechanoreceptor modulators, e. g. Glutamate
	Purinergic modulators
	Proteosome inhibitors
	Intracellular signalling targets, e. g. SMADs

tonin, prostaglandins, growth factors and cytokines. However, the remodelling process is always initiated by osteoclast activation.

Osteoclast formation. Osteoclasts are large, multinucleated cells derived from bone marrow macrophages of the haematopoietic lineage. Osteoclast formation is controlled by circulating hormones such as PTH, 1,25-dihydroxyvitamin D_3 and estrogens, as well as by growth factors (e.g. TGFβ) and cytokines generated in the bone marrow microenvironment. Interestingly, this control is mostly indirect as the receptors for the majority of these factors are located on the ▶ osteoblast surface. Osteoblasts therefore control osteoclast formation through the expression of various stimulatory and inhibitory factors. For example, osteoblasts and stromal cells express macrophage colony stimulating factor (M-CSF) which is a potent activator of osteoclast precursors. Another pathway to induce differentiation and fusion of osteoclast precursors is the binding of an osteoblast-derived ligand called RANKL (or TRANCE) to the osteoclast receptor activator of nuclear factor κ (RANK). Conversely, osteoprotegerin (OPG), a soluble member of the TNF receptor superfamily and a decoy receptor for RANKL, is a potent inhibitor of osteoclast formation (2) (Fig. 1). Other inhibitors of osteoclast differentiation include IL1-ra, IL-4,-10, -12, -18, αINF and TGFβ. Apoptosis of osteoblasts may be induced by estrogens (through TGFβ) and, pharmacologically, by bisphosphonates.

Osteoblast formation. Osteoblasts are derived from mesenchymal (stromal) cells that first differentiate into pre-osteoblasts and then into mature, bone matrix-producing osteoblasts. The processes involved in osteoblast formation are still somewhat obscure. Important stimulators of osteoblast formation and differentiation are circulating hormones such as PTH and PTH-related peptide (PTHrP), 1,25-dihydroxyvitamin D_3 (calcitriol), sex and other steroid hormones, but also locally active factors such as growth factors (TGFβ, IGF1 and 2, FGF), leukaemia inhibiting factor (LIF), various ▶ bone morphogenetic proteins (BMPs) and certain cytokines. Some of these factors are produced by the osteoblasts themselves and deposited in the bone matrix. It is assumed that these factors are released upon bone resorption, thus activating osteoblast precursors in the area of the resorption pit. Another important factor inducing osteoblast differentiation is Cbfa1 (osf2), a recently discovered transcription factor (3) (Fig. 2).

Inactivated or "resting" osteoblasts become "lining cells" and thus a reservoir for bone forming cells to be activated at the next remodelling cycle. Osteoblasts trapped and embedded in the mineralised matrix are called osteocyts, and are important for many properties of living bone. Apoptosis of osteoblasts is associated with the mineralisation of the organic bone matrix and with the expression of cFos, cJun, BAX, p53 and MSX-2.

The bone remodelling cycle. In the mature skeleton and under normal conditions, bone formation and resorption are closely coupled to each other, thus maintaining a stable bone mass and sufficient bone strength. In contrast, metabolic bone diseases are characterised by more or less pronounced imbalances in bone turnover ("uncoupling"). The long term result of such imbalances in bone turnover are often changes in bone mass and structure, which either become clinically symptomatic (i.e. fracture, deformity) or may be detected by means of radiographic or densitometric techniques. Bone remodelling occurs discontinuously at distinct sites, the so-called "bone remodelling units" (BRU) or "basic multicellular units" (BMU). In the mature skeleton and at any given time, approximately 2 million of these BRUs are active, replacing about 5–10% of the existing bone per year. The cellular events always occur in the same sequence and are usually described as a cycle of approximately 100 days: (i) chemotaxis, proliferation, differentiation and activation of osteoclasts, (ii) resorption of bone (approx. 10 days), (iii) reversal, (iv) chemotaxis, proliferation, differentiation and activation of osteoblasts, and formation of new bone in amounts equal to the amount of bone resorbed (approx. 90 days), (v) resting (4) (Fig. 3).

To resorb bone, osteoclasts first adhere to the mineralised surface via specific adhesion molecules (integrins). The cell membrane facing bone then forms a ruffled surface, hydrogen ions generated intracellularly by carbonic anhydrase type II are pumped across the membrane to produce a low pH and to release the mineral. At the same time, proteolytic enzymes are discharged into the resorption area and a resorption pit forms. By mechanisms not understood, osteoclasts stop when a certain resorption depth is reached and move on to other sites. After reversal, osteoblasts move into the resorption pit, probably attracted and stimulated by local factors released during bone resorption. The small cuboid, mononuclear cells produce the organic matrix (also called "osteoid"), which later becomes mineralised. The mechanisms of mineralisation are highly complex and the precise pathways are still not fully understood.

Calcium homeostasis

Bone is the most important reservoir for body calcium. Ionised plasma calcium, which represents ~50% of the total plasma calcium pool, is essential for countless metabolic functions and its therefore tightly controlled through 3 major circulating hormones; PTH, 1,25-dihydroxyvitamin D_3 and, to a much lesser extent, calcitonin. To keep serum ionized calcium levels stable, these regulators act on 3 major tissues; bone, the intestine and the kidney.

The secretion of PTH by the parathyroid glands is directly stimulated through a decrease in plasma levels of ionised calcium. Within very short time, PTH increases plasma calcium levels by activating osteoclasts and thus mobilising calcium from the mineral store. It also increases renal tubular reabsorption of calcium (and the excretion of phosphate). Through the activation of 1α-hydroxylase, i.e. the generation of 1,25-dihydroxyvitamin D_3, PTH also helps to increase intestinal calcium absorption.

The steroid hormone 1,25-dihydroxyvitamin D_3 (calcitriol) slowly increases both intestinal calcium absorption and bone resorption, and is also stimulated through low calcium levels. In contrast, calcitonin rapidly inhibits osteoclast activity and thus decreases serum calcium levels. The relevance of calcitonin in human calcium homeostasis is not well established, and is probably minor.

B

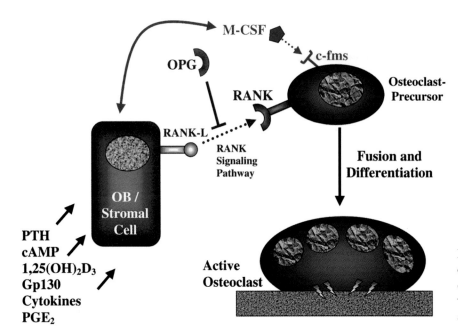

Fig. 1 Mechanisms of osteoclast activation. For details, see text. Modified with permission from a slide by T. Jack Martin.

Pharmacological Intervention

A number of pharmacologic strategies have been developed to modulate osteoclast or osteoblast formation and/or activity in ▶ osteoporosis, cancer-induced osteopathies, Paget's and other diseases of bone. In recent years, an even greater number of potential drugs have been explored (Table 1). Although inhibitors of osteoclast formation/ activity are generally being distinguished from stimulators of osteoblast formation/ activity, some compounds, such as vitamin D, the statins, oestrogens etc. seem to influence both processes.

Estrogens
Estrogens reduce bone loss by inhibiting the generation of new osteoclasts, reducing activation frequency and promoting apoptosis of mature osteoclast via a mechanism not well understood. Some of the effects of estrogen seem to be mediated via the modulation of certain growth factors and cytokines, while others are associated with binding to at least two different estrogen receptors (ERα, ERβ). The presence of different ERs is also, among other facts, the basis for the development and understanding of the so called ▶ Selective Estrogen Receptor Modulators (short ▶ SERMs). While Tamoxifene, a triphenylethylene compound used in the treatment of breast cancer, has long been known to moderately inhibit bone loss, the more recent synthetic compound Raloxifene in postmenopausal women clearly prevents bone loss and reduces fracture risk by 40%. The mechanism of action is probably the same as the one suspected in estrogens, i.e. the inhibition of cytokines that are responsible for osteoclast recruitment and differentiation. Estrogens and SERMs are not potent enough to inhibit the grossly exaggerated osteoclast activity in malignant and Paget's disease of bone. Hormone replacement therapy has been shown to effectively reduce the risk of osteoporotic fractures, but is associated with significant increase in the risk of breast cancer and cardiovascular morbidity.

Calcitonin
Calcitonin is a natural hormone secreted by the clear cells of the thyroid. All calcitonins inhibit osteoclast activity by increasing the intracellular cyclic AMP content via binding to a specific cell surface receptor, thus causing a contraction of the resorbing cell membrane. Long-term treatment with calcitonin leads to down-regulation of its receptors (escape phenomenon). Over the past decade, the availability of more potent drugs with less side effects, and the lack of clear data on the anti-fracture efficacy of calcitonin, has lead to a decline in its clinical use.

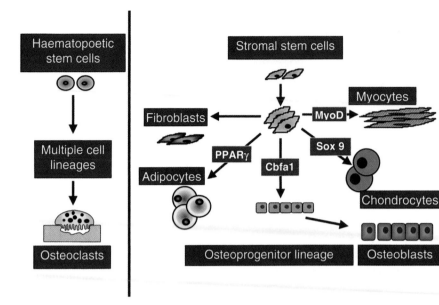

Fig. 2 Differentiation pathways of osteoclasts and osteoblasts. Modified with permission from a slide by Graham Russell.

Bisphosphonates

Bisphosphonates (BP) over the last years have become one of the first line treatments of benign and malignant bone diseases. Being pyrophosphate analogues, BP accumulate in bone and are taken up by osteoclasts. Once in the cell, the nitrogen-containing BP (N-BP) such as Alendronate, Risedronate, Ibandronate and Zoledronate effectively inhibit osteoclast resorption and induce cell apoptosis by inhibiting farnesyl diphosphate synthetase, an enzyme of the mevalonate pathway (Fig. 4). This in turn leads to a reduction in geranylgeranyl diphosphate and in the prenylation of GTP-binding proteins essential to osteoclast organisation and survival. Non-aminobisphosphonates such as Clodronate or Etidronate are incorporated into intracellular analogues of ATP and cause cell death.

▶ Statins

Statins lower plasma cholesterol levels by inhibiting HMG-CoA reductase in the mevalonate pathway (Fig. 4). Recent research has shown that certain statins (but not all) stimulate BMP-2 expression in osteoblasts, increase bone formation and mimic N-BP in that they inhibit bone resorption. The use of statins in osteoporosis is presently being investigated.

For reasons described above (see section on Basic Mechanisms), the following compounds are presently being investigated as anti-resorptive drugs; specific inhibitors of cytokines, H^+-ATPase/proton pumps, metalloproteinases, cathepsin K, and adhesion molecules ($\alpha_v\beta_3$ integrins), as well as nitric oxide modulators and, last but not least, osteoprotegerin.

Fluoride ions

Fluoride ions stimulate bone formation by a direct mitogenic effect on osteoblasts mediated via protein kinase activation and other pathways. Further to these cellular effects, fluorides alter hydroxyapatite crystals in the bone matrix. In low doses, fluorides induce lamellar bone, while at higher doses, abnormal woven bone with inferior quality is formed. The effect of fluorides on normal and abnormal (e.g. osteoporotic) bone therefore depends on the dose administered.

Parathyroid hormone

Parathyroid hormone (PTH) has, for reasons not yet known, a dual effects on bone cells: given intermittently, PTH stimulates osteoblast activity and leads to substantial increases in bone density. When secreted continuously at relatively high doses (as seen, for example, in patients with primary hyperparathyroidism), PTH stimulates osteoclast-mediated bone resorption and suppresses osteoblast activity. Further to its direct effects on bone cells, PTH also enhances renal calcium re-

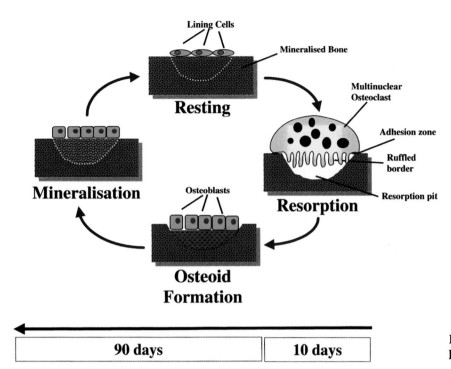

Fig. 3 The bone remodelling cycle.

absorption and phosphate clearance, as well as renal synthesis of 1,25-dihydroxyvitamin D_3. Both PTH and 1,25-dihydroxyvitamin D_3 act synergistically on bone to increase serum calcium levels and are closely involved in the regulation of the calcium/phosphate balance. The anabolic effects of PTH on osteoblasts are probably both direct and indirect via growth factors such as IGF-1 and TGFβ. The multiple signal transduction pathways mediating the effects of PTH on bone cells include activation of cyclic AMP, intracellular protein phosphorylation, activation of phospholipase C, protein kinase C, tyrosine kinase c-src and the generation of inositol 1,4,5-triphosphate (IP3). Intermittend treatment with PTH (1-34) has been shown to effectively lower the risk of osteoporetic fractures in post-menopausal women with osteoporosis.

Oral calcium

Oral calcium has long been used for the treatment of osteoporosis, both in the form ofdietary and pharmacologic supplements. In patients with calcium deficiency, oral calcium at doses of 500–1500 mg per day corrects a negative calcium balance and suppresses PTH secretion. Sufficient calcium intake is most important for the accrual of peak bone mass in the young, but is also considered the basis of most anti-osteoporotic regimes. In the frail elderly, supplementation with oral calcium and vitamin D reduces the risk of hip fracture by about 30–40%.

Vitamin D and its metabolites

Vitamin D and its metabolites are also widely used for the treatment of osteoporosis. Vitamin D (or cholecalciferol) is synthesised in the skin through UV radiation (sun exposure!) and is then metabolised in the liver to 25-hydroxyvitamin D_3 (calcidiol). The latter has little biologic activity. The active form of Vitamin D is generated in the kidney through the hydroxylation at position C_1, leading to 1,25-dihydroxyvitamin D_3. This last step is tightly controlled by a number of regulators such as PTH and serum phosphate levels. 1,25-dihydroxyvitamin D_3 is a potent steroid hormone with almost countless effects throughout the body. Most of these effects concern the differentiation of immature cells. As regards bone, 1,25-dihydroxyvitamin D_3 has differentiation-inducing as well as activating effects on both osteoblasts and osteoclasts. It also increases the absorption of calcium

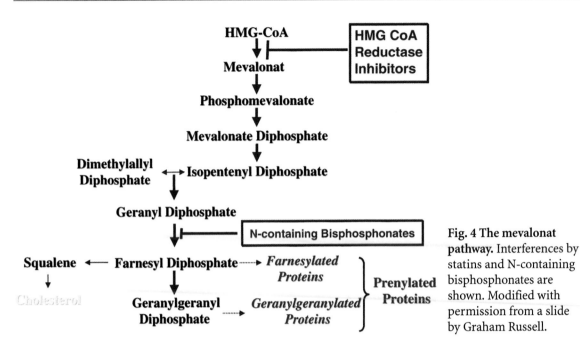

Fig. 4 The mevalonat pathway. Interferences by statins and N-containing bisphosphonates are shown. Modified with permission from a slide by Graham Russell.

from the gut. Data from clinical trials show that the daily supplementation with 500–1200 mg of calcium plus 700–1000 IU of oral Vitamin D reduces the rate of bone loss in postmenopausal women by 50% and reduces the number of hip and non-vertebral fractures in elderly men and women by 30–70%. Data on vertebral anti-fracture efficacy are sparse, but the available evidence indicates moderate efficacy at least in populations with sub-clinical vitamin D deficiency (= more then 80% of the European/ US population aged >70 years). In contrast, "active" vitamin D metabolites are still controversial in regard to their therapeutic use in postmenopausal and/ or age-related ("senile") osteoporosis. There is still no reliable scientific data supporting the hypothesis that in postmenopausal and/ or age-related osteoporosis, vitamin D metabolites such as 1α or $1,25$- dihydroxyvitamin D_3 are more efficacious with regard to bone loss or fractures reduction then native vitamin D given in equivalent doses. There is, however, some consensus that $1,25$-dihydroxyvitamin D_3 might be more efficacious in secondary osteoporosis such as glucocorticoid induced osteoporosis. While native vitamin D has a broad therapeutic window with few or no adverse effects, vitamin D metabolites are characterised by a narrow therapeutic window with hyercalciuria (kidney stones) and hypercalcaemia being the most serious problem.

Strontium salts

Strontium salts have long been under investigation as anabolic agents for bone. In animals, strontium stimulates bone formation and substitutes for calcium in hydroxyapatite crystals. In humans, small studies have shown an increases bone mass (after correction of BMD values for strontium content) and possibly a reduction in vertebral fractures. The mechanism of action is largely unknown and may involve modulation of the calcium receptor or calcium channels.

For reasons deducible from the mechanisms described earlier (see "Basic Mechanisms"), PTHrP and PTHrP analogues, certain growth factors, prostaglandins and prostaglandin mimetics are presently being investigated as anabolic drugs (see also Table 1).

Further Reading

Lian JB and Stein GS (1999) The Cells of Bone. In: Dynamics of Bone and Cartilage Metabolism. Seibel MJ, Robins SP and Bilezikian JP (eds), Academic Press, San Diego, pp. 165–186

Martin TJ, Findlay DM, Moseley JM (1996) Peptide hormones acting on bone. In: Marcus R, Feldman D and Kesley J (eds) Osteoporosis, Academic Press, San Diego, pp.185–204

Rizzoli R and Bonjour JP (1999) Physiology of calcium and phosphate homeostasis. In: Dynamics of Bone and Cartilage Metabolism. Seibel MJ, Robins SP and Bilezikian JP (eds), Academic Press, San Diego, pp. 247–260

References

1. Schenk RK and Olah AJ (1980) Histomorphometrie. In: Handbiuch der Inneren Medizin Bd. IV, Knochen, Gelenke, Muskeln. Kuhlencordt F and Bartelheimer H (eds.), Spinger, Berlin, p437
2. Yasuda H, Shima N, Nakagawa N et al. (1997) Osteoclast differentiation factor is a ligand for osteoprotegerin/osteoclastogenesis-inhibiting factor and is identical to TRANCE/ RANKL. Proc Natl Acad Sci USA 95:3597–602
3. Ducy P, Zahng R, Geoffrey V, Ridall AC, Karsenty G (1997) Osf2/Cbfa1: a transcriptional activator of osteoblast differentiation. Cell 89:747–54
4. Frost HM (1964) Dynamics of Bone Remodelling. Boston. Little & Brown

Bone Morphogenetic Proteins

Bone morphogenetic proteins (BMPs) comprise a family of 15 cytokines involved in the growth and differentiation of various tissues and organs such as bone, heart, kidney, eyes, skin and teeth. The members of this family which influence bone remodelling stimulate the differentiation of bone marrow stem cells into bone forming cells. BMPs are currently being tested in clinical trials for their potential to promote union of fractures and healing of bone defects. Among the BMPs being tested, is BMP-7, which also stimulates the production of erythropoietin (EPO). EPO is produced in the kidney and stimulates the generation of erythrocytes from precursor cells. In the clinic, it is used for the treatment of anemia caused by chronic renal failure.

Bone Remodelling

Bone remodelling is the continuous and life-long process of renewing bone through the balanced processes of bone resorption and bone formation. Bone remodelling is stimulated by biomechanical and biochemical influences and tightly controlled through circulating osteotropic hormones and local mediators.

▶ Bone Metabolism

Bone Resorption

Bone resorption is the removal of mineralised bone by osteoclasts. Bone resorption, which is part of the bone remodelling process, includes the release of mineral (mostly calcium and phosphate) and subsequent proteolysis of organic matter (mostly collagen).

▶ Bone Metabolism

Botulinum Toxin

▶ Bacterial Toxins

Botulism

Botulism is a disease caused by ingestion of foods contaminated with *Clostridium botulinum* (foodborne botulism) or, very rarely, by wound infection (wound botulism) or colonization of the intestinal tract with *Clostridium botulinum*(infant botulism). The toxins block the release of acetylcholine. Botulism is characterized by generalized muscular weakness, which first affects eye and throat muscles and later extends to all skeletal muscles. Flaccid paralysis can lead to respiratory failure.

▶ Bacterial Toxins

Bradykinesia

Bradykinesia is slowness and poverty of movement.

▶ Anti-parkinson Drugs

Bradykinin

Bradykinin is a nonapeptide enzymatically produced from kallidin in the blood, where it is a potent agent of arteriolar dilation and increased capillary permeability. Bradykinin is also released from mast cells within damaged tissues. It produces inflammation and activates nociceptors via bradykinin B1 and B2 receptors.

▶ Kinins

Brain Derived Neurotrophic Factor

▶ Neurotrophic Factors

Brain Natriuretic Peptide

▶ Natriuretic Peptides

Breast Cancer

Breast cancer is cancer of the breast tissues. The major part of this cancer in women is dependent on the female sex hormones for their growth. An estrogen antagonist can therefore be used in the treatment of breast cancer to limit the growth of the tumor.

▶ Selective Sex-steroid Receptor Modulators

Bronchial Asthma

Bronchial asthma is characterized by reversible narrowing of the airways. The underlying causes are inflammatory processes in the airways, leading to "bronchial hyperreactivity" and bronchoconstriction. One group of drugs used in the treatment of bronchial asthma are bronchodilators which reduce bronchoconstriction. First-line drugs are β_2-adrenoceptor agonists such as salbutamol, terbutaline and salmeterol (▶ β-adrenergic system); second-line drugs are xanthins (theophylline) and muscarinic-receptor antagonists (ipratropium bromide). Inflammation is treated by ▶ glucocorticoids, administered by inhalation (beclomethasone, budesonide and fluticasone) or systemically (prednisolone, hydrocortisone). Sodium cromoglycate and nedocromil sodium are used in the treatment of allergic forms of asthma. They appear to inhibit inflammatory cells. However, their precise mechanism of action is not clear.

▶ Allergy
▶ Immune Defense
▶ β-Adrenergic System
▶ Glucocorticoids
▶ Leukotrienes

Bronchodilators

Bronchodilators act by reducing the tone of bronchial smooth muscle. Clinically important bronchodilators are β_2-adrenergic receptor agonists and xanthines.

▶ Bronchial Asthma
▶ Allergy
▶ β-adrenergic System

Btk

Btk (Bruton's tyrosine kinase) is a phosphatidylinositol 3'-kinase sensitive cytoplasmic tyrosine kinase. Germline loss of function mutations of Btk cause X-linked agammaglobulinaemia in human and X-linked immunodeficiency in mice.

▶ Phospholipid Kinases
▶ Tyrosine Kinases

Butyrophenones

▶ Antipsychotic Drugs

Butyrylcholinesterase

▶ Cholinesterase

C

C2 Domain

C2 domains (phosphokinase C conserved 2 domains) mediate membrane targeting of diverse peripheral proteins. A C2 domain consists of approximately 130 residues and was first discovered as the Ca^{2+}-binding site in conventional phosphokinase Cs.

▶ Phospholipid Kinases

C-fibres

▶ Nociception

Ca^{2+}-ATPase

The Ca^{2+}-ATPase transports Ca^{2+} ions into endoplasmic reticulum or out of the cell from the cytoplasm, using the energy of ATP hydrolysis.

Ca^{2+} Channels

▶ Voltage-dependent Ca^{2+} Channels.

Ca^{2+} Channel Blockers

J. STRIESSNIG
Institut für Pharmazie, Abteilung
Pharmakologie und Toxikologie,
Leopold-Franzens-Universität Insbruck,
Innsbruck, Austria
joerg.striessnig@uibk.ac.at.

Synonyms

Ca^{2+} channel antagonists

Definition

Ca^{2+} is an important intracellular second messenger that controls cellular functions including muscle contraction in smooth and cardiac muscle. Ca^{2+} channel blockers inhibit depolarization-induced Ca^{2+} entry into muscle cells in the cardiovascular system causing a decrease in blood pressure, decreased cardiac contractility and antiarrhythmic effects. Therefore, these drugs are used clinically to treat hypertension, myocardial ischemia and cardiac arrhythmias.

▶ Antihypertensive Drugs
▶ Voltage-dependent Ca^{2+} Channels

Mechanism of Action

Voltage gated Ca^{2+} channels are Ca^{2+}-selective pores in the plasma membrane of electrically excitable cells, such as neurons, muscle cells, (neuro)endocrine cells and sensory cells. They open in response to membrane depolarization

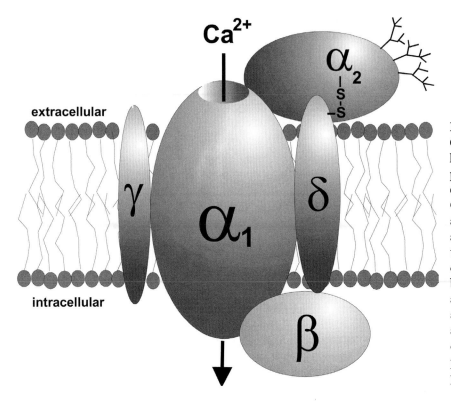

Fig. 1 Most voltage gated Ca²⁺ channels exist as a hetero-oligomeric complex of several subunits. $\alpha 1$ subunits form the Ca²⁺-selective ion pore and contain the voltage-sensors of the channel. In the case of L-type Ca²⁺ channels, they also carry binding sites for Ca²⁺ antagonist drugs. The accessory $\alpha 2$-δ, β and γ subunits stabilize Ca²⁺ channel function and support its targeting to the plasma membrane.

(e.g. an action potential) and permit the influx of Ca²⁺ along its electrochemical gradient into the cytoplasm.

Ca²⁺ Channel Physiology

The resulting increase in intracellular free Ca²⁺ triggers and/or modulates important physiological processes. Ca²⁺ influx into nerve terminals, sensory or endocrine cells initiates neurotransmitter and hormone release, respectively (stimulus-secretion coupling). Ca²⁺ entry into the soma and proximal dendrites of nerve cells leads to the activation of intracellular pathways affecting gene transcription (excitation transcription coupling) and neuronal plasticity. In smooth muscle and cardiac myocytes Ca²⁺ influx through these channels induces muscle contraction (excitation contraction coupling).

Ca²⁺ Channel Function

Like other ► voltage-gated cation channels, Ca²⁺ channels exist in at least three states: A resting state stabilized at negative potentials (such as the resting potentials of most electrically excitable cells) that is a closed state from which the channel can open. The open state is induced by depolarization. Channels do not stay open indefinitely because they are "turned off" during prologend depolarization by transition into an inactivated state. Once the cell repolarizes, inactivated channels return to the resting state and are now again available for opening. Ca²⁺ channel blockers can inhibit Ca²⁺ flux not only by obstructing the pore but also by "allosterically" stabilizing the inactivated closed state. By delaying its transition to the resting state after repolarization drugs can also increase the refractory period of these channels.

Ca²⁺ Channel Types

In order to accomplish these diverse physiological tasks described above, nature has created at least five different types of Ca²⁺ channels. These are termed L-, N-, P/Q-, R- and T-type. Although they are all structurally similar (Fig. 1) they differ with respect to their biophysical properties. Some of them need only weak depolarizations to open and inactivate fast (e.g. most T-type Ca²⁺ channels), whereas others require strong depolarizations and inactivate more slowly (e.g. P- or L-type Ca²⁺ channels). Channel types also differ with respect to their sensitivity to drugs. This selectivity is exploited for pharmacotherapy.

L-Type Ca²⁺ Channel Blockers

At present, only organic blockers of L-type Ca^{2+} channels (also termed "Ca^{2+} antagonist") are licensed for clinical use. They belong to the most frequently prescribed drugs worldwide. L-type Ca^{2+} channels are the major channel type in muscle cells mediating contraction. Although they do not elicit fast neurotransmitter release from nerve terminals under physiological conditions these channels provide Ca^{2+} influx for neurotransmitter release in sensory (cochlear hair cells, retinal photoreceptors) and endocrine cells (insulin secretion in ▶ pancreatic β cells). Despite these multiple functions, *in vivo* L-type Ca^{2+} channel block by therapeutic concentrations only causes pharmacological effects in the cardiovascular system.

The signalling pathways controlling cardiac and smooth muscle contraction are depicted in Fig. 2 and Fig. 3. By blocking L-type channels in arterial smooth muscle they reduce Ca^{2+} influx during depolarisation. Thus less Ca^{2+} is available for activation of calmodulin, which activates myosin-light chain kinase and thereby turns on actin-myosin interaction (Fig. 2). Note that smooth muscle also contracts after stimulation of receptor-activated pathways. Agonists of angiotensin AT1 (e.g. angiotensin II) and α1-adrenergic receptors (e.g. noradrenaline) release Ca^{2+} from intracellular IP_3-sensitive stores (Fig. 2). Noradrenaline-induced contractions are much less sensitive to Ca^{2+} channel blockers. The differential contribution of depolarization-induced and receptor-activated contraction in different types of smooth muscle and under different pathophysiological conditions is one of the explanations why Ca^{2+} channel blockers are not effective muscle relaxants in other diseases states (such as bronchial muscle in asthma or uretral spasms). In the heart, Ca^{2+} entering through L-type channels during the action potential serves as a trigger ("trigger Ca^{2+}") for further Ca^{2+} release from the sarcoplasmic reticulum which initiates contraction (Fig. 3). β-adrenergic receptor activation increases inotropy at least in part by cAMP-dependent phosphorylation of L-type channels thereby increasing Ca^{2+} entry.

Three different chemical classes of organic Ca^{2+} channel blockers can be distinguished: Dihydropyridines (DHPs; prototype nifedipine), phenylalkylamines (prototype verapamil) and benzothiazepines (prototype diltiazem). Despite their different structure they all bind within a single drug binding region close to the pore of the channel. All these drugs reversibly interact with this binding domain in a stereoselective manner and with ▶ dissociation constants in the nanomolar range (0.1–50 nM).

DHPs. Widely used DHPs are nifedipine, amlodipine, nitrendipine, nisoldipine, nicardipine and isradipine. They directly bind to and stabilize the inactivated state of the channel and do not require the channel to open in order to access the binding domain. Inactivated channels are more likely to exist in arterial vascular smooth muscle because depolarizations are longer lasting than in cardiac muscle. Moreover, the arterial smooth muscle channel differs slightly from the cardiac isoform (▶ alternative splicing of α1 subunits) which facilitates channel block by DHPs. As a consequence, DHPs block the channels in arterial smooth muscle at lower concentrations than cardiac muscle. Their clinical use is therefore related to their vasodilating properties in arterial smooth muscle (including the coronary arteries) and not to direct actions on the myocardium and the conduction system (i.e. antiarrhythmic and cardiodepressive effects) which are observed at higher concentrations *in vitro* or at toxic plasma levels.

Phenylalkylamines. Verapamil is the most widely used phenylalkylamine. The more active methoxyverapamil (gallopamil) is also licensed for clinical use in some countries. Verapamil mainly gets access to the binding domain when the channel is open. As an organic cation it blocks the channel by interfering with Ca^{2+} ion binding to the extracellular mouth of the pore. Once bound to the open state it can promote the inactivated channel conformation. Verapamil also slows the recovery of channels from inactivation. This increases the refractory period of the drug bound channel. As a consequence, the number of channels available for Ca^{2+} influx decreases when the time between depolarizations shortens (i.e. when stimulation

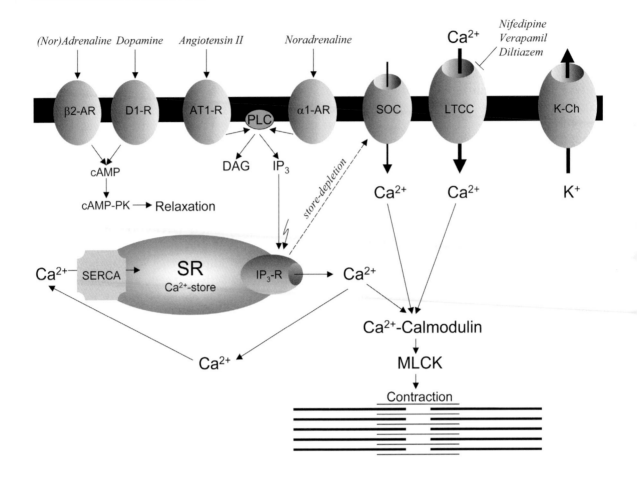

Fig. 2 Simplified view of the pharmacological action of L-type Ca²⁺ channel blockers in arterial smooth muscle: In contrast to cardiomyocytes, action potentials are not carried by fast sodium channels in smooth muscle and depolarzations are more long lasting. Contraction requires the binding of Ca^{2+} to calmodulin, which then activates myosin light chain kinase (MLCK). MLCK phosphorylates the light chain of myosin, which turns on contraction. The Ca^{2+} for activation of this pathway can enter through L-type Ca^{2+} channels in response to depolarization. Ca^{2+} channel blockers inhibit this pathway through concentration-dependent block of Ca^{2+} entry. Alternatively, Ca^{2+} can be released from intracellular stores after activation of membrane receptors (e.g. of angiotensin II AT1 or α1-adrenergic receptors) coupled to IP_3 production. IP_3 opens IP_3 receptor channels, RyR related Ca^{2+} release channels in the SR. This process does not involve L-type Ca^{2+} channels and is not inhibited by Ca^{2+} channel blockers. Store-depletion also triggers the activation of "store-operated channels" (SOC) in the plasma membrane, which are also not sensitive to Ca^{2+} channel blockers. Receptor-mediated activation of cAMP-dependent protein kinase (cAMP-PK) results in muscle relaxation through different mechanisms. D1-R, dopamine1 receptor; AR, adrenergic receptor; PLC, phospholipase C.

frequency increases). The open channel block and slowing of recovery explains why inhibition by a given verapamil concentration increases at higher heart rates. Like the lidocain block of voltage-gate sodium channels, the verapamil block of Ca^{2+} channels becomes more pronounced during tachyarrhythmias. These antiarrhythmic effects of

phenylalkylamines are exploited in addition to its vasodilating and cardiodepressive actions.

Benzothiazepines. Diltiazem is the only benzothiazepine in clinical use. Its molecular mechanism of action as well as its pharmacological effects closely resemble those of phenylalkylamines.

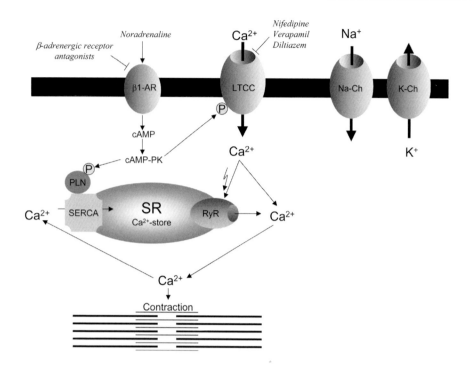

Fig. 3 Simplified view of the pharmacological action of L-type Ca²⁺ channel blockers in cardiac myocytes: In cardiac myocytes, L-type Ca²⁺ channels open when the plasma membrane is depolarised by an action potential carried along the muscle cells by the opening of voltage-gated sodium-channels (Na-Ch). The action potential is terminated (an its duration is determined) by the opening of potassium channels (K-Ch). Ca²⁺ influx triggers massive release of Ca²⁺ from intracellular stores by opening ryanodine-sensitive Ca²⁺ channels (ryanodine receptors, RyR) in the sarcoplasmic reticulum, resulting in an intracellular Ca²⁺ transient. Ca²⁺ influx and released Ca²⁺ directly initiate contraction. Contraction is terminated by the rapid uptake into the SR by SR Ca²⁺ ATPases (SERCA). β-adrenergic receptor stimulation increases inotropy by phosphorylation (P) of phospholamban (PLN) and L-type channels through cAMP-dependent protein kinase (cAMP-PK). The resulting stimulation of Ca²⁺ influx and Ca²⁺-pump activity increases the load of Ca²⁺ in the SR stores. This leads to enhanced Ca²⁺ transients upon depolarization. Inhibition of Ca²⁺ influx through L-type Ca²⁺ channels by Ca²⁺ channel blockers causes decreased Ca²⁺ entry and SR load. Less Ca²⁺ influx and release results in smaller Ca²⁺ transients and a decrease in contractile force.

All three classes also inhibit depolarisation-induced contraction of venous smooth muscle *in vitro*. However, venous relaxation does not contribute to the hemodynamic actions of Ca²⁺ channel blockers.

Clinical Use (incl. side effects)

DHPs are potent arterial vasodilators. They act on resistance vessels and therefore reduce peripheral vascular resistance, lower arterial blood pressure, and antagonize vasospasms in coronary or peripheral arteries. By reducing afterload, DHPs also reduce cardiac oxygen demand. Together with their antivasospastic effect, this explains most of the beneficial actions of DHPs in angina pectoris. Most DHPs are only licensed for the therapy of hypertension, some of them also for the treatment of angina pectoris and vasospastic (Prinzmetal) angina.

The DHP-induced lowering of blood pressure can result in compensatory sympathetic activation and a subsequent increase in heart rate and cardiac oxygen demand. This unfavourable effect has been mainly associated with the use of short-acting DHPs, such as non-retarded formulations of nifedipine, nitrendipine or nicardipine. The use of such formulations that cause fluctuations in plasma levels is discouraged. Instead, formulations with slower onset and longer duration of action (e.g. slow release nifedipine, nisoldipine, amlodipine) are recommended. Due to their vasodilating properties in the absence of negative inotropic actions, DHPs have also been evaluated as vasodilators for the treatment of congestive heart failure in addition to standard therapy. Although long acting DHPs seem to be safe in these patients, no clear benefit could be established for this indication.

In addition to the vasodilatory and antispastic properties, therapeutic doses of verapamil and diltiazem also exert negative inotropic, dromotropic and chronotropic actions. As a consequence, compensatory tachycardia does not occur and heart rate may even decrease. Similar to β-adrenergic antagonists, verapamil and diltiazem also inhibit exercise-induced increases in heart rate and myocardial oxygen consumption. Due to their cardiodepressive effects they are more suitable for the treatment of angina pectoris than DHPs. Both drugs are licensed for the treatment of angina, vasospastic angina and hypertension. Their negative dromotropic and antiarrhythmic properties (see above) can be expoited to slow AV-conduction and to treat supraventricular arrhythmias. In patients with normal contractile function, the negative inotropic action of verapamil is partially compensated by the decreased afterload and improved myocardial perfusion. However, verapamil may decrease left ventricular function in patients with congestive heart failure. Unlike β-adrenergic blockers, Ca²⁺ antagonists are not recommended for early treatment or secondary prevention of myocardial infarction.

DHPs are also used to treat vasospasms of peripheral arteries (e.g. ▶ Raynaud's phenomenon) and ▶ pulmonary hypertension.

Side Effects
Many unwanted effects are related to the vasodilatory effects of Ca²⁺ channel blockers, such as flushing, headache, dizziness, and hypotension. DHPs frequently cause edema and ankle swelling upon chronic use. Constipation is a frequent side effect of verapamil due to its inhibitory action on intestinal smooth muscle. Bradycardia, atrioven-

tricular block or a decrease in left ventricular function are observed with verapamil (and to a lesser degree diltiazem), especially in patients taking β-adrenergic blockers or who have preexisting cardiac disease (impaired left ventricular function, atrioventricular block). Worsening of angina has also been observed with DHPs. This is most likely due to their pronounced effect on coronary resistance resulting in coronary steal in the presence of hypoperfused regions. It may also be caused by the reactive sympathetic activation with increase in heart rate and cardiac oxygen consumption.

Epidemiological and case-control studies suggested that Ca²⁺ channel blockers cause increased risk for myocardial infarction, cancer and gastrointestinal bleeding. The increased cardiovascular morbidity was again associated with short-acting DHPs and fast release forms of verapamil and diltiazem. It was explained by the unfavourable hemodynamic effects of short-acting drugs. Enhanced cardiovascular morbidity has not been consistently shown for long-acting formulations. The increased risk of cancer and gastrointestinal bleeding was not confirmed in other large trials. Although Ca²⁺ channel blockers are not considered first-line agents for the treatment of angina and hypertension, they can be safely used in such patients when they are clearly indicated.

Ca²⁺ channel blockers cause no side effects expected from channel block in other tissues. In cochlear inner hair cells, retinal photoreceptors or neurons, a decreased glucose-tolerance may be observed resulting from a block of pancreatic β-cell L-type chanels and decrease of insulin secretion. However, this side effect plays a minor role in clinical practice. The reason for the absence of these actions can be explained by the lower sensitivity of L-type channels in sensory cells and/or lower bioavailability in these tissues.

Other Pharmacological Actions of Ca²⁺ Antagonists
Some DHPs (such as nifedipine) and verapamil inhibit ▶ p-glycoprotein-mediated drug transport. P-glycoprotein is a drug efflux pump that can confer multidrug resistance to tumor cells. Structural analogues with potent p-glycoprotein but weak Ca²⁺ channel blocking activity were therefore developed but are of no clinical benefit for the treatment of cancer. However, inhibition of transport (and excretion) of other p-glycoprotein sub-

strates, such as digoxin, explains the decrease of their body clearance by Ca^{2+} channel blockers.

In vitro nifedipine inhibits proliferation of colon cancer cells with a DNA mismatch repair defect that are resistant to 5-fluorouracil. Whether this also translates into clinical efficacy in such tumors remains to be determined.

Nimodipine, but not other DHPs, is also a potent inhibitor of nucleoside transport with actions similar to known nucleoside transport inhibitors such as dipyridamol. It is likely that this mechanism also contributes to the potent vasodilating properties of this DHP.

BAYK8644 is a DHP with Ca^{2+} channel activating properties. Although some therapeutic effects can be envisaged for such drugs (such as stimulation of insulin secretion, positive inotropy), severe side effects are also predicted from animal studies (dystonic neurobehavioural syndrome, hypertension, arrhythmias) which currently prevents their clinical development.

References

1. Abernethy DR, Schwartz JB (1999) Ca^{2+}-antagonist drugs. N Engl J Med 341:1447–1457
2. Betkowski AS, Hauptman PJ (2000) Update on recent clinical trials in congestive heart failure. Curr Opin Cardiol 15:293–303
3. Cutler JA (1998) Ca^{2+}-channel blockers for hypertension – uncertainty continues. N Engl J Med 338:679–681
4. Pahor M, Psaty BM, Alderman MH, Applegate WB, Williamson JD, Cavazzini C, Furberg CD (2000) Health outcomes associated with Ca^{2+} antagonists compared with other first-line antihypertensive therapies: a meta-analysis of randomised controlled trials. Lancet 356:1949–1954
5. Striessnig J, Grabner M, Mitterdorfer J, Hering S, Sinnegger MJ, Glossmann H (1998) Structural basis of drug binding to L Ca^{2+} channels. Trends Pharmacol Sci 19:108–115

Ca^{2+}-induced Ca^{2+} Release

▶ CICR
▶ Ryanodine Receptor

Ca^{2+} Release Channel

▶ Ryanodine Receptor
▶ Table appendix: Membrane Transport Proteins

Ca^{2+} Spark

A Ca^{2+} spark is a discrete, transient, very localized increase in Ca^{2+} concentration around Ryanodine receptors *in situ*.

▶ Ryanodine Receptor

Ca^{2+} Transient

A Ca^{2+} transient is a transient increase in intracellular Ca^{2+} concentration, which is detected by a Ca^{2+} indicator. The increased Ca^{2+} levels are due to Ca^{2+} release from intracellular Ca^{2+}-stores and to Ca^{2+} influx from the external medium.

▶ Ryanodine Receptor

Cadherins

▶ Cadherins/Catenins
▶ Table appendix: Adhesion Molecules

Cadherins/Catenins

JÜRGEN BEHRENS
Nikolaus-Fiebiger-Center for Molecular
Medicine, Erlangen, Germany
jbehrens@molmed.uni-erlangen.de

Synonyms

γ-Catenin is a synonym for plakoglobin

Definition

Cadherins (Calcium-dependent adhesion proteins) are transmembrane proteins, which consist of an extracellular domain composed of cadherin-repeats, a transmembrane domain, and a cytoplasmic domain that interacts with catenins and/or other cytoplasmic proteins.

Catenins are defined as cytoplasmic interaction partners of cadherins that form a chain of proteins ("catena", latin for chain), which connects cadherins to the actin cytoskeleton.

▶ Anti-integrins, therapeutic and diagnostic implications

Basic Characteristics

Structural Characteristics

Cadherins are a superfamily of Ca^{++}-sensitive cell-cell adhesion molecules, which cause homophilic cell interactions. Cadherins can be divided into different subfamilies, namely, classical cadherins, desmosomal cadherins, protocadherins and non-conventional cadherins (7TM cadherins, T-cadherin, FAT). Classical cadherins are often denoted by a prefix reflecting their principal expression domains; e.g. E- is epithelial, N- is neuronal, and P- is placental cadherin. However, this classification is not stringent, as for instance E-cadherin can also be found in certain neuronal tissues and N-cadherin is also found in epithelial cells. Among the desmosomal cadherins, two subfamilies can be distinguished, the desmocollins- 1, 2, and 3 and the desmogleins- 1, 2, and 3.

The extracellular domain of cadherins consists of a variable number of a repeated sequence of about 110 amino acids. This sequence is termed the "cadherin repeat" and resembles in overall structure but not in sequence the Ig-like domains. The cadherin repeat is the characteristic motive common to all members of the cadherin superfamily. Classical and desmosomal cadherins contain five cadherin repeats, but as many as 34 repeats have been found in the FAT cadherin (see below). Cadherins are calcium-dependent cell adhesion molecules, which means that removal of Ca^{++}, e.g. by chelating agents such as EDTA, leads to loss of cadherin function. The Ca^{++}-binding pockets are made up of amino acids from two consecutive cadherin repeats, which form a characteristic tertiary structure to coordinate a single Ca^{++} ion (1).

The classical cadherins are translated as precursors that are N-terminally cleaved to reveal the mature proteins. This processing is required to activate the cell adhesion function of cadherins. Cadherins interact in trans (i.e. from opposite cells) via the most N-terminal cadherin repeats. A short amino acid sequence within this repeat, histidine-alanine-valine (HAV), has been implicated in mediating cell-cell contacts as HAV peptides can disrupt cadherin-dependent cell adhesion. Besides the trans-interactions of cadherins, the extracellular domains are also capable of forming cis-dimers through lateral amino acid contacts between cadherin molecules on one cell. This dimerization again mainly involves the first cadherin repeat. A zipper model for the adhesive interactions has been proposed based on the pattern of alternating cis- and trans-dimers. The resulting clustering of cadherin molecules is thought to greatly enhance their adhesive capacity. It is not known whether the desmosomal cadherins or the protocadherins also form cis-dimer (1).

Several non-conventional cadherins have been described that contain cadherin repeats but have specific features not found in the classical cadherins (1). The cadherin Flamingo, originally detected in *Drosophila*, contains seven transmembrane segments and in this respect resembles G-protein coupled receptors. The extracellular domain of Flamingo and its mammalian homologs is composed of cadherin repeats as well as EGF-like and laminin motifs. The seven transmembrane span cadherins have a role in homotypic cell interactions and in the establishment of cell polarity. The

C

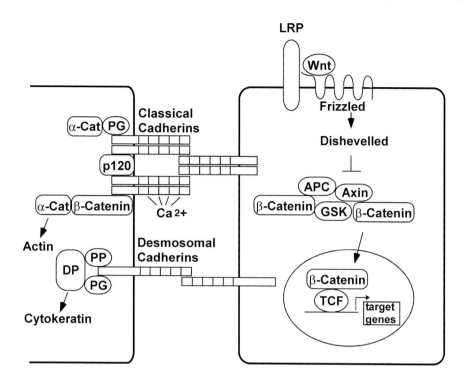

Fig. 1 Overview of cadherin-mediated cell adhesion and the Wnt signaling pathway. Schematic representation of classical and desmosomal cadherins showing extracellullar cadherin repeats and Ca++ binding sites, and cytoplasmic interaction partners (the latter being depicted in the left cell only). The cadherin zipper, which is made up of consecutive cis- and trans-dimers is indicated. The basic outline of the Wnt pathway is shown in the right cell. LRP (lipoprotein receptor-related protein) is a coreceptor for Wnts. PG, plakoglobin, PP, plakophilin.

FAT related cadherins are characterized by a large number of cadherin repeats (34 in FAT and 27 in dachsous). Their cytoplasmic domains can bind to catenins. In *Drosophila*, in which these cadherins have been originally described, Fat functions as a tumor suppressor gene and dachsous is involved in thorax, leg and wing development. Several human and mouse FAT homologs have been identified but their function is as yet unknown. T- (= truncated-) cadherin differs from other cadherins in that it has no transmembrane domain but is attached to the cell membrane via a ▶ glycosyl-phosphatidylinositol anchor.

Cytoplasmic Interactions of Cadherins

The cytoplasmic domains of cadherins bind to various proteins. The most C-terminal portion of classical cadherins directly associates with either β-catenin or the structurally related γ-catenin (more commonly called plakoglobin). β-Catenin/

plakoglobin in turn bind to α-catenin, which is related to the cytoskeletal protein vinculin and associates with actin binding proteins. Thus, β-catenin and α-catenin provide a link of cadherins to the actin cytoskeleton. Another catenin, p120^{ctn} binds to the cytoplasmic juxtamembrane domain of cadherins and appears to be involved in the cis-dimerization and clustering of cadherins. Based on their structure, β-catenin, plakoglobin and p120^{ctn} belong to a protein superfamily, called the armadillo repeat family (2). These proteins contain repeats of about 40 amino acid that were initially identified in armadillo, the *Drosophila* homolog of β-catenin. The armadillo repeats are built up of three α-helices that form a superhelix. The number of repeats varies between different members of the family; for instance, β-catenin contains 12 consecutive armadillo repeats. More distantly related members of the armadillo family include non-junctional proteins, such as the importins, which are involved in nuclear protein import, and the tumor suppressor APC. p120^{ctn} is the founding member of a subfamily of armadillo proteins that include the plakophilins- 1 and 2, ARVCF and the nervous system specific δ-catenin; the latter two bind to the same region of cadherins as p120^{ctn}. Interestingly, the p120^{ctn} related proteins are also found in the cell nucleus, but their function in this compartment is not known. The desmosomal cadherins also associate with plakoglobin but not with β-catenin, and in addition they bind to plakophilins. Plakoglobin and plakophilins connect desmosomal cadherins to the desmosome specific component ▶ desmoplakin, which links the complexes to the intermediate filament network (mainly ▶ cytokeratins in epithelial cells).

The cytoplasmic domains of protocadherins are unrelated to those of classical cadherins. They do not bind catenins and it is not clear whether they are associated with the cytoskeleton (1,3). Some protocadherins interact with the c-src-related kinase ▶ Fyn, indicating a role in signal transduction (see below).

Gene Organization
Several classical cadherin genes (e.g. E-, P-, VE-cadherin and others) are found in a cluster on human chromosome 16 or on the syntenic mouse chromosome 8. The gene clustering is even more pronounced in the case of the desmosomal cadherin, which are all located on human chromosome 18q12 in relatively close vicinity to each other. Interestingly, the desmocollin and desmoglein genes (termed *DSC* and *DSG*) form two subclusters that have opposite transcriptional orientation. Protocadherins show a particularly striking genome organization. Subfamilies of protocadherins can be defined that share a common intracellular domain but differ in their extracellular domains. Each extracellular domain is encoded by a single exon while the intracellular domain is encoded by three exons. Generation of diverse transcripts from these clusters may be achieved by gene rearrangement and/or alternative splicing, which is reminiscent of the mechanisms of diversification of immunoglobulins and T-cell receptors. Which of these mechanisms is indeed relevant in the generation of protocadherins remains to be determined (1).

Functional Characteristics
Classical and desmosomal cadherins are constituents of different types of intercellular junctions. E-cadherin, the classical cadherin of epithelial cells, is part of the adherens junction (zonula adherens), which is attached to a belt of actin via the catenins. As the name suggests, desmosomal cadherins are part of the desmosomes, which are rivet-like structures that make focal connections between cells. Desmosomes are characterized by a prominent intracellular plaque structure, which serves as an attachment point for intermediate filaments.

Functional studies have demonstrated the adhesive role of cadherins (4). For example, cell-cell adhesion *in vitro* can be blocked by treatment of cultured cells with anti-cadherin antibodies, resulting in dissociation of the cell monolayer. Conversely, forced expression of cadherins by cDNA transfection in cells lacking these molecules leads to establishment of intercellular contacts. Thus, cadherins act as an adhesive glue that efficiently holds cells together. However, they may also have signaling function, as several *in vitro* studies show that cadherins influence differentiation and growth of cells. Cadherins act in a very specific manner. *In vitro*, cadherins can mediate the **sorting out** of cells, i.e. cells transfected with different cadherins separate from each other and form homotypic aggregates. Accordingly, a main function of cadherins might be in the delineation of tissue boundaries. Gene knock-out experiments have revealed essential and cell type specific functions of cadherins *in vivo*. The knock-out of the E-cadherin gene results in the dissociation of cells of blastocyst-stage mouse embryos. The α-catenin knock-out has a similar phenotype, while loss of plakoglobin leads to defects in cell adhesion of heart muscle cells. The knock-out of β-catenin does not affect cell junctions but rather has a Wnt signaling phenotype (see below), which is manifested at early stages of embryonic development. Apparently, plakoglobin which is also present in the affected cells, can overtake the adhesive function of β-catenin under these circumstances. The mutation of desmosomal cadherins frequently leads to the disruption of skin layers. These phenotypes resemble those of the ▶ pemphigus blistering diseases in humans, which are caused by autoantibodies against desmocollins and desmoplakins. E-cadherin appears to play a major role in

cancer as its expression is frequently downregulated in dedifferentiated, metastasizing tumors. E-cadherin inhibits invasion of tumor cells in *in vitro* systems and prevents tumor progression in *in vivo* animal models. Moreover, loss-of-function mutations of the E-cadherin gene occur in gastric carcinomas and certain types of breast tumors. The function of cadherins can be modulated by signaling pathways involving tyrosine kinases, which disrupt cell contacts. Moreover, cadherins themselves might be signaling components as they resemble ligand receptor pairs in many aspects. However, a genuine signal transduction pathway originating from cadherins has not been defined in molecular terms so far (4).

It is not clear whether protocadherins are true cell adhesion molecules since some of them show only moderate activity in classical cell aggregation assays (3). However, in *Xenopus* embryos, expression of a dominant-negative mutant of NF-protocadherin leads to disruption of the embryonic ectoderm indicating a role of this protocadherin in maintaining tissue integrity. Biochemical and embryological evidence indicates that protocadherins also have a role in intercellular signalling. A subfamily of protocadherins, termed CNRs (cadherin-related neuronal receptors) associate with ▶ Fyn, a cytoplasmic tyrosine kinase related to ▶ c-src. The extracellular matrix protein ▶ reelin binds to these CNRs and activates the Fyn kinase, which leads to phosphorylation of a downstream signaling protein, mDAB. This pathway appears to be important for certain steps in cortical neuron development, as antibodies to the reelin-binding domain of CNRs perturb the arrangement of cortical neurons. Since there are so many members of the protocadherin family, which are mostly expressed in the nervous system, it has been speculated that protocadherins play discrete roles in setting up neuronal networks (1,3).

β-Catenin in the Wnt Pathway

Besides its role in cell adhesion β-catenin has an important function as a central signal transduction component in the Wnt pathway (4,5). Wnts are a family of secreted glycoproteins that regulate a variety of developmental processes. Binding of Wnts to Frizzled receptors, which are ▶ seven transmembrane span proteins, induces stabilization of β-catenin. This pool of β-catenin is not associated with cadherins but accumulates in the cytoplasm and eventually enters the nucleus, where it teams up with transcription factors of the TCF family. TCFs bind to specific DNA sequences in Wnt target promoters via an HMG box but lack transactivation domains. In the absence of β-catenin TCFs behave as transcriptional silencers, in part because they bind to diverse transcriptional repressors. β-Catenin lacks DNA binding activity but contains strong transactivating sequences in its N- and C-terminal domains. Thus, when β-catenin binds to TCFs a bipartite transcription factor is formed in which DNA binding and transactivation domains reside on separate molecules. The TCF/β-catenin complexes can activate specific Wnt-target genes involved in determining cell fate and differentiation and inducing cancer (see below). For a list of Wnt target genes see www.stanford.edu/~rnusse/wntwindow.html.

In the absence of Wnts, cytoplasmic "free" β-catenin is targeted for degradation by a multiprotein complex containing the scaffold component axin or the related protein conductin, the ▶ tumor suppressor APC (adenomatous polyposis coli) and the serine/threonine kinase GSK3β. When β-catenin binds to axin it becomes phosphorylated by GSK3β. Hyperphosphorylated β-catenin is recognized by the E3 ligase βTrCP/slimb, a component of the ubiquitination machinery, becomes ubiquitinated and finally degraded in proteasomes (4). APC has several β-catenin and axin binding sites and may function by sequestering free β-catenin and delivering it to the axin complex (5). Thus, APC acts as a safeguard to prevent aberrant accumulation of β-catenin. Mutations of APC occur in about 80% of all colorectal carcinomas and lead to the formation of truncated APC proteins that are no longer able to interact with axin/conductin and to induce degradation of β-catenin. Therefore, these mutations result in the stabilization of β-catenin and in the formation of constitutive TCF/β-catenin complexes, which activate transcription of oncogenic target genes in a Wnt-independent fashion. In some colorectal tumors, and more frequently in other tumor types (e.g. hepatoblastomas), stabilization of β-catenin occurs through mutations of the critical serine or threonine residues normally phosphorylated by GSK3β. Thus both genetically and functionally β-catenin behaves as an oncogene and the Wnt pathway has a major role in tumorigenesis. Interestingly, the Wnt-1 gene can be activated in mice by insertion of the mouse mammary tumor virus LTR, which leads to the formation of mammary tumors.

Drugs

There are a several potential approaches for pharmacological interference with the cadherin/catenin system. The HAV peptides, often in circular form, have been shown to disrupt cell-cell adhesion in experimental systems. A potential therapeutic application could lie in the use of such compounds to transiently loosen cell contacts, for instance in order to regulate the permeability of the blood-brain barrier. Drugs that upregulate E-cadherin in tumors could be of potential benefit as part of a differentiation strategy to "normalize" epithelial cancers and to prevent metastasis formation. Finally, drugs that affect components of the Wnt patway, e.g. by blocking the interaction of TCFs with β-catenin are candidates for interference with tumor growth.

References

1. Angst BD, Marcozzi C, Magee AI (2001) The cadherin superfamily: diversity in form and function. J Cell Sci 114:629–641
2. Peifer M, Berg S, Reynolds AB (1999) A repeating amino acid motif shared by proteins with diverse cellular roles. Cell 1994 76:789–791
3. Suzuki ST (2000) Recent progress in protocadherin research. Exp Cell Res 261:13–18
4. Behrens J (1999) Cadherins and catenins: role in signal transduction and tumor progression. Cancer Metastasis Rev 18:15–30
5. Polakis P (2000) Wnt signaling and cancer. Genes Dev 14:1837–1851

cADP-ribose

cADP-ribose (cyclic ADP-ribose) has been shown to trigger the release of calcium from the endoplasmic reticulum *via* ▶ ryanodine receptors (calcium release channels). Cyclic ADP-ribose is enzymatically formed and appears to act as a second messenger, which mediates a sustained increase in cytosolic calcium in various activated eucaryotic cells including T lymphocytes.

cAK

▶ cAMP- and cGMP-dependent Protein Kinases

Calcineurin

▶ Immunosuppressive Agents

Calcitonin

Calcitonin is a peptide hormone which rapidly inhibits osteoclast activity. The relevance of calcitonin in human calcium homeostasis is not well understood. Calcitonin has been used for the treatment of osteoporosis, although due to the availability of more potent drugs with fewer side effects and the lack of clear data on the anti-fracture efficacy of calcitonin, its clinical use has been steadily declining.

▶ Bone Metabolism

Calcitonin Gene Related Peptide

Calcitonin gene related peptide (CGRP) is one of the numerous peptides found in neurons and acting as co-transmitters. It is derived from the gene encoding calcitonin by alternative splicing of mRNA and by proteolytic processing of a precursor peptide. It is mainly found in sensory neurons of the central nervous system. Its prime target is the CGRP receptor, a member of the family of ▶ G protein-coupled receptors. In contrast to calcitonin, which is involved in calcium homeostasis and bone remodeling, CGRP causes vasodilatation and vascular leakage. It is also expressed in C-fiber sensory neurons. It works as a stimulatory (pronociceptive) neurotransmitter when it is released centrally, and as a proinflammatory mediator when it is released peripherally. The central role of CGRP in primary headaches has led to a search for suitable antagonists of CGRP receptors

Calmodulin

Calmodulin is a protein that binds calcium and is present in all cells having a nucleus. Calmodulin controls the activity of many enzymes.

cAMP

▶ AMP, cyclic

cAMP- and cGMP-dependent Protein Kinases

Cyclic AMP- and cGMP-dependent protein kinases (syn.: cAKs, pKAs or cAMP kinases; cGKs, PKGs or cGMP kinases) are enzymes activated by the binding of cyclic AMP or cyclic GMP. When activated, cAKs and cGKs phosphorylate specific serine or threonine residues in target proteins and thereby control the activity of these proteins.

cAMP-binding Guanine Nucleotide Exchange Factors

In the cAMP-bound conformation, cAMP-binding guanine nucleotide exchange factors (cAMP-

GEFs) specifically bind to Ras-like small G proteins and activate these proteins by profoundly accelerating the exchange of GDP for GTP.

▶ Small GTPases

cAMP-GEFs

▶ cAMP-binding Guanine Nucleotide Exchange Factors
▶ Small GTPases

Campothecins

Campothecins (topotecan, irinotecan) are chemotherapeutic agents used for the treatment of cancer (ovarian cancer, lung cancer, colon cancer). Campothecins bind to and inhibit topoisomerase I, an enzyme that prevents DNA tangling during replication by producing transient single-strand breaks.
▶ Antineoplastic Agents

Cancer, molecular mechanisms of therapy

FRED BUNZ
The Sidney Kimmel Comprehensive Cancer Center at Johns Hopkins, The John Hopkins School of Medicine, Baltimore, USA
bunzfre@mail.jhmi.edu

Synonyms

Malignant tumor, malignant neoplasm

Definition

Cancers are tumors that have acquired the ability to invade and disrupt surrounding normal tissues. Such lesions can arise in any tissue of the human body, and so cancers represent a heterogeneous group of diseases that have certain biological features in common.

A tumor begins as an outgrowth of a clonal population of cells that follows a loss of tissue homeostasis, and progresses into a cancer as it grows in size and becomes invasive. During the later stages of cancer progression, cancer cells can enter the bloodstream or lymphatic system and grow in distant sites. This process is known as metastasis. The invasive and metastatic properties of cancers lead to the lethal destruction of normal tissues.

▶ Antineoplastic Agents

Basic Mechanisms

Many anticancer agents currently in use, including chemotherapeutic drugs and radiation, are potent inducers of ▶ apoptosis and ▶ cell-cycle arrest. It is believed that induction of these molecular pathways is central to the efficacy of such agents (1). Genetic and epigenetic alterations that contribute to tumorigenesis often disable the pathways that lead to apoptosis and growth arrest and therefore affect the way that cancer cells respond to therapy. Recent advances in the understanding of how cellular pathways of growth and death work has led to insights as to how therapy might be optimized.

The regulatory apparatus that controls the cell division cycle is the frequent target of inactivating mutations, and some of these mutated genes can be inherited in cancer-prone families. Similarly, mutations can affect apoptotic pathways. Many cancer-derived cell lines demonstrate a resistance to experimental apoptotic stimuli and recent evidence supports the idea that alterations in genetically defined apoptotic pathways are actively selected for during tumor development. It thus appears that inactivation of the pathways that lead to cell-cycle arrest and apoptosis confer a selective growth advantage.

The relative contributions of cell-cycle arrest and apoptosis to the death of tumor cells following therapy remain a point of controversy (2). *In vitro*, cell death triggered by anticancer agents can occur as a result of an immediate apoptotic program or,

alternatively, following a substantial delay as a result of dysregulated cell-cycle arrest. These pathways and the drugs that trigger them have been experimentally defined in a colon cancer cell system (see Figure). At present it appears likely that different pathways dominate in different cell types. Furthermore, it is important to understand that the experimental systems currently in use are imperfect representations of tumors and these no doubt fail to fully represent complex cellular responses of human cancers. The development of model systems that better emulate cancers *in situ* will likely aid in understanding how death pathways can work in a clinical setting.

Apoptosis

A substantial amount of indirect evidence supports the contention that the induction of apoptosis in tumor cells is critical to successful therapy. Cancer therapy might therefore be viewed as an attempt to induce apoptosis in a population of cells that have undergone selection for apoptotic defects. If correct, this hypothesis would suggest why cancer therapy is in many cases unsuccessful. However, recent studies indicate that this fundamental problem can be circumvented. Progress in the identification of molecules key to the cell death pathways has led to a growing understanding of how apoptosis occurs (3). It has become clear that pathways to apoptosis are numerous and often interconnected. A solution to the clinical problem of therapeutic resistance, then, may lie in the fact that there appears to be multiple ways that a cell death program can be implemented.

Apoptosis occurs as a result of a cascade of proteolysis that culminates in the destruction of the cell. Apoptotic proteolysis is catalyzed by the ▶ caspase family of proteases and can occur via the activation of one of two major pathways. In the intrinsic, or mitochondrial apoptotic pathway, an intracellular death signal causes the disruption of mitochondria, which liberates into the cytoplasm proteins that facilitate caspase activation. Proapoptotic members of the *Bcl2* family appear to play a central role in the physical disruption of the mitochondrial membranes. An extrinsic apoptotic pathway uses the same downstream effector proteases as the intrinsic pathway, but in this case the death signal originates from the cell surface. External death-inducing ligands bind a family of

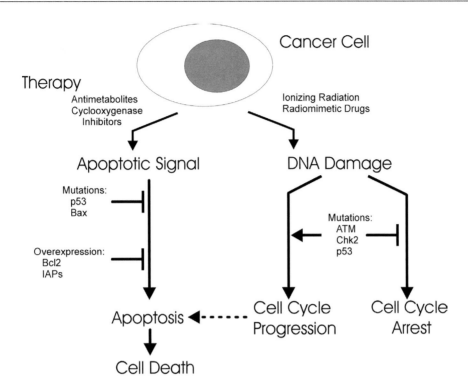

Fig. 1 Cancer therapy and cell death. There are at least two pathways by which therapeutic and preventive agents can cause the death of colon cancer cells. A. Antimetabolites and cyclooxygenase inhibitors can trigger apoptotic signals. The apoptotic signalling pathways can be disrupted in different stages by a number of cancer-related gene mutations and overexpressed proteins, leading to relative therapeutic resistance. B. Therapeutic agents that damage chromosomal DNA can activate a signal transduction pathway that normally results in a protective arrest of the cell cycle. When disrupted by cancer-related mutations, this pathway can fail resulting in progression of the cell cycle, which leads to the dysregulated replication and segregation of damaged chromosomes. Cells that escape cell-cycle arrest are subsequently eliminated by apoptotic effector proteins, resulting in relative therapeutic sensitivity.

death receptors such as CD95 (also known as Fas and Apo-1), tumor necrosis factor receptor 1 and TRAIL (also known as DR5 and KILLER). Ligand binding induces multimerization of these receptors that results in caspase activation.

Negative regulation of apoptosis is effected by Inhibitor of Apoptosis Proteins. Another means of controling apoptosis is by altering the stabilization of mitochondria, which is largely determined by the interplay between the pro- and anti-apoptotic members of the *Bcl2* family (4).

Alterations to the *P53* gene are the most common genetic defects known in cancer (5). The protein product of *P53* is involved in a number of pathways that directly and indirectly lead to apop-

tosis. Many genes that are involved in apoptosis can be induced by this protein, which is a transcriptional transactivator. The emerging hypothesis is that p53 is a central node of a complex apoptotic network that may function differently in diverse cell types and tissues. For example, *Bax*, the prototype proapoptotic member of the *Bcl2* family, can be transcriptionally induced by p53 in certain, but not all, cell types. Like *p53*, *Bax* can modulate the extent to which cells are sensitive to apoptosis caused by therapeutic agents.

Cell-Cycle Regulation

Ionizing radiation and radiomimetic drugs that cause DNA damage are among the most frequently used anticancer agents. In the presence of damaged chromosomes, cellular pathways are triggered which bring to the progression of the cell-cycle to a halt, a status known as cell-cycle arrest. Cell-cycle arrest is mediated by the activation of checkpoints. Checkpoints block specific processes that occur during cell growth. In this way, cells with intact checkpoints prevent the replication and segregation of damaged chromosomes. In cells that have disrupted checkpoint pathways, DNA damage can lead to the aberrant progression of the cell-cycle, which can result in lethal reduplication of genomic DNA and inappropriate timing of cell division. Analysis of genetic alterations that occur in hereditary cancers suggests that the G_2 checkpoint, which prevents the entry of cells with damaged chromosomes into mitosis, is a particularly important target of mutational inactivation during carcinogenesis.

In addition to its role as an mediator of apoptosis, the p53 protein is part of a checkpoint mechanism that causes arrest of the cell-cycle. Whether p53 activation causes apoptosis or cell-cycle arrest depends upon the stimulus applied and upon the cell type being observed (5). In response to DNA damage, p53 can be activated by the Chk2 kinase, which is in turn activated by the ATM (Ataxia Telangiectasia Mutated) kinase. The checkpoint functions of these tumor suppressor genes, which are mutated in a broad spectrum of sporadic and inherited cancers, supports the idea that the inactivation of the G_2 checkpoint is a frequent event during carcinogenesis and that many tumors are likely to be checkpoint defective. An understanding of how cancer cells differ from normal cells in their responses to DNA damage appears likely to prove useful in devising therapy of maximal efficacy.

Pharmacological Intervention

Most of the therapeutic anticancer agents currently in use were developed empirically, without any prior knowlege of apoptotic or cell-cycle control mechanisms. Subsequently, it has become apparent that apoptosis and cell-cycle arrest are triggered upon exposure of tumor cells to these agents. Recent advances in our understanding of the molecular mechanisms of apoptosis and cell-cycle regulation have illuminated the mode of action of many of the common anticancer agents and suggested why some cancers are resistant to therapy.

Therapeutic Induction of Apoptosis

Many of the agents currently in use for the therapy of cancer can trigger apoptosis in cancer cells. Cancer-associated alterations of the genes that regulate apoptosis would therefore be predicted to affect sensitivity to these agents.

One commonly used agent is the ▶ antimetabolite 5-fluorouracil (5-FU), which is frequently used as an adjuvant therapy in conjunction with surgical excision in the treatment of solid tumors. p53 can directly trigger apoptosis in cells exposed to 5-FU *in vitro* (1). In addition, there is a substantial amount of clinical evidence that suggests that *p53* status may be predictive of the response of patients to 5-FU therapy.

The pro- and anti-apoptotic members of the *Bcl2* family affect cellular sensitivity to apoptosis and thus to many chemotherapeutic agents (4). For example, overexpression of the anti-apoptotic genes *Bcl2* and *Bcl-XL* in some cell lines and tumors can confer resistance to apoptosis triggered by ionizing radiation. Conversely, overexpression of pro-apoptotic *Bax* in experimental tumors can induce apoptosis directly or render such tumors more sensitive to cisplatin and 5-FU.

Nonsteroidal anti-inflamatory drugs, such as sulindac and indomethacin, are important chemopreventive agents for patients genetically predisposed to colorectal cancer. This class of compounds, which bind and inhibit ▶ cyclooxygenases, have been found to cause apoptosis in cultured gastrointestinal epithelial cells. Strikingly, the experimental deletion of the *Bax* gene in tumor-derived colon cancers has been found to disrupt the apoptotic response to this class of drugs, demonstrating the potential importance of this pathway in chemoprevention.

Therapeutic Activation of Cell-Cycle Checkpoints

While induction of apoptosis is the most well recognized molecular mechanism of action of anticancer agents, it is becoming clear that many agents can exploit the checkpoint defects that often occur during cancer development. In fact, ionizing radiation and ▶ radiomimetic drugs such as doxorubicin and bleomycin that cause DNA damage are among the most frequently used anti-cancer agents.

Exposure of many types of normal cells to DNA damaging agents result in the activation of cell-cycle checkpoints, which implement a protective cell-cycle arrest. In cancer cells that have check-point defects, such treatment would be predicted to lead to arrest failure, cell-cycle dysregulation, and eventual cell death. The observed sensitivity of cancer cells, then, is thought to result from their failure to undergo a protective cell-cycle arrest in response to treatment. Ultimately, the cell death that follows cell-cycle dysregulation may occur through apoptotic pathways, demonstrating a complex relationship between these fundamental processes.

Though DNA damage-based therapies have been in use for many years, it has remained unclear why such treatment often causes the selective death of tumor cells while sparing adjacent normal tissue. The genetic alterations that occur in cancers that alter the DNA damage reponse may explain why such therapy can be efficacious.

References

1. Bunz F (2001) Cell death and cancer therapy. Curr Opin Pharmacol 1:337–341
2. Brown JM, Wouters BG (1999) Apoptosis, p53, and tumor cell sensitivity to anticancer agents. Cancer Res 59:1391–1399
3. Zornig M, Hueber A, Baum W, Evan G (2001) Apoptosis regulators and their role in tumorigenesis. Biochim Biophys Acta 1551:1–37
4. Gross A, McDonnell JM, Korsmeyer SJ. (1999) BCL-2 family members and the mitochondria in apoptosis. Genes Dev 13:1899–1911
5. Vogelstein B, Lane D, Levine AJ (2000) Surfing the p53 network. Nature 408:307–310

Cannabinoid Receptor

Group of G-protein coupled receptors which mediate the effects of cannabinoids like Δ^9-tetrahydrocannabinol (THC) as well as of endogenous can-nabinoids (endocannabinoids) like anandamide or 2-arachidonylglycerol (2-AG).

▶ Endocannabinoid System

Cannabinoids

Group of compounds which naturally occur in the hemp plant, *Cannabis sativa*. Most of them are unsoluble in water. The most abundant cannabinoids are Δ^9-tetrahydrocannabinol (THC), its precursor cannabidiol and cannabinol, which is formed spontaneously from THC. Cannabinoids exert their effects through G-protein coupled cannabinoid receptors (CB_1/CB_2).

▶ Endocannabinoid System

Cannabis

▶ Endocannabinoid System

Capsaicin

Capsaicin, also known as N-Vanillyl-8-methyl-6-(E)-noneamide, is the most pungent of the group of compounds called capsaicinoids: It is a common ingredient in varieties of pepper such as habanero, Thai, tabasco, cayenne etc. One target with which capsaicin interacts is the capsaicin receptor, an ion channel belonging to the superfamily of TRP channels. Because of the structural relation to other TRP channels and because the vanilloid moiety is an essential component of capsaicin, the capsaicin receptor is also called TRPV1 or vanilloid receptor (VR1). It is involved in heat and pain perception.

▶ Nociception
▶ TRP Channels

Capsid

A capsid is a proteinaceous shell encasing the viral genome. Viral capsids are polymeric, ordered structures composed of one or more virus encoded subunits.

▶ Antiviral Drugs

CAR

The constitutive androstane receptor (CAR) is a nuclear receptor which forms complexes with the retinoid X receptor (RXR) and mediates the body's response to a variety of xenobiotics.

▶ Constitutive Androstane Receptor

Carbon Monoxide

Carbon monoxide (CO) has a high affinity to and reacts with hemoglobin (forming carboxyhemoglobin). As compared to hemoglobin, carboxyhemoglobin has a strongly reduced capacity to carry oxygen. This explains the toxic effect of CO (tissue anoxia). Endogenously, CO is formed enzymatically in neurons and other cells and may function as a modulator of functions of the central nervous system. Similar to NO, it activates ▶ guanylyl cyclases.

Carbonic Anhydrase

Carbonic anhydrase (CA) is a zinc-containing enzyme that facilitates the interconversion of CO_2 and HCO_3. More than 10 carbonic anhydrase isozymes have been identified, some of which are cytoplasmic, such as CA I and CA II, some membrane-bound, such as CA IV, and some mitochon-drial, such as CA V. CA VI is secreted into saliva. CAs have a wide distribution and participate in all physiological processes that deal with CO_2 and HCO_3 handling, such as cellular pH regulation, and acid and ion transport. Highest expression levels are found in red cells (CA I and CA II), but CA activity is also present in lung, endothelial cells, muscle, kidney, ciliary body and lens, pancreatic ducts, salivary gland acini, choroid plexus, osteoclasts and other tissues and cells. The observation that sulfanilamide inhibited renal HCO_3 absorption by inhibition of CA led to the development of the sulfonamide class of diuretics that includes thiazides and loop diuretics. CA II deficiency syndrome is an autosomal recessive disorder characterized by osteopetrosis, renal tubular acidosis and cerebral calcification and mental retardation, while CA VI deficient patients show loss or impairment of taste and smell sensations.

▶ Diuretics

Carcinogens

▶ Cancer, molecular mechanisms of therapy

Carcinogenesis

▶ Cancer, molecular mechanisms of therapy

Cardiac Glycosides

WERNER NICKL, MICHAEL BÖHM
Medizinische Klinik und Poliklinik III,
Homburg/Saar, Germany
wanickl@web.de,
boehm@med-in.uni-saarland.de

Synonym

Digitalis

Definition

Cardiac glycosides (CG) are potent and highly specific inhibitors of the intrinsic plasma membrane Na^+/K^+-ATPase, also known as the sodium pump. They modulate electrophysiological properties of the heart and its contractile functions.

▶ Antiarrhythmic Drugs

Mechanism of Action

The molecular target of cardiac glycosides is the Na^+/K^+-ATPase (EC 3.1.6.37), which maintains the high sodium and potassium gradients across the plasma membrane, coupled to the hydrolysis of the high-energy phosphate ATP. The gradient is required for the regulation of cell volume, active transport of molecules or the creation and propagation of the action or resting potential of electrically excitable cells. Such are cardiac cells, with a high density of Na^+/K^+-ATPase in the ▶ sarcolemma. While potassium is pumped into the cytoplasm, sodium is transported into the extracellular space in a stoichiometric ratio of $3Na^+:2K^+:1ATP$.

Inhibition of the Na^+/K^+-ATPase leads to a loss of potassium and an increase of sodium within the cell. Secondary intracellular calcium is increased via the Na^+/Ca^{++}-exchanger. This results in a positive inotropic effect in the myocardium, with an increase of peak force and a decrease in time to peak tension. Besides this, cardiac glycosides increase vagal activity by effects on the central vagal nuclei, the nodose ganglion and increase in sensitivity of the sinus node to acetylcholine.

Molecular Structure of Cardiac Glycosides

Cardiac glycosides are found in several plants and certain toads. Common to these substances is an aglycone-portion (genine) with a steroid structure, a 17β-unsaturated lactone ring, a glycone-portion (sugar) in 3β-position and an OH-group in postion 14. Glycosides with a 5-numbered lactone ring are classified as cardenolides, those with a 6-numbered ring bufadienolides. The aglycone portion is essential for pharmacological activity. Its basic structure is a cyclopentanoper hydrophenandrene nucleus in a cis-trans-cis-configuration that makes CG distinct from bile acids, sterol or steroid hormones. Saturation of the lactone ring attenuates activity.

The number of sugar residues linked to the aglycone-portion (one to four) or the hydroxyla-

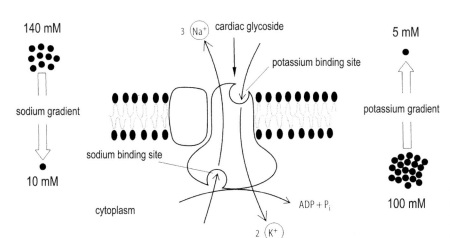

Fig. 1 Cardiac Glycosides – Schematic representation of the Na^+/K^+-ATPase (6).

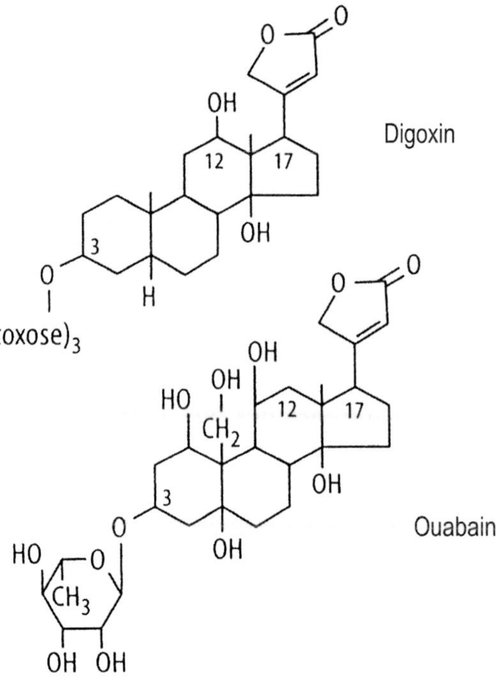

Fig. 2 Cardiac Glycosides – Molecular structure of digoxin and ouabain. Digoxin contains an additional hydroxy group in position 12 compared to digitoxin (6).

tion of the aglycone markedly influences water and lipid solubility, protein binding, metabolic disposition, duration of action and elimination (Table 1).

Intestinal absorption of digoxin is less complete compared to digitoxin. In order to improve absorption, acetylated- and methylated digoxin derivates were developed. Digitoxin is metabolised in hepatic microsomal enzymes and can be cleared independently from renal function. The therapeutical serum level of digoxin is 0.5–2.0 ng/ml and 10–35 ng/ml of digitoxin. Steady state plateau of therapeutic plasma concentrations is reached after 4–5 half-life times using standard daily dosis [1].

Molecular Properties of the Na^+/K^+-ATPase

The pharmacological receptor of cardiac glycosides is the sarcolemmal Na^+/K^+-ATPase expressed on most eucaryotic membranes. It was characterised biochemically in 1957 by J. Skou,

who was awarded with the Nobel Prize in chemistry 1997. The sodium pump belongs to a widely distributed class of P-type ATPases forming a phosphorylated aspartyl residue during the catalytic process. Ions migrate through a narrow 'access channel', and are bound, occluded, and transported by cycling between two different cation-dependent conformations.

Structure and Subunit

The sodium pump is an oligomer composed of two major subunit polypeptides: A catalytic α-unit (MW 110 kD) and a glycosylated β-unit (MW 40–60 kD, depending on degree of glycosylation). The α-unit spans the cell membrane 10 times. Both the NH_2- and the COOH-termini face the cytoplasm. It is responsible for the catalytic and transport characteristics of the ATPase. The α-unit contains binding sites for cardiac glycosides, ATP, sodium or potassium and the phosphorylation site. The β-unit is a modulator of the transport characteristics and proper membrane insertion of the Na^+/K^+-ATPase and crosses the membrane once. The COOH-terminus is located at the large ectodomain of the β-subunit. The NH_2-terminus is exposed to the cytoplasm. A third protein, termed the γ-subunit, can modify the pump activity, yet its physiological significance is unknown [4].

Isoforms

Na^+/K^+-ATPase is expressed as several isozymes (4 α, 3 β subtypes) that are encoded, on different genes. The degree of identity across different species is ~92% for α1 and α2 –► isoforms and ~96% for the α 3-isoform. Within one species the ►homology of α1-, α2- and α3-isoform is ~87%. It is 78% between the α4- and α1-isoform. The highest structural variability among the isoenzymes occurs at the NH_2-terminus, the ouabain-binding site between transmembrane segments 1 and 2, and the region between amino acids 403 and 503. The greatest similarities exist in the cytoplasmic middle region where the ATP binding and phosphorylation sites are located, in the transmembrane hydrophobic regions and in the carboxy-terminal region. Canine vascular smooth muscle utilizes alternative RNA processing of the α1- isoform gene to express a structurally distinct 65 kD isoform, named α1-T (truncated) that lacks 40% of the carboxy-terminal sequence, though retains the

Tab. 1 Cardiac Glycosides

	Ouabain	Digoxin	Digitoxin
Intestinal absorption	3.00 %	60–80 %	> 98 %
Protein binding	3.00 %	25 %	90–100 %
Renal elimination	> 90 %	70–80 %	60 %
Oral daily maintainance dose	--	0.1–0.25 mg	0.07–0.1 mg
Disposition half-time		1.6 days	7–9 days

ATP binding and phosphorylation site. Short variants of the α1-peptide suggest a cation-selective gate close to the NH_2-terminus. In β-subunits, inhibition of glycosylation by tunicamycin or mutation of the β-subunit renders an active enzyme with catalytically competent sodium pumps and normal affinity for ouabain, yet removal of disulfide bonds abolishes assembly of α/β subunits. Truncated β-subunits have been described. Different affinities of the isoenzymes for cations and ATP may be essential in adapting cellular Na^+/K^+-ATPase activity to specific physiological requirements. Its expression of isoforms is species- and tissue specific and can be altered during development and by hormones. The α1/β1-isoenzyme is expressed ubiquitously, whereas the other isoenzymes may play tissue-specific roles. In neuron cells α1- and α2-isoforms seem to maintain the basal ionic gradients. The α3-subunit, because of its low affinity for cations, might serve as a spare pump to help restore the resting membrane potential. The significant role of certain isoforms remains to be established.

The reactivity of the sodium pump isoforms toward ouabain can significantly differ between certain isoenzymes. The α1-isoform from rat is reported to be 100-fold more resistant to ouabain than α2- or α3-isoform. In other species like rabbit, pig, dog or human these differences are not as distinct as in rat, due to a more sensitive α1-isoform. At least two different types of ouabain binding sites are reported for the Na^+/K^+-ATPase [2].

Interactions with the cytoskeleton seem to be responsible for the processing and the targeting of the Na^+/K^+-ATPase to the appropriate compartment structures. Protein kinases are considered to play an essential role in modulation of the sodium pump.

Clinical Use

The main clinical indications of cardiac glycosides are tachyarrhythmic ▶ atrial fibrillation or flutter, as well as severe heart failure (NYHA III-IV) due to systolic dysfunction. In atrial fibrillation or flutter, the properties of digitalis are the reduction of ventricular heart rate at rest by suppression of the AV-node conduction. By this mechanism digitalis is heart rate limiting, without converting atrial fibrillation into ▶ sinus rhythm. In heart failure, digitalis leads to a reduction of enddiastolic filling pressure and volume, decrease in myocardial wall tension and oxygen consumption, with no evidence of desensitisation or tachyphylaxis. Whereas digitalis enhances vascular tone in healthy subjects by direct action on smooth muscle cells, in heart failure patients baroreflex responsiveness is restored, sympathetic nerve activity is decreased in skeletal muscle and vascular blood flow is increased. Furthermore, cardiac glycosides decrease plasma norepinephrine and renin activity [5].

Clinical Trials

A decrease in exercise capacity, left ventricular ejection fraction and increase in clinical symptoms after withdrawal of cardiac glycoside medication in patients with mild to moderate heart failure (NYHA II-III) could be shown in the RADIANCE and PROVE trial. To investigate the digitalis therapy in concern to mortality in patients with chronic heart failure and sinus rhythm who were receiving diuretics and an angiotensin-converting enzyme inhibitor (ACE) the DIG (digitalis investigation group) trial was started.

This trial includes about 6800 patients with decreased cardiac ejection fraction (<45%). The follow up was 37 months. As a result, there was no difference in mortality in both groups, but fewer hospitalizations in the digitalis arm, and a benefit was observed in clinical symptoms in addition to maximum therapeutic regime. A decrease in mor-

Tab. 2 Cardiac Glycosides

Increased digitalis effects	Mechanism of action	Reduced digitalis effects
Hypokalaemia	Sodium receptor interaction	Hyperkalaemia
Hypercalcemia	Sodium receptor interaction	Hypocalcemia
Hypomagnesia	Sodium receptor interaction	Hypermagnesia
Hypothyreosis	Sodium receptor interaction	Hyperthyreosis
Renal failure	Reduced elimination, electrolyte derangements	
Diuretics, laxatives, diarrhea, emesis	Electrolyte derangements	
	Diminished resorption	Cholestyramine
	Diminished resorption	Neomycin
	Diminished resorption	Sulfasalazine
Erythromycine, tetracycline	Increased resorption	
Quinidine	Diminished renal and nonrenal excretion	
Verapamil, diltiazem, amiodarone	Diminished renal and nonrenal excretion	
	Induction of microsomal enzymes	Phenytoin, rifampin

tality in patients with severe heart failure was suggested by subgroup analysis [3].

Interactions and Adverse Effects

Cardiac glycosides have a small ratio of toxic to therapeutic concentration. Possible adverse effects are nausea, vomiting, abdominal pain, diarrhoea, fatigue, headache, drowsiness, colour vision disturbances, sinus bradycardia, premature ventricular complexes, AV-block, bigeminy, atrial tachycardia with AV-Block, ventricular fibrillation. There are several mechanisms relevant for their toxic action (Table 2).

Digoxin is more rapidly eliminated and thereby, possible adverse or toxic effects last for a shorter time.

References

1. Erdmann E., Greef K. J.C.Skou (1986) Cardiac Glycosides 1785–1985. Steinkopff Verlag Darmstadt, Springer-Verlag NY.
2. Blanco G et al. (1998) Isozymes of the Na^+-K^+-ATPase: heterogeneity in structure, diversity in function. Am J Physiol. Nov 275(5 Pt 2):F633–50
3. Gheorghiade M (1997) Digitalis Investigation Group (DIG) trial: a stimulus for further research. Am Heart J. 134(1):3–12
4. Glitsch HG (2001) Electrophysiology of the sodium-potassium-ATPase in cardiac cells. Physiol Rev. 81(4):1791–826
5. Hauptman PJ, Kelly RA. (1999) Digitalis. Circulation 99(9):1265–70
6. Erdmann (Hrg, 2000) Klinische Kardiologie, Springer-Verlag, 5. Auflage

CART

CART (cocaine- and amphetamine-regulated transcript) is a hypothalamic peptide that inhibits both normal and starvation-induced feeding when injected into cerebral ventricles of rats. CART is co-localized with the anorexigenic peptide α-melanocyte-stimulating hormone in neurons of the arcuate nucleus. Secretion of CART is stimulated by leptin and CART may be an endogenous inhibitor of food intake.

▶ Appetite Control
▶ Psychostimulants

Caspase

Caspases (cystinoaspartic acid specific proteases) are a family of cysteine proteases that cleave the target proteins at aspartic acid residues in the defined cascade sequence. Caspases have been shown to be involved in the classical apoptotic form of cell death, which involves both Stage I and Stage II DNA fragmentation. Of the family of caspases, caspases 3, 6 and 7 are considered effector caspases and caspases 2,8,9 and 10 are activator caspases. For example, caspase 9 increases the diffusion limit of nuclear pores allowing the effector caspase 3 to enter the nucleus by diffusion.

▶ Apoptosis

Catabolism

Catabolism is any metabolic process whereby cells break down complex substances into simpler, smaller substances such as amino acids.

▶ Glucocorticoids

Catecholamines

Catecholamines are biogenic amines with a catechol (o-dihydroxy-benzol) structure. They are synthesized in nerve endings from tyrosine and include ▶ dopamine, noradrenaline (norepinephrine) and ▶ adrenaline (▶ epinephrine).

▶ Norepinephrine/Noradrenalin

Catechol-O-Methyltransferase and its Inhibitors

PEKKA T. MÄNNISTÖ
Department of Pharmacology and Toxicology, University of Kuopio, Kuopio, Finland
Pekka.Mannisto@uku.fi

Synonyms

Abbreviations used: COMTase, COMT, EC 2.1.1.6

Definition

Catechol O-methyltransferase (COMT) is a widespread enzyme that catalyzes the transfer of the methyl group of ▶ S-adenosyl-L-methionine (AdoMet) to one of the phenolic group of the catechol substrate (Fig. 1). High COMT activity is found in the liver, kidney and gut wall. A single *COMT* gene codes for two separate enzymes, soluble (S-COMT) and membrane bound (MB-COMT) forms. S-COMT contains 221 amino acids. MB-COMT has an additional amino-terminal extension of 43 (rat) or 50 (man) amino acids. The

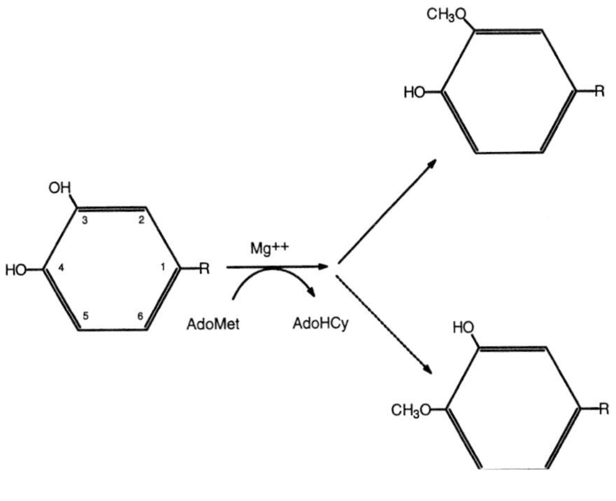

Fig. 1 **The basic function of COMT.** Enzymatic O-methylation of the catechol substrate to 3-methoxy (major route) or 4-methoxy (minor route) products in the presence of Mg^{2+} and S-adenosyl-methionine (AdoMet).

hydrophobic 17 and 24 amino acid residues in rat and man, respectively, form an α-helical transmembrane domain that serves as a membrane anchor; otherwise the two proteins are similar. Synthesis of recombinant S-COMT in *E. coli* and MB-COMT in insect cells, using baculovirus vectors, has helped to clarify the biochemistry, physiology and pharmacology of COMT. The active site of COMT consists of the AdoMet-binding domain and the catalytic site. The catalytic site is formed by a few amino acids that are important for the binding of the substrate, water and Mg^{++}, and for the catalysis of O-methylation. The Mg^{++}, which is bound to COMT only after AdoMet binding, improves the ionization of the hydroxyl groups. The lysine residue (Lys144), which accepts the proton of one of the hydroxyls, acts as a general catalytic base in the nucleophilic methyl transfer reaction.

▶ **α-Adrenergic System**
▶ **β-Adrenergic System**
▶ **Synaptic Transmission**

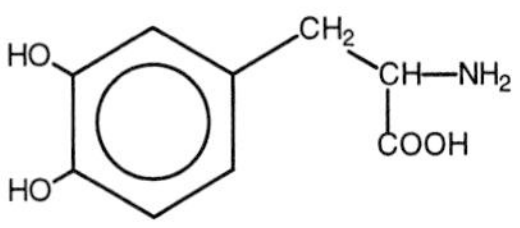

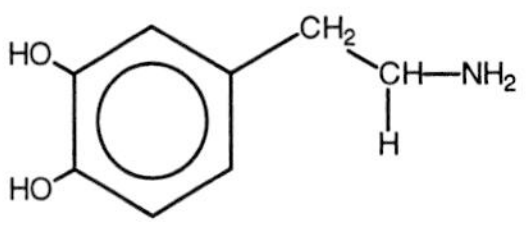

Fig. 2 Some substrates of COMT.

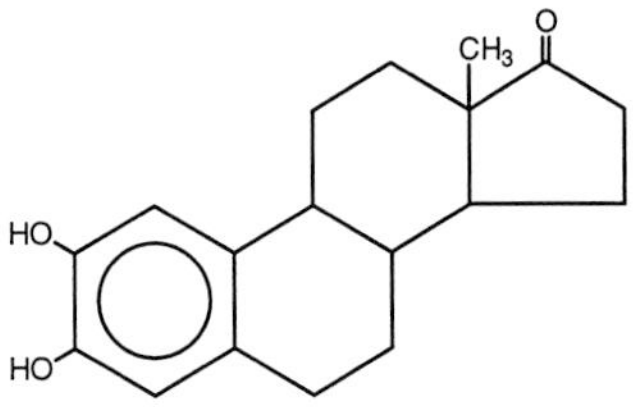

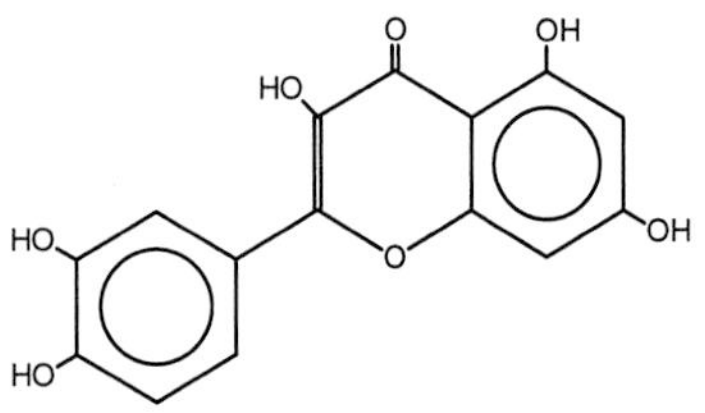

Mechanism of Action

COMT O-methylates ▶ catecholamines and other compounds having a catechol structure including catecholestrogens (Fig. 2). The two isoforms of COMT may have distinct roles: MB-COMT, a high-affinity isoform of COMT, is supposed to be partially responsible for the termination of dopaminergic and noradrenergic synaptic neurotransmission. S-COMT, on the other hand, is a high capacity enzyme isoform being mainly responsible for the elimination of biologically active or toxic, particularly exogenous, catechols and some hydroxylated metabolites. During the first trimester of pregnancy, COMT present in the placenta protects the developing embryo from hydroxylated compounds. COMT also acts as an enzymatic detoxicating barrier between the blood and other tissues, shielding against the detrimental effects of hydroxylated xenobiotics. COMT may serve some unique or indirect functions in the kidney and intestine tract by modulating the dopaminergic tone. The same may be true in the brain: COMT activity may regulate the amounts of active dopamine and noradrenaline in various part of the brain and therefore be associated with mood and other mental processes.

Early COMT inhibitors, like gallates, tropolone and U-0521 (3',4'-dihydroxy-2- methyl-propiophenone) have ▶ IC_{50} and ▶ K_i values in the micromolar range or higher but may still be practical *in vitro* tools. However, owing to unfavourable ▶ pharmacokinetics and toxicity their clinical use is not possible.

Second generation COMT inhibitors were developed by three laboratories in the late 1980s. Apart from CGP 28014, nitrocatechol is the key structure of the majority of these molecules (Fig. 3). The current COMT inhibitors can be classified as follows: 1) mainly peripherally-acting nitrocatechol-type compounds (entacapone, nitecapone, BIA 3-202), 2) broad-spectrum nitrocatechols having activity both in peripheral tissues and the brain (tolcapone, Ro 41-0960, vinylphenylketone), and 3) atypical compounds, pyridine derivatives (CGP 28014, 3-hydroxy-4-pyridone and its derivatives), some of which are not COMT inhibitors *in vitro* but inhibit catechol O-methylation by some other mechanism. The common features of the most new compounds are excellent

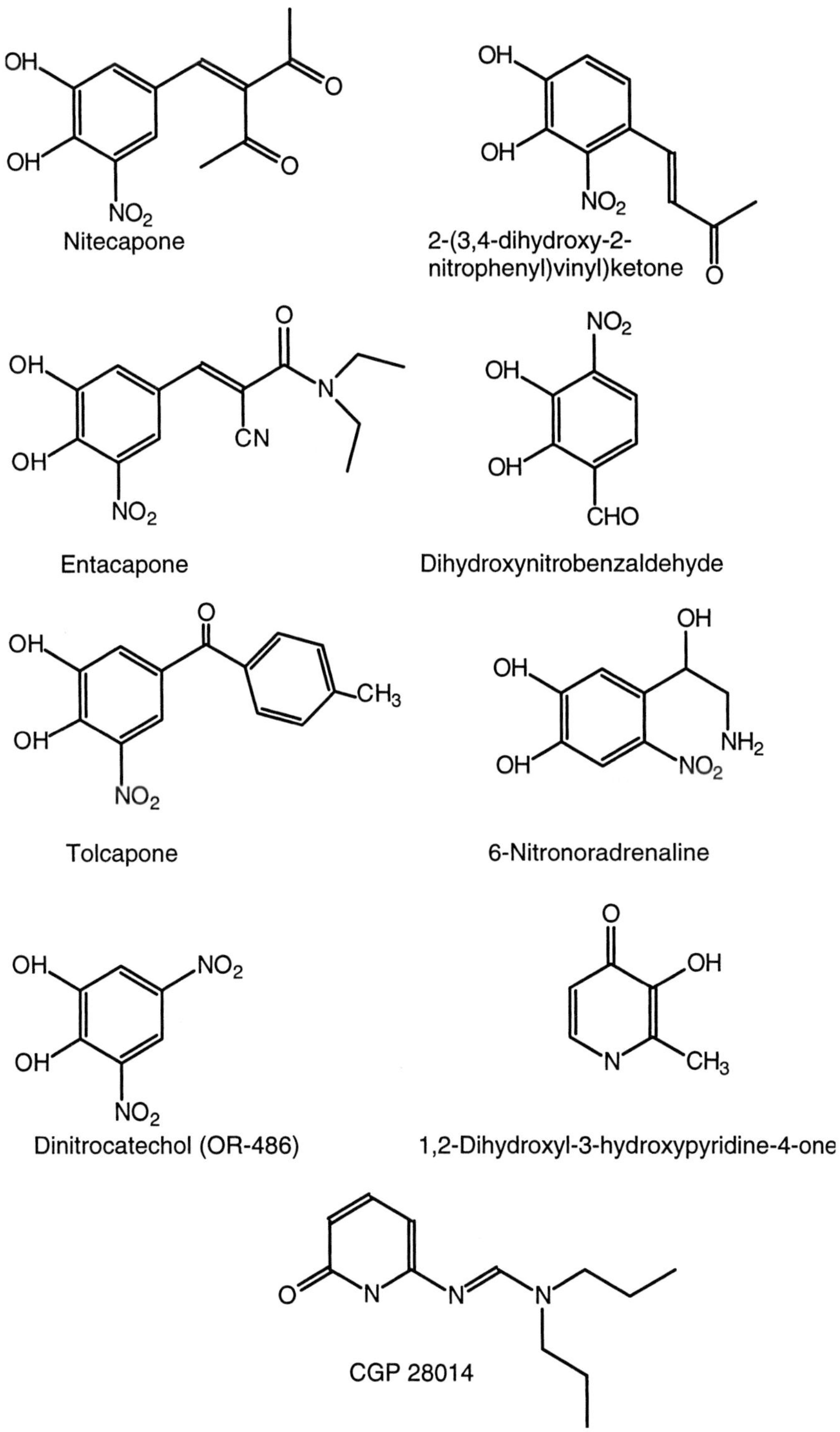

Nitecapone

2-(3,4-dihydroxy-2-nitrophenyl)vinyl)ketone

Entacapone

Dihydroxynitrobenzaldehyde

Tolcapone

6-Nitronoradrenaline

Dinitrocatechol (OR-486)

1,2-Dihydroxyl-3-hydroxypyridine-4-one

CGP 28014

Fig. 3 Chemical structures of some inhibitors of catechol O-methylation.

potency, low toxicity and activity through oral administration. Their biochemical properties have been fairly well characterized. Most of these com-pounds have an excellent selectivity in that they do not affect any other enzymes studied.

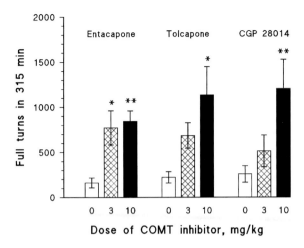

Fig. 4 Rat model of Parkinson's disease. Comparison of entacapone, tolcapone and CGP 28014 in the rat turning model of Parkinson's disease.
Statistics: * P < 0.05 and ** P < 0.01 vs. corresponding controls (data from reference 6).

Tolcapone and Ro 41-0960 are longer acting than entacapone and nitecapone in *in vivo* studies in rats. All types of COMT inhibitors prolong the L-dopa-induced turning behaviour of rats having unilateral nigral lesions (Fig. 4). This has generally been used as a reliable rat model of ▶ **Parkinson's disease**. It is noteworthy that the peripherally-acting compound entacapone is practically as effective as the broad-spectrum compound tolcapone. This suggest that the majority of the beneficial action is peripheral in origin, evidently through enhanced ▶ **bioavailability** of L-dopa.

Clinical Use (incl. side effects)

The main clinical use of COMT inhibitors is as adjunct (or additional adjunct) in the therapy of Parkinson's disease. The standard therapy of Parkinson's disease is oral L-dopa (as a drug ▶ **levodopa**) given with a ▶ **dopa decarboxylase** (DDC) inhibitor (e.g., carbidopa and benserazide), which does not reach the brain. When the peripheral DDC is inhibited, the concentration of 3-O-methyldopa (3-OMD), a product of COMT, in plasma is many times that of L-dopa. Since the ▶ **half-life** of 3-OMD is about 15 h, compared to about 1 h for L-dopa, the concentration of 3-OMD

remains particularly high during chronic therapy, especially if new slow release L-dopa preparations are used. A triple therapy (L-dopa plus DDC inhibitor plus COMT-inhibitor) will evidently substitute the present double therapy in the coming years.

COMT inhibitors rescue ▶ **L-dopa** and improve the brain entry of L-dopa by decreasing 3-OMD formation in peripheral tissues. The dose of L-dopa could be decreased, compared to the present combination therapy. Dose interval of L-dopa could also be prolonged. Further, COMT inhibitors should decrease fluctuations of dopamine formation in the brain.

Clinical studies, available only for entacapone and tolcapone, support preclinical findings. A dose-dependent (100–800 mg) inhibition of the COMT activity of the erythrocytes can be seen after nitrocatechols. However, effective and sufficient dose levels of both entacapone and tolcapone, given concomitantly with L-dopa and DDC inhibitors to patients with Parkinson's disease, appear to be 100–200 mg. However, the treatment strategies of entacapone and tolcapone differ: entacapone is a short-acting compound that is given with each dose of L-dopa, and COMT activity may even recover between the doses. Tolcapone, as a longer-acting compound, is given three times a day, and the aim is keep COMT inhibited most of the time.

Since several ▶ **adrenergic drugs**, having a catechol structure, are also COMT substrates, it is possible to prolong or even potentiate in some cases their actions by COMT inhibitors. Such drugs include bronchodilating compounds (adrenaline, isoprenaline, rimiterol), dopamine agonists (dobutamide, fenoldopam, apomorphine) and antihypertensive drugs (α-methyldopa). It is possible to potentiate interactions with endogenous catecholamines during stress and exercise and adverse drug interactions with, e.g., exogenous ▶ **noradrenaline** and the drugs mentioned above. Fortunately, interaction studies in animals and man have not been able to substantiate this threat. Evidently, the capacity of S-COMT in the peripheral tissues is so high that only a minor general COMT inhibition can ever been achieved. ▶ **Estrogens** are easily hydroxylated to catecholestrogens, which serve as COMT substrates. The consequences of preventing the major metabolic pathway of catecholestrogens by COMT inhibitors requires further studies; it is possible that quinone-forming pathways are activated.

In patients having Parkinson's disease, both entacapone and tolcapone potentiate the therapeutic effect of L-dopa and prolong the daily ON time by 1–2 h. In the clinic COMT inhibitors have been well tolerated, and the number of premature terminations has been low. In general, the incidence of adverse events has been higher in tolcapone-treated patients than in entacapone-treated patients. The main events have comprised of dopaminergic and gastrointestinal problems.

Dopaminergic overactivity causes an initial worsening of levodopa-induced ▶ dyskinesia, nausea, vomiting, orthostatic hypotension, sleep disorders and hallucinations. Tolcapone has been associated with diarrhoea in about 16–18% of cases and entacapone in less than 10% of cases. Diarrhoea has led to discontinuation in 5–6% of patients on tolcapone and in 2.5% of those on entacapone. Urine discolouration to dark yellow or orange is related to the colour of COMT inhibitors and their metabolites. Elevated liver transaminase levels are reported in 1–3% of patients treated with tolcapone but very rarely, if at all, in patients treated with entacapone. Three cases of acute, fatal fulminant ▶ hepatitis have been described in association of tolcapone where more than 100,000 patients have been treated. In addition, a few potentially fatal neurological adverse reactions, including ▶ neuroleptic-like malignant syndrome, have described. Because of these serious adverse drug reactions, tolcapone marketing was suspended in Europe and Canada in 1999. In early 2003, no restrictions of the use of entacapone have been proposed.

Use of COMT Inhibitors in Positron Emission Tomography (PET)

An additional benefit of COMT inhibitors can be found in PET studies. In PET, using 6-[^{18}F]-fluoro-L-dopa (6-FD) to visualize the brain dopamine metabolism, the peripheral formation of 3-O-methyl-6-[^{18}F]-fluoro-L-dopa (3-OMFD) by COMT is harmful. 3-OMFD contaminates the brain radioactivity analyzed since it, like 3-OMD, is easily transported to the brain. COMT inhibition would reduce the formation of 3-OMFD and improve PET analysis. Since 3-OMFD formation continues in the brain, central COMT inhibition may be assumed to offer a further advantage.

References

1. Guldberg HC, Marsden CA (1975) Catechol-O-methyl transferase: pharmacological aspects and physiological role. Pharmacol Rev 27:135–206
2. Männistö PT, Ulmanen I, Taskinen J, Kaakkola S (1993). Catechol O-methyltransferase (COMT) and COMT inhibitors (Ch. 12). In: Sandler M, Smith HJ (eds) Design of Enzyme Inhibitors as Drugs. vol 2. Oxford University Press, Oxford, pp.623–646
3. Männistö PT, Kaakkola S (1989) New selective COMT inhibitors: Useful adjuncts for Parkinson's disease? Trends Pharmacol Sci 10:54–56
4. Männistö PT, Kaakkola S (1999) Catechol-O-methyltransferase (COMT). Biochemistry, molecular biology, pharmacology, and clinical efficacy of the new selective COMT inhibitors. Pharmacol Rev 51:593–628
5. Guttman M, Leger G, Reches A, Evans A, Kuwabara H, Cederbaum JM, Gjedde A (1993) Administration of the new COMT inhibitor OR-611 increases striatal uptake of fluorodopa. Movement Disord 8:298–304
6. Törnwall M, Männistö PT (1993) The effect of three types of COMT inhibitors on L-dopa-induced circling behaviour in rats. Eur J Pharmacol 250:77–84

Cathepsins

Cathepsins are intracellular proteinases that reside within lysosomes or specific intracellular granules. Cathepsins are used to degrade proteins or peptides that are internalised from the extracellular space. Some cathepsins such as cathepsin-G or cathepsin-K may be released from the cell to degrade specific extracellular matrix proteins. All cathepsins except cathepsin-G (serine) and cathepsin-D (aspartyl) are cysteine proteinases.

▶ Non-viral Proteases

Causalgia

Causalgia is burning pain evoked by the activation of sympathetic efferent fibers. The likely mechanism underlying this syndrome involves ectopic expression of α-adrenoceptors on nociceptive afferents following peripheral injury or disease.

▶ Nociception

Caveolae

Caveolae are invaginations of the plasma membrane. They contain the protein caveolin and are rich in certain phospholipids. Similar to coated pits, they bud off internally forming endocytic vesicles. Caveolae play an important role in the internalization of certain cell surface receptors.

CCK

▶ Cholecystokinin
▶ Appetite Control

CD26

CD26 is a synonym for ▶ Dipeptidylpeptidase IV.

cdk

Cdk stands for cyclin-dependent kinase

▶ Cell-cycle Control

Cell Adhesion Molecule

Integrins, selectins, cadherins and other cell adhesion molecules are involved in the interaction of cells with other cells or with extracellular matrix proteins. Most of them also serve as "receptors" by inducing outside-in or additional inside-out signalling.

▶ Anti-integrins, therapeutic and diagnostic implications
▶ Cadherins/Catenins

Cell-cycle Arrest

Cell-cycle arrest is the status of a cell population in which progression through the cell division cycle has been halted as a result of checkpoint activation.

▶ Cell-cycle Control

Cell-cycle Checkpoints

Cell-cycle checkpoints are mechanisms which control cell-cycle transitions. They are signal transduction pathways comprising a sensor detecting cellular damage or improper cell-cycle transition, a signal transduction cascade for amplifying the signal generated by the sensor and a target which initiates gene transcription leading to cell-cycle arrest, initiation of repair programs or apoptosis. Alternatively, the target can induce cell-cycle arrest directly. One distinguishes DNA replication, DNA damage and spindle assembly checkpoints.

▶ Cell-cycle Control

Cell-cycle Control

Holger Bastians, Rolf Müller
Institute of Molecular Biology and Tumor
Research (IMT), Philipps-University Marburg,
Germany
bastians@imt.uni-marburg.de,
mueller@imt.uni-marburg.de

Synonyms

Cell division cycle, cell proliferation, cell multiplication

Definition

The eukaryotic somatic cell cycle is defined by a sequential order of events that are obligatory for ordered cell division: the cell must grow, replicate its DNA, segregate its chromosomes, and finally divide. The cell cycle can be divided into four discrete phases. ▶ DNA replication is restricted to S phase (DNA synthesis phase) and is preceded by a gap phase called G_1 and followed by a gap phase called G_2. During ▶ mitosis (M phase) the sister chromatids are segregated into two new daughter nuclei and mitosis is completed by the division of the cytoplasm, a process termed ▶ cytokinesis (Fig. 1).

▶ Ubiquitin/Proteasome System

Basic Mechanisms

Upon mitogenic stimulation cells can enter the cell cycle which lasts, in the case of a typical human cell, about 20–50 hours. During a single cell cycle a cell accomplishes growth, DNA replication, chromosome segregation and cell division, of which chromosome segregation during mitosis takes only about 30 minutes. How a cell regulates the cell cycle and how tumor cells can override these regulatory mechanisms is only partly understood and still subject of intense research. However, it has become clear in recent years that the basic mechanisms mediating cell-cycle control are remarkably conserved throughout evolution involving:

a) reversible protein phosphorylation
b) regulated ubiquitin dependent protein degradation
c) transcriptional control mechanisms
d) regulation by CDK inhibitors
e) checkpoint control mechanisms

Cell-cycle Regulation by Protein Phosphorylation

The early discovery of a dominant activity designated as the "mitosis (or maturation) promoting factor" (MPF) that drives interphase cells into mitosis led to the idea that certain oscillating activities are responsible for the initiation of mitosis and for driving the different phases of the cell cycle. Biochemical purification of MPF from sea urchin eggs, frog eggs and mammalian cells as well as a large number of genetic experiments in *Saccharomyces cerevisiae* and *Schizosaccharomyces pombe* using the "cell division cycle (cdc) mutants" revealed that MPF represents a heterodimeric protein kinase consisting of a catalytic subunit, a cyclin dependent kinase (CDK1, cdc2 or $p34^{cdc2}$), and a positive regulatory subunit, termed cyclin B (1). The CDK1-cyclin B kinase represents the key trigger for entry into mitosis. In G_2 cyclin B binds to CDK1, thus forming a pre-activated kinase complex. This complex is immediately inactivated by reversible phosphorylation of the CDK1 moiety at residues threonine-14 and tyrosine-15 (in mammals) by the protein kinases Myt1 and Wee1, respectively. This inactive phosphorylated CDK1-cyclin B complex is called the pre-MPF and can be activated just prior to mitosis by removing both inhibitory phosphorylations by the action of the dual specificity phosphatase Cdc25C (Fig. 2). The inactivating kinases Myt1 and Wee1 as well as the activating phosphatase Cdc25C are themselves part of a complex regulatory network involving other important upstream kinases and phosphatases including different MAP kinase pathways. The activated CDK1-cyclin B kinase finally phosphorylates a large number of proteins, thus effecting the hallmarks of mitosis: chromosome condensation, nuclear envelope breakdown, spindle assembly and chromosome segregation (1).

Meanwhile at least ten different CDKs and at least ten different cyclins are known, and most members of these protein families play important roles at different cell-cycle transitions (Fig. 1, also

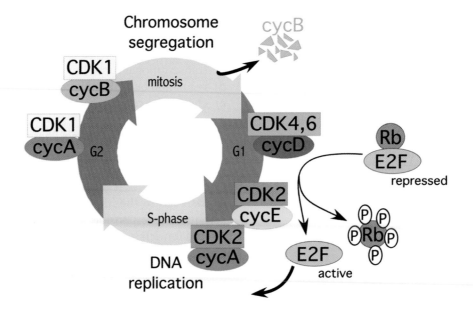

Fig. 1 Basic regulation of the cell cycle. The key regulators of the eukaryotic cell cycle are the cyclin-dependent kinases (CDKs), which consists of a catalytic (CDK) and a regulatory (cyclin) subunit. Different CDK complexes function at different transitions of the cell cycle. In G1 phase, cyclin D- and cyclin E-containing kinases phosphorylate the Rb protein, which releases active E2F transcription factor leading to the transcription of S phase genes required for entry into S phase.

see below). CDKs can be seen as the key players in cell-cycle regulation. Each CDK acts as a specific kinase at different cell-cycle transition points. However, many of the relevant target proteins remain to be defined.

Cell-cycle Regulation by Ubiquitin-mediated Protein Degradation

Cyclins are positive regulatory subunits of CDKs. They represent a family of oscillating proteins that are able to bind to and activate specific CDKs in a cell cycle phase-dependent manner. Each cyclin has certain specificities to activate particular CDKs. The expression of most cyclins is strictly regulated in a phase-specific fashion. The oscillating protein concentrations result from regulatory events at the level of transcription, translation, mRNA stability and in particular protein stability. The cyclin B gene is transcriptionally down-regulated during G_1 phase and becomes activated during S and G_2. Cyclin B protein accumulates continuously throughout S and G_2 phase, binds and activates CDK1 in late G_2 and during the early stages

of mitosis (Fig. 2). Once metaphase to anaphase transition is achieved, cyclin B levels drop dramatically leading to an irreversible inactivation of CDK1 which is required for exit from mitosis. This decrease in cyclin B levels after metaphase to anaphase transition is due to regulated ubiquitin-mediated protein degradation by the 26S proteasome. The ubiquitination of cyclin B, as a prerequisite for its degradation, requires three enzymatic activities: an ubiquitin-activating enzyme (E1), an ubiquitin-conjugating enzyme (E2) and an ubiquitin ligase activity (E3). The latter two provide the substrate specificity of the ubiquitin pathway. While the activity of E1, E2 and the proteasome are not cell-cycle regulated, the activity of the E3 ligase is the cell-cycle regulated component restricting ubiquitination of cyclin B to the M/G_1 phase of the cell cycle. For cyclin B, the ligase activity is part of a large 20S complex that is termed the anaphase-promoting complex or cyclosome (APC/C). Interestingly, the inactivation of the APC/C leads not only to the stabilization of mitotic cyclins but also to the stabilization of vari-

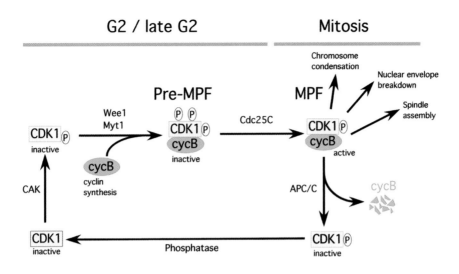

G2 / late G2   **Mitosis**

Fig. 2 Regulation of MPF by reversible phosphorylation. In late G2, CDK1 is phosphorylated by a CDK-activating kinase (CAK), followed by the binding of cyclin B. A pre-formed MPF complex is kept inactive by two inhibitory phosphorylations carried out the Wee1 and Myt1 kinases. Just prior to mitosis, MPF is activated through dephosphorylation of CDK1 by Cdc25C leading to different mitotic events. After anaphase, MPF is inactivated by APC/C-mediated ubiquitin-dependent proteolysis allowing exit from mitosis.

ous other mitotic target proteins, including proteins regulating spindle structure and sister chromatid separation during anaphase (2).

In addition to protein proteolysis during mitosis, ▶ ubiquitin-mediated protein degradation is also required at the G_1 to S transition and during S phase. An ubiquitin ligase complex termed SCF (Skp1-Cdc53-F box protein), which is distinct but related to APC/C, ubiquitinates several substrate proteins including the CDK inhibitor $p27^{Kip1}$, cyclin E and the transcription factor E2F-1. SCF-mediated ubiquitination is essential for proper G_1 to S transition (2). It is thus clear that ubiquitin-mediated protein degradation is an important regulatory mechanism throughout the cell cycle for an irreversible inactivation of various cell-cycle regulators, including cyclins, mitotic regulators, CDK inhibitors and transcription factors.

G_1/S Transition, DNA Replication and Transcriptional Control

Although mitogenic growth factors are required for cells to enter the cell cycle, their presence is no longer required for completion of the cell cycle once the cell has progressed beyond a certain stage in late G_1 – the restriction point, when the cell

becomes committed to enter S-phase. This transition is, at least in part, driven by G_1 cyclins activating various CDKs (1). When cells enter the cell cycle from quiescence (G_0), D-type cyclins (D1, D2, D3), cyclin E and cyclin A are synthesized sequentially. Cyclins A and E activate preferentially CDK2, whereas D type cyclins activate CDK4 and CDK6 (Fig. 1). Several of the regulatory principles described for CDK1-cyclin B in G_2/M also apply to the cyclin-CDK complexes functioning at the G_1/S transition. For example, activation of cyclin A/E-CDK2 and cyclin D-CDK4/6 complexes are subject to two inhibitory phosphorylations that are removed around the G_1/S transition by the cdc25C-related cdc25A phosphatase.

When cells enter the cell cycle cyclin D-dependent CDK4 and CDK6 activity is first detected in mid-G_1 phase and increases when cells approach the G_1/S transition. The best understood function of cyclin D-CDK complexes is phosphorylation of the retinoblastoma protein (Rb). Rb functions as a transcriptional repressor of the E2F family of DNA-binding transcription factors (E2F). E2F binding sites are found in the promoters of many genes that are important for DNA replication and therefore for initiation of, and progression through, S phase (e.g. cyclin E, DNA polymerase α, dihydrofolate reductase, thymidine kinase, thymidylate synthase). In early to mid-G_1 phase Rb is hypophosphorylated and bound to E2F, thereby repressing its transcriptional activity and inhibiting entry into S phase (3). When G_1 phase progresses, cyclin D-dependent CDK activity increases, followed by an induction of cyclin E-dependent kinase activity. Both kinases act in concert to effect the hyperphosphorylation of Rb. The phosphorylated form of Rb can no longer bind to E2F and its transcriptional activity is restored. This leads to the activation of E2F target genes allowing initiation of S phase (3, Fig. 1). Later in S-phase, E2F activity is down-regulated by phosphorylation mediated by cyclin A-CDK2 complexes, and transcription of E2F target genes required for G_1/S transition is turned off.

During S phase the genome must be replicated completely and reliably and only once per cell cycle in order to maintain genomic integrity. Genomic DNA in eukaryotes is organized into multiple chromosomes and replication initiates from multiple origins on these chromosomes. Replication initiates at specific DNA sequences, referred to as autonomously replicating sequences (ARS). According to a current model, a chromatin-associated pre-replication complex including the CDC6, ORC and MCM proteins is formed during G_1 phase. Upon entry into S phase the pre-replication complex is rearranged, chain elongation factors are recruited and replication forks are established. DNA replication induces the dissociation of MCM proteins from chromatin and their reloading onto chromatin during S-phase progression is blocked by CDK2 activity, thereby preventing a second round of replication from the same origin (1).

G_1 Control by CDK Inhibitors

The activity of cyclin-CDK complexes is controlled by a family of negative cell-cycle regulators, termed CDK inhibitors (CKIs). CKIs are small proteins that can be subdivided into two distinct groups: the INK4 proteins (inhibitors of CDK4) include p16[INK4a], p15[INK4b], p18[INK4c] and p19[INK4d], which specifically bind to and inactivate the catalytic subunit of CDK4 and CKD6 (4). The second group of CKIs comprises the Kip/Cip family of CDK inhibitors including p27[Kip1], p21[Cip1] and

p57[Kip2] that display a broader range of substrate specificity.

The signals that lead to induction of synthesis of the INK4 proteins are only partly understood. The ability of TGF-β to induce a cell-cycle arrest in G_1 is, at least in part, brought about by the induction of p15[INK4b], a consequence of the TGF-β-mediated inhibition of Myc recruitment to the p15 promoter. p16[INK4a] in turn accumulates during the ▶ senescence-associated G_1 arrest, and p18[INK4c] and p19[INK4d] may have functions during terminal differentiation (4).

Kip/Cip proteins are induced by signals resulting from cellular damage, metabolic dysfunctions or other stress that makes it necessary for the cell to halt cell-cycle progression. The best studies example in this context is the transcriptional activation of the p21[Cip1] gene by p53 (see below). p53-induced p21[Cip1] binds directly to cyclin A- and cyclin E-CDK2 and inhibits their activity leading to an inhibition of G_1/S transition (4).

Another quite different function of Kip/Cip proteins has been recognized in a different scenario. Kip/Cip proteins are instrumental for the ability of INK4 proteins to induce a G_1 arrest. In this setting the Kip/Cip proteins do not act as CDK inhibitors, but facilitate the formation of cyclin D-CDK4/6 complexes. This leads to the sequestration of the Kip/Cip protein in ternary cyclin CDK – CKI complexes, thus preventing the Kip/Cip proteins from inhibiting cyclin E and cyclin A containing kinases . Upregulation of INK4 proteins is followed by their binding to CDK4/6 kinases, inhibition of their activity and competition with the pre-bound Kip/Cip proteins. This results in a release of Kip/Cip inhibitors that then inhibit cyclin E and cyclin A kinases. The inactivated cyclin D-CDK4/6 kinase can no longer phosphorylate Rb and hypophosphorylated Rb inhibits E2F activity which is essential for entry into S phase.

There is a growing body of evidence suggesting that CKIs exert an essential role as tumor suppressor proteins in human cells. Disruption of p16[INK4a] is a common event in human cancer and low levels of p27[Kip1] caused by enhanced protein degradation appear to be associated with poor prognosis. This is also underscored by observations made with heterozygous p27[Kip1] knockout mice which show a haplo-insufficiency for tumor suppression.

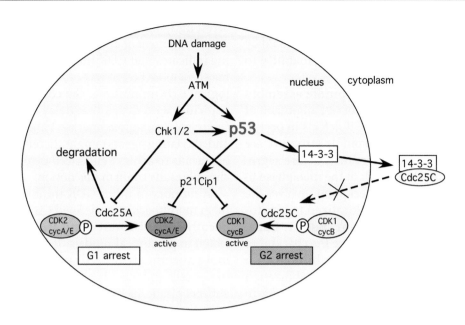

Fig. 3 Checkpoint control of the cell cycle upon DNA damage. After detection of DNA damage a kinase cascade including the ATM and Chk1 and Chk2 kinases are activated leading to the phosphorylation of p53 at multiple sites. These phosphorylations induce the labile protein to accumulate and activate its function as a transcription factor (e.g. by the recruitment of transcriptional co-activators). A large number of proteins including p21Cip1 and 14-3-3 are induced resulting in cell-cycle arrest at G1 or G2 phases.

Checkpoint Control of the Cell Cycle

The survival and integrity of cells is dependent on their ability to transmit the genetic information faithfully into two daughter cells, which involves the completion of DNA replication during S phase, the integrity of the genome during DNA replication and the equal distribution of the chromatids during mitosis. The cell has therefore installed checkpoints at different stages of the cell cycle that can halt cell-cycle progression in case of, for instance, incomplete DNA replication, DNA damage or mitotic spindle damage. The best known example is a checkpoint activated upon DNA damage (5) that is, at least in part, dependent on the tumor suppressor protein p53 (Fig. 3). After exposure to DNA damaging agents, cells activate a stress signaling pathway leading to the activation of the ATM kinase. As a result, the checkpoint kinases Chk1 and Chk2 are phosphorylated and activated. Both, Chk and ATM kinases are able to phosphorylate the transcription factor p53 leading to its cellular accumulation and activation. p53

activates a large number of target genes including p21^{Cip1}, which is instrumental in halting the cell cycle at both the G$_1$/S and the G$_2$/M transition by inactivating CDK2 and CDK1 kinases, respectively. p53 also induces the transcription of DNA repair genes and genes responsible for the induction of ▶ **apoptosis**. The latter guarantees that a damaged cell will choose to die rather than transmitting mutated DNA onto the next generation. p53 plays an essential role as a genomic guardian which is, for example, illustrated by the failure of cells lacking functional p53 to undergo cell-cycle arrest or apoptosis upon DNA damage (5).

The activation of ATM and Chk kinases also results in a p53 independent cell-cycle arrest at G$_2$/M by directly phosphorylating and inactivating the dual specificity phosphatase Cdc25C. The phosphorylated Cdc25C phosphatase is bound by 14-3-3 proteins and thereby sequestered into the cytoplasm (Fig. 3). As a result Cdc25C is unable to dephosphorylate and activate CDK1 at G$_2$/M, thus causing a cell-cycle arrest prior to mitosis.

Similarly, phosphorylation of Cdc25A upon DNA damage leads to its inactivation mediated by protein degradation resulting in an inability to enter S phase (Fig. 3).

By activating the mitotic spindle assembly checkpoint, cells monitor the correct alignment of chromosomes during mitosis. If defects in proper chromosome alignment or spindle structure are detected cells will arrest in mitosis before segregating their sister chromatids at the metaphase to anaphase transition. This checkpoint involves the function of several proteins localized to kinetochores (e.g. Mad1, Mad2, Bub1, BubR1, Bub3, Cenp-E in mammalian cells). Once the checkpoint is activated, APC/C activity is inhibited by a poorly defined pathway, leading to a stabilization of anaphase inhibitors and cyclin B and thereby to a mitotic arrest prior to anaphase.

Pharmacological Intervention

A hallmark of cancer is the loss of cell-cycle control due to unconstrained CDK activities. A promising therapeutic strategy is, therefore, the inactivation of CDK activities by small molecule drugs (6). Prolonged cell-cycle arrest results in induction of apoptosis and elimination of tumor cells.

In addition, cell-cycle checkpoints can be targeted by anticancer drugs (6). Cells damaged by genotoxic agents or spindle poisons activate one or more checkpoints and halt the cell cycle until the damage is repaired. When these checkpoints are compromised, cells enter mitosis or S phase inappropriately prior to repair of the genotoxic damage leading to cell death. Drugs abrogating cell-cycle checkpoints may therefore be able to sensitize cells to chemotherapy and radiation.

Pharmacological CDK Inhibitors
A prototype CDK inhibitor currently in clinical trials is flavopiridol (6). Flavopiridol specifically inhibits the activity of all known CDKs and arrests cells at G_1/S, S and G_2/M, followed by the induction of apoptosis. Flavopiridol is tolerated by most patients relatively well but its anti-tumor effects have been rather modest when used in a monotherapeutic setting. In some tumor cell lines, flavopiridol treatment does not lead to G_1 arrest but induces a delay in S phase followed by more efficient apoptosis. Thus, it appears that failure to

arrest in G_1 in response to CDK inhibitors result in an enhancement of apoptotic responses. This finding indicates that CDK inhibition during S phase may be a more potent way of action for pharmacological CDK inhibitors. The combination of flavopiridol with drugs that delay S-phase transit (e.g. cisplatin, topoisomerase I and II inhibitors, and alkylating agents) might therefore be a suitable means to achieve enhanced cytotoxicity. First clinical results confirm this notion.

A number of other CDK inhibitors, many of them more specific for defined CDKs, have subsequently been discovered and are currently being tested in preclinical models. It is hoped that that more specific drugs will preferentially affect tumor cells and thus show improved efficiencies as anti-neoplastic agents.

Pharmacological Checkpoint Abrogation
The induction of cell-cycle transition in the presence of genomic or spindle damage is one of the most promising new approaches in anti-tumor drug development. In tumor cells, the introduction of DNA damage by genotoxic agents leads to the activation of the DNA damage checkpoint and a cell-cycle block in G_1 and G_2. Overriding the arrest and inappropriate induction of S phase and mitosis, respectively, can result in cell death. Thus, drugs abrogating checkpoint control might sensitize cells to chemotherapy and radiation. One prime target in this context is the ATM kinase, which is activated upon DNA damage and is essential for p53-dependent and independent responses to DNA damage. The inactivation of ATM by methylxanthine-derived drugs (e.g. caffeine and pentoxifylline) indeed leads to inappropriate entry into S phase and mitosis after DNA damage (Fig. 3), but the pharmacological side effects of these compounds limit their use in patients. Another drug, UCN-01, has been shown to compromise DNA damage checkpoints by inactivating the Chk1 kinase, thereby inducing entry into mitosis in the presence of DNA damage (Fig. 3) (6).

The spindle assembly checkpoint is another potentially interesting target with respect to chemosensitization. Chemotherapeutic agents like taxol activate this checkpoint by damaging the mitotic spindle, which might be counter-intuitive in a therapeutic setting. It will be intriguing to design small molecule drugs that inactivate the spindle checkpoint. It is anticipated that these drugs might induce an inappropriate exit from mitosis followed by apoptosis. However, the pathways and mechanisms of spindle assembly checkpoint regulation are only partly understood. It is therefore of paramount importance to identify the crucial components of this checkpoint machinery which are likely to provide new promising targets of future cancer therapy.

References

1. Murray A, Hunt T (1993). The cell cycle – an introduction. Oxford University Press, Oxford.
2. Koepp DM, Harper JW, Elledge SJ (1999). How the cyclin became a cyclin: regulated proteolysis in the cell cycle. Cell 97:431–434
3. Harbour JW, Dean DC (2000). The Rb/E2F pathway: expanding roles and emerging paradigms. Genes and Development 14:2393–2409
4. Sherr CJ, Roberts JM (1999). CDK inhibitors: positive and negative regulators of G_1-phase progression. Genes and Development 13:1501–1512
5. Zhou BB, Elledge SJ (2000). The DNA damage response: putting checkpoints in perspective. Nature 408:433–439
6. Shapiro GI, Harper JW (1999). Anticancer drug targets: cell cycle and checkpoint control. Journal of Clinical Investigation 104:1645–1653

Cellular Immmunity

In a strict sense the term cellular immunity describes the T-lymphocyte mediated arm of adaptive immunity. T-lymphocytes recognize antigens in form of peptides presented by cells on major histocomaptibility antigens (MHC molecules) indicating the phagocytosis of bacteria (presentation of antigen on MHC class II) or infection of a cell by a virus (presentation on MHC class I). T-lymphocytes become activated and clonally expand to become T- helper cells which can induce an inflammatory response *via* soluble mediators (cytokines), which can activate the phagocytic system or induce specific antibody production. Alternatively, T-helper cells can acti-

vate cytotoxic T cells, which kill virus infected cells or tumor cells.

▶ Immune Defense

Central Diabetes Insipidus

In central diabetes insipidus a hypophysial malfunction, caused by different diseases as well as head injuries, neurosurgery, or genetic disorders, leads toarginine vasopressin (AVP) hyposecretion. This type of ▶ diabetes insipidus can successfully be treated by the exogenous administration of AVP or an AVP analogues (desmopressin).

▶ Vasopressin/Oxytocin

Centrosome

Centrosomes, also called the microtubule organizing center, are protein complexes which contain 2 centrioles (ringlike structures) and γ tubulin. They serve as nucleation points for microtubular polymerisation and constrain the lattice structure of a microtubule to 13 protofilaments.

▶ Cytoskeleton

Cephalosporins

Like penicillins, cephalosporins are β-lactam antibiotics and interfere with bacterial cell wall synthesis. A very large number of cephalosporins are available for clinical use. They differ in their route of administration and clinical use.

▶ β-lactam Antibiotics

CFTR

CFTR, the Cystic Fibrosis Transmembrane Conductance Regulator, is the only member of the large ABC transporter gene family that is known to function as an ion channel. Its 'ATP Binding Cassettes' are thought to regulate the opening and closing of the pore, rather than provide energy (by ATP hydrolysis) for active transport. Another important mechanism of regulation is provided by cyclic AMP (cAMP)-dependent phosphorylation of residues in the intracellular 'R-domain'. This renders CFTR into a cAMP-activated chloride channel.

CFTR has a single-channel conductance of about 8 pS. It is present in the apical membranes of many epithelia. Its mutation leads to the potentially lethal disease cystic fibrosis. In addition to acting as a chloride channel, CFTR is also thought to regulate e.g. the epithelial sodium channel ENaC, a molecularly unknown outwardly-rectifying chloride channel, and possibly also potassium channels and water channels. Some of these potential regulatory processes, however, are controversial. CFTR also acts as a receptor for bacteria.

▶ Cl⁻ Channels

CG

▶ Chorionic Gonadotropin
▶ Epithelial Na⁺ Channel

cGK

▶ cAMP- and cGMP-dependent Protein Kinases

cGMP

▶ GMP, cyclic
▶ Guanylyl Cyclase

cGMP Kinase

Cyclic GMP(cGMP)-dependent protein kinase is encoded by two genes that encode for cGMP kinase Iα and Iβ and cGMP kinase II. cGMP kinase Iα and Iβ are isozymes that differ only at the amino terminus. The amino terminus controls the activity of the enzyme and interacts very specifically with different targets.

▶ cAMP- and cGMP-dependent Protein Kinases
▶ Smooth Muscle Tone Regulation

cGMP-regulated Phosphodiesterases

Phosphodiesterases represent a multi-gene family of enzymes that hydrolyze the second messengers cGMP and cAMP. The hydrolytic activity of several subfamilies of these enzymes is regulated in an allosteric manner by the binding of cGMP. The cyclic nucleotide binding site present in cGMP-regulated phosphodiesterases is not homologous to that found in most other cyclic nucleotide-binding proteins.

▶ Phosphodiesterases

CGRP

▶ Calcitonin Gene Related Peptide

Channelopathies

Channelopathies refer to a class of diseases caused by ion channel dysfunction. Channelopathies can be due to autoimmune, drug, toxic or genetic mechanisms. Mutations in genes encoding ion channel proteins that alter channel function are common mechanisms underlying channelopathies. Examples of channelopathy include some forms of ▶ Bartter's Syndrome (Kir1.1), Andersen syndrome (Kir2.1), Weaver Mouse Phenotype (Kir3.2), Persistent Hyperinsulinemic Hypoglycemia of Infancy (PHHI) (Kir6.2/SUR) and Long QT Syndrome (▶ Voltage-dependent Na$^+$ Channels and ▶ K$^+$ Channels).

Channels, ion

▶ Ion Channels

Chaperone Protein

▶ Molecular Chaperones

Chemical Library

A chemical library is a precisely defined collection of different chemical compounds. Chemical libraries can be either prepared by parallel synthesis or by split-and-recombine synthesis.

▶ Combinatorial Chemistry

Chemical Neurotransmission

Chemical neurotransmission is the way in which neurons communicate by releasing chemical substances that are received by the receptors in the next neuron (or the target) and excite or inhibit it. About 50% or more of drug mechanisms are based on modification of chemical neurotransmission.

▶ Synaptic Transmission

Chemokine Receptors

RICHARD HORUK
Department of Immunology, Berlex Biosciences, Richmond, CA, USA
horuk@pacbell.net

Synonyms

Chemoattractant receptors, chemokine receptors, ▶ G-protein-coupled Receptors

Definition

Chemokine receptors are members of the G-protein coupled receptor (GPCR) superfamily (1). At the latest count well over 600 members of this GPCR superfamily have been identified and classified into families. Six CXC, ten CC and one CX3C and XC chemokine receptors have been cloned so far. Receptor binding initiates a cascade of intracellular events mediated by the receptor-associated heterotrimeric G-proteins. These G-protein subunits trigger various effector enzymes that leads to the activation not only of ▶ chemotaxis but also to a wide range of functions in different leukocytes such as an increase in the respiratory burst, degranulation, ▶ phagocytosis and lipid mediator synthesis (1).

▶ Cytokines
▶ Immune Defense

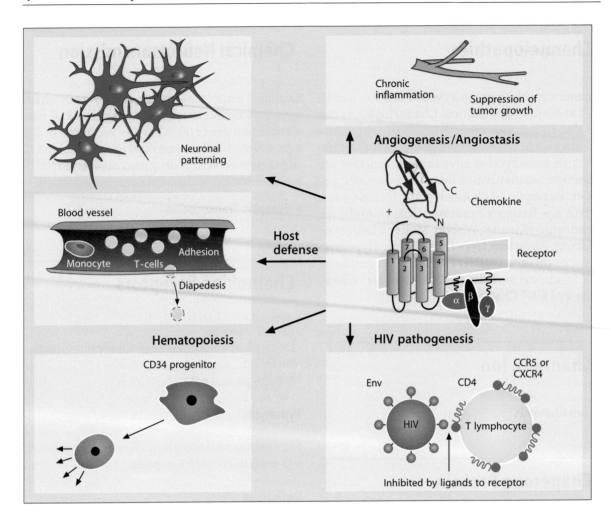

Fig. 1 Biological functions of chemokine receptors as exemplified by the chemokine receptor CXCR4.

Basic Characteristics

Chemokines belong to a large family of small, chemotactic cytokines characterized by a distinctive pattern of four conserved cysteine residues (2). They are divided into two major (CXC and CC) and two minor (C and CX3C) groups dependent on the number and spacing of the first two conserved cysteine residues. Although originally identified on the basis of their ability to regulate the trafficking of immune cells, the biological role of chemokines goes well beyond this simple description of their function as chemoattractants; they have been shown to be involved in a number of biological processes, including growth regulation, hematopoiesis, embryologic development, angiogenesis and ▶ HIV-1 infection (2) (Fig. 1).

Chemokines have been shown to be associated with a number of autoinflammatory diseases including ▶ multiple sclerosis, ▶ rheumatoid arthritis, atherosclerosis, dermatitis and organ transplant rejection (3). Evidence, reviewed below, is mounting that chemokines may play a major role in the pathophysiology of these diseases and thus chemokine receptor ▶ antagonists could prove to be useful therapeutics in treating these and other pro-inflammatory diseases.

Chemokine Receptors

Although leukocytes continue to be the major site of expression of chemokine receptors, several studies have recently demonstrated chemokine receptor expression on neurons in the CNS.

A number of chemokine receptors including CXCR2, CXCR4, CCR1, CCR5 and DARC have been demonstrated in either adult or fetal brain. Not only were these receptors present on the cell surface but they were also functional. Clearly, the role of these receptors on CNS neurons must be very different from their role on immune cells. Given that human astrocytes can be stimulated with cytokines to upregulate the expression of chemokines, it is tempting to speculate that *in vivo* during CNS development, chemokines secreted by astrocytes might engage specific receptors expressed on neurons and may play a role in the directed migration of specific subsets of neurons to distinctive regions of the brain.

Genetic mutations of receptors, both natural and induced (by targeted gene disruption), can help to unravel their biological roles. Nature has been generous in this regard by providing us with two naturally occurring examples of gene inactivation for chemokine receptors. Humans homozygous for inherited inactivating mutations of the Duffy (DARC) gene and the CCR5 gene have been identified and appear to be phenotypically normal and healthy. Indeed, these gene inactivations appear to be beneficial to their hosts, rendering them resistant to certain infectious diseases. For example, DARC-negative individuals are resistant to malaria induced by *Plasmodium vivax*, which utilizes DARC to attach to and enter erythrocytes. CCR5-negative individuals are resistant to HIV-1, which utilizes this chemokine receptor as a co-receptor for invasion (see section role of receptors in HIV infection).

Analysis of receptor-inactivated individuals can also be useful in clarifying the role of these receptors in disease. For example, it is known that MIP-1a (CCL3) appears to play an important role in multiple sclerosis. This chemokine is a potent ► agonist for both CCR1 and CCR5 receptors, opening the possibility that either of these receptors could be involved in mediating the development of the pathophysiological changes seen in this disease. However, analysis of a large group of individuals, comprising both normal subjects and those suffering from relapsing/remitting multiple sclerosis, showed that there was no significant difference in the allele frequency of the CCR5 mutation between the groups. These studies indicate that CCR5 is not an essential component in the expression of multiple sclerosis and implicates CCR1 in the disease.

Role in Immune Response

Chemokines are potent chemoattractants that provide directional cues to summon leukocytes. Leukocyte recruitment is a three-step process that involves the formation of solid phase chemokine gradients generated by the binding of chemokines to extracellular matrix proteins like glycosaminoglycans, which decorate the cell surface of endothelial cells. These gradients then attract immune cells that first undergo selectin-mediated rolling along the endothelial cells. Chemokine-mediated upregulation of CD11/18 complexes then results in a much firmer adherence of immune cells to the endothelium and this culminates in diapedesis of leukocytes across the endothelial space into tissues.

By regulating the movement of different subsets of leukocytes from the peripheral blood to extravascular sites such as organs, skin or connective tissue, chemokines play a critical role in the maintenance of host defence as well as in the development of the immune response. However, sometimes these molecules can inappropriately target immune cells to attack their own tissues and organs leading to inflammation and cellular destruction. Indeed, strong evidence supports the idea that chemokines play an important role in the pathogenesis of a number of autoimmune diseases such as multiple sclerosis and rheumatoid arthritis.

Rheumatoid arthritis is a chronic inflammatory disease characterized in part by a memory T lymphocyte and monocyte infiltrate. The interaction of the same cell types also play a major role in the demyelinating processes that culminate in multiple sclerosis. Recent studies using neutralizing antibodies have provided strong *in vivo* concept validation for a role of chemokines in animal models of both diseases. For example, in an adjuvant-induced arthritis (AIA) model in the rat, antibodies to CCL5 were able to abrogate the development of the disease by greatly reducing the infiltration of mononuclear cells into tissue joints. Similarly, antibodies to CCL3 prevented the development of both initial and relapsing paralytic disease as well as infiltration of mononuclear cells into the central nervous system of a mouse experimental autoimmune encephalomyelitis (EAE) model of multiple sclerosis. These results strongly suggest that chemokines play important roles in T-cell mediated autoimmune diseases.

In contrast to the role of T cells and monocytes in chronic inflammation, the primary hallmark of acute inflammatory diseases, such as empyema, acute lung injury, acute respiratory distress syndrome (ARDS) and dermatitis, is tissue infiltration by neutrophils. Thus, neutrophil-activating CXC chemokines like CXCL8 are most often associated with these diseases. Clear evidence for a role of CXCL8 in acute lung injury and pleurisy has been provided by the finding that antibodies to CXCL8 dramatically increases the survival time of rabbits in models of disease. Not only did the antibodies increase the alveolar-arterial oxygen difference of the animals, increasing the oxygenation of the blood and therefore decreasing breathing difficulties, but they also affected a significant reduction in the infiltration of neutrophils into the lung.

Based on the demonstrated role of chemokines in disease, the generation of small molecule chemokine receptor antagonists have received great interest from pharmaceutical companies as attractive therapeutic approaches. GPCR's like chemokine receptors have in the past been an extremely fertile source of biological targets in the pharmaceutical industry, and compound library screening has proven successful in the discovery of antagonists for a number of these receptors i.e. CCK and neurotensin antagonists. Using similar approaches several drug companies have now identified potent small molecule antagonists of a number of chemokine receptors, which should find broad utility in a variety of acute and chronic inflammatory diseases.

Drugs

Insight into the physiological and pathophysiological roles of chemokine receptors have been provided by studies with potent receptor antagonists for CCR1, CCR2, CCR3, CCR5, CXCR2, CXCR3 and CXCR4, reviewed in Horuk and Ng (4). A number of these antagonists, CCR1, CCR5 and CXCR4, are in human clinical trials. For example, the CCR5 and CXCR4 antagonists are in phase I and II clinical trials, respectively, for the treatment of AIDS. In addition, the CCR1 antagonist is in phase I clinical trials for multiple sclerosis.

The utility of chemokine receptor antagonists as therapeutic agents in disease can be exemplified by the CCR1 antagonist BX 471. BX 471 has been shown to be a potent functional inhibitor specific for CCR1 based on its ability to inhibit a number of CCR1-mediated effects including CCL3- and CCL5-mediated increases in Ca^{2+} mobilization and extracellular acidification rate, CD11b expression and leukocyte migration. In addition, BX 471 demonstrates a greater than 10,000 fold selectivity for CCR1 compared with 28 different GPCR's. Pharmacokinetic studies demonstrated that BX 471 was orally active with a bioavailability of 60% in dogs.

In a rat EAE model of multiple sclerosis, BX 471 dose-responsively decreased the clinical score. At the highest dose of 50 mg/kg, BX 471 reduced the clinical score by around 50%. The much higher doses of BX 471 that are required to be effective in rat EAE are due to the fact that the compound has an IC50 of 121 nM for inhibition of CCL3 binding to rat CCR1, compared with an IC50 of 1–2 nM for human CCR1. Based on these considerations, it is likely that much lower doses of BX 471 (500 µg/kg or less) would be required to be therapeutically effective in treating multiple sclerosis in humans.

The CCR1 receptor antagonist BX 471 is also efficacious in a rat heterotopic heart transplant rejection model. Animals treated with BX 471 and a sub-therapeutic dose of cyclosporin (2.5 mg/kg), which is by itself ineffective in prolonging transplant rejection, was much more efficacious in prolonging transplantation rejection than animals treated with either cyclosporin or BX 471 alone. Immunohistology of the rat hearts for infiltrating monocytes confirmed these data. Three days after transplantation the extent of monocytic graft infiltration was significantly reduced by the combined therapy of BX 471 and cyclosporin. Thus, BX 471 given in combination with cyclosporin resulted in a clear increase in efficacy in heart transplantation compared to cyclosporin alone. These data were in line with the observed effects of BX 471 in dose-responsively blocking the firm adhesion of monocytes triggered by CCL5 on inflamed endothelium. Together, these data demonstrate a significant role for CCR1 in allograft rejection. The promise of highly specific therapies for a number of devastating diseases is on the horizon thanks to the identification of chemokine receptor antagonists, and we can look forward with anticipation to the day when these drugs are finally marketed as potent therapeutics.

Chemokine Receptors in Pathogen Infection

A number of viruses, including those in the Herpes and Pox families, express chemokine-like or chemokine receptor-like molecules that presumably help them to survive immune attack and proliferate. In addition to these strategies, chemoattractant receptors have themselves been targeted as vehicles of cellular invasion by a wide variety of microbes. These range from the Duffy blood group antigen, a promiscuous chemokine receptor on human erythrocytes which serves as a binding protein for the malarial parasite *Plasmodium vivax*, to the fractalkine receptor, CX3CR1, which is a portal of entry for the respiratory synctial virus, and the HIV-1 virus which utilizes the chemokine receptors CXCR4 and CCR5 as coreceptors for cellular entry. CCR5 is an entry cofactor for M-tropic isolates of HIV-1 and is important in the early proliferative part of the disease, while CXCR4 is a coreceptor for T-tropic isolates of HIV-1 whose emergence in infected individuals usually correlates with accelerated disease progression.

HIV-1 resistance exhibited by some exposed but uninfected individuals is due, in part, to a 32 base pair deletion in the CCR5 gene (CCR5D32) which results in a truncated protein that is not expressed on the cell surface. About 1% of Caucasians are homozygous for the CCR5D32 allele and appear to be healthy with no untoward signs of disease. In fact, recent findings suggest that homozygosity for the CCR5D32 alleles confers other selective advantages to these individuals, rendering them less susceptible to rheumatoid arthritis and asthma and prolonging survival of transplanted solid organs.

References

1. Thelen M (2001) Dancing to the tune of chemokines. Nature Immunology. 2:129–34
2. Mackay CR (2001) Chemokines:immunology's high impact factors. Nature Immunology. 2:95–101
3. Gerard G, Rollins BJ (2001) Chemokines and disease. Nature Immunology. 2:108–115
4. Horuk R, Ng HP (2000) Chemokine receptor antagonists. Med. Res. Rev. 20:155–168

Chemokines

Chemokines are protein factors that have been identified as attractants of different types of blood leukocytes to sites of infection and inflammation. They are produced locally in the affected tissues and act on leukocytes through selective chemokine receptors. Chemokines help to control leukocyte maturation, traffic and homing of lymphocytes and the development of lymphoid tissues.

▶ Chemokine receptors
▶ Inflammation

Chemoreceptor Trigger Zone

The chemoreceptor trigger zone (CTZ) is a group of neurons in the area postrema of the medulla. Once stimulated, it activates the vomiting center, which is also located in the medulla, thereby causing emesis. The CTZ is sensitive to a variety of chemical stimuli. Syrup of ipecac (synonym ipecacuanha) and apomorphine are direct stimulators of the CTZ. Clinically they are used to provoke emesis after oral ingestion of a poison. The CTZ is also stimulated by other drugs, e.g. ▶ cardiac glycosides, morphine (▶ opioid system) and ▶ antineoplastic agents.

▶ Emesis

Chemotaxis

Chemotaxis is the detection of and coordinated movement toward a chemical compound by a cell or organism, e.g. neutrophils move towards an area of infection because of chemicals released by infected tissues.

▶ Chemokine Receptors
▶ Hematopoietic Growth Factors

Chemotherapy

Chemotherapy was initially defined by Paul Ehrlich as "the use of a drug to combat an invading parasite without damaging the host". It now commonly refers to the treatment of cancer using drugs that are selectively toxic for the cancerous cells.

▶ Cancer, molecular mechanisms of therapy
▶ Antineoplastic Agents

Cholecystokinin

Cholecystokinin (CCK) is produced in the intestine and the brain. It appears to be an important mediator of anxiety. It also stimulates vasopressin secretion and slows gastric emptying. In addition, it is an important humoral satiety signal (appetite control). Various antagonists have been developed and are currently being investigated with regard to their therapeutic potential.

▶ Appetite Control

Cholegraphic Contrast Agents

Cholegraphic contrast agents are ionic (acidic) iodinated molecules, which reversibly bind to albumen and are actively excreted into the bile.

▶ Radiocontrast Agents

Cholera Toxin

Cholera toxin is a protein toxin of *Vibrio cholerae*. It ADP-ribosylates the α-subunit of the G_s heterotrimeric G-protein at an arginine residue which is involved in GTP hydrolysis. ADP-ribosylation thus leads to constitutive activation of G_s.

▶ Bacterial Toxins

Cholesterol

Cholesterol is a widely distributed sterol found free or esterified to fatty acids. It is an important intermediate in the biosynthesis of steroid hormones and the principal component of cell plasma membranes and the membranes of intracellular organelles.

▶ HMG-CoA-Reductase Inhibitors

Cholinergic Transmission

Cholinergic transmission is the process of synaptic transmission which uses mainly acetylcholine as a transmitter. Cholinergic transmission is found widely in the peripheral and central nervous system, where acetylcholine acts on nicotinic and muscarinic receptors.

▶ Nicotinic Receptor
▶ Muscarinic Receptors

Cholinesterase

In mammals, there are basically 2 types of cholinesterases, acetylcholinesterase (AChE) and butyrylcholinesterase (BChE). AChE plays a critical role e.g. in terminating the action of acetylcholine at the post-synaptic membrane in the neuromuscular junction and elsewhere. Both AChE and BChE exist as polymers of catalytic subunits and are closely related in molecular structure. A soluble, hydrophilic form of BChE, consisting of a tetramer, represents 95% of the activity found in plasma. A similar tetramer of AChE can be found in the cerebrovascular fluid. In tissues, the catalytic units are linked to a collagen-like tail or to glycolipids, through which they are tethered to the cell membrane or the basal membrane of various sites. AChE is bound to the basement membrane in the synaptic cleft at cholinergic synapses at the motor endplate, where it hydrolyzes the released transmitter acetylcholine. In the central nervous system, a tetrameric form of AChE linked to a lipid anchor is the main form. AChE has also been shown to have proteolytic activity, but the physiological significance of this is not clear. BChE is widely distributed and not particularly associated with cholinergic synapses. The form found in plasma is synthesized mainly in the liver. While AChE has a high specificity for acetylcholine and closely related esters such as methacholine, BChE hydrolyses acetylcholine as well as many other esters such as procaine, suxamethonium or propanidid. Its physiological function is not clear. BChE is also called "pseudocholinesterase", or "non-specific cholinesterase". Genetic variants of BChE have been described, which partly account for the variability in the duration of action of e.g. suxamethonium.

Both, AChE and BChE are serine hydrolases, in which the catalytic hydrolysis occurs by transfer of the acetyl group to a serine of the active site. This results in acetylated enzyme and a molecule of free choline. The serine acetyl group spontaneously hydrolyses very rapidly. AChE has an extremely high turnover number resulting in the hydrolysis of more than 10,000 molecules of acetylcholine per second by a single active site.

Various drugs inhibit AChE and BChE by interaction with the active site of the enzyme. Some of them, like edrophonium, or the centrally acting substances tacrine and donepezil, interact reversibly with the substrate binding pocket of the enzyme. The so called "indirect parasympathomimetics" (e.g. neostigmine, physostigmine, pyridostigmine) also reversibly bind to the active site of the enzyme but lead to a transient covalent modification of the enzyme. These drugs possess strongly basic groups, which bind to acetylcholinesterase. They are carbamyl and not acetyl esters. The carbamyl group is transferred to the serine of the active site but the carbamylated enzyme is very slow to hydrolyze it, taking minutes rather then microseconds. Reversible cholinesterase inhibitors are used in anaesthesia to reverse the action of non-depolarising neuromuscular-blocking drugs. They are also used for the treatment of myasthenia-gravis and glaucoma and in Alzheimer dementia.

In contrast to the reversible cholinesterases, irreversible cholinesterase inhibitors are pentavalent phosphorus compounds, which covalently modify the serine by the phosphorus atom. Organophosphate compounds were developed as pesticides as well as war gases (e.g. sarin, soma, tabun).

Cholinesterase inhibitors affect the autonomic cholinergic system, resulting in parasympathomimetic effects. In large doses cholinesterase inhibitors can cause twitching of muscles, and may cause paralyses due to depolarization block at the neuromuscular junction. Centrally acting cholinesterase inhibitors, which can penetrate the blood-brain barrier can cause initial excitation, convulsions, central depression, unconsciousness and respiratory failure.

Chorionic Gonadotropin

Chorionic gonadotropin (CG) is produced in the placenta. Together with the pituitary hormones, luteinizing hormone (LH) and follicle-stimulating hormone (FSH), it constitutes the glycoprotein family of ▶ gonadotropins. The actions of CG are mediated by the LH receptor.

▶ G-protein Coupled Receptors
▶ Contraceptives

Chromosomal Translocations

The presence of chromosomal translocations is a consistent feature of many leukaemias, lymphomas and certain solid tumours. At the genetic level, these events can either deregulate an intact gene by disruption or removal and replacement of the adjacent controlling elements or create a new fusion gene that expresses the N-terminus of one protein fused to the C-terminus of another protein.

▶ Antisense Oligonucleotides

Chromosomes

Double helical DNA is organized in all cells into structures generically referred to as chromosomes. Chromosomes contain most of the genetic information of a cell, although bacterial cells may also have plasmids and eukaryotic cells may also have episomes (extrachromosomal elements). In most bacterial cells, the bacterial chromosome is organized as a single circular loop. Most multicellular organisms have several chromosomes that are linear instead of circular. Sexually reproducing organisms have two copies of each chromosome, one from each parent.

Chymase

Chymase (mast cell protease type II), a chymotrypsin-like protease, is a serine protease found in mucosal mast cells which catalyzes the conversion of angiotensin I to angiotensin II and of big endothelin1 (ET1) to ET1(1-31).

▶ Endothelins

Chymotrypsin-like Proteinases

Chymotrypsin-like proteinases are serine proteinases that recognize peptide residues with aromatic side chains (phyenylalanyl or tyrosyl residues) and that effect hydrolysis of the polypeptide chain on the carboxy-terminal side of these residues. Examples of chymotrypsin-like proteinases are chymotrypsin and cathepsin-G.

▶ Non-viral Proteases
▶ Cathepsins

CICR

CICR (Ca^{2+}-induced Ca^{2+} release) is a Ca^{2+} release triggered by a Ca^{2+} increase from no more than $0.1\,\mu M$ (at rest). CICR is stimulated by less than $0.1\,mM$ Ca^{2+}, ATP and caffeine and inhibited by higher Ca^{2+}, Mg^{2+} or procaine. RyR1-3 can induce CICR. It is notable that native RyR1 in the sarcoplasmic reticulum (SR) suppresses CICR activity, which is removed after purification.

▶ Ryanodine Receptor

Ciliary Neurotrophic Factor

▶ Neurotrophic Factors

Circadian Rhythm

Circadian rhythm is mainly influenced by input from the retina. Melatonin, a derivative of serotonin, is synthesized in the pineal, an endocrine organ which plays an important role in establishing circadian rhythms. The production of melatonin is high at night and low during day-time. Melatonin exerts its effects through ▶ G-protein coupled receptors found in the brain and in the retina, but also in the periphery. How melatonin acts is currently not well-understood. Melatonin is used to treat jet-lag and to improve the performance of night-shift workers.

Circumventricular Organs

The circumventricular organs are brain structures bordering the 3rd and 4th ventricles and are unique since they lack a ▶ blood-brain barrier. Therefore, they are recognized as important sites for communication between the brain and peripheral organs via blood-borne products. They include the median eminence, subfornical organ, area postrema, subcommissural organ, and organum vasculosum of the lamina terminalis.

Class I Antiarrhythmic Drugs

Antiarrhythmic drugs are antagonists of the fast Na^+ channel which slow the propagation of the cardiac action potential. Class I drugs suppress the fast upstroke of the action potential.

▶ Antiarrhythmic Drugs

Class II Antiarrhythmic Drugs

Class II antiarrhythmic drugs are β-adrenoceptor antagonists such as propranolol, metoprolol or atenolol. β-adrenoceptor antagonists slow sinus rate and atrioventricular conduction and exert negative inotropic effects.

▶ Antiarrhythmic Drugs

Class III Antiarrhythmic Drugs

Class III antiarrhythmic drugs are drugs which act as K^+ channel antagonists and result in action potential prolongation without effect on the upstroke of the action potential.

▶ Antiarrhythmic Drugs

Class IV Antiarrhythmic Drugs

Class IV antiarrhythymic drugs are Ca^{2+} channel blockers, which predominatly slow sinus rate and atrioventricular conduction and thus are used in the treatment of supraventricular tachyarrhythmias. These drugs exert a pronounced negative inotropic effect.

▶ Antiarrhythmic Drugs

Classic Cadherins

▶ Cadherins/Catenins
▶ Table appendix: Adhesion Molecules

Clathrin

Clathrin is a protein complex composed of three heavy and three light chains, which assemble in a so called triskelion.

▶ Intracellular Transport

Clathrin-coated Vesicle

Clathrin coated vesicles mediate transport within the late secretory and the endocytic pathways. Their major coat constituents are clathrin and various adaptor complexes.

▶ Intracellular Transport

CLC

CLC is a gene family of *CL-C*hannels. Originally identified by the expression cloning of ClC-0 from the electric organ of the marine ray *Torpedo*, CLC genes are now known to be present in all kingdoms of life, with nine genes in humans alone. CLC proteins have 17 helices in the membrane plane, several of which, however, do not cross the width of the membrane and therefore do not qualify as transmembrane domains. In CLCs of higher organisms (and also in some, but not all bacteria) CLCs have a large cytoplasmic tail with two conserved CBS domains of largely unknown function. CLC channels function as dimers with two largely independent pores ('double-barreled' channel). Each pore is entirely contained within each monomer, and not at the interface between these. All CLC channels that could be functionally expressed have a Cl>I conductance sequence. Gating is often voltage-dependent and depends on anions, resulting in a model in which anions serve as the gating charge.

▶ Cl⁻ Channels

Cl⁻ Channels

THOMAS J. JENTSCH
Institut für Molekulare Neurobiologie Hamburg, Universität Hamburg, Hamburg, Germany
jentsch@plexus.uke.uni-hamburg.de

Synonyms

Anion channels

Definition

Chloride channels are membrane proteins that allow for the passive flow of anions across biological membranes. As chloride is the most abundant anion under physiological conditions, these channels are often called chloride channels instead of anion channels, even though other anions (such as iodide or nitrate) may permeate better.

▶ Table appendix: Membrane Transport Proteins

Basic Characteristics

Chloride channels are transmembrane proteins with several transmembrane domains, which form a pore that allows for the passive flow of anions along their electrochemical gradient. Like other channels, chloride channels can be opened or closed by a process called gating. Gating can be influenced by several factors, e.g. by the transmembrane voltage in voltage-gated chloride channels, by intracellular Ca in Ca-activated chloride channels, by extracellular ligands such as glycine or GABA as in ligand-gated chloride channels, by cAMP-dependent phosphorylation, or by cell swelling.

Chloride channels may be present in the plasma membrane or in the membranes of intracellular organelles.

Classification of Chloride Channels

Chloride channels can be classified by their biophysical characteristics (e.g. single-channel conductance), regulation (e.g. voltage-dependent, ligand-gated, swelling-activated, Ca-activated), or by their sequence (gene families). The latter classification is the most logical one. However, many classes of chloride channels characterized in native tissues have not yet been cloned, raising the possibility that entire gene families of chloride channels remain to be discovered. Therefore, a molecular classification does not yet cover all chloride channels.

Gene Families of Chloride Channels

There are three well established molecular classes of chloride channels: ▶ CLC chloride channels, ligand-gated chloride channels (GABA- and glycine-receptors), as well as ▶ CFTR, the Cystic Fibrosis Transmembrane Conductance Regulator which belongs to the ABC-transporter family. Other proposed gene families include the CLIC proteins and the CaCC proteins, whose function as chloride channels, however, has not yet been proven.

CFTR is the only member of the very large ABC-transporter gene family that is known to function as a chloride channel. Most other members of this gene family (like mdr) probably function as ATP-dependent pumps and not as channels. CFTR is regulated by intracellular ATP and cAMP. cAMP acts through phosphorylation by protein kinase A, resulting in a cAMP-activated chloride channel. CFTR is expressed in many epithelia, e.g. in apical membranes in the lung, pancreas and intestine. Mutations in CFTR underlie cystic fibrosis, a potentially lethal disease with transport defects in the lung, pancreas and colon. In addition to working as a chloride channel, several other important functions (such as the regulation of other ion channels) have been attributed to CFTR. CFTR has 12 transmembrane domains and may function as a monomer.

GABA$_A$- and glycine receptors are ligand-gated chloride channels that belong to a gene superfamily that also includes cation channels (e.g. nicotinic acetylcholine receptors). These ion channels are involved in synaptic transmission and are mostly inhibitory in the adult due to the direction of the chloride concentration gradient. These ligand-gated channels are important pharmacological targets, but cannot be discussed in detail here. These channels function as pentamers of identical or homologous subunits, with four transmembrane spans each.

CLC chloride channels form a large gene family with members in bacteria, archae and eukaryotes.

Many CLCs gate in a voltage-dependent manner. In mammals, there are nine different CLC genes. CLC channels are present in the plasma membrane and in intracellular organelles. They function as dimers, with each monomer having its own pore ('double-barreled' channels). The structure of a bacterial CLC protein has recently been determined by X-ray crystal structure analysis. Some CLC channels have accessory β-subunits.

The CLC Family of Chloride Channels in Mammals

There are nine different CLC genes in mammals. Based on homology, they can be classed into three branches. The first branch includes channels that reside predominantly in the plasma membrane. This includes ClC-1, a skeletal muscle chloride channel, ClC-2, a very broadly expressed channel, and ClC-Ka and ClC-Kb, which are expressed predominantly in the kidney but also in the ear.

The physiological roles of these channels are apparent from human diseases or mouse models in which these genes are disrupted.

Mutations in ClC-1 lead to ▶ myotonia, a muscle stiffness that is associated with a hyperexcitability of the muscle plasma membrane. Thus, the high resting chloride conductance in muscle is necessary for its electrical stability. ClC-1 shows a distinct voltage-dependence and is activated by depolarisation. It is blocked in a voltage-dependent manner by iodide.

The disruption of ClC-2 in mice leads to male infertility and blindness, and was attributed to a defect in transepithelial transport in these tissues. ClC-2 yields currents that slowly activate upon hyperpolarization. It is also activated by cell swelling and by extracellular acidification. Structural determinants that are essential for these types of activation were identified by mutagenesis.

Mutations in ClC-Kb lead to ▶ Bartter's syndrome, a disease associated with severe renal salt loss. This demonstrates that ClC-Kb is essential for the basolateral efflux of chloride from cells of the renal thick ascending limb of Henle. The disruption of ClC-K1 (the species orthologue of ClC-Ka) in mice leads to a syndrome resembling nephrogenic diabetes insipidus, and it was shown that it is essential for the establishment of high osmolarity in kidney medulla. ClC-Kb and ClC-Ka need barttin, a protein with two transmembrane domains, as a β-subunit for functional expression.

Mutations in barttin lead to Bartter syndrome with deafness. It has been shown that barttin associates with ClC-Ka and ClC-Kb in the basolateral membrane of the stria vascularis of the inner ear. In this tissue, ClC-K/barttin heteromeric channels are necessary for the basolateral recycling of chloride that is taken up by a basolateral NaK2Cl cotransporter. Barttin mutations lead to deafness because K-secretion by the stria into the scala media of the cochlea is impaired. In the kidney, ClC-Ka/barttin channels are present in the thin limb of Henle's loop, while ClC-Kb/barttin is present in the thick ascending limb of Henle's loop and some more distal segments (e.g. acid-secreting intercalated cells). Currents of both ClC-Ka/barttin and ClC-Kb/barttin show a rather linear voltage-dependence, are augmented by raising extracellular Ca, and inhibited by extracellular acidification. Given the important role of ClC-K/barttin in renal salt and fluid reabsorption, they are attractive candidate targets for the development of diuretics. In contrast to diuretics that target channels or transporters of apical membranes of the nephron (such as amiloride or furosemide), drugs inhibiting ClC-K/barttin may also be useful in conditions of renal failure.

All members of this CLC branch have a $Cl^->I^-$ permeability and conductance sequence.

ClC-3, -4 and -5 form the second branch of the CLC gene family. These proteins are 80% identical, and with the exception of ClC-5, which is most highly expressed in kidney and intestine, show a broad expression pattern. ClC-3 to ClC-5 reside in intracellular membranes of the endocytotic pathway. Disruption of ClC-5 leads to a defect in endocytosis in mouse models as well as in human Dent's disease, a disorder associated with proteinuria and kidney stones. ClC-5 currents are necessary to balance the current of the electrogenic proton pump of endosomes. Therefore, the disruption of ClC-5 leads to a defect in endosomal acidification, which impairs endocytosis. The defect in proximal tubular endocytosis leads to secondary changes in calciotropic hormones, leading to tertiary changes such as hyperphosphaturia, hypercalciuria and kidney stones.

Similar to ClC-5, ClC-3 is present in endosomes. It is also found in synaptic vesicles. In both instances, and similar to ClC-5, it is necessary for the efficient intravesicular acidification. The acidification of synaptic vesicles is particularly important as their uptake of neurotransmitters depends on the electrochemical proton gradient. Surprisingly, the disruption of ClC-3 in mice resulted in a drastic degeneration of the hippocampus and the retina. Much less is known about ClC-4, which, however, also appears to be present in endosomal compartments.

All three members of this branch give currents with a $NO_3^->Cl^->I^-$ conductance sequence. Currents are very strongly outwardly rectified (opening at voltages more positive than +20 mV), which is enigmatic as this voltage range seems not to be attained *in vivo*. Their currents can be inhibited by extracellular (intravesicular) acidification. The fact that currents can be obsreved shows that ClC-3, -4 and -5 are not exclusively present in endosomes, but can also come to the surface upon heterologous expression. It is currently unclear whether this occurs under physiological conditions as well.

ClC-6 and ClC-7 define the third branch of the CLC family. These proteins are only about 45% identical to each other and are very broadly expressed; in fact, are probably expressed in every cell, although to different extents. It proved impossible to obtain plasma membrane chloride currents with either ClC-6 or ClC-7. This is due to the fact that both channels reside in intracellular organelles under most circumstances.

ClC-6 is still poorly understood. Much more is known about ClC-7. It is expressed in late endosomal/lysosomal compartments, where it probably contributes to their acidification. The disruption of ClC-7 in mice and man leads to severe ▶ osteopetrosis and retinal degeneration. ClC-7 is highly expressed in osteoclasts. In these cells, it is inserted together with the proton pump into the specialized plasma membrane ('ruffled border') that faces the reabsorption lacuna. ▶ Osteoclasts are still present in ClC-7 knockout mice and can still attach to bone. However, they cannot acidify their reabsorption lacuna, resulting in a severe defect of bone resorption. Thus, similar to the roles of other intracellular CLCs, ClC-7 is essential for acidification of certain compartments by electrically balancing the current of the proton pump. This accounts entirely for the osteopetrotic phenotype observed upon ClC-7 disruption. ClC-7 may be an interesting target for the treatment of osteoporosis as its partial inhibition might increase bone mass. This notion is indirectly supported by the observation that patients that are heterozygous for dominant negative ClC-7 mutations (a situation expected to lead only to a partial inhibition of ClC-7) present with a milder form of osteopetrosis in which retinal degeneration is absent.

Drugs

Unfortunately, the pharmacology of chloride channels is poorly developed. Specific and highly useful inhibitors or modulators (e.g. strychnine, picrotoxin, diazepams) are only available for lig-and-gated chloride channels (but these are covered in a different chapter). There are several 'chloride channel inhibitors' such as the stilbene-disulfonates DIDS and SITS, 9-antracene-carboxylic acid (9-AC), arylaminobenzoates such as DPC and NPPB, niflumic acids and derivates, sulfonylureas, and zinc and cadmium. All of these inhibitors, however, are not very specific. Several of these inhibitors (e.g. DIDS) inhibit many chloride channels only partially even at millimolar concentrations.

Tamoxifen and DIDS have been used to inhibit endogenous swelling-activated chloride channels whose molecular identity is still unclear. Glibenclamide has been used to inhibit CFTR, which is quite resistance to DIDS. Endogenous (probably not yet cloned) Ca-activated chloride channels are often sensitive to fenamates such as flufenamic acid and niflumic acid. CLC channels are quite insensitive to DIDS, but can often be inhibited by zinc or cadmium in a submillimor range. 9-AC is a quite specific inhibitor for the muscle channel ClC-1, and its inhibitor binding site has been mapped recently by mutagenesis. ClC-1 can also be inhibited by clofibric acid derivates.

References

1. Jentsch TJ, Stein V, Weinreich F, Zdebik AA (2002) Molecular structure and physiological function of chloride channels. Physiological Reviews 82(2):503-68
2. Piwon N, Günther W, Schwake M, Bösl MR, Jentsch TJ. (2000) ClC-5 Cl- channel disruption impairs endocytosis in a mouse model for Dent's disease. Nature 408:369–373
3. Stobrawa SM, Breiderhoff T, Takamori S, Engel D, Schweizer M, Zdebik AA, Bösl MR, Ruether K, Jahn H, Draguhn A, Jahn R, Jentsch TJ (2001) Disruption of ClC-3, a chloride channel expressed on synaptic vesicles, leads to a loss of the hippocampus. Neuron 29:185–196
4. Kornak U, Kasper D, Bösl MR, Kaiser E, Schweizer M, Schulz A, Friedrich W, Delling G, Jentsch TJ (2001) Loss of the ClC-7 chloride channel leads to osteopetrosis in mice and man. Cell 104:205–215
5. Dutzler R, Campbell EB, Cadene M, Chait BT, MacKinnon R (2002) X-ray structure of the ClC chloride channel at 3.0 A resolution: molecular basis of anion selectivity. Nature 415:287–294

Clearance

Clearance is defined as the volume of plasma cleared of a substance in unit time. It is used to quantify the rate of drug elimination. Routinely, renal clearance is used. It can be calculated from the plasma concentration of a substance, its urinary concentration and the rate of flow of urine.

▶ Pharmacogenetics

Clonal Selection

T- and B-lymphocytes are the only cells in the body which carry antigen receptors on their plasma membrane. Each individual lymphocyte possesses one type of antigen receptor with specificity for one antigen, which has been created during ontogeny of the cell by irreversible random genetic rearrangement of certain sequences of the DNA. Thus a very large diversity of antigen specifities (possibly $> 10^8$) is generated, which allows the specific immune system to cope with all potentially harmful pathogens or substances in the environment. Pathogens invading an organism 'select' (are recognized by) one of the millions of lymphocytes which is then activated in a tightly controlled process and starts to proliferate. It clonally expands in order to create enough T- or B-lymphocyte effector cells capable of coping with the pathogen.

▶ Immune Defense

Clostridial Neurotoxins

Clostridial neurotoxins are bacterial protein toxins that consist of a heavy and a light chain connected by a disulfide bond and non-covalent interactions. They include tetanus toxin (TeNT) and the seven serotypes of botulinum toxins termed BoNT/A, BoNT/B, BoNT/C1, BoNT/D, BoNT/E, BoNT/F and BoNT/G. The heavy chain binds to the surface of peripheral neurons and mediates cell entry. After endocytotic uptake, the light chain is released into the cytoplasm. The difference between the clinical effects of tetanus and botulinal neurotoxins is due to the fact that tetanus toxin, while being sequestered by peripheral motoneurons in parallel with the BoNTs, is only inefficiently released into the cytoplasm but rather transported retrogradely into the spinal cord. There it is released by the dendrites of the motoneurons and inhibits predominantly presynaptic glycinergic interneurons, causing overexcitation and muscle cramps.

The light chains of the clostridial neurotoxins are metalloproteases with exclusive specificity for neuronal SNAREs. TeNT, BoNTs B,D,F, and G cleave synaptobrevin, BoNTs A and E SNAP-25, and BoNT/C1 syntaxin, and to a lesser extent also SNAP-25. Cleavage of any of the SNAREs causes complete and irreversible block of synaptic transmission.

▶ Bacterial Toxins

Clostridium Botulinum Toxin

▶ Botulinum Toxin
▶ Bacterial Toxins

Clotting

▶ Coagulation/Thrombosis

CMV

Cytomegalovirus (CMV) is a herpesvirus, which causes an inapparent infection in immunocompetent persons. Worldwide, approximately 40% of people are infected wih CMV. In immunocompromised patients, transplant recipients and neonates, CMV can cause serious and potentially lethal disease manifestations like pneumonia, retinitis and blindness, hepatitis, infections of the digestive tract, deafness or mental retardation.

▶ Antiviral Drugs

CNBD

▶ Cyclic Nucleotide-binding Domain

CNG Channels

Stands for cyclic nucleotide gated channels.

▶ Cyclic Nucleotide-regulated Cation Channels

CNTF

▶ Ciliary Neurotrophic Factor
▶ Neurotrophic Factors

CO

▶ Carbon Monoxide

Coactivators

▶ Transcriptional Co-activators

Coagulation/Thrombosis

ANDREAS GREINACHER AND BERND PÖTZSCH
Ernst-Moritz-Arndt-Universität Greifswald,
Greifswald, and Universitätsklinikum Bonn,
Bonn, Germany
greinach@mail.uni-greifswald.de

Synonyms

Blood clotting, hemostasis, vessel occlusion

Definition

Coagulation summarizes the mechanisms
involved in stopping bleeding due to an injured or
defective vessel wall. Coagulation is characterized
by procoagulatory and anticoagulatory factors
that are in balance under normal conditions. Vessel injuries are occluded by the coagulation system
and spontaneous vessel occlusions dissolved by
the fibrinolytic cascade.

Thrombosis is an imbalance towards the clotting capacity of the blood that leads to vessel
occlusion by a clot. The clot prohibits further
blood flow and can so cause pathological sequelae
dependent on its localization.

▶ Anticoagulants
▶ Antiplatelet Drugs
▶ Fibrinolytics

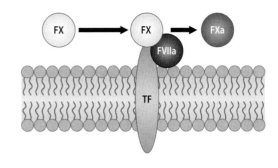

C

Fig. 1 Coagulation/Thrombosis

Mechanism of Action

The different pro- and anticoagulatory systems are
complex regulated cascades involving blood cells
(platelets, monocytes, endothelial cells), enzymes,
cofactors, phospholipids and calcium, which interact with each other and are further influenced by
physical conditions such as blood flow velocity,
turbulences or viscosity.

Coagulation Factors
Coagulation factors are glycoproteins named by
roman numbers (the numbers being ascribed at
the time of the components' definition, not
sequence of activation) (Table 1). Besides von Willebrand factor (vWF), the coagulation factors are
synthesized in the liver. They have very different
half-lifes and different concentrations in the
plasma. Several coagulation factors are stored in
platelets and endothelial cells and can be released
during activation of these cells, which can result in
a much higher local concentration of the respective factor (e.g. vWF).

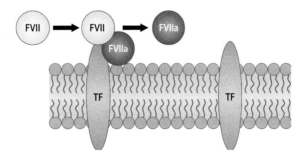

Fig. 2 Coagulation/Thrombosis

Tab. 1 Coagulation/Thrombosis

Name	Abbreviation	Molecular Weight	Plasma Concentration [mg/l]	Plasma Concentration [mmol/l]
Fibrinogen	-	340,000	3000	8800
Prothrombin	-	72,000	100	1400
Factor X	FX	56,000	10	180
Factor IX	FIX	56,000	5	90
Factor VII	FVII	50,000	0.5	10
Factor VIII	FVIII	330,000	0.1	0.3
Factor V	FV	330,000	10	30
Factor XI	FXI	160,000	5	30
Factor XII	FXII	80,000	30	400
Von-Willebrand-factor	vWF	225,000[a]	10	40
Tissue factor	TF	37,000	0.0	-
High molecular kininogen	HK	110,000	70	600
Prekallikrein	PreKK	88,000	40	500

[a] : molecular weight of the smallest subunit

Besides FXIII, all clotting enzymes are serine proteases (FII, FVII, FIX, FX, FXI, FXII). They usually circulate in their inactive form (proenzyme) and become only activated during clotting. In this respect, FVII is an exception as about 1% of FVII circulates in its active form, FVIIa, in plasma without activation of the clotting cascade. Its enzymatic activity is strongly enhanced by binding to its cofactor tissue factor, which under normal conditions is not exposed on cells having direct contact with blood. FV and FVIII are not enzymes but they are required as cofactors to form complexes with activated factors X and IX, respectively.

FVIII circulates in blood complexed to vWF. In the absence of vWF, or in case of impaired binding to vWF, FVIII is degraded.

Activation of the Coagulation Cascade
During activation of the coagulation cascade, coagulation factors form multimolecular (often trimolecular) complexes. The appropriate sterical orientation of the complex partners is usually pro-

vided by a surface of negatively charged phospholipids. The complexes consist of the enzyme, its cofactor and the respective substrate.

The FVIIa/TF-complex is the main activator of the clotting cascade. Under normal conditions TF is not exposed on the surface of cells being in contact with blood but is expressed in high concentra-

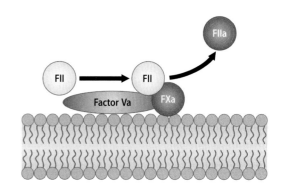

Fig. 3 Coagulation/Thrombosis

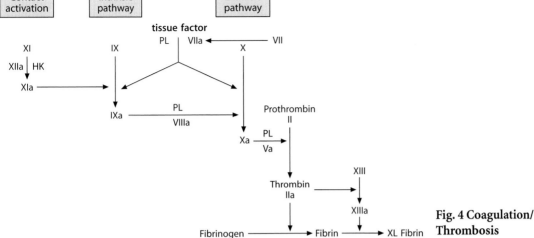

Fig. 4 Coagulation/Thrombosis

tions by all other cells. When flowing blood comes into contact with TF-bearing cells, TF binds the already circulating FVIIa (Fig. 1). This complex activates the serine proteases FX and FIX, and autocatalyzes activation of FVII (Fig. 2). On the surface of negatively charged phospholipids FXa together with its cofactor Va and the zymogen prothrombin (FII) form the prothrombinase complex, which results in the generation of FIIa (thrombin) (Fig. 3). Within this complex, the activity of FXa to generate FIIa is 300,000× enhanced as compared to the activity of uncomplexed FXa. As activated platelets provide a phospholipid surface rich in negatively charged phospholipids, and as platelets release the reaction determining FV during activation, platelets and clotting factors both contribute to the amplifica-

tion of the clotting cascade. Activated FIX enhances the initial activation of the clotting cascade by formation of a FX-activating complex together with its cofactor VIII. The importance of this amplifier loop is demonstrated by the bleeding tendency of patients showing inherited FVIII-(hemophilia A) or FIX-deficiencies (hemophilia B). Thrombin by itself contributes to its self-amplifying loop by activating FXI, FVIII and FV.

Formerly, the clotting cascade had been divided into an extrinsic and intrinsic pathway. Although useful for didactic purposes, both pathways are not separated but linked by tissue factor/FVIIa activation (Fig. 4).

While the extrinsic pathway starts with FVIIa binding to TF, the intrinsic pathway is characterized by activation through binding of contact factors (Factor XII, Prekallikrein, high molecular weight kininogen) to negatively charged surfaces. This leads to a conformational change and activation to FXIIa and kallikreine. Factor XIIa is a serine protease that activates FXI to FXIa (Fig. 5). This system is not of physiologic relevance since patients with hereditary deficiencies of factor XII, prekallikrein, and high-molecular weight kininogen do not present with bleeding symptoms.

Vitamin K-dependent Coagulation Factors

Factors VII, IX, X, and II belong to the group of vitamin K-dependent coagulation enzymes. This group of enzymes binds to phospholipid surfaces via Gla-domains, which are generated in the mole-

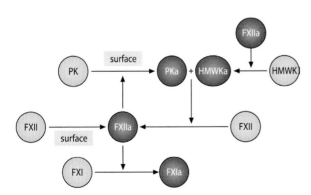

Fig. 5 Coagulation/Thrombosis

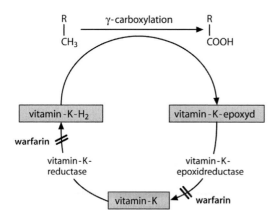

Fig. 6 Coagulation/Thrombosis

cule by γ-carboxylation of glutamic acid residues (Fig. 6). This molecular mechanism explains the therapeutic principle of vitamin K-antagonists, such as warfarine or other coumarines. However, the synthesis of the anticoagulant proteins C and S is also vitamin K-dependent (for clinical consequences see paragraph protein-C-pathway).

Generation of Fibrin
Fibrin is a high molecular polymer. The liver synthesizes its precursor, the protein fibrinogen. It consists of three peptide chains (α-, β-, γ-chain). Catalyzed by thrombin, the N-terminal fibrinopeptides A and B are cleaved from the α- and β-chain. The remaining peptide chains undergo a conformational change that allows end-to-end-polymerisation of the fibrin monomers. Stabilization of the fibrin monomers requires cross-linking by the formation of covalent links between the γ- and the α-chains. These links are catalyzed by the transglutaminase factor XIIIa (FXIIIa). FXIIIa is generated from FXIII by thrombin. Fibrin is also linked by FXIIIa to subendothelial proteins like collagen and fibronectin and to adhesive proteins such as vWF and vitronectin. Both, the covalent crosslink within the polymer and the interaction of the fibrinpolymer with the vessel wall provide a stabile clot. Noteworthy, patients with a FXIII deficiency present with an intact primary haemostasis but bleeding complications after a time delay of several hours due to instable clot formation.

Regulation of the Clotting Process
Without effective control mechanisms, the basic principle of self-enhancing amplification loops within the clotting cascade would lead to complete vessel occlusions (thrombosis) once a vessel wall defect occurs, or activated clotting factors would be transported from the side of a vessel injury with the blood stream to other areas causing unwanted clotting there. The anticoagulant mechanisms controlling the clotting process either inactivate clotting factors directly (e.g.: FXa, FIIa), or inactivate cofactors (e.g.: FVa).

Tissue Factor Pathway Inhibitor
Primarily, tissue factor pathway inhibitor (TFPI) binds to and inactivates FXa. In a second step TFPI/FXa complexes bind to and neutralize tissue factor/FVIIa complexes, the key starting point of the extrinsic clotting cascade (see above) (Fig. 7). Heparin is able to enhance this reaction by direct binding to the complex and by releasing TFPI from the unaltered vessel wall, which then can access the TF-exposing surface.

Antithrombin-heparan sulfate/Heparin System
Antithrombin (AT) is synthezised by the liver. It forms 1:1 complexes with FXa and FIIa (Fig. 8). Although AT binds to the active centre of the clotting factors FXa and FIIa (thrombin) it is not degraded by these proteases, but forms covalently linked complexes (pseudosubstrate). These AT-clotting factor complexes are degraded in the reticulo-endothelial system. Under physiological conditions, AT is catalyzed by endothelial-cell-surface-bound heparansulfate, which binds to AT.

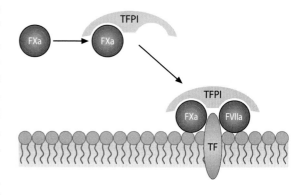

Fig. 7 Coagulation/Thrombosis

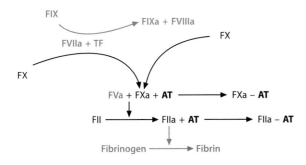

Fig. 8 Coagulation/Thrombosis

Catalyzation of AT is the major priciple of anti-coagulatory treatment with heparin. The length of high molecular weight heparins (>18 glucose units) allows formation of a trimolecular complex of AT and FIIa (thrombin) or FXa in which heparin is binding to both molecules, catalyzing thrombin inactivation. Smaller heparin molecules (low molecular weight heparins or the even smaller pentasaccharide) bind only to AT. This still enables inactivation of FXa but no longer inactivation of thrombin.

Besides AT, heparin cofactor II (HCII) is an anticoagulatory protein enhanced by heparin. HCII inactivates thrombin and the non-clotting-enzymes cathepsin-G and chymotrypsin.

Whereas patients with AT deficiency present clinically with a high risk for thrombosis, HCII deficient patients do not.

Protein-C Pathway

The protein-C pathway is one of the most important anticoagulant mechanisms. It is activated by thrombin. Thrombin binds to a cofactor in the membrane of endothelial cells, thrombomodulin (TM). TM bound thrombin no longer activates clotting factors or platelets but becomes an effective protein C (PC) activator. Activated PC (APC) forms a complex with Protein S, which inactivates FVIIIa and FVa. Hereby generation of FIIa by the prothrombinase complex is inhibited (Fig. 9). Thus, the PC-pathway controls thrombin generation in a negative feed-back manner.

In about 30–40% of patients with suspected inherited thrombophilia the PC-pathway is disturbed by a mutation of FV (FV-Leiden). The FV-Leiden mutation affects one of the APC cleavage sites within the FV molecule. As a consequence, mutated FVa becomes resistant to rapid APC inactivation (APC resistance). About 4–7% of the middle European population carry this polymorphism of FV. Inborn deficiencies of Protein-S or Protein-C are much less frequent (<<1% and 0.2–0.4%, respectively).

Iatrogenic PC deficiency always occurs at the beginning of oral anticoagulation with vitamin-K antagonists. Due to the short half-life of PC, its plasma concentrations decline within one day, whereas the procoagulatory clotting factors are still present in high concentrations. This makes it mandatory to start vitamin K-antagonist treatment only under parallel parenteral anticoagulation with heparin for about 5 days (Fig. 10).

A new aspect of the PC-pathway is the efficacy of recombinant-APC in reducing mortality in patients with septic schock. Whether this is related to the inhibition of thrombin generation or due to other biological activities of APC is currently under investigation.

Fibrinolysis

Lysis of clots is another system for regulation of the clotting system. Plasmin is the key enzyme of the fibrinolytic system. Its proenzyme plasminogen is synthesized by the liver as a one-chain protein. Tissue-type plasminogen activator (t-PA) and urokinase-type plasminogen activator (u-PA) activate plasminogen by cleavage. The remaining two chains are linked by disulphide bounds and undergo auto-catalytic cleavage at the N-terminus; thus, plasmin self-enhances its fibrinolytic activity.

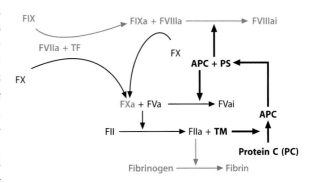

Fig. 9 Coagulation/Thrombosis

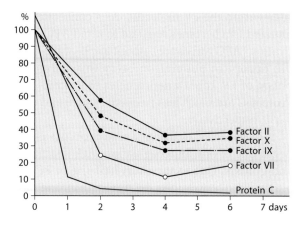

Fig. 10 Coagulation/Thrombosis

Plasmin cleaves fibrin at different positions. Of high clinically practical relevance is the cleavage of the fibrin γ-chain that results in D-Dimers (Fig. 11). D-Dimers are specific for fibrin-cleavage by plasmin. They can easily be detected by commercially available assays and are used to exclude a thrombosis. A negative test for D-Dimer has a high negative predictive value for a thrombosis. Therapeutically t-PA and urokinase are the most important drugs for fibrinolytic therapy (myocardial infarction, stroke, massive pulmonary embolism). This treatment is associated with an enhanced risk of bleeding complications.

Regulation of the Fibrinolytic System
Generation of plasmin is inhibited by the plasmin-activator inhibitor (PAI). PAI is secreted by

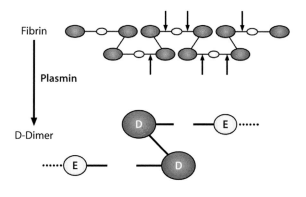

Fig. 11 Coagulation/Thrombosis

endothelial cells. It neutralizes t-PA and u-PA by forming 1:1 complexes.

Non-fibrin bound, free plasmin is inactivated by α_2-anti-plasmin by an irreversible, covalent 1:1 complex.

References

1. Müller-Berghaus G, Pötzsch B, Hämostaseologie, Springer Verlag, Berlin, 1998
2. Colman R.W., Hirsh J., Marder V.J., Salzman E.W. Hemostasis and Thrombosis, 4.ed. J.B. Lippincott Company Philadelphia, 2002
3. Gresele P., Page C., Fuster V., Vermylen J., Platelets in thrombotic and non-thrombotic disorders. Cambridge University Press, 2002

Coatomer

Coatomer is the major coat component of COPI vesicles. The Coatomer complex consists of seven different subunits (α-ζ COP).

▶ Intracellular Transport

Cocaine- and Amphetamine-regulated Transcript

▶ CART
▶ Appetite Control
▶ Psychostimulants

Co-dominant

A co-dominant is a heritable trait in which both alleles of a polymorphism are expressed and are reflected in the phenotype. The phenotype of heterozygous carriers is in between the phenotypes of the two homozygous genotypes.

▶ Pharmacogenetics

Coenzyme Q$_{10}$

Coenzyme Q$_{10}$ (ubiquinone) is a coenzyme in the mitochondrial respiratory chain. It has a side chain made up of 10 isoprene units. Its synthesis can be inhibited by HMG-CoA reductase inhibitors (statins). This effect has been suggested to account for some of the side effects of statins like myositis or rhabdomyolysis.

▶ HMG-CoA Reductase Inhibitors

Coincidence Detection

Coincidence detection describes the ability of the NMDA receptor to function as a sensor for synchronous activity states of the pre- and postsynaptic cell. Around resting membrane potential, NMDA receptors contribute little to fast signal transmission, due to a Mg^{2+} block of the channel pore, this block is released in depolarized cells and the channel can be fully activated.

▶ Ionotropic Glutamate Receptors

Colitis

Colitis is inflammation of the colon often involving ulceration of the mucosa.

▶ Immunosuppressive Agents

Collagen

Collagen is a major component of connective tissue that becomes exposed at the subendothelium of injured blood vessels. It contributes to platelet adhesion and also plays a role in platelet activation by binding to several receptors on platelets such as integrin α2β1 or glycoprotein VI (GP VI).

▶ Antiplatelet Drugs

Colony-stimulating Factors

Colony-stimulating factors (CSFs) belong to the group of cytokines, and function as haematopoietic factors [e.g. GM-CSF (filgrastim, lenograstim), GM-CSF (molgramostim, sargramostim)]. Colony-stimulating factors stimulate the growth and differentiation of haematopoietic progenitor cells.

▶ Hematopoietic Growth Factors

Combination Oral Contraceptive

A combination oral contraceptive contains both an estrogenic and a progestational component to achieve contraception.

▶ Contraceptives

Combinatorial Chemistry

JÖRG RADEMANN
Institut für Organische Chemie, Universität Tübingen, Tübingen, Germany
joerg.rademann@uni-tuebingen.de

Synonyms

Concepts and Methods for Tasks of Molecular Optimisation.

Definition

Combinatorial chemistry constitutes a branch of the molecular sciences, providing an array of concepts and methods to solve molecular optimisation problems (in drug research and beyond) more rapidly and efficiently than classical synthetic approaches.

▶ High-throughput Screening
▶ NMR-based Ligand Screening

Description

Combinatorial chemistry started with an attempt to mimic biological evolution cycles of synthesis and selection in the chemical laboratory. Since specific molecular interactions between proteins and their ligands have been recognized as the molecular basis of most biological processes including disease, it became possible to study and optimise the interactions between drugs and their target proteins on a molecular level. Thus, drug development has turned into a systematic and rational task of optimisation. During the 1990s in the pharmaceutical industry, synthetic chemistry became evident as the major bottleneck in drug development. Combinatorial chemistry was the answer of the synthetic chemistry community. The term `combinatorial` is derived from the mathematical discipline combinatorics dealing with the statistics of element combinations. Combinatorics are employed in chemistry to calculate the number of possible combinations of m chemical building blocks in n synthetic cycles (n^m, see Fig. 1). For example, the 20 native amino acids can be combined to form 20^6 different linear hexapeptides.

Centerpieces of combinatorial concepts include the synthesis of compound libraries instead of the preparation of single target compounds. Library synthesis is supplemented by approaches to optimise the diversity of a compound collection (diversity-oriented synthesis) and by efforts to create powerful interfaces between combinatorial synthesis and bioassays.

These conceptual goals are attained by several combinatorial methods and tools. Characteristic for combinatorial chemistry is the synthesis on solid support or by polymer-supported synthesis, allowing for much higher efficiency in library production. Synthesis can be conducted either in automated parallel synthesis or by ▶ split-and-recombine synthesis. Centerpieces of combinatorial methods further include specific analytical methods for combinatorial chemistry and computer-aided methods for combinatorial chemistry.

Library Synthesis

Precisely defined collections of different chemical compounds are denominated as chemical libraries that can be efficiently prepared by methods of combinatorial chemistry. Each chemical compound owes specific structural, steric, and electronic properties that determine all possible interactions of the small molecule with a given protein or receptor. The molecule's properties are based on the steric arrangement of functional groups, including the conformations that can be attained by a specific structure.

Complex optimisation of the ligand-protein interactions require to scan large areas of the property space. Thus, the combinatorial chemist aims not at the preparation of single compounds but of chemical libraries. Chemical libraries can be produced as collections of single compounds or as defined mixtures.

Diversity-oriented Synthesis

An important criterion of a compound library is its chemical diversity, a term describing the similarity or dissimilarity of all library compounds. Thus, chemical diversity expresses how well a library represents all chemical possibilities of the theoretical library. A library with low chemical diversity contains molecules that are relatively similar, thus covering a small area of the accessible property space. On the contrary, a library with a large chemical diversity will contain relatively dissimilar molecules, covering a large volume of the property space. The diversity of a library is a major criterion of its quality and its possible applications. Large diversity is required mainly in the early stages of drug development (lead search), whereas defined small diversity (focussed libraries) is needed for lead optimisation. Even a large library, however, cannot contain all possible combinations of building blocks as it is impossible to synthesize all individual compounds. Thus, in any case the choice of synthesized compounds has to be considered in order to optimize the diversity. Contrary to classical organic synthesis which was directed at the preparation of a single target compound, diversity-oriented synthesis aims at providing libraries with defined chemical diversity,

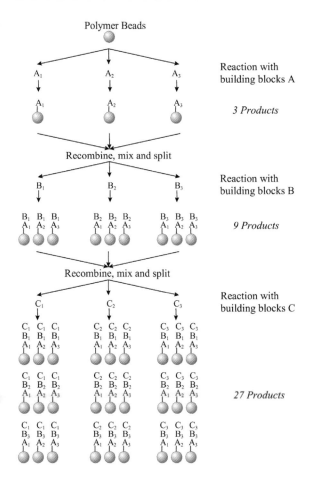

Polymer Beads

A$_1$ A$_2$ A$_3$ Reaction with building blocks A

A$_1$ A$_2$ A$_3$ 3 Products

Recombine, mix and split

B$_1$ B$_2$ B$_3$ Reaction with building blocks B

B$_1$ B$_1$ B$_1$ B$_2$ B$_2$ B$_2$ B$_3$ B$_3$ B$_3$
A$_1$ A$_2$ A$_3$ A$_1$ A$_2$ A$_3$ A$_1$ A$_2$ A$_3$ 9 Products

Recombine, mix and split

C$_1$ C$_2$ C$_3$ Reaction with building blocks C

C$_1$ C$_1$ C$_1$ C$_2$ C$_2$ C$_2$ C$_3$ C$_3$ C$_3$
B$_1$ B$_1$ B$_1$ B$_1$ B$_1$ B$_1$ B$_1$ B$_1$ B$_1$
A$_1$ A$_2$ A$_3$ A$_1$ A$_2$ A$_3$ A$_1$ A$_2$ A$_3$

C$_1$ C$_1$ C$_1$ C$_2$ C$_2$ C$_2$ C$_3$ C$_3$ C$_3$
B$_2$ B$_2$ B$_2$ B$_2$ B$_2$ B$_2$ B$_2$ B$_2$ B$_2$
A$_1$ A$_2$ A$_3$ A$_1$ A$_2$ A$_3$ A$_1$ A$_2$ A$_3$ 27 Products

C$_1$ C$_1$ C$_1$ C$_2$ C$_2$ C$_2$ C$_3$ C$_3$ C$_3$
B$_3$ B$_3$ B$_3$ B$_3$ B$_3$ B$_3$ B$_3$ B$_3$ B$_3$
A$_1$ A$_2$ A$_3$ A$_1$ A$_2$ A$_3$ A$_1$ A$_2$ A$_3$

Fig. 1 Combinatorial chemistry provides an array of concepts and methods to solve molecular optimisation problems. Chemical libraries are prepared either by parallel synthesis or by the split-and-recombine method. In the latter case, coupling m building blocks in n synthetic cycles on a beaded polymer carrier generates a combinatorial library with m^n individual compounds and one compound per bead.

with the help of combinatorial methods and tools described herein.

Solid Phase Synthesis vs. Polymer-supported Synthesis in Solution

The evolution of combinatorial methods was closely linked to the development of polymer-supported synthesis, which opened efficient access to diversity-oriented synthesis. In ▶ solid phase synthesis, forming the backbone of most combinatorial methods, insoluble organic or inorganic matrices are employed as carriers for the construction of product molecules. Using insoluble polymer supports is advantageous, strongly facilitating the isolation of intermediates and products attached to the polymer support. By-products formed in each stage of the synthesis are easily removed by washing the polymer support, thus each isolation step is reduced to simple filtration. By employing reagents in high excess, complete conversion can be attained on the solid phase in reactions that form mixtures in solution. The relative isolation of reactive sites on the polymer supports can be exploited for specific synthetic effects such as favouring cyclisation and the reduction of by-products. Finally, the compartmentalised structure of polymers supports allows for split-and-recombine synthesis.

Under certain condition, however, reactions are still preferably conducted in solution. This is the case e.g. for heterogeneous reactions and for conversions, that deliver complex product mixtures. In the latter case, further conversion of this mixture on the solid support is not desirable. In these instances, the combination of solution chemistry with polymer-assisted conversions can be an advantageous solution. Polymer-assisted synthesis in solution employs the polymer matrix either as a scavenger or for polymeric reagents. In both cases the virtues of solution phase and solid supported chemistry are ideally combined allowing for the preparation of pure products by filtration of the reactive resin. If several reactive polymers are used sequentially, multi-step syntheses can be conducted in a polymer-supported manner in solution as well. As a further advantage, many reactive polymers can be recycled for multiple use.

Parallel Synthesis and Automation

If small or medium libraries for lead optimisation are demanded and all synthetic products are to be screened individually, most often parallel synthesis is the method of choice. Parallel syntheses can be conducted in solution, on solid phase, with polymer-assisted solution phase syntheses or with a combination of several of these methods. Preferably, parallel syntheses are automated, either employing integrated synthesis robots or by automation of single steps such as washing, isolation or identification. The latter concept often allows a more flexible and less expensive automation of parallel synthesis.

Split-and-recombine Synthesis for the Preparation of Large Libraries

If large or very large libraries are demanded and if a powerful interface to a subsequent bioassay is available, split-and-recombine synthesis can be the method of choice. Split-and-recombine synthesis is mostly conducted on solid phase. During each coupling step the resin is divided into one reactor for each coupled building block (split). Following the coupling reaction with m building blocks, all resin beads are pooled and mixed (recombine) (see Fig. 1). Consequently, after n coupling steps m^n different compounds are obtained in theory, the real number of individual compounds is only limited by the number of available resin beads. As in each coupling step only one building block is coupled per reaction vessel, in the end on every bead only one compound is produced (one bead-one compound).

Introduced in the early 1990s, the split-and-recombine concept contributed much to the early success of combinatorial chemistry. Often, all combinatorial methods were identified with this concept. Split-and-recombine synthesis offered easy access to large numbers of individual compounds in few steps. If conducted on polymer beads, these are easily separated mechanically and can be identified subsequent to a screening step.

Though split-and-recombine techniques make available many compounds in few steps, the concept possesses significant limitations as well. A well-defined synthesis requires employing reliable reactions for all of the different starting materials. This requirement is fulfilled only for few reaction types, such as acylations of amines, reductive aminations, substitution of α-halogeno carbonyl compounds. If however, the products of a split-and-recombine synthesis are not obtained purely, it becomes increasingly difficult to ascribe a biological signal unambiguously to an individual compound.

Analytical Methods in Combinatorial Chemistry

Essential prerequisites for the evolution of combinatorial methods was the progress in reaction monitoring and analytics. Of specific importance was the analytics of structures attached to a polymeric support (▶ on-resin-analysis) as well as the analytics of cleaved compounds in solution (off-resin-analysis).

For on-bead analysis vibrational spectroscopy (▶ IR-spectroscopy) can be employed; attenuated total reflection is a method allowing fast and non-destructive on-bead analysis of small samples (single bead analysis) without significant sample preparation. Solid phase ▶ NMR is the method of choice if complex structural analysis is intended on the support. Spatially resolved analysis on the resin is possible with microscopic techniques.

For off-bead analysis, coupling between chromatographic separation and mass spectrometric detection has proven especially powerful. The combination between high performance liquid chromatography (HPLC) and ▶ electrospray ionisation mass spectrometry has the advantage that purity of product mixtures can be coupled on-line with the product identification.

Integration of Combinatorial Synthesis and Screening

The potency of combinatorial chemistry is optimally exploited by efficiently integrating combinatorial synthesis with a subsequent bioassay. This integration is especially yielding if large libraries of synthetic compounds can be screened simultaneously. If the synthetic chemistry is controlled well, it becomes possible through the integration of synthesis and screening to first select the most active compounds, analyse and resynthesise them for verification. By this method the enormous effort necessary for the screening of large libraries is significantly reduced. This concept was especially successful for the on-bead screening of split-and-recombine libraries. Hits (i.e. the most active compounds) are preferably visualized by fluorescence or colour, can be separated by manual or automated selection and subsequently analysed. Identification of hits is effected by non-covalent binding of fluorophor-labelled proteins or, in the case of polymer-based protease inhibitor assays, by a fluorescent dye that is formed dependent on the inhibitor activity. Identification of hit structures is facilitated by tagging of the beads with easily detectable structures that code for the synthesized molecule on one individual bead.

Computer-aided Combinatorial Chemistry

Until the 1980s rational drug design was propagated as the method of choice of medicinal chemistry. One reason for the initial popularity of combinatorial methods was the dissatisfaction with and the limited success of rational molecular design. Meanwhile, it has been recognized that combinatorial chemistry can profit strongly from computer-aided methods. It became obvious that all possible combinations of building blocks cannot be prepared synthetically due to limited physical resources and for cost reasons. Thus, the chemist has devised criteria for selecting prepared compounds from a theoretically available virtual library.

In the easiest case, these criteria are provided by filters that were constituted by statistically analysing all orally available drugs accessible in the word drug index. Similarity filters are usually applied in the early stages of drug development.

During advanced stages of the drug development, especially for the synthesis of focussed libraries, a number of computer-aided methods are available that exploit the acquired information about the target protein and/or the tested compounds. Starting from protein structures or a structural model of the protein binding site, variations of the lead structure can be evaluated by virtual docking. Alternatively, *de-novo* design of potential ligands with the help of a virtual binding site is possible.

Pharmacological Relevance

Combinatorial chemistry is the branch of the molecular sciences providing concepts and methods for solving problems of molecular optimisation fast and efficiently.Since drug development has turned into a systematic and rational task of optimising molecules and their interactions with proteins, cells, and organisms, combinatorial chemistry has become a significant part of this endeavour. Combinatorial methods are mainly employed in the initial (preclinical) stages of drug development.

References

1. Jung G (ed.) (1999) Combinatorial Chemistry - Synthesis, Analysis, and Screening, Weinheim.
2. Nicolaou K C, Hanko R, Hartwig W. (eds.) (2002) Handbook of Combinatorial Chemistry, 2 volumes, Weinheim.
3. Zaragoza Dörwald F. (2000) Organic Synthesis on Solid Phase, Weinheim.
4. Rademann J, Jung G (2000) Integrating combinatorial synthesis with bioassays. Science 287:1947–1948

Compartment

A compartment is an anatomical space in the body into which a drug or metabolite, or a chemical derivative or metabolite formed from the parent drug may distribute.

▶ Pharmacokinetics

Competitive Antagonists

By definition, competitive antagonists compete with the agonist for the same binding domain on the receptor. Therefore, the relative affinities and the relative concentrations of the agonist and antagonist dictate which ligand dominates. Under these circumstances, the concentration of agonist can always be raised to the point where the concomitant receptor occupancy by the antagonist is insignificant. When this occurs, the maximal response to the agonist is observed, i.e. surmountable antagonism results.

▶ Drug-receptor Interaction

Complement System

The complement system is a cascade of proteins of the immune response that can be triggered by antigen-antibody complexes and by the innate immune system (eg exposure to microbial polysaccharides) to raise the immune response. Complement proteins can detect and bind to foreign material or immune complexes and label them for phagocytosis. They can also cause inflammation by directly degranulating mast cells and releasing chemokines to recruit other immune cells into the affected area.

▶ Immune Defense
▶ Allergy
▶ Inflammation
▶ Histaminergic System

Compound Libraries

A compound library is a compound collection. The compound libraries of large pharmaceutical and screening companies can exceed 1 million samples. Libraries are synthesized and stored as either individual samples or as combinations.

▶ Combinatorial Chemistry
▶ High-throughput Screening

Computerized Tomography

Slices of the body are irradiated from one side. X-ray detectors quantify the remaining intensity of the X-rays after passing through the various tissues. The X-ray tube and the detectors are rotating around the body. The data are used to calculate images of the corresponding slice which reflect the absorption of X-rays in a great number of pixels of an individual slice.

▶ Radiocontrast Agents

COMT

▶ Catechol-O-Methyl-Transferase

Conditioned Place Preference

The conditioned place preference paradigm is widely used in order to measure the rewarding properties of drugs of abuse (secondary reinforcement). In general, individuals are injected with either the drug or the vehicle solution and placed in boxes with floors of different texture (i.e. either perforated or bar). In this way, the association between the administration of the drug and a particular floor texture (or place) is established. On the final day of the experiment, individuals are left untreated and placed in conditioning boxes that have the two different floor types. To determine the rewarding effects of the drug, the time that each individual stays on the floor type paired with the drug is measured. If the drug has rewarding properties, the individual shows a preference to the side that has been paired with drug administration.

▶ Drug Addiction/Dependence

Conditioned Withdrawal

Individuals experiencing drug withdrawal can become conditioned to environmental situations. Previously neutral stimuli can elicit many of the symptoms of drug withdrawal, and this "conditioned withdrawal" has motivational significance, especially in alcohol and opiate addiction. Thus conditioned withdrawal may trigger craving and relapse in a particular situation.

▶ Drug Addiction/Dependence

Conjugative Plasmid

A plasmid is termed conjugative if it has the capacity to transfer itself from one cell to the other. They can be either self-transmissible or mobilizable (the latter necessitate the presence of a self-transmissible plasmid that supplies missing transfer functions). The *tra* genes encode among other proteins the subunits that form a sex pilus required to mediate the first contact between the donor and the recipient cell (in case of plasmids of gram-negative bacteria). Both cells then come into close contact and form a stable mating pair. The plasmid DNA in the donor cell is then cleaved at an *ori*T site (origin of transfer) and unwound and one strand is transferred into the recipient cell. Complemetary DNA strands are synthesized and recircularized.

▶ Microbial Resistance to Drugs

Conjugative Transposon

Conjugative transposons are self-transmissible large DNA elements (up to 150 kb pairs) located in the donor chromosome. After excision, a circular intermediate is formed that is unable to replicate autonomously. It is nicked at an origin of transfer site and one strand is then transferred to the recipient cell. After generating a doublestranded circle, the transposon integrates into the recipient's chromosome.

▶ Microbial Resistance toDrugs

Conotoxins

Conotoxins are the venoms of the marine cone snails. The >500 *Conus* species produce >10,000 different toxins. All are cysteine-rich peptides of 10 to 30 amino acids. Many act on their target molecules with high selectivity. The α-conotoxins are competitive antagonists at nicotinic acetycholine receptors$_{(a1)}$. The μ-toxins block voltage-sensitive Na^+ channels. The ω-toxins block Ca^{2+} channels. Synthetic ω-conotoxin MVIIA (ziconotide) has been introduced into therapy for spinal administration in chronic pain. Like morphine (but by direct channel blockade rather than through a G

protein pathway) it inhibits transmitter release from nociceptive afferents.

▶ Voltage-dependent Na^+ Channels

Constitutive Activity

▶ Constitutive Receptor Activity

Constitutive Androstane Receptor

The constitutive androstane receptor (CAR) is a nuclear receptor, which binds a variety of endogenous substances as well as xenobiotics (e.g. 3α, 5α-androstanol, phenobarbital). CAR forms heterodimers with the retinoid X receptor, RXR and induces the expression of a variety of enzymes and transporters including the cytochrome P450 monooxygenase CYP2B.

Constitutive Receptor Activity

▶ G-protein-coupled receptors are thought to exist in at least two states; (1) an inactive state and (2) an active state where the receptor can bind to its G-protein and elicit a functional response. Under basal conditions, the equilibrium between the two states of the receptor is substantially in favour of the inactive state. Agonists normally bind with higher affinity to the active form of the receptor and alter the equilibrium in a manner to increase the proportion of receptors in the active state. Sometimes, however, there is sufficient active receptor present under basal conditions to produce a measurable response in the absence of agonist. In this situation the receptor is termed to have constitutive activity.

▶ Transmembrane Signalling

▶ Drug-Receptor Interaction
▶ Inverse Agonist
▶ Histaminergic System

Contact Inhibition

Contact inhibition is observed in the process of wound healing and describes the ability of a tissue to stop cell proliferation again after cellular multiplication has filled up the defect caused by a wound.

▶ Antineoplastic Agents

Contraceptives

THOMAS GUDERMANN
Philipps-Universität Marburg, Marburg, Germany
guderman@mailer.uni-marburg.de

Synonyms

Hormonal contraceptives, oral contraceptives

Definition

Hormonal contraceptives belong to the most widely prescribed and most efficacious drugs that have a profound impact on western societies since their inauguration in the 1960s. In women, oral hormonal contraceptives are used to prevent fertilization or implantation in cases of unplanned pregnancies. Apart from these primary objectives, there are significant additional medical benefits contributing to a substantial improvement of reproductive health in women.

▶ Selective Sex-steroid Receptor Modulators
▶ Sex Steroid Receptors

Mechanism of Action

The most frequently used oral contraceptives are composed of varying combinations of ▶ estrogens and ▶ progestins, which belong to the large family of ▶ steroid hormones. Steroids interact with intracellular receptors functioning as ligand-activated transcription factors to control the expression of a wide array of specific genes. The receptors for estrogens and progestins are members of a superfamily of approximately 150 structurally related nuclear receptors that bind ligands such as steroid hormones, retinoids, vitamin D_3, eicosanoids and thyroid hormones (1). Members of this receptor superfamily share a common architecture of mainly four conserved functional domains: The N-terminal transactivation domain (activation function, AF-1) is the most variable in the superfamily of receptors. The subsequent DNA-binding domain also participates in receptor dimerization, whereas nuclear localization is determined by the neighbouring hinge region. The C-terminal hormone-binding domain comprises a ligand-dependent transcriptional activation function (AF-2) and provides the sites for the binding of chaperones like heat shock proteins that prevent dimerization and DNA binding of unliganded receptors.

Upon hormone binding, steroid hormone receptors undergo a conformational change, dissociate from heat shock proteins and translocate into the nucleus where they interact as dimers with specific DNA regulatory sequences of target genes. The transcriptional regulation by steroid hormone receptors is mediated by co-regulatory proteins that either positively (▶ co-activators) or negatively (▶ co-repressors) influence steroid hormone-induced transcriptional activity. A complementary mode of steroid hormone receptor action relies on direct protein-protein interactions with other transcription factors such as AP-1, Sp-1, and NF-κB, thus providing an explanation for the well known observation that steroid hormone receptors are able to regulate genes lacking consensus response elements in their non-coding 5′ region (2).

Most nuclear receptors are phosphoproteins, and their function can be influenced by phosphorylation events that are initiated by membranous receptors like receptor tyrosine kinases or G-protein-coupled receptors. Thus, steroid hormone receptors are embedded in complex signalling networks that may give rise to ligand-independent activation of nuclear receptors. In addition to the well-understood nuclear events set in motion by steroid hormones, rapid non-genomic effects have been reported for estrogens and progesterone. These rapid effects of sex steroids that are often initiated at the plasma membrane, may result from receptor-independent alterations of plasma membrane fluidity or from steroid effects on membranous receptors other than classical steroid hormone receptors. In particular, the rapid engagement of the MAP kinase cascade by estrogen has been studied in great detail, and it is quite likely that cardinal estrogenic effects like cell proliferation and survival are not primarily brought about by genomic actions of classical nuclear receptors but by rapid, non-genomic mechanisms (3).

At present, two distinct nuclear estrogen receptors, ERα and ERβ, are known. The receptors differ in their tissue distribution, ligand binding profile and transcription activation functions in that ERβ is devoid of AF-1. In cells that express both estrogen receptors, ERβ appears to oppose the transcriptional activity of ERα. Due to two distinct estrogen-dependent promoters in the single progesterone receptor (PR) gene, two isoforms of the progesterone receptor, PR-B and the N-terminally shortened PR-A, are generated. The biological activities of PR-A and PR-B are distinct and depend on the target tissue in question. In the reproductive system, progesterone acting through its respective nuclear receptors, PR-A and PR-B, serves the role of a physiological negative regulator of estrogen action by causing depletion of estrogen receptors. In addition, the major role of PR-A may be to inhibit transcriptional activity of other steroid receptors like ERα. Although one aspect of the biological relationship between estrogen and progesterone may be called functional antagonism, a concerted, sequential action of estrogen and progesterone is required in reproductive tissues like the endometrium and the breast to yield the desired complex biological response.

Estrogen and progesterone play a central role in the neuroendocrine control of the female menstrual cycle. In the early follicular phase estrogen exerts an inhibitory effect on the pulsatile secretion of ▶ gonadotropins from the pituitary (Fig. 1). Thus, the gradual increase in the peripheral estradiol concentration during the follicular phase is accompanied by a reduced release of luteinizing hormone (LH) and follicle-stimulating hormone (FSH) from the gonadotropes. At midcycle, a different set of regulatory interactions becomes dominant. A sustained elevation of estradiol (150 to 200 pg/ml for approximately 36 hours) induces a positive feedback on the anterior pituitary to trigger the ovulatory surge of LH. The underlying mechanism is a sensitisation of the pituitary gonadotropes towards hypothalamic gonadotropin-releasing hormone (GnRH). Progesterone decreases the frequency of GnRH release from the hypothalamus resulting in a marked decrease of the frequency of gonadotropin pulses in the luteal phase (Fig. 1). At the same time, progesterone increases the amount of LH released per pulse (i. e. the pulse amplitude).

The main mechanism of action of a ▶ combination oral contraceptive is to prevent ovulation by inhibiting gonadotropin secretion via an effect on both pituitary and hypothalamic centers. The progestational component primarily suppresses the surge-like LH release required to induce ovulation, while the estrogenic agent suppresses FSH secretion and thus prevents selection of a dominant follicle. Therefore, both estrogenic and progestational components of an oral contraceptive synergistically contribute to the contraceptive efficacy. However, even if follicular growth were not sufficiently inhibited, the progestational agent alone would suffice to abrogate the ovulatory LH surge. The estrogenic component, however, serves at least two other important purposes. It is responsible for the stability of the endometrium, thus minimizing events of irregular and unwanted breakthrough bleeding. In addition, estrogen action provides for a sufficient concentration of progesterone receptors. In aggregate, a small pharmacologic estrogen level is necessary to maintain the efficacy of the combination oral contraceptive.

As under most circumstances progesterone action will hold primacy over estrogenic effects, the cervical mucus, endometrium, and probably the fallopian tubes reflect progestational stimulation. The cervical mucus becomes thick and viscous and thus impervious to spermatozoa. The

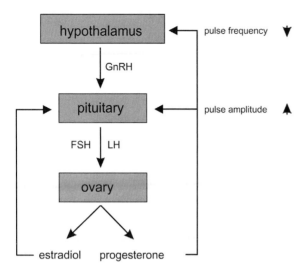

Fig. 1 Regulation of hypothalamic and pituitary function by ovarian steroid hormones. Estrogen exerts a negative feedback on the pituitary and decreases the secretion of follicle-stimulating hormone (FSH) and luteinizing hormone (LH) during most of the menstrual cycle. Yet, it triggers the LH surge at midcycle by sensitising the pituitary to hypothalamic gonadotropin-releasing hormone (GnRH). Progesterone increases the amplitude of gonadotropins released from the pituitary and at the same time decreases the GnRH pulse frequency at the level of the hypothalamus. These feedback controls give rise to fairly frequent LH pulses of low amplitude during the follicular phase of the cycle and less frequent pulses with a higher amplitude in the luteal phase.

endometrium is in a state that is not receptive for implantation of a fertilized egg. Probably, the progestational impact on the secretory activity and peristalsis in the fallopian tubes also assists the general contraceptive effect. It is difficult, however, to assess the relative contribution of the various effects to the contraceptive efficacy, because combination oral contraceptives suppress ovulation very effectively.

The progestin-only minipill contains a small dose of a progestational agent which is sufficient to block ovulation in only 60–80% of cycles. The contraceptive effect is largely dependent on endometrial and cervical mucus effects, as gonadotropins are not reliably suppressed. Because of the low dose of progestins, the minipill must be taken every day at the same time with great accuracy.

Long-acting methods of hormonal contraception are even more effective than oral methods. Two effective systems are available: a sustained-release method of levonorgestrel using implanted steroid-permeable silastic tubing and depot injections of medroxyprogesterone acetate. The mechanism of action is similar to the progestin-only minipill. However, in addition, the long-acting methods yield progestin plasma levels high enough to prevent ovulation in basically all patients.

Large doses of estrogen to prevent implantation were used for emergency postcoital contraception. It was soon appreciated that the extremely large estrogen doses used (25–50 mg/day of diethylstilbestrol or ethinyl estradiol) entailed a high rate of gastrointestinal untoward effects. Clinical trials have ushered the use of combination oral contraceptives for emergency postcoital contraception. In principle, high-dose oral contraceptives are adiministered within 72 hours of intercourse, followed by a second dose 12 hours later. Such a regimen reduces the risk of pregnancy by approximately 75%. Multiple mechanisms appear to contribute to the treatment efficacy, for instance inhibition of ovulation, endometrial receptivity, cervical mucus composition, and tubular transport of spermatozoa. It is important to note that emergency contraceptives are not used as medical abortifacients to interrupt an established pregnancy defined to begin with implantation.

Clinical Use (incl. side effects)

After the seminal observation by Gregory Pincus and colleagues in the 1950s that progestins prevented ovulation in women, initial trials on humans were conducted using progestins like norethynodrel that were contaminated with about 1% mestranol. When subsequent efforts to provide a more pure progestin lowered the estrogenic component but provoked breakthrough bleeding, it was decided to keep the estrogen. Thus, the principles of combined estrogen-progestin oral contraception were established.

A major obstacle to the use of naturally occurring estrogens for the purpose of contraception was extensive first-pass hepatic metabolism and hence inactivation of the compounds when given orally. The addition of an ethinyl group at the 17 position made estradiol orally active. Ethinyl estradiol is a potent oral estrogen and represents one of the two forms of estrogens used in oral contraceptive pills. The other estrogenic compound is the 3-methyl ether of ethinyl estradiol, mestranol which is converted to ethinyl estradiol in the body.

The progestins used in oral contraceptives are 19-nor compounds of the estrane and gonane series (Fig. 2). Each compound possesses various degress of androgenic, estrogenic and antiandrogenic activities, thereby determining the scope of side effects. Animal and human studies showed, however, that only norethindrone, norethynodrel, and ethynodiol diacetate have estrogen activity. Replacement of the 13-methyl group of norethindrone with a 13-ethyl moiety gives rise to the gonane norgestrel, which is a potent progestin with reduced androgenic activity (Fig. 2). More recently developed compounds like desogestrel (Fig. 2), norgestimate and gestoden display the least androgenic characteristics when compared with other 19-nor substances. Although norgestimate is a "newer" progestin, its activity is believed to be largely mediated by levonorgestrel or related metabolites. Therefore, epidemiologists do not generally include combination contraceptives containing norgestimate in the group of third generation compounds.

In epidemiologic studies, all products containing less than 50 µg ethinyl estradiol per pill are summarized as ▸ low-dose oral contraceptives. The first generation of oral contraceptives includes products with 50 µg or more of ethinyl estradiol. The second generation of oral contraceptives comprises formulations of norgestrel (0.3–0.5 mg), levonorgestrel (0.1–0.15 mg), norgestimate (0.25 mg), ethynodiol diacetate (1 mg) and other members of the northethindrone family in conjunction with 30 or 35 µg ethinyl estradiol. Desogestrel (0.15 mg) or gestodene (0.075 mg) are progestins in third generation contraceptives that are combined with 20 or 30 µg ethinyl estradiol. Most notably, the first oral contraceptive available contained 150 µg mestranol and 10 mg norethynodrel. It is nowadays commonly believed that the formulations of third generation oral contraceptives are very close to the lowest hormone levels which can be used without sacrificing contraceptive efficacy.

Combination oral contraceptives are the most frequently used agents and are characterized by a high therapeutic efficacy. Carefully controlled clinical studies with highly motivated subjects achieve an annual failure rate of 0.1%. The typical use effectiveness, however, amounts to 97 to 98%. Combination oral contraceptives are used as monophasic, biphasic, triphasic, and sequential preparations. In ▸ monophasic preparations (Fig. 3), a fixed estrogen/progestin combination is present in each pill which is administered daily for 21 consecutive days followed by a 7-day hormone-free period (usually the pills for the last 7 days of a 28-day pack contain only inert ingredients). In the bi- and triphasic preparations (Fig. 3) varying amounts and ratios of estrogen to progestin are present in order to mimic most closely the sex steroid levels throughout a normal menstrual cycle. In addition, the total amount of steroids administered can be reduced when taking multiphasic oral contraceptives. ▸ Sequential preparations (Fig. 3) contain only estrogens for the first 7 to 11 days followed by a fixed estrogen/progestin combination in the remainder of the 21-day hormone application period. Phasic and sequential preparations were developed mainly to reduce the amount of progestins due to their untoward effects on the cardiovascular system.

Progestin-only contraceptives (Fig. 3) contain low doses of progestins (e. g. 350 µg norethindrone or 75 µg norgestrel) that have to be administered daily without interruption. The lowest expected failure rate during the first year of use is 0.5%, while the typical failure rate amounts to 3%. Subdermal implants of norgestrel (216 mg) for sustained release provides for long-term (for up to 5 years) contraceptive effects characterized by failure rates of only 0.05%. Reliable contraception for 3 months can be achieved by an intramuscular injection of a crystalline suspension of 150 mg medroxyprogesterone acetate (Fig. 2) (failure rate 0.3%).

The main purpose of healthy women taking oral contraceptives is to prevent unwanted pregnancies. "Primum non nocere" applies particularly to preventive health care measures and therefore, untoward effects of oral contraceptives have to be monitored and assessed with great scrutiny. Shortly after the introduction of oral contraceptives approximately 40 years ago they soon

pregnanes:

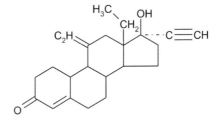

progesterone   medroxyprogesterone acetate

estranes:

19 - nortestosterone   norethindrone

gonanes:

norgestrel   desogestrel

Fig. 2 Examples of progestins derived from progesterone (pregnanes), 19-nortestosterone (estranes), and norgestrel (gonanes).

became one of the most widely used drugs throughout the world. Hence, it is not surprising that reports on adverse effects began to appear rather quickly. Most of the untoward effects appeared to be dose-dependent, thus spurring on researchers to develop the current low-dose preparations. The most worrying adverse effects can be summarized in two main categories: the cardiovascular system and cancer.

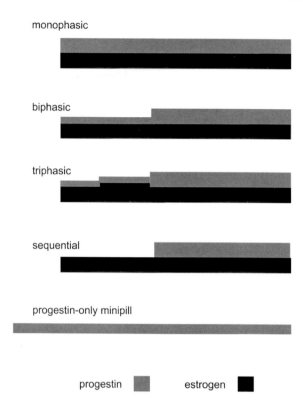

monophasic

biphasic

triphasic

sequential

progestin-only minipill

progestin   ▮   estrogen   ▮

Fig. 3 Principal composition of various forms of oral contraceptives.

Synthetic estrogens like ethinyl estradiol have a profound effect on the production of fibrinogen and clotting factors VII, VIII, X, and XII in the liver. In parallel, the concentrations of anticoagulation factors like protein C, S, and antithrombin III are diminished. This procoagulatory effect leads to an increased risk of thromboembolism in healthy women taking oral estrogens. In 1995 several studies reported on a two-fold increase in the risk of venous thromboembolism when third generation oral contraceptives containing desogestrel and gestoden were compared with older preparations mostly containing levonorgestrel. This highly contentious issue was finally resolved when further analyses were able to explain the divergent results by confounding variables.

The effects of oral contraceptives on thrombosis can be surmised as follows: All low-dose oral contraceptives, regardless of the type of progestin, have an increased risk of venous thromboembolism. Smoking has no effect on the risk of venous

thrombosis. However, smoking and estrogen administration have an additive effect on the risk of arterial thrombosis. Oral contraceptive-induced hypertension was previously observed in users of higher dose pills. An increased risk of clinically significant hypertension, however, has not been reported for low-dose oral contraceptives, including those containing the third generation progestins. Preexisting hypertension is an important additive risk factor for stroke in oral contraceptive users. Most notably, recent clinical studies fail to find any substantial risk of myocardial infarction or stroke in healthy, non-smoking women, regardless of age, who take low-dose oral contraceptives. The vast majority of myocardial infactions and strokes in oral contraceptive users occur when women over the age of 35 and cardiovascular risk factors take high-dose products (more than 50 µg ethinyl estradiol per pill). By meticulous screening for the presence of smoking and cardiovascular risk factors, especially hypertension, in older women, the risk of thromboembolic disease associated with low-dose oral contraceptives can virtually be annihilated.

In 1996 a metaanalysis of 54 epidemiologic studies indicated that women had a slightly increased risk of breast cancer while taking oral contraceptives when compared to non-users (relative risk = 1.24). The increased risk diminished steadily after cessation of medication and was not found elevated 10 years after discontinuation. However, a recent population based case-control study of more than 4,500 women with breast cancer and nearly 4,700 controls showed no association between past or present use of oral contraceptives (4). Due to the large study, subgroups of women, e.g. those taking a formulation with a high estrogen content, duration of oral contraceptive use, initiation of use during adolescence, history of breast cancer in a first-degree relative, could be analysed. None of these subgroups had a significantly increased risk of breast cancer. In light of these reassuring data, one has to conclude that oral contraceptive use is not associated with an increased risk of breast cancer. Such a conclusion contrasts sharply with the outcome of the Women's Health Initiative (WHI), the first randomised primary prevention trial on the effect of combined estrogen plus progestin (0.625 mg conjugated equine estrogen and 2.5 mg medroxyprogesterone acetate per day) on healthy postmeno-pausal women. The latter study was terminated early, chiefly because women receiving the active drug had an increased risk of breast cancer and the overall assessment was that the treatment was causing more harm than good (5). It is therefore important to note that because of differences in doses and specific agents used, it is not justified to extrapolate adverse side effects of hormone replacement therapy to oral contraceptives or vice versa.

Thus, our attention should shift from the concern of potential adverse effects to the health benefits imparted by hormonal contraceptives. The use of oral contraceptives for at least 12 months reduces the risk of developing endometrial cancer by 50%. Furthermore, the risk of epithelial ovarian cancer in users of oral contraceptives is reduced by 40% compared with that on nonusers. This kind of protection is already seen after as little as 3 to 6 months of use. Oral contraceptives also decrease the incidence of ovarian cysts and fibrocystic breast disease. They reduce menstrual blood loss and thus the incidence of iron-deficiency anemia. A decreased incidence of pelvic inflammatory disease and ectopic pregnancies has been reported as well as an ameliorating effect on the clinical course of endometriosis.

Future efforts should be directed at optimising current formulations to finally come up with an ideal oral contraceptive which would reduce the risk of breast, ovarian and endometrial cancer whithout any cardiovascular complications.

References

1. Gruber CJ, Tschugguel W, Schneeberger C, Huber JC (2002) Production and actions of estrogens. N Engl J Med 346:340–352
2. McDonnell DP, Norris JD (2002) Connections and regulation of the human estrogen receptor. Science 296:1642–1644
3. Cato AC, Nestl A, Mink S (2002) Rapid actions of steroid receptors in cellular signaling pathways. Sci STKE 2002:RE9.
4. Marchbanks PA, McDonald JA, Wilson HG, Folger SG, Mandel MG, Daling JR, Bernstein L, Malone KE, Ursin G, Strom BL, Norman SA, Wingo PA, Burkman RT, Berlin JA, Simon MS, Spirtas R, Weiss LK (2002) Oral contraceptives and the risk of breast cancer. N Engl J Med 346:2025–2032
5. Writing Group for the Women's Health Initiative Investigators (2002) Risks and benefits of estrogen plus progestin in healthy postmenopausal women: principal results From the Women's Health Initiative randomized controlled trial. JAMA 288:321–333

Contracture

Contracture is muscular contraction without accompanying action potential.

▶ Ryanodine Receptor

Convulsant Drugs

Convulsant drugs are a group of drugs, which can induce seizures. These drugs include antagonists of glycine receptors (e.g. strychnine) and antagonistst of the $GABA_A$-receptor (e.g. bicuculline, picrotoxin).

▶ Glycine Receptor
▶ $GABA_A$-Receptor

Convulsions

▶ Seizures
▶ Antiepileptic Drugs

Co-operativity Factor

An allosteric ligand has an effect on a receptor protein mediated through the binding of that ligand to the allosteric binding domain. The intensity of that effect, usually a change in the affinity of the receptor for other ligands or the efficacy of a ligand for the receptor, is quantified by the co-operativity factor. Denoted α, a positive value for α defines a potentiation, a fractional value an inhibition. Thus if $\alpha=0.1$, a maximal ten-fold decrease in the affinity of a tracer ligand for the receptor would be produced by the allosteric modulator.

▶ Drug-Receptor Interaction

COPI Vesicle

COPI vesicles mediate anterograde transport from the intermediate compartment to the Golgi, transport within the Golgi apparatus and retrograde transport back from the Golgi to the ER by the recruitment of soluble proteins from the cytoplasm, the GTP-binding protein ARF1 and the coat protein complex coatomer that lead to budding of COPI-coated vesicles.

▶ Intracellular Transport

COPII Vesicle

COPII vesicles are transport intermediates from the endoplasmic reticulum. The process is driven by recruitment of the soluble proteins that form the coat structure called COPII from the cytoplasm to the membrane.

▶ Intracellular Transport

Co-repressors

The antagonist-induced conformation of steroid hormone receptors attracts co-repressors like Nco/SMRT (nuclear hormone receptor corepressor/silencing mediator of retinoid and thyroid receptors) which further recruit other nuclear proteins with histone deacetylase activity. Their action leads to chromatin condensation, thus preventing the general transcription apparatus from binding to promoter regions.

▶ Contraceptives
▶ Gluco-/Mineralocorticoid Receptors
▶ Sex Steroid Receptors

Cortico-medullary Solute Gradient

While the osmotic concentration of renal cortical tissue is isotonic, interstitial solute concentration begins to rise at the border between renal cortex and renal medulla to reach maximum concentrations at the tip of the renal papilla. This rise in tissue osmolarity, the cortico-medullary osmotic gradient, is a consequence of the countercurrent multiplication along the loops of Henle driven by active NaCl retrieval across the water-impermeable ascending limb. The interstitial solutes are about half NaCl and half urea. The medullary hypertonicity permits the generation of a hypertonic urine when the collecting duct epithelium is water-permeable under the influence of vasopressin.

▶ Diurectics

Corticosteroids

▶ Glucocorticoids
▶ Mineralocorticoids
▶ Steroids

Corticosterone

▶ Glucocorticoids

Corticotropin

▶ ACTH

Corticotropin Releasing Hormone

▶ CRH

Co-stimulatory Molecules

Co-stimulatory molecules are cell surface proteins (e.g. CD80, CD86) present on antigen-presenting cells. In addition to the MHC-restricted presentation of foreign antigens, presence of co-stimulatory molecules is essential for the activation of T-cells.

▶ Immune Defense

Cotransmission

Cotransmission is transmission through a single synapse by means of more than one transmitter. For example, to elicit vasoconstriction, postganglionic sympathetic neurones release their classical transmitter noradrenaline (which acts on smooth muscle α-adrenoceptors) as well as ATP (which acts on smooth muscle P2-receptors) and neuropeptide Y (which acts on smooth muscle Y_1-receptors).

▶ Synaptic Transmission

Coumarins

▶ Anticoagulants

COX-1

▶ Cyclooxygenases
▶ Non-steroidal Anti-inflammatory Drugs

COX-2

▶ Cyclooxygenases
▶ Non-steroidal Anti-inflammatory Drugs

Coxibs

Coxibs are a class of drugs that effect their action by selectively inhibiting the activity of cyclooxygenase-2. They have potent analgesic, antipyretic and anti-inflammatory properties, and have reduced adverse gastrointestinal side effects.

▶ Non-steroidal Anti-inflammatory Drugs
▶ Cyclooxygenases

CpG Dinucleotide Motif

CpG stands for cytosine phosphate guanine dinucleotide in a particular sequence context. CpG motifs are responsible for proliferative effects of antisense oligonucleotides, particularly with respect to B-lymphocytes. The optimal immune-stimulatory consensus sequence surrounding CpG is R1R2CGY1Y2 where R1 is a purine (mild preference for G), R2 is a purine or T (preference for A) and Y1 and Y2 are pyrimidines (preference for T).

▶ Antisense Oligonucleotides

CPI-17

CPI-17 protein kinase C potentiates protein phosphatase 1 inhibitory protein, a smooth muscle specific inhibitor of myosin phosphatase.

▶ Smooth Muscle Tone Regulation

Crack

Crack is the free base form of cocaine which in contrast to cocaine, the salt form, can be smoked. This inhalative application results in a very rapid, intense effect.

▶ Psychostimulants

Craving

There are opposing views in the field regarding the term "craving", as to whether it describes a physiological, subjective or behavioural state, if it is necessary at all to explain addictive behaviour or is an epiphenomenon which is not necessary for the production of continued drug use in addicts. The World Health Organization agreed on the definition of craving as "the desire to experience the effect(s) of a previously experienced psychoactive substance". Behavioural researches conceptualize craving within the framework of incentive motivational theories of behaviour and modify the definition of craving as "incentive motivation to self-administer a psychoactive substance". Such an operational definition of craving has the advantage of making the phenomenon of craving accessible to experimental investigation and making it measurable.

▶ Drug Addiction/Dependence

Cre/loxP

Cre is a bacterial recombinase (cre = **c**auses **re**combination), which recognizes loxP sites of bacteriophage P. If two loxP (loxP = **lo**cus of **x**-ing over of bacteriophage **P**) sites have a parallel orientation, the DNA segment between these sites will be deleted by the action of the Cre recombinase.

▶ Transgenic Animal Models

CREB

CREB stands for cyclic-AMP response element (CRE) binding protein and is a transcription factor. When phosphorylated, it binds to gene promoters that contain a specific binding site. After binding, the respective transcription activity is modulated.

▶ Antidepressant Drugs

CRH

CRH (Corticotropin releasing hormone) is expressed in the nucleus paraventricularis of the hypothalamus and drives the stress hormone system by activating synthesis and release of corticotropin at the pituitary and in turn corticosteroid from the adrenal cortex. CRH is also expressed at many other brain locations not involved in neuroendocrine regulation, e.g. the prefrontal cortex and the amygdala. Preclinical studies have shown that CRH also coordinates the behavioral adaptation to stress (e.g. anxiety, loss of appetite, decreased sleepiness, autonomic changes, loss of libido).

▶ Antidepressant Drugs

Cromones

Cromones are drugs used topically in the treatment of allergic reactions. They inhibit the activation of mast cells and basophils and the subsequent mediator release by a yet unknown molecular mechanism.

▶ Allergy

Cross Tolerance

Cross tolerance is a form of tolerance which may develop to the effects of pharmacologically related drugs, particularly to those acting at the same receptor.

▶ Tolerance

Crosslinks

Crosslinks result from the reaction of a bifunctional electrophilic species with DNA bases and imply a covalent link between two adjacent DNA strands which inhibits DNA replication. Primary targets within bases are N7 and O6 in guanine and N3 in cytosine. The initial lesions are removed by the suicide enzyme alkyltransferase, whereas nucleotide excision repair is needed for fully established crosslinks.

▶ Antineoplastic Agents

Cross-packaging

Cross-packaging is the packaging of viral genomes into the virion shell of other viruses.

▶ Gene Therapy

CSFs

▶ Colony-stimulating Factors
▶ Hematopoietic Growth Factors

CTLs

▶ Cytotoxic T-cells
▶ Immune Defense

Curare

Curare is a generic term for various South American arrow poisons. Curare has been used for centuries by the Indians along the Amazon and Orinoco rivers for immobilizing and paralyzing wild animals used for food. Preparations of curare are derived from *Strychnos* species, which contain quaternary neuromuscular alkaloids like tubocurarine. Tubocurarine is a potent antagonist at the nicotinic acetylcholine receptor.

▶ Nicotinic Acetylcholine Receptor

Current-voltage Relationship (I-V)

The current-voltage relationship is a plot of the current through a channel versus the voltage of the membrane potential.

▶ Voltage-dependent Ca^{2+} Channels
▶ Voltage-dependent Na^+ Channels

Cyclic-AMP Response Element Binding Protein

▶ CREB
▶ Antidepressant Drugs

Cyclic Nucleotides

Cyclic nucleotides (cAMP and cGMP) are formed enzymatically from the corresponding triphosphates. As ubiquitous second messengers, they mediate many cellular functions which are initiated by first (extracellular) messengers. Their prime targets in eucaryotic cells are protein kinases (cyclic AMP-dependent protein kinase, cyclic GMP-dependent protein kinase) and ion channels.

▶ Adenylyl Cyclases
▶ Cyclic Nucleotide-gated Channels
▶ Guanylyl Cyclases
▶ Transmembrane Signalling
▶ AMP, cyclic
▶ GMP, cyclic

Cyclic Nucleotide-binding Domain (CNBD)

In cyclic nucleotide-regulated channels, the cyclic nucleotide-binding domain (CNBD) serves as a high-affinity binding site for 3'-5' cyclic monophosphates. The CNBD of channels has significant sequence similarity to the CNBDs of most other classes of eukaryotic cyclic nucleotide receptors and to the CNBD of the prokaryotic catabolite activator protein (CAP). The primary sequence of CNBDs consists of approximately 120 amino acid residues forming three α-helices (αA-αC) and eight β-strands (β1-β8).

▶ Cyclic Nucleotide-regulated Cation Channels

Cyclic Nucleotide-gated Channels

▶ Cyclic Nucleotide-regulated Cation Channels.

Cyclic Nucleotide-regulated Cation Channels

MARTIN BIEL
Department Pharmazie, Zentrum für Pharmaforschung, Ludwig-Maximilians-Universität München, München, Germany
mbiel@cup.uni-muenchen.de

Synonyms

CNG channels and HCN channels

Definition

Cyclic nucleotide-regulated cation channels are ion channels whose activation is mediated by the binding of cyclic AMP or cyclic GMP to a cyclic nucleotide-binding domain (CNBD)in the channel protein. Two families of channels regulated by cyclic nucleotides have been identified, the cyclic nucleotide-gated (CNG) channels (1,2) and the hyperpolarization-activated cyclic nucleotide-gated (HCN) channels (3–5). CNG channels require the obligatory binding of a cyclic nucleotide in order to be activated. In contrast, HCN channels are activated by membrane hyperpolarization. Cyclic nucleotides enhance HCN channel activity by affecting the voltage-dependence of channel activation.

▶ Table appendix: Membrane Transport Proteins

Basic Characteristics

Cyclic nucleotides exert their cellular effects by binding to four major classes of cellular receptors: ▶ cAMP- and cGMP-dependent protein kinases, cGMP-regulated phosphodiesterases, cAMP-binding guanine nucleotide exchange factors and cyclic nucleotide-regulated cation (CNG and HCN) channels. Cyclic nucleotide-regulated cation channels are unique among these receptors because their activation is coupled to the influx of extracellular cations into the cytoplasm and to the depolarization of the plasma membrane. Unlike HCN channels which conduct only monovalent cations CNG channels pass both Na^+ and Ca^{2+} ions. By providing an entry pathway for Ca^{2+}, CNG channels control a variety of cellular processes that are triggered by this cation.

CNG and HCN channels belong to the superfamily of ▶ voltage-gated cation channels. The proposed structure of the channels is shown in Fig. 1. The transmembrane channel core consists of six α-helical segments (S1–S6) and an ion-conducting pore loop between the S5 and S6. The amino- and carboxy-termini are localized in the cytosol. CNG and HCN channels contain a positively charged S4 helix carrying three to nine regularly spaced arginine or lysine residues at every third position. In HCN channels, as in most other members of the channel superfamily, the S4 helix functions as "voltage-sensor" confering voltage-dependent ▶ gating. In CNG channels, which are only slightly voltage-dependent, the specific role of S4 is not known. In the carboxy-terminus, CNG and HCN channels contain a CNBD that is homologous to CNBDs of cAKs, cGKs and cAMP-GEFs. In CNG channels, the binding of cGMP or cAMP to the CNBD initiates a sequence of allosteric transitions that lead to the opening of the ion-conducting pore (2). In HCN channels, the binding of cyclic nucleotides is not required for activation.However, cyclic nucleotides shift the voltage-dependence of channel activation to a more positive membrane potential and thereby facilitate voltage-dependent channel activation. Native CNG and HCN channels are tetramers consisting either of identical (homomeric channels) or different (heteromeric) subunits.

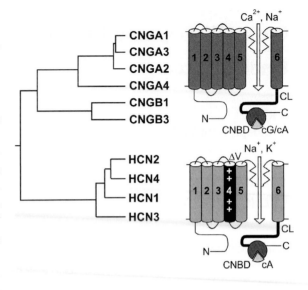

Fig. 1 Phylogenetic tree and structural model of cyclic nucleotide-regulated cation channels. The CNG channel family comprises six members, which are classified into α subunits (CNGA1-4) and β subunits (CNGB1 and CNGB3). A "CNGB2" subunit does not exist. The HCN channel family comprises four members (HCN1-4). CNG and HCN channels share the same transmembrane topology, consisting of six transmembrane segments (1–6), a pore loop and a cyclic nucleotide-binding domain (CNBD). CNG channels conduct Ca^{2+} and Na^+ whereas HCN channel conduct Na^+ and K^+ but not divalent cations. CNG channel are activated *in vivo* by binding of either cAMP (cA) or cGMP (cG), depending on the channel type. HCN channels activate on membrane hyperpolarization (ΔV), and are enhanced by binding of cAMP. The positively charged amino acid residues in the S4 segment of HCN channels are indicated by + symbols. CL, C-linker involved in activation gating of CNG and HCN channels.

CNG Channels

CNG channels are expressed in retinal photoreceptors and olfactory neurons and play a key role in visual and olfactory signal transduction. In addition, CNG channels are found at low density in some other cell types and tissues such as brain, testis and kidney. While the function of CNG channels in sensory neurons has been unequivocally demonstrated, the role of these channels in other cell types where expression has been observed remains to be established. Based on their phylogenetic relationship, the six CNG channels identified in mammals are divided in two subfamilies, the A-subunits (CNGA1-4) and the B-subunits (CNGB1 and CNGB3). When expressed in ▶ heterologous expression systems, A-subunits, with the exception of CNGA4, form functional homomeric channels. In contrast, B-subunits do not give rise to functional channels when expressed alone. However, together with CNGA1–3 they confer novel properties (e.g. single channel flickering, increased cAMP sensitivity) that are characteristic of native CNG channels. In native tissues, CNG channels are heterotetramers with different heteromers displaying distinct nucleotide sensitivity, ion selectivity and modulation by Ca^{2+}. The physiological role and subunit composition is known for three native channels: the rod and cone photoreceptor channels and the olfactory channel. The CNG channel of rod outer segment consists of the CNGA1 subunit and a long isoform of the CNGB1 subunit (CNGB1a). The cone photoreceptor channel consists of the CNGA3 and the CNGB3 subunit. CNG channels control the membrane potential and the calcium concentration of photoreceptors. In the dark both channels are maintained in the open state by a high concentration of cGMP. The resulting influx of Na^+ and Ca^{2+} ("dark current") depolarizes the photoreceptor and promotes synaptic transmission. Light-induced hydrolysis of cGMP leads to the closure of the CNG channel. As a result the photoreceptor hyperpolarizes and shuts off synaptic glutamate release. Mutations in human CNG channel genes have been linked to retinal diseases. Mutations in the CNGA1 and CNGB1 subunits have been identified in the genome of patients suffering from ▶ retinitis pigmentosa. The functional loss of either the CNGA3 or the CNGB3 subunit causes total color blindness (achromatopsia) and degeneration of cone photoreceptors.

The olfactory CNG channel consists of three different subunits: CNGA2, CNGA4 and a short isoform of the CNGB1 subunit (CNGB1b). The channel is activated *in vivo* by cAMP which is synthesized in response to the binding of odorants to their cognate receptors. The olfactory CNG channel almost exclusively conducts Ca^{2+} under physiological ionic conditions. The increase in cellular Ca^{2+} activates a Ca^{2+}-activated Cl^- channel which further depolarizes the cell membrane. Ca^{2+} is not only a permeating ion of the olfactory CNG channel, it also represents an important modulator of this channel. By forming a complex with calmodulin, which binds to the CNGA2 subunit, Ca^{2+} decreases sensitivity of the CNG channel to cAMP. The resulting inhibition of channel activity is the principal mechanism underlying odorant adaptation.

HCN Channels

A cation current that is slowly activated by membrane hyperpolarization (termed I_h, I_f or I_q) is found in a variety of excitable cells including neurons, cardiac pacemaker cells and photoreceptors. The best understood function of I_h is to control heart rate and rhythm by acting as "pacemaker current" in the sinoatrial (SA) node. I_h is activated during membrane hyperpolarization following the termination of an action potential and provides an inward Na^+ current that slowly depolarizes the plasma membrane. Sympathetic stimulation of SA node cells raises cAMP levels and increases I_h by a positive shift of the current activation curve, thus accelerating diastolic depolarization and heart rate. Stimulation of muscarinic receptors slows down heart rate by the opposite action. In the brain I_h fulfills diverse functions: (1) controls the activity of spontaneously spiking neurons ("neuronal pacemaking"), (2) is involved in the determination of resting potential, (3) provides, in photoreceptors, rebound depolarizations in response to pronounced hyperpolarizations, (4) is involved in the transduction of sour taste and (5) is involved in the control of synaptic plasticity and the integration of synaptic inputs.

HCN channels represent the molecular correlate of the I_h current. In mammals, the HCN channel family comprises four members (HCN1–4) that share about 60% sequence identity to each other and about 25% sequence identity to CNG channels. The highest degree of sequence homology between HCN and CNG channels is found in the CNBD that is also highly conserved in cAKs, cGKs and cAMP-GEFs. When expressed in heterologous systems all four HCN channels generate currents displaying the typical features of native I_h: (1) activation by membrane hyperpolarization, (2) permeation of Na^+ and K^+ with a permeability ratio P_{Na}/P_K of about 0.2, (3) positive shift of voltage-dependence of channel activation by direct binding of cAMP, (4) channel blockade by extracellular Cs^+.

HCN1-4 mainly differ from each other with regard to their speed of activation and the extent by which they are modulated by cAMP. HCN1 is the fastest channel, followed by HCN2, HCN3 and HCN4. Unlike HCN2 and HCN4, whose activation curves are shifted by about +15 mV by cAMP, HCN1 is only weakly affected by cAMP (shift of less than +5 mV).

Site-directed mutagenesis experiments have provided initial insight into the complex mechanism underlying dual HCN channel activation by voltage and cAMP. Like in other voltage-gated cation channels, activation of HCN channels is initiated by the movement of the positively charged S4 helix in the electric field. The resulting conformational change in the channel protein is allosterically coupled by other channel domains to the opening of the ion-conducting pore. Major determinants affecting channel activation are the intracellular S4–S5 loop, the S1 segment and the extracellular S1–S2 loop. The CNBD fulfils the role of an auto-inhibitory channel domain. In the absence of cAMP the cytoplasmic carboxy-terminus inhibits HCN channel gating by interacting with the channel core and, thereby, shifting the activation curve to more hyperpolarizing voltages. Binding of cAMP to the CNBD relieves this inhibition. Differences in the magnitude of the response to cAMP among the four HCN channel isoforms are largely due to differences in the exent to which the CNBD inhibits basal ▶ gating. It remains to be determined if the inhibitory effect of the CNBD is confered by a direct physical interaction with the channel core domain or by some indirect pathway. There is initial evidence that the so-called C-linker, a peptide of about 80 amino acids that connects the last transmembrane helix (S6) to the CNBD plays an important role in this process. The C-linker was also shown to play a key role in the gating of CNG channels, suggesting that the functional role of this domain has been conserved during channel evolution (2).

HCN channels are found in neurons and heart cells. In mouse and rat brain all four HCN isoforms have been detected. The expression levels and the regional distribution of the HCN channel mRNAs vary profoundly between the respective channel types. HCN2 is the most abundant neuronal channel and is found almost ubiquitously in the brain. In contrast, HCN1 and HCN4 are enriched in specific regions of the brain such as thalamus (HCN4) or hippocampus (HCN1). HCN3 is uniformly expressed throughout the brain, however at very low levels. HCN channels have also been detected in the retina and some peripheral neurons such as dorsal root ganglion neurons. In SA node cells, HCN4 represents the predominantly expressed HCN channel isoform. In addition, minor amounts of HCN2 and HCN1 are also present in these cells.

Drugs Acting on CNG Channels

Several drugs have been reported to block CNG channels, although not with very high affinity. The most specific among these drugs is L-*cis* diltiazem which blocks CNG channels in a voltage-dependent manner at micromolar concentrations. The D-*cis* enantiomer of diltiazem, which is an important therapeutic blocker of the L-type calcium channel, is much less effective than the L-*cis* enantiomer in blocking CNG channels. High affinity binding of L-*cis* diltiazem is only seen in heteromeric CNG channels containing the CNGB1 subunit. CNG channels are also moderately sensitive to blockage by some other inhibitors of the L-type calcium channel (e.g. nifedipine), the local anaesthetic tetracaine and calmodulin antagonists. Interestingly, LY83583 [6-(phenylamino)-5,8-quinolinedione] blocks both the soluble guanylyl cyclase and some CNG channels at similar concentrations. H-8 [N-2-(methylamino)ethyl-5-isoquinolinesulfonamide], which has been widely used as a non-specific cyclic nucleotide-dependent protein kinase inhibitor, blocks CNG channels, though at significantly higher concentrations than needed to inhibit protein kinases. Thus, a careful pharmacological analysis will be required to dissect processes mediated by the activation of CNG channels from those mediated by cyclic nucleotide-dependent protein kinases or soluble guanylyl cyclase.

Drugs Acting on HCN Channels

Given the key role of HCN channels in cardiac pacemaking, these channels are promising pharmacological targets for the development of drugs used in the treatment of cardiac arrhythmias and ischemic heart disease. HCN channels are not expressed in vascular and airway smooth muscle. As a consequence, specific HCN channel blockers are expected to have no side effect on the peripheral resistance. Most importantly, unlike the well-established β-adrenoceptor blockers, HCN channel blockers would not impair pulmonary function in patients with asthma or obstructive pulmonary disease. The most extensively studied blocker of native I_h is the drug ZD7288 [4-(N-ethyl-N-phenylamino)-1,2-dimethyl-6-(methylamino)pyrimidinium chloride]. ZD7288 blocks I_h in the low micromolar range and reduces heart rate in a variety of species including man. Unfortunately, ZD 7288 also blocks I_h in photoreceptors and thereby induces visual disturbances that have prevented therapeutic use of the drug. Another blocker of I_h is the drug ivabradine (S16257). Like ZD7288, ivabradine is a bradycardic agent, but seems to have much less pronounced, if any, side effects on vision. Ivabradine is currently under investigation in clinical trials. Studies with expressed HCN channels indicate that ivabradine preferentially blocks the HCN4 channel that is highly enriched in pacemaker cells of the SA node. Two other blockers of I_h, alinidine and zatebradine, show insufficient specificity and selectivity, and have not been introduced as therapy.

References

1. Kaupp UB, Seifert R (2002) Cyclic nucleotide-gated ion channels. Physiol Rev 82:769-824
2. Flynn GE, Johnson JP, Zagotta WN (2001) Cyclic nucleotide-gated channels: shedding light on the opening of a channel pore. Nature Rev 2:643–651
3. Pape HC (1996) Queer current and pacemaker: the hyperpolarization-activated cation current in neurons. Annu Rev Physiol 58:299–327
4. Biel M, Schneider A, Wahl C (2002) Cardiac HCN channels: structure, function andmodulation. Trends Cardiovasc Med 12:206-213
5. Kaupp UB, Seifert R (2001) Molecular diversity of pacemaker ion channels. Annu Rev Physiol 63:235–257

Cyclin

▶ Cell-cycle Control

Cyclin-dependent Kinases

▶ Cell-cycle Control

Cyclooxygenases

REGINA BOTTING, JACK BOTTING
William Harvey Research Institute, School of Medicine and Dentistry, St. Bartholomew's and Royal London, London, UK
r.m.botting@qmul.ac.uk

Synonyms

Prostaglandin H_2 synthase (PGHS); EC 1.14.99.1; COX-1; COX-2

Definition

Cyclooxygenase (COX) is the enzyme that catalyses the conversion of arachidonic acid to the highly active group of lipid mediators, the prostaglandins and thromboxane. These end products are involved in a multitude of diverse pathophysiological processes ranging from the induction of the vascular inflammatory response to tissue damage or infection, fever, pain perception, ▶ haemostasis, cytoprotection of the gastric mucosa from the erosive effects of gastric acid, the induction of labour and the regulation of kidney function. Thus, inhibition of COX can result in alleviation of the symptoms of many diseases, particularly inflammatory joint disease such as ▶ rheumatoid arthritis. However, this often occurs with the generation of severe side effects, such as gastrotoxicity due to the inhibition of physiological functions.

In 1971 inhibition of COX was established as the mode of action of the archetypal non steroid anti-

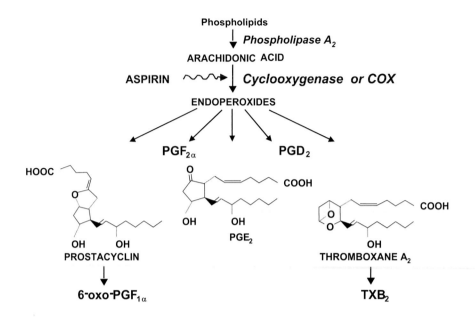

Fig. 1 Pathways for the Formation of Prostanoids from Arachidonic Acid. Arachidonic acid is converted by cyclooxygenase to endoperoxides, which are acted upon by various synthesases to form the prostanoids. Prostacyclin and thromboxane are relatively unstable and break down rapidly to form the inactive metabolites 6-oxo-$PGF_{1\alpha}$ and thromboxane B_2 respectively.

inflammatory drug (NSAID) aspirin, thus resolving an enigma that had puzzled researchers since the synthesis of salicylate in the mid-nineteenth century. The realisation that inhibition of COX was the general mode of action of the large number of marketed NSAIDs also explained why the common toxic effects of these drugs, such as gastro- and nephrotoxicity, prolongation of bleeding time and delayed labour, could not be divorced from their beneficial analgesic, antipyretic and anti-inflammatory actions.

▸ Inflammation
▸ Non-steroidal Anti-inflammatory Drugs
▸ Prostanoids

Basic Characteristics

COX possesses two catalytic sites. The cyclooxygenase active site converts arachidonic acid substrate, mobilised from membrane phospholipid by a phospholipase, to the prostaglandin endoperoxide, PGG_2. The endoperoxide is then converted by a peroxidase active site to form prostaglandin H_2

(PGH_2). PGH_2 is then acted upon by various synthases to form the active ▸ prostanoids, the most important of which are prostaglandin E_2 (PGE_2), thromboxane A_2 (TXA_2), prostacyclin (PGI_2), prostaglandin D_2 (PGD_2) and prostaglandin $F_{2\alpha}$ ($PGF_{2\alpha}$). COX is widely distributed in tissues; indeed, prostanoids can be synthesised and released by any mammalian cells except erythrocytes. The stages in the production of the prostanoids are summarised in Fig. 1. The main actions of these mediators are listed in Table 1.

By the late 1980s it became obvious that there were two forms of COX, one that was constitutive, i.e. permanently present in many tissues, and a second form that could be induced over time by mitogens or pro-inflammatory agents; this induction being inhibited by anti-inflammatory steroids such as dexamethasone. In 1991 it was established that there were in fact two distinct COX enzymes encoded by two distinct genes. The constitutive enzyme was designated COX-1, the inducible enzyme COX-2. In general, COX-1 is responsible for the synthesis of PGs that serve physiological or so-called "house-keeping" functions, whereas COX-2 synthesises PGs involved in pathological processes which are responsible for symptoms such as the swelling and pain of inflammatory conditions.

The two isozymes are both homodimers composed of approximately 600 amino acids and possess approximately 60% homology. The three-dimensional structures of COX-1 and COX-2 are very similar. They each consist of three independent units; an epidermal growth factor-like domain; a membrane binding section and an enzymatic domain. The catalytic sites and the residues immediately adjacent are identical but for two small but crucial variations that result in an increase in the volume of the COX-2 active site, enabling it to accept larger inhibitor molecules than could be accomodated in the COX-1 molecule.

The identification of the two COX isozymes explained why some NSAIDs had the same efficacy as other drugs, but apparently were marginally less likely to produce the common side effect of gastrotoxicity manifested by perforations, ulcers or bleeding from the gastric mucosa. Of greater significance, the establishment of differences in the volume of the active site of COX-2 also raised the possibility of the synthesis of inhibitors tailor-made to fit the COX-2 site without the capacity to inhibit COX-1. Such drugs would prevent the formation of PGs responsible for pain, fever and inflammatory reactions, with minimal or no action on the synthesis of the beneficial or "housekeeping" PGs (Fig. 2).

Drugs

Aspirin has been remarkably successful in the treatment of the pain and swelling of inflammatory disease. Indeed, an estimated 45,000 tons are consumed each year. This success resulted in the synthesis of many other "aspirin-like drugs", now referred to as NSAIDs. Aspirin however, continues to have a unique use in the prevention of thrombosis. Since it produces irreversible inhibition of COX-1 by acetylation of serine at position 530 in the active site, a low daily dose of aspirin will cause a cumulative inhibition of COX-1 in platelets in the portal circulation. A gradual inhibition of platelet aggregation occurs, reducing the possibility of occlusion of coronary or cerebral vessels by platelet thrombi. However, there are no systemic

Tab. 1 Actions of the common prostanoids.

Actions of the common prostanoids	
PGE_2	Vasodilatation (decrease in blood pressure); inhibits platelet aggregation; decreased gastric secretion; bronchodilatation; hyperalgesia; fever; contraction of intestinal and uterine smooth muscle. (Mediates inflammation, fever, pain, protects gastric mucosa)
PGI_2	Vasodilatation (decrease in blood pressure); inhibits platelet aggregation; decreased gastric secretion; bronchodilatation; hyperalgesia. (Mediates pain, protects gastric mucosa, antithrombogenic)
$PGF_{2\alpha}$	Vasodilatation/vasocostriction; bronchoconstriction; contraction of intestinal and uterine smooth muscle. (Important functions in ovulation and parturition)
PGD_2	Vasodilatation; inhibits platelet aggregation; decreases fever; relaxes intestinal smooth muscle. (Released mainly in brain and mast cells, induces sleep)
TXA_2	Increases blood pressure; platelet aggregation; vasoconstriction; bronchoconstriction. (Important in haemostasis)

Putative pathophysiological functions placed in parenthesis

toxic effects since the small dose of aspirin is destroyed by hepatic metabolism.

NSAIDs are used as the first-line treatment of rheumatoid arthritis, ▶ osteoarthritis, systemic lupus erythematosis and other inflammatory diseases, and are thus amongst the most widely used drugs in the developed world. This widespread use inevitably entailed a considerable associated morbidity, in particular a high incidence of gastric toxicity. In the USA alone perforations, ulcers and bleeds lead to the hospitalisation of 100,000 patients per year, and about 15% of these die in intensive care

NSAIDs are of diverse chemical structures: salicylates (aspirin, sulphasalazine), indole acetic acids (indomethacin, etodolac), heteroaryl acetic acids (diclofenac), arylpropionic acids (ibuprofen, naproxen), anthranilic acids (mefenamic acid) and enolic acids (piroxicam, meloxicam).

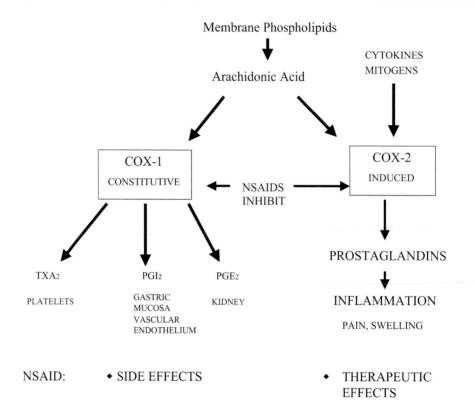

Fig. 2 Mechanism of the therapeutic and toxic actions of NSAIDs. The induced cyclooxygenase (COX-2) produces the pro-inflammatory prostaglandins responsible for the swelling and pain associated with inflammation. COX-1 produces the prostanoids responsible for protective physiological actions: thromboxane A_2 (TX)A_2 causes platelet aggregation, PGI_2 prevents intravascular aggregation and is protective for the gastric mucosa, and PGE_2 maintains renal blood flow (from Botting, 1999, with permission).

The identification of COX-2 as the enzyme responsible for the synthesis of PGs involved in pathology led to the examination of the relative activities of the established NSAIDs on COX-1 and COX-2. Various test systems have been used for this purpose and it is now generally accepted that the whole blood assay (3) is the preferred method since it uses the human enzymes in platelets (COX-1) and activated mononuclear cells (COX-2) in the presence of the plasma proteins, thus allowing for the participation of protein binding that is significant for some NSAIDs.

Three established NSAIDs were found to inhibit COX-2 in lower concentrations than those required to inhibit the constitutive enzyme. These were nimesulide, etodolac and meloxicam. Epidemiological studies showed that at therapeutic doses these drugs induced less gastro-intestinal toxicity than NSAIDs such as indomethacin, naproxen and ketorolac, which are more potent at inhibiting COX-1 compared to COX-2. The proof that selective inhibitors of COX-2 are efficacious antiinflammatory agents with minimal or no toxic side effects stimulated several commercial groups to develop, through knowledge of the differences in the shape of the catalytic sites of the isozymes, highly selective inhibitors of COX-2, some of which are 1000-fold more potent against COX-2 than COX-1.

Two such compounds, celecoxib and rofecoxib have been marketed and subjected to in depth clinical trials. Both compounds are as effective as standard NSAIDs in rheumatoid arthritis, osteoarthritis and for pain following orthopaedic or dental surgery. Gastro-intestinal side effects were far fewer than with comparator drugs and in fact were no more common with the ▶ coxibs than with placebo treatment.

Possible Future Uses of Selective COX-2 Inhibitors.

Cancer. The possibility of prolonged use of COX-2 inhibitors in the absence of marked toxicity, and the recent focus on the pathophysiological significance of this enzyme have exposed possible further indications for these drugs. Epidemiological observations have shown that regular aspirin users have a lower incidence of colon cancer. COX-2, but not COX-1, is expressed in human and animal colon cancer cells, and COX-2 levels are high in human colon adenocarcinomas but are absent in adjacent normal tissue. Patients with the inherited condition familial adenomatous polyposis (FAP), who develop many colorectal polyps that eventually progress to tumours, have their polyp number considerably reduced by the NSAID, sulindac. In the mutant Apc mouse, an animal model of FAP, the development of polyps is markedly reduced in COX-2 gene deleted mice or those on prolonged treatment with a COX-2 selective NSAID. This evidence strongly suggests that selective COX-2 inhibitors may have a use in colon cancer prevention. A clinical trial of celecoxib in patients with FAP has shown a 30% reduction in polyps, and this indication for the drug has been allowed by the Food and Drug Administration, USA. COX-2 overexpression has recently been demonstrated in cancer tissue of the breast, prostate, pancreas, liver and stomach, indicating that COX-2 selective inhibitors may have a major use in general cancer prophylaxis.

Alzheimer's Disease. Development of ▶ Alzheimer's disease is less in regular NSAID users than in the general population. Post mortem studies reveal that mRNA for COX-2 is higher in brains of Alzheimer's disease patients than in control groups. Trials are therefore ongoing with selective COX-2 inhibitors in patients with minimal cognitive impairment to examine if COX-2 selective NSAIDs may be valuable in prophylaxis against Alzheimer's disease.

Premature Labour. Labour is induced partly through the uterotonic effect of PGs synthesised presumably by COX-2, since mRNA for COX-2 increases in the amnion and placenta before and during labour. The COX-2-selective nimesulide has been used successfully to treat premature labour and prevent miscarriage. Non-selective NSAIDs such as indomethacin also delay premature labour but are contraindicated for this condition since they also cause early closure of the ductus arteriosus through inhibition of COX-1 which is responsible for synthesis of PGs maintaining patency of the ductus.

References

1. Vane JR, Botting RM (2001) Formation and actions of prostaglandins and inhibition of their synthesis. In: Vane JR, Botting RM (eds) Therapeutic Roles of Selective COX-2 Inhibitors. William Harvey Press, London. 1–48
2. Vane JR, Bakhle YS, Botting RM (1998) Cyclooxygenases 1 and 2. Annu. Rev. Pharmacol. Toxicol 38:97–120.
3. Patrignani P, Panara MR, Greco A, Fusco O, Natoli C, Iacobelli S, Cipollone F, Gauci A, Creminon C, Maclouf J, Patrono C (1994) Biochemical and pharmacological characterization of the cyclooxygenase activity of human blood prostaglandin endoperoxide synthases. J. Pharmacol. Exp Ther 271:1705–1712
4. Botting JH (1999) Nonsteroidal antiinflammatory agents. Drugs of Today 35:225–235

CYP

CYP is also known as P450 or cytochrome P450.

▶ P450 Mono-oxygenase System

CYP Enzyme

CYP enzymes are cytochrome P-450 isozymes, a superfamily of monooxygenases, which are mostly found in liver. There are many subfamilies such as CYP1A, CYP2B, CYP2C, CYP3A and CYP2D. These enzymes oxidize various chemicals. Depending on the chemical structure, each enzyme subfamily has different affinity and metabolizes in different ways.

▶ P450 Mono-oxygenase System

Cysteine Proteinases

Cysteine proteinases are proteinases that utilize the terminal sulfhydral moiety of the side chain of cysteine to effect peptide bond hydrolysis.

▶ Non-viral Proteases

Cysteinyl Leukotrine

Cysteinyl leukotrie is a compound synthesized from arachidonic acid in inflammatory cells that contains an amino-acid side chain.

▶ Leukotrienes

Cystic Fibrosis

Cystic fibrosis is a common autosomal recessive disorder caused by mutations in the gene encoding the cystic fibrosis transmembrane conductance regulator (CFTR) protein. The CFTR protein is a cAMP-regulated chloride channel belonging to the ABC transporter family. The main symptoms of cystic fibrosis are a progressive obstructive lung disease and pancreatic insufficiency. Patients suffer from the increased production of viscous mucus which leads to severe respiratory infections. About 70% of the patients carry the $\Delta F508$ mutation which leads to an intracellularly-retained CFTR protein.

▶ Epitelial Na^+ Channel

Cytochalasins

Cytochalasins B and D are used as tools to study F-actin. Cytochalasins bind to the barbed end of F-actin and block the addition as well as dissociation of G-actin at that end. When applied to cultured cells micromolar concentrations of cytochalasins remove stress fibers and other F-actin structures.

▶ Cytoskeleton

Cytochrome P450

Cytochrome P450 (CYP) is a family of hemeprotein monooxygenase enzymes that plays a central role in the oxidative metabolism of structurally diverse lipophilic steroids, fatty acids, drugs and environmental chemicals. P450-catalyzed biotransformation of drugs is primarily carried out by 10-15 distinct human P450 enzymes, each encoded by a separate P450 gene.

▶ P450 Mono-oxygenase System

Cytochrome P450 2C19

Cytochrome P450 2C19, also termed S-mephenytoin hydroxylase, is a mixed-function oxidase localized in the endoplasmic reticulum which is responsible for the biotransformation of S-mephenytoin, some barbiturates, almost all proton pump inhibitors such as omeprazole, diazepam and others.

▶ Pharmacogenetics
▶ P450 Mono-oxygenase System

Cytochrome P450 2C9

Cytochrome P450 2C9 is a mixed-function oxidase localized in the endoplasmic reticulum which is responsible for the biotransformation of several nonsteroidal anti-inflammatory drugs, S-warfarin, several sulfonylurea antidiabetics and other drugs.

▶ Pharmacogenetics
▶ P450 Mono-oxygenase System

Cytochrome P450 2D6

Cytochrome P450 2D6, also termed debrisoquine-sparteine hydroxylase, is a mixed-function oxidase localized in the endoplasmic reticulum which is responsible for the biotransformation of several tricyclic antidepressants, antipsychotics, beta-blockers, opioids, and many other drugs.

▶ Pharmacogenetics
▶ P450 Mono-oxygenase System

Cytochrome P450 Induction

P450 induction is the process whereby cellular and tissue levels of one or more cytochrome P450 enzymes are increased in response to treatment of cells, or a whole organism, with certain drugs or environmental chemicals referred to as P450 inducers. P450 induction leads to an increase in the cell's capacity for P450-catalyzed oxidative metabolism of many xenochemicals, as well as endogenous steroidal and fatty acid P450 substrates.

▶ Pharmacogenetics
▶ P450 Mono-oxygenase System

Cytokeratin

Cytokeratins are members of the intermediate filament class of cytoskeletal proteins. Cytokeratins are a large protein family comprising two subfamilies of polypeptides, i.e. acidic (type I) and basic (type II) ones. Cytokeratins form tetramers, consisting of two type I and two type II polypeptides arranged in pairs of laterally aligned coiled coils. The distribution of the different type I and II cytokeratins in normal epithelia and in carcinomas is differentiation-related and can be used for cell typing and identification.

▶ Cadherins/Catenins
▶ Cytoskeleton

Cytokine Receptors

Cytokine receptors are a group of structurally related receptors, which couple to the JAK-STAT pathway. Cytokine receptors function as homodimers or heterooligomers. They are divided into two main subclasses, class I, which contains receptors for a variety of hematopoietic growth factors and interleukins and class II, which contains receptors for interferons and interleukins 10, 20/24 and 22.

▶ Cytokines
▶ JAK-STAT Pathway
▶ Table appendix: Receptor Proteins

Cytokines

MICHAEL KRACHT, HELMUT HOLTMANN
Medizinische Hochschule Hannover, Hannover,
Germany
Kracht.Michael@MH-Hannover.de,
Holtmann.Helmut@MH-Hannover.de

Synonyms

No true synonyms. Related terms/subgroups: lymphokines, monokines, interleukins, chemokines, interferons, growth factors

Definition

Cytokines are a large and heterogenous group of small polypeptides, most of them with an Mr between 8–30 kD. They are mostly soluble extracellular mediators (some exist in membrane-associated form) and function through high affinity cell surface receptors. Released by cells of hematopoietic origin (reflected in the terms "lymphokines" and "monokines") as well as by a wide variety of non-hematopoietic cells, cytokines are critical for the normal functioning of the immune defence, which they coordinate by communicating between participating cells.

"My private metaphor was that of a zoo of factors in a jungle of interactions surrounded by deep morasses of acronyms and bleak deserts of synonyms" (4).

▶ Chemokine Receptors
▶ Immune Defense
▶ JAK-STAT Pathway

General Characteristics and Function

Historically, many cytokines were discovered by means of their immunoregulatory properties, hence the term interleukins. However, cytokines regulate not only functions of the specific immune system, but also many aspects of infection and inflammation. At the cellular level they control proliferation, differentiation, functional activity and apoptosis. As a whole, they are synthesized by a broad variety of different cell types. This also holds true for many cytokines individually (e. g.

IL-6, IL-8, IFN-β, for further information on individual cytokines see ref. 4), whereas synthesis of others is restricted to one or few cell types (e. g. IL-2, IL-4, IFN-γ). In general, their biosynthesis is rapidly and highly inducible by changes in the cell microenvironment. Cytokines often have a short half-life and production is restricted to potentially pathological conditions. Uncontrolled synthesis results in chronic inflammatory or other diseases. All cytokines act locally in an autocrine or paracrine manner, but some may also act systemically. Examples for the latter are the induction of fever by IL-1 and ▶ TNF, and the induction of acute phase proteins in the liver by IL-6. Cytokines can therefore also be regarded as hormones. Cytokines are pleiotropic, i.e. they control multiple biological responses. There is considerable functional overlap between certain cytokines (e.g. TNF and IL-1). In general, activation of a cell by a cytokine results in reprogramming of the cell's gene expression profile.

Mechanism of Action

Most cytokines – in particular the ones that are in clinical use – bind to high affinity receptors on the plasma membrane. These receptors fall into different classes, those with enzymatic tyrosine kinase activity (e. g. the receptors of certain hematopoietic growth factors (M-CSF, SCF), G-protein-coupled receptors (chemokine receptors) and several groups that bind to other intracellular adaptor proteins (IL-1-, TNF-, interferon- and hematopoietic cytokine receptor families). Ligand-dependent receptor clustering activates several intracellular signalling patwhays. These pathways consist of consecutive interactions between protein components that in part involve enzymatic activities. The activity of many proteins in a given cytokine-activated pathway is regulated by reversible phosphorylation. The ▶ MAP kinase cascades and the ▶ JAK/STAT pathways are intensively studied examples. Certain receptors (of the TNF-R family) can activate caspases; a family of proteases that executes programmed cell death. Other protein synthesis-independent effects of cytokines include cytoskeletal changes and modulation of cell surface receptors and adhesion molecules. Most cytokine-activated intracellular pathways ultimately turn on expression of genes whose prod-

Tab. 1   Structural/functional groups of cytokines (examples).

Interferons	IFN-α, β, γ
Hematopoietic cytokines/colony-stimulating factors	IL-3, IL-5, IL-6, IL-7, erythropoietin, GM-CSF, G-CSF, M-CSF, thrombopoietin
IL-1 family	IL-1α, IL-1β, IL-18, IL-1RA
TNF family	TNF-α, TNF-β, CD40 ligand, CD95 ligand, TRAIL
Chemokines	IL-8, MIP-1-α, RANTES
Immunoregulatory cytokines	IL-2, IL-4, IL-10, IL-12

ucts change the biological function of the same or a neighbouring cell. These include cytokines (hence the term "cytokine network"), cell surface receptors and adhesion molecules, enzymes involved in degradative processes (e. g. collagenases) and in formation of small molecular weight mediators (e. g. cyclooxygenase II, inducible NO-synthase).

Cytokines and Therapy

Knowledge on cytokines has been exploited to improve the therapy of many diseases, basically in two ways:

1. Application of cytokines as drugs. Several examples will be given below. In general, treatment with cytokines turned out to be problematic due to their pleiotropic nature of function. Thus tumor necrosis factor, apart from its antitumoral effect, has severe systemic side effects as manifestations of its activity, which largely precludes its use as anticancer drug. Similar toxicity has been observed for several other inflammatory cytokines. Recombinant cytokines can be used to boost immune reactions during infection and cancer (interleukin-2, interferons) or to substitute cytokine deficiencies (hematopoietic growth factors, erythropoietin).

2. Interference with cytokine action. Inhibition of cytokine synthesis has turned out to be a major component of the activity of anti-inflammatory drugs, glucocorticoids being a prominent example. Because for many cytokines the molecular mechanisms of their actions have been worked out in detail, rational strategies for interfering with their biological activities have been or are being developed. The action of cy-

tokines can be suppressed pharmacologically by different means: 1. Inhibition of their synthesis by drugs (cyclosporin-IL-2 synthesis); 2. Prevention of their interaction with cell surface receptors by soluble receptors (TNF-RI extracellular domain), anti-cytokine or -cytokine receptor-antibodies (anti-TNF, anti-IL-2R antibodies), or natural antagonists (IL-1R antagonist); 3. Blockade of specifc events in the intracellular signalling pathways (protein kinase inhibitors). Clinically used cytokines or cytokine antagonists are proteins. Repeated application, especially for those of non-human origin, bears the risk of recognition by the immune system and antibody production against them with subsequent loss of efficacy. Therefore the proteins are often genetically engineered, i.e. humanized (see Humanized Monoclonal Antibodies) to be as homologous as possible to human proteins.

Clinical Use (incl. side effects)

Examples of Recombinant Cytokines Currently in Use

Interferons. Interferon alfacon-1 (Inferax®), interferon alfa-2b (IntronA®) and interferon alfa-2a (Roferon®-A) are effective in the treatment of chronic hepatitis B and C and some malignancies, especially hairy cell leukemia. IFN-α proteins induce the expression of antiviral, antiproliferative and immunomodulatory genes.

Interferon beta-1a (AVONEX®), interferon beta-1b (Betaferon®) and interferon beta (Fiblaferon®) are applied for the treatment of severe viral infections and of multiple sclerosis to reduce both frequency and severity of disease inci-

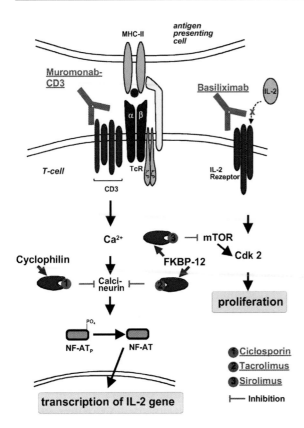

Fig. 1 Inhibition of cytokine synthesis during activation of the specific immune system. The monoclonal antibodies Muromonab and Basiliximab are specific for the CD3 complex of the T-cell receptor, and for the IL-2 receptor on lymphocytes, respectively. Cyclosporin and Tacrolimus inhibit activation of cytoplasmic NF-AT, a transcription factor essential for activation of the IL-2 gene. Sirolimus interferes with mTOR signaling and inhibits IL-2 dependent proliferation. Red: pharmaka, blue: target proteins.

dents. IFN-β proteins modulate the destruction of myelin in the cause of the autoimmune reaction.

Interferon gamma-1b (Imukin®) is effective in the treatment of chronic granulomatosis by an unknown mechanism.

Common side effects of interferons are flu-like symptoms, fever, myelosuppression and skin-reactions.

Human Recombinant Colony-stimulating Factors.
Molgramostim (rhu GM-CSF, Leucomax®), Filgrastim (r-metHuG-CSF, Neupogen®), and Lenograstim (rHuG-CSF, Granocyte®) promote

the differentiation of pluripotent bone marrow stem cells to leukocytes. GM-CSF induces proliferation in cells of the macrophage, neutrophil and eosinophil lineages, while G-CSF acts primarily on neutrophil precursors. They are effective in treatment of congenital and aquired neutropenias during chemotherapy of cancer or bone marrow transplantation. Side effects include bone pain, fever and myalgia.

Interleukin 2 (Aldesleukin, Proleukin®) is a major growth factor and activator of cytotoxic and other T-lymphocytes. It is applied in the therapy of metastasing renal carcinoma and melanoma. Side effects include hypotension, arrhythmias, edema, pruritus, erythema, central nervous symptoms, fever and many others.

Erythropoietin (Eprex®) is physiologically produced in the kidney and regulates proliferation of committed progenitors of red blood cells. It is used to substitute erythropoietin in severe anemias due to end stage renal disease or treatment of cancer with cytostatic agents. Side effects include hypertension and increased risk of thrombosis.

Inhibitors of Cytokine Action
Inhibition of hematopoietic growth factors: Imatinib (Glivec®) is applied to treat chronic myeloic leukemia in Philadelphia-chromosome positive patients. In these patients translocation of parts of chromosomes 9 and 22 results in the expression of a fusion protein with increased tyrosine kinase activity, called Bcr-Abl. Imatinib is a small Mw inhibitor selective for the tyrosine kinase activity of Bcr-Abl. Thereby, it inhibits the Bcr-Abl-induced cell-cycle progression and the uncontrolled proliferation of tumor cells.

Inhibition of immunomodulatory cytokines (Fig. 1): Anti-T-cell receptor antibodies: Muromonab (OKT3, Orthoclone®) binds to the CD3 complex of the T-cell receptor and induces depletion of T-lymphocytes. It is applied to prevent acute rejection of kidney, liver and heart allografts. Rapid side effects (within 30–60 min) include a cytokine release syndrome with fever, flu-like symptoms and shock. Late side effects include an increased risk of viral and bacterial infections and an increased incidence of lymphproliferative diseases due to immunosuppression.

Humanized recombinant anti-IL-2 receptor antibodies (Basiliximab, Simulect® and Daclizu-

C

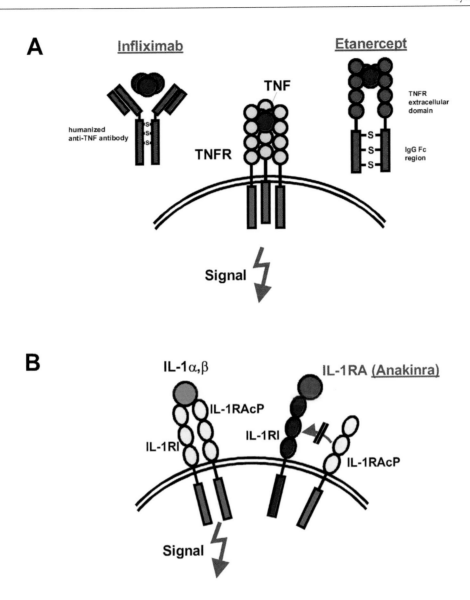

Fig. 2 Cytokines. Strategies directed against TNF or IL-1 in anti-inflammatory therapy. A. TNFRI-IgGFc fusion proteins or monoclonal anti-TNF antibodies capture TNF and prevent its binding to cell surface receptors. B. The IL-1 receptor antagonist (IL-1Ra) is a natural ligand that occupies the IL-1 receptor type I (IL-1RI). Thereby it prevents the IL-1-induced formation of a signal-inducing heterodimeric complex with the IL-1 receptor accessory protein (IL-1RAcp).

mab Zenapax®). These antibodies bind with high affinity to the IL-2 receptor on T-lymphocytes and prevent activation and clonal expansion of anti-allograft T-lymphocytes by endogenous IL-2. They are used to prevent kidney allograft rejection. The main side effect is immunosuppression.

Intracellular inhibition of interleukin-2 production and activity: The immunosuppressants Ciclosporin (Sandimmune®), Tacrolimus (Prograf®) and Sirolimus (Rapamune®) are used for the prophylaxis of allograft rejection. Ciclosporin binds to the intracellular protein cyclophilin, Sirolimus binds to the intracellular protein FKBP12. The resulting complexes inhibit a serine-threonine phosphatase, calcineurin, which is required for T-lymphocyte activation and for IL-2 gene expression. Sirolimus also binds to FKBP12, however the complex inhibits a different enzyme, the protein kinase mTOR (mammalian target of rapamycin); thereby it inhibits IL-2-dependent progression of activated T-lymphocytes through the cell cycle. All three drugs suppress clonal expansion of antigen-activated T-lymphocytes. Ciclosporin and Tacrolimus are nephrotoxic, and Sirolimus causes hyperlipidemia. For further details see ▶ Immunosuppressive Agents.

Inhibition of inflammatory cytokines (Fig. 2): Humanized monoclonal anti-TNF antibodies (Infliximab, Remicade®) bind with high selectivity to human TNF-α and neutralize its activity. Thereby, Infliximab decreases the effects of enhanced TNF levels during inflammatory disease such as production of proteases, chemokines, adhesion molecules, cycloxygenase products (prostaglandins) and pro-inflammatory molecules such as interleukin-1 and - 6. It is used to treat Crohn's disease and rheumatoid arthritis. Side effects include immunosuppression and increased risk of infections.

Recombinant soluble TNF-RI-IgG1 fusion protein (Etanercept, Enbrel®). This is a chimeric molecule consisting of the extracellular domain of the TNF receptor I (TNF-RI) and the Fc portion of human IgG1. Two Fc domains are bound to each other via disulfide-bonds, thereby yielding dimers with two binding sites for the TNF trimer. Etanercept binds with high affinity to extracellular TNF and reduces TNF activity. Indications and side effects are as for Infliximab.

Recombinant human IL-1 receptor antagonist (Anakinra, Kineret®): Anakinra blocks the biological activity of interleukin-1 by competitively inhibiting IL-1 binding to the interleukin-1 type I receptor (IL-1RI), which is expressed in a wide variety of tissues and organs. Thereby it reduces the pro-inflammatory activities of IL-1 including cartilage destruction and bone resorption. Side effects include an increased risk of infections and neutropenia.

References

1. Dinarello CA (2000) The role of the interleukin-1-receptor antagonist in blocking inflammation mediated by interleukin-1. N Engl J Med 343:732–734
2. Feldmann M, Maini RN (2001) Anti-TNF α therapy of rheumatoid arthritis: what have we learned? Annu Rev Immunol 19:163–196
3. Pascual M, Theruvath T, Kawai T, Tolkoff-Rubin N, Cosimi AB (2002) Strategies to improve long-term outcomes after renal transplantation. N Engl J Med 346:580–590
4. Ibelgaufts H. Cytokines Online Pathfinder Encyclopaedia. Free online information at http://www.copewithcytokines.de

Cytokinesis

Cytokinesis is the division of the cytoplasm at the end of mitosis after re-establishment of the cell nuclei, resulting in two independent daughter cells.

▶ Cell-cycle Control

Cytoskeleton

DIETER K. MEYER
Institut für Experimentelle und
Klinische Pharmakologie und Toxikologie,
Albert-Ludwigs-Universität Freiburg,
Freiburg, Germany
dieter.meyer@pharmakol-uni-freiburg.de

Synonyms

F-actin = actin filaments = microfilaments

Definition

▶ Microtubules, ▶ F-actin (microfilaments) and ▶ intermediate filaments form the cytoskeleton. These polymeric structures are highly dynamic and respond to extracellular signals. Thus, they mediate the adaptation of the cellular architecture to functional changes. They are essential for cell attachment, motility and proliferation, and organize the intracellular transport and compartments. In addition, cytoskeletal elements anchor receptors and ion channels in the cell membrane and organize the subsequent signal transduction pathways. Several drugs are known that specifically affect microtubules and microfilaments, whereas the specific pharmacological manipulation of intermediate filaments is presently not possible. Therefore, the present chapter will not deal with intermediate filaments.

▶ Bacterial Toxins
▶ Small GTPases

Basic Characteristics

Organisation of Microtubules (MTs)

The globular polypeptides α and β ▶ tubulin have molecular weights of about 50 kD. Whereas both tubulins bind GTP, only the GTP bound by β tubulin is exchangeable. Higher eukaryotes have up to 7 isoforms of α and β tubulin, which are encoded by different genes. α and β tubulins associate to heterodimers that polymerise head to tail to form protofilaments, 13 of which make up a hollow tube of 25 nm diameter, a microtubule (MT) (Fig. 1A). These polarized structures have GTP binding β tubulins at the plus ends and α tubulins at the minus ends. β tubulins within the protofilament are in the GDP binding state. Heterodimers can be added or released during processes called "dynamic instability" and "treadmilling". Dynamic instability is characterized by abrupt stochastic transitions among phases of growing, shortening and pause, whereas treadmilling is a net addition of tubulin heterodimers at the plus end and the balanced net loss from the minus end.

MT associated proteins (MAPs) are attached to MTs *in vivo* and play a role in their nucleation, growth, shrinkage, stabilization and motion. Of the MAPs, the tau family proteins have received special attention as they are involved in the pathophysiology of Alzheimer's disease.

MTs are stabilized at their minus ends by the ▶ centrosome (also called microtubule organizing center, MTOC). Centrosomes are protein complexes containing among other proteins 2 centrioles (ring-like structures) and α tubulin. Centrosomes serve as nucleation points for microtubular polymerisation and constrain the lattice structure of an MT to 13 protofilaments. Centrosome-independent nucleation is possible and may be

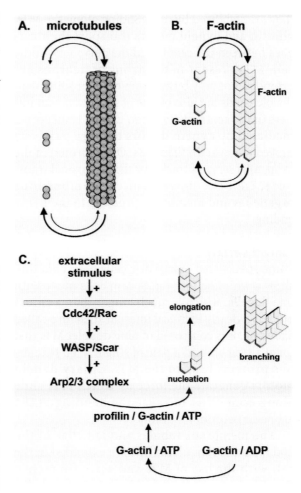

Fig. 1 Cytoskeleton – see text for further explanation.

induced by DNA or proteins such as cadherin. At the plus end, capping proteins such as mDIA can stabilize MTs. Stable MTs often are acetylated at lysine-40 of α tubulin and detyrosinated at the C-terminal of the β tubulin.

▶ Motor proteins move along MTs in an ATP-dependent manner. Members of the superfamily of kinesin motors move only to the plus ends and dynein motors only to the minus ends. The respective motor domains are linked via adaptor proteins to their cargoes. The binding activity of the motors to MTs is regulated by kinases and phosphatases. When motors are immobilized at their cargo binding area, they can move MTs.

MTs extend from the centrosome throughout the cytoplasm to the plasma membrane, where they are stabilized by caps. Sliding along the MTs, kinesin and dynein motors transport their cargoes between the center and the periphery of the cell. MTs present in the axons of neurons are extended not only by addition of heterodimers to the plus ends but also by use of short MTs that initiate in the centrosome. Their axonal transport is mediated by dynein motors that are passively moved along actin filaments. Once formed in the axon, MTs serve as tracks for the fast axonal transport, i.e., the movement of membranous organelles and membrane proteins to the nerve ending.

Functions of MTs

Some specialized eukaryotic cells have cilia that show a whiplike motion. Sperm cells move with one flagella, which is much longer than a cilium but has a nearly identical internal structure called axoneme. It is composed of nine doublet MTs that form a ring around a pair of single MTs. Numerous proteins bind to the MTs. Ciliary dynein motors generate the force by which MTs slide along each other to cause the bending of the axoneme necessary for motion.

The membrane tubules and lamellae of the endoplasmic reticulum (ER) are extended in the cell with the use of MTs and actin filaments. Kinesin motors are required for stretching out the ER, whereas depolymerization of microtubules causes the retraction of the ER to the cell centre in an actin-dependent manner. Newly synthesized proteins in the ER are moved by dynein motors along MTs to the Golgi complex (GC), where they are modified and packaged. The resulting vesicles move along the MTs to the cell periphery transported by kinesin motors. MTs determine the shape and the position also of the GC. Their depolymerization causes the fragmentation and dispersal of the GC. Dynein motors are required to rebuild the GC.

When cells enter mitosis, the interphase array of MTs is dismantled. The centrosome duplicates, and the daughters move to opposite poles of the nucleus. After disassembly of the nuclear envelope, MTs emanating from both centrosomes show pronounced dynamic instability. They grow and shorten and thus probe the cytoplasm until they find attachment sites at the condensed chromosomes, the ▶ kinetochores. Dynein motors are

involved in the attachment and in the subsequent segregation of the two sets of chromosomes. In some cells, spindles are formed in the absence of centrosomes. Here, microtubular nucleation is initiated at the kinetochores by DNA itself with the help of the GTPase Ran and/or the microtubule-destabilizing factor stathmin. Kinesin and dynein motors then bundle and focus the MTs at their minus ends (1).

Organization of Actin Filaments (F-actin)

Globular actin (▶ G-actin) has a molecular weight of about 42 kD. In higher vertebrates 6 isoforms of G-actin are expressed in a cell specific manner and contain 374/375 residues. They are present in striated muscle cells (skeletal and cardiac isoforms), smooth muscle cells (vascular and visceral isoforms) and in non-muscle cells (2 isoforms). All isoforms are N-terminally acetylated and bind ATP/ADP. F-actin is a double-stranded, right-handed helix with 14 actin molecules per strand and turn. F-actin has a diameter of 8 nm and is polarized with a pointed (minus) and a barbed (plus) end. The length of F-actin is regulated by dynamic instability and treadmilling (Fig. 1B). Within the F-actin polymer the ATP of an actin protomer is hydrolysed to ADP. Once the inorganic phosphate is dissociated from the actin-ADP complex, the actin molecule will ultimately dissociate from the pointed end. After exchange of ADP to ATP G-actin binds to the protein profilin and is ready for the next cycle (Fig. 1C).

Numerous ▶ actin binding proteins (ABPs) influence the turnover of F-actin. They are regulated in their activity via membrane receptors and thus transmit extracellular stimuli to the actin cytoskeleton (3). The small GTPases of the Rho family RhoA, Rac1 and Cdc42 are important mediators in the signal transduction pathway (Fig. 1C). Upon stimulation they activate proteins of the WASP/Scar family that bind to and activate the Arp2/3 complex. Subsequently ATP-G-actins bound to profilin are nucleated, i.e., two ATP binding G-actins self–assemble side by side and further G-actins are added in a head to tail fashion (Fig. 1C). Alternatively, branches may be formed on existing actin filaments. Capping proteins that bind to the barbed end can block further elongation. Proteins of the ADF/cofilin family can sever and depolymerize ADP actin filaments (4).

Functions of F-actin

The interaction with myosin motors enables F-actin to transport molecules as well as to change or maintain the shape of the cell by exerting tension. Thus, myosin-I motors move to the barbed end and can transport cargoes such as vesicles. When immobilized at the cargo site they can move actin filaments. Two myosin-II motors can assemble in an antiparallel manner. Attached to antiparallel F-actin, they can slide the actin filaments over each other and thus cause contractions. Such actomyosin interactions are essential for skeletal muscle contraction. Also, the contractile ring formed in the telophase of the cell cycle is an actomyosin structure that separates the filial cells during cytokinesis. In addition, actomyosin interactions play critical roles in the regulation of the morphology, adhesion and migration of non-muscle cells. Obviously, drugs that destroy F-actin have profound effects on cell shape and proliferation. In addition, F-actin plays an important role in cell adherence and motility.

Drugs

Drugs with Actions on MTs

The alkaloids vinblastine and vincristine extracted from the plant *Catharantus roseus* (also called *Vinca rosea*) and the semisynthetic derivatives vindesine, vinorelbine, and vinflunine can block mitosis and are clinically used for cancer treatment. When used at micromolar concentrations, the alkaloids bind with 1:1 stochiometry to β-tubulin in a region between residues 175 and 213. The bound disassembled tubulin heterodimers can no longer polymerize to MTs and form paracrystalline tubulin-*Vinca* alkaloid arrays. Pre-existent MTs are subsequently depolymerised. Chromosomes are no longer separated but dispersed or clumped in the cytoplasm. The cells undergo apoptosis. When used at nanomolar concentrations, *Vinca* alkaloids may block mitosis at the metaphase-anaphase transition by inhibiting the dynamic instability and treadmilling of MTs, without affecting microtubular mass (2). The cytostatic agent estramustin has similar effects. It blocks heterodimer polymerisation at micromolar concentrations and inhibits dynamic instability at nanomolar concentrations.

In contrast, paclitaxel (from the bark of the Western yew tree) and its more potent analogue docetaxel bind to microtubules when used at nanomolar concentrations. By attaching to β-tubulin between amino acids 239 and 254, the agents block the release of heterodimers from MTs and prevent the dynamic instability necessary for the capturing of chromosomes without affecting microtubular mass. Both taxols are used for cancer treatment. Labelled paclitaxel is also used for the immunocytochemical localization of MTs.

The alkaloid colchicine (from *Colchicum autumnale*) blocks tubulin polymerisation by binding to heterodimeric β-tubulin between amino acids 239 and 254. Since it inhibits the MT-dependent migration of granulocytes into areas of inflammation and their MT-dependent release of pro-inflammatory agents, it is used to treat attacks of gout. Its antimitotic effect in the gastrointestinal system induces diarrhoea. Nocodazole competes for the binding site of colchicine and has similar effects on heterodimeric β-tubulin.

In addition to their clinical use, the drugs are excellent experimental tools for the analysis of the cellular role of MTs.

Drugs with Actions on F-actin

Several agents affect the turnover of F-actin. They are not used therapeutically but serve as experimental tools to study the role of F-actin in cell function.

The ▶ cytochalasins A, B, C, D, E, and H are found in various species of mould. Mainly cytochalasin B and D are used as experimental tools. Cytochalasin D is 10 times more potent, acting at concentrations between 2 and 35 nM in cell free systems. Cytochalasins bind to the barbed end of F-actin and block the addition as well as dissociation of G-actin at that end. At micromolar concentrations, cytochalasin D can bind to G-actin and actin dimers and thus block additional polymerization. When applied to cultured cells, micromolar concentrations of cytochalasins remove stress fibers and other F-actin structures.

Swinholide A, isolated from the marine sponge *Theonella swinhoei*, sequesters actin dimers and induces their formation. One molecule of swinholide A binds to one dimer. In addition, swinholide A can sever F-actin by binding to the neighbouring protomers. Increased depolymerization of F-actin has been also reported.

Latrunculins A and B are macrolides from the sponge *Latrunculia magnifica*. Latrunculin A ($\geq$50 nM) binds close to the nucleotide binding site of G-actin and blocks the assembly with F-actin without promoting disassembly.

Phalloidin and phallacidin are cyclic peptides from the mushroom *Amanita phalloides* that stabilize F-actin. Phalloidin binds to residues 114–118 of an actin protomere and blocks nucleotide exchange without interfering with nucleotide hydrolysis. It enhances the rate of nucleation as well as that of elongation. It slowly penetrates the cell membrane and is used for immunocytochemical localization of F-actin.

In contrast, jasplakinolide, a cyclodepsipeptide from the marine sponge *Jaspis johnstoni*, rapidly penetrates the cell membrane. It competes with phalloidin for F-actin binding and has a dissociation constant of approximately 15 nM. It induces actin polymerization and stabilizes preexisting actin filaments. Dolastatin 11, a depsipeptide from the mollusk *Dolabella auricularia*, induces F-actin polymerisation. Its binding site differs from that of phalloidin or jasplakinolide.

References

1. Karsenti E, Vernos I (2001) The mitotic spindle: a self made machine. Science 294:543–547
2. Ngan VK, Bellman K, Panda D, Hill BT, Jordan MA, Wilson L (2001) Novel actions of the antitumor drugs vinfluvine and vinorelbine on microtubules. Cancer Res. 60:5045–5051
3. Geiger B, Bershadsky A, Pankov R, Yamada KM (2001) Transmembrane extracellular matrix-cytoskeleton crosstalk. Nature Reviews Mol Cell Biol 2:793–805
4. Pollard TD, Blanchoin L, Mullins RD (2001) Actin dynamics. J Cell Science 114:3-4

Cytotoxic Agents

▶ Antineopolastic Agents

Cytotoxic T-cells

Cytotoxic T-cells, or cytolytic T-cells (CTLs), are effector cells of the immune system that carry the CD8 surface marker. These cells are able to recognize autologous cells expressing foreign antigens (e.g. virus infected cells). Recognition is depending on the recognition of the MHC-I molecule by the T-cell receptor present on CTLs. This interaction of CTLs and target cells can lead to the lysis of the target cell.

▶ Immune Defense

D

Databank

In the biosciences, a databank (or data bank) is a structured set of raw data, most notably DNA sequences from sequencing projects, e.g. the EMBL and GenBank databases, respectively http://www.ebi.ac.uk/embl/ and http://www.ncbi.nlm.nih.gov/Genbank/index.html

▶ Bioinformatics

Database

A database (or data base) is a collection of data that is organized so that its contents can easily be accessed, managed, and modified by a computer. The most prevalent type of database is the relational database which organizes the data in tables; multiple relations can be mathematically defined between the rows and columns of each table to yield the desired information. An object-oriented database stores data in the form of objects which are organized in hierachical classes that may inherit properties from classes higher in the tree structure.

In the biosciences, a database is a curated repository of raw data containing annotations, further analysis and links to other databases. Examples of databases are the

SWISSPROT database for annotated protein sequences: http://www.ebi.ac.uk/swissprot/or the FlyBase database of genetic and molecular data for *Drosophila melanogaster*: http://flybase.bio.indiana.edu/

▶ Bioinformatics

2DE

▶ Two-dimensional Electrophoresis
▶ Proteomics

Death Receptor

Death receptors are proteins that belong to the tumor necrosis factor (TNF) receptor superfamily and are expressed on the cell surface. When ligated, they transduce a signal into the cytoplasm resulting in the activation of caspases and the induction of apoptosis. Examples of death receptors include CD95/Fas, TNF receptor I, and TNF receptor related, apoptosis inducing ligand (TRAIL) receptors.

▶ Apoptosis
▶ TNF Receptor Superfamily
▶ Multidrug Transporter

Delayed-rectifier K⁺ Channels

Delayed-rectifier potassium channels activate with a delay and mediate outwardly-rectifying potassium currents. These channels may make a significant contribution to the repolarizing phase of nervous action potentials.

▶ K⁺ Channels

Delayed Type Hypersensitivity Reaction

Delayed type hypersensitivty (DTH) reactions (synonym type IV allergic reactions) are exaggerated, T-lymphocyte mediated, cellular immune reactions to foreign substances, which require one to two days to manifest clinical symptoms.

▶ Allergy

Dendritic Cells

Dendritic cells are antigen-presenting cells, that is cells capable of retaining antigen-antibody complexes for an extended period of time, which are involved in immune defense of the body.

▶ Immune Defense

Dependence

Dependence is a somatic state which develops after chronic administration of certain drugs. This condition is characterized by the necessity to continue administration of the drug to avoid the appearance of withdrawal symptoms. Withdrawal symptoms are relieved by the administration of the drug upon which the body was "dependent". Psychological dependence is due to (e.g. social) reinforcement processes in the maintenance of drug-seeking behavior.

▶ Drug Addiction / Dependence

Depolarization-induced Ca²⁺ Release

▶ DICR

Depolarization-induced Suppression of Inhibition

Depolarization-induced suppression of inhibition (DSI) is a rapid synaptic feedback mechanism which regulates the strength of transmission of both excitatory and inhibitory synapses. Recent studies indicate that endocannabinoids act as retrograde messengers at central synapses and can mediate DSI.

▶ Endocannabinoid System

Depression

▶ Antidepressants

Dermatomycoses

Dermatomycosis is an illness of the skin caused by fungi.

▶ Anti-fungal Drugs

Dermatophytes

Dermatophytes are a special type of fungi, invading the skin and able to grow on keratin as a sole nutrient base.

▶ Anti-fungal Drugs

Descending Inhibitory Pathway

The descending inhibitory pathway is an endogenous pain-suppressing system, which becomes activated especially under pathological conditions, when stress is present. A key part of this system is an area of the midbrain, called the "periaqueductal grey" (PAG). The PAG is rich in enkephalin-containing neurons. It receives inputs from many other brain regions, including the hypothalamus, cortex and thalamus. These connections may represent the mechanism whereby cortical and other inputs control pain perception. Activation of PAG neurons leads to the activation of neurons in the rostroventral medulla, which includes the *nucleus raphe magnus*. From the *nucleus raphe magnus*, serotonin- and enkephalin-containing neurons project to the *substantia gelatinosa* of the dorsal horn of the spinal cord and exert their inhibitory influences on nociceptive transmission. There is also a noradrenergic pathway, which originates from the *locus ceruleus*, which also has an inhibitory effect on the nociceptive transmission in the dorsal horn. The PAG and the *substantia gelatinosa* are especially rich in enkephalin-containing neurons, suggesting that opioid peptides function as transmitters in this system. The antinociceptive effects of opioids are believed to be at least partly mediated by effects on the descending inhibitory pathway.

▶ Nociception
▶ Periaqueductal Grey

Desensitization

Desensitization is the rapidly attenuation of receptor activation as a result of stimulation of cells and occurs in seconds to minutes. Receptor phosphorylation by G-protein-coupled receptor kinases and second-messenger-regulated kinases as well as receptor/G-protein uncoupling contribute to this process. In the continued presence or at high concentrations of agonistic ligands, ligand gated ion channels may undergo desensitization by entering a permanently closed state. While the ligand binding domain is occupied by the agonist, the desensitized channel is unable to re-open. For ligand gated ion channels, the structural basis of desensitization is not understood. For voltage dependent potassium channels, the 'ball and chain' model suggests a mechanism of ion channel desensitisation.

▶ Tolerance and Desensitization

Desmoplakin

Desmoplakin is the most abundant desmosomal component that plays a critical role in linking intermediate filament networks to the desmosomal plaque. Desmoplakin forms rod-like dimers that bind to intermediate filaments and to the cadherin-associated proteins, plakoglobin and plakophilin. Gene knock-out experiments have revealed an essential role for desmoplakin in establishing cell-cell contacts in early mouse embryos.

▶ Cadherins/Catenins
▶ Cytoskeleton

DHOD

Dihydroorotate dehydrogenase (DHOD) represents the key enzyme in the *de novo* pyrimidine nucleotide biosynthesis that is required for the proliferation of activated lymphocytes.

DHPR

▶ Dihydropyridine Receptor

Diabesity

Obese people are predisposed to diabetes and cardiovascular disease. The term diabesity (sometimes referred to as 'syndrome X' or 'metabolic syndrome') reflects the intricate association between these disorders.

▶ Diabetis Mellitus

Diabetes Insipidus

Diabetes insipidus is a disease in which the kidney is unable to concentrate urine. It is characterized by hypostenuria, polyuria and polydipsia. There are two mayor forms of diabetes insipidus, central and nephrogenic. This type of diabetes is not related to diabetes mellitus (insulin deficiency or resistance), where large amounts of urine and glucose are excreted by the kidney. Other types of diabetes insipidus are the dipsogenic (neurological origin) and gestational diabetes insipidus (during pregnancy).

▶ Vasopressin/Oxytocin

Diabetes Mellitus

Hans-Georg Joost, Annette Schürmann
German Institute of Human Nutrition,
Potsdam-Rehbrücke, Germany
joost@mail.dife.de, schuerman@mail.dife.de

Synonyms

None

Definition

Diabetes mellitus is defined as hyperglycemia (fasting >7 mM and/or 2 h postprandial >11.1 mM) due to absolute or relative lack of insulin. The most common forms are type 1 diabetes (prevalence 0.25%), with absolute lack of insulin, and type 2 diabetes (prevalence 4–6%) which is due to the combination of insulin resistance and insufficient insulin secretion.

▶ Appetite Control
▶ Glucose Transporters
▶ Insulin Receptor
▶ Oral Antidiabetic Drugs

Basic Mechanisms

Type 1 diabetes (previously insulin-dependent diabetes mellitus, IDDM, or juvenile diabetes): Progredient destruction of insulin-secreting β-cells by an autoimmune mechanism during a period of several years (1). The diagnosis is confirmed by detection of antibodies against β-cell proteins (glutamic acid decarboxylase, tyrosine phosphatase IA-2, insulin). Islet cell destruction is probably mediated by activated T lymphocytes. The pathogenesis has a polygenic basis; seven susceptibility loci (Iddm1-7) have been mapped. However, genetic and epidemiological data indicate a strong environmental factor in the pathogenesis. An unknown viral infection has been implicated in the triggering of the autoimmune process, but is not proven.

Type 2 diabetes (previously non insulin-dependent diabetes mellitus, NIDDM): Type 2 diabetes is a frequent consequence of the ▶ metabolic

Tab. 1 Pharmakokinetic characteristics of the most commonly used insulin preparations and analogs.

	Onset of action:	Maximum:	Duration of action:
Short acting insulins:			
Insulin lispro	15 min	1 h	2–5 h
Insulin aspart	15 min	1 h	2–5 h
Regular insulin	30 min	2–4 h	6–8 h
Intermediary insulin:			
NPH insulin	30–60 min	2–9 h	16–20 h
Long acting insulin:			
Insulin glargine	60 min	4–12 h	>22 h

syndrome (obesity, insulin resistance, dyslipidemia, hypertension). Obesity causes insulin resistance that is initially compensated by hyperinsulinemia. In the course of insulin resistance, the β-cell function deteriorates and insulin secretion is reduced, leading to relative insulinopenia. In particular, the initial response (first phase) of the pancreas to a glucose load is impaired during the first stages of the disease. Fasting hyperglycemia is preceded by a variable period of impaired glucose tolerance (IGT) during which secondary complications (micro- and macrovascular) start to develop. Thus, in most type 2 diabetics, secondary complications can be diagnosed at the time of the detection of hyperglycemia; these are accelerated and aggravated by other components of the metabolic syndrome (dyslipidemia, hypertension).

Obesity and insulin resistance appear to be due to a heterogenous combination of genes involved in the control of appetite and thermogenesis (▶ Thrifty Gene Constellation). Several genes have been identified that are involved in the regulation of food intake and of body weight (e.g. leptin, the leptin receptor, melanocortin receptors; see chapter on appetite control). However, the genes responsible for polygenic obesity are largely unknown. Data obtained from rodent models indicate that islet cell failure is produced by a different set of genes; obesity is a necessary condition for their effects on the pancreas (2). This cooperation of two different genetic constellations (obesity and diabetes genes) explains the heterogeneity of the type 2 diabetes with regard to its association with body weight.

The molecular pathology of the β-cell destruction in the course of insulin resistance is largely unknown. It has been suggested that the constant hyper-stimulation of the β-cell by glucose ('glucose toxicity') or elevated fatty acids ('lipotoxicity') may lead to cell damage.

Pharmacological Intervention

Type 1 diabetes always requires treatment with insulin. The preferred therapeutic regimen is the 'intensified conventional therapy' (ICT) that combines 1–2 daily injections of a retarded insulin (usually NPH insulin) with 3–4 injections of a short-acting insulin (e.g. regular insulin) at mealtimes. ICT requires 4–5 daily blood sugar determinations and adjustment of the dose to (preprandial) blood sugar and (estimated) carbohydrate content of meals. If the complicated ICT regimen is not feasible, a conventional regimen (CT) may be employed that comprises two daily injections of a combination of NPH with regular insulin (two thirds of the daily dose before breakfast, one third before dinner). CT usually applies constant doses of insulin and requires a stricter adherence to the diet than ICT, i.e. meals that contain a controlled carbohydrate content and are timed according to the profile of the insulin injections.

Insulin preparations (Table 1): Recombinant human insulin obtained from genetically engineered *E. coli* or yeast is used predominantly. Retarded preparations are generated by addition of protamine (NPH-insulin, neutral protamine Hagedorn) that may provide the 'basal' supply in both ICT and CT. Three insulin analogs with altered amino acid sequence and different pharmacokinetic characteristics are available: insulin lispro (swap of B28 proline and B29 lysine) and insulin aspart (exchange of B29 lysine for aspartate) exhibit a more rapid onset and a shorter duration of action because of a faster dissociation of the hexameric insulin-zinc-phenol complex. Insulin glargine is a long acting analog that is soluble at low pH because of two additional arginines at B31 and B32. After injection, the analog precipitates from its solution and forms a long-acting depot; its absorption kinetics appears to be steadier than that of NPH insulin.

Mechanism of insulin action: Binding of insulin to its receptor stimulates receptor autophosphorylation and phosphorylation of substrates (IRS1, IRS2) on tyrosine residues. Subsequently, ▶ PI 3-kinase is activated by binding to the phosphorylated IRS, and generates phosphatidyl inositol phosphates that activate PDK1. The serine kinase PDK1 phosphorylates and activates ▶ PKB/Akt. Some effects of insulin on gene expression are then triggered by PKB-dependent phosphorylation of the transcription factor FKHR and of its subsequent export from the nucleus; this effect leads to repression of genes encoding gluconeogenic enzymes. PKB also phosphorylates and inactivates glycogen synthase kinase; these two effects represent the molecular basis of the reduction of glucose output from the liver. In adipose and muscle tissue, activation of PKB/Akt triggers the translocation of vesicles containing the glucose transporter GLUT4 from an intracellular pool to the plasma membrane (3). Proteins that are thought to be involved in docking and fusion of the vesicles are VAMP2, SNARE, syntaxin 4, SNAP23, and Synip (Fig. 1). Insulin appears to release Synip from its binding to syntaxin 4, thereby presumably initiating the fusion process.

Type 2 diabetes: After clinical diagnosis, weight normalization by hypocaloric, low fat diet and exercise may normalize glucose homeostasis for a period of several years. Accordingly, this intervention markedly delays the onset of overt hyperglycemia when employed at the stage of IGT. Because the 'lifestyle changes' are difficult to maintain, and because of the progression of the islet cell failure, pharmacological intervention will usually become inevitable and has to be intensified throughout the course of the disease. Initially, normalization of blood sugar can be accomplished with oral antidiabetics. Lateron, a combination of oral antidiabetics with insulin or insulin alone (preferably ICT) will be required.

β-Cytotropic agents: These agents enhance the effect of glucose on the secretion of insulin (4). Commonly used drugs are sulfonylurea derivatives and the more recently introduced benzoic acid derivatives repaglinide and nateglinide. Their receptor is a membrane protein (SUR, ▶ Sulfonyurea Receptor) that regulates the activity of the ATP-dependent potassium channel of the pancreatic β-cell (Kir 6.2). Binding of ATP or a sulfonylurea to SUR reduces the potassium current and causes membrane depolarization, subsequently opening voltage-gated calcium channels, and calcium-stimulated exocytosis of insulin-containing granules (Fig. 2). Lack-of-function mutants of SUR are chacterized by an increased secretion of insulin (congenital hypoglycemia). The effect of the β-cytotropic agents on the channel is antagonized by the 'potassium channel openers' diazoxide and minoxidil.

Two isotypes of SUR have been cloned, SUR1 and SUR2. In addition, 2 splicing variants of SUR2, distinguished by 42 C-terminal amino acids, have been identified. SUR1 is mainly expressed in β-cells. SUR2B is expressed in vascular smooth muscle, heart, skeletal muscle and brain, whereas expression of SUR2A is restricted to heart and skeletal muscle. Sulfonylureas exhibit a higher affinity for SUR1. Block of SUR2 by minoxidil or diazoxide produces vasodilation, stimulation of SUR2 by high, non-therapeutic concentrations of glibenclamide produces vasoconstriction. A potential effect of sulfonylureas on the cardiac SUR2, producing cardiac arrhythmia in particular under ischemic conditions, has been a matter of debate. However, clinical studies failed to demonstrate an increased cardiac mortality in patients treated with glibenclamide or chlorpropamide.

To date, the commonly used sulfonylureas are the long-acting derivatives glibenclamide (US syn-

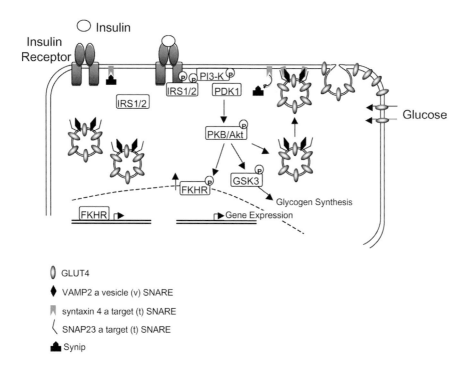

Fig. 1 Mechanism of insulin action. The binding of insulin to its receptor initiates phosphorylation of the insulin receptor, recruitment and phosphorylation of the insulin receptor substrates IRS1 and 2, and activation of PI 3-kinase. The subsequent 3-phosphorylation of phosphinositides recruits and activates PDK1, which then phosphorylates and activates PKB/Akt. Activation of PKB/Akt results in the translocation of GLUT4-containing vesicles to the plasma membrane. VAMP2 (a vesicle (v) SNARE) is present in the GLUT4 vesicles and participates in the formation of a fusion complex with the plasma membrane targets (t) SNAREs, syntaxin 4 and SNAP23. Under basal conditions, syntaxin 4 interacts with Synip, and is released from this complex upon stimulation with insulin. Activated PKB/Akt phosphorylates the transcription factor FKHR, stimulates its translocation to the cytoplasm, which results in repression of insulin-controlled genes. PKB/Akt also phosphorylates and inactivates glycogen synthase kinase-3 (GSK3), leading to the dephosphorylation and activation of glycogen synthase.

onym: glyburide) and glimeripide. Glimepiride is believed to have a somewhat longer duration of action than glibenclamide, and to exert additional extrapancreatic effects. The mechanism of these potential extrapancreatic effects is not defined and their clinical relevance is unclear. The non-sulfonylurea potassium channel blockers repaglinide and nateglinide have been shown to act by the same mechanism of action as the sulfonylureas. The duration of action of repaglinide and nateglinide is short because of their rapid metabolism and/or excretion. These pharmakokinetic parameters are thought to allow a specific reduction of postprandial glucose excursions. However, because the effects of the potassium channel open-

ers largely depend on plasma glucose levels, both long- and short-acting agents mainly stimulate a postprandial insulin secretion. A potential advantage of the short-acting derivatives might be a reduced risk of hypoglycemias.

Metformin: The biguanide metformin lowers blood sugar mainly by the inhibition of glucose output from the liver. It is generally accepted that this effect reflects a marked inhibition of gluconeogenesis, presumably through reduction of pyruvate transport into the mitochondria. The 'receptor' of metformin and its specific molecular function is unknown. Other effects of metformin (stimulation of glucose transport in muscle, inhibition of intestinal glucose absorption) require

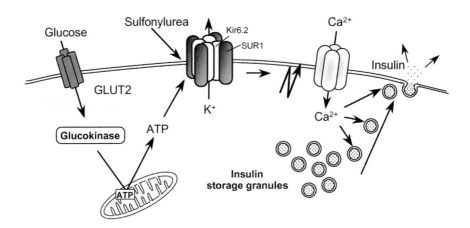

Fig. 2 Mechanism of insulin secretion from pancreatic β-cell. Glucose enters the β-cell via GLUT2, is phosphorylated by glucokinase, and generates ATP. A rise in the ATP-ADP ratio results in closure of ATP-dependent K^+ channels, membrane depolarization and opening of voltage-gated Ca^{2+} channels. The Ca^{2+} influx activates the exocytosis of insulin-containing secretory granules. The ATP-dependent K^+ channel consists of Kir6.2 (a K^+ inward rectifier) and SUR (sulfonylurea receptor). Sulfonylureas block the ATP-dependent K^+ channels by enhancing the effect of ATP.

higher concentrations and appear to contribute little to the *in-vivo* effect.

Under certain circumstances, and very rarely, the inhibition of gluconeogenesis by metformin may suppress lactic acid metabolism and precipitate a potentially fatal lactic acidosis. Impairment of renal function, liver disease, alcoholism, conditions that give rise to increased lactate production (e.g. congestive heart failure, infections) are therefore contraindications for the application of metformin.

Oral formulations of metformin are rapidly and completely absorbed. The agent is poorly bound to plasma proteins; its duration of action is determined exclusively by renal elimination. Higher concentrations of metformin than in most tissues are found in the intestinal mucosa, giving rise to common side effects (irritation, diarrhea).

Acarbose and Miglitol: These agents are specific inhibitors of intestinal glucosidases and reduce the conversion of sucrose and starch to glucose. Their main effect is a delay, not a complete inhibition, of the absorption of carbohydrates. Postprandial blood sugar excursions are effectively reduced. Because a small portion of the carbohydrates enters the colon, their microbial degradation frequently causes flatulence or meteorism.

Acarbose produces a somewhat lower reduction of HbA_{1c} levels than glibenclamide and metformin, but may enhance the effect of these agents. Interestingly, when given to patients with impaired glucose tolerance, acarbose reduces the progression of the disease to overt hyperglycemia by 30%.

Thiazolidinediones (PPARγ-agonists): Thiazolidinediones lower blood glucose levels in animal models of insulin resistance and also in insulin resistant patients. They enhance the effect of insulin, reduce serum insulin levels, and are therefore considered 'insulin sensitizers' (5). Clinically used agents are rosiglitazone and pioglitazone; earlier derivatives (ciglitazone or troglitazone) have not been introduced into the clinic or were withdrawn because of unacceptable side effects.

The ▶ peroxisome proliferator-activated receptor γ (PPARγ) is a transcription factor that controls the expression of enzymes and proteins involved in fat and glucose metabolism. More importantly, stimulation of this receptor induces differentiation of preadipocytes to adipose cells. It is believed that the formation of additional, small fat cells lowers free fatty acids, thereby correcting insulin resistance. Such a mechanism is based on the assumption that insulin resistance is mainly due to the effect of fatty acids on glucose metabolism.

References

1. Atkinson MA, Eisenbarth GS (2001) Type 1 diabetes: New perspectives on disease pathogenesis and treatment. Lancet 358:221–229
2. Plum L, Kluge R, Giesen K, Altmüller J, Ortlepp JR, Joost HG (2000) Type 2 diabetes-like hyperglycemia in a backcross model of New Zealand obese (NZO) and SJL mice: Characterization of a susceptibility locus on chromosome 4 and its relation with obesity. Diabetes 49:1590–1596
3. Holman GD, Sandoval IV (2001) Moving the insulin-sensitive glucose transporter GLUT4 into and out of storage. Trends Cell Biol. 11:173–179
4. Aguilar-Bryan L, Bryan J (1999) Molecular biology of adenosine triphosphate-sensitive potassium channels. Endocrine Rev. 20:101–135
5. Murphy GJ, Holder JC (2000) PPAR-γ agonists: Therapeutic role in diabetes, inflammation and cancer. Trends Pharmacol. Sci. 21:469–474

Diacylglycerol

Diacylglycerol is glycerol esterified to two fatty acids at the sn-1 and sn-2 positions. It is a product of phospholipase C action and an activator of ▶ protein kinase C. It is also an intermediate in the biosynthesis of triacylglycerol, phosphatidylethanolamine and phosphatidylcholine.

▶ Phospholipases

Dicer

Dicer represents the key enzyme in the RNAi pathway. Dicer is also known as Helicase with RNAse motif, heRNA, Helicase-moi, K12H4.8-like, or KIAA0928. Dicer cleaves long double stranded RNA into small pieces of about 21-23 nucleotides. These so-called siRNA duplexes produced by the action of action of Dicer contain 5'-phosphates and free 3'-hydroxylgroups.

▶ Antisense Oligonucleotides

▶ RNA Interference

DICR

DICR (depolarization-induced Ca^{2+} release) is Ca^{2+} release triggered by depolarization of the sarcolemma. In skeletal muscle, conformational change in the voltage sensor (α1S subunit of the dihydropyridine receptor) in the T-tubule is directly transmitted to the ryanodine receptor (RyR1), resulting in Ca^{2+} release through RyR1. $Ca2^{+}$-induced $Ca2^{+}$ release (CICR) in the skeletal muscle is too slow to make a significant contribution to DICR. In cardiac muscle, in contrast, Ca^{2+} influx through the α1C subunit of DHPR triggers CICR. Consistently, contraction of skeletal muscle is independent of the external Ca^{2+}, whereas cardiac muscle contraction is dependent on it.

▶ Ryanodine Receptor

Differential Display

Differential display is a method for identifying differentially expressed genes, using anchored oligo-dT, random oligonucleotide primers and polymerase chain reaction on reverse-transcribed RNA from different cell populations. The amplified complementary DNAs are displayed and comparisons are drawn between the different cell populations.

▶ Gene Expression Analysis
▶ Microarray Technology

Dihydrofolate Reductase

Dihydrofolate reductase is required for the sythesis of tetrahydrofolate, a co-factor required for the transfer of single carbon groups. Inhibition of dihydrofolate reductase blocks the synthesis of DNA and RNA (thymidylate and purines). The enzyme inhibitors include antibacterial and -parasitic drugs (pyrimethamine, trimethoprim) and the antineoplastic agent methotrexate.

▶ Antineoplastic Agents
▶ Vitamins, watersoluble

Dihydropyridine Receptor

The dihyropyridine receptor (DHPR) is the L-type voltage dependent Ca^{2+} channel which specifically binds dihydropyridine (DHP) derivatives and is inhibited by the ligand. It is composed of 5 subunits ($\alpha 1$, β, $\alpha 2/\delta$, and γ): $\alpha 1$ forms the main part of the Ca^{2+} channel and voltage sensor, and the other subunits are modulatory. $\alpha 1S$ is the isoform specific to the skeletal muscle where it serves as the voltage sensor rather than a Ca^{2+} channel, and $\alpha 1C$ to the cardiac muscle where it plays the critical role as a Ca^{2+} channel. By electron microscopic observation of the freeze-fractured sarcolemma, it is identified as a large intramembranous particle.

▶ Voltage-dependent Ca^{2+} Channels
▶ Ca^{2+} Channel Blockers

Dihydropyridines

Dihydropyridines are a large family of compounds which block HVA calcium channels.

▶ Voltage-dependent Ca^{2+} Channels

Dimer, Trimer, Oligomer

These terms denote a physical association (covalent or noncovalent) between two (dimer), three (trimer), or ... several (oligo) proteins. *Homo*mers

are composed of two identical proteins. *Heteromers* are associations of different proteins.

Dioxins

Dioxins are prominent members of the class of polychlorinated hydrocarbons that also includes dibenzofuran, biphenyls and others. Dioxins are highly toxic environmental contaminants. Like others small planar xenobiotics, some dioxins bind with high affinity to the arylhydrocarbon (Ah) receptor. Dioxins activate the receptor over a long time period, but are themselves poor substrates for the enzymes which are induced via the Ah-receptor. These properties of the dioxins and related xenobiotics may be important for the toxicity of these compounds. Dioxins like 2,3,7,8-tetrachloro-p-dibenzodioxin can cause persistent dermatosis, like chloracne and may have other neurotoxic, immunotoxic and carcinogenic effects.

▶ Arylhydrocarbon Receptor
▶ Nuclear Receptor Regulation of Drug-metabolizing P450 Enzymes

Dipeptidylpeptidase IV

Dipeptidylpeptidase IV (also known as CD26) cleaves ▶ neuropeptide Y and ▶ peptide YY to generate their subtype-selective fragments NPY_{3-36} and PYY_{3-36}.

Discharge

Discharge is the electrical signal of an activated neuron or a group of neurons. During a discharge or 'action potential', neurons lose their negative intracellular potential and become positively charged for a fraction of a second (1-4 milliseconds). This excitation is conducted to the nerve terminals which form ▶ synapses with other cells and can thereby facilitate action potential generation in these target cells (at excitatory synapses) or impede action potential generation (inhibitory synapses).

Dissociation Constant

The dissociation constant (Kd) is the concentration of free ligand that results in occupancy of 50% of the receptors for this ligand available in the system.

▶ Drug-receptor Interaction

Dissociative Anesthetic

Dissociative anesthetic is a term applied to phencyclidine and ketamine which induce a peculiar subjective state of dissociation from the environment, together with sedation, immobility, amnesia, analgesia, and ultimately coma.

▶ Psychotomimetic Drugs

Distribution of Drugs

▶ Pharmacokinetics

Diuretics

JÜRGEN SCHNERMANN
National Institutes of Health, Bethesda, USA
jurgens@intra.niddk.nih.gov

Synonyms

Natriuretics, antinatriferics

Definition

Diuretics promote the urinary excretion of sodium (Na) and water by inhibiting the absorption of filtered fluid across the renal tubular epithelium. The ensuing reduction in Na reabsorption reduces the Na content of the body, the critical determinant of extracellular and plasma fluid volumes. Thus, the use of diuretics is primarily indicated in the treatment of edematous diseases and of arterial hypertension.

▶ Antihypertensive Drugs
▶ Epithelial Na$^+$ Channel

Mechanisms of Action

The mammalian kidney generates its excretory product, the urine, in a two-step process where filtration of a large volume of plasma-like fluid across the glomerular blood capillaries is followed by the absorption and secretion of solutes and water across the tubular epithelial cell wall. Transcellular absorption of filtered Na is achieved by apical Na uptake along a favorable electrochemical gradient, and by basolateral Na extrusion through the energy consuming action of Na/K-ATPase. The renal tubule is cytologically and functionally heterogeneous along its longitudinal axis. One expression of the functional heterogeneity is the type of transport protein responsible for apical Na uptake. As a general rule, currently available diuretics inhibit a specific apical Na transporter, and their action therefore displays tubule segment-specificity.

Na uptake in the proximal tubule, a segment in which about 2/3 of the filtered Na is reabsorbed, is mediated by a Na/H exchanger (NHE3) and a number of other transporters that typically carry a second solute in a Na-dependent cotransport mode. Along the thick ascending limb of the loop of Henle Na uptake occurs mostly through the electroneutral ▶ Na/K/2Cl-cotransporter (NKCC2) in a process that accounts for roughly 25% of total renal Na absorption. Na uptake in the distal convoluted tubule is mediated by a ▶ NaCl cotransporter (NCC), and this segment accounts for about 5% of Na absorption. Finally, electrogenic Na absorption through the ▶ epithelial Na channel (ENaC) is the uptake mode across the cor-

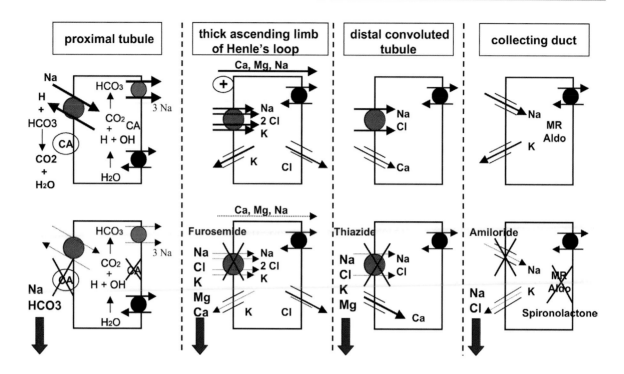

Fig. 1 Schematic representation of four cells representative for the proximal tubule, the thick ascending limb of the loop of Henle, the distal convoluted tubule, and the collecting duct. The upper diagrams show the normal functional state of these cells whereas the lower diagrams show the effect of the segment-specific diuretics. Circles indicate transport proteins, and double lines represent channels. Arrows indicate the normal direction of net transport, and the boldness of the arrows is a qualitative index of transport rate. Only those cellular features are shown that are relevant to understanding the action of the diuretic agents. CA carbonic anhydrase; MR Aldo mineralocorticoid receptor aldosterone complex.

tical collecting duct, a process that may be responsible for 2–3% of Na absorption. Na transport through ENaC is regulated by the adrenal gland steroid aldosterone.

Proximal Tubule Diuretics

Inhibition of ▶ carbonic anhydrase (CA) causes inhibition of NaHCO$_3$ absorption in the proximal tubule. Apical Na uptake through NHE3 requires the delivery of H ions to the intracellular binding site of the transporter and of HCO$_3$ to the basolateral 3Na/ HCO$_3$ cotransporter. The generation of H and HCO$_3$ at appropriate rates from H$_2$O and CO$_2$ is dependent upon catalysis by intracellular carbonic anhydrase (type II CA). In addition, carbonic acid dehydration in the tubular lumen is catalyzed by a CA located in the luminal membrane of proximal tubules (type IV CA). Both enzymes must be functional for reabsorption of Na HCO$_3$ in

the proximal tubule to proceed at normal rates. CA inhibitors (acetazolamide, benzolamide, methazolamide and others) cause Na HCO$_3$ absorption to decrease by about 40–80% and urinary Na HCO$_3$ excretion to increase by about 25–30%. Efficacy of CA inhibitors is reduced by a consistent reduction in ▶ glomerular filtration rate.

Loop of Henle Diuretics

The so-called loop diuretics (sulfonamide derivatives like furosemide, bumetanide, torsemide and others, and phenoxyacetic acid derivatives like ethacrynic acid) augment the excretion of NaCl through inhibition of the electroneutral NKCC2 cotransporter in the apical membrane of the thick ascending limb of the loop of Henle. Loop diuretics directly interact with the transport protein, presumably by binding to a region that is also critical for binding of a chloride ion. By collapsing the normally lumen-positive transepithelial potential difference, loop diuretics abolish the electrical driving force that is responsible for the paracellular absorption of Na and other cations such as Ca and Mg. Since NaCl transport across the TAL causes the accumulation of medullary solutes, loop diuretics lead to a dissipation of the ▶ cortico-medullary solute gradient, and thereby disable the urinary concentrating mechanism. Renal blood flow and glomerular filtration rates are usually not affected by loop diuretics. While some of the natriuretic actions of loop diuretics is due to direct inhibition of NKCC2, another part is the secondary consequence of simultaneous stimulation of PGE_2 production. Blockade of cyclooxygenases, particularly of cyclooxygenase-2, has been shown to reduce loop diuretic-induced natriuresis by about 50% through mechanisms that are not fully understood. Since PGE_2 generated by cyclooxygenase-2 under conditions of reduced NaCl transport is also a main factor in macula densa stimulation of renin secretion, loop diuretics are typically associated with an increase in renin secretion and greatly elevated plasma renin levels. Loop diuretics act from the luminal aspect of the tubule. Because of their intense protein binding, these agents are not filtered effectively, and gain access to the tubule lumen by secretion. Loss-of-function mutations in the NKCC2 gene are the cause of ▶ Bartter syndrome type I, and the symptoms of this disease are comparable to those caused by loop diuretics including salt and water loss, calciuria, magnesiuria, hypokalemia, metabolic alkalosis, hyperreninemia and hyperprostaglandinuria.

Distal Convoluted Tubule Diuretics

Electroneutral NaCl transport in the distal convoluted tubule is inhibited by the class of thiazide diuretics (chlorothiazide, hydrochlorothiazide, metolazone, chlorthalidone and others). Thiazides interfere with the Cl binding site of NCC and cause a relatively small increase in Na excretion. Inhibition of NCC is not associated with persistent and marked changes in renal hemodynamics. Like the loop diuretics, thiazides act from the luminal side and gain access to it by tubular secretion. Loss-of-function mutations in the NCC gene have been identified as the cause of ▶ Gitelman's syndrome, an electrolyte disorder characterized by hypokalemic metabolic alkalosis, magnesium wasting, and hypercalcemia.

Collecting Duct Diuretics

Na uptake through ENaC in cortical and probably also in inner medullary collecting ducts is inhibited by the so-called K-sparing diuretics (amiloride and triamterene). The natriuretic effect of this class of diuretics is small, commensurate with the small fraction of filtered Na normally absorbed along the collecting duct. Clinically more important than their natriuretic effects is the inhibition of K secretion that results from a reduced Na flux through ENaC. Inhibition of electrogenic Na absorption causes a hyperpolarization of the apical membrane and therefore a reduction in the electrochemical driving force for K secretion. The result is a reduction in K secretion and K excretion since the tubular site of ENaC expression overlaps with that of the K channel responsible for the secretory cell to lumen K flux. Loss-of-function mutations in the ENaC gene are the cause of ▶ pseudohypoaldosteronism type I, a salt losing nephropathy, and gain-of-function mutations cause ▶ Liddle's syndrome, a salt retaining state with severe hypertension.

A second diuretic acting along the collecting duct is spironolactone, a steroid that antagonizes the action of aldosterone. Spironolactone competes with aldosterone for the mineralocorticoid receptor and prevents the nuclear translocation of the receptor-ligand complex that is required for its genomic actions. Like amiloride, spironolactone causes mild natriuresis and a reduction in K secretion.

Clinical Use

CA Inhibitors

The use of CA inhibitors as diuretics is limited by their propensity to cause metabolic acidosis and hypokalemia. Their use can be indicated in patients with metabolic alkalosis and secondary hyperaldosteronism resulting for example from aggressive use of loop diuretics. Furthermore, CA inhibitors are effective drugs to produce a relatively alkaline urine for the treatment of cystine and uric acid stones as well as for the accelerated excretion of salicylates. Perhaps the most common use of CA inhibitors is in the treatment of glaucoma.

Loop Diuretics

Loop diuretics are the drugs of choice for the treatment of edematous patients with congestive heart failure, cirrhosis of the liver, and nephrotic syndrome. Excretion of Na is helpful only to the extent that some of the excess interstitial fluid is mobilized and shifted into the intravascular space. Aggressive diuretic therapy is only necessary in pulmonary ► edema resulting from left ventricular heart failure. In all edematous conditions, the diuretic treatment addresses a symptom, not the cause of the disease, and it is therefore not the therapeutic mainstay. Other clinical situations where loop diuretics are indicated include hypercalcemia, hyperkalemia and hypermagnesemia. Loop diuretics have also been found to be advantageous in the treatment of asthma.

Adverse side effects of loop diuretics are mainly the consequence of the altered absorptive function along the loop of Henle. The most common side effect of diuretic treatment is the loss of potassium that may result in ► hypokalemia. K loss is a consequence of malabsorption along the TAL due to the direct inhibition of NKCC2, and of increased K secretion due to the increased tubular fluid flow along the K secreting cortical collecting duct, and to the increase in plasma aldosterone that results from diuretic-induced hypovolemia. Furthermore, loop diuretics can cause metabolic alkalosis and the urinary loss of calcium and magnesium. Presumably because NKCC2 is involved in maintaining the ionic composition of the endolymph, loop diuretics, especially ethacrynic acid, can cause hearing impairment that is typically reversible, but can also lead to permanent deafness.

Thiazide Diuretics

Interference with Na absorption in the distal convoluted tubule by thiazide-like diuretics is effective in the therapy of arterial hypertension. On average, about half of patients with essential hypertension respond to thiazide monotherapy with a blood pressure reduction of more than 10%. While the initial reduction in blood pressure appears to be a consequence of a reduced plasma volume, venous return and cardiac output, the prolonged effect of thiazides to reduce blood pressure is related to a reduction in total peripheral resistance. The cause for this long term adjustment is multifactorial. The hypotensive effect of thiazides is enhanced by a low NaCl diet, and by combination with other blood pressure lowering drugs. Often in combination with loop diuretics, thiazides are also used in the treatment of edematous diseases. Like loop diuretics, thiazides can cause K loss and hypokalemia, hyponatremia and urinary magnesium wasting, while they usually reduce the excretion of calcium. This characteristic feature to stimulate Ca absorption makes thiazides a useful drug in the prevention of calcium stone formation in idiopathic hypercalciuria. Thiazides have also been described to diminish the occurrence of bone loss, hip fractures and osteoporosis.

K-Sparing Drugs

Amiloride, triamterene or spironolactone are typically not used to augment the excretion of Na but to counteract the kaliuretic effect of loop diuretics and thiazides as an alternative to dietary K supplements. Thus, K-sparing drugs often accompany treatment with loop diuretics and are useful in other K-wasting states such as primary hyperaldosteronism or Bartter's syndrome. Another beneficial effect of amiloride is a stimulation of calcium and magnesium absorption along distal tubules and collecting ducts, an action that counteracts the Ca and Mg wasting of loop diuretics and the Mg wasting of thiazides. Spironolactone requires functional adrenal glands and is most effective in patients with elevated plasma aldosterone levels such as those with cirrhosis of the liver and ascites. Interestingly, spironolactone has been found to have beneficial effects as an adjuvant therapy in the treatment of heart failure.

References

1. Okusa MD, Ellison DH (2000) Physiology and pathophysiology of diuretic actions. In: Seldin DW, Giebisch G (eds) The Kidney. Physiology and Pathophysiology. Lippincott Williams & Wilkins, Philadelphia 2877–2922
2. Taylor SH (2000) Diuretic therapy in congestive heart failure. Cardiol Rev 8:104–114
3. Brater DC (2000) Pharmacology of diuretics. Am J Med Sci 319:38–50

4. Kaplan NM (1999) Diuretics: correct use in hypertension. Sem Nephrol 19:569–574
5. Lifton RP, Gharavi AG, Geller DS (2001) Molecular mechanisms of human hypertension. Cell 23:545–556

DNA Fragmentation

DNA fragmentation occurs in two stages. Firstly, endonucleolytic activity cleaves the DNA into high molecular weight fragments leading to the morphological picture of chromatin condensation characteristic of apoptosis. The second stage involves a calcium-magnesium endonuclease which catalyses the further fragmentation of the DNA into oligonucleosomal fragments, which give rise to the pattern of DNA base pairing which shows up as the classical DNA ladder pattern by electrophoresis. In several populations of lymphocytes, namely B lymphocyte populations in the germinal centre of lymph nodes, immature thymocytes, and cytotoxic T lymphocytes, it has been noted that only the first stage of DNA fragmentation is occurring.

▶ Apoptosis

DNA Methylation

In higher eukaryotes, most of the chromosomal DNA carries 5-methyl-cytidine residues located in CpG sequence motifs. There is a close correlation between transcriptional inactivation and methylation. Moreover, considerable evidence shows that regions of DNA that are actively engaged in transcription lack 5-methylcytidine nucleotides in CpG motifs. Hence DNA methylation is a means by which cells regulate gene expression.

DNA Replication

DNA replication is DNA synthesis during the S phase of the cell cycle which results in a doubling of the genomic DNA. Replication can be subdivided into three distinct phases: initiation, elongation and termination.

▶ Cell-cycle Control

DNA Response Elements

DNA response elements are generally found a short distance upstream of promoters in selected genes. They are specific for selective transcription factors and thereby control the expression of genes regulated by these factors. The response elements often consist of small sequence repeats (or inverted repeats) separated by a variable number of DNA base pairs.

▶ Glucocorticoids

Domain

A domain is a part of a larger protein which has distinctive structural or functional properties.

Dopa Decarboxylase

Dopa decarboxylase is an enzyme catalyzing the synthesis of dopamine from L-dopa or of serotonin (= 5-hydroxytryptamine) from L-tryptophan. Inhibitors of this enzyme, which do not pass through the blood-brain barrier (e.g. carbidopa), reduce the toxicity and peripheral side-effects of L-dopa during treatment of Parkinson's disease.

▶ Antiparkinson Drugs

Dopamine

Dopamine is a neurotransmitter in dopaminergic nerves as well as being a precursor for the synthesis of noradrenaline.

▶ Dopamine System

Dopamine-β-hydroxylase

Dopamine hydroxylase synthesizes norepinephrine (Nor-adrenalin) from dopamine.

▶ α-Adrenergic System

Dopamine System

James N. Oak, Hubert H.M. Van Tol
Centre for Addiction & Mental Health,
University of Toronto, Toronto, Canada
james.oak@utoronto.ca;
hubert.van.tol@utoronto.ca

Synonyms

Dopamine: 3,4-dihydroxyphenylethylamine

Definition

The dopamine system constitutes the cellular and biochemical network that is involved in the synthesis, release and response to dopamine. In general this involves cells that express significant levels of ▶ tyrosine hydroxylase (TH) and limited amounts of dopamine β-hydroxylase (1). Dopamine-responsive cells express receptors specifically activated by this neurotransmitter, which are known as dopamine D1, D2, D3, D4 and D5 receptors (2, 3).

▶ Anti-parkinson Drugs
▶ Antipsychotic Drugs

▶ Neurotransmitter Transporters

Characteristics and Basic Mechanisms

Anatomy and Function

Dopamine is one of the main neurotransmitters in the central nervous system (CNS), but has also been reported to play a role in the periphery. In the CNS, dopamine-synthesizing neurons have been found in a number of discreet cell groups in the mid- and forebrain, designated as A8-A10 (mid brain areas), A11-A15 (hypothalamic areas), A16 (olfactory bulb) and A17 (retina). The main dopaminergic neurons are found in the substantia nigra pars compacta and in the ventral tegmental area, which are also designated as the A9 and A10 cell groups and constitute the nigrostriatal and mesocortical/mesolimbic systems, respectively.

The nigrostriatal system is predominantly involved in motor control, which is particularly evident in ▶ Parkinson's disease (PD), where a progressive loss of these neurons results in loss of motor function. In the early stages of the disorder, the motor impairment can be reversed by the administration of the dopamine precursor ▶ L-DOPA (L-3,4-dihydroxyphenylalanine), which bypasses the need for TH in dopamine synthesis (1). The mesocortical and mesolimbic systems play important roles in reward, emotion and cognition. This is exemplified by the addictive properties of dopamine stimulants, such as cocaine and amphetamine, as well as the therapeutic properties of drugs that block the D2 class of dopamine receptors, which control the psychotic symptoms of ▶ schizophrenia (see below). Dopaminergic hypothalamic neurons in the arcuate nucleus (A12) and A14 cell groups form the tuberoinfundibular system. These neurons project to the median eminence and control the release of prolactin through the hypophysial portal system. More dorsally located dopamine neurons in the hypothalamus (A11, A13) project to autonomic areas of the lower brain stem and preganglionic sympathetic neurons of the spinal cord. Dopamine in the retina has been found in the amacrine and interplexiform cells, and is involved in light and dark adaptation.

In the periphery, potential physiological roles of dopamine are less well established. The main

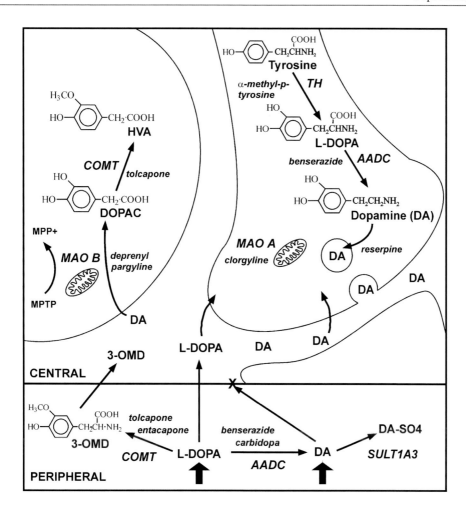

Fig. 1 Dopamine synthesis and metabolism in humans. The enzyme tyrosine hydroxylase (TH) catalyzes the formation of L-DOPA from tyrosine in presynaptic catecholaminergic neurons. L-DOPA (L-3,4-dihydroxyphenylalanine) is converted to dopamine by AADC (aromatic amino acid decarboxylase) and taken up by vesicles through the vesicular monoamine transporter (VMAT). After the release of vesicular dopamine into the synapse, signaling is terminated by the reuptake of dopamine into the presynaptic terminal by the dopamine transporter (DAT). Dopamine that leaves the synapse is primarily inactivated by the sequential action of monoamine oxidase (MAO) B and catecholamine-O-methyl transferase (COMT), which catalyze the formation of DOPAC (3,4-dihydroxyphenylacetic acid) and HVA (homovanillic acid), respectively. MAO B also catalyzes the formation of the neurotoxin MPP$^+$ from MPTP. Although MAO A can also oxidize dopamine, it does not appear to carry out this role in humans. In the periphery, dietary dopamine is primarily inactivated by the action of the phenyl sulfotransferase SULT1A3. Dopamine sulfate (DA-SO4) is the predominant form of dopamine in human plasma. In Parkinson's disease patients, L-DOPA treatment results in a large increase in peripheral dopamine metabolites such as DA-SO4 and 3-OMD (3-O-methyldopa). Drugs such as carbidopa, benserazide, tolcapone and entacapone are used clinically to increase the brain availability of L-DOPA. The selective MAO B inhibitor deprenyl is used to delay the progression of PD symptoms and enhance the effectiveness of L-DOPA therapy.

roles for peripheral dopamine appear in the control of blood pressure. Dopamine affects vasodilation by sympathetic and renal mechanisms involving hemodynamic and direct effects on the nephron as well as effects on renin secretion. Furthermore, dopamine can modulate the secretion of aldosterone from the adrenals. Peripheral dopamine is also postulated to function in the gastrointestinal system. In this respect, it is important to note the antiemetic effects of the peripheral D2 class blockers, such as domperidone. These drugs presumably act via interaction with receptors in the chemoreceptor trigger zone. The origin of peripheral dopamine is not entirely resolved. Most of the dopamine in the circulation is in an inactivated form conjugated to sulphate or glucuronide. Origins of peripheral dopamine are thought to be from the sympathetic neurons, mesenteric organs and adrenals.

Genetic disruption of dopamine synthesis in mice lacking TH shows that dopamine is not essential for development. However, dopamine deficient mice do not survive long after weaning unless treated with L-DOPA. These mice display severe aphagia and adipsia and loss of motor function. While these mice have a major reduction in dopamine levels some residual dopamine can be detected that is generated through the action of tyrosinases.

Dopamine Synthesis and Metabolism
The rate-limiting step in dopamine biosynthesis is the conversion of L-tyrosine to L-DOPA by the enzyme tyrosine hydroxylase (TH) (1). TH is expressed in catacholaminergic neurons in the brain, sympathetic ganglia and adrenal medulla. The monoxygenase activity of TH is dependent on the co-factor tetrahydropterin (BH4), and nigrostriatal neurons are particularly sensitive to BH4 levels. Genetic mutation in GTP cyclohydrolase I, which regulates production of BH4, is the cause of HPD (hereditary progressive dystonia). In catecholaminergic neurons, the enzyme aromatic amino acid decarboxylase (AADC) (also known as dopamine decarboxylase) catalyzes the formation of dopamine from L-DOPA. Dopamine is taken up into vesicles by the vesicular monoamine transporter (VMAT). In humans, peripheral dopamine formed from L-DOPA or absorbed intestinally is rapidly converted to inactive dopamine sulfate by the phenol sulfotransferase SULT1A3. In some species such as rats, the major form of dopamine in plasma is glucuronide conjugated (4).

The principal mechanism for terminating dopamine signalling is reuptake by the presynaptic neuron via the dopamine transporter (DAT).

Dopamine that is not taken up is metabolized by the enzymes ▶ monoamine oxidase (MAO) and ▶ catechol-O-methyl transferase (COMT) (5, 6). MAO is a FAD (flavin adenine dinucleotide)-dependent enzyme with two distinct forms, MAO A and MAO B. Both occur on the outer mitochondrial membrane but they have distinct localization and substrate specificity. MAOs are involved in inactivating neuroactive amines in the brain and periphery as well as detoxification of xenobiotics. Low levels of MAO A have been observed in dopaminergic neurons. However, dopamine oxidation in humans occurs primarily through MAO B, which is located in serotonergic neurons and glial cells. The distinction between the sites of dopamine biosynthesis and MAO B expression suggests that its role is to prevent dopamine from affecting non-dopaminergic neurons. MAO A is selectively inhibited by clorgyline and moclobemide while MAO B is blocked by the reversible inhibitor deprenyl. Deprenyl also protects nigrostriatal neurons from the PD-like effect of the drug MPTP (1-methyl-4-phenyl-1,2,3,6-tertrahydropyridine). MAO B activity is required to catalyze the formation of neurotoxic MPP^+ (1-methyl-4-phenylpyridinium ion), which is selectively taken up by nigrostriatal neurons resulting in Parkinsonism. MAO B activity increases with aging, and deprenyl has been shown to delay the progression of PD, although its precise mechanism of action is currently unknown.

MAO converts dopamine to DOPAC (3,4-dihydroxyphenylacetic acid), which can be further metabolized by COMT to form HVA (homovanillic acid). HVA is the main product of dopamine metabolism and the principal dopamine metabolite in urine. Increased neuronal dopaminergic activity is associated with increases in plasma concentrations of DOPAC and HVA. COMT preferentially methylates dopamine at the 3'-hydroxyl position and utilizes S-adenosyl-L-methionine as a methyl group donor. COMT is expressed widely in the periphery and in glial cells. In PD, COMT has been targeted since it can convert L-DOPA to inactive 3-OMD (3-O-methyl-dopa). In the presence of an AADC inhibitor such as carbidopa, 3-OMD is the major metabolite of L-DOPA treatment.

Dopamine Receptors

To date, 5 different dopamine receptors have been identified in and cloned from mammalian organisms (2, 3). These are classified as dopamine D1 (D1a), D5(D1b), D2, D3 and D4 receptors. The genes for the D1 and D5 receptors have 2 exons and are intronless in the coding sequence, while the D2, D3 and D4 receptors have eight, six and four exons, respectively. Through alternative splicing of the sixth exon (fifth in coding sequence) the human D2 receptor gene can generate two forms of the receptor, which are called D2long (D2L, D2(443)) and D2short(D2S, D2(414)). The dopamine receptors belong to the superfamily of ▶ G protein-coupled receptors (GPCR). Most structural data on dopamine receptors has been derived from mutagenesis studies, by analogy with the structure of other catecholamine receptors and from structural information on the protoypic class I GPCR, rhodopsin. Critical amino acid residues for dopamine binding and receptor activation are an aspartate in transmembrane domain three, which serves as counterion for the primary amine of dopamine, and the two serine residues in transmembrane domain five, which are involved in hydrogen bonding with the hydroxyl groups of the catechol ring. Dopamine has access to these residues through a hydrophilic pocket that is presumably formed through the counter-clockwise orientation of the transmembrane domains. To date there are no crystallographic data on the dopamine receptors. As with other GPCR, it has been shown that dopamine receptors, particularly D2 receptors, can form homo- and hetero-oligomeric structures. Whether the receptor exists as monomeric or oligomeric form *in vivo*, or whether this is regulated in a functionally dynamic fashion is still unknown.

Functionally, the D1-like receptors (D1, D5) are coupled to the G protein Gαs and thus can stimulate adenylyl cyclase. The D2-like receptors (D2, D3 and D4) couple to pertussis toxin sensitive ▶ G proteins (Gαi/o), and consequently inhibit adenylyl cyclase activity. While the D1-like receptors almost exclusively signal through Gαs-mediated activation of adenylyl cyclase, the D2-like receptors have been reported to modulate the activity of a plethora of signalling molecules and pathways. Many of these actions are mediated through the Gβγ subunit. Some of these molecules and pathways include the calcium channels, potassium channels, sodium-hydrogen exchanger, arachidonic acid release and mitogen-activated protein kinase pathways.

Direct interactions of dopamine receptors with signalling, regulatory and structural molecules have also been reported. This includes the interaction of D1 receptors with calcyon, D5 receptors with GABAa channel subunits, D2 receptors with spinophilin and actin-binding protein (ABP-280) and D2-like receptors with SH3 domain-containing proteins. Dopamine receptors may be substrates for GPCR kinases (GRK) and arrestins, regulating the activity of the receptors through GRK-mediated phosphorylation and subsequent increased affinity for arrestins. Repeated and/or extended activation of many GPCRs, including dopamine receptors, results in reduced responsiveness. This desensitization process is mediated by the association of arrestin to GPCR. Regulation of dopamine receptors by GRK and arrestins is shown for D1 and D2 receptors, but not yet extensively studied. Most of the functional activities have been examined *in vitro* and in heterologous expression systems using recombinant receptors. The particular use of any signalling pathway/molecule *in vivo* is largely dependent on the cellular phenotype of these cells.

Dopamine receptors are widely expressed in the brain. The main areas of D1 receptor expression are the caudate nucleus, putamen and accumbens, with lower levels in the neocortex, hippocampus and amygdala. The D5 receptor is expressed at very low levels in the brain, predominantly in limbic areas. The D2 receptor is also expressed highly in the caudate nucleus, putamen, accumbens and islands of Calleja. D2 receptor levels in the neocortex, amygdala and hippocampus are in the same order of magnitude as D1 receptor levels. Expression of the D2 receptor in the dopamine neurons of the substantia nigra and ventral tegmental indicate that it serves as a so-called dopamine autoreceptor. Unlike the D1 receptor, the D2 receptor is expressed in the pituitary gland, most notably in the mammotrophic cells of the anterior pituitary. It has been reported that the alternatively spliced short form (D2S) is preferentially expressed in the dopaminergic neurons of the substantia nigra, while the long isoform (D2L) is expressed in postsynaptic areas. The

D

D3 receptor is expressed at intermediate levels in brain, most notably in the shell region of the accumbens and Islands of Calleja, and at lower levels in dopaminergic neurons. The D4 receptors are widely expressed through the brain at intermediate to low levels. D4 receptor expression has been observed in the retina, neocortex, hippocampus and amygdala.

Clearly, the highest levels of expression of D1 and D2 receptors are seen in the striatum. The levels of expression are at least one order of magnitude higher than in any other brain region or for any of the other receptors. The D1 and D2 receptors are expressed in the medium spiny neurons of this region. The majority of these receptors are not co-localized in this region and form, respectively, the so-called direct and indirect pathways to the output neurons of the basal ganglia. In cortical areas, dopamine receptors are found in the pyramidal neurons and interneurons. D2 receptors have also been found in cortical astroglia. The dopamine receptors are found in the terminal fields of dopaminergic projections and a significant proportion of dopamine-mediated modulation is via "volume-control".

In the periphery, dopamine receptor levels are generally lower than those observed in brain, particularly in comparison to striatal dopamine receptor levels. Due to these low levels, knowledge of receptor distribution in the periphery is not yet comprehensive. Nevertheless, D1-like receptors have been reported in the parathyroid gland and in the tubular cells of the kidney. D2-like dopamine receptors have also been observed in the kidney. In addition, dopamine D2 and D4 receptors have been found in the adrenal cortex, where they modulate aldosterone secretion. The dopamine D4 receptor has been detected at relatively high levels in the cardiac atrium. Furthermore, D1- and D2-like receptors have been reported in various arterial beds (including renal, coronary, pulmonary, and cerebral arteries), the carotid body, sympathetic neurons and the gastrointestinal tract.

The physiological roles of the different dopamine receptors in the CNS have been investigated by pharmacologic and genetic means. Pharmacologically, D1 and D5 receptors cannot be distinguished. However, D1-like receptor blockade can induce catalepsy, while mice in which the D1 receptors are genetically ablated display only minor motor control problems. However pharmacological and genetic evidence suggests a role for D1 receptors in mediating the action of psychostimulants. D5-deficient mice have only been generated recently and no major phenotypes have yet been reported.

Drugs that block D2 receptors and D2 receptor-deficient mice have both demonstrated that these receptors have a major role in motor control, reward mechanisms and endocrine control. Clinical pharmacological evidence indicates that the majority of antipsychotic medications mediate their effects through this receptor. While there are several D3 receptor preferring ligands, no truly selective ligands for this receptor have been identified to date. Nevertheless, pharmacological and genetic studies do not indicate a major role for this receptor in motor control, although a possible role in the response to psychostimulants is emerging. Similarly, the D4 receptor appears to play no major role in motor control. However, pharmacological evidence combined with the use of mice deficient for D4 receptors indicate that D4 receptors are involved in the response to psychostimulants and novel stimuli. Human genetic studies have provided evidence that the D3 receptor gene is a factor in the development of neuroleptic-induced tardive dyskinesia, while D4 receptors may be a genetic factor contributing to the development attention deficit hyperactivity disorder (ADHD). D1 and D3-deficient mice develop hypertension, indicating a role for dopamine receptors in blood pressure control.

Pharmacology, Drugs and Clinical Uses

The dopamine D1-like receptor family has preferential affinity for ligands of the benzazepine class. Currently, there are no ▸ antagonists or agonists that can distinguish between D1 and D5 receptors. However, the antagonist SCH23390 and agonist SKF38393 are selective for the D1-class of receptors, although no major clinical applications for D1 receptor-selective ligands have been identified.

The antipsychotic activity of ▸ neuroleptics (D2-like receptor antagonists) has led to the development of many different ligands for the D2 receptor. These drugs are used to control the psychosis that is seen in schizophrenia, as well as Huntington's disease and Alzheimer's disease. The major drug classes are the phenothiazines, butyrophenones and benzamides, of which chlorpromazine, haloperidol and sulpiride are examples frequently used in the clinic. Many of the so-called classic neuroleptics display an increased propensity for motor side effects (Parkinsonian-like effects), particularly when used at too high doses (over 80% D2 receptor occupancy). Atypical ▸ antipsychotics, like clozapine, risperidone and olanzapine, display a limited propensity for motor side effects. These drugs have a more complex pharmacological profile that includes antagonism of 5HT, muscarinic and α-adrenergic receptors, as well as D2 receptor block. Most of the common antipsychotics also block the D3 and D4 receptors, but the antipsychotics raclopride and sulpiride have a poor affinity for D4 receptors. Selective ligands for D3 and D4 receptors have been developed, but have no clinical use thus far. D2-like receptor blockers that cannot cross the blood-brain barrier, like domperidone, are frequently used as antiemetic/prokinetic to combat nausea and dyspepsia.

Dopamine D2-like receptor ▸ agonists include quinpirole, bromocryptine and pergolide. Selective agonists, like bromocryptine, are used in the control of prolactinomas and its associated hyperprolactinaemia. Dopamine agonists like pergolide are used in the treatment of PD. Because of their vasodilatory and renal effects, dopamine receptor agonists, including dopamine itself, have been used in the treatment of heart failure.

The dopamine precursor L-DOPA (levodopa) is commonly used in th treatment of the symptoms of PD. L-DOPA can be absorbed in the intestinal tract and transported across the blood-brain barrier by the large neutral amino acid (LNAA) transport system, where it taken up by dopaminergic neurons and converted into dopamine by the activity of TH. In PD treatment, peripheral AADC can be blocked by carbidopa or benserazide to increase the amount of L-DOPA reaching the brain. Selective MAO B inhibitors like deprenyl (selegiline) have also been effectivly used with L-DOPA therapy to reduce the metabolism of dopamine. Recently, potent and selective nitro-catechol-type COMT inhibitors such as entacapone and tolcapone have been shown to be clinically effective in improving the bioavailability of L-DOPA and potentiating its effectiveness in the treatment of PD.

References

1. Nagatsu T, Stjärne, L (1998) Catecholamine synthesis and release. Adv. Pharmacol. 42:1–14
2. Schwartz J-C, Carlsson A, Caron M, Civelli O, Kebabian JW, Langer SZ, Scatton B, Sedvall G, Seeman P, Sokoloff P, Spano PF, Van Tol HHM (2000) Dopamine Receptors. In: The IUPHAR Compendium of Receptor Characterization and Classification 2000, Second Edition, 171–181
3. Emilien G, Maloteaux J-M, Geurts M, Hoogenberg K, Cragg S (1999) Dopamine receptors – Physiological understanding to therapeutic intervention potential. Pharmacol. Ther. 84:133–156
4. Kopin IJ (1985) Catecholamine metabolism: Basic aspects and clinical significance. Pharmacol. Rev. 37 (4):333–364
5. Männistö PT, Kaakkola S (2000) Cetechol-O-methyltransferase (COMT): Biochemistry, molecular biology, pharmacology, and clinical efficacy of the new selective COMT inhibitors. Pharmacol. Rev. 51(4):593–628
6. Shih JC, Chen K, Ridd MJ (1999) Monoamine oxidase: From genes to behavior. Annu. Rev. Neurosci. 22:197–217

Dose-response Curves

▸ Drug-Receptor Interaction

Double Stranded (ds) RNA

Double stranded (ds) RNA is not a constituent of normal cells but is produced during replication of many RNA and DNA viruses either as an obligatory intermediate or as a side product. As a foreign molecule, double stranded RNA induces the secretion of interferon (IFN) from lymphocytes, neutrophils and fibroblasts.

▸ Interferons

Drug Addiction/Dependence

RAINER SPANAGEL
Central Institute of Mental Health, Mannheim, Germany
spanagel@zi-mannheim.de

Definition

Drug addiction is defined as a syndrome in which drug use (e.g. psychostimulants, opiates, alcohol) pervades all life activities of the user. Life becomes governed by the drug and the addicted patient can lose social compatibility (e.g. loss of partner and friends, loss of job, crime). Behavioural characteristics of this syndrome are compulsive drug use, ► craving and chronic relapses that can occur even after years of abstinence.

Drug addiction is a pathological behavioural syndrome that has to be strictly separated from ► physical dependence. An individual can be physically dependent on a drug without being addicted to it and vice versa. Transient neuroadaptive processes underlie physical dependence and ► tolerance to a drug, whereas persistent changes within specific neuronal systems underlie addictive behaviour.

- ► Ethanol
- ► Psychostimulants
- ► Psychotomimetic Drugs
- ► Tolerance and Desensitization

Basic Mechanisms

1. Acute Drug Action/ Drug Reinforcement and the Mesolimbic Dopamine System

The ► mesolimbic system is thought to serve as a final common neural pathway for mediating drug reinforcement and reward processes (1). Drugs of abuse have different primary pharmacological targets (e.g. monoamine transporters, opioid receptors, cannabinoid receptors) but ultamitely they all activate dopamine neurons. Although drug-induced activation of mesolimbic dopamine neurons has an important function in the acquisition of behaviour reinforced by drug stimuli, the subjective rewarding actions of drugs of abuse are more likely to be mediated via activation of opioidergic systems. Thus a variety of drugs of abuse including alcohol and psychostimulants stimulate endorphin release in the nucleus accumbens (2).

Psychostimulants. Both d-amphetamine and cocaine elevate extracellular dopamine concentrations in the terminal region of midbrain dopamine neurons, especially in the nucleus accumbens. Microdialysis experiments examining the dopaminergic response to cocaine in self-administering rats with high-time resolution demonstrate that responses to cocaine are regulated by changes in extracellular dopamine levels in the nucleus accumbens. Since cocaine-induced increases in extracellular dopamine concentrations are due to the blockade of presynaptic dopamine transporters (DAT), disruption of DAT should attenuate the reinforcing effects of cocaine; however, DAT knockout mice acquire self-administration of cocaine. Thus, the reinforcing actions of cocaine do not depend solely on cocaine-induced increases in synaptic dopamine. It has been found that serotonin transporters (SERT) are also involved in acute reinforcement processes of cocaine.

Opioids. *In vivo* microdialysis data demonstrate that acute systemic or intracerebroventricular administration of μ- or δ-opioid receptor agonists increase dopamine release in the nucleus accumbens. Opioid agonists increase extracellular dopamine levels within the nucleus accumbens by inhibiting GABA interneurons in the ventral tegmental area. Activation of μ-opioid receptors on GABAergic interneurons hyperpolarizes these interneurons and concomitantly inhibits dopamine cell firing. These inhibitory actions of opioid receptor agonists are restricted to the ventral tegmental area since direct application of μ-opioid receptor agonists into the midbrain increases mesolimbic dopamine activity whereas intra-nucleus accumbens infusions do not alter extracellular dopamine levels in this structure. Opiate reward as measured by the ► conditioned place preference method depends on midbrain dopamine mechanisms. Microinjections of opioid receptor agonists into the ventral tegmental area, but not nucleus accumbens, induce conditioned place preference.

Alcohol. Alcohol given intravenously increases firing of dopamine neurons in the ventral tegmental area, and acute administration of alcohol results in preferential release of dopamine from the nucleus accumbens shell region. Similar to opioid-induced stimulation of dopamine release, alcohol is thought to decrease the activity of GABAergic neurons in the ventral tegmental area which leads to a inhibition of mesolimbic dopamine neurons. However, alcohol might also have some local effects in the nucleus accumbens. Indeed, the activation of dopamine neurons by ethanol may involve an interaction with endogenous opioids in the ventral tegmental area since the suppression of alcohol intake by non-selective opioid receptor antagonists has been linked to interference by these agents with the dopamine-stimulatory actions of ethanol. Rats will self-administer ethanol directly into the ventral tegmental cell body region of mesolimbic dopamine neurons, and both dopamine D1 and D2 antagonists administered either systemically or locally into the nucleus accumbens decrease home cage drinking and operant responding for alcohol showing that alcohol reinforcement depends on the mesolimbic system.

2. Molecular Mechanisms of Physical Dependence
Chronic administration of opiates and alcohol leads to physical dependence; a phenomenon which is only weakly expressed following chronic administration of psychostimulants. Physical dependence results from neuroadaptive intracellular changes to an altered pharmacological state. Abstinence from chronic opiate or alcohol use leads to a variety of physiological and psychological withdrawal symptoms based on these adaptations of the neuronal system.

Opioids. The opiate withdrawal symptoms in humans and experimental animals are generally the same: Elevation of temperature and blood pressure, alteration of pulse rate, restlessness, diarrhoea, weight loss, anxiety and depression. Most of the physiological aspects of opiate withdrawal are based upon an over-excitability of the noradrenergic system. The locus coeruleus is the major noradrenergic nucleus in the brain and is thought to be involved in physical dependence. Chronic opiate exposure results in an up-regulation of the cAMP system. This up-regulated or "hypertrophied" cAMP system in the locus coeruleus and other brain stem nuclei is a compensatory, homeostatic response to the inhibition from chronic opiate treatment. cAMP up-regulation results in the activation of the transcription factor cAMP response binding element (CREB). The up-regulated cAMP system has been shown to contribute to the increase in the electrical excitability of locus coeruleus neurones associated with opiate withdrawal, and transgenic mice deficient in CREB exhibit attenuated withdrawal signs compared to wild-type mice.

Alcohol. Chronic administration of ethanol leads to a variety of adaptive responses within the central nervous system that become uncovered during withdrawal. Especially, hyperexcitability and susceptibility to seizures during withdrawal are thought to be due to adaptive responses within the glutamatergic system in the hippocampus. Assuming that acute ethanol induces a reduction in glutamate release, adaptive responses such as changes in the number and affinity of synaptic glutamate receptors and glutamate transporters occur in order to keep physiological homeostasis of the glutamatergic system (3). During withdrawal these adaptive responses become visible. Indeed, microdialysis studies within the nucleus accumbens and the hippocampus, which were performed in alcohol-dependent rats after withdrawal, show that glutamate levels increase 2–3 fold approximately 6 h after withdrawal, which is the time associated with the commencement of seizures and hyperexciatbility, and reach a peak at 12 h then decline to baseline values at 24 to 36 h from the interruption of the chronic alcohol treatment. It is important to note that these changes in glutamate are observed in occurrence with overt physical withdrawal signs.

3. Molecular Mechanisms of Addictive Behaviour
Chronic drug use and abuse leads to ▶ sensitization processes within the mesolimbic system. In the case of psychostimulants and opioids, *in vivo* measurements of extracellular dopamine levels provide direct evidence that these drugs, when administered under an intermittent injection schedule, can lead to a more pronounced increase in dopamine levels as compared

to acute administration of these drugs. A major hypothesis postulates that the activation of a sensitized dopaminergic system by conditioned stimuli is directly involved in drug craving. Changes within the mesolimbic dopaminergic system and behavioural abnormalities that characterize drug addiction are long lasting, and it is thought that regulation of neural gene expression is involved in the process by which drugs of abuse cause a state of addiction. The transcription factor ΔFosB represents one mechanism by which drugs of abuse can produce relatively stable changes in the brain that contribute to drug-induced sensitization processes and ▶ reinstatement of drug-seeking behaviour in mice and rats (4). ΔFosB, a member of the Fos family of transcription factors, accumulates within a subset of neurons of the nucleus accumbens after repeated administration of many kinds of drugs of abuse. Thus, ΔFosB can be seen as a "molecular switch" that gradually converts acute drug responses into relatively stable adaptations that may contribute to the long-term neural and behavioural changes underlying addiction.

Psychostimulants and Opioids. Dopaminergic mechanisms also play a role in relapse as measured by reinstatement of cocaine and heroin self-administration after extinction. Selective dopamine receptor antagonists attenuate reinstatement of heroin self-administration induced by heroin priming injections but failed to attenuate stress-induced reinstatement of heroin self-administration. This finding argues against a role of dopamine in stress-associated heroin-seeking behaviour and shows that different molecular pathways are involved in relapse behaviour.

Alcohol. The neurobiological and molecular basis of alcohol craving and relapse is still not well understood, however, preclinical as well as clinical data strongly imply that craving and relapse for alcohol can be induced through different mechanisms. A first pathway may induce alcohol craving and relapse due to the mood enhancing, positive reinforcing effects of alcohol consumption. This pathway seems to involve opioidergic and dopaminergic systems in the ventral striatum. The role of the dopaminergic system may lie in the direction of attention towards reward-indicating stimuli, while the induction of euphoria and posi-

tive mood states may be mediated by opioidergic systems. Associative learning may, in turn, transform positive mood states and previously neutral environmental stimuli into alcohol-associated cues that acquire positive motivational salience and induce reward craving. A second and potentially independent pathway may induce alcohol craving and relapse by negative motivational states, including conditioned withdrawal and stress. This pathway seems to involve the glutamatergic system and the corticotropin releasing hormone (CRH)-system. Chronic alcohol intake leads to compensatory changes within these systems. During withdrawal and abstinence increased glutamatergic excitatory neurotransmission as well as increased CRH release leads to a state of hyperexcitability that becomes manifest as craving, anxiety and autonomic dysregulation. Moreover, cues associated with prior alcohol intake that are not followed by actual drug consumption may induce ▶ conditioned withdrawal.

Pharmacological Relevance

Treatment of drug addicts can be separated into two phases: detoxification and relapse prevention. Detoxification programs and treatment of physical withdrawal symptoms, respectively, is clinically routine for most drugs of abuse. However, pharmacological intervention programs for relapse prevention are still not very efficient.

1. Detoxification

Alcohol. Cessation of prolonged heavy alcohol abuse may be followed by alcohol withdrawal or life-threatening alcohol withdrawal delirium. Typical withdrawal symptoms are autonomic hyperactivity, increased hand tremor, insomnia and anxiety, and are treated with benzodizepines and thiamine. Alcoholism is the most common cause of thiamine deficiency and can lead in its extreme form to the ▶ Wernicke's syndrome that can be effectively treated by high doses of thiamine.

Opioids. Opiate overdose is a medical emergency that can result in respiratory and CNS depression. The opioid receptor antagonist naloxone immediately reverses cardiorespiratory depression. However, repeated naloxone administration is

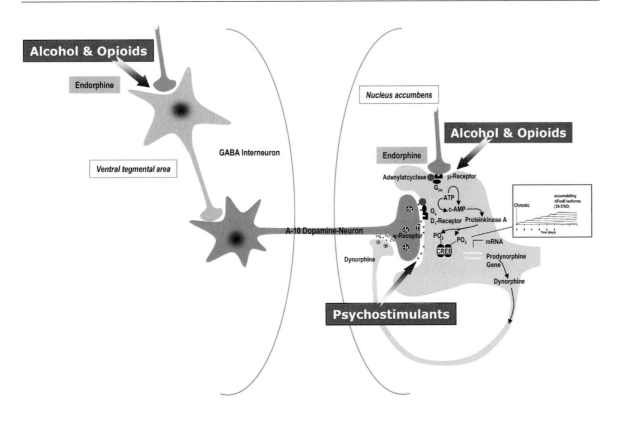

Fig. 1 Actions of drugs of abuse on dopaminergic neurons. Acute and long-lasting effects of alcohol, opioids and psychostimulants on mesolimbic dopaminergic neurons. Nicotine, cannabinoids and other drugs of abuse also affect these neurons in order to produce their reinforcing and long-lasting effects. Note that all drugs of abuse enhance either directly or indirectly dopamine release in the nucleus accumbens. Activation of neurons within the nucleus accumbens by chronic drug use leads to long-lasting changes in gene expression (e.g. pro-dynorphine gene) as indicated by accumulated ΔFosB isoforms (small inlet).

required, since the effects of naloxone last for 30 minutes, while opioid agonists can remain at potentially lethal blood levels for several hours.

2. Relapse Prevention

Alcohol. Anti-relapse compounds have recently been registered for relapse prophylaxis in weaned alcoholics in various European countries and in the United States. Acamprosate, the Ca^{2+} salt of N-acetyl-homotaurinate, interacts with the glutamatergic system in various brain regions and reduces Ca^{2+} fluxes through voltage-dependent ion channels. The opioid receptor antagonist naltrexone interferes with alcohol-induced reinforcement via blockade of opioid receptors. Ondansetron, a selective 5-HT$_3$-antagonist, shows promise for decreasing drinking and increasing abstinence rates among early onset alcoholics who respond poorly to psychosocial treatment alone. In the future low-affinity, non-competitive NMDA-receptor antagonists such as memantine are seen as a new generation of anti-relapse compounds (5).

It is important to note that only a small percentage of alcoholic patients can be effectively treated with these compounds indicating that there are different neurobiological phenotypes involved in alcoholism. Thus specific medications in combination might further enhance the effectiveness of relapse prevention as has been recently demonstrated with a naltrexone/acamprosate combination.

Opioids. Some opiate addicts might benefit from naltrexone treatment. One idea is that patients should undergo rapid opiate detoxification with naltrexone under anaesthesia which then allows further naltrexone treatment to reduce the likelihood of relapse. However, the mode of action of rapid opiate detoxification is obscure. Moreover, it can be a dangerous procedure and some studies now indicate that this procedure can induce even more severe and long-lasting withdrawal symptoms as well as no improvement in relapse rates than a regular detoxification and psychosocial relapse prevention program.

References

1. Spanagel R, Weiss F (1999) The dopamine hypothesis of reward: past and current status. Trends Neurosci 22:521–527
2. Olive MF, Koenig HN, Nannini MA, Hodge CW (2001) Stimulation of endorphin neurotransmission in the nucleus accumbens by ethanol, cocaine, and amphetamine. J Neurosci 21:1–5
3. Tsai GE, JT Coyle (1998) The role of glutamatergic neurotransmission in the pathophysiology of alcoholism. Annu Rev Med 49:173–184
4. Nestler EJ, Barrot M, Self D (2001) ΔFosB: A sustained molecular switch for addiction. Proc Natl Acad Sci USA 98:11042–11046
5. Spanagel R, Zieglgänsberger W (1997) Anti-craving compounds: new pharmacological tools to study addictive processes. Trends Pharmacol Sci 18:54–59

Drug Discovery

Drug discovery is the identification and optimization of compounds for further development of drugs.

▶ High-throughput Screening

Drug Interactions

KIYOMI ITO AND YUICHI SUGIYAMA
Kitasato University, Tokyo; University of Tokyo, Tokyo; Japan
itok@pharm.kitasato-u.ac.jp,
sugiyama@mol.f.u-tokyo.ac.jp

Synonyms

Drug-drug interaction, pharmacokinetic and/or pharmacodynamic interaction, pharmacokinetic and/or pharmacodynamic consequence of multiple drug therapy.

Definition

Drug interactions can occur when two drugs are administered together, one affecting the pharmacological and/or adverse effects of the other. One or both of the drugs could be affected leading to either clinically beneficial interactions (e.g. increased pharmacological effects or reduced adverse effects) or harmful interactions (e.g. reduced pharmacological effects or increased adverse effects).

▶ Drug-Receptor Interaction
▶ Pharmacokinetics

Basic Mechanisms

Pharmacokinetic Interactions
Interactions resulting from a change in the amount of drug reaching the site of action are called ▶ pharmacokinetic interactions (Fig. 1). A co-administered drug can affect any of the processes of absorption, distribution, metabolism, and excretion of the original drug, which are determinants of its pharmacokinetic profile (1–3).

Drug Interactions During Absorption

Changes in Gastrointestinal pH. Following oral administration, drug molecules in their lipophilic non-ionic form are more easily absorbed by ▶ simple diffusion through the gastrointestinal mucosa. Therefore, the alteration in the fraction of

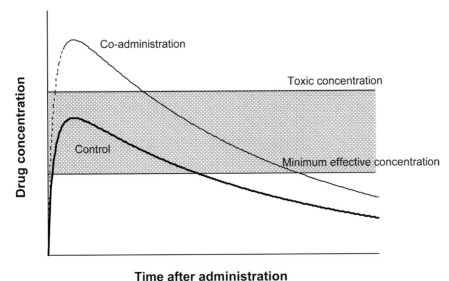

Fig. 1 Increase in drug concentration caused by pharmacokinetic interactions. Shadow represents the therapeutic range.

D

non-ionic form caused by gastrointestinal pH changes due to co-administered drugs, such as antiacids, can lead to a change in drug absorption.

Adsorption, Chelation and Complex Formation. Charcoal, which is used as a detoxicant in overdosage etc., is able to adsorb drugs, thereby causing a reduction in drug absorption. Absorption of new quinolone antibiotics is reduced by forming an insoluble chelate with secondary or tertiary cations, such as Mg^{2+} or Al^{3+}, found in many antiacids. The cholesterol lowering agent, cholestyramine, which is an anion-exchange resin, reduces the absorption of drugs like warfarin by binding to them.

Changes in Gastrointestinal Motility. Because the majority of orally administered drugs are absorbed mainly from the upper part of the small intestine, an alteration in ▶ gastric emptying rate caused by co-administered drugs can lead to alterations in drug absorption. For example, anticholinergic drugs such as propantheline delay gastric emptying by reducing gastrointestinal motility, causing the reduced absorption rate of acetaminophen etc., while metoclopramide has the opposite effect.

Effects on Transporters. ▶ P-glycoprotein (P-gp) works as a transporter at the intestinal mucosa to pump drugs out into the lumen. Absorption of P-

gp substrates, such as digoxin, cyclosporine etc., can be increased by inhibitors of P-gp and reduced by inducers.

Drug Interactions During Distribution

Displacement from Plasma Protein Binding Sites. In general, only the free molecules which are not bound to plasma proteins, such as albumin and α_1-acid glycoprotein, cross biological membranes and exhibit pharmacological effects. Therefore, displacement from plasma protein binding sites by co-administered drugs can cause an increase in the unbound fraction of the original drug in plasma, possibly leading to increased pharmacological effects.

Effects on Transporters. The tissue distribution of substrates of P-gp, which regulates the uptake of drugs into the brain, tumor cells etc., and those of other transporters involved in the ▶ active transport into or out of tissues can be affected by the co-administration of inhibitors and/or inducers of such transporters.

Drug Interactions During Metabolism

Enzyme Inhibition. Following concurrent administration of two drugs, especially when they are metabolized by the same enzyme in the liver or small intestine, the metabolism of one or both

Tab. 1 Examples of clinically important drug interactions due to enzyme inhibition.

Substrate	Inhibitor	Inhibited enzyme	Possible clinical outcome
Theophylline	Ciprofloxacin, Fluvoxamine etc.	CYP1A2	Theophylline toxicity
Phenytoin	Chloramphenicol, Isoniazid etc.	CYP2C9, CYP2C19	Phenytoin intoxication
Tolbutamide	Sulfaphenazole	CYP2C9	Hypoglycaemia
Warfarin	Fluconazole, Metronidazole etc.	CYP2C9	Haemorrhage
Astemizole, Terfenadine	Ketoconazole, Erythromycin etc.	CYP3A4	Ventricular Arrhythmia
Cyclosporine, Tacrolimus	Ketoconazole, Erythromycin etc.	CYP3A4	Cyclosporine/tacrolimus toxicity
Lovastatin, Simvastatin	Ketoconazole, Erythromycin etc.	CYP3A4	Rhabdomyolysis
Azathioprine, Mercaptopurine	Allopurinol	Xanthine oxidase	Azathioprine/ mercaptopurine toxicity

drugs can be inhibited, which may lead to elevated plasma concentrations of the drug(s) and increased pharmacological effects. The types of enzyme inhibition include reversible inhibition, such as ▶ competitive or noncompetitive inhibition, and irreversible inhibition, such as ▶ mechanism-based inhibition. The clinically important examples of drug interactions involving the inhibition of metabolic enzymes are listed in Table 1 (1,4).

Enzyme Induction. The co-administration of drugs that induce the metabolic enzymes in the liver or small intestine can reduce the plasma concentrations of drugs which are substrates of the enzyme, leading to reduced drug effects. For example, the plasma concentrations of many drugs that are substrates of the enzyme CYP3A4, such as cyclosporine, are decreased by co-administration of rifampicin, which is an inducer of CYP3A4.

Drug Interactions During Excretion

Changes in urinary pH. As in gastrointestinal absorption, the lipophillic non-ionic form of a drug is more susceptible to re-absorption from the renal tubules by simple diffusion. Therefore, re-absorption of weakly acidic drugs can be enhanced (or inhibited) by co-administration of drugs that reduce (or elevate) the urinary pH, leading to elevated (or reduced) plasma concentrations. The opposite effects are observed for weakly basic drugs.

Effects on renal tubular secretion. The co-administration of drugs that inhibit the transporters involved in renal tubular secretion can reduce the urinary excretion of drugs which are substrates of the transporter, leading to elevated plasma concentrations of the drugs. For example, probenecid increases the plasma concentration and the duration of effect of penicillin by inhibiting its renal tubular secretion. It also elevates the plasma concentration of methotrexate by the same mechanism, provoking its toxic effects.

Effects on biliary excretion. The co-administration of drugs that inhibit the transporters involved in biliary excretion can reduce the biliary excretion of drugs which are substrates of the transporter, leading to elevated plasma concentrations of the drugs.

Pharmacodynamic Interactions

▶ Pharmacodynamic interactions are drug interactions involving alterations in drug effects following co-administration of drugs, without alterations in the drug concentrations at the site of action. They include direct interactions, such as two drugs exhibiting their pharmacological effects via binding to the same receptor, and indirect interactions, in which the drug effects are affected by biochemical or physiological changes due to the co-administered drug.

Additive or ▶ Synergistic Interactions. When two drugs with similar pharmacological and/or adverse effects are administered simultaneously, an additive or synergistic increase in their effects can be observed. These include the increased sedative effects seen in the central nervous system following co-administration of alcohol and benzodiazepine hypnotics/anxiolytics and the increased risk of bleeding following co-administration of the anticoagulant, warfarin, and the non-steroidal anti-inflammatory drug, aspirin.

Antagonistic Interactions. The pharmacological and/or adverse effects of a drug can be reversed by co-administration of drugs that compete for the same receptor. For example, an opioid receptor antagonist naloxone is used to reverse the effects of opiates. Drugs acting at the same site with opposite effects also can affect each other e.g. the reduction in the anticoagulant effect of warfarin by vitamin K.

Pharmacological Relevance

Drug interactions can cause serious problems in clinical practice especially when the affected drug has the potential to be highly toxic. Furthermore, pharmacokinetic interactions are clinically important if the affected drug has a narrow therapeutic range (i.e. small difference between the minimum effective concentration and the toxic concentration; Fig. 1) and a steep concentration-response curve (i.e. significant alterations in pharmacological and/or adverse effects caused by small changes in blood concentration).

Although drug interactions involving plasma protein binding and drug metabolism are often evaluated in *in vitro* studies, the interactions observed *in vitro* are not necessarily observed *in vivo* or are clinically relevant. For example, even when the plasma unbound fraction of a drug is increased by protein binding displacement, kinetic theory (clearance concept) indicates that the steady-state plasma unbound concentration may not change because the unbound drug is subject to metabolism and excretion. Therefore, this type of drug interaction is unlikely to be clinically significant unless a high clearance drug is administered intravenously. However, a transient increase in the plasma unbound concentration can be observed under non-steady-state conditions, especially for drugs with small volumes of distribution. It should be taken into account that such a transient increase may cause some side effect of drugs.

In the case of drug interactions involving metabolic inhibition, little increase in the substrate concentration is expected when the inhibition constant (Ki) determined in *in vitro* studies using human liver samples is larger than the inhibitor concentration *in vivo*. Various approaches have been adopted using mathematical models in attempts to quantitatively predict *in vivo* drug interactions from *in vitro* data (5).

References

1. Stockley I (1991) Drug interactions, 2nd edition, Blackwell Scientific Publications, Oxford.
2. Rowland M and Tozer TN (1995) Clinical pharmacokinetics, concepts and applications, Williams & Wilkins, Baltimore.
3. Kusuhara H and Sugiyama Y (2001) Drug-drug interactions involving the membrane transport process. In: Rodrigues AD (ed) Drug-Drug Interactions. Marcel Dekker, New York, p123–188
4. Hansten PD and Horn JR (2000) The top 100 drug interactions: a guide to patient management, H&H Publications, Edmonds.
5. Ito K, Iwatsubo T, Kanamitsu S, Ueda K, Suzuki H, Sugiyama Y (1998) Prediction of pharmacokinetic alterations caused by drug-drug interactions. Pharmacol Rev 50:387–411

Drug Metabolism

The metabolism of foreign compounds (xenobiotics) often takes place in two consecutive reactions, classically referred to as phases one and two. Phase I is a functionalization of the lipophilic compound that can be used to attach a conjugate in Phase II. The conjugated product is usually sufficiently water-soluble to be excretable into the urine. The most important biotransformations of Phase I are aromatic and aliphatic hydroxylations catalyzed by cytochromes P450. Other Phase I enzymes are for example epoxide hydrolases or carboxylesterases. Typical Phase II enzymes are UDP-glucuronosyltransferases , sulfotransferases , N-acetyltransferases and methyltransferases e.g. thiopurin S-methyltransferase.

▶ P450 Mono-oxygenase System

Drug Reinforcement

In its reinforcing capacity, a drug of abuse increases the frequency of preceding responses, and accordingly is called a reinforcer. All drugs of abuse are primary reinforcers and lead to self-administration.

▶ Drug Addiction/Dependence

Drug-Receptor Interaction

TERRY P. KENAKIN
Receptor Biochem Glaxo Wellcome Research,
Research Triangle Park, NC, USA
tpk1348@GlaxoWellcome.com

Synonyms

Drug Receptor Theory, Quantification of Drug Effect

Definition

Mathematical models of the interaction between drugs and ▶ receptors, based on ▶ Michaelis-Menten enzyme kinetics, are utilized to create the quantitative tools currently used in receptor pharmacology to quantify drug effect in biological systems. Such tools are necessary since drugs almost always are tested in surrogate systems until they are known to be sufficiently active and safe for therapeutic use. The aim of receptor pharmacology is to define the molecular properties of ▶ affinity and ▶ intrinsic efficacy of drugs; these can be used to predict drug effect across different biological systems.

▶ Drug Interactions
▶ G-protein-coupled Receptors
▶ Tolerance and Desensitization

Basic Mechanisms

A basic premise in receptor pharmacology is that all drugs have affinity for receptors (the chemical property that unites the drug with the receptor), and some drugs have efficacy, the chemical property that causes the receptor to change its behavior toward its host cell. Drugs that have efficacy produce concentration-dependent responses in physiological systems, characterized by a concentration-response curve (also often referred to as a dose-response curve).

Drugs that produce pharmacological activation of a system are called *agonists*, those that inhibit activation of a receptor system are called *antagonists*, and those that reverse spontaneously active receptor systems (▶ Constitutive Receptor Activity) are called *inverse agonists* (Fig. 1). This latter class of drugs reduce elevated basal responses. Agonism is the observed effect of a ligand producing stimulus to a receptor. The host cellular system processes that stimulus and yields an observable response.

The common currency of drug receptor pharmacology is the dose-response curve, as it defines the relationship between concentrations of drug and the resulting effect. Dose-response curves have three basic properties with which they can be described: threshold abscissal value, slope and maximum asymptote. The location parameter of

AGONISM

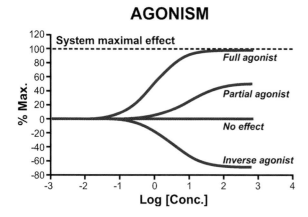

Fig. 1 Dose-response curves to drugs that have direct effects on physiological systems. A drug that produces the maximal effect capable from the system is a **full agonist.** A sub-maximal effect is produced by a **partial agonist.** Drugs may not produce directly observable effects but may be present on the receptor to produce antagonism (see Fig. 2). If a system is constitutively active and shows an actively elevated basal response, then a drug that reduces this is termed an **inverse agonist.**

the dose response characterizes drug potency; most often this is quantified as the EC_{50} or the molar concentration of drug producing half the maximal effect. Given tissue systems have maximal capabilities to return drug response. When an agonist produces a maximal response that is equal to the system maximal response it is referred to as a *full agonist* (Fig. 1). If an agonist produces a sub-maximal system response it is called a *partial agonist* (Fig. 1). While the potency of an agonist is quantified by the location parameter of the dose-response curve (EC_{50}), a reflection of (but not a direct measure of) the intrinsic efficacy of an agonist is given by its maximal response.

The inhibition of agonist response is termed antagonism. The effect that a given antagonist has on the dose-response curve to an agonist can be a clue to the mechanism of action of that antagonists' interaction with the receptor. In the presence of an antagonist, more agonist must be present in the receptor compartment to produce a response than would be necessary in the absence of the antagonist. A singular characteristic of an antagonist is its effect on the maximal capability of an

agonist to overcome the presence of the antagonist and produce the system maximal response. If enough agonist can be added to produce the agonist maximal response in the presence of the antagonist, the antagonism is referred to as surmountable antagonism (see Fig. 2). If no amount of agonist will produce the maximal response, the antagonism is referred to as insurmountable (see Fig. 2).

A basic concept in receptor pharmacology is the idea of orthosteric and allosteric interaction. Orthosteric interaction occurs when two molecules compete for a single binding domain on the receptor. With allosteric interactions two molecules each have their own binding domain on the receptor and the two interact through effects on the protein (conformational change). Thus, with orthosteric interactions only one molecule may occupy the receptor at any one instant whereas with allosteric interactions both molecules can bind to the receptor at the same time. There are implications for pharmacological activity, especially for antagonists, that arise from these two molecular mechanisms (*vide infra*).

There are certain molecular mechanisms of antagonism associated with these observed patterns on dose-response curves. Thus, ▶ competitive antagonists produce parallel shifts to the right of agonist dose-response curves with no diminution of maximal response through an orthosteric interaction of antagonist and agonist (Fig. 2A). Theoretically, there is no limit to the degree of dextral displacement a given competitive antagonist can produce on a dose-response curve. ▶ Schild analysis is used to measure the affinity of competitive antagonists. This same pattern of response also can occur with ▶ allosteric modulators (Fig. 2B) but in this case the shift of the agonist dose-response curve is limited to a maximal value defined by the molecular ▶ co-operativity factor of the antagonist. Thus, a hallmark of allosteric inhibition is that it is saturable and reaches a maximal asymptotic value. In some cases, ▶ irreversible antagonists can produce parallel shifts to the right of dose-response curves if there is a ▶ receptor reserve for the agonist (Fig. 2C). This latter mechanism can be detected with increasing concentrations of irreversible antagonist since these eventually cause depression of the maximal response.

ANTAGONISM

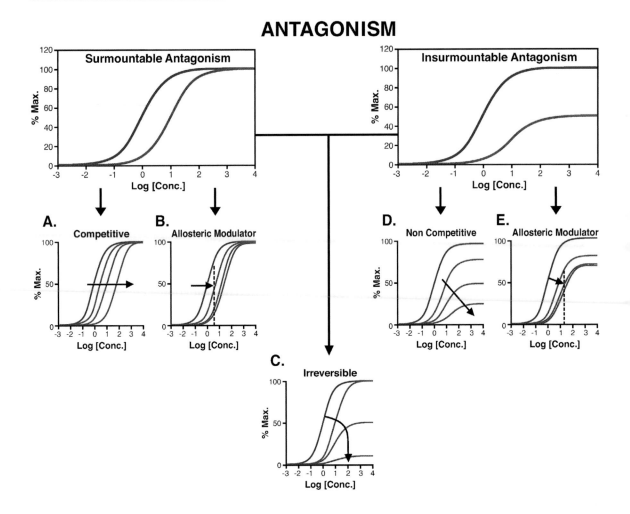

Fig. 2 Various patterns of antagonism of drug effect. Antagonism is classified according to effects on the dose-response curve to the agonist (blue lines). Two general classifications are surmountable antagonism (maximal response to the agonist retained-top left panel) or non-surmountable antagonism (depressed maximal response to the agonist-top right panel). These general patterns can be the result of different molecular mechanisms. **A)** Orthosteric competition between the agonist and antagonist for the same binding site on the receptor. **B)** Binding of an allosteric modulator to its own binding site to modify the affinity or efficacy of the agonist in a saturable manner. **C)** Irreversible blockade of receptors in a system with receptor reserve (parallel shift to the right followed by depression of the maximal response at higher concentrations of antagonist). **D)** Blockade of receptor function or access of agonist to the receptor either orthosterically or allosterically in a system with little receptor reserve for the agonist. **E)** Saturable allosteric modulation of receptor function by an antagonist in a system with little receptor reserve for the agonist.

In cases where insurmountable antagonism is observed, this can be evidence of ▶ non-competitive antagonism. This can result from an inhibiiton of receptor function (either orthosteric or allosteric) or be due to antagonist-mediated modification of receptor reactivity to the agonist (Fig. 2E). The **method of Gaddum** (▶ Gaddum, Method of) is used to measure the affinity of non-competitive antagonists for receptors. Parenthetically, similar effects on dose-response curves are produced by irreversible antagonists when there is no receptor reserve for the agonist.

Pharmacological Relevance

An important tenet of receptor pharmacology states that the molecular properties of a drug, namely affinity and intrinsic efficacy, are interpreted and reflected by physiological systems and that this process *controls* what is observed as drug effect. For example, a physiological system requires a certain sensitivity to return response from stimulation by a weak agonist, i.e. the receptor coupling of that system must be of sufficient efficiency to amplify the stimulus into an obervable response. When the same weak agonist is tested in a physiological system of lower sensitivity, it might be an antagonist. Thus, it can be seen that the monikers of agonist and antagonist can be system dependent and unreliable as molecular labels for drugs. In the same manner that a system must be of sufficient sensitivity to detect efficacy and return response, it also can be overloaded by a strong stimulus. When this occurs, the system returns the system maximal response and the agonist demonstrates full agonism. A series of agonists of differing intrinsic efficacy may all overload a given system and all return the same (system) maximal response (all be full agonists); this does not imply that these agonists are of equal efficacy but only that the system was unable to discern different efficacies beyond a certain level. For this reason, the labels of full and partial agonist are also system dependent and not useful for molecular characterization of drugs.

Since drugs are tested in many surrogate systems, it is necessary to develop methods to quantify drug effect in a system-independent manner. Absolute scales are not practical, or in some cases, even possible, in this process. As discussed previously, while an absolute potency for an agonist can be determined by the EC_{50}, the magnitude of this value depends on the sensitivity of the particular measuring system and thus it cannot be extrapolated to other systems. Rather, the relative potency of agonists (ratios of EC_{50} values) is used to quantify agonist power to induce response. This process utilizes the null method and isolates only the intrinsic ability of the agonists to produce response at the receptor level. This allows for the resulting potency ratios to be a measure of relative agonist activity that is comparatively independent of the system in which the measurement is made. This ratio transcends the particular system in which it is measured and is applicable to all systems in which the agonists produce maximal response. Under optimal conditions, the therapeutic profile of the standard agonist will be known in humans, therefore the agonist potency ratio can be used to gauge the expected activity of the experimental agonist in the therapeutic arena.

In the case of antagonists, absolute measures of potency are theoretically possible since these are chemical terms describing the affinity of the drugs for receptor protein. However, physiological systems can also control the observed antagonism. For example, a non-competitive antagonist will produce a diminution of the maximal response to an agonist in a system where the response is linearly related to the receptor occupancy (Fig. 2D). However, if the receptors in a system are coupled with high efficiency and the agonist has high efficacy, then maximal responses may be achieved with less than maximal agonist receptor occupancy, i.e. there may be a ▶ receptor reserve for the agonist. Under these circumstances the agonist may still produce the maximal response even when the antagonist completely inactivates a portion of the receptors. When this occurs the antagonism resembles competitive antagonism at low concentrations and non-competitive antagonism at higher concentrations (resembling the profile in Fig. 2C). This would be system dependent and not necessarily indicative of the molecular mechanism of the antagonist.

Another example of where the setpoint of the physiological system can change the observed behavior of drugs is the absence of direct effects of inverse agonists in non-constitutively active receptor systems. A receptor system must be constitutively active (elevated basal response) to detect inverse agonism (Fig. 1). In non-constitutively active receptor systems, inverse agonists behave as simple competitive antagonists.

In general, receptor theory uses indirect mathematical models to estimate descriptors of drug effect. These descriptors still must be used with the proviso that biological systems may still modify drug effect in a system-dependent manner and thus predictions of therapeutic effect must be made with caution across different systems.

References

1. Black JW, Leff P (1983) Operational models of pharmacological agonism. Proc. Roy. Soc. Lond. B. 220:141–162
2. Colquhoun, D. (1998) Binding, gating, affinity and efficacy: The interpretation of structure-activity relationships for agonists and of the effects of mutating receptors. Br. J. Pharmacol. 125:924–947
3. Ross EM, Kenakin TP (2001) Pharmacodynamics: Mechanisms of drug action and the relationship between drug concentration and effect. In The Pharmacological Basis of Therapeutics, ed. By Hardman JG, Limbird LE, Gilman AG. 10th edition McGraw-Hill publishing Co., New York pp. 31–43

DSI

▶ Depolarization-induced Suppression of Inhibition
▶ Endocannabinoid System

DTH

▶ Delayed Type Hypersensitivity Reaction
▶ Allergy

Dyskinesias

Dyskinesias are abnormal movements, usually caused by neurological diseases or by drugs used to treat neurological (e.g., levodopa) or psychiatric diseases (e.g., neuroleptics).

▶ Anti-parkinson Drugs
▶ Antipsychotic Drugs
▶ Tardive Dyskinesia

Dyslipidemia

Dyslipidemia is change in the normal lipid concentrations in the blood. In particular, hypercholesterolemia is a major cause of increased atherogenic risk, leading to atherosclerosis and atherosclerosis-associated conditions, such as coronary heart disease, ischemic cerebrovascular disease and peripheral vascular disease. Both genetic disorders and diets enriched in saturated fat and cholesterol contribute to the elevated lipid levels in a considerable part of the population of developed countries. Hypertriglyceridemia, when severe, may cause pancreatitis. Moderately elevated levels of triglycerides are often associated with a syndrome distinguished by insulin resistance, obesity, hypertension and substantially increased risk of coronary heart disease. Hypercholesterolemia, especially, requires treatment either by diet and/or with lipid-lowering drugs (e.g. statins, anion exchange resins).

▶ Statins
▶ Anion Exchange Resins
▶ Fibrates

Dysrhythmias

▶ Antiarrhythmic Drugs

E

EC$_{50}$

The EC$_{50}$ is the concentration of a drug required to achieve a half-maximal effect.

▶ Drug-Receptor Interaction

ECaC

ECaC stands for epithelial calcium channel.

▶ Epithelial Ca^{2+} Channel 1

EC Coupling

▶ Excitation-contraction Coupling

ECE

▶ Endothelin Converting Enzyme
▶ Endothelins

Ecogenetics

Ecogenetics is the study of genetically determined inter-individual variation within one species with respect to the response to environmental chemicals or physical environmental factors.

▶ Pharmacogenetics

Ecstasy

▶ Methylenedioxymethamphetamine
▶ Psychostimulants

ED$_{50}$

The ED$_{50}$ is the dose of a drug required to achieve a half-maximal effect.

▶ Drug-Receptor Interaction

Edg Receptors

Edg receptors are a group of recently discovered G-protein coupled receptors, which mediate the action of lysophospholipids (sphingosine-1-phosphate, lysophosphatidic acid).

▶ Lysophospholipids

EEG

EEG is the abbreviation for Electroencephalogram. An EEG is the electrophysiological recording of changes in the electric potential of neurons in the brain.

Effector

Receptors induce a signal transduction process upon binding of an extracellular signal. The receptor-protein domain or receptor-linked protein whose activities are altered in order to generate the earliest signals in a signalling cascade are called effectors. Enzymes or ion channels can be receptor-controlled effectors.

▶ Transmembrane Signalling

Efficacy

Efficacy is a parameter which describes the "strength" of a single drug-receptor complex in evoking a response from the cell or tissue. The intrinsic efficacy of a drug is a proportionality constant that defines the power of the drug to induce a response.
Potency

▶ Intrinsic Efficacy
▶ Drug-Receptor Interaction

EGF

▶ Epidermal Growth Factor
▶ Growth Factors

Eicosanoids

Eicosanoids are any of the collection of oxygenated metabolites of arachidonic acid that are the products of cyclooxygenase, cytochrome P450 or lipoxygenase pathways, e.g., prostaglandins, thromboxanes, HETEs, and leukotrienes. They exert a multitude of cardiovascular and inflammatory actions immediately at the site of synthesis.

▶ Leukotrienes
▶ Prostanoids

Elastase-like Proteinases

Elastase-like proteinases are serine proteinases that recognized peptide residues with linear aliphatic side chains (alanyl, valyl, leucyl or isoleucyl residues) and that effect hydrolysis of the polypeptide chain on the carboxy-terminal side of these residues. Examples of elastase-like proteinase are: pancreatic elastase, neutrophil elastase and proteinase-3.

▶ Non-viral Proteases

Electrochemical Driving Force

The net electrochemical driving force is determined by two factors, the electrical potential difference across the cell membrane and the concentration gradient of the permeant ion across the membrane. Changing either one can change the net driving force. The membrane potential of a cell is defined as the inside potential minus the outside, i.e. the potential difference across the cell membrane. It results from the separation of charge across the cell membrane.

Electrospray Ionization Mass Spectrometry

Electrospray ionization mass spectrometry (ESI-MS) is an analytical method for mass determination of ionised molecules. It is a commonly used method for "soft" ionization of peptides and proteins in quadrupole, ion-trap, or time-of-flight mass spectrometers. The ionization is performed by application of a high voltage to a stream of liquid emitted from a capillary. The highly charged droplets are shrunk and the resulting peptide or protein ions are sampled and separated by the mass spectrometer.

▶ Proteomics

Elimination Half-life

▶ Half-life /Elimination Half-life
▶ Pharmacokinetics

Elimination of Drugs

The elimination of a drug is its removal from the body, either by chemical modification through metabolism or by removal from the body through the kidney, the gut, the lungs or the skin.

▶ Pharmacokinetics

Emesis

F. MITCHELSON
Department of Pharmacology, The University of Melbourne, Victoria, Australia
fjmitc@unimelb.edu.au

Synonyms

Vomiting

Definition

Emesis is the forceful involuntary expulsion of the stomach contents through the mouth. It is a reflex response that may be initiated by a number of stimuli.

Nausea is an unpleasant sensation of a desire to vomit or of an impending vomiting episode. When prolonged it may occur in waves and may not always be followed by vomiting.

Retching is the process of emesis but without the actual expulsion of any of the stomach contents.

▶ Dopamine System
▶ Histaminergic System
▶ Muscarinic Receptors
▶ Serotoninergic System

Basic Mechanisms

The vomiting reflex is controlled by the vomiting centre, a diffuse area in the medullary region of the brainstem. There are a number of ways to initiate the reflex (Fig. 1), including stimulation of sensory receptors in the alimentary canal, activation of the chemoreceptor trigger zone (CTZ) in the ▶ area postrema and excessive motion or other disturbances of the labyrinth. Pregnancy, exposure to radiation, psychological or visual stimuli and various disease states such as migraine, diabetes or uraemia may also cause vomiting.

In the gastrointestinal tract, drugs or toxins as well as mechanical stimulation induce emesis by activation of sensory receptors on afferent neurons in the vagus and sympathetic nerves. Information is relayed to the vomiting centre *via* the

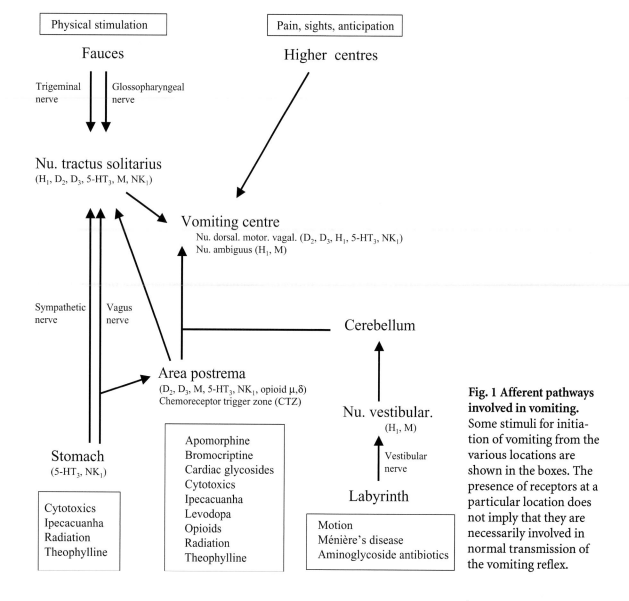

Fig. 1 Afferent pathways involved in vomiting. Some stimuli for initiation of vomiting from the various locations are shown in the boxes. The presence of receptors at a particular location does not imply that they are necessarily involved in normal transmission of the vomiting reflex.

nucleus tractus solitarius (NTS) in the medulla. The area postrema lacks a ▶ blood-brain barrier and is accessible to emetogens in the bloodstream. Neuronal pathways extend from the CTZ to the NTS and the vomiting centre.

Impulses from the vestibular apparatus in the labyrinth are conducted *via* the vestibular nucleus and cerebellum to the vomiting centre. Abnormal stimulation of the vestibular apparatus is involved in motion sickness and emesis associated with Ménière's disease.

Nausea and vomiting may also be induced by stimuli affecting higher centers of the brain, presumably the cortex, from unpleasant sights and smells as well as pain. Anticipatory vomiting also may occur during cancer chemotherapy. The act of ▶ vomiting involves contraction of the diaphragm and abdominal muscles to increase intragastric pressure. Also, retroperistaltic contractions of the intestine move the contents back into the stomach. Relaxation of the oesophagus and the cardiac sphincter at its lower end then allows the stomach contents to be vomited. The role of the stomach is passive, as active contraction is inhibited preceding emesis.

Nausea is often assumed to be a low level stimulation of the vomiting reflex. However, vomiting occurs without nausea in intestinal obstruction and in space motion sickness. Elevated plasma levels of ▸ vasopressin as well as tachygastria may play a role in nausea development.

Several neurotransmitters and ▸ autacoids are involved in initiating and conducting the vomiting reflex, including ▸ acetylcholine, ▸ dopamine, ▸ histamine, ▸ serotonin (vomiting), ▸ substance P and possibly ▸ prostaglandins. Receptors for the neurotransmitters are known to occur in many central areas associated with pathways for initiating emesis (Fig. 1). However the presence of receptors may not always be indicative of their involvement. For example, muscarinic receptors in the area postrema are probably not involved in motion sickness since all muscarinic receptor antagonists that are active as antiemetics have a non-quaternary structure suggesting that they must be capable of crossing the blood-brain barrier. Dopamine D_2 receptors are involved in some emetic responses, but recent studies have also suggested that activation of D_3 receptors in the area postrema may either produce vomiting or enhance that elicited by D_2 receptor activation.

Release of serotonin from enterochromaffin cells in the gastrointestinal tract with activation of serotonin 5-HT_3 receptors on vagal afferents has an important role in the initiation of vomiting by anticancer drugs, exposure to radiation and in postoperative vomiting after abdominal surgery, and may cause the vomiting seen on oral ingestion of hyperosmolar solutions of sodium chloride or after intravenous injection of erythromycin. Peripheral as well as central sites may also be involved in the emetic action of substance P. It is present in sensory nerves in the gut as well as being co-localised with serotonin in some enterochromaffin cells.

Clinical Aspects of Emesis

Drug-Induced. Emetogenic drugs may be of value in treating cases of acute poisoning, but usually nausea and vomiting induced by a drug are unwanted effects occurring in addition to its therapeutic action.

Emetics for Poisoning – Ipecacuanha
The most widely used emetic is syrup of ipecac, which contains the alkaloids emetine and cephaëline. Emetine induces vomiting by activation of sensory neurons in the vagus and sympathetic nerves to the stomach and centrally in the medulla, possibly at the CTZ. The release of serotonin may be involved as 5-HT_3 receptor antagonists prevent emesis induced by ipecacuanha. The use of syrup of ipecac in the treatment of poisoning is declining as activated charcoal is equally or more effective with fewer complications.

Cytotoxics
The incidence of vomiting in cancer chemotherapy is variable; the highly emetogenic cisplatin affects >99% of patients but some with low emetogenic potential such as vincristine affect <25%. The time course of emesis also varies; cyclophosphamide induces a single phase that persists for 24 h whereas cisplatin produces a biphasic pattern; an acute phase peaking at 6 h and a less intense second phase peaking at day 2–3. Patients on repeated courses of chemotherapy often develop anticipatory vomiting and nausea, commencing several hours before treatment is given, subsequent to the initial course. This appears to be due to associative learning together with psychological stress from the drug regimen. Cytotoxics cause cellular damage and the release of serotonin and other mediators from enterochromaffin cells. There is conflicting evidence as to whether 5-HT_3 receptors in the medulla are activated during chemotherapy and contribute to production of emesis. Currently the weight of evidence favours peripheral 5-HT_3 receptors with minor involvement of central receptors. Cytotoxics also cause an elevation of dopamine levels in the area postrema in animal studies and may release prostaglandins and inhibit enzymes such as enkephalinases to allow increased levels of enkephalins to activate opioid δ receptors on dopaminergic nerves. The delayed phase of vomiting with cisplatin may involve the release of substance P.

Dopamine Receptor Agonists
Parkinsonian patients receiving the dopamine precursor levodopa, or dopamine receptor agonists such as bromocriptine and apomorphine may experience nausea and vomiting due to stimulation of dopamine D_2 receptors in the CTZ.

E

Opioids

Opioids act on the area postrema and/or the NTS *via* μ or δ receptors to produce emesis. Also, ambulatory patients receiving opioids are more affected than those confined to bed, suggesting a vestibular component in the effect. The emetic action of opioids is complicated by an antiemetic action, possibly involving μ_2 receptors at the NTS or the vomiting centre.

Morning Sickness and Hyperemesis Gravidarum

Morning sickness is experienced by many expectant mothers during the first 3 months of gestation. Symptoms usually consist of nausea and retching rather than vomiting but a few women experience protracted vomiting (hyperemesis gravidarum). The basis for morning sickness is not known but has been variously considered to involve psychosomatic, endocrine, allergic and metabolic aspects. It may be a protective mechanism against ingestion of toxins or harmful chemicals in foodstuffs. Endocrine studies show hyperemesis gravidarum is associated with elevated serum levels of human chorionic gonadotrophin.

Motion Sickness

Motion sickness arises in the vestibular apparatus. Stimulation of the semicircular canals or the utricles by unfamiliar accelerating movement may cause a mismatch between the sensory information reaching the brain centres controlling balance and posture, with that anticipated. Motion sickness may be avoided by reducing 'sensory conflict'; fixing vision on a stable reference point such as the horizon may be effective. Cortical centers may also contribute; memories of previous travel or the sight and sounds of others being affected often increases susceptibility.

Postoperative Vomiting

The incidence of postoperative nausea and vomiting is variable depending on a number of factors including the nature of the operation, the sex and age of the patient, women and children being more prone, the anaesthetic and other drugs used. For example, opioid administration increases the incidence. Intra-abdominal operations and eye, ear, nose or throat surgery have a high likelihood of nausea and vomiting. Overall incidence has recently been estimated as ca 20–30%.

Pharmacological Intervention

Dopamine D2-like Receptor Antagonists

Several D_2-like receptor antagonists are used as anti-emetics. They include phenothiazines (metopimazine, perphenazine, prochlorperazine, thiethylperazine), butyrophenones (droperidol, haloperidol), metoclopramide and domperidone. Metoclopramide also raises tone in the lower oesophagus and increases gastrointestinal motility, and in high concentrations causes blockade of serotonin 5-HT_3 receptors. Domperidone does not readily cross the blood-brain barrier. It is particularly useful in controlling emesis associated with levodopa and dopamine receptor agonists used in Parkinsonism as it will not affect their beneficial action in the basal ganglia. The D_2-like receptor antagonists are useful in emesis occurring postoperatively and for cancer chemotherapy or radiotherapy but are not effective in motion sickness. Metoclopramide used in high doses is more effective than other D_2 receptor antagonists in emesis due to cancer chemotherapy but its usefulness is limited by ▶ extrapyramidal effects. It is effective in vomiting associated with migraine and uraemia but its value in postoperative nausea and vomiting is variable. Metoclopramide and domperidone also reduce nausea and vomiting associated with diabetic gastroparesis.

Histamine H1 Receptor Antagonists

Several histamine H_1 receptor antagonists are effective in treating motion sickness, Ménière's disease, morning sickness, uraemia and postoperative vomiting. They are not effective against cytotoxics. Antagonists with piperazine-based structures (chlorcyclizine, cinnarazine, cyclizine, meclozine) or ethanolamine-based (dimenhydrinate, diphenhydramine, doxylamine) as well as promethazine are effective and appear to depend on central inhibition of histamine H_1 receptors and possibly also on an ability to inhibit muscarinic receptors. The non-sedating H_1 receptor antagonist, astemizole, is not effective in motion sickness. There has been considerable controversy as to whether H_1 receptor antagonists pose a teratogenic risk when used to treat morning sickness but a recent meta-analysis concluded that they can be used safely in pregnancy if nausea and retching cannot be controlled adequately by dietary modification.

Muscarinic Receptor Antagonists

These include atropine, scopolamine (hyoscine), trihexyphenidyl (benzhexol) and benzatropine. They block central muscarinic receptors involved in various afferent pathways of the vomiting reflex (Fig. 1). They have been used to control motion sickness, emesis in Ménière's disease and postoperative vomiting. Currently, hyoscine is largely restricted to the treatment of motion sickness where it has a fast onset of action but a short duration (4–6 h). Administration of hyoscine by transdermal patch produces a prolonged, low level release of the drug with minimal side effects. To control postoperative vomiting, it should be applied >8 h before emesis is anticipated.

Corticosteroids

Steroids, usually dexamethasone or methylprednisolone, are useful in cytotoxic-induced vomiting, possibly by inhibiting central prostaglandin formation. They are used either alone for low emetogenic risk chemotherapy or in combination with 5-HT$_3$ receptor antagonists to improve control for moderate to highly emetogenic chemotherapy. Steroids been found useful in the delayed as well as acute phase of cisplatin-induced emesis. They can also be combined with metoclopramide and other dopamine receptor antagonists to enhance control of cytotoxic-induced vomiting. Combination with ondansetron, but not with droperidol or metoclopramide, has improved control of postoperative vomiting.

Cannabinoids

Dronabinol (tetrahydrocannabinol), the active principle from cannabis and synthetic cannabinoids, nabilone and levonantradol are effective in treating nausea and vomiting in cancer chemotherapy. The mode of action is unclear but appears to involve cannabinoid CB$_1$ receptors. Cannabinoids have been shown to reduce acetylcholine release in the cortex and hippocampus and have been suggested to inhibit medullary activity by a cortical action. Inhibition of prostaglandin synthesis and release of endorphins may also be involved in the antiemetic effect. A recent review of trials of dronabinol, nabilone or levonantradol

concluded that while the cannabinoids were superior to placebo or dopamine receptor antagonists in controlling emesis due to moderate emetogenic cancer chemotherapy, they produced harmful adverse effects more frequently.

Lorazepam

The benzodiazepine lorazepam acts allosterically on GABA$_A$ receptors to facilitate the actions of GABA. Lorazepam has some antiemetic activity in cancer chemotherapy but is currently used only in combination therapy where it does not appear to add to antiemetic control but may contribute to a reduction in anxiety.

Pyridoxine

Pyridoxine is used in morning sickness. Its mechanism of action remains unclear and several reviews of the use of pyridoxine have failed to find conclusive evidence of effectiveness. A recent double blind trial found pyridoxine to be of benefit in reducing nausea only. Some clinicians use pyridoxine as the first drug on the basis that it is the least likely to be toxic to the foetus.

Serotonin 5-HT3 Receptor Antagonists

Those developed for clinical use as antiemetics include dolasetron, granisetron, ondansetron and tropisetron. They are the most effective antiemetics for vomiting induced by cytotoxics and are also effective against radiation-induced and postoperative vomiting. Preliminary evidence suggests they may also limit binge-vomiting in bulimics, and ondansetron has been shown to reduce nausea following intraduodenal infusion of lipids. The 5-HT$_3$ receptor antagonists are ineffective against motion sickness.

Neurokinin NK1 Receptor Antagonists

Animal studies have shown that non-peptide selective NK$_1$ receptor antagonists (CP-99994, CP-122721, GR205171, L-758298, MK-869) inhibit emesis produced by the neurokinin, substance P and other emetogens such as apomorphine, morphine, ipecacuanha, cytotoxics and radiation. They have a central site of action but a new peptide NK$_1$ antagonist, sendide, appears to act *via* a peripheral site. Clinical trials with the non-peptide antagonists have relieved nausea and vomiting after gynaecological surgery and after cisplatin, especially for the delayed phase of vomiting. Combination of NK$_1$ receptor antagonist with a 5-HT$_3$ receptor antagonist and steroid produced the most effective control of both acute and delayed emesis after cisplatin.

References

1. Andrews PLR (1992) Physiology of nausea and vomiting. British Journal of Anaesthesia 69 (suppl. 1):2S–19S
2. Fauser AA, Fellhauer M, Hoffmann M, Link H, Schlimok G, Gralla RJ (1999) Guidelines for antiemetic therapy: Acute emesis. European Journal of Cancer 35:361–370
3. Lucot JB (1998) Pharmacology of motion sickness. Journal of Vestibular Research 8:61–66
4. Scott-Walker TM, Ball PA, Berry PR (2000) A review of the prophylaxis and treatment of postoperative nausea and vomiting. Australian Journal of Hospital Pharmacy 30:157–164
5. Watcha MF, White PF (1992) Postoperative nausea and vomiting. Anesthesiology 77:162–184

ENaC

▶ Amiloride-sensitive Na$^+$ Channel
▶ Epithelial Na$^+$ Channel

Endocannabinoid System

Derivatives of the hemp plant *Cannabis sativa* such as marijuana, hashish, bhang etc. have been used medicinally and recreationally for thousands of years. The identification of Δ^9-▶ Tetrahydrocannabinol (Δ^9-THC) as the main active compound led to the synthesis of high-affinity cannabinoid ligands which in turn enabled the identification of cannabinoid receptors. The discovery of Δ^9-THC and its receptors also suggested the presence of an endogenous signalling system that utilizes these widely expressed receptors. Several arachidonic acid derivatives that activate the cannabinoid receptor were isolated, including arachidonylethanolamide (anandamide) and 2-arachidonylglycerol (2-AG). The formation of these endogenous cannabinoids (endocannabinoids) is stimulated by calcium. The formation of anandamide in response to elevated intracellular calcium concentration is likely to proceed from breaking up a phospholipid precursor, N-arachidonylphosphatidylethanolamine (NAPE), by phospholipase D (PLD). Newly formed anandamide is released from the membrane to outside the cell. 2-AG, which occurs also in the brain and which shares many properties with anandamide, is formed through a biosynthetic pathway distinct from that producing anandamide and possibly involves phospholipase C and diacylglycerol lipase. Moreover, cells can actively take up endocannabinoids using a hitherto unknown transport system. Both anandamide and 2-AG are cleaved by the intracellular enzyme fatty-acid amide hydrolase (FAAH).

The physiological effects of cannabinoids are mediated by specific receptors that belong to the group of 7-transmembrane domain G-protein-coupled receptors. The highest levels of cannabinoid binding in the vertebrate brain are found in basal ganglia, cerebellum, hippocampus, and cortex. The cannabinoid receptor which is prominently expressed in the central nervous system has been termed the CB$_1$ receptor. A second cannabinoid receptor, mainly expressed in the immune system and absent from the neuronal system, became known as the CB$_2$ receptor. On the cellular level, CB$_1$ receptors are mainly found in presynaptic fibres and terminals. In contrast, CB$_1$ expression is not as prominent in the cell bodies and dendrites of neurons. Outside the nervous system, CB$_1$ receptor expression has been described in the adrenal gland, bone marrow, heart, lung, prostate, testes, thymus, tonsils, and spleen. The CB$_2$ receptor has been described to be expressed in spleen, thymus, tonsils, bone marrow, pancreas, splenic macrophage/monocyte preparations, mast cells and in peripheral blood leukocytes. Recent data suggest that there may be a third cannabinoid receptor ("CB$_3$"), based on the finding that some of the cannabinoid effects in the central nervous system are still present in CB$_1$-deficient mice.

Receptor-mediated actions of cannabinoids in the central nervous system include the inhibition

E

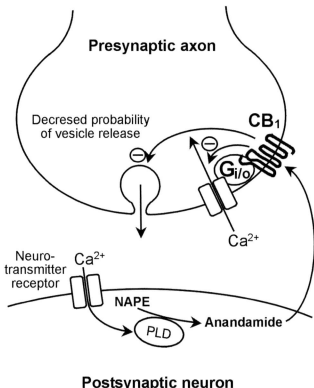

Fig. 1 Retrograde signalling by endocannabinoids like anandamide. Postsynaptic depolarization results in Ca^{2+} influx. Ca^{2+} stimulates the synthesis of endocannabinoids which are released and activate presynaptic CB_1 receptors leading to the inhibition of neurotransmitter release. This rapid retrograde suppression of synaptic transmission may underly phenomena like "depolarization-induced suppression of inhibition" (DSI). See text.

of both N-type and P/Q-type calcium channels and the activation of G-protein coupled inward rectifier K^+ (GIRK) channels through G-proteins of the G_i/G_o family. Actions of cannabinoids are predicted to have an inhibitory effect on neurons in most cases. Whereas the inhibition of presynaptic calcium channels reduces neurotransmitter release, the activation of postsynaptic potassium channels, suppresses action potential firing.

In contrast to classical neurotransmitters, endogenous cannabinoids can function as retrograde synaptic messengers. Released from postsynaptic neurons they travel backwards across synapses, activate CB_1 receptors on presynaptic axons and suppress neurotransmitter release. Cannabinoids may affect memory, cognition, and pain perception (see below) by this cellular mechanism.

The retrograde signalling property of cannabinoids has recently been linked to a phenomenon called ▶ depolarization-induced suppression of inhibition (DSI) (fig) which occurs following depolarization of a postsynaptic neuron and is characterized by a transient presynaptic suppression of inhibitory postsynaptic currents (IPSC). DSI appears to be triggered in response to a rise in postsynaptic calcium levels and involves a retrograde messenger that is released by the postsynaptic cell. In many cases this appears to be an endocannabinoid-like substance e.g. anandamide. Endocannabinoid signalling, therefor, appears to provide a temporarily distinct feedback mechanism to regulate the synaptic strength. Although retrograde signalling by endocannabinoids has so far only been described in the cerebellum and hippocampus it most likely occurs also in other brain regions.

Cannabinoids have been shown to affect a variety of physiological and pathological processes which most likely involve the endocannabinoid system. Cannabinoid agonists are, for example, effective in a wide range of acute and chronic pain models including thermal and chemical-induced nociception. Cannabinoid receptors are located in the trigeminal ganglion, the dorsal horn, capsaicin-sensitive and large-diameter primary afferent fibres, and non-primary afferent fibres. Cannabinoid receptors are also present in the periaqueductal gray area and dorsal raphe nucleus, areas critical for nociceptive signalling. It is currently not clear whether the endocannabinoid system tonically controls sensory perception or whether it is only activated under pathophysiological conditions. It has long been recognized that marijuana consumption in humans as well as in laboratory animals strongly affects cognitive functions and can produce disturbances in various aspects of learning and memory. Most consistently it has been shown that the activation of CB_1 receptors leads to the disruption of short-term memory while long-term memory is largely unaffected. There is little question that CB_1 receptors located in the hippocampus are crucially involved in cannabinoid actions on cognition and that other forebrain areas are also likely to be involved. However, it remains an open question whether endocannabinoids tonically modulate the neural pathways that underlie cognition. There are also many reports describing anticonvulsant effects of cannabinoids which can be explained on the basis of the inhibitory effects exerted by cannabinoids in the central nervous system (see above). There are also ample clinical data that demonstrate antiemetic effects of cannabinoids. It is, however, not clear whether endocannabinoids are primary mediators of emesis or whether they have a modulatory influence on the processes underlying nausea and vomiting. One of the most prominent effects of cannabis and synthetic cannabinoids is their stimulatory effect on appetite. Activation of cannabinoid receptors has clearly been shown to result in a stimulation of food intake. Again, it is currently not clear whether the endocannabinoid system plays an active role in the regulation of feeding behaviour. Finally, cannabinoids produce vasodilatation,

hypotension, and tachykardia in humans. Vascular dilation in response to cannabinoids may be due to the inhibition of transmitter release from sympathetic nerve terminals, direct effects on vascular smooth muscle cells or effects on endothelial cells.

Cannabinoids have a well established clinical value in the treatment of nausea and emesis, anorexia and weight loss especially in tumour patients. Relatively well established are their effects in the treatment of pain, spasticity, asthma, and glaucoma, while many other suggested indications are less well established. Cannabinoids such as THC are relatively safe in overdose, producing drowsiness and confusion, but no respiratory or cardiovascular effects that threaten life. Already at low doses, however, cannabinoids produce euphoria and drowsiness which are sometimes accompanied by sensory distortion and halluzinations. These effects, together with the legal restrictions on the use of cannabinoids, preclude the widespread therapeutic use of cannabinoids. THC has been reported to produce teratogenic and mutagenic effects in animals and to affect endocrine functions in humans. There is ongoing controversy about the question whether cannabinoids are of medicinal value in terminally ill patients suffering from pain, nausea/emesis and anorexia.

Endogenous Opioid Peptides

Endogenous opioid peptides are the wide variety of endogenous peptides isolated since 1975 which are the natural ligands for the opioid receptors. The peptides derive from three precursor molecules (proopiomelanocortin, proenkephalin, prodynorphin). each encoded by a separate gene. The discovery of the endomorphins, two amidated tetrapeptides which do not derive from the three precursor molecules, indicate the existence of additional opioid peptide genes which, however, have not yet been identified.

▶ Opioid System
▶ Analgesics

Endoplasmic Reticulum

The endoplasmic reticulum (ER) is a system of membrane enclosed cisternae in the cytoplasm. The ER is continuous with the outer membrane of the nuclear envelope. The part of the ER coated with ribosomes is called rough ER, the other part is called smooth-surfaced ER. The rough ER is the first compartment of the secretory pathway. Here, membrane proteins are integrated into and secretory proteins translocated across the ER membrane. Furthermore, protein folding is established and checked by a quality control system. From the ER, proteins are delivered in vesicles to the endoplasmic reticulum/Golgi intermediate comparment (ERGIC).

▶ Protein Trafficking and Quality Control

Endorphins

Endorphins belong to the group of ▶ endogenous opioid peptides.

▶ Analgesics
▶ Opioid System

Endothelial Cells

Endothelial cells are the cells in the inner intimal layer of blood vessels.

Endothelin Converting Enzyme

Endothelin COncerting Enzymes (ECEs) belong to the family of metalloproteases that catalyze the proteolytic activation of big endothelins.

▶ Endothelins

Endothelins

ALEXANDER OKSCHE
Freie Universität Berlin and Forschungsinstitut für Molekulare Pharmakologie (FMP), Berlin, Germany
oksche@fmp-berlin.de

Definition

Endothelins comprise a family of three vasoactive isopeptides of 21 amino acids that have an essential role in the regulation of the vascular and bronchiolar tone and the control of natriuresis in the kidney.

▶ Blood Pressure Control

Basic Characteristics

Endothelin and endothelin-converting enzymes. In 1985 a peptide was described in the supernatants of endothelial cells that mediated vasoconstriction. This peptide, was isolated, sequenced and the was cDNA cloned. According to its origin from endothelial cells it was named endothelin.

To date, three endothelin isoforms are known (ET1, ET2, ET3), encoded by different genes. Endothelins are synthesized as prepropolypeptides of approximately 200 amino acids (Table 1). The biological active endothelins are generated in a two-step proteolytic process (Fig. 1). In the first step, ▶ furin-like proteases generate big-endothelins (big-ETs) of 38 to 41 amino acids that are biologically inactive. In a second step specific ▶ endothelin-converting enzymes (ECEs) specifically cleave big-ETs between tryptophan 21 and valine/isoleucine 22, thereby producing the mature endothelins. Big-ET1 was also found to be cleaved by mast cell ▶ chymase and ▶ matrix metalloproteinase 2 (gelatinase A) resulting in biologically active ET1(1–31) and ET1(1–32), respectively (Fig. 1).

ECEs are ▶ metalloproteinases that are homologous to the ▶ neutral endopeptidase (NEP, E-24.11, neprilysin); unlike NEP, however, they form disulfide-bonded homodimers. In man, with ECE-1 and ECE-2, two isoforms are known, which are

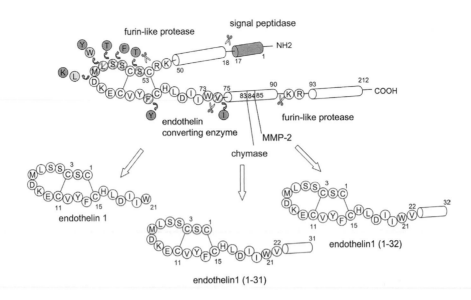

Fig. 1 Processing of prepro-ET1. ET1 is generated as a preprohormone consisting of 212 amino acids. Amino acids 53 to 90 represent big-ET1, amino acids 53 to 73 mature ET1. Amino acids that vary between the three endothelin isoforms are depicted by hatched circles (only variant amino acids of the mature ET1 moiety and of the ECE-cleavage site are indicated). The amino acids present in ET2 and ET3 are depicted by light or dark grey circles respectively. The signal peptide (grey cylinder) is cleaved off in the endoplasmic reticulum by the signal peptidase. Big-ET1 is generated by proteolytical processing (furin-like proteases), which recognize dibasic amino acids motifs. Mature ET1 is formed after processing through the endothelin converting enzyme. Mast cell chymase and matrix metalloprotease-2 (MMP-2) also generate biologically active peptides.

encoded by two separate genes. For ECE-1 four different variants have been identified (ECE-1a–d), which are generated by the use of alternative promoters (Table 2). For ECE-2, a single gene product has been described in man, whereas in mouse and calf two splice variants have been identified. In calf, an ECE-3 isoform has been isolated from iris microsomes and the choroid plexus, which is specifically involved in the conversion of big-ET3 to ET3. A human homologue of bovine ECE-3 has not yet been identified.

The ECE isoforms show different subcellular distributions and enzymatic characteristics (Table 2). ECE-1a and ECE-1c are mainly expressed at the plasma membrane, whereas ECE-1b, ECE-1d and ECE-2 are expressed intracellularly. Plasma membrane-bound ECE cleaves bigET1 circulating in the blood, whereas intracellular ECE isoforms are involved in the generation of mature endothelins.

Human umbilical vein endothelial cells (HUVEC) express the isoforms ECE-1a, -1b,-1d and ECE-2. In these cells, ET1 is secreted *via* both a constitutive and a regulated pathway. The ratio of released ET1:big ET1 is 4:1. About 80% of the ET1 is secreted at the abluminal membrane of endothelial cells. ECE-isoforms are abundantly expressed on the cell surface of endothelial cells and to a lower level also on vascular smooth muscle cells. In atherosclerotic lesions of vessels, however, ECE expression in smooth muscle cells is upregulated. It is likely that the ECE-isoforms expressed in smooth muscle cells contributes significantly to the generation of mature ET in normal and in particular atherosclerotic vessels.

Endothelial cells are the major source of ET1-synthesis. ET1 is also produced by astrocytes, neurons, hepatocytes, bronchial epithelial cells, renal epithelial and mesangial cells. Physiological stimuli of ET1-synthesis in endothelial cells are angi-

Tab. 1 Human endothelin isoforms.

| | Number of Amino Acids in | | Chromosome | Diseases |
	prepro-ET1	big ET1		
hET1	212	38	6p23-24	
hET2	178	38	1p34	
hET3			20q13.2-13.3	Hirschsprung's disease,
	238	41		Waardenberg syndrome, type 4

E

otensin II, catecholamines, thrombin, growth factors, insulin, hypoxia and shear stress. Inhibitors of ET1 synthesis are atrial natriuretic peptide, ET3, prostaglandin E2 and prostacyclin. ET2 is mainly synthesized in kidney, intestine, myocardium and placenta and ET3 is predominantely produced by neurons, astrocytes and kidney epithelial cells.

Endothelin receptors. Endothelins exert their diverse actions *via* two G protein-coupled receptors named endothelin A (ET_A) and endothelin B (ET_B) receptor, which share an identity of about 64% in their amino acid sequences. Both receptors display a signal peptide that is required for the correct biogenesis. After the N terminus is accessible in the ER lumen, the signal peptide is cleaved off (comprises 20 and 26 amino acids in ET_A and ET_B receptors, respectively). Further post-translational modifications are ▶ **Asn-linked glycosylation** of the extracellular N terminus (hET_A: Asn29, Asn 62; hET_B Asn 59) and ▶ **palmitoylation** of cysteine residues in the intracellular C terminus. Mass spectometry of the bovine ET_B receptor revealed that cysteine residues 402 and 404 are palmitoylated. The palmitoylation of endothelin receptors is essential for the activation of G proteins, since palmitoylation-deficient ET_A and ET_B receptors fail to stimulate $G_{q/11}$ and G_i proteins, respectively. The significance of the N-terminal glycosylation for receptor function remains elusive. Disulfide bonds between the highly conserved cysteine residues of the 1st (ET_A: Cys158, ET_B: Cys174) and the 2nd extracellular loop (ET_A: Cys239, ET_B: Cys255) are also likely. Whether cysteine residues in the extracellular N terminus (ET_A: Cys69, ET_B: Cys90) and the 3rd extracellular loop (ET_A: Cys341, ET_B: Cys359) also form disulfide bonds has not been clarified.

The endothelin receptor subtypes show differences in their signal transduction, ligand binding and tissue distribution. The ET_A receptor is isopeptide-selective and binds ET1 and ET2 with the same and ET3 with 70–100 fold lower affinity. The ET_B receptor binds all three isoforms with the same affinity. Pharmacological studies provided evidence for two subtypes of ET_A (ET_{A1}, ET_{A2}) and ET_B receptors (ET_{B1}, ET_{B2}), although genetic studies revealed only two different genes. Thus, the additional receptor subtypes may be derived from i) alternative splicing, ii) differences in post-translational processing or iii) protein-protein-interactions. For the ET_B receptor splice variants have been described. However, these isoforms most likely do not account for the postulated second receptor subtype. One splice variant harbours 10 additional amino acids in the 3rd intracellular loop and has normal binding characteristics and functional activity (IP and cAMP formation). The second splice variant, which carries a completely altered intracellular C terminus, has normal binding properties but lacks functional activity.

The ET_A receptor activates G proteins of the $G_{q/11}$ and $G_{12/13}$ family. The ET_B receptor stimulates G proteins of the G_i and $G_{q/11}$ family. In endothelial cells, activation of the ET_B receptor stimulates the release of NO and prostacyclin (PGI_2) *via* pertussis toxin-sensitive G proteins. In smooth muscle cells, the activation of ET_A receptors leads to an increase of intracellular calcium *via* pertussis toxin-insensitive G proteins of the $G_{q/11}$ family and to an activation of Rho proteins most likely *via* G proteins of the $G_{12/13}$ family. Increase of intracellular calcium results in a calmodulin-dependent activation of the myosin light chain kinase (MLCK, Fig. 2). MLCK phosphorylates the 20 kD myosin light chain (MLC-20), which then stimu-

Tab. 2 Properties of the different isoforms of endothelin-converting enzymes.

	Subcellular Localization	pH Optimum	Amino Acids (in human)	Species
ECE1a	pm	6.8-7.2	758	human, bovine, rat
ECE1b	i.c.	6.8-7.2	770	human, bovine, rat
ECE1c	pm late endosomes / multivesicular bodies	6.8-7.2	754	human
ECE1d	i.c. recycling endosomes	6.8	767	human, rat
ECE2a	i.c.	5.5	787	human, mouse, bovine
ECE2b	?	?	-	mouse/bovine
ECE3	?	6.6	-	bovine

pm: plasma membrane, *i.c.*: intracellular

lates actin-myosin interaction of vascular smooth muscle cells resulting in vasoconstriction. Since activated Rho inhibits the myosin light chain phosphatase *via* Rho-kinase, the dephosphorylation of the MLC-20 is blocked. The dual action of the ET_A receptor signaling on MLC-20 results in a robust vasoconstriction of vessels. Beside the short-term effects such as vasodilation and vasoconstriction, endothelin receptors also stimulate long-term events (cell growth and differentiation). Both endothelin receptor subtypes activate ERK1/2 and thereby mediate mitogenic responses as shown for cardiomyocytes, cardiac fibroblasts, vascular smooth muscle cells and renal mesangial cells.

ET1 also stimulates anti-apoptotic signal cascades in fibroblasts, vascular smooth muscle and endothelial cells (*via* phosphatidylinositol-3-kinase and Akt/protein kinase B). In prostate, ovarial and colorectal cancer, upregulation of endothelin synthesis and ET_A receptors has been associated with a progression of the disease. The inhibiton of ET_A receptors results in a reduced tumor growth. In malignant melanoma, ET_B receptors are associated with tumor progression. Endothelins can also stimulate apoptosis in stretch-activated vessels *via* the ET_B receptor, which contrasts the above mentioned effects. The molecular basis for these differential anti- and pro-apoptotic reactions mediated by endothelins remains elusive.

Activation of matrix metalloproteinases (MMP) is also involved in vascular and cardiac remodelling. For example, the fibrillar collagen matrix of the heart maintains the shape of the left ventricle. If the delicate balance between matrix deposition and degradation is altered, cardiac fibrosis (increase of collagen synthesis) or left ventricular remodelling (increase of degradation) occurs. Activation of ET_A receptors leads to a stimulation of MMP-1,-2 and -9 in isolated myocytes and in the myocardium. The endothelin-mediated activation of MMPs is essentially involved in ventricular remodeling after myocardial infarction in the rat: inhibiton of ET_A receptors by the selective ET_A receptor antagonist sitaxsentan prevents MMP activation and consequently left ventricular dilation.

Sites of endothelin receptor expression. ET_A receptors are expressed in the smooth muscle cells of the vascular medial layer and the airways, in cardial myocytes, lung parenchyma and airway epithelial cells. ET_B receptors are expressed in endothelial cells, in airway smooth muscle cells, vascular smooth muscle cells of certain vessels (e.g. saphenous vein, internal mammary artery), in the renal proximal and distal tubule, the renal collecting duct and in the cells of the atrioventricular conducting system.

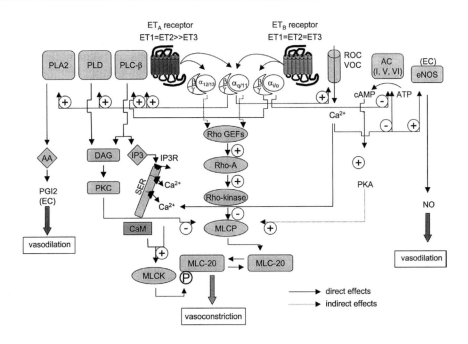

Fig. 2 Summary of short-term signaling events mediated by endothelin. In endothelial cells (EC) the activation of the ET_B receptor leads to the formation of prostacyclin (PGI_2) and NO and mediates vasodilation of vessels. In vascular smooth muscle cells activation of the ET_A receptor results in a robust vasoconstriction by a dual regulation of the 20 kD myosin light chain (MLC-20). *AA*: arachidonic acid, *AC*: adenylyl cyclase, *ATP*: adenosine triphosphate, *CaM*: Calmodulin, *cAMP*: cyclic adenosine monophosphate, *DAG*, diacyl glycerol, *eNOS*: endothelial NO synthase, *IP3*: inositol-3,4,5-phosphate, *MLC-20*: 20 kD myosin light chain, *MLCP*: myosin light chain phosphatase, *Rho-GEF*: Rho-guanine nucleotide exchange factor, *SER*: smooth endoplasmic reticulum, *IP3R*: IP3 receptor, *PKA*: protein kinase A, *PKC*: protein kinase C, *PLA*: phospholipase A, *PLC*: phospholipase C, *PLD*: phospholipase D.

In addition, ET_B receptors are upregulated in vessels with atherosclerotic lesions and in pulmonary vessels of patients with severe pulmonary hypertension. The upregulation can be attributed to increased ET_B receptor expression in smooth muscle cells and to ET_B receptors expressed on infiltrating macrophages.

In the vascular system, endothelial ET_B receptors mediate a transient vasodilation, whereas ET_A receptors cause a long-lasting vasoconstriction. The role of ET_B receptors expressed on smooth muscle cells remains elusive. In some vessels, ET_B receptor stimulation causes vasoconstriction which is, however, only of transient nature and quantitatively much lower than that following ET_A receptor activation. In the kidney, ET_A receptors, which are almost exclusively expressed in vessels, regulate renal circulation, whereas ET_B receptors,

expressed in the proximal and distal tubule and in the collecting duct are involved in natriuresis and diuresis. The main natriuretic action occurs most likely *via* the inhibition of the ▶ amiloride-sensitive sodium channel (ENaC). In the lung, endothelin causes long-lasting vaso- and bronchoconstriction. The contribution of each receptor subtype to the endothelin-evoked pulmonary responses is still controversial. The current data suggest that in the healthy lung ET_A receptors are involved primarily in pulmonary vasoconstriction and ET_B receptors in bronchoconstriction. In the central nervous system, ET_A receptors are expressed on smooth muscle cells of large and small cerebral arteries. In addition, ET_A receptors were also found to be expressed on endothelial cells isolated from capillaries and larger microvessels of the brain, but the physiological need for the ET_A receptor expression

Tab. 3 Summary of clinical trails with endothelin receptor antagonists or ECE-inhibitors.

Drug	Company	Antagonist/Inhibitor of	Approval/Clinical study
Bosentan (Tracleer®)	Actelion, Switzerland	ET_A / ET_B receptor	pulmonary hypertension (approved in USA); CHF (III)
TBC11251 (Sitaxsentan®)	Texas Biotechnology, USA	ET_A receptor	pulmonary hypertension (IIb/III)
Ro-61-0612 (Tezosentan®)	Actelion, Switzerland	ET_A / ET_B receptor	AHF (III)
ABT-627 (Atrasentan®)	Abbott Laboratories, USA	ET_A receptor	prostate cancer (III)
LU135252 (Darusentan®)	Aventis, Germany	ET_A receptor	CHF (III, discontinued)
S-0139	Shionogi, Japan	ET_A receptor	Cerebrovascular ischemia (II, Japan)
BSF208075 (Ambrisentan®)	Myogen, USA	ET_A receptor	CHF (II), CRF (II), pulmonary hypertension (II)
SLV306	Solvay, Germany	NEP/ECE (dual inhibitor)	CHF (II), hypertension (II)

AHF: acute heart failure, *CHF*: chronic heart failure, *CRF*: chronic renal failure, *NEP*: neutral endopeptidase, *ECE*: endothelin converting enzyme.

in endothelial cells in the brain remains elusive. Neurons, particular those of the level III and IV of the cortex predominately express ET_B receptors. In isolated astrocytes, both receptor subtypes were found to be expressed at the cell surface.

Genetic studies and human diseases

Mice homozygous for an ET_A receptor gene disruption show craniofacial malformations, such as cleft palate, micrognathia, microtia and microglossia. ET_A (-/-) mice die shortly after birth due to respiratory failure. Mice with an ET1-null mutation show the same cranciofacial malformations and, in addition, cardiovascular disorders (e.g. septal defects, abnormal cardial outflow tract, aortic arch and subclavian arteries).

Mice with a disruption of the ET3 or the ET_B receptor gene display pigment disorder and a megacolon. The former resembles the congenital megacolon (Morbus Hirschsprung) associated with pigment disorders and cochlear hearing problems (Waardenberg syndrome) or the isolated congenital megacolon (Hirschsprung's disease) observed in man. Hirschsprung's disease and Waardenberg syndrome can be caused by several

different gene mutations, among others inactivating mutations in the ET3 and the ET_B receptor gene (about 5% of the patients with Hirschsprung's disease have ET_B receptor mutations). The lack of ET3/ET_B receptor results in the absence of parasympathic ganglionic neurons in the myenteric plexus (Auerbach). Mice with an ET3/ET_B receptor disruption die within two weeks after birth. In transgenic mice, in which the expression of the ET_B receptor is driven by the dopamine-β-hydroxylase promoter, normal myenteric plexus are present and no enteric disorder develops. These mice, however, show a salt-sensitive hypertension, which can be efficiently treated with amiloride, indicating that ET_B receptors are involved in the regulation of natriuresis *via* the amilorid-sensitive sodium channel ENaC.

The genetically engineered disruption of the ECE1 gene causes craniofacial and cardiovascular malformations (ET1/ET_A receptor phenotype), congenital megacolon and pigment disorders (ET3/ETB receptor phenotype). The ECE-2 (-/-) mice do not display any abnormality, indicating that ECE-1 is of crucial importance in embryonic development. Strikingly, ECE-1 (-/-) mice and

ECE-1 (-/-)/ECE-2 (-/-) mice still have about 60% of wild-type ET1 levels. This result indicates that alternative pathways in the generation of mature ET1 exist (e.g. NEP). This alternatively generated ET1, however, cannot compensate for the embryogenic defects.

Drugs

Clinical Use

As endothelins mediate potent vasoconstrictor effects, ECE-inhibitors and endothelin receptor antagonists were developed for the treatment of cardiovascular diseases, such as acute and chronic heart failure, pulmonary hypertension and subarachnoid hemorrhage. In addition, ET_A receptors have potent mitogenic responses and are upregulated in ovarial and prostate cancer. Thus ET_A receptors are also considered as a potential targets for anti-tumor activity.

A great number of ECE-inhibitors and mixed and selective ET_A and ET_B receptor antagonists have been developed in the past. For specific inhibitors of ECE, however, only very limited effects on the endothelin system were found. The limited potency of ECE inhibition might be due to the generation of mature ET1 from big-ET1 by other proteases such as neutral endopeptidase or other currently unidentified proteases.

In the case of receptor antagonists, it is still unknown whether mixed antagonism of endothelin receptors or selective blockade of ET_A receptors is of greater benefit in the treatment of diseases. Several clinical trials have been launched involving the treatment of heart and renal failure, pulmonary hypertension, subarachnoid hemorrhage and prostate cancer (Table 3). The majority of the studies is performed with selective ET_A receptor antagonists. At present, however, only the mixed endothelin receptor antagonist Tracleer (Bosentan) is approved for treatment (pulmonary hypertension).

References

1. Yanagisawa M, Kurihara H, Kimura S, Tomobe Y, Kobayashi M, Mitsui Y, Yazaki Y, Goto K, Masaki T (1988) A novel potent vasoconstrictor peptide produced by vascular endothelial cells. Nature 332:411–415

2. Handbuch der Experimentellen Pharmakologie. Band 152: Endothelin and its inhibitors. Editor: T.D. Warner. Springer Verlag, Berlin, Heidelberg, New York. 2001.

3. Gohla A, Schultz G, Offermanns S. (2000) Role for $G_{\alpha 12}/G_{\alpha 13}$ in agonist-induced vascular smooth muscle cell contraction. Circ Res 87:221–227

4. Yanagisawa H, Hammer RE, Richardson JA, Emoto N, Williams SC, Takeda S, Clouthier DE, Yanagisawa M (2000) Disruption of ECE-1 and ECE-2 reveals a role for endothelin-converting enzyme-2 in murine cardiac development. J Clin Invest 105:1373–1382

5. Goto K (2001) Basic and therapeutic relevance of endothelin-mediated regulation. Biol Pharm Bull 24:1219–1230

Endotoxin

Endotoxins are the lipopolysaccharides (LPS) of the outer membrane of Gram-negative bacteria. They trigger inflammatory reactions in the infected organism, activate complement and cause fever or even a septic shock. They act on ▶ toll-like receptors.

Enkephalin

Enkephalins belong to the group of ▶ endogenous opioid peptides.

▶ Analgesics
▶ Opioid System

Entamoeba Histolytica

Entamoeba histolytica is an anaerobic rhizopod that occurs in tropical and subtropical areas. It can cause intestinal and extraintestinal manifestations. It is transmitted orally by ingestion of cysts that develop into trophozoites in the large intestine. Amebic trophozoites release several cytolytic factors, e.g. amoebapore, which enable the parasite to invade tissue. In intestinal amoebiasis, *E. histolytica*trophozoites invade the intestinal mucosa, causing a form of ulcerative colitis with bloody and mucous diarrhoea. Extraintestinal manifestation of amebiasis results in abscess formation, usually in the liver but sometimes in the brain.

▶ Antiprotozoal Drugs

Envelope

In some viruses, the capsid is surrounded by a lipid membrane (envelope), which is derived from the host cell membrane at the site of virus budding. The membrane contains viral envelope glycoproteins as well as host cell membrane proteins.

▶ Antiviral Drugs

Enzyme

Enzymes are biocatalysts for all the biochemical reactions needed in a living organism.

Eosinophil

▶ Allergy
▶ Immune Defense

Eotaxin

An eotaxin is a chemokine of the CC-family, which stimulates the migration of eosinophils. Eotaxin effects are mediated by the chemokine receptor CCR3. Eotaxin may play a role as a chemoattract-

ant for eosinophils in the lungs of asthmatic patients.

▶ Chemokine receptors

Eph Receptor Tyrosine Kinase

▶ Angiogenesis and Vascular Morphogenesis
▶ Table appendix: Receptor Proteins

Ephrin-B

Ephrin-B molecules are ligands of Eph-B receptor tyrosine kinases, which regulate the differentiation of arteries and veins through bidirectionally acting signal transduction mechanisms.

▶ Angiogenesis and Vascular Morphogenesis

Ephrins

Ephrins are a group of membranous ligands, which function through a family of receptor tyrosine kinases (Ephs). Ephrin/Eph-mediated signaling processes are involved in morphogenetic processes taking place e.g. during the development of the nervous system or the vasculature.

▶ Angiogenesis and Vascular Morphogenesis

Epidermal Growth Factor

▶ Growth Factors

Epidermal Growth Factor Receptor Family

The epidermal growth factor (EGF) receptor family, also called the "ErbB-receptor family", consists of 4 receptor family members ErbB1 (EGFR), ErbB2 (Neu, HER2), ErbB3 (HER3) and ErbB4 (HER4). ErbB-receptors can form heterodimers and mediate the actions of a variety of factors including epidermal growth factor (EGF), epiregulin or neuregulins. ErbB2-containing receptors are highly upregulated in a variety of tumors. Antibodies targeting ErbB2 (e.g. Trastuzumab) are used as antineoplastic agents.

▶ Growth Factors
▶ Receptor Tyrosine Kinases
▶ Table appendix: Receptor Proteins

Epidural (Space)

The epidural space surrounds the dura mater of the spinal cord. It is bounded by the pedicles of the vertebral arches and by the anterior and posterior ligaments connecting the bony vertebral column. The epidural space contains nerve roots, fat and blood vessels.

▶ Local Anaesthetics

Epigenetic

An epigenetic change influences the phenotype without altering the genotype.

Epilepsy

Epilepsy is a heterogeneous group of syndromes characterised by abnormal, rhythmic electrical activity of the brain or parts of the brain. The term 'epilepsy' is reserved for chronic diseases, while a single, isolated ▶ seizure does not justify the diagnosis of epilepsy.

▶ Antiepileptic Drugs

Epinephrine

▶ Adrenaline

Episodic Ataxia/Myokymia

Episodic ataxia is an autosomal dominant disorder that causes brief episodes of ataxia can be triggered by physical or emotional stress. The symptom can occur several times during the day, lasts for seconds to minutes, and is associated with dysarthria and motor neuron activity, which causes muscle rippling (myokymia) between and during attacks.

▶ Voltage-dependent Ca^{2+} Channels

Episome

An episome is nuclear DNA that is maintained without integrating into chromosomes.

▶ Gene Therapy

Epithelial Ca^{2+} Channel 1

Epithelial calcium channel 1 (ECaC1), synonym TRPV5, is a member of the TRP family of ion channels, implicated in vitamin D-dependent transcellular Ca^{2+} transport in epithelial cells of the kidney, placenta and the intestine.

▶ TRP Channels

Epithelial Na$^+$ Channel

L. SCHILD, B.C. ROSSIER
Institut de pharmacologie et de toxicologie de l'Université, Lausanne, Switzerland
Laurent.Schild@ipharm.unil.ch,
Bernard.Rossier@ipharm.unil.ch

Definition

The epithelial Na$^+$ channel (ENaC or amiloride-sensitive Na$^+$ channel) is the highly selective sodium channel expressed in epithelia. The ENaC channel is a heteromeric channel made of homologous α β γ ENaC subunits. The human genes encoding the α β γ ENaC named *SCNN1A,SCNN1B* and*SCNN1G* are located in chromosomes 12 (α) and 16 (β γ), respectively. The mouse genes encoding the α β γ ENaC named *Scnn1a,Scnn1b* and*Scnn1g* are located on chromosomes 6 (α) and 7 (β γ), respectively (1).

▶ Table appendix: Membrane Transport Proteins
▶ Diuretics
▶ Voltage-dependent Na$^+$ Channels

Basic Characteristics

ENaC belongs to a recently discovered family of ionic channels that include, in mammals, the neuronal acid-sensing ion channels (ASICs) and, in the worm,*C.elegans*, the degenerin channel family (Mec4, Mec10), involved in mechanosensation (2). The homologous α β γ subunits of ENaC are made of two transmembrane domains and arranged

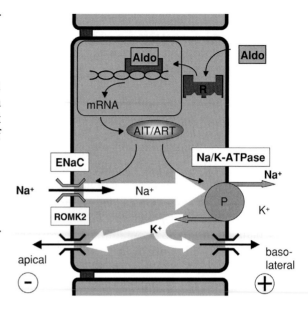

Fig. 1 Transepithelial ion transport in a principal cell of the cortical collecting duct (CCD). ENaC mediates Na$^+$ entry from the tubule lumen at the apical membrane and the Na$^+$/K$^+$ ATPase extrudes Na$^+$ at the basolateral side. K$^+$ channels are present on the basolateral and apical membrane. K$^+$ channels at the apical membrane mediate K$^+$ secretion into the tubular lumen.

The ENaC is located in the apical membrane of polarized epithelial cells where it mediates Na$^+$ transport across tight epithelia (3). The most important tight epithelia expressing ENaC include the distal nephron of the kidney, the respiratory epithelium and the distal colon. The basic function of ENaC in polarized epithelial cells is to allow vectorial transcellular transport of Na$^+$ ions. This transepithelial Na$^+$ transport through a cell basically involves two steps, as illustrated in Fig. 1. The large electrochemical gradient for Na$^+$ ions existing across the apical membrane provides the driving force for the entry of Na$^+$ into the cell. Active Na$^+$ transport across the basolateral membrane is accomplished by the ▶ Na$^+$/K$^+$-ATPase.

ENaC mediates Na$^+$ entry from the tubular lumen at the apical membrane and the Na$^+$/K$^+$ ATPase extrudes Na$^+$ at the basolateral side. K$^+$ channels are present on the basolateral and apical membrane. K$^+$ channels at the apical membrane mediate K$^+$ secretion into the tubular lumen.

In the distal nephron, ENaC activity controls Na$^+$ absorption, in order to balance urinary Na$^+$ excretion with the daily intake. The Na$^+$ absorption in the distal nephron is coupled to K$^+$ secretion *via* K$^+$ channels (ROMK2) located at the apical membrane. ENaC activity is under the control of ▶ aldosterone and ▶ vasopressin that are secreted in response to stimuli such as extracellular volume contraction, dehydration or hyperkalemia. Aldosterone binds to intracellular mineralocorticoid receptors (MR receptors); the ligand-receptor complex is translocated to the nucleus and induces the expression of ENaC and the Na$^+$/K$^+$-ATPase proteins *via* aldosterone-induced transcripts (AITs) and/or aldosterone-repressed transcripts (ARTs). Vasopressin binds to the G-protein-coupled V2 receptor and activates ENaC *via* the c-AMP-dependent pathway.

The role of ENaC is crucial for the maintenance of the extracellular fluid volume and blood pressure (4). The recent identification of mutations in genes encoding the epithelial sodium channel (ENaC), the mineralocorticoid receptor (MR) and the ▶ 11β-hydroxysteroid dehydrogenase (11β-HSD-2) that causes monogenic forms of hypertension, strongly supports this notion. Mutations of ENaC associated with an increased Na$^+$ absorption in the distal nephron leading to a low aldosterone and low plasma renin hypertension (▶ Liddle syndrome or pseudoaldosteronism), are activating mutations. These mutations remove a conserved proline-rich motif in the intracytoplasmic region of ENaC, important for channel endocytosis and degradation. Conversely, loss of function mutations causes Na$^+$ losing nephropathy with dehydration, hyperkalemia, elevated plasma renin and aldosterone levels characteristic of the recessive form of pseudohypoaldosteronism Type 1 (recessive PHA-1).

In the lung, ENaC is important for the ionic composition and the clearance of the airway surface liquid (ASL) (5). The activity of ENaC is inversely coupled to that of Cystic Fibrosis Transmembrane Regulator (▶ CFTR), responsible for chloride secretion at the apical membrane or airway epithelium. In cystic fibrosis, CFTR activity is lost and ENaC activity enhanced, causing an increased fluid reabsorption of ASL and increased mucous viscosity, preventing a normal mucociliary clearance. Conversely, loss of function muta-

tions of ENaC, as observed in recessive PHA-1, causes an increase of mucociliary clearance and a decrease in mucous viscosity. ENaC activity in the lung is developmentally regulated and plays a critical role at birth for a rapid and normal fluid reabsorption from the lung which turns from a secretory (fetal) to a reabsorptive (adult) mode. Respiratory distress syndrome (RDS) observed in premature newborn can, in part, be due to ENaC immaturity. In the fetal lung, ENaC maturation is controlled by glucocorticoids and, at birth, by sympatheticomimetics and pO$_2$. In the adult distal lung, ENaC activity is primarily controlled by β ▶ adrenergic agonist and pO$_2$. It plays an important role in the pathophysiology of high altitude pulmonary edema (HAPE), which can be greatly prevented by administration of β adrenergic drugs.

In the skin, ENaC is expressed in keratinocytes of the epidermis and in hair follicles. It could play a role in terminal differentiation by modulating keratinocyte calcium signaling. The skin expresses MR, GR and 11βHSD2, but the role of aldosterone and glucocorticoids on ENaC activity and keratinocyte differentiation is not yet understood.

In the tongue, ENaC is expressed in taste bude-pithelial cells. The expression of α, β and γ subunits at the apical membrane of taste buds is observed under low salt diet, known to greatly increase plasma aldosterone. This observation suggests that ENaC could play a significant role in the transduction of salt sensation.

In the inner ear, ENaC is expressed in supporting cells surrounding hair cells and is postulated to play a role in the low sodium concentration of endolymph, critical for proper mechano-transduction and hearing.

Drugs

ENaC is blocked from the tubular lumen of the distal nephron by amiloride at a submicromolar concentration. By blocking ENaC activity at the apical membrane of the target cell of the distal nephron, the electrochemical gradient favoring the passive secretion of potassium through ROMK2 (or other apically located K channels) is dissipated and potassium secretion blocked. Unlike loop diuretics (furosemide and analogues) or distal convoluted diuretics (i.e. thiazide diuretics), which cause potassium secretion and ▶ hypokalemia, amiloride and analogues cause potassium retention (and ultimately ▶ hyperkalemia) and are currently used as K^+-sparring diuretics. Spironolactone, a competitive antagonist of aldosterone for the mineralocorticoid receptor, inhibits epithelial sodium transport and potassium secretion and belongs to the same class of diuretic. Obviously, it is mostly effective when plasma aldosterone is elevated (▶ Primary or Secondary Aldosteronism), whereas amiloride is effective even in the presence of low circulating aldosterone. The biophysical characteristics of the block of ENaC by amiloride including voltage-dependence, competitive interaction with permeant cations, such as Na^+ or Li^+ ions, strongly suggest that amiloride is a pore blocker which, upon binding to its receptor on the channel, physically occludes the ion permeation pathway. The binding site for amiloride is located in the extracellular vestibule of the channel pore close to the ion selectivity filter and involves specific amino acid residues on each of the extracellular domain of the α β γ ENaC subunits. Amiloride shares its binding site on ENaC with triamterene which blocks the channel with a lower affinity.

Since the distal nephron under physiological conditions reabsorbs less than 10% of the filtered load of sodium, blockade of ENaC results only in a slight increase in urinary excretion of sodium. Consequently, amiloride is usually used in association with other diuretics. As suggested by genetic forms of hypertension associated with ENaC gain of function mutations, amiloride should be efficient in the treatment of low-renin, salt-sensitive hypertension but, unfortunately, its potency is markedly lowered by salt intake. The development of "non-competitive" antagonists of ENaC (i.e. potent in the presence of high luminal sodium) would be a useful addition to the drugs available today.

The development of amiloride analogues targeted to block selectively ENaC in the lung could be useful in the treatment of ▶ cystic fibrosis (CF) patients or more generally of patients suffering from chronic bronchitis, a condition in which an increased mucociliary clearance is highly desirable. Channel activators are presently not available but will be useful for the treatment of RDS in the newborn or HAPE in the adult, or, eventually, lung edema in congestive heart failure.

References

1. Rossier BC, Pradervand S, Schild L, Hummler E (2002) Epithelial sodium channel and the control of sodium balance: interaction between genetic and environmental factors. Annu. Rev. Physiol. 64:877–897.
2. Kellenberger S, Schild L (2002) Epithelial sodium channel/degenerin family of ion channels: a variety of functions for a shared structure. Physiol. Rev. 82:735–767.
3. Palmer LG, Garty H (2000) Epithelial Na Channels. In: Lippincott Williams & Wilkins (eds) The Kidney: physiology & pathophysiology, Third ed., volume 1, Philadelphia, p 251–276.
4. Lifton RP, Gharavi AG, Geller DS (2001) Molecular mechanisms of human hypertension. Cell 104:545–556.
5. Knowles MR, Boucher RC (2002) Mucus clearance as a primary innate defense mechanism for mammalian airways. J. Clin. Invest. 109:571–577.

EPS

▶ Extrapyramidal Side Effects
▶ Antipsychotic Drugs
▶ Dopamine System

EPSP

A postsynaptic potential or PSP is the voltage response of a postsynaptic neuron to a neurotransmitter released by a nerve terminal. The response may be depolarizing, in which case the voltage shift is in a positive direction causing an excitatory effect or EPSP, or hyperpolarizing, in which case the voltage shift is in a negative direction causing an inhibitory effect or IPSP.

▶ Ionotropic Glutamate Receptors

ER

ER can stand for the following

▶ Endoplasmatic Reticulum
▶ Estrogen Receptor

ERT

Stands for Estrogen Replacement Therapy.

▶ Hormone Replacement Therapy

ERGIC

▶ ER/Golgi Intermediate Compartment
▶ Protein Trafficking and Quality Control

ER/Golgi Intermediate Compartment

The endoplasmic reticulum (ER)/Golgi intermediate compartment (ERGIC) is composed of highly mobile tubovesicular structures (also known as VTCs = vesicular tubular clusters) located in the vicinity of the Golgi apparatus and also in the periphery of the cell. The ERGIC receives proteins from the ER and delivers them to the Golgi apparatus. The ERGIC concentrates proteins in the secretory pathway and is also part of the quality control system.

▶ Protein Trafficking and Quality Control

ErbB Receptor Family

▶ Epidermal Growth Factor Receptor Family
▶ Growth Factors
▶ Table appendix: Receptor Proteins

E

Erectile Dysfunction

Erectile dysfunction is treated by local or systemic application of vasodilator drugs. The most effective is sildenafil, a phosphodiesterase-type 5 inhibitor.

▶ Phosphodiesterases
▶ Smooth Muscle Tone Regulation

Ergot Alkaloids

Ergot alkaloids occur naturally in the fungus *Clavicepts purpurea* which infects cereal crops. Contaminated grain has caused epidemics of ergot poisoning for centuries. The key symptom of ergot poisoning is irreversible, painful peripheral vasoconstriction leading to peripheral gangrene (St. Anthony's fire). Ergot alkaloids are a rather heterogeneous group acting on adrenoceptors, dopamine receptors and 5-HT (serotonin)-receptors. Examples are ergotamine, dihydroergotamine, bromocryptine and methysergide. They are used in the prophylaxis and treatment of migraine, the treatment of parkinsonism and in the prevention of postpartum haemorrhage.

▶ α-Adrenergic System
▶ Dopamine System
▶ Serotoninergic System

Erythropoietin

Erythropoietin is a growth factor produced by interstitial cells of the kidney in response to hypoxia. Erythropoietin stimulates haematopoiesis in the bone marrow. Recombinant human erythropoietin is used to treat anemias, e.g. anemia caused by chronic renal failure and anemia in AIDS and cancer patients.

▶ Hematopoietic Growth Factors
▶ Cytokines

ESI-MS

▶ Electrospray Ionization Mass Spectrometry

EST

An EST is a short DNA sequence usually representing the most terminal regions of a cDNA clone.

▶ Microarray Technology

Estrogen Receptor

The estrogen receptor (ER) is the nuclear receptor for the hormone estrogen.

▶ Sex Steroid Receptors
▶ Selective Sex-Steroid Receptor Modulators

Estrogen Replacement Therapy (ERT)

▶ Hormone Replacement Therapy
▶ Selective Sex-Steroid Receptor Modulators
▶ Sex Steroid Receptors

Estrogens

Estrogens are 18-carbon steroids based on the estrane nucleus. In the non-pregnant female, they are mainly produced in the ovary.

▶ Sex Steroid Receptor
▶ Contraceptives
▶ Selective Sex-Steroid Receptor Modulators

Ethanol

HANS ROMMELSPACHER
University Hospital Benjamin Franklin,
Department of Clinical Neurobiology,
Free University Berlin, Germany
hans.rommelspacher@medizin.fu-berlin.de

Synonyms

Ethyl alcohol

Definition

C_2H_5OH, ▶ ethanol is formed by bacteria in the gastrointestinal tract in low amounts. Most of the ethanol of bacterial source is metabolized during the first liver passage yielding acetaldehyde and subsequently acetic acid.

▶ Drug Addiction/Dependence

Mechanism of Action

The main target structures in the brain that are affected by ethanol are ▶ GABA$_A$-receptors and glutamate- ▶ NMDA receptors. The action of the neurotransmitter γ-amino-butyric acid (▶ GABA) is facilitated, and the function of the NMDA-receptor is reduced by physiologically relevant concentrations of ethanol (10–50 mM). Therefore, this essay focuses on GABA and glutamate. Somewhat higher doses of ethanol affect other neuronal systems, among them endogenous opioids, dopamine and serotonin. Furthermore, second messenger and other intracellular mechanisms are altered after both acute and chronic exposure. Chronic ethanol abuse causes severe health problems. This essay does not deal with these aspects.

▶ GABA$_A$ receptor: The inhibitory GABA$_A$ and strychnine-sensitive glycine receptors are modulated positively by ethanol. Site-directed mutagenesis techniques have identified amino acid residues important for this action. Mutation of a single amino acid in specific transmembrane domains (TM2 (Ser270) and TM3) of the α$_2$ and β subunits of GABA$_A$ and glycine (TM2) receptors abolish the action of ethanol. Initial studies of transgenic mice with a reduced sensitivity to ethanol as measured by loss of righting reflex revealed an ethanol-resistant α$_1$-subunit of the glycine receptor (2). The corresponding mutations introduced into the γ subunit of GABA$_A$ -R had less effect. These findings indicate that in the GABA$_A$ receptor, ethanol may bind in a cavity formed between TM2 and TM3, and that binding to the α or β subunit may be more critical than to the γ subunit.

In an attempt to visualize the site of action of ethanol, tryptophan mutation at position S270, TM2 and TM3 domains of the GABA$_A$ α$_2$ subunit were modeled as antiparallel α-helices. The model showed that the region between S270 TM2 and TM3 contains a small cavity that may not be filled by side chains of adjoining helices. In contrast, the model of the S270W mutation demonstrated that the side chain of tryptophan completely occupied this cavity, which could eliminate occupation of the putative cavity by ethanol.

These findings were unexpected because previous studies had demonstrated that the γ$_2$ subunit is required for potentiation of GABA$_A$ receptor function by low concentrations of ethanol (2). The γ$_2$ subunit gene is located within a definitely mapped quantitative trait locus (QTL) for acute alcohol withdrawal on mouse chromosome 11 (1). Allelic variation was genetically correlated with acute alcohol withdrawal, ethanol-conditioned taste aversion, ethanol-induced motor incoordination and ethanol-induced hypothermia (1).

Furthermore, the γ$_2$ subunit of GABA$_A$-R is the most abundant subunit in the central nervous system (CNS) and is required for localization to synapses. The γ$_2$ subunit exists as two spliced variants, the long version (γ$_{2L}$) containing an additional eight amino acids in the large TM3/4 intracellular loop, relative to the short version (γ$_{2S}$). The extrapeptide sequence contains a consensus sequence for ▶ protein kinase C (PKC) phosphorylation. The γ$_{2L}$ subunit was at one time claimed to be essential for ethanol modulation of GABA$_A$-R function, presumably related to the unique PKC substrate on this subunit. Differential functions for γ$_{2L}$ and γ$_{2S}$ might involve rapid regulation of GABA$_A$-R channels by PKC. Another possibility is regulation of GABA$_A$-R subcellular targeting, trafficking, or turnover, presumably involving interactions with other proteins. Chronic ethanol induced a drop in the γ$_{2L}$/γ$_{2S}$ ratio, e.g. lower levels of the γ$_{2L}$ splice variant. This might favor production of α$_4$β$_2$γ$_{2S}$ receptor composition. This subtype differs markedly in various properties (compared to α$_4$βγ$_{2L}$) including sensitivity to zinc inhibition, channel kinetics, and possibly sensitivity to positive modulation by neurosteroids. PKC involvement in ethanol pharmacology and interactions with GABA$_A$-R is also supported by changes in ethanol sensitivity of mice lacking PKCγ and other subtypes of PKC. PKC$_\gamma$ null mutant mice displayed reduced sensitivity to the effects of ethanol on loss of righting reflex and hypothermia, and abolished the ethanol-enhancement of GABA$_A$ receptor agonist muscimol stimulated ^{36}Cl-uptake, demonstrating at least the link between behavioral actions of ethanol, PKC phosphorylation, and GABA receptor function (2).

PKC$_\varepsilon$ knockout mice are supersensitive to acute low-dose hyperlocomotor and high-dose sedative effects of ethanol and other drugs such as diazepam and pentobarbital, which allosterically activate GABA$_A$ receptors. In addition, these mice voluntarily consume 75% less alcohol than wild-

E

type mice when tested by using a two-bottle choice paradigm. They also showed about 50% less alcohol-reinforced operant responses than wild-type mice and reduced relapse drinking after a period of alcohol deprivation. These findings were not associated with metabolic changes of ethanol nor with receptor binding affinity or density in cerebral cortex, striatum or cerebellum. These findings suggest that PKC_ε regulates sensitivity to ethanol intoxication and thereby influences alcohol consumption. $GABA_A$ receptors from PKC_ε-null mice were more sensitive to activation by muscimol (GABA agonist) plus ethanol or flunitracepam. PKC_ε might regulate sensitivity of GABA receptors to allosteric activators possibly by phosphorylating the polypeptide.

Furthermore, PKC_ε is required for nerve growth factor-induced activation of mitogen-activated protein kinases and neurite outgrowth by ethanol. It is also required for ethanol-induced increases in N-type voltage-gated calcium channels in PC12 neural cells.

In several studies, chronic ethanol treatment has been associated with PKC up-regulation. In PC12 cells, increased levels of PKC_δ and ε were found (25 to 200 mM ethanol, 2 to 8 days of treatment) which was associated with increased PKC-mediated phosphorylation.

The possibility that acute ethanol directly activates PKC would seem to be ruled out by the lack of such effect occurring in various *in vitro* systems that have been studied. One possibility is the activation of a phosphatase, others are the modulation of the availability and type of activator. It is also possible that ethanol could modify the sensitivity of the ion channel to the effect of PKC phosphorylation or its proteolytic down-regulation.

Overall, our understanding of the precise location and substrates for the different PKC isoforms and protein-protein interactions involving PKC is still in its infancy.

Subunit changes are other mechanisms that alter the physiology of GABA synapses and account for plastic changes seen following chronic ethanol treatment.

Dependent on the various treatment regimes (continuous administration, chronic intermittent administration with multiple ethanol withdrawal, CIE) chronic ethanol produced reduced $GABA_A$-R mediated synaptic inhibition, hyperexcitability and seizure susceptibility. The α_6 subunit polypeptide was increased in cerebellum after both regimes, although there was no significant increase in α_6 mRNA in CIE in contrast to continuous ethanol paradigms and a decrease in α_1 subunit mRNA. A 20–30% increase in α_4 subunit mRNA was detected in hippocampal formation in CIE treatment paradigm. Thus, the cerebellar changes occur with chronic ethanol no matter which paradigm is used and are transient. They might contribute to short-term plasticity such as tolerance to motor impairment. Reduced function and altered pharmacological properties of GABA-R in the hippocampus of CIE rats were more persistent, lasting at least 2 days in some cases up to 40 days. Thus, the changes in this region such as increased α_4 and γ_{2S} subunits might be more important in the altered behaviour of CIE rats. Continuous ethanol also produced an increase in diazepam-insensitive binding (involving α_4 and α_6 subunits) in the cortex (specifically α_4 because α_6 is not found in cortex).

NMDA-glutamate receptor. The other important molecular target of ethanol is the ▶ N-methyl-D-apartate receptor (NMDA-R), which is acutely inhibited although the mechanism is not clear. It was speculated that at least in some brain region the coactivating glycine sites are involved and/or the coactivating polyamine sites. The receptors containing the NMDA-R2B subunits are the most ethanol-sensitive (4). The subunit has a fyn-kinase phosphorylation site that may rapidly render NMDA-R1 insensitive to ethanol during the development of acute tolerance.

NMDA-R play a major role in various aspects of chronic ethanol action, e.g. withdrawal and drug-dependent reorganization of neural circuitry (5). Long-term potentiation (LTP) and long-term depression (LTD) are important candidate mechanisms for the drug-induced reorganization of neural circuitry that occurs during addiction. Both processes require activation of NMDA-R. One exception is the dorsal striatum in which the rise in Ca^{2+} mediates the LTD by the activation of voltage dependent Ca^{2+} channels. It is interesting to note that the numbers of both the NMDA-R and the voltage-dependent Ca^{2+} channels (L-type, PKC_δ-dependent, N-type, PKC_ε-dependent) are increased after chronic ethanol (4). This is paralleled by an increase in NMDA-R function as measured by an NMDA-induced increase in $[^{21}Ca]$ influx. These events are present after 7 days of withdrawal and seem to be associated with lowered seizure threshold.

Distinct alterations in neural gene expression of NMDA-R1 splice variants and the NMDA-R2B subunit are observed after long-term ethanol ingestion. Increased mRNA levels of the NMDAR1-1 splice variant can be detected in all brain regions that expressed this isoform. On the other hand, the NMDA-R2B subunit decreases dramatically both at the mRNA and protein levels. However, 24 hrs after onset of withdrawal NMDA-R2B mRNA and hippocampal protein levels are elevated dramatically. Furthermore, NMDAR1-4 splice variant expression of mRNA and protein are elevated in the hippocampus 24 h after ethanol withdrawal. One may speculate that cells that express heterodimeric NMDA-R1/2B receptors are highly susceptible to ethanol. Another study found increases (~35%) in NR1, NR2A, and NR2B protein levels in homogenates from the cortex and hippocampus of rats exposed to intragastric infusions of ethanol for 6 days. There are consistent findings that during withdrawal, NMDA-Rs are overactivated pathologically by increased glutamate release and that this effect is accentuated by the interaction of polyamines acting *via* the 2B subunit.

AMPA receptor subunits GluR1, GluR2/3 and the kainate receptor subunits GluR5, GluR6 and KA2 are unaltered after 16 days of ethanol exposure. No adaptive changes of NMDA-R subunits are found in a recent study (6). Therefore maladaptive changes in brain ionotropic glutamate receptor levels do not underlie, in all cases, the neurobiological consequences of chronic ethanol exposure.

Opioid peptides

▶ Opioid systems in the brain are important for the reinforcing effects of ethanol. Selective μ-opioid receptor antagonists reliably decrease ethanol drinking in rats.

Chronic free-choice ethanol consumption causes increased β-endorphine immunoreactivity in the hypothalamus and septum of alcohol-preferring mice (C57BL/6), and Met-enkephalin in the nucleus accumbens of ethanol-prefering AA rats.

Continuous-access ethanol consumption caused a significant decrease in preproenkephalin mRNA expression in the nucleus accumbens and olfactory tubercle and a significant increase in mRNA in nuclei of the amygdala of fawn-hooded rats. Ethanol consumption had no significant effect on preprodynorphin mRNA. Thus, ethanol seems to negatively regulate enkephalin expression *in vivo*. The increase of preproenkephalin mRNA in the amygdala may be caused by the facilitating effect of ethanol on gabaergic neurones.

Cyclic AMP

Acutely, ethanol has been shown to potentiate G_S-stimulated cAMP accumulation. Conversely, brain tissue and cell culture treated chronically with ethanol have decreased levels of adenylyl cyclase activity (5). Tolerance to chronic ethanol is accompanied by a fall in the levels of $G_{\alpha S}$-proteins and $G_{\alpha S}$-mRNA in NG108-15 neuroblastomaxglioma cells and an increase in $G_{\alpha i2}$-proteins, in blood platelets from alcoholics up to 6 months after ethanol withdrawal (3). However, the contention that an increased level of $G_{\alpha i}$ and a reduced level of $G_{\alpha S12}$, respectively, are the cause of ethanol-induced tolerance was disputed in recent studies. Others have demonstrated a reduced catalylic activity of the ▶ adenylyl cyclase after 4 weeks ethanol in most but not all brain regions. The changes were not reflected by altered levels of the enzyme (3). Among the nine isoforms of adenylylcyclase, the type VII was activated by acute ethanol (50 mM) and prostaglandin E_1 (10 μM) 2–3-fold greater than that seen with the other tested adenylyl cyclases. PKC_δ is involved in ethanol modulation of AC activity. Ethanol could promote a conformational change in AC that provides or enhances availability of a site(s) for PKC_δ-mediated phosphorylation, or ethanol could promote the association of AC with PKC_δ within a transducisome complex. In the presence of ethanol the more phosphorylated form of AC7 becomes more sensitive to activated $G_{s\alpha}$. The increased levels of cAMP during such a signalling process will produce a greater effect of PKA and a greater modification of downstream effectors dependent on cAMP signalling (5).

Clinical Use (incl. side effects)

No clinical use, used in some medicinal drugs to solubilize active compounds.

References

1. Buck KJ, Metten P, Belknap JK, Crabbe JC (1997). Quantitative trait loci involved in genetic predisposition to acute alcohol withdrawal in mice. J. Neurosci. 17:3946–3955
2. Harris RA, Blednov Y, Findlay G, Mascia MP (2001). Can a single binding site account for actions of alcohols on $GABA_A$ and glycine receptors? Alcohol Clin. Exp. Res. 25:Suppl., 79S–80S
3. Lichtenberg-Kraag B, May T, Schmidt LG, Rommelspacher H (1995). Changes of G-protein levels in platelet membranes from alcoholics during short-term and long-term abstinence. Alcohol Alcohol 30:455–464
4. Lovinger DM (2000). Examination of ethanol spermine and acamprosate actions on native and recombinant NMDA receptors. Alcohol Clin. Exp. Res. 24:183A.
5. Tabakoff B, Nelson E, Yoshimura M, Hellevuo K, Hoffman PL (2001). Phosphorylation cascades control the actions of ethanol on cell cAMP signalling. J. Biomed. Sci. 8:44–51
6. Ferreira VM, Frausto S, Browning MD, Savage DD, Morato GS and Valenzuela CF (2001). Ionotropic glutamate receptor subunit expression in the rat hippocampus: lack of an effect of a long-term ethanol exposure paradigm. Alcoholism Clin Exp Res. 25 1536-41

Euglycaemia

Euglycaemia (normoglycaemia) is a blood glucose concentration within the normal range, e.g. fasting blood glucose 3.5–6.5 mmol/l; postprandial blood glucose 5–11 mmol/l (reference ranges vary between laboratories).

▶ Diabetes Mellitus
▶ Insulin Receptor
▶ Oral Antidiabetic Drugs

Eukaryotic Expression Cassette

The eukaryotic expression cassette is the part of an expression vector that enables production of a protein in a eukaryotic cell. The cassette consists of an eukaryotic promoter for mRNA transcription, the gene and a mRNA termination and processing signal (Poly-A signal).

Excitability

Excitability refers to the capacity of nerves and other tissues to generate and sometimes propagate action potentials, i.e. signals that serve to control intracellular processes, such as muscle contraction or hormone secretion. Examples of excitable cells and tissues include neurons and glia, muscle and endocrine tissues. Examples of non-excitable cells and tissues include blood cells, most epithelia and connective tissue.

▶ Ionotropic Glutamate Receptors
▶ Voltage-dependent Na^+ Channels
▶ Inward Rectifier K^+ Channels

Excitation-contraction Coupling

Excitation-contraction coupling (EC coupling) is the mechanism underlying transformation of the electrical event (action potential) in the sarcolemma into the mechanical event (muscle contraction) which happens all over the muscle. In other words, it is the mechanism governing the way in which the action potential induces the increase in the cytoplasmic Ca^{2+} which enables the activation of myofibrils.

▶ Ryanodine Receptor

Excitatory Amino Acids

▶ Glutamate

Excitotoxicity

Excitotoxicity is the over-activity of the glutamatergic system responsible for the large number of dead neurons observed after ischemia or epileptic seizures. This neuronal death is due to an over-excitation of the neurons and the massive Ca^{2+} entry resulting from the depolarization. Because of their large Ca^{2+} permeability, the NMDA iGlu receptors play a major role in the excitotoxic effect of glutamate.

▶ Ionotropic Glutamate Receptors

Exocytosis

R. JAHN, T. LANG
Max-Planck-Institut für biophysikalische
Chemie, Göttingen, Germany
rjahn@gwdg.de, tlang@.gwdg.de

Synonyms

(Constitutive, regulated, neuronal) secretion

Definition

Cellular secretion from (macro)-molecules mediated by fusion of vesicles with the plasma membrane

▶ Bacterial Toxins
▶ Intracellular Transport
▶ Small GTPases
▶ Synaptic Transmission

Basic Mechanisms

Constitutive and Regulated Exocytosis

During exocytosis, intracellular vesicles fuse with the plasmalemma. As a consequence, the vesicle components are incorporated into the plasma membrane and the vesicle content is released into the extracellular space. We distinguish constitutive and regulated exocytosis.

Constitutive exocytosis/secretion takes place in all eukaryotic cells and is essential for cell viability and growth. Trafficking vesicles destined for constitutive exocytosis originate from the trans Golgi-network and contain secretory macromolecules derived from the biosynthetic pathway. They are transported along microtubules to the cell surface and fuse with the plasma membrane. Constitutive secretion leads to the continuous release of secretory products and to the incorporation of membrane constituents into the plasmalemma. Hence, constitutive cargo is not stored within the cell. Excess plasma membrane is retrieved by endocytosis. The balance between exocytosis and endocytosis ensures ordered cell growth during proliferation and maintains a constant surface area in non-dividing cells. Proteins secreted by constitutive exocytosis include immunoglobulins, serum and milk proteins, and proteoglycans. In addition to vesicles derived from the biosynthetic route, recycling vesicles derived from endocytic precursor organelles (mostly endosomes) also fuse constitutively with the plasma membrane, thus returning endocytosed membrane constituents to the surface.

Regulated exocytosis differs from constitutive exocytosis in that secretion-ready vesicles are stored in the cytoplasm, often in large numbers, and that they require a stimulus for fusion with the plasma membrane. Regulated secretory cells include, for instance, exocrine and endocrine cells, mast cells, platelets, large granular lymphocytes, neutrophils and neurons. Depending on the cell type, exocytosis can be triggered by a variety of physiological stimuli that exert their action by means of receptor activation or electrical excitation. Release kinetics range from milliseconds in neurons to many minutes in exocrine and certain endocrine glands. All stimuli ultimately cause the transient rise of an intracellular second messenger, in most cases calcium. Calcium either directly

E

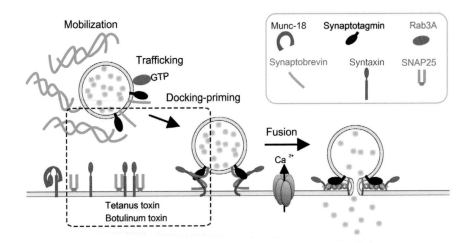

Fig. 1 Model for protein-mediated membrane fusion in neuronal exocytosis. Syntaxin and SNAP-25 form a complex on the plasma membrane that interacts with synaptobrevin on the synaptic vesicle membrane. The assembly of the resulting ternary complex forces the opposing membranes into close apposition. Such complex assembly may be enough to induce constitutive exocytosis. For neuronal exocytosis, fusion requires calcium that enters the cell via voltage-gated calcium channels. Triggering of fusion involves probably Ca^{2+}-induced interactions implicating synaptotagmin. A network of cytoskeletal elements controls the availability of secretory vesicles at the plasma membrane, and targeting of synaptic vesicles to docking sites may be carried out by Rab-GTPases. Tetanus and Botulinum toxins block exocytosis by specifically cleaving the neuronal SNAREs.

activates exocytosis or it operates in conjunction with cAMP and protein kinases that potentiate the effect of calcium. In some systems, calcium ions are only permissive, and the triggering stimulus involves other second messengers and signaling cascades. In electrically excitable cells, the intracellular calcium concentration rises after depolarization by calcium entry through voltage-gated calcium channels. In cells lacking regulated calcium influx pathways, hormones, acting mostly through G-protein-coupled receptors, cause the release of calcium from intracellular stores. Regulated exocytosis also differs from constitutive exocytosis in that secretory products are often packaged at high concentrations within the secretory vesicles. Thus secretory cells are capable of rapidly discharging large amounts of secretory products in a short time without the need for concomitant product biosynthesis.

In addition to secretory cells, many non-secretory cells are capable of regulating exocytotic fusion of transport vesicles that are derived from endosomal precursors. For instance, vesicles enriched in plasma membrane transport proteins are incorporated in a regulated manner in order to alter metabolite fluxes. Examples include the glucose transporter GLUT-4 in muscle and fat tissues, a key element in the control of serum glucose levels, and the vacuolar proton ATPase and aquaporins in the kidney that are essential for pH and water homeostasis. Last not least, regulated fusion of intracellular vesicles is used by many cells to repair tears in the plasma membrane.

Molecular Mechanisms of Exocytosis
Before exocytosis, the vesicle first moves from the cytoplasm to the plasmalemma. Second, the vesicle becomes attached to the plasma membrane, a process often referred to as docking. Third, activation involving metabolic energy, also referred to as priming, is required to achieve fusion competence. Finally, the vesicle and plasma membranes merge (see Figure). Each of these steps involves a multitude of proteins that operate by complex protein-protein and protein-phospholipid interaction networks. Although we are still far from a comprehensive molecular description, it is becoming clear that these steps are mediated by sets of com-

mon proteins that belong to evolutionary conserved protein families. While these proteins appear to operate in all intracellular fusion events (probably with the exception of mitochondria and peroxisomes), they are controlled by additional factors specific for a given fusion event or a given cell type.

Transport of vesicles occurs along microtubular tracks with the aid of kinesin motor proteins. In contrast, interactions with the actin-based microfilament network are thought to regulate the availability of vesicles for fusion, and they are also involved in certain types of vesicle movement. For instance, in neurons synaptic vesicles are thought to be attached to the actin cytoskeleton by crossbridges of synapsins that bind both to synaptic vesicles and to actin. Upon activation, synapsins are phosphorylated by calcium- and cAMP-dependent protein kinases, resulting in a weakening of binding affinities and the release of the vesicles from the cytoskeleton.

The initial contact between the vesicle and the plasma membrane is mediated by protein complexes that appear to be essential for ensuring that only appropriate membranes fuse. While more is known about the proteins involved in the "homotypic" docking of intracellular transport vesicles than in docking of vesicles to the plasma membrane, similar mechanisms may be involved. A key role has been assigned to Rab proteins, a family of Ras-related small GTPases. Apparently, each fusion step is controlled by a specific family member that resides on the vesicle membrane and appears to play a key role in recruiting docking proteins to the vesicle surface. Like ras, Rabs operate as molecular switches that are active in the GTP-form and inactive in the GDP-form. Active rabs recruit a variety of structurally diverse effector proteins to the vesicle that may then bridge the membranes destined to fuse. Protein recruitment may also be assisted by the phospholipid phosphatidylinositol bisphosphate (PIP2). Several Rab effectors possess characteristic PIP2-binding domains, and it is known that interference with the metabolism of PIP2 inhibits exocytosis in some systems.

Membrane fusion itself is probably the best understood step in the sequence of events leading to exocytosis, although many questions remain. Essential for fusion are the ▶ SNAREs, a super-family of small membrane proteins. Appropriate sets of three to four SNAREs spontaneously assemble from unstructured precursors into tight α-helical complexes that need metabolic energy for disassembly, and the assistance of the chaperone-like ATPase ▶ NSF, with additional cofactors for disassembly. Different sets of SNAREs are required for the various intracellular fusion steps. When appropriate SNAREs on the membranes destined to fuse contact each other, assembly is thought to pull the opposing membranes tightly together, a process that may suffice to initiate membrane fusion (see Figure). After fusion, the spent SNARE complexes are regenerated by ATP and NSF.

While the basic features of SNARE assembly and disassembly provide a convenient framework for explaining how membrane fusion works, both the regulation of SNAREs and the molecular details of fusion are not well understood. Most is known about the neuronal SNAREs that mediate regulated membrane fusion of synaptic vesicles and of secretory granules in neuroendocrine cells. They include synaptobrevin2, localized to the synaptic vesicle, and SNAP25 (▶ SNAPs) and syntaxin1A, both of which are localized to the plasma membrane. Several proteins are known that bind to these proteins and thus may regulate their activity. They include Munc-18, a syntaxin-binding protein, complexins that bind only to the fully assembled SNARE complex, and tomosyn which possesses a SNARE-like domain and competes with synaptobrevin. Genetic and physiological studies assign essential roles to these proteins in exocytosis, although their mechanism of action remains to be established.

While the steps described above are common to all exocytotic events, regulated secretion is distinguished by an additional layer of control proteins. Principally, each of the steps may be subject to regulation and thus control the overall rate of exocytosis, and there appears to be a large variety of mechanisms that is reflected in a kinetic range covering several orders of magnitude. Even for the universal second messenger calcium there seems to be no universal mechanism of action. In chromaffin cells and possibly also neurons, calcium controls the rate of several distinct and consecutive steps, the last being directly linked to membrane fusion. A prime candidate for the neuronal calcium receptor in the last step is

E

▶ synaptotagmin, a transmembrane protein of synaptic and secretory vesicles. Synaptotagmin possesses two calcium-binding modules (referred to as C2–domains) that interact in a calcium-dependent manner both with phospholipids and with SNAREs. Deletion of synaptotagmin largely abolishes calcium-dependent exocytosis whereas exocytosis can still be elicited by calcium-independent pathways. In other cells, however, the control of the exocytotic rate appears to occur at an earlier stage, e.g. by regulating vesicle availability through cytoskeletal interactions. Identifying and characterising such control mechanisms remains one of the most urgent tasks for future research.

While recent attention has been largely on proteins, it should be borne in mind that membrane fusion ultimately involves the merger of phospholipid bilayers. However, little is known about the specific membrane lipid requirements. When membranes fuse, energetically unfavourable transition states are generated that may require specific lipids and lipid domains for stabilization. Although there is some evidence for a specific influence of lipids on exocytosis, it is still unclear whether specific lipid metabolites are needed or even generated at the site of membrane merger.

Pharmacological Intervention

Exocytosis represents the final step in a multistep pathway involving vesicle formation and storage, transport to the plasma membrane by microtubule dependent transport, possibly involving additional cytoskeletal elements (e.g. the actin-myosin system), vesicle attachment to the plasma membrane, vesicle activation ("priming"), and finally membrane fusion. Each of these steps is probably regulated, but the details of such regulation have only been worked out in a few cases. Exocytosis can be regulated by many membrane receptors, dependent on the cell type, *via* second messengers or by electrical activity. Accordingly, regulated exocytosis can be controlled by appropiate receptor agonists and antagonists, by drugs influencing second messenger levels (e.g. Ca-channel blockers) or by reagents interfering with the cytoskeleton. However, most of the second messenger targets in exocytosis remain to be identified, and it is conceivable that they may emerge as

attractive drug targets. For instance, there is evidence that protein phosphorylation by protein kinases potentiates calcium-dependent exocytosis and in some cases suffices to induce exocytosis by itself, but it is not known which of the phosphorylated proteins are rate-limiting. Furthermore, the release of calcium from internal stores by second messengers may be an interesting point to control exocytosis by externally applied drugs. For example, hormones from pituitary gonadotropes are secreted in response to gonadotropin-releasing hormones. The gonadotropin releasing hormone receptor couples to a G-protein, which activates the phospholipase C cascade with production of inositol trisphosphate and oscillatory release of calcium from intracellular stores. Hormone secretion may be controled by interfering specifically with one of the steps in the cascade. Several biological toxins are known to directly affect exocytosis. Best characterized are the botulinal and tetanus neurotoxins, proteinaceous AB-toxins with a heavy chain mediating cell entry and a light chain that carries the catalytic activity. All light chains are proteases that cleave one of the three neuronal SNAREs and some of their close relatives. As a result, neuronal exocytosis is irreversibly inhibited. While extremely toxic upon systemic application, local application of botulinum neurotoxin A has become the treatment of choice for blepharospasm, hemifacial spasm, cervical dystonia and laryngeal dystonia. The toxin also alleviates pain and may be used in therapeutic trials for prediction of the response to surgical elongation. New toxin serotypes are now being tested. There are also cosmetic uses of Botulinum neurotoxin A. Local injections are used to diminish the undesirably negative and expressive wrinkles of the face by producing a reversible weakness of the hyperfunctional mimetic muscles of facial expression. In addition, several animal toxins block neurotransmission but the mechanism is different. These toxins cause massive exocytosis until the synaptic vesicle pool is exhausted. Best studied among these toxins is α-latrotoxin, the active ingredient of black widow spider venom, and probably also some snake toxins (e.g. crotoxin, taipoxin). Their mechanism of action, however, is not understood.

References

1. Burgess, T.L. and Kelly, R.B. (1987) Constitutive and regulated secretion of proteins. Annu Rev Cell Biol 3:243–293
2. Hille, B., Billiard, J., Babcock, D.F., Nguyen, T. and Koh, D.S. (1999) Stimulation of exocytosis without a calcium signal. J Physiol 520:23–31
3. Jahn, R. and Südhof, T.C. (1999) Membrane fusion and exocytosis. Annu Rev Biochem 68:863–911
4. Chen, Y.A. and Scheller, R.H. (2001) SNARE-mediated membrane fusion. Nat Rev Mol Cell Biol 2:98–106

Exon

An exon is a length of DNA in a gene that is transcribed into mRNA and translated into the final protein product.

▶ Intron

Exportins

Exportins are transport receptors at the ▶ nuclear pore complex needed for the selective export of proteins from the nucleus into the cytoplasm. They recognize nuclear export signal sequences of cargo proteins.

▶ Small GTPases

Extrapyramidal Side Effects

Extrapyramidal side effects (EPS) are adverse effects of D_2-receptor antagonists acting on the nigrostriatal system. EPS include parkinsonism (stiffness, slow movements, stooped posture, and tremor of extremities), akathisia (an inner sense of restlessness or need to move), and dystonia (spasm of a muscle group, most commonly involving the neck, extraocular muscles, and the tongue). Dose adjustment is often sufficient in managing these side effects, though use of other medications such as beta blockers (e.g. propranolol for akathisia), anticholinergic medications (e.g. benztropine for dystonia and parkinsonism), and amantadine (for parkinsonism), may sometimes be necessary.

▶ Antipsychotic Drugs
▶ Dopamine System

F

F-actin

F-actin (also called microfilament or actin filament) is a double-stranded, right-handed helix with 14 actin molecules per strand and turn. F-actin has a diameter of 8 nM and is polarized with a pointed (minus) and a barbed (plus) end.

▶ Cytoskeleton

Fab Fragments

Fab fragments are variable (specific) regions of antibodies.

▶ Humanized Monoclonal Antibodies

Factor IIa

▶ Thrombin
▶ Coagulation/Thrombosis
▶ Anticoagulants

FAD

▶ Flavin Adenine Dinucleotide
▶ Vitamins, watersoluble

Familial Persistent Hyperinsulinemic Hypoglycemia of Infancy

Familial persistent hyperinsulinemic (PHHI) is a rare, heterogenous metabolic disorder of neonates and infants characterized by severe hypoglycemia due to inappropriate and excessive insulin secretion. Different phenotypes of PHHI are associated with mutations of the SUR1 or the Kir6.2 gene that give rise to various recessive forms. Mutations in the glucokinase and glutamate dehydrogenase genes that result in mild, dominantforms of PHHI have also been identified.

▶ ATP-dependent K^+ Channels

Farnesyl Transferase Inhibitors

▶ Lipid Modifications

FasL

FasL is part of the tumour necrosis factor receptor super family, which are a family of proteins that share significant similarities in their extracellular ligand binding domains and in the intracellular effector or death domains. FasL or CD95L is a cell surface receptor ligand, which is involved in the transduction of signals for apoptosis. FasL- or CD95L-mediated apoptosis can be blocked by naturally occurring protein inhibitors, which can prevent apoptosis by serving as non-cleavable substrates for caspases.

▶ Apoptosis

Favism

Favism is the haemolysis observed after eating *Vica fava*. This reaction is observed in individuals with glucose-6-phosphate dehydrogenase deficiency. This common deficiency is also responsible for haemolysis in response to the antimalarial drug primaquine and others.

▶ Pharmacogenetics

Fever

Body temperature is controlled by the hypothalamus. Under normal conditions, the core body temperature is maintained at 37°C. Fever (Pyrexia) is an elevation of body temperature, following an increase in the hypothalamic set point. Substances causing an elevation of body temperature are called pyrogens. Exogenous pyrogens are, e.g., microbacterial products or toxins. They induce the release of endogenous pyrogens (pyrogenic ▶ cytokines) from monocytes, neutrophils and lymphocytes. Pyrogenic cytokines increase prostaglandin E_2 (PGE_2) production in the hypothalamus. PGE_2 binds to and activates four different ▶ G-protein coupled receptors (▶ prostanoids). Activation of only one of the four receptors, the EP-3 receptor, appears to be crucial for the increase in body temperature. Receptor activation results in an increased formation of cyclic AMP. The elevation of cyclic AMP appears to be responsible for the increase in the hypothalamic set point.

Antipyretic agents are drugs used for the treatment of fever. Commonly used antipyretic agents are acetaminophen (synonym paracetamol) and aspirin. Non-steroidal anti-inflammatory drugs are also effective antipyretics. All these agents act by inhibiting the constitutively expressed enzyme cyclooxygenase and thereby the synthesis of PGE_2 in the hypothalamus.

Fibrates

Fibrates are fibric acid derivatives, including e.g. bezafibrate, gemfibrozil, fenofibrate or clofibrate. Fibrates cause a marked reduction in circulating very low density lipoproteins (VLDL) as well as a modest (10%) reduction in low density lipoproteins (LDL) and an approximately 10% increase in high density lipoproteins (HDL). Many of the effects of fibrates on blood lipids are mediated by their interaction with ▶ peroxisome proliferator activated receptor (PPAR), which regulates gene-transcription in a variety of organs. Fibrates bind to the α-isotype of PPAR (PPARα), which is expressed primarily in the liver and brown adipose tissue and to a lesser extend in kidney, heart and skeletal muscle. Fibrates reduce triglycerides through PPARα-mediated stimulation of fatty acid oxidation, increased lipoprotein lipase synthesis and reduced expression of apoC-III. A major side-effect of fibrates is myositis, which is rare but can be severe. Fibrates are clinically used to treat elevated levels of triglycerides.

Fibrin

Fibrin is an elastic filamentous protein elaborated from its precursor, fibrinogen, which is present in plasma at high concentration. Fibrin is formed in response to the actions of thrombin. Thrombin cleaves small peptides from the fibrinogen molecule, forming fibrin monomers that will begin to polymerize and become crosslinked.

► Coagulation/Thrombosis
► Fibrinolytics

Fibrinogen

Fibrinogen is a 340 kD protein with an overall homodimeric structure, that is present at high concentrations in the plasma. Proteolytic cleavage of 4 small peptides by thrombin results in its polymerization to fibrin. The homodimeric structure allows fibrinogen to cross-bridge activated integrin $\alpha_{IIb}\beta_3$ integrin molecules on adjacent platelets, the crucial step in platelet aggregation.

► Coagulation/Thrombosis
► Fibrinolytics
► Antiplatelet Drugs

Fibrinolysis

► Fibrinolytics

Fibrinolytics

CHRISTOPHER F. TOOMBS
Amgen Inc., Thousand Oaks, USA
ctoombs@amgen.com

Synonyms

Thrombolytics

Definition

Fibrinolytic agents manipulate the function of the endogenous fibrinolytic system, which plays an important role in the maintenance of hemostasis by mediating the dissolution of ► fibrin clots and ► thrombus. The formation of fibrin clots and thrombus are important hemostatic responses to vascular injury that serve to prevent significant blood loss. In settings where fibrin clot and thrombus formation jeopardizes blood flow to a critcal organ such as the heart, fibrinolytic drugs can be used to dissolve the thrombus and restore blood flow.

► Anticoagulants
► Coagulation/Thrombosis

Mechanism of Action

In contrast to the function of ► platelets and the ► coagulation cascade, the endogenous fibrinolytic system can prevent a hemostatic response from both inappropriately propagating beyond the site of injury and can also effect clot dissolution. This occurs through the stimulation of the endogenous fibrinolytic system. The fibrinolytic system utilizes the plasminogen conversion into ► plasmin, whereby an inactive precursor molecule (plasminogen) is converted into an active serine protease (plasmin), which is capable of proteolytically degrading fibrinogen or fibrin into soluble fragments. The plasmin that is recruited for fibrinolysis may arise from either circulating- or clot-associated plasminogen. As a result, fibrinolysis can occur from within a clot and on its surface, thereby effecting clot dissolution. Under physiologic conditions, the endogenous fibrinolytic system is intimately involved in the maintenance of vascular patency and the clearance of hemostatic fibrin deposits, which occur with minor vascular injury.

The endogenous fibrinolytic system can be activated by any of several possible initiating events. For instance, activation of the fibrinolytic system can occur in response to vascular stasis, a condition that can be recognized by the endothelial lining of blood vessels. In response to stasis, the endothelium can release an enzyme, known as ► tissue plasminogen activator or tPA, which is a serine protease than can cleave plasminogen and liberate plasmin. In addition, plasmin can be generated in reponse to the formation of activated factor XII (XIIa) or by kallikrein, both of which are involved in the initiation of coagulation through contact activtion.

The inhibitors of the endogenous fibrinolytic system include α−2 antiplasmin, which forms a

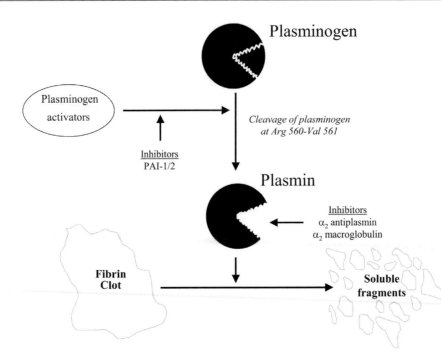

Fig. 1 Plasminogen is the inactive precursor molecule that is converted into the active serine protease, plasmin. The plasminogen activators effect this conversion by promoting cleavage of plasminogen at an arginine-valine bond. The plasminogen activators can be antagonized by their endogenous inhibitor, plasminogen activator inhibitor 1 or 2 (PAI-1/2). Once formed, plasmin mediates the breakdown of insoluble fibrin clot into soluble fragments. However, plasmin can be antagoized by the actions of alpha-2 antiplasmin or alpha-2 macroglobulin.

complex with and inhibits the activities of plasmin. In addition, endogenous tPA can be inhibited by plasminogen acivator inhibitor, of which there are two isoforms (PAI-1 and PAI-2).

The specific fibrinolytic agents include those derived from both bacterial and mammalian origin. For example, streptokinase is a natural product of group C hemolytic *streptococci* and commercial preparations of streptokinase are purified forms of the protein. The name streptokinase is a bit of a misnomer since an enzymatic activity is implied by the suffix "-ase". However, streptokinase does not enzymatically activate plasminogen to plasmin, rather, it forms a noncovalently associated (1:1) complex with plasminogen. While streptokinase alone does not possess enzymatic activity, the complex it forms is referred to as the "streptokinase:plasminogen activator complex" because it is capable of generating plasmin.

Anistreplase is related to streptokinase and is a commercial preparation of the streptokinase:plasminogen activator complex. The product is derived from the combination of streptokinase (from bacterial sources) and anisoylated lys-plasminogen (from human plasma). The anisoylation of the plasminogen renders the streptokinase:plasminogen complex inactive. Upon administration, anistreplase becomes active as spontaneous deacylation of the complex occurs *in vivo*, liberating an active streptokinase:plasminogen complex.

Among the first mammalian derived fibrinolytic agent is urokinase. Urokinase is produced in the kidneys where it is normally responsible for the dissolution of thrombus or fibrin clot that may have formed in the renal vasculature. Urokinase can be purified from urinary sources or can be prepared from primary cell culture of fetal kidney tissue.

Alteplase is the recombinant version of the tPA that is released from the endothelium in the endogenous fibrinolytic system. Alteplase is a poor plasminogen activator on its own. However in the presence of fibrin, alteplase binds to fibrin through an association at the finger domain of the tPA molecule and, as a result, its enzymatic activity is greatly enhanced. The "fibrin specificity" of alteplase was thought to be the basis of the added clinical benefit obtained with alteplase (versus streptokinase) in patients with acute myocardial infarction as demonstrated in the landmark GUSTO study (1).

Through molecular biology, mutations of tPA have also been produced. Reteplase is a derivative of alteplase, which involves deletion of the finger, EGF and kringle-1 domains of the native tPA molecule. In this deletion, the finger domain (fibrin binding) and the EGF domain (hepatic binding) are removed. This has the net effect of prolonging the half-life of reteplase (due to reduced hepatic clearance) while at the same time reducing the fibrin specificity of the molecule.

Tenecteplase is a genetically engineered mutation of alteplase where specific amino acid substitutions have been made in three positions on the native tPA molecule. Collectively, these amino acid substitutions serve three purposes: 1) increasing the circulating half-life of tenecteplase; 2) increasing the fibrin specificity of tenecteplase, and 3) reducing tenecteplase's susceptibility to its principal inhibitor molecule, plasminogen activator inhibitor (PAI-1).

Despite the modifications to reteplase and tenecteplase, which alter the pharmacologic activity of these agents, in large scale trials where these agents have been compared with native tPA, the efficacy results are very similar (2,3).

Clinical Use (incl. side effects)

Fibrinolytic agents are used clinically when dissolution of fibrin clot and thrombus is needed to restore blood flow to a critical organ vascular bed. One of the earliest uses of urokinase was for treatment of massive pulmonary embolism (one or more lobes affected) or where pulmonary embolism is accompanied by hemodynamic instability. Pulmonary angiography or lung scanning, prior to the initiation of thrombolytic therapy is recommended to confirm the diagnosis of pulmonary embolism. In cases of successful lysis, thrombolytic therapy can be expected to improve capillary wedge pressure and improve ventilatory capacity.

The more widely practiced use of fibrinolytics is in the treatment of acute myocardial infarction, as shown in the GISSI trial (4) that evaluated streptokinase. Over the past two decades, the benefit of fibrinolysis in Q-wave myocardial infarction has been repeatedly demonstrated, using virtually all of the available fibrinolytic drugs. As a result, fibrinolysis is indicated for treatment of acute myocardial infarction, and therapy should be administered as soon as possible following the onset of symptoms. Successful lysis can be expected to improve ventricular function and reduce the incidence of congestive heart failure and mortality associated with acute myocardial infarction.

More recently, fibrinolytics have gained an indication for use in the management of acute ischemic stroke, although alteplase is the only agent approved in this indication. The diagnosis of acute ischemic stroke must be confirmed by computerized tomography (CT) scanning in order to differentiate ischemic stroke from hemorrhagic stroke, which might be worsened by the administration of a fibrinolytic drug. Therapy should only be initiated within the first 3 hours following the onset of symptoms and where successful, fibrinolysis is effective in improving neurologic recovery and reducing the incidence of disability.

During pharmacologic induced fibrinolysis, the endogenous inhibitors of the fibrinolytic system are overwhelmed by pharmacologic dosages of fibrinolytic agents. As a result, fibrinolytic activity occurs throughout the entire cirulatory system and often results in an excessive generation of plasmin and the creation of a systemically fibrinolytic state, termed plasminemia. Unfortunately, the plasmin cannot differentiate between a pathologic thrombus (such as one whcih has precipitating a myocardial infarction) and a thrombus that is beneficial for the healing process following minor trauma or injury. As a result, clot dissolution can occur systemically and this forms the basis for the contraindication and side effects that can occur with fibrinolytic therapy.

The absolute contraindications to fibrinolytic therapy are generally consistent across the specific agents and are related to either the presence of bleeding or a bleeding phenotype or any conditions where, should bleeding occur, the outcome would be catastrophic. Examples of the contraindications include: known bleeding diathesis, active internal bleeding, history of cerebrovascular accident, recent intracranial or intraspinal surgery, recent trauma, intracranial neoplasm, arteriovenous malformation, aneurysm or severe, uncontrolled hypertension.

The most common adverse reaction to thrombolytic therapy is bleeding. Bleeding is generally classified as major or minor and is dependent upon the location and severity of the bleeding event. Examples of major bleeding events would include intracranial hemorrhage, gastrointestinal bleeding, genitourinary bleeding or retroperitoneal bleeding. Examples of minor bleeding would include minor hematoma formation or bleeding at catheterization and recent venipuncture sites.

While bleeding is the principle complication of thrombolytic therapy, other adverse events have been observed. Anaphylactic reactions to thrombolytic agents are very rare but have been reported. More moderate allergic reactions can occur with streprokinase, anistreplase and urokinase and can present as fever, chills and shaking. The incidence of allergic-like reactions appears to be greatly reduced for the tissue-type plasminogen activator molecules.

During fibrinolytic therapy, significant alteration of the hemostatic system occurs in order to accomplish clot dissolution. The typical laboratory findings can be expected to reveal several changes in plasma and serum values, including decreased coagulation factors (factors V, VIII, IX, XI and XII), prolonged coagulation times, elevated plasmin and consumption of fibrinogen.

Significant drug interactions are also possible when using fibrinolytic therapy. The anticoagulant agents such as heparin (unfractionated and low molecular weight) and the vitamin K antagonists are capable of causing bleeding when used by themselves. In addition, antiplatelet agents such as aspirin, dipyridamole, ADP receptor antagonists and fibrinogen receptor antagonists are also associated with an increased risk of bleeding. As such, the concomitant use of anticoagulant and antiplatelet agents can increase the risk of bleeding associated with thrombolytic therapy. Careful laboratory monitoring of hemostatic parameters is warranted when these agents are used in combination with thrombolysis.

References

1. The GUSTO Investigators (1993) An international randomized trial comparing four thrombolytic strategies for acute myocardial infarction. New Engl J Med. 329:673
2. ASSENT-2 Investigators (1999) Single-bolus tenecteplase compared with front-loaded alteplase in acute myocardial infarction: the ASSENT-2 double-blind randomised trial. Lancet 354:716–22
3. The GUSTO III Investigators (1997) A comparison of reteplase with alteplase for acute myocardial infarction. New Engl J Med. 337:1118–1123
4. GISSI. (1986) Effectiveness of intravenous thrombolytic treatment in acute myocardial infarction. Gruppo Italiano per lo Studio della Streptochinasi nell'Infarto Miocardico (GISSI) Lancet 1:397–402

Fibroblast Growth Factors

Fibroblast growth factors (FGFs) are a group of about 20 growth factors, which function through a group of receptor tyrosine kinases (FGF-R-1, -2, -3 and -4). They play multiple roles in the morphogenesis and growth of higher organisms.

▶ Growth Factors

First-order Kinetics

First order kinetics describes the most common time course of drug elimination. The amount eliminated within a time-interval is proportionate to the drug concentration in the blood.

▶ Pharmacokinetics

First-pass (presystemic) Metabolism

First-pass metabolism is the elimination of an orally administed drug by the liver or sometimes the gut wall, before it reaches the systemic circulation. First-pass metabolism results in a decreased systemic bioavailability.

▶ Pharmacokinetics

Flare

Flare is the surrounding redness caused by the vasodilatation of local blood vessels in the skin (hyperaemia). Histamine released at the site of contact acts on sensory nerve endings in the skin. Impluses travel along the axon to other peripheral branches of the same neuron to cause release of vasodilataory peptide neurotransmitters from nerve endings serving a wider area of skin than the initial contact point. Impluses reaching the CNS are interpreted as itch and pain.

▶ Histaminergic System

Flavin Adenine Dinucleotide

Flavin Adenine Dinucleotide (FAD) ($C_{27}H_{33}N_9O_{15}P_2$) is a coenzyme that acts as a hydrogen acceptor in dehydrogenation reactions in an oxidized or reduced form. FAD is one of the primary cofactors in biological redox reactions.

▶ Vitamins, watersoluble

Flavin Mononucleotide

Flavin Mononucleotide (FMN) ($C_{17}H_{21}N_4O_9P$) is a phosphoric ester of riboflavin that constitutes the cofactor of various flavoproteins.

▶ Vitamins, watersoluble

Flp/FRT

Flp/FRT is a system analogous to the cre/loxP system. Flp is a yeast enzyme which recognizes FRT sites. If two FRT sites have a parallel orientation, the DNA segement between these sites will be deleted by the action of the Flp recombinase.

▶ Transgenic Animal Models

Fluorides

Fluoride is a mineral ion that stimulates bone formation by protein kinase activation-mediated effects on osteoblasts. Fluorides have been used in the treatment of osteoporosis, but their anti-fracture effect is not undisputed.

▶ Bone Metabolism

Fluoroquinolones

A fluorine atom in position 6 of the basic structure of quinolones enhances the antimicrobial activity considerably. All widely used quinolones are fluorinated in position 6 and the term "fluoroquinolones" is often used to describe these drugs. However, some new quinolones with similar antimicrobial activity are not fluorinated in position 6 (e.g. garenoxacin, PGE9262932) and therefore the term "quinolones" is more appropriate to describe this group of antimicrobial agents.

▶ Quinolones

FMN

▶ Flavin Mononucleotide
▶ Vitamins, watersoluble

Folate

▶ Folic Acid
▶ Dihydrofolate Reductase

Folic Acid

▶ Vitamines, watersoluble

Follicle-stimulating Hormone

FHS
▶ Contraceptives

Follitrophin

▶ Follicle-stimulating Hormone

Force Fields / Molecular Mechanics

Force field methods, also called molecular mechanics, are empirical approaches to calculate molecular geometries and energies. The general aim of a force field calculation is to find that conformation of the three-dimensional structure of a molecule or complex with the minimal energy. The acting forces between the atoms are described by analytical functions with customisable parameters. Covalent as well as non-covalent forces are considered.

The basic idea of force fields is the assumption that bond length and bond angles adjusts whenever possible to standard values. Steric hindrance of non-bonded atoms can cause non-ideal values of bond length and angle. The repulsive interaction is called van der Waals interaction. A force field equation to calculate the energy of the structure for a molecule contains at least the terms van der Waals interaction, bond length stretching, angle deformation and torsion angle deformations. Many force fields contain additional terms like electrostatic attraction and others. The derived force field for each term is achieved by calibration on experimental structural data, quantum-chemical calculation and, if included, charge-type calculations. There are a variety of different force fields calibrated for certain type of molecules and solutes. Among the force fields for proteins the AMBER force field is suitable for protein calculations in vacuum and water, the GROMACS force field is suitable for proteins in water and lipid environments.

▶ Molecular Modelling
▶ Bioinformatics

Forskolin

Forskolin is a diterpene derivative from the Indian plant *Coleus forskohlii* . It activates all isozymes of adenylyl cyclase except types IX and X. Active derivatives of forskolin include:
7-deacetyl-forskolin (EC_{50} ~20µM), 6-acetyl-7-deacetyl-forskolin (EC_{50} ~40µM),
7-deacetyl-7-O-hemisuccinyl-forskolin (EC_{50} ~50µM). The last of these has been used as an immobilized affinity chromatography ligand for the purification of adenylyl cyclases from tissues.

▶ Adenylyl Cyclases

Frontal Cortex

The frontal cortex consists of 3 main structures: 1. motoric regions (including the Broca area and ocular areas), 2. the prefrontal cortex and 3. the orbital cortex. The prefrontal cortex is associated with attention, arousal and expectation, the orbital cortex with motivation.

▶ Psychostimulants

FSH

▶ Follicle-stimulating Hormone
▶ Contraceptives

F-type ATPase

▶ Table appendix: Membrane Transport Proteins

Functional Genomics

Functional genomics (sometimes refered to as functional proteomics) aims at determining the function of the proteome (the protein complement encoded by an organism's entire genome). It expands the scope of biological investigation from studying single genes or proteins to studying all genes or proteins at once in a systematic fashion, using large-scale experimental methodologies combined with statistical analysis of the results.

▶ Bioinformatics
▶ Gene Expression Analysis
▶ Microarray Technology
▶ Pharmacogenetics

Functional Proteomics

▶ Functional Genomics

Fungi

Fungi (Mycophyta, Mycota, Eumycetes) are chlorophyll-free plants, eukaryotic cells growing in hyphae or yeasts and causing diseases in plants, animals and humans.

▶ Antifungal Drugs

Fungicidal Effect

A fungicidal effect is that which kills the fungal cell.

▶ Antifungal Drugs

Fungistasis/Fungistatic

Fungistasis is the inhibition of fungal growth without killing the fungal cell.

▶ Antifungal Drugs

Funicular Myelitis

The neurological disorder associated with severe vitamin B12 deficiency is termed funicular myelitis. Vitamin B12 deficiency leads to disturbed choline, phospholipid and nucleic acid syntheses, resulting in spinal marrow damage. Disturbed myelin synthesis finally causes irreversible neurological failure. In addition, there are psychiatric disturbances (disturbed memory, apathy).

▶ Vitamins, watersoluble

Furin

Furin, also known as paired basic amino-acid-cleaving enzyme (PACE), is a membrane bound subtilisin-like serine protease of the trans-Golgi compartment. It is ubiquitously expressed and mediates processing of many protein precursors at Arg-X-Lys/Arg-Arg sites.

So far, seven mammalian precursor convertases (PCs) have been identified: furin, PC1, PC2, PC4, PC5, PACE4 and PC7.

▶ Somatostatin

Furin-like Protease

Furin-like protease is a prohormone convertase, a pro-protein-processing enzyme with cleavage selectivity for paired basic amino acid residues.

▶ Endothelins

Fyn

Fyn is a non-receptor tyrosine kinase related to Src that is frequently found in cell junctions. The protein is N-myristoylated and palmitoylated and thereby becomes associated with caveolae-like membrane microdomains. Fyn can interact with a variety of other signaling molecules and controls a diversity of biological processes such as T cell receptor signaling, regulation of brain function, and adhesion mediated signaling.

▶ Tyrosine Kinases

FYVE Domain

The FYVE domain is a phosphatidylinositol-3-phosphate-binding module of approximately 60 to 80 amino acids. It was named after the first four proteins, where this domain was described (Fab1p, YOTB, Vac1p and EEA1).

▶ Phospholipid Kinase

G

GABA

GABA$_A$ Receptor

GABA$_A$ receptors are pentameric complexes on the postsynaptic membrane with a central pore with selectivity for chloride ions. Benzodiazepines increase the GABA-induced chloride currents, which lead to hyperpolarization of the postsynaptic membrane.

GABA$_B$ Receptors

GABA$_B$ receptors mediate the slow and prolonged physiological effects of the inhibitory neurotransmitter GABA. Functional GABA$_B$ receptors are comprised of two subunits, GABA$_B$R1 and GABA$_B$R2. Both subunits are G-protein-coupled receptors, which couple to the Gi/o family and are densely expressed at spinal nociceptive synapses.

GABAergic System

UWE RUDOLPH
Institute of Pharmacology and Toxicology,
University of Zürich, Zürich, Switzerland
rudolph@pharma.unizh.ch

Definition

GABA (γ–aminobutyric acid) is an amino acid with mostly inhibitory functions in the mammalian central nervous system. Structures involved in releasing or binding GABA as a neurotransmitter constitute the GABAergic system. The GABAergic system is involved in the regulation of vigilance, anxiety, muscle tension, epileptogenic activity and memory functions.

Basic Characteristics

GABA is the major inhibitory neurotranmitter in the mammalian central nervous system. It is synthesized in presynaptic terminals from glutamate by the action of the enzyme glutamic acid decarboxylase, stored in vesicles and released upon the arrival of an action potential. GABA binds to and mediates its effects via postsynaptic ionotropic GABA$_A$ receptors and pre- and postsynaptic metabotropic GABA$_B$ receptors (Fig. 1). Whereas the GABA$_A$ receptors mediate fast responses, the GABA$_B$ receptors mediate slow responses. GABA is removed from the synaptic cleft by GABA trans-

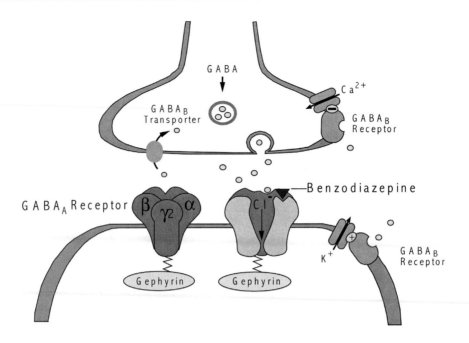

Fig. 1 GABAergic synapse. Schematic of a GABAergic synapse, depicting the major elements of signal transduction. Postsynaptic GABA$_A$ receptors are pentameric ligand-gated ion channels assembled from various types of subunits. On the cytoplasmatic site they are indirectly linked to gephyrin. GABA$_B$ receptor occur pre- and postsynaptically and are coupled to calcium or potassium channels.

porters and metabolized in a transamination reaction.

GABA$_A$ Receptors

GABA$_A$ receptors are pentameric membrane protein complexes that operate as GABA-gated chloride channels (1). They belong to the superfamily of ligand-gated ion channels. They have an extracellular N-terminal domain, four putative transmembrane domains and an extracellular C-terminal domain. The third intracellular loop contains consensus sequences for phosphorylation by protein kinases. The second transmembrane domain presumably lines the channel. On the cytoplasmic side, most GABA$_A$ receptors are indirectly linked to the cytoskeletal protein gephyrin via the γ2 subunit; these two components have been shown to play a role in synaptic clustering of defined GABA$_A$ receptors. The GABA$_A$ receptor subunits are drawn from seven classes with mostly multiple variants (α1–α6, β1–β3, γ1–γ3, ρ1–ρ3, δ, ε, θ). The α subunits share greater than 70% amino acid sequence identity, whereas from one subunit class

to the other, e.g. α and β, the amino acid sequence identity is in the range of ca. 30–40%. Most GABA$_A$ receptors are composed of α, β and γ subunits with α1β2,3γ2 being the most abundant receptor subtype. Some evidence suggests that the pentamers may contain two α subunits, two β subunits and one γ subunit. GABA$_A$ receptors are responsible for the fast synaptic inhibition. Binding of GABA to the receptor is followed in a matter of milliseconds by a chloride influx, leading – in most cases – to hyperpolarization and thus functional inhibition of the postsynaptic neuron. GABA$_A$ receptors are of physiological relevance because they play an essential role in the regulation of the excitability of the brain. They are, in addition, of pharmacological relevance since their activity is modulated by a variety of therapeutic agents. These include benzodiazepines, barbiturates, neurosteroids and general anesthetics (Fig. 2). A subset of GABA$_A$ receptors is frequently referred to as "GABA$_C$" receptor (2). These receptors are composed of ρ subunits, which only assemble with each other and are

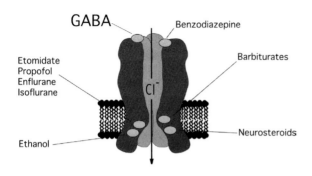

GABA

Benzodiazepine

Etomidate
Propofol
Enflurane
Isoflurane

Barbiturates

Cl⁻

Neurosteroids

Ethanol

Fig. 2 Model of a GABA$_A$ receptor and its binding sites. In addition to the binding site for the neurotransmitter GABA, GABA$_A$ receptors have modulatory binding sites for a variety of ligands including benzodiazepines, barbiturates, neurosteroids, ethanol and general anaesthetics such as isoflurane, enflurane, etomidate and propofol. The positioning and size of the binding sites is arbitrary. One subunit has been removed to visualize the pore.

found primarily in the retina. In contrast to the typical GABA$_A$ receptors, these receptors are insensitive to the classical GABA$_A$ receptor antagonist bicuculline. In the IUPHAR nomenclature (3) these receptors are classified as GABA$_A$ receptors.

GABA$_A$ receptors are widely expressed in the central nervous system (4), balancing the excitatory neurotransmission. The GABA$_A$ receptor subtypes display a differential distribution. The $\alpha 1$ subunit, which is by far the most abundant α subunit, is expressed e.g. in cerebral cortex, hippocampus and thalamus, the $\alpha 2$ subunit e.g. in hippocampus, striatum and amygdala, the $\alpha 3$ subunit e.g. in monoaminergic and serotonergic neurons of the brain stem, in basal forebrain cholinergic neurons and in the reticular nucleus of the thalamus, the $\alpha 4$ subunit e.g. in the thalamus, the $\alpha 5$ subunit e.g. in the hippocampus, and the $\alpha 6$ subunit in cerebellar granule cells. Among the β subunits, the $\beta 2$ subunit is the most abundant, followed by the $\beta 3$ and $\beta 1$ subunits. The by far most abundant γ subunit is $\gamma 2$, whereas $\gamma 1$ and $\gamma 3$ are rare. In some instances, receptors contain a δ subunit presumably instead of a γ subunit. The GABA binding site is most likely located at the interface between α and β subunits. The binding site for modulatory benzodiazepines is, however, most likely located at the interface between α and γ subunits. Recombinant receptors consisting of α and β subunits are only activated by GABA, but not modulated by benzodiazepines. The GABA$_A$ receptors containing the $\alpha 1$, $\alpha 2$, $\alpha 3$ and $\alpha 5$ subunits (in addition to β and γ subunits) are sensitive to modulation by classical benzodiazepines such as diazepam, whereas receptors containing the $\alpha 4$ and $\alpha 6$ subunits are not. The latter receptors are also referred to as "diazepam-insensitive" GABA$_A$ receptors. Whereas the diazepam-sensitive α subunits $\alpha 1$, $\alpha 2$, $\alpha 3$ and $\alpha 5$ contain a histidine residue at a conserved position in the N-terminal extracellular region (postions $\alpha 1$-H101, $\alpha 2$-H101, $\alpha 3$-H126 and $\alpha 5$-H105), the diazepam-insensitive $\alpha 4$ and $\alpha 6$ subunits contain an arginine residue in the corresponding position ($\alpha 4$-R99 and $\alpha 6$-R100). Mutational analysis revealed that the presence of a histidine residue or an arginine residue at this position in the α subunit determines whether the respective GABA receptor is diazepam-sensitive or diazepam-insensitive, respectively. Depending on their sensitivity to CL218872, GABA$_A$ receptors can be further classified into those having a high affinity for CL218872 ($\alpha 1\beta x\gamma 2$) and those having a low affinity for CL218872 ($\alpha 2\beta x\gamma 2$, $\alpha 3\beta x\gamma 2$ or $\alpha 5\beta x\gamma 2$). A glycine in position 201 of the $\alpha 1$ subunit has been found to be necessary for high affinity binding of CL218872 to the respective receptor. The imidazopyridine zolpidem, which binds to the benzodiazepine site, has intermediate affinity for different GABA$_A$ receptor subtypes: It has a high affinity for $\alpha 1\beta x\gamma 2$, $\alpha 2\beta x\gamma 2$ and $\alpha 3\beta x\gamma 2$ receptors, but essentially no affinity for $\alpha 5\beta x\gamma 2$ receptors. The rare $\gamma 3$ subunit may also confer zolpidem-insensitivity to GABA$_A$ receptors.

Pharmacological Intervention

Several groups of CNS active drugs exert all or some of their clinical effects by their action on the GABAergic system.

Benzodiazepines

▶ Benzodiazpines act by shifting the GABA dose-response curve to the left and thus increases the affintiy of the receptors for GABA. At a given concentration of GABA in a synapse the chloride current will be increased. Benzodiazpines have no action in the absence of GABA (use-dependence)

G

and cannot increase maximal physiological stimulation by a high concentration of GABA, i.e. their action is self-limiting, which most likely contributes to the safety of these drugs with respect to overdoses. They are used as anxiolytics, sedatives, hypnotics, anticonvulsants and central muscle relaxants. At the molecular level, benzodiazepines increase the opening frequency and thus the number of channels that are opened by a given concentration of GABA.

By introducing histidine to arginine point mutations in the $\alpha 1$, $\alpha 2$ and $\alpha 3$ subunits the respective $GABA_A$ receptors are rendered diazepam-insensitive. Thus, it was found that the sedative, the anterograde amnesic and in part the anticonvulsant actions of diazepam are mediated by $GABA_A$ receptors containing the $\alpha 1$ subunit, whereas its anxiolytic and muscle relaxant actions are mediated by $GABA_A$ receptors containing the $\alpha 2$ subunit (5). The anxiolytic action is observed at much lower concentrations than the muscle relaxant action.

Barbiturates

The binding site for ▶ barbiturates on the $GABA_A$ receptor is less well defined. Barbiturates act by increasing the conductance level. In contrast to benzodiazepines, they also display direct agonistic action on $GABA_A$ recptors. Also in contrast to benzodiazepines, their action is not self-limiting, i.e. they can activate the $GABA_A$ receptor to higher levels than high concentrations of GABA alone. These features may be responsible for the fact that overdoses of barbituarates are life-threatening.

General Anaesthetics

Both volatile and intranvenous anesthetics have been shown to modulate the activity of the $GABA_A$ receptor, and the assumption is reasonable that these actions may contribute to at least some of the clinical effects of general anaesthetics. Though a binding site for general anesthetics on the $GABA_A$ receptor is still elusive, several mutations in the second and third transmembrane regions of α and β subunits have been identified that can abolish or inhibit the action of general anesthetics. These include the volatile anesthetics isoflurane and enflurane and the intravenous anesthetics propofol, etomidate and also barbiturates. Interestingly, these mutations may affect the agonistic and the modulatory actions of general anesthetics independently. Whereas mutations in both α and β subunits inhibit the actions of isoflurane and enflurane on the $GABA_A$ receptor, only mutations in the β subunits inhibit the actions of propofol and etomidate. Since many general anaesthetics, in particular the volatile anaesthetics also act on other excitatory and inhibitory neurotransmitters and also on two-pore domain potassium channels (background channels), the contribution of the $GABA_A$ receptor system as a whole and specific $GABA_A$ receptor subtypes in particular to certain anesthetic endpoints is not known and may be different for each drug. In recombinant systems, the ε subunit, which is found in amygdala and thalamus and which is particularly abundant in the subthalamic nucleus, confers insensitivity of recombinant $\alpha\beta\varepsilon$ $GABA_A$ receptors to general anaesthetics.

Neurosteroids

▶ Neurosteroids prolong the mean open time of recombinant $GABA_A$ receptor channels. Whereas, at least in recombinant systems, the identity of the α and β subunits has little or no effect on neurosteroid action, substitution of the γ subunit by a δ subunit suppresses the GABA-modulatory activity of the neurosteroids.

$GABA_A$ Receptor Mutants as Models for Disease

Several animal models based on the generation of targeted mutations (see also chapter "Transgenic Animal Models") in $GABA_A$ receptor subunits have been developed. Mice carrying point mutations in certain α subunits rendering the respective receptors GABA-sensitive but diazepam-insensitive have already been discussed in this chapter. They have provided information about pharmacological and at least indirectly also physiological roles of individual $GABA_A$ receptor subtypes.

Mice lacking the $\gamma 2$ subunit die shortly after birth presumably due to a lack of receptor clustering. However, mice heterozygous for the $\gamma 2$ knockout allele display a limited reduction of $GABA_A$ receptor function, visualized by decreased ligand binding and receptor clustering, notably in hippocampus and cortex. In addition, these mice display enhanced reactivity to naturally aversive stimuli such as novelty, exposed space and brightly illuminated areas, representing anxiety-related responses thought to include the activity of the septo-hippocampal system. Furthermore, the heterozygous mice display a heightened fear response in assessing the negative association of an ambiguous stimulus in cue discrimination learning; these mice perceived a partial stimulus as threatening as a fully conditioned stimulus (6). They represent a genetic model of anxiety and represent a correlate of the GABA$_A$ receptor deficit identified in patients with panic disorder.

Deletion of the gene encoding the β3 subunit resulted in a loss of half of the GABA$_A$ receptors at birth. Most homozygous knockout mice died in the perinatal period, perhaps in part due to a cleft palate, and the few survivors were interbred on a hybrid background and grew to normal body size. They displayed various neurological impairments including hyperresponsiveness to sensory stimuli, strong motor impairment and epileptic seizures, which might be due to the lack of GABA$_A$ receptors containing the β3 subunit that act as "desynchronizers" of neuronal activity. In these mice, the immobilizing actions of halothane and enflurane are also reduced.

Mice lacking the δ subunit, which is mainly expressed in cerebellum and thalamus, display an attenuation of sleep time following the administration of the neurosteroids alphaxalone and pregnanolone, while the responses to propofol, etomidate, ketamine and the benzodiazepine midazolam were unaffected. This demonstrates the role of GABA$_A$ receptors containing the δ subunit for neurosteroid action.

Mice lacking the α6 subunit display no change in the response to pentobarbital, general anesthetics or ethanol, but are more sensitive to the motor-impairing action of diazepam in an accelerated rotarod test, though in a limited dose range only. These mice display significant compensatory changes in GABA$_A$ receptor subunit composition and also GABA$_A$ receptor expression levels in the forebrain. A selective posttranslational loss of the δ subunit revealed a close association of the α6 and δ subunits *in vivo*. In these mice, a compensatory upregulation of two-pore domain potassium channel, TASK-1, was found.

Mice lacking the α1 subunit have also been generated, as well as mice lacking the β2 subunit. Given the fact that these are the most abundant α and β subunits respectively, it is surprising that these animals survive, presumably indicating the presence of compensatory mechanisms. A thourough behavioral analysis has not been reported so far.

The GABA$_B$ Receptor

The GABA$_B$ receptor is a heterodimer of GABA$_B$R1 and GABA$_B$R2. GABA$_B$R1 exists in two isoforms that differ at the N-terminus, GABA$_B$R1a and GABA$_B$R1b. GABA$_B$ receptors are coupled to second messenger systems via G proteins. Presynaptic GABA$_B$ receptors influence neurotransmission by suppression of neurotransmitter release, presumably by inhibiting Ca^{2+} channels. Postsynaptic GABA$_B$ receptors hyperpolarize neurons by activating an outward K^+ current that underlies the late inhibitory postsynaptic potential (▶ IPSP), presumably mediated by inwardly rectifying potassium channels of the Kir3 type.

Currently, baclofen is the only clinically used GABA$_B$ receptor agonist. It is used as a muscle relaxant for treatment of spasticity in spinal injury and multiple sclerosis. The cloning of GABA$_B$ receptors has renewed the interest in the search for more selective drugs and novel therapeutic indications.

References

1. Sieghart W (1995) Structure and Pharmacology of γ-aminobutyric acidA receptor subtypes. Pharmacol Rev 47:181–234
2. Bormann J (2001) The "ABC" of GABA receptors. Trends Pharmacol. Sci. 21:16–19
3. Barnard EA, Skolnick P, Olsen RW, Mohler H, Sieghart W, Biggio G, Braestrup C, Bateson AN, Langer SZ (1998) International Union of Pharmacology. XV. Subtypes of γ-aminobutyric acidA receptors: classification on the basis of subunit structure and receptor function. Pharmacol Rev 50:291–313
4. Fritschy J-M, Mohler H (1995) GABAA-receptor heterogeneity in the adult rat brain: differential regional and cellular distribution of seven major subunits. J Comp Neurol 14:154–94
5. Rudolph U, Crestani F, Möhler H (2001) GABAA recpetor subtypes: dissecting their pharmacological functions. Trends Pharmacol Sci 22:188–194

6. Crestani F, Lorez M, Baer K, Essrich C, Benke D, Laurent JP, Belzung C, Fritschy J-M, Lüscher B, Mohler H (1999) Decreased GABAA-receptor clustering results in enhanced anxiety and a bias for threat cues. Nat Neurosci 2:833–839

G-actin

G-actin has a molecular weight of about 42 kD. In higher vertebrates, 6 isoforms of G-actin, which contain 374/375 residues, are expressed in a cell-specific manner, . They are present in striated muscle cells (skeletal and cardiac isoforms), smooth muscle cells (vascular and visceral isoforms) and in non-muscle cells (2 isoforms).

▶ Cytoskeleton

Gaddum, method of

The method of Gaddum compares equiactive concentrations of agonist in the absence and presence of a concentration of non-competitive antagonist that depresses the maximal agonist response. These concentrations are compared in a double-reciprocal plot (or variant thereof) to yield the equilibrium dissociation constant of the non-competitive antagonist-receptor complex (chemical measure of the potency of the antagonist).

▶ Drug-receptor Interaction

Galanin

Galanin is a biologically active neuropeptide containing 30 amino acids and a non-amidated C-terminus in humans; galanin from other species contains 29 amino acids and C-terminal amidation.

▶ Galanin Receptors

Galanin Receptors

MARY W. WALKER, KELLI E. SMITH
Synaptic Pharmaceutical Corporation,
Paramus, USA
mwalker@synapticcorp.com,
ksmith@synapticcorp.com

Synonyms

Galanin receptor type 1, galanin receptor type 2, galanin receptor type 3, Galanin receptor-1, Galanin receptor-2, Galanin receptor-3, Galanin-R1, Galanin-R2, Galanin-R3, Gal-R1, Gal-R2, Gal-R3, GalR1, GalR2, GalR3, GAL1, GAL2, GAL3

Definition

The ▶ galanin receptors form a distinct subfamily of G protein-coupled receptors (GPCRs). Three ▶ receptor subtypes have been cloned and characterized: GAL1, GAL2, GAL3 (1). Structurally, each receptor is a typical ▶ GPCR, i.e. a monomeric serpentine protein with seven helical transmembrane domains, an extracellularly directed N-terminus and an intracellularly directed C-terminus. Functionally, each receptor is coupled to ▶ heterotrimeric G proteins. These galanin receptors are thought to mediate various effects of galanin, such as those associated with cognition, emotion, pain, growth and metabolism. Other GPCRs which are similar at the amino acid level (30–38%) include the somatostatin sst_4 and sst_5 receptor subtypes, the ORL1 (nociceptin) receptor and the GPR54 (KiSS-1) receptor.

Basic Characteristics

Galanin Overview

Galanin was first described in 1983 by Tatemoto *et al.* as a 29-residue C-terminally amidated peptide isolated from a porcine intestinal extract. The name "galanin" was assigned to reflect the presence of glycine and alanine in the N- and C-terminal positions, respectively. The N-terminal sequence galanin-1–14 is highly conserved across species, with 100% identity for example in porcine, human, rat and mouse. Structure-activity

Tab. 1 Galanin receptor subtype relationships (% amino acid identity).

receptor	human GAL1	human GAL2	human GAL3	rat GAL1	rat GAL2	ratGAL3
human GAL1	100 %					
human GAL2	42 %	100 %				
human GAL3	38 %	58 %	100 %			
rat GAL1	92 %	41 %	38 %	100 %		
rat GAL2	40 %	87 %	58 %	40 %	100 %	
rat GAL3	37 %	58 %	92 %	36 %	55 %	100 %

Overall amino acid identity values were generated with the GAP program (GCG, Inc., Madison, USA).

G

analyses indicate the N-terminal region is the primary peptide pharmacophore involved in receptor recognition. The C-terminus is relatively less conserved across species; human galanin is particularly distinguished in this region for terminating at position 30 with an unamidated serine.

Galanin has a widespread distribution in regions such as brain, spinal cord and gastrointestinal tract. Galanin modulates physiological processes such as neurotransmitter release, neuroendocrine release, nerve growth and regeneration, seizure, cognition, emotion, food consumption, cardiovascular and gastrointestinal function. Transgenic mice overexpressing galanin exhibit cognitive defects resembling those seen in ▶ Alzheimer's disease; they also display an elevated threshold for thermal ▶ nociception, suppressed seizure in response to hippocampal kindling, and elevated release of central monoamines (such as norepinephrine and serotonin) after a forced swim stress. Transgenic mice with a loss-of-function mutation in the *galanin* gene exhibit defects in nociception, spinal reflex and nerve regeneration in various models of pain and nerve injury; they also have fewer cholinergic neurons in the basal forebrain. Female *galanin* (-/-) mice show defects in prolactin secretion and lactotroph proliferation.

Galanin and related peptide analogs have historically provided the means for characterizing putative or cloned receptor subtypes. Peptides can be generally described as follows: 1) galanin peptides containing modified and/or unnatural amino acids, such as D-Trp^2-galanin-1-29; 2) peptide fragments or extensions such as galanin-3-29,

galanin-1-15, galanin-1-16, galanin-(-7-29) and galanin-(-9-29); 3) chimeric peptides in which the N-terminus of galanin (commonly galanin-1-13) is fused with a C-terminus comprised of a novel sequence, or a fragment of a bioactive peptide such as NPY, bradykinin, substance P (well known examples are M15, M32, M35, C7 and M40); and 4) combinations of the above such as the GAL1/GAL2 agonist AR-M961 ([Sar^1-D-Ala^{12}]-Gal(1-16)-NH$_2$) or the GAL2-selective agonist AR-M1896 (GAL(2-11)-Trp-Thr-Leu-Asn-Ser-Ala-Gly-Tyr-Leu-Leu-NH$_2$) (2).

Recently Discovered Galanin-like Peptide

In 1999, Ohtaki *et al.* reported the purification of a novel 60-residue peptide from a fraction of porcine hypothalamic extract, on the basis of functional activity in a GAL2 receptor assay. Residues 9–21 of the 60-residue peptide shared 100% sequence identity with galanin-1-13, thereby prompting the name "galanin-like peptide", or GALP. ▶ GALP is more discretely localized than galanin; mRNA for GALP in rat and mouse brain is limited to hypothalamus (arcuate), median eminence and pituitary neural lobe, with additional expression observed in rat gut. GALP binds and activates cloned GAL1 and GAL2 receptors (K_i=4.5 nM and 0.24 nM, respectively). Therefore, GALP might also interact with endogenous galanin receptors, at least in part.

The GAL1 Receptor

The cloned human GAL1 receptor cDNA encodes a protein of 349 amino acids (1). Human GAL1 shares 42% amino acid identity with human GAL2 and 38% with human GAL3 (Table 1). GAL1 receptor homologs have also been cloned from rat and mouse, with amino acid identities of 92% and 93%, respectively, relative to human (Table 1). The human *GAL1* gene on chromosome 18q23 has an unusual intron/exon organization for a GPCR, with a coding region interrupted by 2 introns. The mouse *GAL1* gene has been mapped to chromosome 18E4, syntenic with the human *GAL1* gene, and has a similar intron/exon organization.

The cloned human GAL1 receptor binds porcine $[^{125}I]$-$[Tyr^{26}]$galanin and is functionally coupled to G_i/G_o-type G proteins or related pathways. Specific examples of ▶ second messenger effects measured *in vitro* include reduction of forskolin-stimulated cAMP accumulation and stimulation of MAP kinase activity. The cloned GAL1 receptor activates G protein-coupled inwardly rectifying K^+ channels (▶ GIRKs) when transfected into *Xenopus* oocytes. Thus, native GAL1 receptors on mammalian neurons are likely to hyperpolarize and inhibit neurotransmitter release.

A pharmacological signature for GAL1 was based on rank order of binding affinity for galanin and derivatives: human galanin, rat galanin, porcine galanin> porcine galanin-1-16> porcine galanin-2-29> porcine D-Trp^2-galanin > galanin-3-29 (1). Among the chimeric galanin peptide constructs, the rank order of binding affinity is M32, M35, C7, M15>M40 (1). All peptides with measurable binding activity are agonists *in vitro*. The pharmacological profile is similar to that derived for the native GAL1 receptor in the Bowes melanoma cell line.

Human GAL1 receptor mRNA has been detected in multiple cell and tissue samples including Bowes melanoma cells, brain, gastrointestinal tract (from esophagus to rectum), heart, prostate and testes. Rat GAL1 mRNA was detected in olfactory regions, many hypothalamic nuclei (including supraoptic nucleus), amygdala, ventral hippocampal CA fields, dorsomedial thalamic areas, brainstem (medulla oblongata, locus coeruleus and lateral parabrachial nucleus), spinal cord (dorsal horn) and pancreas-derived cells (RIN-14b). Rat GAL1 mRNA distribution and expression level were essentially constant when examined from embryonic day 20 to postnatal day 70, suggesting that GAL1 receptors in the CNS function broadly in normal synaptic transmission (3). Under certain circumstances, however, GAL1 mRNA is up- or down-regulated, as in the following examples: 1) GAL1 mRNA was elevated in rat locus coeruleus after precipitated withdrawal from chronic morphine treatment. 2) GAL1 mRNA was also elevated in rat hypothalamic nuclei after treatment with metabolic inhibitors (the glucose anti-metabolite 2-deoxy-glucose or the fatty acid anti-metabolite sodium mercaptoacetate, both of which stimulate feeding) or by salt loading. 3) Hypothalamic GAL1 mRNA was decreased by hypophysectomy and also by lactation. 4) Hypothalamic GAL1 mRNA was variable across the estrous cycle in female rats, and decreased in males by castration except when testosterone was administered. 5) GAL1 mRNA was decreased in the dorsal horn after inflammation or peripheral nerve injury.

Based on current knowledge, the GAL1 receptor is likely to transmit multiple actions of galanin. Potential targets include feeding, nociception, neuroendocrine release, cognition, emotion, stress response, morphine withdrawal, metabolism and gastrointestinal function. The following examples provide support: 1) In a study of rat feeding behavior, the galanin-induced feeding response was attributed either to GAL1 or a GAL1-like receptor, based on similarity between the *in vitro* pharmacological profile for GAL1 and the *in vivo* actions of various peptides when injected icv. (Galanin produced a stronger feeding response than galanin-2-29, galanin-3-29 or galanin-1-16). 2) In a study of the nociceptive reflex pathway in rat, intrathecal administration of a cell-penetrating peptide nucleic acid complimentary to GAL1 attenuated the inhibitory effect of galanin on the flexor reflex, suggesting a role in pain processing. 3) In an allodynic Bennett rat model, a GAL2-selective peptide AR-M1896 was inactive whereas a GAL1/GAL2-selective peptide AR-M961 increased the threshold for mechanical ▶ allodynia. Based on these data the GAL1 receptor was considered a potential target for the treatment of neuropathic pain. 4) In human colonic cells, GAL1 mRNA was upregulated by the inflammatory nuclear transcription factor NF-κB and also by pathogenic *E. coli*, resulting in an increase in Cl^- secretion; thus GAL1 may be partly responsible for excessive fluid secretion during infectious diarrhea. In a separate study of guinea pig ileum, GAL1 antagonists blocked galanin-induced inhibition of electrically-induced contraction (4). 5) In a study of rat brain cortical slices, GAL1 antagonists blocked galanin-induced inhibition of acetylcholine release, consistent with a role in cognitive function (4). 6) Children with the 18q- syndrome exhibit a growth hormone insufficiency phenotype and display a common 2-megabase deletion in chromosome 18q resulting in loss of the *GAL1* gene; these data suggest a possible role for GAL1 in growth and development.

The GAL2 Receptor

The cloned human GAL2 receptor cDNA encodes a protein of 387 amino acids (1). Human GAL2 shares 42% amino acid identity with human GAL1 and 58% with human GAL3 (Table 1). The human *GAL2* gene, located on chromosome 17q25.3, has a single intron interrupting the coding region just after TM3. The cloned rat GAL2 receptor homolog has 15 fewer amino acids in the C-terminus and shares only 87% amino acid identity with human GAL2 (Table 1). The mouse GAL2 receptor has been cloned and mapped to chromosome 11.

The cloned human GAL2 receptor binds porcine [^{125}I]-[Tyr^{26}]galanin and couples readily to G_q/G_{11}-type G proteins or related pathways *in vitro*. Under certain conditions, GAL2 also appears to couple with G_i/G_o- and G_{12}-type proteins (1, 2). Specific examples of second messenger effects measured *in vitro* include inositol phosphate hydrolysis, intracellular calcium mobilization, stimulation of MAP kinase activity, reduction of forskolin-stimulated cAMP accumulation, and induction of stress fiber formation. The cloned GAL2 receptor activates Ca^{++}-dependent Cl^- channels when transfected into *Xenopus* oocytes. Native GAL2 receptors in H69 small lung cell carcinoma cells are proposed to activate the monomeric GTPase RhoA, which functions in cell migration.

A pharmacological signature for GAL2 was based on rank order of binding affinity for galanin and derivates: human galanin, rat galanin, porcine galanin, porcine galanin-2-29, porcine galanin-1-16> porcine D-Trp^2-galanin> galanin-3-29 (1). A distinguishing feature of GAL2 is its relatively high preference for porcine galanin-2-29. Among the chimeric galanin peptide constructs,

the rank order of binding affinity is M32 > M35, C7, M15, M40 (1). All peptides with measurable binding activity are agonists *in vitro*.

Human GAL2 receptor mRNA has a widespread distribution in several central and peripheral tissues including hippocampus, kidney, liver, small intestine and retina; depending on the study GAL2 mRNA has also been found in hypothalamus and pituitary. In rat brain, GAL2 mRNA was found in anterior and posterior hypothalamus (including POMC neurons of the arcuate), dentate gyrus of the hippocampus, amygdala, pyriform cortex, dentate gyrus, raphe and spinal trigeminal nuclei, mammillary nuclei, cerebellar cortex (Purkinje cells) and discrete brainstem nuclei including dorsal motor nucleus of the vagus. Interestingly, GAL2 mRNA was relatively more widespread and abundant in neonatal rat brain studied on postnatal days 0–7 than in the adult, with highest levels in neonatal neocortex and thalamus. These data suggest that GAL2 may have distinct functions related to establishment of synaptic connections in the developing brain, with implications for neural damage and repair in the adult nervous system (3). In rat periphery, rat GAL2 mRNA was found in vas deferens, prostate, uterus, ovary, stomach, large intestine, dorsal root ganglia and anterior plus intermediate lobes of the pituitary as well as pancreas-derived cells (RIN-m5f).

Based on current knowledge, the GAL2 receptor is likely to transmit multiple actions of galanin. Potential targets include neurotransmitter and neuroendocrine release, growth, reproduction, seizure, cognition, emotion, nociception, nerve regeneration, peripheral metabolism and gastrointestinal motility. Support is provided by the following examples: 1) In a study of rat jejunal contraction, the galanin-dependent contractions were attributed to GAL2 based on the abundance of GAL2 mRNA in the jejunum, and on the relative efficacy of galanin-2-29 and galanin-1-16 compared to galanin and galanin-3-29. 2) GAL2 mRNA levels are modulated by nerve injury. Three days after peripheral tissue inflammation in the rat a peak elevation of GAL2 mRNA was observed in dorsal root ganglia. Seven days after facial nerve crush in the rat a peak elevation in GAL2 and galanin mRNA was observed in motor neurons of the ipsilateral facial nucleus. Conversely, GAL2 mRNA in dorsal root ganglia was down-regulated after axotomy. 3) In a study of normal rats, intrathecal administration of the GAL2-selective peptide AR-M1896 produced mechanical and cold allodynia; thus GAL2 was proposed to mediate sensory processing in the spinal cord(2). 4) In the Morris swim maze, rats injected with galanin in the dorsal and ventral dentate gyrus (an area of GAL2 mRNA expression) displayed a significant spatial learning deficit while maintaining normal swim speed and performance (5), consistent with a role for GAL2 in learning and acquisition. 5) *Galanin (-/-)* mice were found to have approximately 30% fewer cholinergic neurons in the basal forebrain than wild type counterparts, suggesting that galanin normally exerts a trophic effect in this region. In people with Alzheimer's disease, the dwindling population of cholinergic neurons in basal forebrain is hyperinnervated by neuronal fibers expressing galanin, prompting speculation that trophic effects mediated by a GAL2-like receptor might counteract the degenerative process. 6) The *GAL2* gene is localized on chromosome 17q25 in a region associated with two diseases (hereditary neuralgic amyotrophy and Russel-Silver syndrome) that are characterized by short stature and low birth weight dwarfism, respectively, in addition to developmental defects. This relationship suggests a possible role for GAL2 in growth and development.

The GAL3 Receptor

The cloned GAL3 receptor cDNA encodes a protein containing 368 amino acids (1). As shown in Table 1, the human GAL3 receptor is more closely related to the human GAL2 receptor (with 58% amino acid identity) than GAL1 (with 38% amino acid identity). The human *GAL3* gene is located on chromosome 22q12.2-13.1 and has the same intron/exon organization as *GAL2*, with a single intron interrupting the coding region just after TM3. The intron/exon pattern suggests a common evolutionary origin for GAL2 and GAL3, and a convergent evolutionary relationship to GAL1. The intron in human *GAL3* contains a Pst 1 restriction site polymorphism of unknown significance. Rat GAL3 shares 92% amino acid identity with the human homolog (Table 1). A mouse GAL3 homolog has been cloned and mapped to chromosome 15.

The cloned human GAL3 receptor binds porcine [^{125}I]-[Tyr^{26}]galanin and is functionally coupled to G_i/G_o-type G proteins. The cloned GAL3 receptor inhibits forskolin-stimulated cAMP accumulation (3). The cloned GAL3 receptor activates GIRKs when transfected into *Xenopus* oocytes (1). Thus native GAL3 receptors on mammalian neurons are likely to inhibit neurotransmitter secretion, as proposed previously for native GAL1.

A pharmacological signature for GAL3 was based on binding affinity for galanin and derivates: porcine galanin, rat galanin> human galanin, porcine galanin 2-29> porcine galanin-1-16> porcine D-Trp^2-galanin, galanin 3-29 (1). A distinguishing feature of the GAL3 receptor is that human galanin binds with slightly lower affinity than rat and porcine galanin. Among the chimeric peptides, the rank order of binding affinity is M32, M35, C7> M15, M40 (1). All peptides with measurable binding activity are agonists *in vitro*. A native GAL3 receptor has not yet been pharmacologically characterized.

Human GAL3 mRNA was detected centrally in regions such as cerebellum, amygdala, cerebral cortex, occipital lobe, frontal lobe, temporal lobe, putamen, caudate nucleus and spinal cord. Human GAL3 receptor mRNA was also detected in peripheral tissues such as thyroid, adrenal gland, skeletal muscle, pancreas, gastrointestinal tract and testes. Rat GAL3 mRNA was found in discrete regions of the CNS such as cerebellum, amygdala, hypothalamus (ventromedial, arcuate, paraventricular and supraoptic nuclei), olfactory pathways, cerebral cortex, hippocampus, caudate putamen, central gray, medulla oblongata and spinal cord. Rat GAL3 transcripts were also detected in peripheral tissues such as pituitary (a particularly rich source), liver, kidney, stomach, testes, adrenal cortex, lung, adrenal medulla, spleen and pancreas. In general, human and rat GAL3 transcripts were widely distributed and more overlapping with GAL2 than GAL1.

Based on current knowledge, it is plausible that GAL3 transmits multiple effects of galanin. Potential targets include nociception, neuroendocrine release, cognition, emotion and metabolism. The chromosomal localization of the *GAL3* gene (22q12.2-13.1) places it in a possible susceptibility locus for ▶ bipolar disorder (manic depressive illness). This relationship suggests that GAL3 gene might play a role in depression and related mood disorders. Interestingly, chromosome 22q is also a susceptibility locus for schizophrenia.

Possibility of Additional Receptor Subtypes

The pharmacological profiles of the cloned galanin receptors do not account for all the profiles derived from native cells and tissues. For example, peptide agonist studies provide data for the existence of a receptor preferring galanin-1-15> galanin, and for another receptor which binds to galanin-3-29. Furthermore, chimeric peptides such as M15, M32, M35, C7 and M40 are agonists when tested at cloned receptors, yet they behave as antagonists in many (but not all) *in vivo* assays. While several interpretations are conceivable to explain the discrepant pharmacology, the possibility remains that additional galanin receptor genes have yet to be identified (1).

Drugs

Currently, there are two descriptions of nonpeptidic ligands for galanin (GAL1) receptors. 1) A fungal metabolite SCH202596 (spitocoumaranone with a molecular mass of 353 D) was reported by Chu *et al.* in 1997 (4) to bind the GAL1 receptor in human Bowes melanoma cells with an IC_{50} of 1.7 micromolar. 2) A series of 1,4-dithiin and dithiepine-1,1,4,4-tetroxides with molecular weights ~250 to 450 Da were reported by Scott *et al.* in 2000 to bind human GAL1 in Bowes melanoma cells with affinities (IC_{50} values) ranging from 0.19 to 2.7 micromolar (5). Two of the dithiepines were characterized as human GAL1 antagonists, based on activity in a cAMP accumulation assay and also in a GTPγ^{35}S binding assay.

The two dithiepines of interest also blocked galanin-induced inibition of acetylcholine release from rat cortical brain slices or synaptosomes, as well as galanin-induced inhibition of electrically-induced contraction in the guinea pig ileum.

There are no reports of small molecular weight, nonpeptide, orally available antagonists or agonists with high affinity and selectivity for individual galanin receptors. Such molecules are clearly required to accurately assess the value of galanin receptors as potential therapeutic targets. As work continues in this field, the expectation is that receptor-selective drug candidates will eventually emerge.

References

1. Branchek TA, Smith KE, Gerald C, Walker MW (2000) Galanin Receptor Subtypes. TiPS 21:109–116
2. Wittau N, Grosse R, Kalkbrenner F, Gohla A, Schultz G, Gudermann T (2000) The galanin receptor type 2 initiates multiple signaling pathways in small cell lung cancer cells by coupling to G(q), G(i) and G(12) proteins. Oncogene 19: 4199-209
3. Kolakowski *et al.* (1998) Molecular characterization and expression of cloned human galanin receptors GALR2 and GALR3. J Neurochem 71:2239-51
4. Chu, M. *et al.* (1997) A new fungal metabolite, Sch 202596, with inhibitory activity in the galanin receptor GALR1 assay. Tetrahedron Lett. 38: 6111-6114.
5. Schott MK, Ross TM, Lee DH, Wang HY, Shank RP, Wild KD, Davies CB, Crooke, JJ, Potocki AC, Reitz AB (2000) 2, 3-Dihydro-dithiin and -dithiepine-1, 1, 4, 4-tetroxides: small molecule non-peptide antagonists of the human galanin hGAL-1 receptor. Bioorg Med Chem 8: 1383-1391.

GALP

GALP is a biologically active peptide comprised of 60 residues found in human, rat, mouse and pig. The name is derived from "**galanin-like peptide**", based on structural and functional similarity with galanin.

▶ Galanin Receptors

γ-Aminobutyric Acid

▶ GABAergic System

γ-Glutamyl-transpeptidase

This is the enzyme that converts Leukotriene C_4 (LTC$_4$) to Leukotriene D$_4$ (LTD$_4$) upon its secretion from inflammatory cells.

▶ Leukotrienes

GAPs

▶ GTPase Activating Proteins
▶ Small GTPases

Gastric Emptying Rate

The gastric emptying rate is the rate at which an orally administered drug reaches the small intestine from the stomach. This can be affected by various factors such as food, body position and certain drugs.

▶ Drug Interactions
▶ Pharmacokinetics

Gastric H, K-ATPase

The H, K-ATPase transports H$^+$ ion from cytoplasm to lumen in exchange for extracytoplasmic K$^+$ ion in an electroneutral exchange using the energy of ATP hydrolysis.

▶ Proton Pump Inhibitors

Gastrin

Gastrin is a peptide hormone, which is synthesized in cells of the mucosa of the gastric antrum and duodenum. It is secreted into the portal blood. The main effect of gastrin is the stimulation of secretion of acid by the parietal cells of the stomach. It also increases pepsinogen secretion and stimulates blood flow and gastric motility. The release of gastrin from G-cells in the gastric antrum is controlled by various mechanisms. Vagal stimulation to the antrum causes presynaptic release of acetylcholine, which causes the release of gastrin releasing peptide (GRP) from GRP-postsynaptic neurons, which directly stimulates the endocrine release of gastrin from G-cells. G-cells are also stimulated to release gastrin in response to protein digestion products on the luminal surface. These include amino acids and small peptides, which act directly on the gastrin-secreting cells. The release of ▶ somatostatin from D-cells, which are localized in the vicinity of G-cells has a negative influence on gastrin secretion. Release of somatostatin is enhanced by high luminal acidity, which provides a negative feedback for the endocrine pathway. Release of somatostatin is inhibited by vagal cholinergic neurons. Gastrin exerts its effects by binding to a ▶ G-protein coupled receptor (CCK$_2$), which functions through G-proteins of the G$_{q/11}$-family.

Gastrin Releasing Peptide

▶ Bombesin-like Peptides

Gastroesophageal Reflux Disease

Gastroesophageal reflux disease (GERD) is a digestive disorder. Gastric acid flows back up into the esophagus through the lower esophageal sphincter (LES), which connects the esophagus and stomach. The acid is irritating to the esophagus and causes heartburn.

▶ Proton Pump Inhibitors and Acid Pump Antagonists

Gating

Gating, a property of many ion channels, is the active transition between open and closed states in response to specific signals, such as membrane voltage or the presence of neurotransmitters.

▶ Voltage-dependent Na^+ Channels
▶ Ionotropic Glutamate Receptors

G-CSF

▶ Granulocyte-CSF
▶ Hematopoietic Growth Factors

GDIs

▶ Guanine Nucleotide Dissociation Inhibitors
▶ Small GTPases

GEFs

▶ Guanine Nucleotide Exchange Factors
▶ Small GTPases

Gene Activity Profile

A gene activity profile is a collection of quantitatively determined levels of gene products, found in one tissue or cell type, which is characteristic of the tissue, a disease process, a hormone response, a pharmaceutical intervention, etc.

▶ Gene Expression Analysis

Gene-environment Interaction

Gene-environment interaction is the synergistic or antagonistic effect of polymorphisms and environmental factors with respect to the occurrence of symptoms or diseases.

▶ Pharmacogenetics

Gene Expression

Gene expression is the process by which the information encoded in a gene is converted into RNA and then translated into protein.

▶ Gene Expression Analysis

Gene Expression Analysis

JOHN C. CHERONIS, VICTOR V. TRYON, DAVID B. TROLLINGER, MICHAEL D. ROPER, DANUTE BANKAITIS-DAVIS AND MICHAEL P. BEVILACQUA
Source Precision Medicine, Boulder, CO, USA
jcheroni@SourceMedicine.com

Synonyms

Transcriptional analysis, gene activity profiling, mRNA profiling

Definition

The determination of gene activity through analysis of mRNA.

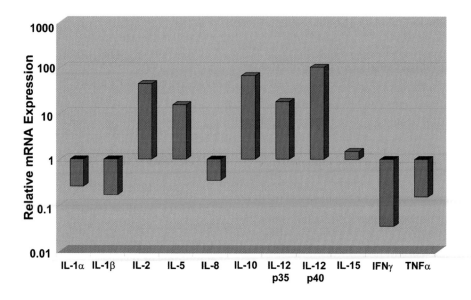

Fig. 1 *In Vivo* **Study: Steroid Treatment Alters mRNA Profiles in Human Blood.**   Precision mRNA profiles were determined on whole blood, drawn from a volunteer before and following a three-day course of prednisone (100 mg daily *per os*). The height of each bar represents the fold increase of the mRNA assayed for the gene listed below the bar. The ordinate of the graph is depicted logarithmically, and values for each bar have been normalized to the level determined for the individual before steroid treatment.

▶ Microarray Technology
▶ Proteomics

Description

Gene activity can be monitored through cellular or tissue concentrations of mRNA. Cellular adaptation is associated with and guided by altered gene expression. The resulting specific mRNA changes are subsequently reflected in the levels of their encoded proteins. These effects follow when cells interact with endogenous agents, such as hormones, as well as exogenous ones, such as pharmaceutically-active compounds. Determination of mRNA concentration in tissues, including whole blood, can thereby provide major pharmacological and pharmacodynamic insights into the action of therapeutic agents. When mRNA changes are measured with high degrees of precision, these effects become striking. For example, as depicted in Fig. 1, a simple 3-day treatment of an individual with oral prednisone results in a substantial

molecular response in blood leukocytes. Moreover, the specific response pattern reveals the drug's anti-inflammatory activity.

Integration of high precision assays, targeted drug-response and disease databases and diagnostic algorithms significantly advances the interpretation of gene expression during drug evaluation. Multiple gene response profiles, stored in appropriately designed databases, facilitate wide-scale comparisons that reveal trends that would otherwise be cryptic. Biomedical algorithms simplify examination of the large amounts of data generated in each study and facilitate comparisons with the data contained in these databases. Fig. 2 represents an implementation of this process.

Analysis of specific mRNA levels is not new. DNA and RNA gel blotting (Southern (1) and Northern (2), hydridization-based approaches, have been practiced worldwide for more than a quarter-century. ▶ Microarray hybridization to large arrays of nucleic acids (often called microarrays) has grown very popular during the last decade [3]. Fig. 3 depicts a microarray comparison of

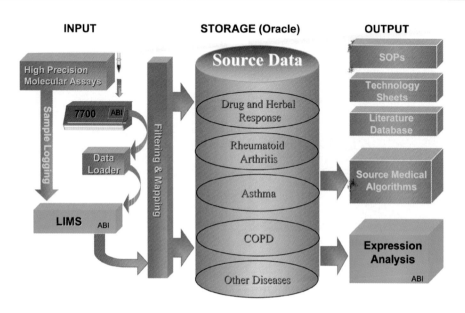

INPUT   **STORAGE (Oracle)**   **OUTPUT**

Fig. 2 Schematic of the Source Precision Profile System. Samples arriving for analysis are first entered into Laboratory Information Management System (LIMS), then analyzed for mRNA using the high precision molecular analysis system, described in the text. Threshold crossing data, obtained from the ABI Prism® 7700 is buffered by the data loader program, then stored in LIMS together with the sample data previously stored. Following preliminary analysis (filtering and mapping), data are entered into the appropriate database, managed by Oracle. These data flow into the appropriate bins, indicated on the figure (Note: the COPD bin refers to chronic obstructive pulmonary disease). System output, derived from the database, include fact sheets such as standard operating practice directives (SOPs), technology descriptions, and literature relevant to the gene loci determined by the analysis. Biomedical algorithms are used to simplify gene expression data, and further information may be obtained from the associated Expression Analysis tool from ABI.
7700: ABI PRISM® 7700 Sequence Detection System, Applied Biosystems, Foster City, CA; **Oracle:** Oracle9*i*™, Oracle Corporation, Redwood Shores, CA; **ABI:** Applied Biosystems, Foster City, CA, a division of Applera Corporation

two different preparations of Echinacea. These hybridization methods can reveal relatively large mRNA concentration swings. Messenger RNA detection by quantitative reverse transcriptase-polymerase chain reaction (quantitative ▶ RT-PCR, or QPCR), an amplification-based approach, has also experienced increased popularity in recent years [4]. Though not as amenable to the measurement of large numbers of transcripts, this method lends itself to the development of more sensitive and precise assays. Subtle, pharmacologically important, up- or down-regulation requires substantial precision to extract meaningful data. This requirement can be met by QPCR, especially properly run can yield a great deal of information,

in light of improved techniques that tighten the coefficients of variation (CV) for the assay.

▶ Quantitative PCR was historically accompanied by CVs between 20 and 50%. These wide variations obscure subtle, pharmacologically relevant differences in gene expression. Recent advances in analytical methods developed by our laboratory reduce these CVs to 1–5%, thereby enabling the detection of small changes in mRNA levels. Currently available equipment and disposables afford measurement of 96 or more separate gene activities in a single run. However, careful selection of candidate genes can often result in high-impact assays using 24 genes or fewer. Samples that are even with small gene panels.

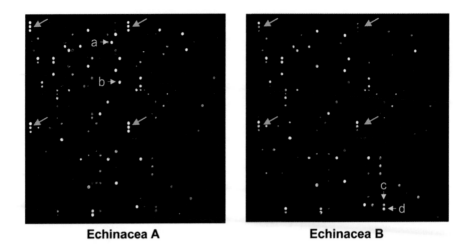

Echinacea A　　　　　　　　**Echinacea B**

Fig. 3 Comparison of two Echinacea Preparations using Microarray. THP-1 cells were stimulated with bacterial lipopolysaccharide (LPS) and incubated with commercial preparations of Echinacea extracted using methanol and water, then lyophilized. Spots represent genes expressed within the limits of the assay. Each microarray is divided into quadrants; blue arrows indicate the calibration gene products (nonhuman control clones EST-91, EST-35, EST-34). Many genes were expressed in common for cells treated with either preparation, with notable exceptions of (a) HSU67733, (b) HSNMCFL1, (c) HSBBC1, and (d) HSLBP.

Sample preparation is also critical to the success of gene activity determination. Many pharmacological applications of gene expression analysis involve RNA determination in whole blood derived from a test subject. In the absence of rigorous experimental protocols, RNA levels may be changed both by gratuitous induction of transcription in living cells and inappropriate degradation by ribonucleases which are active in both living and dead cells. Blood leukocytes are physiologically active for a substantial period of time following collection. Accordingly, blood responds to a wide variety of environmental stressors, including phlebotomy conditions, agitation, and shipping. With the advent of new collection methods, however, these effects can be minimized and meaningful data derived from blood subjected to experimental conditions over a substantial period of time.

Specific protein release following gene activation may exhibit considerable latency. This latency results from RNA transcription, processing, and translocation to the cytoplasm, together with protein translation, transport, maturation and secretion. Steady-state protein levels in circulation, furthermore, depend on clearance rates, which range from minutes to days. Accordingly, mRNA changes significantly precede protein changes in response to pharmaceutical administration.

Pharmacological Relevance

Gene expression analysis facilitates a number of pharmaceutical determinations. Newly developed agents may be compared to the actions of known, established pharmaceuticals, thereby providing an early indication of efficacy and potential side effects. Of equal importance, dose-response studies may be greatly accelerated by analyzing the activities of relevant genes. Gene expression analysis may also be used to better understand the mechanism of action of a new therapeutic agent and to improve the selection of a development path, i.e., selecting the right disease for initial testing of a new compound and using clear-cut, gene expression profile data as part of the entrance criteria.

The technique is applicable in three major study methodologies:

1. In vitro studies in whole blood, cell or tissue model systems for compound screening and benchmarking;

2. Ex vivo studies in whole blood or other tissues taken from human subjects (or animals) that have been administered a therapeutic agent for pharmacodynamic analysis; and

3. In vivo studies for direct clinical study of a compound's effect in normal subjects or patient populations.

In the first of these methods (*in vitro* studies), blood or other tissues are taken from untreated normal subjects or patients and subsequently exposed to drugs and stimuli. These studies can rapidly benchmark a test compound against other candidates and commercially available agents, thereby improving candidate selection. In addition, they yield a rapid assessment of individual subject responses, and allow the preliminary selection of an appropriate panel of gene loci for further studies. Two example studies focused on the effects of NSAIDs and other anti-inflammatory agents on human blood are depicted in Fig. 4.

Ex vivo studies can provide a rapid and effective approach to pharmacodynamic analysis. Blood or other tissues are taken from treated individuals undergoing a well-defined therapeutic regimen (i.e., dose, time and route of administration) and subsequently exposed to various stimuli (e.g. specific cytokines or bacterial endotoxin) or other experimental conditions in culture. These studies can provide excellent pharmacodynamic insights in both normal subjects and patient populations.

Fig. 5 illustrates the effect of oral prednisone treatment (single dose, given prior to blood collection) on the whole blood response to LPS stimulation (performed after blood collection). Administration of prednisone 2 h prior to phlebotomy depressed LPS-stimulated mRNA levels for all 5 genes shown. The effect of the steroid ranged from 10-fold (*IL-1α*) to as much as 100-fold (*IFNγ* and *CSF2*). After 24 h, the anti-inflammatory effects of the steroid disappeared; the gene expression response patterns were again similar to pre-steroid conditions.

In vivo studies with high-precision gene expression analysis, either as stand-alone projects or as part of traditional clinical trials, provide a powerful way to track disease progression and drug efficacy.

In these studies, normal subjects or patients are treated with the therapeutic agent, and blood or other tissues are collected and immediately stabilized for mRNA measurement. Such studies can provide high-quality surrogate markers for tracking. As noted above (Fig. 1), the effect of a three-day regime of glucocorticosteroids on whole blood gene expression is a good example of this type of study. Following a three-day course of glucocorticosteroid treatment, the levels of *IL-1α*, *IL-1β*, *IL-8*, *IFN-γ*, and *TNFα* mRNAs were depressed while the levels of *IL-2*, *IL-5*, *IL-10*, *IL-12-p35*, and *IL-12-P40* mRNAs were elevated. *IL-15* mRNA was found to be only slightly elevated by the steroid. These results are consistent with the established inhibitory effects of glucocorticosteroids on type I cytokines followed by a relaxed inhibition of type II cytokines ([5]). In the three-day course of this study, key cytokine levels were altered. Compared to baseline, *IL-1α*, *IL-1β*, and *IL-8* were depressed 40 to 60%, and *IFNγ* was blocked approximately 95%. In contrast, *IL5* and *IL-12p35* were elevated about 10-fold.

The changes observed in these studies are relatively modest in magnitude, and could be easily obscured by less precise measurement or poor sample conditions. Although the fold increases may appear to be large, they could be entirely hidden by gratuitous induction in blood samples that are not immediately stabilized after collection. Indeed, whole blood specimens often exhibit 10-fold or greater stimulation of mRNA when drawn into standard EDTA tubes and allowed to sit at room temperature even for short periods. Systems that assist in RNA stabilization are now commercially available. Of particular note is the PAXgene™ Blood RNA System (PreAnalytiX, Hombrechtikon, Switzerland). This system, in our hands, provides consistent integration of whole blood collection and stabilization of intracellular RNA for days at room temperature and weeks at 4°C. Precision assays are mandatory for measurement of gene expression, particularly when changes are modest. The combination of highly precise assays and low levels of gratuitous gene activation in the specimens is required to demonstrate meaningful gene expression in test subjects.

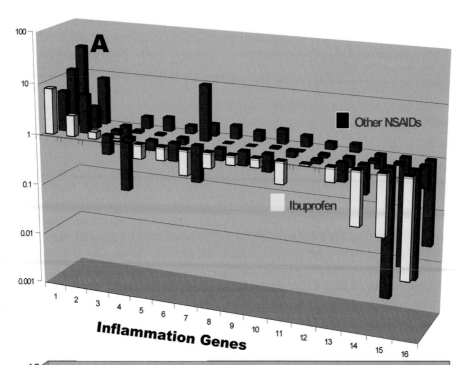

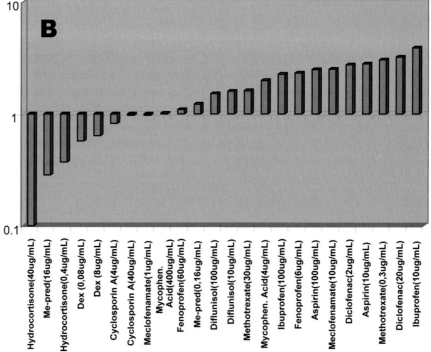

◀ **Fig. 4** *In Vitro* **Effects of Therapeutic Anti-inflammatory Agents on Gene Expression in Whole Blood. A) Pre-clinical Precision mRNA Profiles can be used to compare bioactivity of drugs.** The ibuprofen gene expression profile in LPS-stimulated whole blood was compared electronically to profiles for aspirin, acetaminophen and naproxen resident in the Source Precision inflammation database. Sixteen of 24 genes demonstrated a change in gene expression after drug treatment, with drug-to-drug variation. **B) Effect of 12 anti-inflammatory drugs on IL-1β gene expression in whole blood.** The glucocorticoids tested include dexamethasone, hydrocortisone, and methylprednisolone. These act to modify disease. The non-steroidal anti-inflammatory drugs (NSAIDs), including ibuprofen, diclofenac, meclofenamate, and fenoprofen, do not affect disease but do provide significant patient relief. Interestingly, glucocorticoids significantly reduce IL-1β gene expression, while the NSAIDs increase expression of IL-1β. The importance of this difference in drug-induced gene expression of a key gene locus will require additional investigation, but the observation does demonstrate the potential of gene expression analysis to monitor response to specific drug therapy.

G

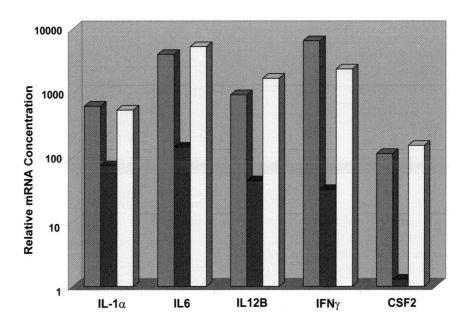

Fig. 5 *Ex Vivo* **Study: Precision mRNA Profiles of Human Whole Blood Reveal the Time-course of Glucocorticosteroid Action in Normal Individuals.** Blood was drawn from a volunteer before (blue bar), 2 h after (red bar) and 24 h after (yellow bar) administration of 60 mg prednisone. All samples were incubated for 6 h with 10 ng LPS/ml prior to assay. Samples were normalized to the mRNA levels found in unstimulated blood (equal to 1.0 on the ordinate). The height of the bar represents the relative level of mRNA corresponding to the gene listed below the bar.

Summary

Gene expression analysis is markedly enhanced through highly precise mRNA analysis, targeted drug-response and disease databases and diagnostic algorithms. Substantially improved handling procedures for whole blood severely curtail or entirely eliminate both inadvertent mRNA degradation and gratuitous gene activation. Together, these mRNA profiling improvements allow more rapid selection of pharmacological model systems, curtail the time spent in preclinical and clinical trials, and should compress the time required to pass from drug candidate to market – a process which has recently been estimated to consume 10 to 15 years and up to $800 million in resources[6]. Lastly, as drug-response and disease databases and diagnostic algorithms based upon gene expression grow and improve in the near future, we will improve our understanding of both the ▶ pharmacodynamics and ▶ pharmacokinetics of new pharmaceutical agents. Comparisons to gene expression profiles of known drugs will allow pharmaceutical companies to evaluate the mechanism of action of drug candidates. Precision gene expression analysis of clinical trial subjects will help companies to quickly and more safely determine the effective doses of these agents, as well as to predict the time the drug is likely to be effective in patients. The pharmacological applications of quantitative gene expression are manifold.

References

1. Southern, EM (1974) An improved method for transferring nucleotides from electrophoresis strips to thin layers of ion-exchange cellulose. Anal Biochem 62:317–318
2. Alwine JC, Kemp DJ, Stark GR (1977) Method for detection of specific RNAs in agarose gels by transfer to diazobenzyloxymethyl-paper and hybridization with DNA probes. Proc Natl Acad Sci U S A. 74:5350–5354
3. Schena, M (1996) Genome analysis with gene expression microarrays. Bioessays 18:427–431
4. Singer-Sam J, Robinson MO, Bellve AR, Simon MI, Riggs AD (1990) Measurement by quantitative PCR of changes in HPRT, PGK-1, PGK-2, APRT, MTase, and Zfy gene transcripts during mouse spermatogenesis. Nucleic Acids Research 18:1255–1259
5. Agarwal, SK, and Marshall, GD (2001) Dexamethasone promotes type 2 cytokine production primarily through inhibition of type 1 cytokines. J Interferon Cytokine Res 21:147–155
6. Tufts Center for the Study of Drug Development, Tufts University (2001) How New Drugs Move through the Development and Approval Process. "Backgrounder" Nov.30, www.tufts.edu/med/csdd/images/StepsInDrugDevelopment.pdf

Gene Gun

A gene gun is a device to introduce DNA into cells *in vivo*. The DNA is attached to gold particles which are introduced under high velocity into the target tissue.

▶ Genetic Vaccination

Gene Products

In the context of gene expression analysis, gene products include proximal products, such as primary transcripts, intermediate products, such as mRNA, tRNA, and rRNA, and distal products including proteins and peptides.

Gene Promoter

The gene promoter is a nucleotide sequence in DNA near the start of a gene, consisting of regulatory elements to which transcription factors and RNA polymerase bind. This leads to activation of the gene promoter and transcription of the corresponding gene.

Gene Therapy

ALEXANDER PFEIFER
University of Munich, Department of Pharmacy, Center for Drug Research, Munich, Germany
alexander.pfeifer@cup.uni-muenchen.de

Synonyms

Genetic therapy, gene based therapy

Definition

Gene therapy is a novel medical technology that is based on a simple prinicipal: genetic material is transfered into a cell and translated into therapeutic gene products (e.g. receptor proteins). The basic form of gene therapy is the introduction of a gene into the patient to correct the defect of a single gene. In addition, gene therapy can be used to treat complex diseases, e.g. by expressing genes that slow down the progression of the disease (for a more detailed overview see (1,2)).

▶ Antisense Oligonucleotides and RNA Interference
▶ Genetic Vaccination

Description

With the progress of the Human Genome Project and the numerous functional genomic projects, the number of genes that could be used as therapeutic agents is increasing at an astonishing pace. However, one of the major obstacles to successful gene transfer are the shortcomings of the presently available gene delivery vehicles. These vehicles can be divided in two basic categories: viral and non-viral vectors.

Compared to viral vectors, non-viral vectors present fewer problems regarding the biosafety. However, the major draw back of the presently available non-viral vectors is the insufficient gene transfer and that, due to the fact that these vectors do normally not integrate into the host genome, the delivered gene is expressed only transiently. In contrast, the hallmark of many viral vectors is that they achieve sustained and high levels of gene expression.

Design of viral vectors

Viral vector design focuses mainly on the efficacy of gene delivery and on the biosafety of the engineered viruses. A prerequisite for the use of a virus as gene therapy vehicle is to identify and eliminate pathological or toxic viral genes. Ideally, all viral genes are deleted from the viral vector and replaced by the gene of interest (also called transgene) (Fig. 1). The viral gene products required for the assembly of infectious viral particles and packaging of the vector into these particles are provided in *trans* by so-called producer/packaging cells, while necessary *cis*-acting factors (like packaging signals) are incorporated into the vector genome.

Viral vectors are usually classified by the characteristics of the parental virus. Based on the viral genome one can distinguish DNA and RNA viruses [for details see (2)].

DNA virus vectors

The most widely used DNA virus vectors are based on adenovirus (Ad) and adeno-associated virus (AAV). Adenoviruses contain a double-stranded DNA of ca. 36 kb and can infect and transduce a broad spectrum of cells including non-dividing cells like hepatocytes and neuronal cells. Ad vectors can be produced at high titers (~10^{14} particle/ml) and efficiently express transgenes in many different cells. However, transgene expression is only short-lived because the Ad chromosome does not integrate into the host genome and is maintained as an ▶ episome. In addition, adenoviral infection causes a humoral and cellular immune response in immune competent hosts. This immune response is not only directed against the viral particles but also against the infected cells. An unbalanced, massive immune response directed against Ad can be live threatening to the patient especially if a high concentration of Ad vectors is administered (1).

One rather new development in the Ad vector field are "gutless" Ad vectors that do not contain viral genes. Transgene expression from these gutless vectors has been reported to be more long lasting and the host immune response less pronounced [for ref. see (1)]. The other promising novelty are replication-competent Ad vectors that preferentially replicate in tumor cells, and are used for viral oncolysis. An example for such a virus is an Ad mutant (ONYX-015) that lacks the Ad E1B protein, which binds to the tumor suppressor p53 [ref. in (2)]. Thus, this Ad mutant replicates only in those cells that are p53-deficient and can be used to target tumor cells.

AAV-derived vectors are becoming ever more popular amongst gene therapists. Adeno-associated viruses are parvoviruses that are non-pathogenic to humans and carry a small genome of only 4.7 kb. Entry of AAV into the cell is mediated by binding to heparan sulfate proteoglycan (integrin avb5 and the fibroblast growth factor receptor 1 act as co-receptors). In the absence of so-called helper viruses (Ad and herpes viruses), AAV integrates into the host genome and establishes a latent infection. The integration of wild-type AAV is site-specific and requires the presence of the viral Rep protein, which is absent from the AAV-derived vectors presently available. Therefore, most of the AAV vector genomes do not integrate into the the

G

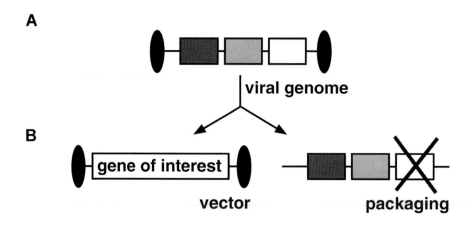

Fig. 1 Design of viral gene therapy vectors. A. Viral genome: The viral genome contains *cis*-acting sequences like packaging signals (black ovals) and the viral genes (squares). **B. Typical viral gene therapy vector with packaging construct:** In the ideal gene therapy vector all viral genes are deleted and replaced by the gene of interest; the vector contains the essential *cis*-acting sequences (left). The viral genes necessary for the production of infectious particles are provided in trans by transfection of helper/packaging cells with the packaging construct (right). Toxic or pathogenic viral genes are deleted from the packaging construct.

genome of the target cell, and in the rare case of integration it is random. *In vivo* analysis of AAV vector integration into murine hepatocytes demonstrated integration in no more than ~10% of the infected cells (3). The major form of recombinant AAV, at least in the liver, is extrachromosomal (3). However, the episomal circular form of AAV vector genomes exhibit long-lasting AAV-mediated gene expression for up to 9 months in brain and muscle [ref. in (2)].

The development of AAV-based gene therapy vectors is presently focused on the analysis of the properties of the different AAV serotypes especially the host range of the virion shells of the different serotypes. By packaging the commonly used AAV vector, which is derived from AAV type 2, into the virion shells of other AAV serotypes (▶ Cross-packaging) one can achieve efficient serotype-specific ▶ transduction of the target cell depending on the AAV receptors expressed on the target tissue. Thereby the host range of AAV vectors can be increased.

Another important issue is the size-limitation of AAV vectors: the optimum size of recombinant AAV genomes is 4.1 to 4.9 kb. To overcome this constraint a dual vector system with split-genome has been developed by several laboratories [ref. in

(2)] the dual vectors are based on trans-splicing of the split-genome after being transcribed from the episomal circular multimers formed by the AAV vector genomes. Theoretically, this simple principal should work if both vectors infect the target cell, however, the efficacy of the dual vector system has been debated.

RNA virus vectors

The principal RNA viruses used to develop gene therapy vectors are the Retroviridae. Retroviruses are enveloped viruses that integrate into the host genome. All retroviruses contain a basic set of three genes: *gag* (the structural virion proteins), *pol* (essential viral enzymes) and *env* (the viral glycoproteins of the envelope). Prototypic retroviruses like murine leukemia virus (MLV) carry only this simple set of genes, while complex retroviruses like the lentiviruses carry additional regulatory genes. The first gene therapy vectors were derived from prototypic retroviruses, and they were the first viral vectors to be used in clinical trials. Retroviral virions can accommodate ~ 7 kb of RNA and after reverse transcription in the target cells, the vector DNA is integrated randomly into the host chromosomes. Although, integration of the vector genome is of advantage if long-term (perhaps even life-long) vector expression is needed, the disadvantage of vector integration is the risk of insertional mutagenesis and activation of proto-oncogenes. To cope with the latter problem, self-inactivating retroviral vectors have been developed that carry deletions of the essential viral promoter/enhancer sequences [ref. in (2)]. An important feature of retroviral vectors is that one can change the ▶ tropism of the virus by pseudo-typing: i.e. the change of the envelope glycoprotein, which binds to receptors expressed by the target cells. A prerequisite for vector integration and transduction of the target cells by prototypic retroviral vectors is cell division, which allows for the passage of the viral ▶ preintegration complex into the nucleus. Therefore, vectors based on prototypic retroviruses can transduce only dividing cells, and many tissues (e.g. liver, muscle, and brain) of the adult are refractory to productive infection with simple retroviral vectors.

To circumvent this problem, vectors have been developed that are based on complex retroviruses, namely lentiviruses. In contrast to prototypic retroviruses, lentiviruses do not require cell-division for integration: the lentiviral preintegration complex is actively transported into the nucleus. Gene therapy vectors have been developed from a broad spectrum of lentiviruses ranging from human immunodeficiency virus (HIV) to visna/maedi virus (sheep virus). Presently, the most advanced lentiviral vector system is based on HIV-1. These vectors can efficiently transduce a broad spectrum of dividing and non-dividing cells including neurons, hepatocytes, muscle cells, and hematopoietic and embryonic stem cells [ref. in (2)]. The biosafety concerns are of utmost importance especially in the case of HIV-1-derived vectors. To address these concerns, self-inactivating lentiviral vectors, and stable packaging cell lines have been developed. Furthermore, the most commonly used HIV-1-derived lentiviral vectors contain only ~10% of the parental genome and no intact viral gene.

Apart from being a promising gene therapy vector, lentiviral vectors are also an important tool for molecular biology. These vectors can be used to transduce non-dividing cells *in vitro* and have been used to generate transgenic mouse and rats by infecting fertilized eggs and embryonic stem cells (4,5). In addition, human embryonic stem cells can be transduced by lentiviral vectors (5).

Regulation of gene expression

Another important problem of gene therapy is the regulation of gene expression in the target cells and tissues. Permanent or even life-long expression of the therapeutic gene is desired only in a minority of diseases (e.g. metastatic cancers). Thus, controlled expression of the foreign gene in a reversible manner would be highly desirable in many cases (e.g. gene therapy for insulin-dependent diabetes mellitus). Regarding the complex task of regulating gene expression within the organs of the patient, the presently available regulatable systems are rather simple. They are either based on naturally occurring inducible promoters that exhibit tissue-specificity or consist of chimeric systems, which contain pro- and eukaryotic elements.

To achieve physiological and/or therapeutical expression profiles new regulatable systems have to be developed that are controlled by endogenous (e.g. hormones) and/or exogenous (e.g. pharmacological agents) factors. In addition, the time course of gene expression and the induction pattern may also be crucial parameters for the therapeutic effect of gene therapy: the transition between the off-state and the on-state of gene expression can be achieved either by a quasi-discontinuous jump ("toggle-switch") or through a sigmoidal induction curve. Once turned on, regulation of transgene expression by the product of the transgene itself via negative or positive feedback mechanisms may also be a wanted feature for some applications.

Pharmacological Relevance

Modern pharmacology relies not only on chemical agents, but is also using biological agents, such as proteins (e.g. antibodies), to elicit therapeutic effects in patients. A new concept is to use DNA and other genetic material as a therapeutic agent. Thus, gene therapy is a form of molecular pharmacology.

Clinical Trials

Recently, the first successful gene therapy trial was published (6): Alain Fischer and colleagues treated children with severe combined immunodeficiency-X1 (SCID-X1) by *ex vivo* infection of the patients hematopoietic stem cells with a MLV-based vector. Presently, hundreds of clinical trials are being conducted in the U.S. and the EU.

A list of human gene therapy trials in the United States is available at the Office of Biotechnology Activities, National Institute of Health (http://www4.od.nih.gov/oba/rdna.htm).

Potential Risks

An important safety issue of viral vectors is whether or not the recombinant viruses are able to replicate in the infected cells. Replication of viral vectors is unwanted in most gene therapy approaches, in order to avoid spreading of the vector. Therefore, replication-defective vectors have been designed, which are able to perform only one initial infectious cycle within the target cell. In addition, replication-competent vectors have been designed – especially for the treatment of cancer – that are able to productively infect the target cell and to spread in the target tissue.

Another concern are immunological reactions of the host to either the delivery vehicle (be it viral or non-viral) or its cargo. The host immune response might not only eliminate the vector particles before they reach the target cells/tissues. In addition, it can also be directed against the product(s) of the genes delivered by the vector, especially if a null-mutation is replaced with a functional copy of the affected gene (in this case no immunological tolerance would exist for the product of the mutated gene) or if genes of other species are introduced.

References

1. Somia, N., and I. M. Verma (2001) Gene therapy: trials and tribulations. Nature Reviews Genetics 1:91–99
2. Pfeifer, A., and I. M. Verma (2001) Gene Therapy: Promises and Problems. Annu. Rev. Genomics Hum. Genet. 2:177–211
3. Nakai, H., S. R. Yant, T. A. Storm, S. Fuess, L. Meuse, and M. A. Kay (2001) Extrachromosomal recombinant adeno-associated virus vector genomes are primarily responsible for stable liver transduction in vivo. J Virol 75(15):6969–6976
4. Lois, C., E. J. Hong, S. Pease, E. J. Brown, and D. Baltimore (2002) Germline transmission and tissue-specific expression of transgenes delivered by lentiviral vectors. Science 295(5556):868–872
5. Pfeifer, A., M. Ikawa, Y. Dayn, and I. M. Verma (2002) Transgenesis by lentiviral vectors: lack of gene silencing in mammalian embryonic stem cells and preimplantation embryos. Proc Natl Acad Sci USA 99(4):2140–2145
6. Cavazzana-Calvo, M., S. Hacein-Bey, G. de Saint Basile, F. Gross, E. Yvon, P. Nusbaum, F. Selz, C. Hue, S. Certain, J. L. Casanova, P. Bousso, F. L. Deist, and A. Fischer (2000) Gene therapy of human severe combined immunodeficiency (SCID)-X1 disease. Science 288(5466):669–672

General Anaesthetics

Keith Wafford
Merck, Sharp & Dohme Research Laboratories, Harlow, UK
keith_wafford@merck.com

Synonyms

Anesthetic

Definition

General anaesthesia can encompass several different end points, the most critical of which can be defined as unconsciousness. A loss of sensation including that of any painful stimulus, and muscle relaxation are also desirable endpoints of general anaesthesia. Modern-day anaesthesia is accomplished using a balanced combination of different drugs to confer these different endpoints.

▶ GABAergic System
▶ Local Anaesthetics

Mechanism of Action

General anaesthetics have been in use for the last 100 years, yet their mechanism of action are still not yet clearly defined. For many years it was thought that general anaesthetics exerted their effects by dissolving in cell membranes and perturbing the lipid environment in a non-specific manner. This theory derived from the observation that for a number of drugs which induced anaesthesia, their potency correlated with their oil-water partition coefficients. This Meyer-Overton correlation was accepted for a number of years, however in the last 15–20 years evidence has shown that a more likely theory is that of specific interactions of anaesthetics with proteins, particularly those within the CNS that mediate neurotransmission (1).

Two methods of anaesthesia are currently in use, the application of inhaled gaseous or volatile anaesthetics such as halothane, sevoflurane and isoflurane to maintain a level of anaesthesia. Older compounds in this category include nitrous oxide and chloroform. The other method used is infusion of intravenous anaesthetics such as propofol, etomidate (for induction) and the barbiturates such as thiopental and pentobarbital. Investigations into the mechanism of anaesthesia have made use of all these compounds in order to identify a common mode of action linked to likely mechanisms within the CNS.

Research on anaesthetic mechanisms over the last 20 years has moved away from the lipid theory and focussed on specific protein interactions. The discovery that anaesthetics have major effects on receptors and channels within the nervous system have provided a clear and rational approach to understanding how anaesthesia is generated. Effects on ligand-gated ion channels currently offer the most likely mechanism of action, however some anaesthetics interact directly with voltage-gated channels (2). In general, activity at voltage-gated ion channels are relatively weak and may not correlate with anaesthetic doses. Similarly, there have been some reports of interactions with G-protein coupled receptors but again at non-clinical concentrations.

Which of the ligand-gated receptors are affected by anaesthetics and are relevant in conferring unconsciousness and loss of sensation? Volatile anaesthetics and alcohols are quite promiscuous in their effects on ligand-gated channels, showing potentiation of inhibitory channels such as ▶ GABA$_A$ and ▶ glycine receptors and inhibition of neuronal nicotinic acetylcholine, AMPA and ▶ NMDA receptors (3). Where investigated these compounds also potentiate kainate and 5-HT3 receptors (alcohols inhibit kainate). Intravenous agents are slightly more selective, potentiating GABA$_A$ and inhibiting neuronal nicotinic

receptors, however, effects on other ion channels are detectable at non-clinical concentrations. Ketamine is unique in having little effect on GABA receptors but strong inhibition of NMDA receptors. Recent studies using enantiomeric isomers of etomidate have suggested that the inhibition of nicotinic receptors is not what underlies the anaesthetic properties of this compound, but these effects are much more likely to be via potentiation of ▶ GABA$_A$ receptors, a feature common to the majority of anaesthetic agents at clinically relevant concentrations. The potency of volatile anaesthetics is expressed as MAC (minimum alveolar concentration) and when expressed as aqueous concentration ranges from 0.2–30 mM in terms of plasma concentration. These values equate well with their potency at GABA$_A$ receptors. Intravenous anaesthetic levels are estimated from measured drug concentrations in plasma during anesthesia and range between 0.3 and 50 μM, however, this may underestimate the true receptor occupancy with the drug.

Many anaesthetics exist as enantiomeric pairs which when seperated show selectivity in terms of anaesthetic potency. Studies on the action of anaesthetics at GABA$_A$ receptors have mimicked this selectivity, again providing evidence that anaesthetic effects are mediated via these receptors. The inhibitory component of all central nervous system transmission is primarily determined by GABA$_A$ receptors, being present at most inhibitory synapses and on the majority of neuronal cell bodies. It is clear that as GABA is such a major inhibitory component, enhancement of GABAergic function will produce pronounced depression of neuronal activity, consistent with that observed during anaesthesia.

A considerable body of data now exists demonstrating that the majority of volatile and intravenous anaesthetics potentiate GABA$_A$ receptor transmission both *in vivo* and *in vitro*. GABA$_A$ receptors comprise of a number of subtypes dependent on the components of a pentameric arrangement of subunits, which combine to form an ion channel selectively permeable to chloride. These are made up of $\alpha, \beta, \gamma, \delta, \epsilon$ and θ, with the majority of receptors comprising of 2α, 2β and a $\gamma2$ subunit. While the subunits all have unique regional distribution the majority of these receptors show sensitivity to anaesthetic agents. One exception to this is etomidate which demonstrates receptor selectivity for those containng a β2 or β3 subunit with little effect at β1 containing receptors. Recent studies combining molecular biology and electrophysiology have addressed the question of the site of action of anaesthetics on the receptor and these have revealed that potentiation by volatile anaesthetics and alcohols are dramatically affected by specific mutations at a serine residue within the second ▸ transmembrane spanning domain of the receptor (4). A second residue, an asparagine in the third transmembrane domain, can also abolish effects of these agents when mutated. Further studies based on these residues have shown that the ▸ anaesthetic cut-off for receptor potentiation can be affected and that photoactivatable anaesthetics can covalently label these residues, suggesting that there may be a binding pocket for these agents within this region of the receptor. Interestingly, the majority of intravenous agents remain unaffected by these mutations indicating that a separate region is involved in the binding of non-volatile agents. The availability of GABA$_A$ receptor subunit knockout mice, and the application of transgenic technology to generate mice containing receptor mutants such as those described above will considerably advance our understanding of anaesthetic mechanisms in the next few years.

Clinical Use (incl. side effects)

General anaesthetics are administered for many surgical procedures where the patient is likely to undergo a severely painful procedure, and complete unconsciousness and immobility is required for the surgery to be performed. The most commonly used volatile anaesthetics are halothane, isoflurane and sevoflurane. Nitrous oxide is also commonly used, particularly during childbirth. Side-effects that may be encountered following administration of these agents are cardiovascular and respiratory depression, post operative nausea and vomiting, hepatotoxicity via metabolite induction of liver enzymes, and occasionally nephrotoxicity from breakdown products.

Intravenous general anaesthetics are becoming increasingly popular due to the ease of application and continuous monitoring. Their rapid recovery has resulted in an increased use of these drugs in ambulatory surgery. They currently represent at least 50% of the total anaesthetic market and are dominated by propofol, followed by thiopental, etomidate and ketamine. A growing method of applying these anaesthetics is by target controlled infusion. This apparatus pumps a continous amount of drug into the blood, allowing the anaesthetist to set a desired plasma concentration, which the software inside the pump produces rapidly, but safely, by automatically controlling the infusion rate according to a continuous measure of either level of compound in the plasma or depth of anaesthesia, continuously monitered by EEG. This method known as TIVA (total intravenous anaesthesia) is becoming popular due to the ease of use and additional level of control it allows. Side effects associated with intravenous anaesthetics are less than the volatiles, particularly in regard to postoperative nausea and vomiting (especially propofol), however, cardiovascular and respiratory depression still cause problems with propofol and the barbiturates. Lack of cardiovascular side effects make etomidate particularly attractive for patients with a compromised heart condition, however, continuous infusion results in cortisol inhibition and adrenal failure, so etomidate can only be used for anaesthetic induction.

References

1. Franks NP, Lieb WR (1994) Molecular and cellular mechanisms of general anaesthesia. Nature 367:607–614
2. Thompson SA & Wafford KA (2001) Mechanism of action of general anaesthetics – new information from molecular pharmacology. Current Opinion in Pharmacology 1:78–83
3. Krasowski MD, Harrison NL (1999) General anaesthetic actions on ligand-gated ion channels. Cell Mol Life Sci. 55:1278–303
4. Mihic SJ, Ye Q, Wick MJ, Koltchine VV, Krasowski MD, Finn SE, Mascia MP, Valenzuela CF, Hanson KK, Greenblatt EP, Harris RA, Harrison NL (1997) Sites of alcohol and volatile anaesthetic action on GABA$_A$ and glycine receptors. Nature 389:385–389

Genetic Polymorphism

A genetic polymorphism is a difference in DNA sequence that has a frequency of at least 1% in a population. Some DNA sequence differences change the expression or function of drug metabolizing enzymes or of drug transporters or of drug target proteins and can therefore affect the disposition and action of drugs and xenobiotics. These are called pharmacogenetic polymorphisms.

▶ Single Nucleotide Polymorphisms
▶ Pharmacogenetics

Genetic Vaccination

Nico Michel, Martin Müller
Deutsches Krebsforschungszentrum Heidelberg
Germany
N.Michel@dkfz.de, Martin.Mueller@dkfz.de

Definition

DNA vaccines induce cellular and/or humoral immune responses upon injection of purified ('naked') plasmid DNA. In a more extended view, nucleic acid vaccination is performed using viral vector systems to increase the efficiency of delivery (for a more comprehensive overview see (1) andhttp://www.dnavaccine.com). The DNA that is used for vaccination contains a eukaryotic promoter that drives expression of a downstream gene encoding the antigen against which an immune response is to be evoked (▶ eukaryotic expression cassette, see Fig. 1). Compared to other vaccines (e.g. purified recombinant proteins, attenuated or inactivated live virus), DNA vaccines are of great simplicity and therefore can be produced easily and are very cost effective. The DNA is administered either via simple injection or with the aid of delivery vehicles (aerosols, liposomes, gold particles in combination with a ▶ gene gun). The choice of the application method has both qualitative and quantitative effects on the induction of an immune response. The major advantage of DNA vaccines is that the expressed protein enters the pathway of ▶ MHC-I presentation and thereby allows the induction of a cytotoxic T-cell response that is otherwise difficult to achieve using conventional vaccines, with the exception of live vaccines. DNA vaccines are currently under clinical investigation with the aim to produce prophylactic as well as therapeutic immune responses against a large variety of human pathogens including *Plasmodium falsiparum*, Human Immunodeficiency virus, Hepatitis B virus.

▶ Antisense Oligonucleotides and RNA Interference
▶ Gene Therapy

Description

Principles of DNA Vaccines, Mechanisms of Action
DNA vaccination was born when eukaryotic expression vectors were injected into the muscle of laboratory animals (2). The authors observed protein expression for more than two months after injection and noted that no special delivery systems was required to obtain this expression. Subsequently, it was demonstrated that antibodies can be induced simply by injecting plasmid DNA into the muscle of mice (3). Subsequent studies found that the injection of expression plasmids also leads to the induction of a cytotoxic T-cell response. In contrast to conventional vaccines, not the antigen itself but a gene encoding the antigen of interest is injected. After injection, the DNA enters cells of the vaccinated host and the encoded gene becomes expressed. This eventually leads to the induction of a cellular cytotoxic T-cell, T-helper and/or humoral (antibody) immune response.

While a humoral immune response is the primary protection against most viral and some bacterial diseases, protective defense against other pathogens such as HIV, plasmodium and tuberculosis requires a cellular, cytotoxic response mediated by $CD8^+$ T-cells (CTL response). Since the introduction of the vaccination concept by Jenner almost 200 years ago, only few vaccines have been developed that are able to induce a CTL response. These vaccines are usually attenuated live vaccines that are accompanied by certain risks and are not readily available for most pathogens. The growing

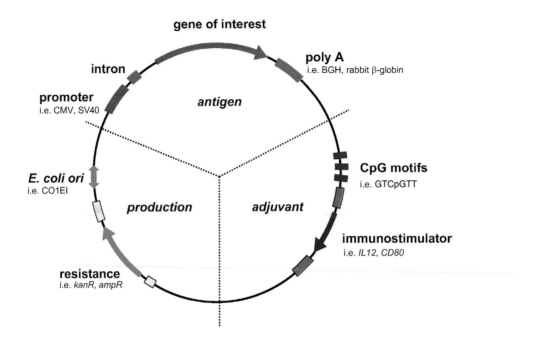

Fig. 1 Plasmid vector for DNA vaccination. Three functionally different regions can be distinguished in a typical vaccination vector. 1. *antigen region:* contains the gene encoding the antigen of interest under the control of either a strong viral, or a tissue type specific cellular promoter. Nuclear export and stability of mRNA require the presence of polyadenylation (poly A) sequences. In many instances, expression can be enhanced by insertion of a small exon upstream of the gene of interest. 2. *adjuvant region:* CpG DNA motifs (cytosine-phoshate-guanosine as part of the sequence: GACpGTC/T) of prokaryotic origin stimulate cytokine production *in vivo.* Optionally, genes for cytokines or co-stimulatory molecules (e.g. IL-4, IL-12, IL-18), can be co-delivered with the antigen gene to improve the immune response. 3. *production unit:* contains elements for the production of the plasmid in bacteria. This unit includes an origin of replication, antibiotic resistance gene or other selectable marker (note: the *ampicillin* resistance gene must not be used in clinical trials on humans).

success of DNA vaccines can be attributed primarily to the fact that they are able to induce long lasting CTL responses. Additionally, since the antigens are expressed in an authentic intracellular environment they have a high probability of assuming a native conformation and thereby induce an effective antibody response. Other advantages of DNA vaccines include (i) their low production costs, (ii) relatively safe use compared to live vaccines, and (iii) high stability not requiring intact cold chains.

Pharmacological Relevance

There are various protocols of administering eukaryotic expression vectors aiming to deliver

(i.e. transfect) the DNA into the cytoplasm of the host cells (see Fig. 2). The DNA is subsequently imported into the nucleus of the transfected cells allowing expression of the encoded antigen. To induce antigen-specific CD8$^+$ ► cytotoxic T-cells, the antigen has to be presented by professional ► antigen-presenting cells (APCs). It is under discussion whether DNA vaccination requires direct ► transfection of APCs (see Fig. 2A) or whether delivery of the DNA into non-immune cells (e.g. muscle cells; Fig. 2B) is sufficient. In the latter scenario, there are a number of pathways that allow transfer of the antigen from non-immune cells to APCs, a process that is called cross-priming.

Depending on the method used for DNA vaccination, the resulting immune response shows

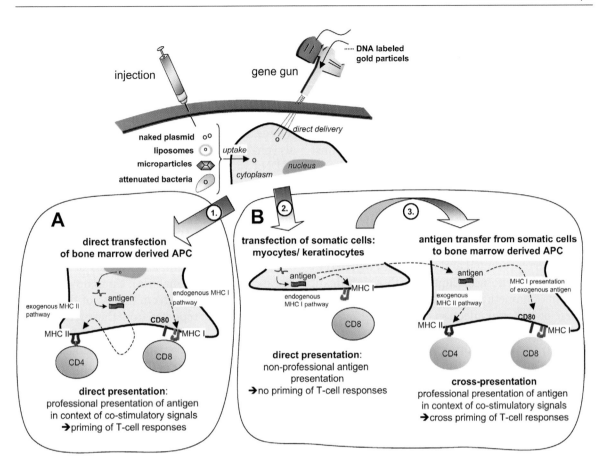

Fig. 2 Mechanisms of DNA vaccination. Via needle injection or with the aid of a gene gun, the expression construct is delivered into the cytoplasm and subsequently the nucleus of cells *in vivo*. Alternatively, non-invasive methods, such as aerosols and viral vectors are under development for improved DNA delivery. Following uptake of the DNA, the gene of interest becomes expressed by the transfected cell. Two major hypotheses have been proposed for the induction of a cellular immune response. A: In this scenario the DNA is delivered directly to specialized immune cells, the professional antigen-presenting cells (APCs). These cells have the ability to process the expressed antigen and present it to $CD8^+$ effector cells of the immune system in the context of the major histocompatibility complex class I (MHC I). The cytotoxic T-cells become efficiently activated since antigen-presenting cells provide the required co-stimulatory signals (i.e. CD80). An alternative mechanism for the induction of a cellular response (called cross-priming) is shown in B. In this setting, the antigen becomes expressed and presented by somatic, non-immune cells. Since these cells lack the co-stimulatory signals, this presentation does not lead to the activation of $CD8^+$ effector cells. It has been, however, postulated that the antigen expressed by the somatic cells can be transferred to APCs, which are able to activate the effector T-cells. Part of the antigen can also be released from cells thereby inducing the production of specific antibodies by circulating B-cells. This humoral immune response is further stimulated by $CD4^+$ T-helper cells that become activated by APCs presenting the antigen through the MHC class II pathway.

qualitative differences. Injection of naked plasmid DNA predominantly leads to the induction of a strong cytotoxic T-cell response. In contrast, if the DNA is delivered via gold-particle bombardment using a gene gun, the immune response is biased towards a humoral response. The reason for these differences is based on the fact that gold particle bombardment is thought to deliver the DNA directly into the cytoplasm of the host cells. This bypasses the interaction of the bacterially-derived vector DNA with specialized ▶ 'toll-like'-receptors present on the surface of many cells.

It has been established that plasmid DNA of prokaryotic origin, as is used in all DNA vaccination protocols, carries by itself an adjuvant effect on the stimulation of an immune response against the vector-encoded antigen but also against other antigens if they are co-administered with the DNA. The reason of this adjuvant effect lies in the presence of so-called CpG (5'-Cytosine-phosphate-Guanosine-3') motifs in the vector backbones. These motifs are, in comparison with prokaryotes, underrepresented and usually methylated in mammalian genomes. Contact with a significant amount of unmethylated ▶ CpG motifs during the course of bacterial infection or following vaccination with plasmid DNA of prokaryotic origin, leads to the activation of certain cells of the immune system and, as a consequence, to the secretion of a number of immuno-modulating ▶ cytokines. Meanwhile, it is known that DNA containing unmethylated CpG motifs are recognized by 'toll-like'-receptors present on a number of different cells of the immune system.

Potential Risks

There are a number of general safety concerns accompanying the use of DNA vaccines in humans: (i) The injected DNA might integrate into the host genome and thereby could cause cancer by insertional mutagenesis. (ii) The injected DNA might induce anti-DNA antibodies known to be key factors in certain autoimmune diseases. (iii) Immuno-regulatory cytokines induced by the CpG motifs present on the DNA vaccine might interfere with the host immune response either leading to autoimmune diseases or inducing tolerance to human pathogens that are present at the time of vaccination. Additional concerns are raised when, in addition to the antigen of interest, genes encoding immuno-stimulatory proteins such as cytokines are co-administered. It has been demonstrated that plasmid DNA can persist for weeks or even years post vaccination. It is as yet unclear what consequences might derive from such long term exposure to foreign antigens. None of the above listed events have yet been observed in existing experimental models. However, long term

consequences of DNA vaccination has to be evaluated carefully, especially since most vaccine applications that are currently in evaluation target newborns or young children.

Clinical Use

A large and rapidly growing number of clinical trials (phase I and pahse II) evaluating the potential of DNA vaccines to treat and prevent a variety of human diseases are currently being performed, however, there is yet no licensed DNA vaccine product available for use in humans. The clinical trials include the treatment of various types of cancers (e.g. melanoma, breast, renal, lymphoma) but also the prevention and therapy of infectious diseases (e.g. AIDS, malaria). Up to now, no principally adverse effects from the use of DNA vaccination have been reported from these trials.

Routes of Administration/Vehicles for Administration

Since the vast majority of DNA molecules become readily degraded by cellular nucleases upon injection of naked plasmid DNA, efforts have been undertaken to increase the number of DNA molecules reaching the nucleus of cells. DNA molecules can be introduced into the cytoplasm of cells by the use of gold particle bombardment via a gene gun. This reduces the amount of DNA required for induction of an immune response to $1/10^{th}$ compared with the injection of plasmid DNA. DNA molecules can also be delivered by liposome formulation and by microencapsulation. In addition, a number of routes of DNA injection (intramuscular, intradermal, intraperitoneal, epidermal, intranasal, intravenous) have been investigated. In most protocols, between 1–100 µg of DNA for small laboratory animals and 100–4000 µg of DNA for humans is used per administration. However, only a minute fraction of the DNA molecules actually arrive in the nucleus and lead to the production of protein in the pico–nanogram range over a time period of weeks to several months. Lastly, it has been demonstrated that oral delivery of a vaccine can be greatly improved by the use of nasal sprays and the use of viral vector systems that are able to target these tissues.

References

1. Gurunathan S, Klinman DM, Seder RA (2000). DNA vaccines: immunology, application, and optimization. Annu Rev Immunol 18:927–974
2. Wolff JA, Malone RW, Williams P, Chong W, Acsadi G, Jani A, Felgner PL (1990). Direct gene transfer into mouse muscle in vivo. Science 247:1465–1468
3. Tang DC, DeVit M, Johnston SA (1992). Genetic immunization is a simple method for eliciting an immune response. Nature 356:152–154

Genome

The genome is the gene complement of an organism. A genome sequence comprises the information of the entire genetic material of an organism.

Genomics

A primary goal of genomics is to determine the complete DNA sequence for all the genetic material contained in an organism's complete genome.

▶ Functional Genomics
▶ Structural Genomics

Genotype

The genotype is the form of a genetic polymorphism measured by molecular genetic methods.

▶ Pharmacogenetics

Gephyrin

Gephyrin is an intracellular membrane trafficking protein implicated in plasma membrane targeting and clustering of inhibitory glycine and GABA$_A$ receptors. The tubulin-binding protein forms oligomers, generating a submembraneous scaffold at the postsynaptic face of inhibitory synapses. This scaffold serves as an anchor to the inhitory glycine receptor and subtypes of the GABA$_A$ receptor, preventing the receptor complexes from lateral diffusion. Additional components of the postsynaptic protein scaffold include the phosphatidylinositol 3,4,5-trisphosphate binding proteins collybistin and profilin. Serving dual functions, gephyrin also contributes to the biosynthesis of the molybdenum cofactor, an essential coenzyme of dehydrogenases.

▶ Glycine Receptors
▶ GABAergic System

GERD

▶ Gastroesophageal Reflux Disease
▶ Proton Pump Inhibitors and Acid Pump Antagonists

GH

▶ Growth Hormone

Ghrelin

Ghrelin is a 28 amino acid peptide predominantly produced by the stomach, with substantially lower amounts derived from bowel, pancreas, kidney, placenta, pituitary and hypothalamus. Ghrelin has a strong ▶ growth hormone (GH)-releasing activity, which is mediated by the type Ia GH secretagogue (GHS Ia) receptor, which also specifically binds to a family of synthetic, peptidyl and non-pepetidyl, GH secretagogues (GHS). Ghrelin receptors are concentrated in the hypothalamus-pituitary unit, but are also distributed in other central and peripheral tissues. Besides its potent GH-releasing action, ghrelin has a variety of activities including stimulation of lactotroph and corticotroph secretion, orexant activity coupled with control of energy expenditure, influence on sleep, control of gastric motility and acid secretion, influence on endocrine pancreatic function and glucose metabolism, cardiovascular actions and anti-proliferative effects. It appears that ghrelin is a hormone controlling metabolic balance and managing the neuroendocrine and metabolic response to starvation.

Giardia Lamblia

Giardia lamblia is a ubiquitous, anaerobic flagellate that is responsible for acute and chronic diarrhoea. The cysts of *Giardia lamblia* are passed out with stool and are then ingested orally. In the small intestine they develop into trophozoites which attach to the mucosa. Giardiasis goes along with steatorroea and, if the infection persists, can cause typical symptoms of malabsorption.

▶ Antiprotozoal Drugs

GIRK

GIRK stands for G protein-regulated inwardly rectifying K^+ channel. GIRK channels are a family of proteins characterised by two membrane spanning domains and a pore-forming domain. GIRK channels are important components of signal transduction pathways regulated by G protein-coupled receptors. Activation of GIRK channels in neurons results in hyperpolarization and inhibition of neurotransmitter release.

▶ K^+ Channels
▶ Inward Rectifier K^+ Channels

Gitelman's Syndrome

A milder clinical course with symptoms usually not apparent before age 5-10, and hypocalciuria with hypomagnesemia has been the clinical distinction between Gitelman's syndrome and true ▶ Bartter's syndrome. The identification of a linkage between NaCl cotransporter (NCC) mutations and the disease provides a justification for this classification, and an explanation for the distinctly different phenotypes.

▶ Diuretics

Glial Cells

Glial cells are cells within the central or peripheral nervous system which are not immediately involved in information processing. Glial cells play an mportant role in the metabolic homeostasis of brain tissue and in nervous system development.

Glomerular Filtration Rate

Glomerular filtration rate (GFR) is the volume of plasma-like fluid that is filtered per unit time across the glomerular capillary membranes to enter the tubular space. Filtrate formation is driven by the net filtration pressure that is equal to the capillary hydrostatic pressure diminished by the sum of capillary oncotic pressure and tubular hydrostatic pressure. Although normally only 1% of the filtered NaCl and water is excreted as urine, reductions in GFR are often accompanied by parallel reductions in urine excretion.

▶ Diuretics

Glucagon

Glucagon is a single chain 21 amino acid polypeptide, which is synthesized mainly in the A-cells of the pancreatic islets as well as in the stomach. Glucagon secretion is stimulated by low, and inhibited by high, concentrations of glucose or fatty acids in the plasma. Sympathetic nerves and circulating adrenaline stimulate glucagon release *via* β-adrenoceptors. ▶ Somatostatin, released from D-cells of the pancreas to the glucagon-secreting A-cells in the periphery of the islets, inhibits glucagon release. One of the main physiological stimuli for glucagon secretion is the concentration of amino acids, in particular arginine, in the plasma. Glucagon acts on the liver to stimulate glycogen breakdown and gluconeogenesis as well as to inhibit glycogen synthesis and glucose oxidation. The net effect is consequently an increase in blood glucose. In liver and fat cells, glucagon induces lipolysis, while in muscle it leads to catabolism of proteins. The actions of glucagon on its major target tissues are thus the opposite of those of ▶ insulin. Glucagon exerts its effects through specific receptors, which belong to the group of ▶ G-protein coupled receptors. The glucagon receptor is coupled to ▶ adenylyl cyclase *via* the G-protein G_s in a stimulatory fashion . Glucagon can be used clinically to treat hypoglycaemia in unconscious patients under emergency conditions.

Glucagon-like Peptide-1

Glucagon, glucagon-like peptide-1 (GLP1), and GLP2 are three peptide hormones generated by cleavage of a common precursor polypeptide (pre-proglucagon). GLP1 stimulates insulin secretion from pancreatic B cells and inhibits feeding in fasted rats when injected into cerebral ventricules.

▶ Glucagon
▶ Insulin Receptor

Gluco-/Mineralocorticoid Receptors

HOLGER M. REICHARDT
Institute of Virology and Immunobiology,
University of Würzburg, Würzburg, Germany
holger.reichardt@mail.uni-wuerzburg.de

Synonyms

Glucocorticoid Receptor: GR; GCR; GRL; Nuclear Receptor Subfamily 3, Group C, Member 1 (NR 3C1); Glucocorticoid Receptor Type II
    Mineralocorticoid Receptor: MR; MCR; MRL; Nuclear Receptor Subfamily 3, Group C, Member 2 (NR3C2); Glucocorticoid Receptor Type I; Aldosterone Receptor

Definition

Glucocorticoid receptor (GR) and mineralocorticoid receptor (MR) are members of the nuclear receptor superfamiliy and mediate an organisms response to cortisol and aldosterone, two steroid hormones synthesized in the adrenal gland (1). GR is ubiquitously expressed and orchestrates a plethora of physiological processes including energy homeostasis, stress response and inflammation. In contrast, expression of MR is largely restricted to epithelial cells in kidney and colon as well as the limbic system of the brain. Consequently, MR mainly controls water homeostasis and cognitive processes. Due to their central roles in many physiological processes, lack of each of the two receptors is incompatible with life.

▶ Glucocorticoids
▶ Retinoids
▶ Sex Steroid Receptors

Basic Characteristics

In the inactive state GR and MR both reside in the cytoplasm bound to a complex of heat shock proteins. Due to their lipophilic nature, the main ligands cortisol and aldosterone can freely cross the cell membrane. Upon hormone binding the recep-

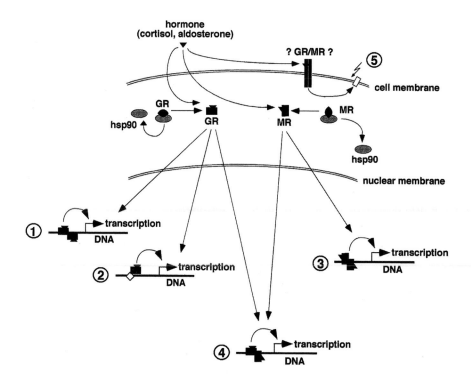

Fig. 1 Molecular modes of glucocorticoid and mineralocorticoid receptor action. After hormone binding GR translocates into the nucleus and modulates transcription either by binding of homodimers to DNA (1) or via protein-protein interaction with other transcription factors such as AP-1 or NF-κB (2). Similarly, hormone-occupied MR translocates into the nucleus and binds to DNA as a homodimer (3). GR and MR may also regulate transcription by forming heterodimers on DNA (4). Finally, glucocorticoids and mineralocorticoids presumably bind to yet uncharacterized membrane receptors and thereby elicit fast responses (5). For more details refer to text.

tor is released and translocates into the nucleus (Fig. 1). Following homodimerization GR and MR bind to specific response elements located in the promoter and enhancer region of responsive genes and thereby induce gene expression. Thus, GR and MR both act as transcription factors. In addition, evidence has accumulated that the two receptors may also heterodimerize, resulting in synergy or inhibition of transcription. Besides these DNA-binding-dependent mechanisms, GR but not MR also interacts with other transcription factors without direct DNA contact itself (4). In this case, GR acts as a corepressor or coactivator of transcription. This second mode of GR-action, also known as cross-talk, plays a particularly pivotal role in the regulation of the immune system. Finally, so-called non-genomic effects have been described for both GR and MR. These fast

responses, occuring within seconds or minutes, are mainly found in the nervous system. However, whether they are mediated by classical GR and MR or via unrelated receptors remains an unsolved issue.

Molecular Characterization of Glucocorticoid and Mineralocorticoid Receptors

The cDNA of GR was first cloned in 1985 (2). GR is a 94kD protein and consists of 777 (α) amino acids in the human. The cDNA of MR was cloned two years later by homology screening and represents a 107kD protein consisting of 984 amino acids in the human (3). GR and MR are formed of a modular structure consisting of three major domains, common to most members of the nuclear receptor superfamily. The central DNA-binding domain is the most conserved one and consists of two zinc-fingers. The first one is responsible for DNA-binding whereas the second one contributes to dimerization of the receptor. The C-terminal region is made of the ligand-binding domain which is responsible for hormone binding and interpretation. Additionally, the hormone-dependent transactivation domain AF-2 and a nuclear-localization signal are located here. The N-terminal domain is the least conserved region and contains the transactivation domain AF-1.

Human glucocorticoid receptor maps to the long arm of chromosome 5 (5q31-5q32) whereas human mineralocorticoid receptor maps to the long arm of chromosome 4 (4q31.1).

Between 5,000 and 100,000 GR molecules are found within almost every cell of an organism. The affinity constant for cortisol is approximately 30 nM, which is in the range of the concentration of free hormone in the plasma under normal conditions. Consequently, receptor occupancy can be expected to be 10–70%. This suggests that changes in cortisol secretion, such as under stress conditions, directly translate into alterations in GR occupancy and thus transcriptional responses.

Although MR also binds glucocorticoids, its main ligand in classical mineralocorticoid target tissues such as kidney and colon is aldosterone (K_d 1.3 nM). This can be attributed to the ability of ▶ 11β-hydroxysteroid dehydrogenase type II (11β-HSD II) to convert active cortisol into its inactive metabolite cortisone in these tissues. Since aldosterone is no substrate for this enzyme it can readily bind to MR, leading to exclusive occupation of the receptor by aldosterone. In contrast, no such mechanism exists in brain, resulting in predominant glucocorticoid binding to MR. Since MR has an approximately 10-fold higher affinity for cortisol than GR, it is almost completely occupied by hormone under basal conditions.

Control of Glucocorticoid Secretion by the Hypothalamus-Pituitary-Adrenal Axis

Synthesis and secretion of glucocorticoids is controlled by a neuroendocrine cascade called the ▶ hypothalamus-pituitary-adrenal (HPA) axis. Stimuli such as stress or infection lead to the release of corticotropin-releasing hormone (CRH) in the hypothalamus. CRH is transported to the anterior pituitary where it induces increased synthesis and secretion of adrenocorticotrope hormone (ACTH). Finally, ACTH stimulates release and production of glucocorticoids in the adrenal cortex. Protection from chronically elevated hormone levels is achieved by a negative feedback loop where glucocorticoids inhibit their own production and secretion by binding to GR, mainly in the pituitary and in the hypothalamus. Further regulation comprises effects of GR and MR on glucocorticoid production exerted via higher brain centers such as the hippocampus. Superimposed on the regulation by the HPA axis, glucocorticoid serum levels show a circadian rhythm with high levels in the morning and low levels in the evening (in the human). Finally, a feedback loop connecting glucocorticoid production with the control of the immune system is operative. Cytokines released during inflammation stimulate glucocorticoid secretion which in turn inhibits cytokine production. This shows that glucocorticoids acting via GR and MR are under complex regulation in the field of tension between the endocrine, immune and central nervous system.

Physiological Functions of Glucocorticoid Receptors

As it can easily be deduced from its name, glucocorticoids play an important role in carbohydrate metabolism. They increase hepatic glycogen and gluconeogenesis, decrease glucose uptake and utilization in peripheral tissues, and cause a tendecy for hyperglycemia and reduced glucose tolerance. Furthermore, energy homeostasis is also influenced via effects on protein and lipid metabolism. An important function of glucocorticoids which is widely employed in clinical therapy is its pronounced anti-inflammatory and immunosuppressive activity. Glucocorticoids inhibit (i) production and release of various cytokines (IL-1, IL-6, TNFα), chemokines (IL-8) and vasoactive agents (prostaglandins, NO), (ii) the movement of leukocytes to inflamed areas, and (iii) the function of immunocompetent cells, such as T-lymphocytes and macrophages (induction of apoptosis, inhibition of proliferation, impairment of phagocytosis). In the central nervous system, glucocorticoids contribute to mood and memory formation. Pathological effects of high glucocorticoid levels include osteoporosis due to enhanced bone resorption as well as hypertension and growth retardation. Further sites of GR action which become important under various circumstances are erythropoiesis, adrenalin synthesis and lung function. This shows that a plethora of physiological processes involves transcriptional regulation by GR, also explaining the variety of symptoms observed in diseases related to GR dysfunction or after genetic manipulation in animals (see below).

Diseases Related to Glucocorticoid Dysregulation

The most common disease related to glucocorticoids is Cushing's syndrome. This disorder is characterized by hypercortisolism due to a pituitary or adrenal tumor. The elevated glucocorticoid levels lead to a large spectrum of symptoms, including obesity, hirsutism, hypertension, muscular weakness, depression, osteoporosis, short stature, facial plethora, fat redistribution and atrophy of the skin. Treatment of Cushing's disease is either achieved by surgical removal of the tumor or by pharmacological interference with ACTH or cortisol hypersecretion. Addison's disease, in contrast, is caused by adrenocortical insufficiency mainly following autoimmune destruction or tuberculosis. Clinical features of hypocortisolism include fatigue, weight loss, anorexia and hypotension. Treatment can only be achieved by life-long replacement therapy with both glucocorticoid and mineralocorticoid hormones. In contrast to the two formerly described syndromes, congenital adrenal hyperplasia (CAH) has a genetic cause. Mutations in genes encoding steroidogenic enzymes impair the production of both glucocorticoid and mineralocorticoid hormones. As a consequence of the missing negative feedback, there is an overproduction of ACTH resulting in enhanced androgen production by the adrenal gland, which also contributes to the clinical features of CAH. Finally, depression is also linked to GR and MR function in a way not fully understood. It has been observed that depressive illnesses are usually accompanied by elevated glucocorticoid levels and a blunted circadian rhythm and that these changes normalize after application of anti-depressants. However, whether glucocorticoids are cause or effect of depression remains to be elucidated.

Clinical Features and Genetic Basis of Glucocorticoid Resistance

Primary glucocorticoid resistance in humans is characterized by elevated plasma cortisol concentrations, a normal circadian pattern set at a higher level and resistance to adrenal suppression by dexamethason in the absence of clinical signs of Cushing's syndrome. The absence of hypercortisolism is presumably due to the fact that glucocorticoid resistance is in balance, with periperal tissues being as resistant to hormone as the central tissues of the HPA axis. In severe forms, primary glucocorticoid resistance is accompanied by an increase in mineralocorticoid secretion leading to hypertension and hypokalemic alkalosis. In women, overproduction of androgens causes signs of hirsutism. The causes of glucocorticoid insensitivity are diverse and not yet fully understood. For example, point mutations in the GR gene leading to reduced hormone binding or transcriptional capacity, reduced number of receptor molecules due to heterozygosity or splice-site mutations, and changes in receptor associated proteins have accounted for the observed clinical symptoms. Additionally, resistance to glucocorticoids can also be aquired as shown in leukemia or asthma patients who have continually been treated with high doses of hormone.

Animal Models for Glucocorticoid Receptor Function

Pepin and coworkers generated transgenic mice in which antisense RNA complementary to GR cDNA led to reduced expression mostly in neuronal tissues. Consequently, reduced GR expression was found to result in impaired behaviour, a defective response to stress as well as obesity. King and coworkers generated transgenic mice where reduced GR expression was limited to the thymus. This led to an altered thymocyte development, changes in the T-cell repertoir and a reduced risk to develop autoimmune diseases.

Cole *et al.* (1995) reported the production of ▶ knock-out mice with a germ-line deletion of GR. They demonstrated that the lack of GR leads to perinatal death, atelectasis of the lung and lack of adrenalin synthesis. To circumvent perinatal lethality, Tronche *et al.* (1999) generated tissue-specific somatic deletions of GR. When restricted to the nervous system this led to reduced anxiety and an altered neuroendocrine response. Due to the upregulation of the HPA axis, high glucocorticoid levels were found in these animals causing symptoms reminescent of those observed in Cushings' disease.

Since GR can influence transcription both through DNA-binding-dependent and -independent mechanisms, Reichardt *et al.* (1998) attempted to separate these two modes of action by introducing a point mutation into GR. This mutation interferes with transactivation while transcriptional regulation via cross-talk with other transcription factors such as AP-1 and NF-κB remains intact (see above). In contrast to mice lacking GR, these GR^{dim} mice are viable, revealing the importance of DNA-binding-independent transcriptional regulation by GR *in vivo*. Mutant mice loose the ability to transactivate gene transcription by cooperative DNA-binding, which results in impaired thymocyte apoptosis, erythropoiesis, gluconeogenesis and memory formation. In contrast, most immunosuppressive and anti-inflammatory effects of glucocorticoids are functional in the absence of DNA-binding by GR.

To study the effect of an increased gene dosage of GR, Reichardt *et al.* (2000) generated mice with four functional GR alleles. This led to an overexpression of GR protein, resulting in a reduced response to stress, increased sensitivity to thymocyte apoptosis and a lower risk to die from experimentally-induced endotoxic shock. These results highlight the importance of tight control of GR expression in target tissues and may explain differences in the susceptibility of humans to inflammatory diseases and stress.

Physiological Functions of Mineralocorticoid Receptors

MR forms an essential component of the ▶ renin-angiotensin-aldosterone system (RAAS) which regulates salt and water homeostasis in the body. In particular, MR mediates an organisms response to aldosterone in tissues such as kidney, colon and salivary gland. In the distal tubules of the kidney it induces enhanced sodium and water retention in response to a reduction in extracellular fluid volume or a fall in blood pressure. Besides its role in salt and water homeostasis, MR appears to play a major role in the limbic system of the brain. Notably, high levels of MR are expressed in hippocampus and amygdala where it modulates the transcriptional response to glucocorticoid hormones in concert with GR. Studies with specific MR ligands as well as analyses of genetically manipulated mice have indicated that MR in the brain is involved in the control of cognitive processes such as learning and memory and in the modulation of mood and anxiety.

Diseases Related to Mineralocorticoid Receptors

Several diseases involving dysregulation of MR function have been described although most of them are not causatively linked to the receptor itself. For example, pseudohypoaldosteronism is a syndrome of mineralocorticoid resistance that is characterized by urinary salt loss and dehydration. However, mutations in the MR gene have rarely been found in these patients. In most cases this syndrome appears to be linked to defects in the subunits of the amiloride-sensitive sodium channel ENaC, a major target of mineralocortiocid action in the kidney.

Patients suffering from hyperaldosteronism usually present with severe hypertension and marked sodium retention due to high levels of circulating aldosterone. Whereas primary forms of this disease are caused by certain tumors of the adrenal cortex resulting in increased hormone production (Conn's disease), secondary forms often can be attributed to enhanced secretion of renin. In contrast, patients with apparent mineralocorticoid excess (AME) show unremarkable levels of aldosterone and cortisol. In fact, this syndrome can be explained by recessive mutations in the gene encoding 11β-HSD II (see above). Diminished or absent activity of the enzyme leads to massive activation of MR in kidney by the comparably high concentrations of circulating cortisol and consequently to strong sodium and water retention.

Animal Models for Mineralocorticoid Receptor Function

Berger and coworkers generated MR knock-out mice by gene targeting. Until day 10 after birth these mice developed normally. Later the mice showed symptoms of pseudohypoaldosteronism characterized by massive loss of renal sodium and water, finally leading to death. The lack of MR caused a severe upregulation of the renin-angiotensin-aldosterone system with a strong increase in most of its components. Using a salt replacement protocol, it was possible to rescue the mutant mice from postnatal death, thus allowing the study of the physiological role of MR in adults. Analyses of the brain revealed that loss of MR caused increased neurodegeneration in the hippocampus accompanied by reactive gliosis and decreased neurogenesis. This observation offers an attractive explanation for the effects of steroid hormones on cognitive functions and anxiety. More detailed analyses on the role of MR in the adult will be conduced using recently developed tissue-specific MR knock-out mice.

Drugs

GR Ligands

Glucocorticoid agonists mainly comprise cortisol, corticosterone, aldosterone and a number of synthetic steroids used in clinical therapy, such as dexamethasone, prednisolone or triamcinolone. Agonists are defined as compounds that bind to a receptor and elicit a transcriptional response. Cortisol and corticosterone have equal affinities for GR, however due to the concentration of circulating hormone, cortisol is the principal glucocorticoid in humans whereas it is corticosterone in rodents. Aldosterone also displays high affinity for GR but since its concentration in plasma is about three magnitudes of order lower than the one of cortisol, aldosterone does not play a physiologically meaningful role for GR activity.

Glucocorticoid antagonists also bind specifically to GR. However, these steroids don't elicit a response but rather compete with agonists for binding and therefore prevent an agonist response. In addition, partial agonists are known that elicit an intermediate reponse of GR. Well known examples of glucocorticoid antagonists are RU486 (Mifepristone), which also binds to progesterone receptor, and the unrelated compound ZK98299, a presumably pure GR ligand. However, RU486 is not a full antagonist since some transcriptional activities of GR cannot be inhibited by this compound.

Synthetic glucocorticoids may be grouped in several classes: First, compounds which are more potent than naturally occurring glucocorticoids due to a higher binding affinity or decreased clearance rate. Due to both of these effects, dexamethasone for example is over 10 times more potent than cortisol. Second, compounds that have less mineralocorticoid activity resulting in a reduced spectrum of MR-mediated side-effects. Third, dis-

sociating compounds that are unable to induce transcriptional responses which are mediated by DNA-binding of GR but which are still functional in modulating transcription by interaction with other transcription factors (see above). This characteristic is expected to be useful in achieving potent anti-inflammatory and immunosuppressive effects (thought to be primarily mediated by interaction with other transcription factors) but lacking some of the adverse effects (presumably mediated by DNA-binding-dependent transcriptional regulation by GR). This principle has recently gained support from an animal model (GR^{dim}, described above) which mimicks this dissociating principle *in vivo*.

MR Ligands

MR has a high affinity for mineralocorticoids such as aldosterone and DOC. In addition, MR also binds glucocorticoids although in mineralocorticoid target tissues this is prevented by the enzyme 11β-HSD II (see above). Since mineralocorticoids are not substrates for 11β-HSD II, due to their cyclic 11,18-hemiacetyl-group, they are able to bind to MR despite the 1000-fold lower concentration in plasma as compared to cortisol.

The main mineralocorticoid agonist in humans is aldosterone. Additionally, cortisol, corticosterone and DOC also have mineralocorticoid agonistic activity. The synthetic steroid fludrocortisone (9α-fluorocortisol) is extremely potent and usually chosen for replacement mineralocorticoid therapy. In contrast, aldosterone and DOC are not useful in oral therapy due to rapid degradation in the liver following absorption.

Mineralocorticoid antagonists include RU26752, spironolactone and progesterone. Whereas endogenous progesterone may only play a role during the third trimester of pregnancy, spironolactone and RU26752 are synthetic drugs which have been developed for the treatment of pathological states of sodium-regulation and hypertension. Both drugs bind to MR with equal affinity as aldosterone but induce an transcriptionally silent state.

References

1. Beato M, Herrlich P, Schütz G (1995) Steroid hormone receptors: many actors in search of a plot. Cell 83:851–857
2. Hollenberg SM, Weinberger C, Ong ES, Cerelli G, Oro A, Lebo R, Thompson EB, Rosenfeld MG, Evans RM (1985) Primary structure and expression of a functional human glucocorticoid receptor cDNA. Nature 318:635–641
3. Arriza JL, Weinberger C, Cerelli G, Glaser TM, Handelin BL, Housman DE, Evans RM (1987) Cloning of human mineralocorticoid receptor complementary DNA: structural and functional relationship with the glucocorticoid receptor. Science 237:268–275
4. Reichardt HM, Kaestner KH, Tuckermann J, Kretz O, Wessely O, Bock R, Gass P, Schmid W, Herrlich P, Angel P, Schütz G (1998) DNA binding of the glucocorticoid receptor is not essential for survival. Cell 93:531–541
5. Cole TJ, Blendy JA, Monaghan AP, Krieglstein K, Schmid W, Aguzzi A, Fantuzzi E, Hummler K, Unsicker K, Schütz G (1995) Targeted disruption of the glucocorticoid receptor gene blocks adrenergic chromaffin cell development and severly retards lung maturation. Genes and Development 9: 1608-1621
6. Tronche F, Kellendonk C, Kretz O, Gass P, Anlag P, Orban PC, Bock R, Klein R, Schütz G (1999). Disruption of the glucocorticoid receptor gene in the nervous system results in reduced anxiety. Nature Genetics 23: 99-103
7. Reichardt HM, Umland T, Bauer A, Kretz O, Schütz G (2000) Mice with an increased glucocorticoid receptor gene dosage show enhanced resistance to stress and endotoxic shock. Molecular and Cellular Biology 20: 9009-9017

Glucocorticoids

Ian M. Adcock
Imperial College, London, UK
ian.adcock@ic.ac.uk

Synonyms

Corticosteroids, Glucocorticoid agonists, Steroids, Asthma Controllers.

Definition

Endogenous glucocorticoids (cortisol) are released from the zona fasiculata of the ▶ adrenal gland in response to stress. When in excess glucocorticoids can cause ▶ catabolism of muscle and release of amino acids; these are subsequently used to increase glucose synthesis by the liver (gluceonogenesis). The most important function of glucocorticoids in disease is to regulate the inflammatory response to exogenous stimuli. Exogenous glucocorticoids have been used clinically for over 50 years and have proved to be indispensable in the regulation of a variety of inflammatory and immune states.

▶ Gluco-/Mineralocorticoid Receptors
▶ Immunosuppressive Agents
▶ Inflammation

Mechanism of Action

Inflammation is a central feature of many chronic lung diseasesincluding ▶ bronchial asthma. The specific characteristics of the inflammatory response and the site of inflammation differ between these diseases, but all involve the recruitment and activation of inflammatory cells and changes in the structural cells of the lung. These diseases are characterised by an increased expression of many mediators including cytokines, chemokines, growth factors, enzymes, receptors and adhesion molecules. Increased inflammatory gene transcription is regulated by pro-inflammatory transcription factors, such as nuclear factor-κB (▶ NF-κB). For example, NF-κB is markedly activated in epithelial cells of asthmatic patients and this transcription

Tab. 1 Glucocorticoid sensitive genes

Increased transcription	Decreased transcription
Lipocortin-1/Annexin-1 (phospholipase A_2 inhibitor)	Cytokines (IL-1, 2, 3, 4, 5, 6, 9, 11, 12, 13, 16, 17, 18, TNFa, GM-CSF, SCF)
β_2-Adrenoceptor	Chemokines (IL-8, RANTES, MIP-1α, MCP-1, MCP-3, MCP-4, eotaxin)
Secretory leukocyte inhibitory protein (SLPI)	Inducible nitric oxide synthase (iNOS)
Clara cell protein (CC10, phospholipase A_2inhibitor)	Inducible cyclooxygenase (COX-2)
IL-1 receptor antagonist	Cytoplasmic phospholipase A_2 (cPLA$_2$)
IL-1R2 (decoy receptor)	Endothelin-1
IκBα (inhibitor of NF-κB)	NK$_1$-receptors, NK$_2$-receptors
CD163 (Scavenger receptor)	Adhesion molecules (ICAM-1, E-selectin)

factor regulates many of the inflammatory genes that are abnormally expressed in ▶ bronchial asthma.

NF-κB is activated by all the stimuli thought to be important in the inflammatory response to allergen exposure seen in asthma and is the major target for glucocorticoids. NF-κB is ubiquitously expressed within cells and is able to not only control the induction of inflammatory genes in its own right but can enhance the activity of other cell- and signal-specific transcription factors. NF-κB is activated by numerous extracellular stimuli including cytokines, such as tumour necrosis factor-α (TNFα) and interleukin-1β (IL-1β), rhinovirus infection and allergen exposure. NF-κB is held within the cytoplasm in an inactive state by an inhibitor protein I-κBα. Phosphorylation of IκBα following cell stimulation leads to the dissociation of IκBα from NF-κB, enabling nuclear translocation and binding to specific DNA response elements within the ▶ regulatory regions of responsive genes.

Due to the large amount of DNA present within the nucleus it must be carefully packaged. In the resting cell DNA is tightly compacted around basic ▶ histone proteins, excluding the binding of the enzyme ▶ RNA polymerase II, which activates the formation of ▶ mRNA. This conformation of the chromatin structure is described as 'closed' and is associated with suppression of gene expression. Expression of genes is associated with enzymatic modification of core histones leading to alterations

in chromatin structure. Specific lysine residues within the N-terminal tails are capable of being post-translationally modified by acetylation. Acetylation of the σ-group on lysines reduces the charge of the histone residues within the tightly wound DNA inducing a relaxed DNA structure and allowing the recruitment of large protein complexes including RNA polymerase II.

Repression of genes is associated with reversal of this process by histone deacetylation, a process controlled by histone deacetylases (HDACs). Deacetylation of histones increases the winding of DNA round histone residues, resulting in a dense chromatin structure and reduced access of transcription factors to their binding sites, thereby leading to repressed transcription of inflammatory genes.

Cytokines such as TNFα and IL-1β, acting via NF-κB, can induce histone acetylation in both a time- and concentration-dependent manner. Upon DNA binding, NF-κB recruits ▶ transcriptional co-activators such as CREB binding protein (CBP) and p300/CBP-associated factor (PCAF) which have intrinsic histone acetyltransferase (HAT) activity.

Glucocorticoids exert their effects by binding to a cytoplasmic receptor (GR). GRs are expressed in almost all cell types. The inactive GR is bound to a protein complex that includes two subunits of the Heat Shock Protein (▶ HSP) 90, which thus act as cytoplasmic inhibitors preventing the nuclear localisation of unoccupied GR. Once the ligand binds to GR, HSP90 dissociates allowing the nuclear localisation of the activated GR-steroid complex and its binding as a homodimer to specific DNA sequences (GREs, GGTACAnnnTGT-TCT) and interaction with ▶ co-activator complexes.

Glucocorticoids produce their effect on responsive cells by stimulating GR to directly or indirectly regulate the transcription of target genes. The number of genes per cell *directly* regulated by glucocorticoids is estimated to be between 10 and 100, but many genes are indirectly regulated through an interaction with other transcription factors and co-activators. Glucocorticoids may suppress inflammation by increasing the synthesis of anti-inflammatory proteins, such as annexin-1, IL-10 and the inhibitor of NF-κB, IκB-α (Table 1). In addition, it is likely that glucocorticoid side effects, such as ▶ osteoporosis, cataracts, skin fragility and Hypothalamic-Preoptic-Adrenal axis suppresion are due to gene activation.

GRs, as with NF-κB and other transcription factors, increase gene transcription through an action on chromatin modifications and recruitment of RNA polymerase II to the site of local DNA unwinding. GR interacts with CBP and other co-activator proteins, including CBP, PCAF and steroid receptor co-activator-1 (SRC-1), which enhance local HAT activity. This raises the question: how can GR, or any other transcription factor, interact with its recognition site when DNA is compacted? GR may bind to a GRE within the linker DNA between nucleosomes or alternatively GR may bind to a GRE when the GRE is wound around histones as long as the GRE residues are facing outwards. Binding to the GRE may then modify the local chromatin structure altering GR access.

There is now clear evidence that GR does not stably associate with DNA but rather it has a 'hit-and-run' mechanism of action. After activation GR resides on DNA for less than 10s before being ejected and replaced by another GR. This ejection may allow binding of additional regulatory factors that enhance gene transcription such as HAT-containing complexes and may also play a role in feedback regulation and subsequent ▶ proteosomal degradation of GR.

In spite of the ability of glucocorticoids to induce gene transcription, the major anti-inflammatory effects of glucocorticoids are through repression of inflammatory and immune genes. The inhibitory effect of glucocorticoids appears to be due largely to an interaction between activated GR and transcription factors, such as NF-κB and activator protein-1 (AP-1, a heterodimer of Fos and Jun proteins), which mediate the expression of inflammatory genes. The interplay between pro-inflammatory transcription factors and GR may reflect differing effects on histone acetylation/deacetylation. Thus, glucocorticoids are able to attenuate the NF-κB-mediated induction of histone acetylation by IL-1β. This occurs by a direct inhibition of NF-κB-associated HAT activity and by active recruitment of HDAC proteins (Fig. 1). Overall, this results in the deacetylation of histones, increased tightening of DNA round histone residues resulting in repression of inflammatory genes.

▶ Mitogen-activated protein kinases (MAPK) play an important role in inflammatory gene expression through the regulation of pro-inflammatory transcription factors and there is increasing evidence that glucocorticoids may exert an inhibitory effect on these pathways. Glucocorticoids reduce the stability of mRNA for inflammatory genes such as cyclooxygenase-2 (▶ COX-2) through an inhibitory effect on p38 MAP kinase, through rapid induction of a specific p38 MAPK phosphatase (MKP-1) and subsequent dephosphorylation of phospho-p38 MAPK. GR has also been shown to prevent serine phosphorylation of c-Jun and, subsequently, AP-1 activation, by blocking the induction of the Jun N-terminal kinase (JNK) signalling cascade. Consistent with this, glucocorticoids also antagonise other JNK-activated transcription factors such as ETS-Like Kinase 1 (Elk-1) and Activating Transcription Factor 2 (ATF-2). Conversely, JNK can phosphorylate GR and thereby attenuate glucocorticoid responsiveness.

The importance of cross-talk in GR actions is indicated by the construction of a GR dimerisation-deficient mutant mouse in which GR is unable to dimerise and therefore bind to DNA, thus separating the DNA-binding (transactivation) and inflammatory gene repression (transrepression) activities of glucocorticoids. In these animals dexamethasone was able to inhibit AP-1- and NF-κB-

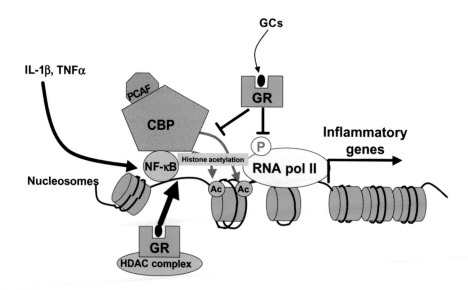

Fig. 1 How glucocorticoids switch off inflammatory genes. Inflammatory genes are activated by inflammatory stimuli, such as interleukin-1β (IL-1β) or tumor necrosis factor-α (TNF-α), resulting in activation of the transcription factor nuclear factor κB (NF-κB). NF-κB translocates to the nucleus and binds to specific κB recognition sites and also to co-activators, such as CREB-binding protein (CBP) or p300/CBP-activating factor (PCAF), which have intrinsic histone acetyltransferase (HAT) activity. This results in acetylation of lysines in histone proteins, resulting in recruitment and phosphorylation of RNA polymerase II and subsequent increased expression of genes encoding inflammatory proteins. Glucocorticoid receptors (GR), after activation by glucocorticoids (GCs), translocate to the nucleus and bind to co-activators thereby inhibiting HAT activity. In addition, GR is able to recruit histone deacetylases (HDAC) to the NF-κB complex leading to suppression of inflammatory genes. GR may also affect the phosphorylation of RNA polymerase II to block inflammatory gene expression.

mediated gene transcription, but the ability to facilitate GRE-mediated effects such as cortisol suppression and T-cell apoptosis were markedly attenuated. This suggests that the development of glucocorticoids with a greater therapeutic window is possible.

Clinical Use (incl. side effects)

Glucocorticoids are widely used to treat a variety of inflammatory and immune diseases. With the recognition that airway inflammation is present even in patients with mild asthma, treatment with glucocorticoids is now the mainstay of asthma therapy. Consequently, by far the most common use of glucocorticoids today is in the treatment of asthma and inhaled glucocorticoids have now become established as first-line treatment in adults and children with persistent asthma, the commonest chronic airway inflammatory disease.

Inhaled glucocorticoids reduce the number of infiltrating mast cells, macrophages, T-lymphocytes, and eosinophils in the airway. Furthermore, glucocorticoids reverse the shedding of epithelial cells and the goblet-cell ► hyperplasia characteristically seen in asthmatic patients (Fig. 2). By reducing airway inflammation, inhaled glucocorticoids reduce ► airway hyperresponsiveness in adults and children with asthma.

Although glucocorticoids are highly effective in the control of asthma and other chronic inflammatory or immune diseases, a small proportion of patients with asthma fail to respond even to high doses of oral glucocorticoids. Resistance to the therapeutic effects of glucocorticoids is also recognised in other inflammatory and immune dis-

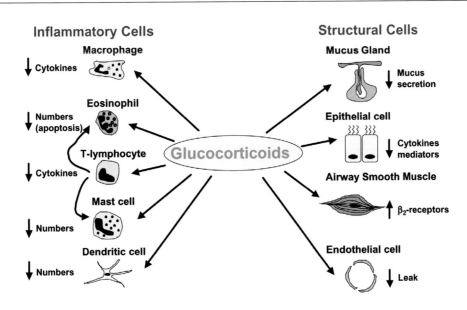

Fig. 2 Cellular effect of glucocorticoids. Glucocorticoids can affect the activation of most resisent and infiltrating cells with the airway suppressing either cell number or mediator release or both. In addition, glucocorticoids are able to decrease vascular permeablility (leak) within the airways that causes oedema and increase the expression of β_2-receptors in smooth muscle cells.

eases, including rheumatoid arthritis and inflammatory bowel disease. Glucocorticoid-resistant patients, although uncommon, present considerable management problems. It is likely that there is a spectrum of glucocorticoid responsiveness, with the rare resistance at one end, but a relative resistance is seen in patients who require high doses of inhaled and oral glucocorticoids (glucocorticoid-dependent asthma). At present the limiting factor to treating these patients with ever increasing doses of glucocorticoids is the side effect profile.

Generally, inhaled glucocorticoids have few side effects, the appearance of which depends on the dose, the frequency of administration, and the delivery system used. The most common side effect is dysphonia (hoarseness), which affects approximately one third of treated patients. Oropharyngeal candidiasis (thrush) may also be a problem for some patients, particularly the elderly, when the drug is given more than twice daily. There has been some concern that inhaled glucocorticoids may cause stunting of growth in children but recent evidence suggests that this is not a problem even in children treated with higher doses of inhaled glucocorticoids for a long period.

Thinning of the skin, telangiectasia, and easy bruising are also classic side effects of both oral and topical glucocorticoids. The easy bruising linked to inhaled glucocorticoids is more frequently seen in elderly patients.

Oral glucocorticoids used to treat severe asthmatic subjects, however, give rise to more serious side effects. Glucocorticoids suppress the hypothalamic-pituitary-adrenal axis by reducing cortisol secretion by the adrenal glands. The degree of suppression depends upon the dose, duration, frequency, and timing of glucocorticoid administration. Oral glucocorticoid therapy also causes osteoporosis with an increased risk of vertebral and rib fractures, but there are no reports suggesting that long-term treatment with inhaled glucocorticoids is associated with an increased risk of fractures. In addition, long-term treatment with oral glucocorticoids increases the risk of posterior subcapsular cataracts; this may be a problem in a few patients taking inhaled glucocorticoids.

Due to the side effect problems seen with high doses of inhaled glucocorticoids resulting from systemic absorption and the use of oral glucocorticoids in severely affected patients, there has been

G

a search for safer glucocorticoids for inhalation and even for oral administration. As discussed above, a major mechanism of the anti-inflammatory effect of glucocorticoids appears to be inhibition of the effects of pro-inflammatory transcription factors (*trans*repression). By contrast, the endocrine and metabolic effects of glucocorticoids that are responsible for the systemic side effects of glucocorticoids are likely to be mediated predominantly via *trans*activation. This has led to a search for novel glucocorticoids that selectively *trans*repress without significant *trans*activation, thus reducing the potential risk of systemic side effects.

Several steroidal and non-steroidal Selective Glucocorticoid Receptor Agonists (SEGRA) have recently been reported to show dissociated properties and some are now in clinical development. This suggests that the development of glucocorticoids and SEGRA with a greater margin of safety is possible and may even lead to the development of oral compounds that do not have significant adverse effects.

Now that the molecular mechanisms of glucocorticoids have been elucidated, this raises the possibility that novel non-steroidal anti-inflammatory treatments might be developed which mimic the actions of glucocorticoids on inflammatory gene regulation. Inhibition of specific HATs activated by NF-κB may prove useful targets, especially if they also repress the action of other pro-inflammatory transcription factors. Many of the anti-inflammatory effects of glucocorticoids appear to be mediated via inhibition of the transcriptional effects of NF-κB and small molecule inhibitors of IκB kinase-2 (IKK2), which activate NF-κB, are now in development. However, glucocorticoids have additional effects so it is not certain whether IKK2 inhibitors will parallel the clinical effectiveness of glucocorticoids and they may have side effects, such as increased susceptibility to infections. Other treatments that have therapeutic potential as glucocorticoid-sparing agents include p38 MAP kinase inhibitors.

References

1. Baldwin AS (2001) Series introduction: the transcription factor NF-kappaB and human disease. J. Clin. Invest. 107:3–6.
2. Barnes PJ (1995) Inhaled glucocorticoids for asthma. N. Engl. J. Med. 332:868–875.
3. Karin M (1998) New twists in gene regulation by glucocorticoid receptor: is DNA binding dispensable? Cell 93:487–490.
4. Umland SP, Schleimer RP, Johnston SL (2002) Review of the molecular and cellular mechanisms of action of glucocorticoids for use in asthma. Pulm. Pharmacol. Ther.15:35–50.
5. Urnov FD, Wolffe AP (2001) A necessary good: nuclear hormone receptors and their chromatin templates. Mol. Endocrinol. 15:1–16.

Glucocorticoids, inhalable

Inhalable glucocorticoids are derivates of the hormone cortisol, which are applied topically in the treatment of (allergic) bronchial asthma. In contrast to systemically applied glucocorticoids, these drugs are metabolized upon first liver passage into inactive forms, thus reducing the systemic side effects of unintentionally swallowed drug. Like all glucocorticoids they exert strong anti-inflammatory and anti-allergic effects.

▶ Allergy
▶ Glucocorticoids

Glucocorticosteroids

▶ Glucocorticoids

Gluconeogenesis

Gluconeogenesis is the synthesis of glucose from glycerol, lactate, and amino acids. This pathway is essential to maintain normal blood glucose during fasting. ▶ Glucagon, the predominant hormone regulating carbohydrate metabolism during fasting, stimulates gluconeogenesis by inducing the expression of two rate-limiting enzymes (pho-

phoenolpyruvate carboxykinase and glucose-6-phosphatase). ▶ Insulin inhibits expression of these enzymes and reduces gluconeogenesis.

▶ Insulin Receptor

Glucose Transport Facilitators

Acronym: GLUT.
▶ Glucose Transporter

Glucose Transporters

HANS-GEORG JOOST, ANNETTE SCHÜRMANN
German Institute of Human Nutrition,
Potsdam-Rehbrücke, Germany
joost@mail.dife.de, schuerman@mail.dife.de

Synonyms

▶ Glucose transport facilitators (GLUT1-12; gene symbols: *SLC2A1-12, solute carrier family 2A1-12*), ▶ Na$^+$-dependent glucose cotransporters, sodium-glucose symporters (SGLT1-3), gene symbols: *SLC5A1-3, solute carrier family 5A1-3*)

Definition

Glucose transporters are integral membrane proteins that catalyze the permeation of sugars into cells along or against a concentration gradient.

▶ Diabetes Mellitus
▶ Insulin Receptor

Basic Characteristics

The Family of Glucose Transport Facilitators (GLUT)

Glucose transport facilitators (GLUT proteins) are uniporters that catalyze the diffusion of glucose into (or out of) cells along a concentration gradient (1). During this process, the proteins are believed to undergo specific conformational changes: Binding of glucose to the outward-facing binding site induces a conformational alteration that moves the substrate through the pore of the GLUT protein. Thereafter, glucose is released from the inward-facing binding site to the cytoplasm, and the transporter undergoes the reverse conformational change (Fig. 1a). Within most cells, glucose is rapidly phosphorylated and metabolized. Thus, under normal conditions the influx of glucose into cells does not alter its concentration gradient. In liver, kidney and intestinal mucosa, GLUT proteins catalyze the efflux of glucose from cells, when the intracellular glucose concentration exceeds the serum glucose concentration.

The family of GLUT proteins comprises 12 structurally-related members, GLUT1–12 (29%–65% identity). Among these, there are glucose (GLUT1–3, 4, 8), fructose (GLUT5) and polyol (GLUT12) transporters (2). At present, the function of the other family members is not completely characterized. The presumed secondary structure of all GLUT proteins is similar, with 12 membrane spanning helices, intracellular N- and C-termini and a large cytoplasmic loop. GLUT proteins carry charged residues at the intracellular surface of the proteins that are believed to provide the proper orientation and anchoring of the helices in the membrane, and to participate in the conformational changes during the transport process. Several sequence motifs, the sugar transporter signatures, are conserved in all family members and are essential for the function of the proteins (Fig. 1b).

According to a comparison of the sequences, the GLUT family can be divided into three subclasses (2). Class I comprises the thoroughly characterized members GLUT1–4 that are distinguished mainly by their tissue distribution (GLUT1: erythrocytes, brain microvessels; GLUT2: liver, pancreatic islet; GLUT3: neuronal cells; GLUT4: muscle, adipose tissue), their affinity to glucose and their hormonal regulation. Class II comprises the fructose-specific transporter GLUT5 (testis, intestine, muscle) and three related proteins, GLUT7 (unknown), GLUT9 (pancreas, kidney) and GLUT11 (heart, muscle). For GLUT11, fructose-inhibitable glucose transport activity has been demonstrated in a system of reconstituted vesicles. Class III comprises 4 isotypes: GLUT6 (brain, spleen, leukocytes), GLUT8 (testis, brain, adipocytes), GLUT10 (pancreas, liver) and GLUT12

G

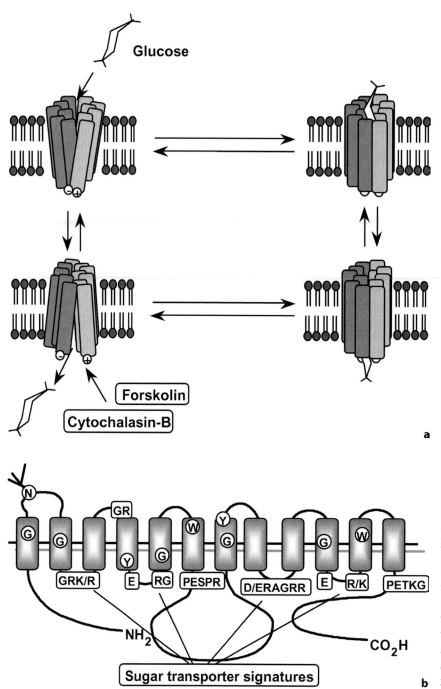

Fig. 1 A: Proposed model of the mechanism of glucose entry into cells by facilitated diffusion. Glucose binds to an out-ward facing site of the GLUT protein and induces a conformational change that moves the hexose through a pore in the protein. After glucose is released from its inward-facing binding site, the GLUT protein undergoes the reverse conformational change. Two inhibitory ligands (cytochalasin B and forskolin) bind to the cytoplasmic site of GLUT proteins. **B: Schematic model of the GLUT proteins with their predicted 12 membrane spanning helices.** The figure highlights motifs that are considered specific for the GLUT family (sugar transporter signatures), and other residues that are highly conserved in all members of the family.

(heart, prostate). Glucose transport activity has been shown for GLUT6 and GLUT8.

Glucose transport activity is regulated through transcriptional and translational control of the GLUT proteins, through their activity and through alterations of their intracellular distribution. Most importantly, GLUT4 continuously cycles between an intracellular, vesicular storage compartment and the plasma membrane of adipose and muscle cells (3). In basal cells, most transporters are sequestered in an intracellular compartment. In the presence of insulin, the translocation of GLUT4-containing vesicles to the plasma membrane is markedly accelerated, resulting in an

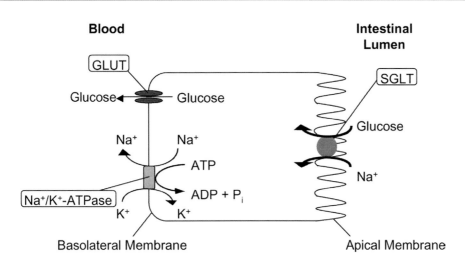

Fig. 2 Transport of glucose in intestinal epithelium. Entry of glucose into the epithelial cells is catalyzed by a sodium-dependent cotransporter (SGLT) located in the apical membrane. The Na^+/K^+ ATPase in the basolateral membrane generates the Na^+ gradient that drives the sodium-glucose co-transport by SGLT against the concentration gradient of glucose. Glucose leaves the cell via a facilitated glucose transporter (GLUT) located in the basolateral membrane.

increase in glucose transport uptake (see chapter Diabetes mellitus). Proteins that presumably participate in this process are VAMP2 (syn. synaptobrevin2; ▶ Exocytosis), ▶ SNARE proteins, syntaxin 4 (▶ Exocytosis), SNAP23 and Synip. In some cells, GLUT1 may also be sequestered through a discrete vesicular pathway and translocated to the plasma membrane in response to energy depletion or lack of glucose.

For some of the GLUT isotypes, the phenotype of null mutants is known. Haploinsufficiency of the GLUT1 in humans causes a syndrome of low glucose levels in the cerebrospinal fluid and drug-resistant seizures. Disruption of the GLUT2 gene in mice leads to impaired insulin secretion and diabetes mellitus. In contrast, hepatic glucose output is normal in GLUT2-null mice, suggesting that an alternative pathway for glucose export from hepatocytes exists. Muscle-specific deletion of the GLUT4 results in a reduction of basal glucose transport and a near absence of the effect of insulin, leading to hyper-insulinemia and impaired glucose tolerance. Furthermore, it is believed that impaired GLUT4 translocation in skeletal muscle is an important factor in the pathogenesis of insulin resistance in obesity and type 2 diabetes. In animal models of morbid obesity, transgenic over-

expression of GLUT4 results in increased glucose uptake in muscle and in improved whole body glucose disposal. Thus, strategies designed to enhance expression and/or translocation of GLUT4 might lead to an effective treatment of insulin resistance and type 2 diabetes (4).

The Family of Sodium-Dependent Glucose Cotransporters (SGLT)

Sodium-dependent glucose cotransporters (SGLT) are located on small intestine and kidney brush-border membranes. SGLT1, SGLT2 and SGLT3 are structurally different sodium-glucose cotransporters with 59%–75% identity and no homology with the glucose transport facilitators (5). They catalyze glucose transport into the cell against a concentration gradient. This transport process is a cotransport of one glucose and of one (for SGLT2) or two (for SGLT1 and SGLT3) Na^+ ions in the same direction. The energetically favored movement of a Na^+ ion through the plasma membrane into the cell, driven both by its concentration gradient and by the membrane potential, is coupled to the movement of the glucose molecule. SGLT proteins exhibit binding sites for glucose and Na^+ on their exofacial surface. The simultaneous binding of Na^+ and glucose to these sites induces a conformational change, generating a transmembrane pore that allows both Na^+ and glucose to pass into the cytosol. After this passage, the proteins revert to their original conformation. In the steady state, Na^+ ions transported from the intestinal lumen into the cells are pumped by a Na^+/K^+-ATPase across the basolateral membrane (Fig. 2). Glucose, concentrated inside the cell by the symport, moves outward through the basolateral membrane via glucose transport facilitators (GLUT).

The secondary structure of SGLT1 differs from that of other members of the family. As compared with SGLT2 and 3, SGLT1 contains a hydrophobic C-terminus that is assumed to form a 14th transmembrane. SGLT1 is a high-affinity transporter that mediates the sodium-glucose cotransport across the intestinal brush-border membrane. SGLT1 is also expressed in the proximal tubule S3 segments of the kidney. Mutations within the SGLT1 gene (*SLC5A1*; on chromosome 22q12.3) are described in patients suffering from glucose/galactose malabsorption.

SGLT2 is a low-affinity, high capacity sodium-glucose cotransporter located in the early proximal convoluted tubule S1 segment. SGLT2 comprises 13 membrane spanning domains. In contrast to SGLT1, SGLT2 does not transport D-galactose. It has been suggested that a defect in the SGLT2 gene (*SLG5A2* on chromosome 16p11.2) is responsible for renal glucosuria.

SGLT3 is also a low-affinity sodium-glucose cotransporter. SGLT3 mRNA was mainly detected in intestine, followed by spleen, liver, kidney and muscle. SGLT3 comprises of 13 membrane spanning domains. SGLT3 has a lower affinity for Na^+ than SGLT2 under identical sugar concentrations.

Drugs

Insulin
At present, the only available drug that stimulates glucose transport is insulin. Insulin increases the abundance of the GLUT4 in plasma membranes of adipose and muscle cells by its recruitment from intracellular storage sites (for a detailed description of its mechanism, see Chapter Diabetes mellitus).

Phlorizin
Phlorizin (phloretin-2'-β-glucoside) is a plant product from the bark of the apple tree that inhibits intestinal glucose absorption and renal reabsorption in proximal tubules by binding to SGLTs. This effect has been used to correct hyperglycemia in experimental, diabetic animals. SGLT2 has a higher affinity for the inhibitor than SGLT1.

Phloretin
Phloretin is the aglycon of phlorizin and inhibits the facilitated diffusion of glucose catalyzed by GLUT1 or GLUT4. It has been used to terminate the uptake of glucose in timed assays with isolated membranes or reconstituted transporters.

Cytochalasin B
Cytochalasin B is a fungal metabolite that binds to the internal site of helices 10 and 11 of the GLUT proteins, and potently inhibits glucose transport in cells or isolated membrane vesicles (K_D=100 nM). Because cytochalasin B binding can be inhibited by glucose in a competitive manner, it is believed that the ligand binds to the internal glucose binding site of the transporter.

Forskolin
The plant product forskolin (from *Coleus forskolii*) is a diterpene that directly stimulates adenylate cyclase. In addition, the agent potently inhibits glucose transport independent from changes in adenylate cyclase activity. Specific binding of forskolin to GLUT1 or GLUT4 is inhibited by glucose and cytochalasin B in a competitive manner, indicating that the ligand binds to a domain involved in glucose binding. Its binding site has been mapped to helix 8–10 of GLUT1/GLUT4 with the aid of the photoreactive 3-[^{125}I]odo-4-azido-phenethylamino-7-O-succinyl-deacetyl-forskolin (IAPS-forskolin).

References

1. Hruz PW, Mueckler MM (2001) Structural analysis of the GLUT1 facilitative glucose transporter. Mol. Membr. Biol.18:183–193
2. Joost H-G, Thorens B (2001) The extended GLUT-family of sugar/polyol transport facilitators – Nomenclature, sequence characteristics, and potential

fuction of ist novel members. Mol. Membr. Biol. 18(4):247-56

3. Holman GD, Sandoval IV (2001) Moving the insulin-regulated glucose transporter GLUT4 into and out of storage. Trends in Cell Biol. 11:173–179

4. Shepherd PR, Kahn BB (1999) Glucose transporters and insulin action: Implications for insulin resistance and diabetes mellitus. N. Engl. J. Med. 341:248–257

5. Turk E, Wright EM (2001) Membrane topology motifs in the SGLT cotransporter family. Mol. Membr. Biol. 159:1–20

GLUT

GLUT stands for Glucose Transport Facilitators.

▶ Glucose Transporters

Glutamate

Glutamate is a small amino acid which constitutes the most important neurotransmitter at excitatory ▶ synapses in the mammalian brain. Glutamate can act on several different types of receptors, many of which are ion channels which mediate influx of Na^+ or Ca^{2+} into the postsynaptic cell. Important glutamate receptor subtypes are AMPA-receptors, NMDA-receptors, kainate-receptors and metabotropic glutamate receptors (the latter are not ion channels, but coupled to intracellular second-messenger pathways).

▶ Ionotropic Glutamate Receptors
▶ Metabotropic Glutamate Receptors

Glutamate Receptors

Glutamate receptors are classified as AMPA, NMDA and mGluR. All three subtypes are highly expressed at nociceptive synapses. AMPA and NMDA receptors are agonist-gated cation channels, which depolarise synaptic membranes upon activation. Ion-channels associated with AMPA receptors demonstrate fast activation and inactivation kinetics and mediate rapid excitatory neurotransmission. Owing to their slow kinetic properties, their high Ca^{2+}-permeability and their blockade by Mg^{2+} under physiological synaptic conditions, NMDA receptors potentiate synapses in several neural pathways, including those involved in chronic pain. mGluRs are G-protein-coupled receptors, which couple to G-proteins of the Gq family or the Gi/o family. Their activation at spinal synapses leads to the facilitation of postsynaptic responses and enhanced neurotransmitter release via calcium-mediated activation of intracellular signalling kinases.

▶ Ionotropic Glutamate Receptors
▶ Metabotropic Glutamate Receptors

Glycine

▶ Glycine Receptor

Glycine Receptors

CORD-MICHAEL BECKER
Universität Erlangen-Nürnberg,
Erlangen, Germany
cmb@biochem.uni-erlangen.de

Synonyms

Inhibitory glycine receptor, ▶ strychnine-sensitive glycine receptor, glycine-gated chloride channel, glycine-gated anion channel.

Definition

The amino acid glycine serves as an important mediator of synaptic inhibition, predominantly in brain stem, spinal cord and retina. Binding of the neurotransmitter to its postsynaptic receptors is antagonized by strychnine, a convulsant alkaloid from nux vomica (1). The inhibitory action of glycine is distinct from its function as a coagonist to glutamate at a strychnine-resistant binding domain of the NMDA receptor. Inhibitory glycine receptors represent a family of ligand-gated chloride channels that exist as pentameric protein complexes which are assembled from ligand-binding α subunits and a structural β polypeptide (2). At the postsynaptic membrane, glycine receptors are clustered by interaction with the tubulin-binding protein▶ gephyrin (4). ▶ Hyperekplexia, a human neurological disorder characterized by exaggerated startle responses and an increased muscle tone, is associated with mutant alleles of the glycine receptor α1 and β subunit genes,*GLRA1* and*GLRB*. Likewise, homologous disease states exist in mutant mouse lines carrying mutations of glycine receptor α1 and β subunit genes (2).

▶ GABAergic System

Basic Characteristics

The glycinergic synapse and its constituents
Glycinergic synapses show a widespread distribution throughout the CNS (1,2). Glycine-mediated inhibition underlies the modulation of brain stem reflexes and the segmental regulation of spinal motoneurons by small interneurons including the Renshaw cells. The neurotransmitter pool of glycine is derived from both metabolic precursors and re-uptake from the synaptic cleft. Synthesis of glycine from its precursor serine is catalyzed by the mitochondrial isozyme of ▶ serine-hydroxymethyltransferase, which is dependent on tetrahydrofolate and pyridoxal phosphate. Finally, glycine is degraded to CO_2 and ammonia by the glycine cleavage system, a mitochondrial enzyme complex. Mutations of its genes cause non-ketotic hyperglycinemia, a devastating neonatal disease characterized by lethargy, seizures, and mental retardation in surviving patients. In the presynaptic terminal, the release fraction of glycine is stored in small synaptic vesicles. Vesicular loading of glycine is mediated by the vesicular inhibitory amino acid transporter (VIAAT or vesicular GABA transporter/VGAT), which is also involved in synaptic vesicular storage of GABA. Inhibitory miniature potentials recorded from rat motoneu-

rons are consistent with the presynaptic vesicular release of the neurotransmitter into the synaptic cleft. The exocytotic release of glycine is a highly regulated process, where the vesicle protein synaptobrevin plays a pivotal role for vesicle fusion with the presynaptic membrane. ▶ Tetanus, a disease caused by the anaerobic, spore-forming rod-*Clostridium tetani*, is associated with a presynaptic block of glycine release. The clostridial protein, tetanus toxin, possesses a protease activity which selectively degrades synaptobrevin. Consistent with a loss of glycinergic inhibition, the hypertonic motor symptoms of tetanus resemble strychnine intoxication. Once released into the synaptic cleft, glycine is rapidly taken up by sodium-dependent transporters characterized by distinct regional distributions. The transporters GLYT1a and GLYT1b represent splice variants of the same gene, differing in N-terminal structure. Both variants show a widespread distribution throughout the CNS, with GLYT1a predominating in the grey matter and GLYT1b in the white matter. In contrast, the transporter GLYT2 colocalizes with the strychnine-sensitive glycine receptor, suggesting a role in the termination of glycinergic inhibition.

Glycine receptor structure and genetics
Receptor-binding of glycine induces the opening of an intrinsic anion channel highly selective for chloride and bicarbonate (2). Depending on the low reversal potential for chloride that prevails in many neurons of the mature CNS, this elicits inward chloride currents and a postsynaptic hyperpolarization. Glycine receptors are derived from a family of highly homologous subunit genes. This group of genes is part of the superfamily of ligand-gated ion channels which also includes the nicotinic acetylcholine, $GABA_A$, and $5-HT_3$ receptors. Glycine receptor subunits assemble into pentameric channels thought to form a rosette-like arrangement surrounding a central ion pore. Glycine receptor isoforms are characterized by distinct developmental and regional expression patterns. The adult isoform, $GlyR_A$, is an oligomeric protein composed of ligand-binding α1 and structural β subunits. The neonatal isoform, $GlyR_N$, prevails in newborn rodents and is replaced by the adult type $GlyR_A$ within two weeks postnatally. The $GlyR_N$ protein appears to be a

homooligomer composed of α2 subunits. In addition to α3 and α4 subunits encoded by distinct genes, further complexity of α subunits results from alternative pre-mRNA splicing.

Glycine receptor α and β subunit variants are characterized by transmembrane topologies common to the superfamily of ligand-gated ion channels (1,2). A large, N-terminal extracellular domain, which in the mature α1 subunit comprises 220 amino acid residues, is followed by four transmembrane regions (TM1 to TM4) spanning the postsynaptic membrane. A fifth hydrophobic region preceding the mature protein represents the cleavable signal peptide. Displaying a rare ability among receptor channel polypeptides, glycine receptor α subunits are self-sufficient in creating homomeric receptor channels when subjected to recombinant expression. Recombinant glycine receptor variants faithfully reproduce pharmacological characteristics of their native counterparts from mammalian CNS. Attempts to elucidate structure-function relationships of glycine receptor subunits have led to the identification of structural motifs involved in distinct steps of ligand-gated ion conductance: (i) As deduced from radio-ligand-binding studies and whole-cell current recordings, glycine and strychnine bind to partially overlapping, but not identical, sites on the receptor. Determinants of ligand-binding and agonist-antagonist discrimination have been assigned to the N-terminal domain, where two stretches of amino acid residues preceding the TM1 domain were identified to contribute to the ligand-binding pocket. A recombinant switch in aromatic hydroxyl groups flanking position α1(160) generated a β-alanine receptor responsive to GABA. (ii) Domains involved in anion translocation include the TM2 region as well as the short loops flanking TM2 at the intracellular and extracellular faces of the plasma membrane. Receptor-gating, i.e. the open-close transition of the ion channel, has been interpreted as an intramolecular motion of TM2, where the flanking loops act as hinges for the conformational transition. While two anion binding sites within the glycine receptor channel have been postulated from electrophysiological analysis, the pathway of chloride permeation across the membrane still awaits elucidation. ▶ Desensitization of glycine receptor ion channels is affected by intracellular determinants positioned within the short loop between TM1 and TM2, as well as within the large loop connecting TM3 and TM4. In particular, the splice variants α3K and α3L which differ in a motif located within the TM3-TM4 loop, also differ in desensitization behavior. (iii) Receptor assembly and heteropentameric subunit stoichiometry are governed by motifs, in particular an eight amino acid sequence, residing within the N-terminal extracellular regions of the receptor subunits.

Excitatory action of glycine receptors in developing CNS

In the embryonic CNS and in dorsal root ganglia, the neuronal reversal potential for chloride is above the membrane potential. Under these conditions, opening of glycine-associated chloride channels will result in depolarizing currents and subsequent excitation, once the neuronal threshold for formation of action potentials is exceeded. During a short postnatal period, glycine receptors are abundantly expressed in rat cerebral cortex which, by immunological criteria, correspond to the $GlyR_N$ isoform. Activation of the cortical glycine receptors results in excitatory impulses and appears to be mediated by nonsynaptically released taurine (2). The functional role of glycine receptor mediated excitation in the developing neocortex remains to be established.

Postsynaptic clustering by gephyrin

Glycine receptors associate with gephyrin, a tubulin-binding protein involved in the formation of postsynaptic receptor clusters (4). Gephyrin is thought to form a submembraneous protein scaffold that dramatically reduces lateral diffusion of the receptor complexes. This interaction increases receptor life-time by stabilizing the protein remaining in its postsynaptic location in the plasma membrane. Receptor stabilization is activity-dependent, resulting in a loss of receptors under conditions of reduced glycinergic transmission, as induced by application of strychnine. Interaction of gephyrin and glycine receptor subunits occurs by means of an 18 amino acid residue motif located within the intracellular loop between TM3 and TM4. Gephyrin also interacts with $GABA_A$ receptors, potentially via the $GABA_A$ receptor associated protein(GAB_ARAP). As additional components of the postsynaptic protein

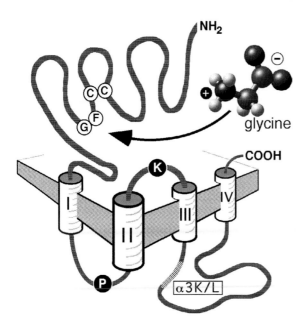

Fig. 1 Transmembrane topology of glycine receptor α subunits. Positions of amino acid exchanges α1(P250T) and α1(K276E) associated with the human neurological disorder hyperekplexia are as indicated by filled circles, amino acid residues involved in ligand binding and discrimination are indicated by open circles. The glycine receptor subunit variant α3L carries a cytoplasmic insertion sequence (box) which is generated by alternative splicing. This insertion is missing from the splice variant α3K.

scaffold, phosphatidylinositol 3,4,5-trisphosphate-binding proteins have been identified, including collybistin and profilin. However, gephyrin also serves dual functions apparently beyond synaptic organization, as it contributes to biosynthesis of the molybdenum cofactor, an essential coenzyme of a variety of dehydrogenases.

Disease mechanisms

Based on its clinical resemblance to subconvulsive strychnine poisoning, glycine receptor dysfunction has long been considered a candidate mechanism of hypertonic motor disorders (1,2). As exemplified in the spontaneous mouse mutants spastic, spasmodic, and oscillator, glycine receptor defects result in hereditary neurological disorders. In the spastic mouse, the intronic insertion of a LINE-1 transposable element into the β subu-

nit gene *Glyrb* results in aberrant splicing and a consecutive loss of receptors. Consistent with a numerical receptor defect, the spastic phenotype is rescued by a transgene expressing β subunit mRNA. The spasmodic mouse carries a missense mutation of the α1 subunit gene, *Glra1(A52S)* that diminishes agonist affinity. The spasmodic locus is linked by synteny homology to the human chromosomal region 5q31.3 carrying the human *GLRA1* gene. In the oscillator mutant, a microdeletion within the *Glra1* gene causes a complete loss of the glycine receptor isoform $GlyR_A$, resulting in lethality. During development, the postnatal appearance of all of these mutant phenotypes coincides with the switch from the unaffected neonatal ($GlyR_N$) to the diminished adult receptor isoform, $GlyR_A$.

Hyperekplexia (startle disease, stiff baby syndrome) is a congenital human motor disorder that follows autosomal-recessive as well as dominant modes of inheritance (2). Affected patients exhibit an exaggerated startle response and increased muscle tone. Hyperekplexia is associated with a variety of *GLRA1* and *GLRB* mutant alleles that affect glycine receptor affinity and ion conductance. In the disease associated α1 subunit variants, the amino acid positions mutated cluster near segment TM2. In particular, the hyperekplexia allele α1(P250T) predicts a substitution in the cytoplasmatic loop TM1-TM2 (Fig. 1). Recombinant α1(P250T) channels show reduced chloride conductance and enhanced desensitization, defining an intracellular determinant of channel-gating. In contrast, the mutation α1(K276E) situated within the extracellular loop TM2-TM3, is without effect on channel conductance, but almost exclusively affects gating. Hyperekplexia mutations of *GLRA1* also give clues to glycine receptor regulation in the human: In a case of recessive hyperekplexia, homozygosity for a null allele of *GLRA1* was found, consistent with a complete loss of gene function. Born to consanguineous parents, the affected child displayed relatively mild symptoms despite this "knockout" situation. In contrast to lethality of the null allele in homozygous oscillator mice, the complete loss of the α1 subunit is tolerated in the human. This suggests that either the loss of glycine receptors is effectively compensated or that subunit regulation substantially differs among these species.

Drugs

The inhibitory glycine receptor still lacks a therapeutic pharmacology. The agonistic properties of glycine are imitated by a series of structurally related amino acids (1,2). In spinal neurons, the relative potency of these agonists decreases in the order of: glycine > β-alanine > taurine > α-alanine > serine. In contrast, the structurally related amino acid GABA is not an agonist at glycine receptors. Recombinant α1 subunit receptors respond to this group of glycinergic amino acid agonists, while recombinant α2 subunit receptors are preferentially activated by glycine and barely respond to β-alanine and taurine. The convulsant alkaloid strychnine is a high affinity antagonist ($K_D \approx 10$ nM) of receptor binding by glycine ($K_D \approx 10$ μM). Consistent with the physiology of glycinergic synapses, sublethal strychnine poisoning causes motor disturbances, e.g. increases in muscle tone and hyperreflexia. Further symptoms include alterations of sensory, visual, and acoustic perception. As a result of dysinhibition in auditory and motor centers, strychnine generates excessive startle responses, while higher doses lead to convulsions and death. Glycine displaceable binding of [³H]strychnine is a highly specific probe of the glycine receptor. High affinity binding of [³H]strychnine has been demonstrated to spinal cord, sensory, and acoustic ganglia of the brain stem as well as to retina. Symptoms of strychnine intoxication correlate to the dysfunction of those CNS regions displaying high [³H]strychnine binding. In addition, numerous drugs and toxins including muscimol analogues, benzodiazepines, convulsant steroids, and picrotoxinin have been shown to exert strychnine-like effects, yet at significantly higher concentrations.

Glycine receptor function is modulated by alcohols and anesthetics (3). Amino acid residue α1(S267) is critical for alcohol potentiation, as mutation to small residues (Gly, Ala) enhance, and mutation to large residues (His, Cys, Tyr) diminish the ethanol effect. Glycine receptor modulation by Zn^{2+} involves structural determinants located within the large N-terminal domain. Additional glycinergic modulators include neuroactive steroids and the anthelmintic, ivermectin, which activates glycine receptors by a novel, strychnine-insensitive mechanism.

References

1. Becker, C.-M. (1992) Convulsants acting at the inhibitory glycine receptor. In: Selective neurotoxicity (Ed.: Herken, H., Hucho, F.), Springer: Heidelberg. Handbook of Experimental Pharmacology 102:539–575.
2. Breitinger, H.-G., Becker, C.-M. (2002) The inhibitory glycine receptor - Simple views of a complicated channel. Chem. Bio. Chem. 4:1042–1052.
3. Harris, R.A. (1999) Ethanol actions on multiple ion channels: Which are important? Alcohol Clin. Exp. Res. 23:1563–1570.
4. Kneussel, M., Betz, H. (2000) Receptors, gephyrin and gephyrin-associated proteins: Novel insights into the assembly of inhibitory postsynaptic membrane specializations. J. Physiol. 525:1–9.

Glycogen Synthase Kinase 3

Glycogen synthase kinase 3 (GSK3) phosphorylates glycogen synthase (GS), the key enzyme for glycogen synthesis, which builds up glycogen by adding UDP-glucose. Phosphorylation of GS by GSK3 leads to inactivation of GS. GSK3 is a substrate of the protein kinase Akt. Stimulation of Akt by insulin leads to phosphorylation of GSK3, to inhibition of its kinase activity, and consequently to activation of GS and glycogen synthesis. Recently, a role of GSK3 in the regulation of insulin-dependent gene expression has also been described.

▶ Insulin Receptor

Glycopeptide Antibiotics

Glycopepetide antibiotics, a group which includes vancomycin and teicoplanin, are primarily active against gram-positive bacteria, including methicillin-resistant staphylococci. They have also been used against resistant enterococci. However, resistance against glycopeptide antibiotics is now emerging rapidly world-wide. Glycopeptide antibiotics inhibit the synthesis of the cell wall in sensitive bacteria by binding with high affinity to the *D*-alanyl-*D*-alanine terminus of cell wall precursor units. The drug is bactericidal for dividing microorganisms. Enterococcal resistance to vancomycin results from the alteration of the *D*- alanyl-*D*-alanine target to *D*-alanyl-D-lactate or *D*-alanyl-*D*-serine, which bind vancomycin poorly.

▶ β-lactam Antibiotics
▶ Ribosomal Protein Synthesis Inhibitors
▶ Quinolones
▶ Microbial Resistance to Drugs

Glycoprotein IIb/IIIa Receptor Antagonists

▶ Antiplatelet Drugs
▶ Anti-integrins, therapeutic and diagnostic implications

Glycoproteins

A glycoprotein is a conjugated protein containing carbohydrate units.

Glycosaminoglycan

A glycosaminoglycan is any one of a number of non-branching, sulfated polysaccharides, consisting of repeating disaccharide units comprised of a uronic acid moiety (glucuronic or iduronic acid) and an amino sugar (glucosamine or galactosamine) that are variably O- and N-sulfated and N-acetylated, and polydisperse (variable chain length). For example, heparin consists of alternating uronic acid (either glucuronic or iduronic acid moieties that are variably 2-O-sulfated) and glu-

cosamine (variably 2-N-sulfated, 3-O-sulfated, 6-O-sulfated, and/or 2-N-acetylated).

▶ Anticoagulants

Glycosides, cardiac

▶ Cardiac Glycosides

Glycosylphosphatidylinositol Anchor

Glycosylphosphatidylinositol (GPI) anchoring is a posttranslational modification occurring in the endoplasmic reticulum where preassembled GPI anchor precursors are transferred to proteins bearing a C-terminal GPI signal sequence. The GPI anchor precursors are synthesized in the endoplasmic reticulum by sequential addition of sugar and other components to phosphatidylinositol. Protein GPI anchors are ubiquitous in eukaryotic cells. In mammalian cells, GPI anchored proteins are often found in lipid rafts, which are subdomains of the plasma membrane containing various signaling components.

▶ Lipid Modifications

Glycylcyclines

Glycylcyclines are a new generation of tetracyclines (e.g. tigilcycline), which have been developed to overcome problems of resistance to common tetracyclines.

▶ Ribosomal Protein Synthesis Inhibitors

GM-CSF

▶ Granulocyte-macrophage-CSF
▶ Hematopoietic Growth Factors

GMP, cyclic

Cyclic GMP (cGMP) ia an intracellular messenger generated by guanylyl cyclase from GTP.

▶ Guanylyl Cyclases
▶ Smooth Muscle Tone Regulation

GnRH

▶ Gonadotrophin-releasing Factor/Hormone

Gold Compounds

Gold compounds such as sodium aurothiomalate or auranofin are used to treat chronic inflammatory diseases like ▶ rheumatoid arthritis. The anti-inflammatory effects develop slowly, with maximum action occurring after 3-4 months. The exact mechanism of action is not understood. However a variety of inflammatory processes such as mitogen-induced lymphocyte proliferation, the activation of lysosomal enzymes, the production of O_2 metabolites, the chemotaxis of neutrophils or the induction of various cytokines have been shown to be inhibited by gold compounds.

Golgi Apparatus

The Golgi apparatus is a stack of flattened vesicles that functions in posttranslational processing and sorting of proteins. The Golgi apparatus receives proteins from the endoplasmic reticulum *via* the endoplasmic reticulum/Golgi intermediate compartment and directs them to endosomes, lysosomes or the plasma membrane. It is organized into a number of stacks of disc like compartments (cisternae).

▶ Intracellular Transport
▶ Protein Trafficking and Quality Control

Gonadorelin

▶ Gonadotrophin-releasing Factor/Hormone

Gonadotropin-releasing Factor/Hormone (GnRH)

GnRH is derived by proteolytic processing of a 92-amino acid precursor peptide to produce mature GnRH, a decapeptide. GnRH is released from neurons in the hypothalamus. GnRH release is intermittent and is governed by a neural pulse generator that is located in the mediobasal hypothalamus, that controls the frequency and amplitude of GnRH release. The GnRH pulse generator is active during fetal life and for about one year after birth, thereafter its activity decreases but increases again during puberty. The intermittent release of GnRH is crucial for the proper synthesis and release of the gonadotropins, which are also released in a pulsatile manner. The gonadotropins, luteinizing hormone (LH) and follicle-stimulating hormone (FSH), are synthesized and secreted by gonadotrophs, which make up about 20% of the hormone-secreting cells in the anterior pituitary. GnRH is the main stimulus which induces secretion of LH and FSH. The continuous administration of GnRH, in contrast to the physiological intermittent action, leads to desensitization and down-regulation of GnRH receptors on pituitary gonadotrophs. This action forms the basis for the clinical use of long-acting GnRH analogs that suppress gonadotropin secretion. These compounds transiently increase LH and FSH secretion, but eventually desensitize gonadotrophs to GnRH, and thereby inhibit gonadotropin release. Synthetic GnRH is termed "gonadorelin". GnRH and a variety of analogs with agonist activity like buserelin, leuprorelin, goserelin or nafarelin can be given in a continuous fashion in order to achieve gonadal suppression through the decreased production of FSH and LH. Gonadal suppression may be desirable to treat endometriosis, precocious puberty, sex hormone-dependent cancers (e.g. advanced prostatic cancer), or hirsutism due to the polycystic ovary syndrome.

▶ Contraceptives

Gonadotropins

The pituitary hormones, luteinizing hormone (LH) and follicle-stimulating hormone (FSH) together with the placental hormone chorionic gonadotropin are collectively called gonadotropins. They are large, glycosylated heterodimers composed of a common α-subunit and a hormone-specific β-subunit.

▶ Gonadotropin-releasing Factor/Hormone (GnRH)
▶ Contraceptives

Gout

Gout is the consequence of hyperuricemia and is characterized by uric acid deposits in joints, bursae, tendons, kidney and urinary tract. In the initial stage, gout is characterized by asymptomatic hyperuricemia. In the second stage, the disease manifests itself by acute gouty arthritis. The third (intercritical) stage is asymptomatic, and the fourth stage is characterized by progressive uric acid deposits in joints, bursae, tendons, kidney and urinary tract.

▶ Anti-gout Drugs

GPIIb/IIIa Receptor Antagonists

▶ Antiplatelet Drugs
▶ Anti-integrins, therapeutic and diagnostic implications

GPCR

▶ G-Protein Coupled Receptors

GPI Anchor

▶ Glycosylphosphatidylinositol (GIP) Anchor
▶ Lipid Modifications

G-protein-coupled Receptors

THOMAS FINSTERBACH, BRIAN K. KOBILKA
Stanford University Medical School,
Stanford, USA
tfinster@cmgm.stanford.edu,
kobilka@pmgm2.stanford.edu

Synonyms

Seven-transmembrane helix receptors, heptahelical receptors, serpentine receptors

Definition

G-protein-coupled receptors (GPCRs) are a large family of plasma membrane receptors. Upon bind-

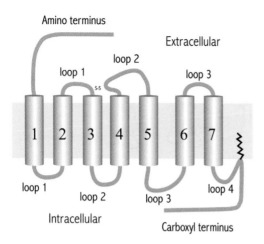
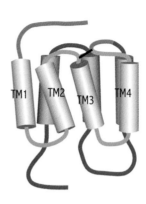

Fig. 1 Diagrams of the structural characteristics of G protein coupled receptors. A. The secondary structure of a generic G protein coupled receptor showing the seven membrane spanning domains and connecting loops. B. A cartoon of the predicated three-dimensional structure of a generic G protein coupled receptor based on the structure of rhodopsin. These diagrams were taken from (1).

ing its agonist, a GPCR activates an intracellular heterotrimeric guanine nucleotide regulatory protein (G protein). The activated G protein modulates the activity of one or more enzymes or ion channels.

▶ Table appendix: Receptor Proteins
▶ Drug-Receptor Interaction
▶ Tolerance and Desensitization
▶ Transmembrane Signalling

Basic Characteristics

Cells receive much of the information about their external environment by way of receptor proteins that span the plasma membrane. G-protein coupled receptors (GPCRs) are the largest family of plasma membrane receptors. These receptors have in common a seven transmembrane topology and functional interactions with heterotrimeric guanine nucleotide binding proteins (G proteins). Over 200 GPCRs, responsive to a large variety of stimuli from photons, ions, amino acids and small organic molecules to peptide and protein hormones, have been identified in the human genome. Several hundred more GPCRs (called orphan GPCRs) for as yet unknown ligands have been identified based on homology to the known GPCRs.

GPCRs as a group constitute the largest family of targets for pharmacological intervention. They are critically involved in virtually every physiological system. A partial list of natural GPCR ligands includes glutamate, calcium, GABA, acetylcholine, histamine, GTP/ATP, adenosine, cAMP, melatonin, epinephrine, seratonin and dopamine. Peptide hormone GPCR activators include angiotensin, vasopressin, bradykinin, calcitonin, FSH, glucagon, somatostatin and a host of chemokines, pheromones, opioids and cannibinoids. Olfactory and gustatory sensory transduction involves GPCRs responsive to a large array of odorants, and vision depends on the light-activated ligand retinal covalently bound to its own GPCR rhodopsin. GPCRs are grouped into five families of which the Rhodopsin like family is by far the most numerous. Smaller families include the secretin-like receptors, metabotropic glutamate/ pheromone-like receptors, fungal pheromone receptors and cAMP receptors (Dictyostelium) Putative new families have been proposed for Frizzled/ Smoothened, vomeronasal and other receptors, and many orphans in each family remain to be characterized.

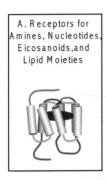

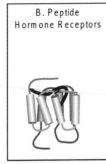

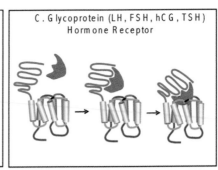

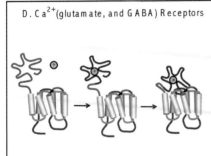

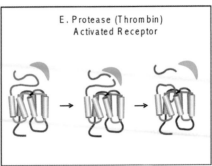

Fig. 2 Diagram illustrating the binding sites for different families of hormones and neurotransmitters on their receptors. Adapted from (1).

Receptor Structure

The structure of only one GPCR, bovine rhodopsin, has been solved at high resolution; however, it is thought that the all GPCRs have the same core structure (Fig. 1) consisting of seven transmembrane (TM) spanning domains with an extracellular amino terminus and an intracellular carboxyl terminus (1). The structures of GPCRs diverge most in the amino terminus, the carboxyl terminus and the intracellular loop between TM5 and TM6. Amino termini are frequently glycosylated and range in size from 7 to 595 amino acids. The intracellular carboxyl terminus is typically tethered to the membrane by a lipid modification such as palmitoylation and ranges in size from 12 to 359 amino acids. The carboxyl terminus and the intracellular loop between TM5 and TM6 often contain sites for phosphorylation by one or more regulatory kinases such as protein kinase A, protein kinase C or a member of the GPCR kinase (GRK) family. A disulfide bond between two highly conserved cysteines links the second and third extracellular loops of most GPCRs.

Ligand Binding

The location of the agonist binding site is highly variable (Fig. 2) (1). Monoamine hormones such as catecholamines, dopamine, serotonin and acetylcholine bind within the TM core (Fig. 2A). Small peptide hormones bind to the amino terminus, the extracellular loops between TM domains and within the TM core (Fig. 2B). Large amino terminal domains form the binding site for glycoprotein hormones (such as follicle stimulating hormone) (Fig. 2C), as well as for ions (the Ca^{2+}-sensing receptor, Fig. 2D) and the neurotransmitters glutamate and GABA. Finally, in protease-activated receptors, the agonist is generated by proteolytic cleavage of the amino terminus of the receptor (Fig. 2E).

G protein Coupling Domains

Mutagenesis studies have identified multiple sites of interaction between GPCRs and their cognate G proteins. These include the intracellular loop 2 between TM3 and TM4, the intracellular loop 3 between TM 5 and TM 6, and loop 4 formed between TM 7 and the lipid modification on the proximal carboxyl terminus (Fig. 1). Agonist binding (Fig. 3A) is thought to lead to subtle changes in the arrangement of the TM domains (2). These conformational changes are transmitted to the associated G protein. In an interaction that has yet to be fully characterized, this movement triggers a G protein heterotrimer ($G\alpha\beta\gamma$) to dissociate into

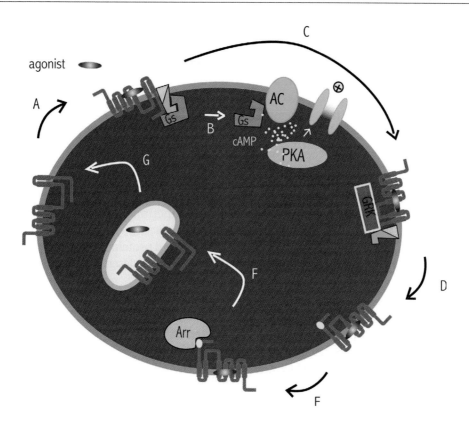

Fig. 3 Signaling cycle for the β_2 adrenergic receptor (β_2AR), a prototypical GPCR. A. The agonist (adrenaline) binds to the β_2AR, which leads to activation of the associated G protein (G_S). **B.** $G_{S\alpha}$ dissociates and activates adenylyl cyclase (AC), which converts ATP to cyclic AMP (cAMP). cAMP activates protein kinase A (PKA) which phosphorylates and activates a channel. **C.** Following G_S activation, a G protein coupled receptor kinase (GRK) associates with the agonist occupied receptor and $G_{\beta\gamma}$. **D.** GRK phosphorylates the receptor. **E.** Arrestin binds to the phosphorylated receptor blocking further interactions with G_S. **F.** Arrestin promotes internalization of the receptor into an endosomal compartment where the phosphate is removed. **G.** The dephosphorylated receptor is recycled back to the plasma membrane.

Gα and G$\beta\gamma$ subunits, thereby unmasking interactive domains on both of the freed G protein subunits and on the receptor itself. Both dissociated Gα and G$\beta\gamma$ subunits are capable of modulating a variety of effecter systems including adenylyl cyclase, phospholipase C and ion channels (Fig. 3). Recent studies suggest that some GPCRs may also signal through G protein independent pathways (3).

Pharmacologic Modulation of Receptor Activity
Ligands that bind to G protein coupled receptors display a broad spectrum of activity ranging from full ▶ agonist, to partial agonists, to neutral ▶ antagonist, to ▶ inverse agonists. Some GPCRs are capable of activating G proteins even in the absence of a ligand. This ligand-independent activity is often referred to as basal or constitutive activity. Inverse agonists suppress this basal activity while neutral antagonists do not alter basal activity. Full and partial agonists increase G protein activation above that attributed to the basal, ligand-independent activity. Perhaps the most widely accepted model used to describe ligand modulation of GPCRs is the extended ternary complex model. In its simplest form, this model proposes that the receptor exists in two functionally distinct states in equilibrium: the inactive (R)

and the active (R^*) state. In the absence of ligands, the level of basal receptor activity is determined by the equilibrium between R and R^*. The efficacy of ligands is thought to be a reflection of their ability to alter the equilibrium between these two states. Full agonists stabilize R^* while inverse agonists stabilize R. The majority of natural hormones and neurotransmitters act as agonists for their associated receptors. However, there is substantial evidence that the agouti-related peptide behaves as an antagonist or possibly an inverse agonist for the melanocortin receptor. While the simple two state model is able to explain many aspects of GPCR function, there is a growing body of evidence for the existence of multiple, ligand-specific receptor states (2). In addition, recent studies suggest that many GPCRs may exist as homodimers and/or heterodimers (4). The functional significance of dimers and their role in G protein activation remains to be determined for most GPCRs. The requirement for GPCR dimers is most convincing for heterodimers such as the functional GABA$_B$ receptor formed by a GBR1/GBR2 heterodimer. The GBR2 behaves as a chaperone bringing the GBR1 to the cell surface. However, while GBR1 contains the main determinants for ligand binding, GBR2 is the major site of G protein coupling. In other cases, heterodimers may create receptors having novel pharmacologic or regulatory properties (4).

Regulation of GPCR Function

GPCR function has been shown to be regulated by several different mechanisms. The number of receptors on the plasma membrane may be regulated by transcription, mRNA stability, biosynthetic processing and protein stability. In addition, the function of receptors in the plasma membrane can be influenced by regulatory phosphorylation and by association with other proteins that determine the subcellular location of receptors relative to other signaling molecules.

One of the most well characterized regulatory pathways for GPCRs is that mediated by the G-protein coupled receptor kinase (GRK) family (5). After a signaling event, a multi-stage desensitization process begins with the agonist-dependent phosphorylation by a GRK of one or more serines or threonines located on intracellular domains of the receptor, particularly in the carboxyl terminus and the third intracellular loop (between TM5 and TM6) (Fig. 3C,D). This phosphorylation promotes the recruitment of an arrestin (Fig. 3E). Arrestins are a family of molecules that bind to agonist-occupied, phosphorylated GPCRs and interfere with G protein coupling. Arrestins may mediate receptor internalization (Fig. 3F) by way of clathrin coated pits or other mechanisms. Internalized receptors may be targeted for degradation (down regulation) or, after being dephosphorylated to restore functionality, they may be redeployed at the cell surface (3G). In addition to GRKs, protein kinase A and protein kinase C have been shown to play roles in the desensitization of several GPCRs.

Drugs

Limited list (Trade Name)

Albuterol (Ventolin®)
Alprenolol
Amthamine
Antihistamines [class]
Atenolol (Tenormin®)
Baclofen (Lioresal®)
β- Blockers [class]
Betaxolol
β-Funaltrexamine
Bisoprolol
Bromocriptine
Caffeine
Candesartan (Atacand®)
Cannibinoids
Carbamazepine (Tegretol®)
Carvedilol (Coreg®)
Cimaterol
Cimetidine (Tagamet®)
Cirazoline
Clemastine
Clenbuterol
Clobenpropit
Clocinnamox
Clonidine (Catapres®)
Clozapine
Corynanthine
DAMGO
Deltorphin
Dihydrexidine
Dihydroergocristine
Dihydroergotamine
Dilazep
Dimaprit
Dobutamine (Dobutrex®)

Doxazosin (Cardura®)
Doxepin
Epinephrine (Adrenalin)
Famotidine Pepcidine
Flavorings
Fluorobenzylspiperone
Fluoxetine (Prozac®)
Formoterol
Guanabenz
Guanfacine
Haloperidol
Hydrocodone (Vicodin®)
Hyoscyamine (Levsin®)
Ibopamine
ICI 118,551
Ifenprodil
Imetit
Immepip
Iodophenpropit
Ipratropium (Atrovent®)
Irbesartan (Avapro®)
Ketotifen
Loratadine (Claritin®)
Losartan (Cozaar®)
Mepyramine
Metoprolol (Toprol-XL®)
Midazolam (Versed®)
Morphine
Naftopidil
Naloxonazine
Naltriben
Naltrindole
Nizatidine (Axid®)
Opioids [class]
Oxymetazoline
Paroxetine (Paxil®)
Pimozide
Pindolol
Piribedil
Practolol
Prazosin
Procaterol
Pronethanol
Propranolol (Inderal®)
Quinpirole
Ranitidine (Zantac®)
Remoxipride
Rilmenidine
Salbutamol
Salmeterol (Serevent®)
Scents
Sotalol
Sulpiride
Sumatriptan (Imitrex, Imigran®)

Tamsulosin (Flomax®)
Terazosin (Hytrin®)
Theophylline (TheoDur®)
Thioperamide
Timolol (Blocadren®)
Tiotidine
Tizanidine (Zanaflex®)
trans-Triprolidine
Valsartan (Diovan®)
Ondansetron (Zofran®)
Zolantidine

References

1. Ji TH, Grossmann M, Ji I (1998) G protein-coupled receptors. I. Diversity of receptor-ligand interactions. J Biol Chem. 273(28):17299–17302
2. Gether U, Kobilka BK (1998) G protein-coupled receptors. II. Mechanism of agonist activation. J Biol Chem. 273(29):17979–17982
3. Lefkowitz RJ (1998) G protein-coupled receptors. III. New roles for receptor kinases and β-arrestins in receptor signaling and desensitization. J Biol Chem. 273(30):18677–18680
4. .Bouvier M (2001) Oligomerization of G-protein-coupled transmitter receptors. Nat Rev Neurosci. 2(4):274–286
5. Krupnick JG, Benovic JL (1998) The role of receptor kinases and arrestins in G protein-coupled receptor regulation. Annu Rev Pharmacol Toxicol. 38:289–319

G-protein-coupled Receptor Kinases

G-protein-coupled receptor kinases (GRKs) are a family of enzymes that catalyze the phosphorylation of threonine or serine residues on G protein-coupled receptors. Characteristically, G protein-coupled receptor kinases (GRKs) only phosphorylate the ligand-activated form of the receptors. Phosphorylation by GRKs usually leads to impaired receptor/G protein coupling.

▶ G-protein Coupled Receptors

G-proteins

▶ Heterotrimeric GTP-binding Protein

GRKs

▶ G-protein-coupled Receptor Kinases
▶ G-protein-coupled Receptors

Granulocyte-CSF

G-CSF.

▶ Hematopoietic Growth Factors

Granulocyte-macrophage-CSF

GM-CSF.

▶ Hematopoietic Growth Factors

Graves' Disease

Graves' disease is an organ specific autoimmune disease. Antibodies against the TSH receptor mimic the action of TSH thereby causing stimulation of thyroid epithelial cells leading to hyperthyroidism. The specific cause of thyroid antibody production is not known at present. Susceptibility to Graves' disease is determined by genetic, environmental and endogenous factors.

▶ Antithyroid Drugs

Growth Factors

BOSE KOCHUPURAKKAL SKARIA,
KEREN SHTIEGMAN, YOSEF YARDEN
Department of Biological Regulation, The Weizmann Institute of Science, Rehovot, Israel,
Bose.Kochupurakkal@weizmann.ac.il,
Keren.Shtiegman@weizmann.ac.il,
Yosef.Yarden@weizmann.ac.il

Synonyms

Cytokines; differentiation factors; lymphokines; mitogens.

Definition

Growth factors are relatively stable, secreted or membrane-bound peptide ligands that mediate short-range cell-to-cell interactions. Growth factors and their cognate receptors function as a module that regulates various cellular processes such as proliferation, differentiation, migration and apoptosis. These modules are evolutionary conserved, and their primary developmental function is determination of cell lineage through heterotypic cellular interactions. Their expression is spatio-temporally regulated, but their concentration in body fluids and intercellular spaces is usually low (sub-nanomolar) and highly regulated.

▶ Hematopoietic Growth Factors
▶ Neurotrophic Factors

Classification

Growth factors are classified based on their structure and the family of receptors they activate. Whereas the definition of growth factors may broadly apply to lymphokines (e.g., interleukins; ILs) and cytokines like members of the tumor necrosis factor (TNF) family, here we will consider only growth factors that bind to receptors harboring an intrinsic tyrosine ▶ kinase domain. Growth factors bind such receptors with high affinity (in the low nanomolar range) and specificity, and they may be accordingly classified as ligands of a specific receptor sub-family (1) (see Table 1). For example, growth factors comprising an epidermal growth factor (EGF) motif bind to the ErbB sub-group of receptor tyrosine kinases (RTKs; also called type I RTKs). We will use this classification to elaborate on the shared mechanism of action of growth factors.

Mechanism of Action

Many growth factors contain a cleavable hydrophobic amino-terminal signal peptide and they are expressed as pre-pro-peptides, primarily as transmembrane proteins or secreted forms (2). The precursors are converted into biologically active peptides by multiple steps of proteolytic cleavage and processing. Yet, some other growth factors, e.g., members of the fibroblast growth factor (FGF) family, typically lack a signal peptide and their secretion or release may involve certain physiological conditions (e.g., cell injury). The receptors are expressed as transmembrane proteins with an extracellular ligand binding domain and an intracellular kinase domain, with specificity to either tyrosine or serine/threonine residues (3). The biochemical series of events that follows binding of a growth factor to the cell surface-localized receptor, and culminating in cellular activation is known as signal transduction (see Fig. 1).

Ligand binding to the extracellular receptor's portion leads to dimerization/oligomerization of receptor molecules within the plane of the plasma membrane (4). In cases where the receptors exist as disulfide-linked dimeric receptors (e.g., receptors for insulin and insulin-like growth factors; IGFs), ligand binding causes a significant change in the juxtaposition of receptors. This event orients the kinase domains of two receptors in a manner that facilitates auto- and trans-phosporylation of residues situated in the activation loop of the kinase domains, as well as other residues in the intracellular region, especially the stretches flanking the kinase domain (5). Phosphotyrosine residues of RTKs serve as docking sites for proteins containing ▶ Src homology 2 (SH2) or ▶ phosphotyrosine-binding (PTB) domains. Many cytosolic kinases, ▶ phosphatases, lipases (▶ phospholipases) and ▶ adaptor proteins containing SH2 or PTB domains are recruited to the receptor, either directly or through specific adaptors and scaffolding proteins with multiple docking sites. Thus, a large multi-protein signaling complex is assembled at the membrane with the receptors as the anchor. Recruited kinases further phosphorylate other proteins resulting in a cascade of protein recruitment and associated amplification of the signal, culminating in the nucleus with activation of transcriptional regulators and gene expression. These events result in multiple branching of the signal and propagation of the extracellular biochemical message to sub-cellular organelles. Though the outcome of signaling events initiated by receptors within a family and between families are distinct, some common themes have emerged.

One of the signaling pathways common to many growth factor receptors is the route leading to stimulation of the mitogen-activated protein kinase [MAPK; (6)]: Grb-2, an SH2 and ▶ SH3 domain containing adaptor protein is recruited to the phosphorylated receptor, and interacts with SOS, a guanine nucleotide exchange factor, through the SH3 domain. Translocation of SOS to a membrane proximal region facilitates its interaction with and activation of Ras, a membrane-anchored protein, by exchanging GDP for GTP. Once Ras is in the GTP-bound form, it can recruit Raf, a cytosolic serine/threonine kinase, which in-turn activates MEK, a dual specificity protein kinase. MEK phosphorylates MAPK (also called Erk) on threonine and tyrosine residues, thereby activating it. Activated MAPK translocates to the nucleus and phosphorylates multiple targets, some of which are responsible for the progression of the cell cycle and subsequent cell proliferation. In a similar manner, the GTP-bound form of Ras can also recruit phosphoinositide 3-kinase (PI3K), which generates specific inositol lipids. A major target of PI3K lipid products is the protein kinase Akt (or protein kinase B; PKB). In quiescent cells, PKB resides in the cytosol in a low-activity conformation. Upon cellular stimulation, PKB is activated through recruitment to cellular membranes by PI3K lipid products and phosphorylation by 3'-phosphoinositide-dependent kinase-1 (PDK1). PKB is a serine/threonine kinase that phosphorylates and inactivates pro-apoptotic proteins like BAD and FKHR-1, a transcription factor, thereby promoting cell survival. PKB also activates the glycogen synthase kinase and phosphofructo kinase,

G

Tab. 1 Summary of a number of growth factor families, the tyrosine kinase receptors they bind, and the major physiological consequences of their interactions. Abbreviations: epidermal growth factor (EGF), transforming growth factor-α (TGF-α), amphiregulin (AR), heparin binding EGF-like growth factor (HB-EGF), neuregulins (NRG), fibroblast growth factors (FGF), platelet derived growth factor (PDGF), hepatocyte growth factor (HGF), glial-cell-line-derived neurotrophic factor (GDNF), neurturin (NRTN), artemin (ARTN), persephin (PSPN), vascular endothelial factor (VEGF), stem cell factor (SCF), nerve growth factor (NGF), brain-derived neurotrophic factor (BNNF), neurotrotrophin-3,-4 (NT-3,4), rearranged during transfection (RET), tyrosine kinase receptor in endothelial cells (TIE), and tyrosine kinase receptor (Trk).

Growth Factor Family	Receptor Tyrosine Kinase Family	Major Physiological Functions
EGF Family and neuregulins (EGF, TGF-α, AR, Epiregulin, HB-EGF, Betacellulin, NRG1, NRG2, NRG3, NRG4)	ErbB Family ErbB1 (EGFR), ErbB2 (Neu, HER2), ErbB3, ErbB4	Development of epithelial organs and nervous system
FGF (22 members) FGFs require heparan sulfate to activate their receptors	FGFR (4 members expressed as a number of splice variants)	Embryo patterning and organogenesis, bone development
PDGF Isoforms consist of homo- and heterodimers of A- and B-polypeptide chains and homodimers of C- and D-polypeptide chains	PDGFR (consists of PDGFR α and β receptors)	Embryonal development, particularly in the formation of the kidney, blood vessels, and various connective tissues
HGF The ligands are heterodimers of alpha and beta subunits linked by a disulfide bond	HGFR (consists of two receptors: MET and RON)	Motogenesis, morphogenesis, angiogenesis, and embryological development
GDNF Family (GDNF, NRTN, ARTN and PSPN)	RET (alternative splicing results in 3 isoforms)	Required for enteric neuron development, kidney development, and spermatogenesis
VEGF Family (VEGF-A, -B, -C, -D, -E, and PlGF)	VEGFR (VEGF receptor-1, -2, and -3)	Formation and maintenance of vasculature
Angiopoietin Family (Ang1, -2)	TIE	Crucial for vessel stabilization
SCF Due to splice variants there are soluble and membrane forms of SCF	KIT/SCFR	Hematopoiesis, gametogenesis, and melanogenesis
NGF family (NGF, BDNF, NT-3 and NT-4)	TRK (TRK-A, -B, -C)	Promotes neurite outgrowth and neural cell survival
Ephrins (2 classes: EphA and EphB, with a number of members within each class)	EPHR (2 classes: EPHRA and EPHRB, with a number of members within each class)	Patterning the developing hind-brain Rhombomeres, axon pathfinding, and guiding neural crest cell migration

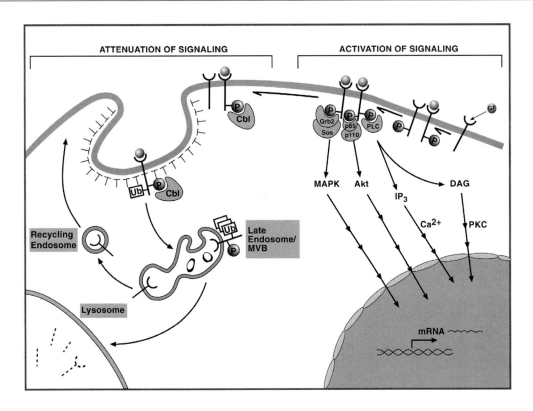

Fig. 1 Mechanisms of cellular activation by a growth factor and their desensitization mode. Upon activation by a growth factor (GF), the receptors undergo dimerization and autophosphorylation. Autophosphorylation of specific tyrosine residues dictate and enable the recruitment of multiple adaptor proteins containing SH2 or PTB domains (for example: Grb2, p85, and PLCγ). Examples of three major signaling pathways initiated at the cell surface and propagated to the nucleus are depicted. Other phosphotyrosine binding proteins that are recruited by tyrosine phosphorylation include Cbl which functions in receptor endocytosis (attenuation of signaling). Activated receptors are ubiquitinated and internalized via clathrin coated pits (symbolized by T letters). These receptors are then subsequently sorted through several endosomal compartments. Recycling of receptors back to the cell surface may occur from most endosomal compartments. However, as a receptor proceeds in the endocytic pathway, the efficiency of recycling declines and the receptors are ultimately degraded in the lysosome.

two enzymes involved in glycolysis and glyconeogenesis.

Phospholipase C-γ, another SH2 domain – containing protein hydrolyzes phosphatidyl 4′, 5′ bisphosphate (PIP_2) to diacylglycerol (DAG) and inositoltriphosphate (IP_3) once recruited to the plasma membrane (7). IP_3, a second messenger, binds to receptors on the membrane of the endoplasmic reticulum resulting in the release of calcium which, in-turn activates Ca^{2+} dependent protein kinases (e.g., the tyrosine kinase Pyk-2) and phosphatases (e.g., calcineurin). On the other hand, DAG binds to PKC, a serine/threonine

kinase, thereby mediating its translocation to the membrane and activation.

Multiple mechanisms exist to regulate and eventually attenuate signaling by activated growth factor receptors. The action of protein and lipid phosphatases, GTPase activating enzymes and inhibitory ligands regulate cellular stimulation by restricting signaling through specific downstream pathways. Proteins lacking apparent enzymatic activity but nevertheless curtail signaling through particular pathways have also been identified (e.g., Sprouty). Concomitant to the activation of signaling pathways, a whole series of proteins is set in motion to remove ligand-activated receptors from the cell surface, and to sort them for degradation in lysosomes (8). As in the case of EGFR and other tyrosine kinase receptors, receptors destined to endocytosis are tagged by conjugation of a 76 amino acid-long molecule called ubiquitin. Tagging is performed by a three-step enzymatic pathway culminating in an ubiquitin ligase called Cbl, which recognizes both the substrate receptor and the ubiquitin donor, an E2 ubiquitin-conjugating enzyme. A series of ubiquitin-binding endocytic adaptors subsequently recognize the ubiquitylated receptor and target it to clathrin-coated regions of the plasma membrane. The latter invaginate to form a clathrin-coated neck that progressively moves inward, eventually generating a coated vesicle. This tiny vesicle shuttles to a vesicular compartment called the early endosome. Through acidification of the endosome's lumen, some ligand-receptor complexes are dissociated, leading to recycling to the plasma membrane, while other complexes remain intact. The latter are handed to the subsequent sorting compartment, the multi-vesicular body, where hydrolases are accumulated. It is in this compartment and the subsequent one, the lysosome, where degradation of the receptor is completed.

Examples of Growth Factor Families

EGF-like factors and neuregulins. The EGF family includes transforming growth factor α, epiregulin, betacellulin, HB-EGF and several neuregulin families. All factors share a motif of 45–60 amino acids, including six cysteines, and their receptors belong to the ErbB family. In addition to their involvement in inductive cell-to-cell interactions in embryogenesis, these factors play an essential role in the development of epithelial organs (e.g., the mammary gland) and in wound healing. Aberrantly expressed forms of the ligands and ErbB proteins are widely implicated in cancer of epithelial and neuronal origins (9).

Fibroblast growth factors (FGFs). Four receptors with a variety of splice variants bind more than twenty types of FGFs (10). Many FGFs require glycosaminoglycan heparin sulfate for receptor binding. FGFs play a critical role in the patterning of the embryo and in organogenesis, including bone development. Many genetic disorders like Chondroplasia, Apert syndrome, Pfeiffer syndrome and Jackson-Weiss syndrome are associated with non-lethal mutations in one of the FGF receptors. FGF receptor activation has been shown to promote migration, proliferation and differentiation of endothelial and other cells, and has been implicated in angiogenesis.

Platelet derived growth factors (PDGFs). Disulfide linked homologous subunits designated A, B, C, and D constitute PDGFs, ligands that bind and activate two receptors, PDGFR-α and PDGFR-β. PDGF-A and PDGFR-α are expressed early while PDGF-B and PDGFR-β are expressed late during embryogenesis. Ablation of either the receptors or the ligands in mice results in embryonic or perinatal lethality with defects in alveogenesis, formation of the glomeruli in the kidney, cardiovascular disorders and hematological abnormalities. PDGFs are potent mitogens for connective tissues and effective chemotactic factors for inflammatory cells responsible for tissue repair and wound healing. Autocrine loops involving PDGFs have been implicated in sarcomas and gliomas, and they function in atherosclerosis, cardiac hypertrophy leading to heart failure, fibrosis of visceral organs, rheumatoid arthritis, glomeruloneptritis and proliferative vitreoretinopathy.

Hepatocyte growth factors (HGFs). The scatter factor (HGF) binds to Met, a single transmembrane protein with an extracellular α subunit and a membrane-spanning β subunit, whereas the macrophage-stimulating protein (MSP) binds to a related receptor called Ron. The ligands are heterodimers of α and β subunits linked by a disulfide bond. The α subunit contains one hairpin loop homologus to the plasminogen activation peptide, four kringle domains and a triple loop cysteine-rich motif. The β subunit is homologus to a serine protease but it has no enzymatic activity. HGF has been implicated in liver development, conversion of mesenchyme to epithelium in orgnogenesis of the kidney, ovary and testes, myoblast migration, axon sprouting and bone development. HGF expression is upregulated in response to liver injury and it was also shown to play a critical role in regulating fat accumulation in hepatocytes. Germ line and somatic mutations in Met were observed in patients with papilary renal carcinomas. Overexpression of Met has been implicated in myeloid malignancies and in carcinomas of the breast and bladder.

Vascular endothelial growth factors (VEGFs). Three tyrosine kinase receptors called VEGFR-1 (Flt-1), VEGFR-2 (KDR/Flk-1) and VEGFR-3 (Flt-4), and Neuropilins (NRP) 1 and 2 are the players at the receptor level. VEGF (also called vascular permeability factor, VPF) and its splice variants, as well as placenta growth factor and its isoforms serve as ligands. Activation by VEGF and semaphorin ligands results in the heterodimerization of VEGFR-2 with neuropilins. Heparin has been shown to play an important role in the signaling by this family. VEGF is predominantly an endothelial cell factor and is a prominent factor in the genesis and maintenance of the vasculature. VEGF and other factors are critical for physiological processes requiring angiogenesis, such as ovulation and menstruation. VEGF is induced by hypoxia and is expressed in tumors where the core is hypoxic. Secreted VEGF stimulates endothelial cells in the vicinity and promote the vascularization of the tumor and consequent tumor growth. VEGFs may also play a role in chronic inflammatory diseases and in diabetic retinopathy, conditions characterized by excessive angiogenesis.

Clinical Use

Growth factors and their respective receptors are emerging as attractive targets for pharmacological intervention. Potential uses include wound healing, artificial organs (including skin replacement) and cell-based therapy. On the other hand, blocking the actions of specific growth factors may be beneficial in hyperproliferative diseases such as psoriasis and in clinical cases like balloon injury-induced stenosis. Other potential uses are in inflammatory diseases such as sepsis, cirrhosis, experimental autoimmune encephalitis and cancer. Recombinant growth factors, humanized monoclonal antibodies to specific growth factors or their receptors, and low molecular weight inhibitors of specific RTKs or their downstream targets are currently in various phases of clinical testing. Examples include tyrosine kinase inhibitors specific to ErbB receptors (e.g., Iressa and CI-1033) or to VEGF receptors (e.g., SU-5416). A humanized monoclonal antibody directed to ErbB-2/HER2 has been approved in 1998 for the treatment of metastasizing breast cancers. Likewise, a chimaeric antibody specific to ErbB-1/EGFR is currently tested in various types of carcinomas. Finally, a monoclonal antibody to VEGF is under development as an anti-angiogenic agent.

References

1. Blume-Jensen P and Hunter T (2001) Oncogenic kinase signaling. Nature 411:355–365
2. Massague J and Pandiella A (1993) Membrane-anchored growth factors. Ann. Rev. Biochem. 62:515–541
3. van der Geer P, Hunter T and Lindberg RA (1994) Receptor protein-tyrosine kinases and their signal transduction pathways. Ann Rev Cell Biol 10:251–337
4. Heldin C-H (1995) Dimerization of cell surface receptors in signal transduction. Cell 80:213–223
5. Hubbard SR and Till JH (2000) Protein tyrosine kinase structure and function. Ann. Rev. Biochem. 69:373–398
6. Marshall CJ (1995) Specificity of receptor tyrosine kinase signaling: transient versus sustained extracellular signal-regulated kinase activation. Cell 80:179–185
7. Kamat A and Carpenter G (1997) Phospholipase C-γ1: regulation of enzyme function and role in growth factor-dependent signal transduction. Cytokine Growth Factor Rev 8:109–117
8. Waterman H and Yarden Y (2001) Molecular mechanisms underlying endocytosis and sorting of ErbB receptor tyrosine kinases. FEBS Lett 490:142–152
9. Yarden Y and Sliwkowski MX (2001) Untangling the ErbB signalling network. Nat Rev Mol Cell Biol 2:127–137
10. Powers CJ, McLeskey SW and Wellstein A (2000) Fibroblast growth factors, their receptors and signaling. Endocr Relat Cancer 7:165–197

G

Growth Hormone

Growth hormone (GH) is synthesized in the anterior pituitary. It belongs to the rather heterogeneous family of ▶ cytokines. Secreted GH is a mixture of polypeptides, the main polypeptide consisting of 191 amino acids. The receptor for GH is widely distributed. Like other members of the cytokine receptor family, it possesses one transmembrane domain. A single GH molecule binds to two receptor molecules and causes their dimerisation. The newly formed dimer provides a binding site for a member of the Janus kinase (JAK) family (▶ JAK-STAT Pathway). Clinically, recombinant human GH is used for the treatment of GH deficiency. GH deficiency in children leads to short stature. GH deficiency in adults has been associated with changes in fat distribution, increases in circulating lipids, decreased muscle mass and increased mortality from cardiovascular causes.

GSK3

▶ Glycogen Synthase Kinase 3
▶ Insulin Receptor

GTPase Activating Proteins (GAPs)

GTPase activating proteins (GAPs) stimulate the intrinsic GTP hydrolysis of GTPases.

▶ Small GTPases

GTPase, small

▶ Small GTPases

Guanine Nucleotide Dissociation Inhibitors (GDIs)

Guanine nucleotide dissociation inhibitors (GDIs) bind to small GTPases and inhibit the dissociation and thus the exchange of the bound nucleotide.

▶ Small GTPases

Guanine Nucleotide Exchange Factors (GEFs)

Guanine nucleotide exchange factors (GEFs) are proteins which catalyse the release of nucleotide bound to small GTPases.

▶ Small GTPases

Guanylyl Cyclase

DORIS KOESLING
Pharmakologie und Toxikologie,
Ruhr-Universität Bochum, Bochum, Germany
koesling@iname.com

Synonyms

Guanylate cyclase, guanyl cyclase

Definition

Guanylyl cyclases (GC) are a family of enzymes (EC 4.6.1.2) that catalyse the formation of the second messenger cyclic GMP (cGMP) from GTP. GCs are subdivided in soluble GCs and GCs that are membrane-bound and linked to a receptor. Activation occurs by nitric oxide (NO) and peptide hormones, respectively (1,2).

▶ Adenylyl Cyclases
▶ NO Synthases
▶ Smooth Muscle Tone Regulation
▶ Phosphodiesterases

Basic Characteristics

Activation of GCs leads to an increase of the intracellular messenger molecule cGMP. cGMP-signalling is mediated by three different groups of cGMP effector molecules: cGMP-activated protein kinases, cGMP-regulated ▶ phosphodiesterases and cGMP-gated ion channels, see Fig. 1. The levels of cGMP is reduced by cGMP-degrading phosphodiesterases. cGMP plays a role in the relaxation of smooth muscle, inhibition of platelet aggregation and in retinal phototransduction. It also participates in signal transduction within the nervous system. Moreover, cGMP is involved in regulation of the water and electrolyte household as well as in bone metabolism. According to their structural features and their regulation, GCs can be divided into NO-stimulated and receptor-linked enzymes.

NO-Stimulated GC

Soluble, NO-stimulated GC (sGC) represents the most important effector enzyme for the signalling molecule NO, which is synthesized by ▶ NO synthases in a Ca^{2+}-dependent manner (3). NO-stimulated GC contains a prosthetic ▶ heme group, which provides the acceptor site for NO. Formation of the NO-heme complex leads to a conformational change, resulting in an increase of up to 200-fold in catalytic activity of the enzyme (1). The organic nitrates (see below) commonly used in the therapy of coronary heart disease exert their effects via the stimulation of this enzyme.

So far two isoforms of the NO-sensitive heterodimeric enzyme have been identified; the ubiquitous $\alpha_1\beta_1$ isoform and the less broadly distributed $\alpha_2\beta_1$ isoform. Although both isoforms show the same regulatory properties, they appear to differ in their subcellular distribution. The N-terminal regions of the subunits are responsible for heme binding and heme coordination, whereas the cyclase catalytic domains are located in the C-terminal regions. The cyclase catalytic domain is conserved in the membrane-bound guanylyl cyclases as well as in the adenylyl cyclases (see below).

Soluble GCs occur in relatively high concentration in vascular smooth muscle cells and platelets as well as in lung, kidney and brain tissues. The NO-induced increase in cGMP causes smooth muscle relaxation and the inhibition of platelet aggregation. Aside from the cardiovascular system, the NO/cGMP cascade has an important function in the nervous system, where it is thought to participate in synaptic plasticity, i.e. the use-dependent change of the efficiency of synaptic transmission.

Besides NO, only few other sGC-activating substances have been reported: Carbon monoxide (CO) is known to bind heme groups with high affinity but has been shown to induce enzyme activity only marginally (3- to 5-fold). A 10-fold increase of activity has been reported for the NO-sensitive GC when using YC-1 ([3-(5'-hydroxymethyl-2'-furyl)-1-benzyl indazole]) as an activator. Moreover, YC-1 induces NO and CO sensitivity of the enzyme. Apart from an increase in the formation of cGMP via the stimulation of sGC, the substance also inhibits phosphodiesterases. In intact cells, YC-1 causes pronounced increases in cGMP levels by preventing cGMP degradation. Thus, YC-1 may represent a new class of drugs that are of potential use in the treatment of cardiovascular diseases. YC-1-related compounds have already been developed and their therapeutic benefits are currently under investigation.

Receptor-linked GC

Membrane-bound GCs belong to the group of receptor-linked enzymes with one membrane-spanning region (2). Although all of these GCs share a conserved intracellular catalytic domain, they differ in their extracellular ligand-binding domains and are activated by different peptide hormones. The guanylyl cyclase A (GC-A) isoform acts as the receptor for the ▶ natriuretic peptides ANP and BNP, two primarily cardiac hormones that are involved in the regulation of blood pressure as well as in the water and electrolyte household. ANP-induced and BNP-induced increases in cGMP levels mediate physiological effects such as smooth muscle relaxation, inhibition of aldosteron secretion in the adrenal cortex and salt and water excretion in the kidney. A sec-

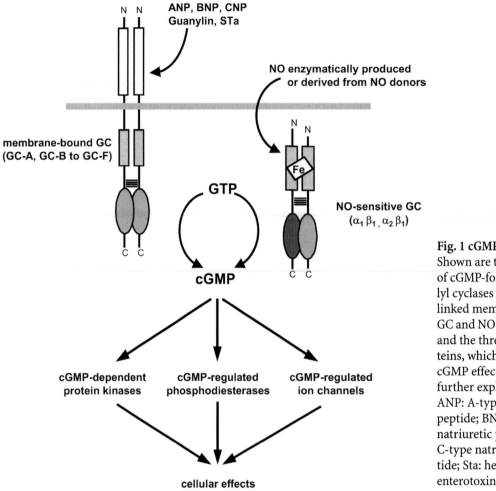

Fig. 1 cGMP-signalling.
Shown are the two groups
of cGMP-forming guany-
lyl cyclases (receptor-
linked membrane-bound
GC and NO-activated GC)
and the three effector proteins, which mediate the
cGMP effect (see text for
further explanation).
ANP: A-type natriuretic
peptide; BNP: B-type
natriuretic petide; CNP:
C-type natriuretic pep-
tide; Sta: heat-stable
enterotoxin of *E. coli*.

ond ANP receptor, containing only a very short intracellular C-terminal region and without any GC activity, has also been identified. As intracellular signalling of this ANP receptor has not been detected, this protein was suggested to function as a 'clearance receptor', removing excess ANP from the circulating blood. Another GC isoform, GC-B, displays the highest affinity for the natriuretic peptide of the C-type (CNP). GC-B is mainly found in the vascular endothelium and is thought to participate in smooth muscle relaxation. However, occurrence of the above GC isoforms and the natriuretic peptides is not limited to the cardiovascular system, they may also play a role in the central nervous system. Further GC isoforms are GC-C, GC-D, GC-E and GC-F. Of these, GC-C

binds the peptide hormone guanylin that occurs mainly in the intestine. It is stimulated by the heat stable enterotoxin of *Escherichia coli*, a fact that, pathophysiologically, can lead to severe diarrhoea. Therefore, GC-C and its ligand are probably involved in regulating the salt and water balance in the intestine. The other receptor-linked GC isoforms are restricted to sensory cells. GC-D is only expressed in olfactory neurons, GC-E and GC-F are exclusively found in the retina. Regulation of these GC isoforms by proteins that interact with the intracellular cGMP-forming domain has been demonstrated. Since no ligand to the N-terminal domain of such isoforms has been identified to date, it is not clear whether cGMP-forming activity is controlled by the receptor domain at all.

Drugs

Drugs Acting on Soluble GC

Clinically, the ▶ organic nitrates glyceryl trinitrate, isosorbide dinitrate and isosorbide mononitrate are mainly used in the treatment of coronary heart disease. They exert their main therapeutic effect by activating sGC via NO (4). None of the nitrates release NO spontaneously, instead they undergo a complex enzymatic bioactivation that either yields NO or bioactive S-nitrosothiols. Enzyme(s) and cofactors required for this biotransformation have not been clearly identified, yet it appears that the activity of certain enzyme(s) and cofactors can vary within different regions of the vascular system. This may cause, or may contribute, to the observed differences in NO sensitivity. Since nitrate-induced vasodilation is more pronounced in veins than in arteries, the organic nitrates cause marked venorelaxation and reduce central venous pressure. In turn, the preload and the cardiac work decrease, resulting in a relief of angina pectoris symptoms. Treatments with organic nitrates that reduce cardiac preload are also used in patients with heart failure. However, direct coronary dilation or redistribution of the blood flow to ischemic regions of the myocardium remains controversial.

In general, nitrates are either used to treat or to prevent acute episodes of angina, or they are employed to provide long-term prophylaxis against episodes of angina in patients with frequent angina attacks. For the appropriate application of organic nitrates, pharmacokinetical and pharmaceutical aspects have to be taken into account. A hepatic high capacity organic nitrate reductase rapidly inactivates organic nitrates by effectively removing nitrate groups. The bioavailability of the traditional organic nitrate glyceryl trinitrate is therefore very low, and for the immediate treatment of angina, the sublingual application of glyceryl trinitrate is preferred. This way the first pass effect is circumvented and a therapeutic blood level of glyceryl trinitrate is rapidly achieved. The nitrate can be efficiently absorbed and exert its antianginal effect within minutes. However, because the drug's duration of effect is very short (15–30 minutes), sublingually applied glyceryl trinitrate is not suitable for maintenance therapy. In such cases, the sublingual application

of isosorbide dinitrate, which is similar to glyceryl trinitrate, is advised. In comparison, isosorbide dinitrate has a slightly delayed onset of activity but its duration of effect (2 hours) is more sustained. For a drug effect that lasts even longer, nitrates such as sustained-release preparations of nitroglycerin, isosorbide dinitrate or isosorbide mononitrate are administered orally at sufficient dosage to provide effective plasma levels after first-pass-degradation. Other options to administer nitroglycerin include transdermal and buccal absorption from slow release preparations. As an active metabolite of isosorbide dinitrate, isosorbide mononitrate is available for clinical use and has a bioavailability of 100%.

A major problem of nitrate-based prophylaxis of angina is the loss of drug efficacy. The continuous application of nitrates for more than a few hours leads to the development of nitrate tolerance. Although the precise mechanisms of this tolerance phenomenon are unknown, it is conceivable that tolerance occurs at the level of the metabolising enzymes and/or the NO receptor GC. Moreover, an increase in the NO-scavenging superoxide ion and other counter-regulatory mechanisms may contribute to the development of tolerance. However, since the marked attenuation of the nitrate effect is rapidly reversible upon discontinuation of the drug, any tolerance development can be controlled and is achieved by allowing a 'nitrate-free' period of about 8 hours (usually at night) within 24 hours.

An option for patients who develop nocturnal angina is molsidomine, another NO containing compound that is believed not to induce tolerance. molsidomine features a similar pharmacological profile as the organic nitrates. As a prodrug, it is bioactivated in the liver and yields SIN-1 that decomposes, enzyme-independently, in a two-step reaction. In the first step, SIN-1 undergoes a base-catalysed ring opening to form SIN-1A. This in turn yields NO and the stable metabolite SIN-1C. As the onset of action of molsidomine is comparatively slow, it is not used to treat acute cases of angina. Furthermore, due to its putative carcinogenic effect, molsidomine should only be considered when treatment with organic nitrates is not sufficient, for example in the 'nitrate-free' interval.

The acute toxicity of the organic nitrates as well as molsidomine is directly related to their therapeutic vasodilation of orthostatic hypotension, tachycardia and throbbing headache.

Apart from the substances mentioned above, there is one other NO-containing compound, sodium nitroprusside (SNP), which effectively reduces ventricular preload and afterload, This powerful vasodilator has to be administered parenterally and is used in intensive care units that deal with emergency patients who exhibit hypertension. In the presence of reducing agents such as glutathione, SNP spontaneously releases NO concomitantly with cyanide. Its most serious adverse effects are therefore related to the accumulation of cyanide.

In low doses, inhaled NO may have a beneficial therapeutic effect, since NO in the inspired air leads to pulmonary vasodilation. In persistent pulmonary hypertension of the newborn, NO inhalation has already been used with some success. NO inhalation as the treatment for acute respiratory distress syndrome, however, has been disappointing. Only transient improvements of oxygenation were detected and the outcome of placebo-controlled trials did not show any improvement

Drugs Acting on Receptor-linked GC

In theory, one could utilize GC-A ligands to lower blood pressure and to reduce blood volume as they increase the excretion of water and salt. The effectiveness of BNP in managing acute congestive heart failure is currently under investigation in clinical trials.

Besides the attempt to substitute natriuretic hormones with the recombinant form of BNP, there is a pharmacological approach to elevate the concentration of natriuretic peptides by inhibiting degradation by the neutral endopeptidase. Of special interest are dual-function inhibitors that block not only the neutral natriuretic peptide-degrading endopeptidase but also the angiotensin-converting enzyme, thereby decreasing the level of angiotensin II.

References

1. Koesling D, Friebe A (1999) Structure and regulation of soluble guanylyl cyclase. Rev Physiol. Biochem. Pharmacol. 135:35–41
2. Wedel, BJ, Garbers DL (2001) The guanylyl cyclase family at Y2K. Annu. Rev. Physiol. 63:215–233
3. Moncada S, Higgs EA (1995) Molecular mechanisms and therapeutic strategies related to nitric oxide. FASEB J. 13:1319–1330
4. Harrison DG, Bates JN (1993) The nitrovasodilators. New ideas about old drugs. Circulation 87:1461–1467

Gyrase

Gyrase is another term for bacterial topoisomerase II. The enzyme consists of two A and two B subunits and is responsible for the negative supercoiling of the bacterial DNA. Negative supercoiling makes the bacterial DNA more compact and also more readily accessible to enzymes that cause duplication and transcription of the DNA to RNA.

▶ Topoisomerase
▶ Quinolones

Gyrase Inhibitors

▶ Topoisomerase
▶ Quinolones

H

Haemostasis

Haemostasis is the mechanism activated after damage to the blood vessel wall that ensures that blood loss is restricted. Blood platelets are are activated and adhere to elements on the damaged lumenal surface of the vessel, eventually forming a platelet plug that stops the leakage of blood. Fibrinolytic mechanisms later produce lysis of the platelet mass when repair of the vessel has occurred.

▶ Coagulation/Thrombosis

Half-life /Elimination Half-life (t1/2 or t1/2β)

Half-life is the time taken to decrease the concentration of a drug to one-half its original value. There may be several phases in the elimination, and the most common is the so-called beta-phase. Alpha-phase is a distribution phase and gamma-phase is the terminal phase when the drug is finally leaving the tissues.

▶ Pharmacokinetics

Haplotype

A haplotype describes a specific set of polymorphisms located on one chromosome. Since most organisms are diploid, elucidation of the haplotypes composed of polymorphisms located a long distance apart provides a major experimental problem. For populations, haplotype frequencies can be calculated by statistical methods.

▶ Pharmacogenetics

Hashish

Cannabinoid System

HCN

Hyperpolarisation-activated cyclic nucleotide-gated-channel.

▶ Cyclic Nucleotide-regulated Cation Channels

HCV (Hepatits C Virus)

▶ Hepatitis C
▶ Antiviral Drugs
▶ Interferons

HDL

▶ High-density-lipoproteins Cholesterol
▶ HMG-CoA-reductase-inhibitors

Heat Shock Protein

Eukaryotes respond to heat shock and other forms of environmental stress by inducing synthesis of heat-shock proteins (HSP). The hsp90 proteins are a group of HSPs with an average molecular weight of 90 Kd. The precise function of hsp90 is unclear. The protein is associated with steroid hormone receptors, tyrosine kinases, eIF2alpha kinase, actin and tubulin. HSPs act as chaperonins with ATPase activity, maintaining the correct 3-D structure of large protein complexes.

▶ Glucocorticoids
▶ Stress Proteins

Helicobacter Pylori

Helicobacter pylori is a spiral shaped bacterium that lives in the stomach and duodenum (the section of intestine just below the stomach). Most bacteria cannot live in the stomach since the environment is too acid to survive. However, *Helicobacter pylori* has large amounts of urease, which converts urea to ammonia and carbon dioxide. Ammonia is used to maintain the periplasmic and cytoplasmic pH of the bacterium at neutrality, so this bacterium can survive.

▶ Proton Pump Inhibitors and Acid Pump Antagonists

Helix Bundle

A helix bundle is a protein composed of a series of rod-like helical domains linked by flexible segments and inserted into a membrane to form a cluster of helices roughly parallel to one another and perpendicular to the plane of the membrane.

Helix-loop-helix Motif

A helix-loop-helix motif is a DNA-binding motif, related to the leucine-zipper. A helix-loop-helix motif consists of a short α helix, connected by a loop to a second, longer α helix. The loop is flexible and allows one helix to fold back and pack against the other. The helix-loop-helix structure binds not only DNA but also the helix-loop-helix motif of a second helix-loop-helix protein forming either a homodimer or a heterodimer.

Helper T Cells

▶ Immune Defense

Hemangioblast

Hemangioblasts are the bipotential precursor cell population from which hematopoietic and angioblastic cells arise.

▶ Angiogenesis and Vascular Morphogenesis

Hematopoiesis

Hematopoiesis is the formation and development of blood cells.

▶ Hematopoietic Growth Factors

Hematopoietic Growth Factors

MARYANN FOOTE, GEORGE MORSTYN
Amgen Inc., Thousand Oaks and UCLA School of Medicine, Los Angeles, USA
mfoote@amgen.com; gmorstyn@amgen.com

Synonyms

Colony-stimulating factors

Definition

Hematopoietic (blood) cells transport oxygen, contribute to host immunity and facilitate blood clotting (1). A complex, interrelated, and multistep process, called ▶ hematopoiesis, controls the production as well as the development of specific marrow cells from immature precursor cells to functional mature blood cells. This well-regulated process also allows for replacement of cells lost through daily physiologic activities. The proliferation of precursor cells, the maturation of these into mature cells, and the survival of hematopoietic cells require the presence of specific growth factors.

▶ Growth Factors
▶ Neurotrophic Factors

Mechanism of Action

Hematopoiesis is mediated by a series of growth factors that act individually and in various combinations involving complex feedback mechanisms. The growth factors are glycoproteins that act through specific receptors found on the cell membrane surface of appropriate cells. All mature blood cells arise from primitive hematopoietic cells in the bone marrow, the pluripotent stem cells. The stem cell pool maintains itself through a process of asymmetrical cell division: when a stem cell divides, one daughter cell remains a stem cell and the other becomes a committed colony-forming cell (CFC). The proliferation and differentiation of CFCs are controlled by hematopoietic growth factors. The hematopoietic growth factors stimulate cell division, differentiation and maturation, and convert the dividing cells into a population of terminally differentiated functional cells (see figure).

More than 20 hematopoietic growth factors have been identified. The chemical properties of these growth factors have been characterized and the gene that encodes for the factor identified and cloned. Several hematopoietic growth factors are commercially available as recombinant human forms, and they have utility in clinical practice. These factors include; the recombinant forms of two myeloid hematopoietic growth factors, granulocyte colony-stimulating factor (G-CSF) and granulocyte-macrophage colony-stimulating factor (GM-CSF); erythropoietin (EPO), the red cell factor; stem cell factor (SCF), an early-acting hematopoietic growth factor; and the platelet factors, thrombopoietin (TPO) and interleukin-11 (IL-1). T lymphocytes, monocytes/ macrophages, fibroblasts and endothelial cells are the important cellular sources of most hematopoietic growth factors, excluding EPO and TPO. EPO is produced primarily by the adult kidney and TPO is produced in the liver and kidney.

Granulocyte colony-stimulating factor (recombinant products: filgrastim, lenograstim, pegfilgrastim) maintains neutrophil production during steady state conditions and increases production of neutrophils during acute situations such as infections (2). Recombinant human G-CSF (rHuG-CSF) reduces neutrophil maturation time from 5 days to 1 day, leading to the rapid release of mature neutrophils form the bone marrow into the blood. rHuG-CSF also increases the circulating half-life of neutrophils and enhances ▶ chemotaxis and ▶ superoxide production. Pegfilgrastim is a sustained-duration formulation of rHuG-CSF that has been developed by covalent attachment of a ▶ polyethylene glycol molecule to the filgrastim molecule.

H

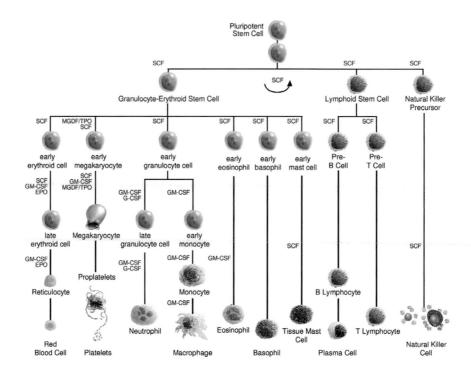

Fig. 1 Schema of hematopoiesis, including some of the growth factors that influence the production of blood cells.

Granulocyte-macrophage colony-stimulating factor (recombinant products: molgramostim, sargramostim) is locally active and remains at the site of infection to localize and activate neutrophils (3). Like G-CSF, GM-CSF stimulates the proliferation, differentiation and activation of mature neutrophils; and enhances superoxide production, ▶ phagocytosis and intracellular killing. GM-CSF, unlike G-CSF, stimulates the proliferation, differentiation and activation of mature monocytes/macrophages.

Erythropoietic factors (recombinant products: epoetinα, epoetinβ, darbepoetinα) increase red blood cell numbers by causing committed erythroid progenitor cells to proliferate and differentiate into normoblasts, nucleated precursor cells in the erythropoietic lineage (4). Tissue ▶ hypoxia resulting from anemia induces the kidney to increase its production of EPO by a magnitude of 10-fold or more. Patients with chronic renal failure are unable to produce adequate levels of endogenous EPO because of loss of renal function and must receive rHuEPO to maintain red blood cell counts. Darbepoetinα is another erythropoietic factor that has an extended half-life due to its increased number of ▶ sialic acid-containing carbohydrate molecules.

Stem cell factor (recombinant product: ancestim) is an early-acting hematopoietic growth factor that stimulates the proliferation of primitive hematopoietic and non-hematopoietic cells (5). *In vitro*, SCF has minimal effect on hematopoietic and non-hematopoietic progenitor cells, but it synergistically increases the activity of other hematopoietic growth factors, such as G-CSF, GM-CSF and EPO. Stem cell factor stimulates the generation of ▶ dendritic cells *in vitro* and ▶ mast cells *in vivo*.

Thrombopoietic factors (recombinant products: TPO, megakaryocyte growth and development factor [MGDF], and IL-11 [oprelvekin]) stimulate the production of megakaryocyte precursors, megakaryocytes and platelets (6). Interleukin-11 has many effects on multiple tissues, and can itneract with IL-3, TPO and SCF.

Clinical Use (incl. side effects)

The use of recombinant hematopoietic growth factors (i.e., the commercially available forms of the native products) has been evaluated in many disorders affecting all types of blood cells. Recombinant human hematopoietic growth factors are identified as "rHu". Not all uses discussed have received regulatory approval in all countries.

The myeloid growth factors rHuG-F and rHuGM-CSF have been tested and are used for the treatment of many neutrophil disorders, particualarly neutropenia caused by ▶ myelosuppressive chemotherapy and other drugs, bone marrow transplantation, severe chronic neutropenia, leukemia and AIDS. Neutropenia is a serious side effect of chemotherapy. Patients with neutropenia have a severely impaired ability to fight infections, and if not treated, neutropenia can be fatal. Peripheral blood progenitor cell transplantation is similar in principle to the more commonly recognized bone marrow transplantation, but collection of peripheral blood progenitor cells is less invasive than collection of bone marrow. rHuEPO is used to treat anemia, the condition of low number of red blood cells. Patients who are anemic often experience fatigue, headaches, shortness of breath, chest pains and depression. Severe anemia can result in congestive heart failure. Anemia can be caused by myelosuppressive chemotherapy, kidney failure, and chronic diseases such as cancer. Another complication of chemotherapy is ▶ thrombocytopenia, an inadequate number of platelets, requiring transfusion. Thrombocytopenia can be caused by exposure to certain drugs and radiation, and can occur as the result of inherited diseases. Patients with thrombocytopenia bruise easily and may have serious internal bleeding that can cause death. rHuTPO and rHuIL-11 both act on bone marrow to produce platelets.

When hematopoietic growth factors are used clinically, they can be associated with adverse effects. Very often patients who require hematopoietic growth factors are quite ill with their disease (i.e., cancer or kidney failure) or from their treatment (i.e., chemotherapy) and it is difficult to determine if a recombinant growth factor is responsible for a given side effect. Both rHuG-CSF and rHuGM-CSF are associated with mild-to-

moderate bone pain. It is possible that rHuGM-CSF can also be associated with fever and allergic-like reactions. In general, rHuEPO (as well as darbepoetinα) is well tolerated, but some patients experience flu-like symptoms, hypertension or headaches. The most common event associated with rHuSCF is injection-site reactions (i.e., ▶ edema or ▶ urticaria). Administration of rHuIL-11, the only commercially available thrombopoietin, is associated with several toxicities, including fluid retension, anemia and cardiac arrhythmias.

New formulations of existing recombinant hematopoietic growth factors are in development and other recombinant hematopoietic growth factors are being developed. The recombinant hematopoietic growth factors have had a significant impact on the treatment of cancer, including prevention of serious infections and anemia.

References

1. Mecalf D (1990) The colony stimulating factors. Discovery, development, and clinical applications. Cancer 65:185–195.
2. Welte K, Gabrilove J, Bronchud MJ, Platzer E, Morstyn G (1996) Filgrastim (r-metHuG-CSF): the first 10 years. Blood 88:1907–1929
3. Armitage JO (1998) Emerging applications of recombinant human granulocyte colony-stimulating factor. Blood 92:4491–4508
4. Jacobson JO, Goldwasser E, Fried W, Plzak L (2000) Role of the kidney in erythropoiesis. J Amer Society Nephrol 11:58–592
5. Broudy VC (1997) Stem cell factor and hematopoiesis. Blood 90: 1345–1364.
6. Kuter DJ, Hunt P, Sheridan W, Zucker-Franklin D, editors (1994) Thrombopoiesis and Thrombopoietins. Totwa, N.J., U.S.A.; Humana Press, Inc., 412 pp.

Heme

Heme ($C_{34}H_{32}O_4N_4Fe$) represents an iron-porphyrin complex that has a protoporphyrin nucleus. Many important proteins contain heme as a prosthetic group. Hemoglobin is the quantitatively most important hemoprotein. Others are cytochromes (present in the mitochondria and the

H

endoplasmic reticulum), catalase and peroxidase (that react with hydrogen peroxide), ▶ soluble guanylyl cyclase (that converts guanosine triphosphate, GTP, to the signaling molecule 3',5'-cyclic GMP) and ▶ NO synthases.

Hemozoin

Hemozoin, also known as malaria pigment, is, in terms of its chemical composition, identical to β-hematin. Hemozoin is formed as a crystallization product of heme under the acidic conditions present in the food vacuole of malarial parasites. In the crystal, the heme molecules are linked into dimers through reciprocal iron-carboxylate bonds to one of the propionate side chains of each porphyrin. The dimers form chains linked by hydrogen bonds.

▶ Antiprotozoal Drugs

Heparin

Pentasaccharide

▶ Anticoagulants

Hepatitis

Hepatitis is acute or chronic inflammation of the liver, which is frequently caused by infection with hepatotropic viruses. Several forms of viral hepatitis (A, B, C, D, E) are known, which result from infection with viruses belonging to separate virus families, differing in their genomic organization, replication strategies, morphology and modes of transmission.

▶ Antiviral Drugs
▶ Interferons

Hepatitis C

Hepatitis C Virus (HCV) is the causative agent of hepatitis C, identified in 1989. HCV is a positive-strand RNA virus of the *Flavivirideae* family, known to infect human liver. Infection may be symptomless but may cause severe liver damage after several years. It is estimated that 1-3% of the world population are infected with HCV. The main route of transmission is parenteral with high incience among intravenous drug users. Other risk factors are tattooing and needle stick injuries, whereas sexual transmission appears to be infrequent. About 20% of HCV cases cannot be associated with risk factors (sporadic infections) but correlate with low socio-economic background and enhanced contact with risk groups. Prior to the identification of the virus, blood transfusions, blood products or renal dialysis could lead to infection, due to unchecked contamination with HCV. Nowadays, reliable diagnostic assays are used to monitor the presence of HCV in blood or blood products and have dimished the chance of infection to less than 1 in a million transfused units.

▶ Antiviral Drugs
▶ Viral Proteases

Heptahelical Domain

Heptahelical domains are protein modules found in all known G-protein coupled receptors. The structure of one of these (rhodopsine) has been recently solved. It is made up of 7 transmembrane helices interconnected by 3 extra and 3 intracellular loops. For most G-protein coupled receptors activated by small ligands, the binding site is located in a cavity formed by transmembrane domains 3, 5, 6 and 7.

▶ G-protein Coupled Receptors

HERG-channels

HERG-channels are voltage-gated K^+ channels which belong to the ether-à-go-go (eag) family of Kv-channels. HERG stands for human eag related gene. Mutations in the human gene are associated with the long QT-syndrome LQT2. Together with MiRP1 (MinK-related peptide 1), HERG constitues the cardiac rapid delayed rectifier K^+ channel (IK_R) which is reponsible for repolarization of cardiac action potential and therefore governs the action potential duration. Many drugs ranging from erythromycin to sotalol may block HERG channels. Certain mutations in HERG channels are associated with drug-induced arrhythmia.

▶ K^+ Channels
▶ Voltage-gated K^+ Channels

Heterologous Desensitization

Heterologous desensitization is a form of desensitization which does not require agonist binding of the receptor. Second messenger dependent kinases such as protein kinase A (PKA) and protein kinase C (PKC) are involved in this form of receptor desensitization. Heterologous desensitization simply depends on the over-all kinase activity which is regulated by many different stimuli.

▶ Tolerance and Desensitization

Heterologous Expression System

Heterologous expression systems are prokaryotic organisms (e.g. *E. coli*) or eukaryotic cells (e.g. yeast, HEK293, *Xenopus* oocytes) that are used to express foreign genes or cDNAs.

Heterotrimeric G-proteins

▶ Heterotrimeric GTP-binding Protein

Heterotrimeric GTP-binding Proteins

Heterotrimeric G-proteins are part of a widely used transmembrane signaling system consisting of G-protein coupled receptors or binding proteins, (GPCRs), heterotrimeric G-proteins and a variety of effectors (enzymes or ion channels). Activation of GPCRs by extracellular ligands leads, via the activation of G-proteins, to the regulation of effectors. Heterotrimeric G-proteins consist of α-, β-, and γ-subunits. In order to convey a signal from an activated receptor to an effector, the heterotrimeric G-protein undergoes an activation-inactivation-cycle, which allows it to function as a regulatory molecular switch. In the basal state, the β/γ-complex as well as the GTP-bound α-subunit are associated, and this complex is recognized by an appropriate activated receptor. Interaction with the receptor results in the dissociation of GDP from the α-subunit and its replacement by GTP. Binding of GTP induces a conformational change, which results in the dissociation of the α-subunit and the β/γ complex. Both, the α-subunit and the β/γ-complex, are now able to regulate effectors. The reassociation of heterotrimeric G-protein is induced by the hydrolysis of GTP to GDP. Two bacterial toxins have been found to specifically interfere with the G-protein activation-inactivation cycle, pertussis toxin blocks the interaction of the activated receptor with several members of the $G_{i/o}$-family of G-proteins whereas cholera toxin leads to the constitutive activation of some G-proteins including G_s. The inactivation of G-proteins is enhanced by various effector molecules as well as by a group of proteins called "regulators of G-protein signaling" (RGS-proteins), which act as GTPase activators. There are four main subfamilies of G-proteins which are classified according to the identity of the their α-subunits. The G_s-

H

family mediates the stimulatory regulation of adenylyl cyclases, whereas the $G_{i/o}$-family mediates the inhibitory regulation of adenylyl cyclases. $G_{i/o}$-family members are also involved in the stimulatory regulation of K^+-channels (GIRK) and the inhibitory regulation of some voltage-dependent Ca^{2+}-channels. The $G_{q/11}$ is involved in the stimulatory regulation of β-isoforms of phospholipase C. The $G_{12/13}$-family couples receptors to the activation of the small GTPase RhoA.

▶ G-protein Coupled Receptors
▶ Table appendix: Receptor Proteins

High-density-lipoprotein-cholesterol

High-density-lipoproteins (HDLs) are believed to carry cholesterol away from the blood vessels and back to the liver. High plasma concentrations are associated with a reduced risk of heart disease. HDL is also some times called "the good cholesterol".

▶ HMG-CoA-reductase-inhibitors

High-throughput Screening

PAUL A. NEGULESCU
Vertex Pharmaceuticals Incorporated,
San Diego, CA, USA
paul_negulescu@sd.vrtx.com

Definition

High-throughput screening (HTS) is the term used to describe the portion of the ▶ drug discovery process in which ▶ compound libraries are tested for an effect in an ▶ assay directed against a molecular ▶ target or biological mechanism. Although there is no precise definition of high-throughput *per se*, any process capable of performing 10,000 or more tests per day is generally considered a high-throughput screen. Achieving this screening rate often involves the use of robotics and automation to perform some or all steps in the assay. Therefore, the fundamental components comprising HTS are an assay, a compound collection, and some automated methods for carrying out the screen. Compounds that are identified as active by HTS are called hits and may be the starting points for further chemical optimization. A target is a protein or protein assembly whose function is believed to be important for promoting health or treating disease. An assay is used to measure the effect of the test compound on the target. There are many different assay formats that are compatible with HTS. However, in order to be suitable for high-throughput screening, an assay should be sensitive, informative, reliable and simple to implement (i.e. relatively few steps). Assay performance can be measured statistically using commonly accepted standards. HTS is an important component of modern drug discovery and an area of active research and development in the pharmaceutical and biotechnology industries.

▶ Combinatorial Chemistry

Description

Types of targets
Any protein whose function is believed to be clinically relevant and suitable for modulation by a drug can be considered a drug target. Targets may be grouped according to their functional class. Historically, many mammalian targets have been cell surface molecules such as receptors, transporters or ion channels. More recently intracellular targets such as kinases and nuclear receptors have received increased attention (1). Many infectious disease targets are genes essential for microbial growth or viral replication.

Types of assays
Broadly defined, assays fall into two major categories: biochemical and cell-based. Biochemical assays are based on isolated protein preparations, while cell-based assays utilize intact cells. Usually, cell-based assays rely on recombinant mammalian cell lines in which the target of interest is heterologously expressed. There are many different types

of target–based assays ranging in complexity and information content. Among the simplest assays are ligand-binding assays that measure displacement of a radiolabeled ligand from a purified protein preparation by a test compound. These assays are best applied when the target has a well-defined binding site. G-protein coupled receptors (GPCRs) represent such a target class. For membrane-bound targets such as GPCRs, these binding assays can be carried out in membrane preparations. Binding assays, while simple, do not provide information on whether a test compound affects the function of a target.

Functional assays provide information as to whether a test compound activates, inhibits or otherwise modulates the target. Functional biochemical assays can be performed on purified proteins such as enzymes (e.g. kinase protease, etc). These assays typically utilize substrates to indicate the turnover rate of the enzyme. The most complex assays are cell-based functional assays. These assays are favored when it is necessary to measure the effect of a compound on target function in a cellular environment. For example, many ion channels are not ligand-regulated and/or require multi-subunit assemblies to function. Therefore, the most practical way to screen these targets is to measure their activity in an intact cell. Measurements of ion flux, ion concentration, or membrane potential are all viable methods to screening these targets. Cell-based functional assays can be developed for most targets and are particularly useful when one is screening for a particular type of modulator. For example, in addition to detecting target activation or inhibition, these assays can identify allosteric modulators of target activity.

Not all cell-based functional assays are directed against a specific molecular target. Indeed many drugs have been identified based on an observed effect of a compound on a cellular phenotype, such as shape, viability or growth. An example of this is cyclosporin, a natural product initially identified for its anti-microbial effects and later found to inhibit T-cell proliferation. Such assays can be considered "phenotypic" in the sense that one is assaying for a change in some measurable cell parameter. The advantage of these types of screens is that they do not introduce a target-centric bias to drug discovery. A challenge for these assays is the difficulty in identifying the molecular mechanism of compound action, and the consequence of developing drugs without full understanding their mode of action. An alternative use of phenotypic assays is to screen for novel targets (2).

Assay Formats

While it is beyond the scope of this article to describe all the assay formats used in HTS, a general description of the types of readouts is pertinent. In general, HTS assays are either end-point or kinetic assays. End-point assays take only a single read from a well (possibly with a pre-read before compound or reagent addition) and allow more flexibility for automation while kinetic assays require more precise processes and timings associated with multiple reads from the same well. Compounds may be pre-incubated or added acutely to the assay. Because HTS is an automated process, assay formats with minimal steps are preferred. The most favored assays are so-called "homogeneous" assays that require only addition steps and lack exchange or separation steps. Most assays utilize either radioactive, absorbent (colored), fluorescent or luminescent reagents to determine the activity of the test compound in the assay. Optical detection methods for both biochemical and cell-based assays have improved in quality, sophistication and ease of use in recent years and have contributed greatly to advances in the field. Because of the importance of the assay in the screening process, competitive advantage may be afforded to those who are proficient in the design and implementation of screening assays. The reader is referred to reviews for more information (3,4).

Screening formats

HTS is usually carried out it multi-well plates and the industry has settled on certain standard formats. One key standard is that most screening assays are carried out in 96 (8×12) or 384 (16×24) well plates with a standard footprint. This standard is important because most automation is optimized for use with these plates and attendant assay volumes in the 100 microliter range. Furthermore, source plates containing test compound are typically stored in a similar configuration, allowing for more efficient transfer of test compound from the source plate to the assay plate. Various types of plates are available to match different assay formats, including opaque plates for scintillation counting and clear plates for absorbance or fluorescence assays. For cell-based assays, plates are available with special surface coatings or treatments to render them suitable for incubation of cells. The industry is experimenting with miniaturization beyond 384 (e.g. 864,1536 and 3456 well plates and assay volumes in the 1–10 microliter range). Although there are promising examples of success in this area, miniaturized formats are not in widespread use as of 2002. This is due in part to the fact that the higher density formats require novel instrumentation and automation processes, and represent a high barrier to entry. The industry is also experimenting with fundamentally different approaches such as flow-based, format-free, or panning methods. These methods face similar or greater barriers to entry as high-density plates. As technologies improve and costs decrease one would expect to see increased use of both high-density plate formats and, perhaps, completely novel HTS formats.

Compound Libraries

The quantity and quality of compound libraries are key considerations and drivers for HTS. The compound libraries of large pharmaceutical and screening companies can exceed 1 million samples, creating the need for significant infrastructure and technologies to complement HTS activities. There has been significant retrospective analysis of biological and chemical descriptors associated with "drug-likeness" (5,6) and many companies are attempting to fill chemical "space" with smaller, more precisely focused compound collections. Nevertheless, drug discovery is still an inexact science and screening libraries in most companies still contain at least 100,000 samples. Libraries are synthesized and stored as either individual samples or as combinations. Individual samples offer the advantage of generally being of higher purity and allow for more rapid follow-up. However, they are costly to generate and this method is not amenable to rapid exploratory chemistry. In the past decade parallel synthesis and other methods have led to the notion of "combinatorial" chemistry in which sets of compounds are generated simultaneously (7). These reactions generate

multiple variants on a chemical theme and these are often stored as mixtures to be tested. Because both methods offer some advantage, many screening libraries are composed of compounds generated by both methods. Historically, most compounds were synthesized in-house, making each library unique. More recently chemistry companies have begun commercializing libraries, so the prospect exists that many companies are screening similar, if not identical compounds against identical targets.

Automation and the Screening Process

With an assay and screening library in hand, automation and instrumentation complete the HTS process. An HTS lab typically consists of at least one automated system capable of moving plates from one task station to another. This is often accomplished by means of a robotic arm with sub-stations arranged in either a linear or radial fashion. A minimum suite of stations consists of an automated pipettor to add assay reagents or compounds, incubators (or racks) to store assay and/or compound plates, and a plate reader to detect the assay results. Additional stations may remove plate lids, change the orientation of plates or read barcodes to keep track of plates. The steps associated with different assays can vary significantly depending on whether compounds are pre-incubated and/or whether the read-out is end-point or kinetic. Because different assays require different processes and timings, the efficiency of the system is maximized by software.

Measuring HTS output: data quality and validated hits

If an assay has been properly designed and executed against an appropriate target and compound collection, the result should be quality data that identifies chemical starting points for further chemical optimization and drug development. Data quality (i.e. assay and screen performance) can be measured by objective statistical criteria based on assay statistical separation of positive and negative controls (8), but the quality and value of hits is less quantitative. Hits are scored and prioritized by biological and chemical criteria. Biological criteria include potency and selectivity against the target while chemical criteria take into account novelty, chemical properties, synthetic tractability and scientific intuition.

Conclusion

HTS is a relatively young field, with some of the earliest references dating to the early 1990s and its impact on the efficiency of the drug discovery has yet to be fully assessed (1). Like most new fields, the value of HTS to drug discovery is the subject of debate. Only time and disclosure by pharmaceutical companies of internal historical data will provide the metrics for long-term assessment of the method of broad screening activities. Indeed, one successful outcome of HTS would be if the generation of large data sets created a more rational basis for predicting which compounds will be appropriate for a given biological target. Thus, one role of HTS is to eventually limit the need for random screening of compound libraries. In an even broader sense, HTS has driven and will continue to influence thinking about the role of engineering and automation at the interface of chemistry and biology. One undisputed legacy of HTS will likely be an increase in the technological sophistication of discovery research.

References

1. Drews J (2000) Drug discovery: a historical perspective. Science 287:1960–1964
2. Mayer TU, Kapoor TM, Haggarty SJ, King RW, Schreiber SL, Mitchison TJ (1999) Small molecule inhibitor of mitotic spindle bipolarity identified in a phenotype-based screen. Science 286:971
3. Macarron R, Hertzberg RP. (2002) Design and implementation of high throughput screening assays. Methods Mol Biol. 190:1–29
4. Gonzalez JE and Negulescu PA (1998) Intracellular detection assays for high-throughput screening. Curr Op Biotech 9:624–631
5. Lipinski CA, Lombardo F, Dominy BW, Feeney PJ (2001) Experimental and computational approaches to estimate solubility and permeability in drug discovery and development settings. Adv Drug Deliv Rev 46(1–3):3–26
6. Walters WP, Murcko MA (2002) Prediction of drug-likeness Adv Drug Deliv Rev 54(3):255–271
7. Dolle RE (2002) Comprehensive survey of combinatirial library synthesis. J Comb Chem 4(5):369-418
8. Zhang JH, Chung TD, Oldenburg KR (1999) A simple Statistical Parameter for Use in Evaluation and Validation of High Throughput Screening Assays, J. Biomolecular Screening 4(2):67–73.

Hippocampus

The hippocampus, which got its name from the Greek word for seahorse, due to its form, is a nucleus in the depth of the ▸ temporal lobe. The hippocampus is important for the integration of sensory information, for spatial orientation and for memory formation. The hippocampal formation contains the 'CA' (cornu ammonis) regions, the dentate gyrus and the subiculum.

▸ Antiepileptic Drugs

Hirudin

Hirudin is a polypeptide derived from the saliva of the leech *Hirudo medicinalis* that binds to the blood serine proteinase, thrombin and thus blocks clot formation.

▸ Anticoagulants

Histamine

Histamine, a metabolite of the amino acid histidine, is stored in vesicles in mast cells and is rapidly released upon activation. By binding to its receptors, histamine causes symptoms of an allergy (rhinitis, itching, etc.).

▸ Histaminergic System

Histaminergic System

STEPHEN J HILL, JILLIAN G BAKER
University of Nottingham, Nottingham, UK
stephen.hill@nottingham.ac.uk,
jillian.baker@nottingham.ac.uk

Definition

Histamine is a biogenic amine that is widely distributed in the body and functions as a major mediator of inflammation and allergic reactions, as a physiological regulator of gastric acid secretion in the stomach, as a neurotransmitter in the central nervous system (CNS) and may also have a role in tissue growth and repair.

▶ Allergy

Basic Characteristics

Histamine is stored within granules of mast cells in almost all tissues of the body and has a major role as a local hormone (▶ autocoid) in the generation of allergic and inflammatory reactions. It is found in particularly high concentrations in mast cells in the lungs, skin and gastrointestinal tract and is also present in circulating basophils. ▶ Allergens and antigens bind to IgE antibodies on the surface of mast cells causing the IgE to crosslink. This conformational change stimulates the release of pre-stored histamine (degranulation) from mast cells. Direct interaction of components of the ▶ complement system (C3a and C5a) with specific cell surface receptors can also trigger mast cell degranulation. A number of clinically used drugs (e.g. morphine, tubocurarine) and neuropeptides (at high concentrations e.g. substance P) can also stimulate histamine release from mast cells directly via non-receptor mechanisms. In the gastric mucosa, histamine from stomach mast cells has an important physiological role in the secretion of gastric acid. Parasympathetic nerve stimulation (acetylcholine via the vagus) and gastrin release from G cells both activate gastric mast cells, releasing histamine. All three stimuli are able to act synergistically to activate the neighbouring parietal cells to produce more gastric acid.

Although mast cells and basophils probably account for >90% of stored histamine in the body, histamine is also present in platelets, enterochromaffin-like cells, endothelial cells and neurons. Histamine can act as a neurotransmitter in the brain. Histaminergic nerves have their cell bodies within a very small area of the brain (the magnocellular nuclei of the posterior hypothalamus) but have axons in most areas of the forebrain. There is also evidence for axons projecting into the spinal cord. Finally, there is evidence that histamine synthesis can be induced in tissues undergoing rapid tissue growth and repair. In certain neonatal tissues (e.g. liver), the rate of synthesis of this unstored diffusable histamine (termed nascent histamine) is profound and may point to a role for histamine is cell proliferation.

Histamine is synthesised from the amino-acid histidine via the action of the specific enzyme histidine decarboxylase and can be metabolised by histamine-N-methyl transferase or diamine oxidase. In its role as a neurotransmitter, the actions of histamine are terminated by metabolism rather than re-uptake into the pre-synaptic nerve terminals.

Receptors for Histamine

Histamine binds to and activates cell surface receptors. Four such receptors for histamine have now been identified so far (H_1, H_2, H_3, H_4) and their structural sequences determined following molecular cloning. All four are members of the G-protein-coupled receptor family and mediate their functional responses by activating specific ▶ heterotimeric G-proteins. H_1-receptors coupled to $G_{q/11}$-proteins and mediate responses primarily via the activation of phospholipase C, which hydrolyses membrane phospholipid phosphatidylinositol-4,5-bis phosphate into the intracellular second messengers inositol 1,4,5-tris phosphate (IP_3) and diacyglycerol. IP_3 is released into the cytosol and stimulates the release of Ca^{2+} ions from intracellular stores, while diacyglycerol remains within the plasma membrane and mediates responses via the activation of protein kinase C. Histamine H_2-receptors couple to G_S-proteins and stimulate the enzyme adenylyl cyclase, which is responsible for the synthesis of the second mes-

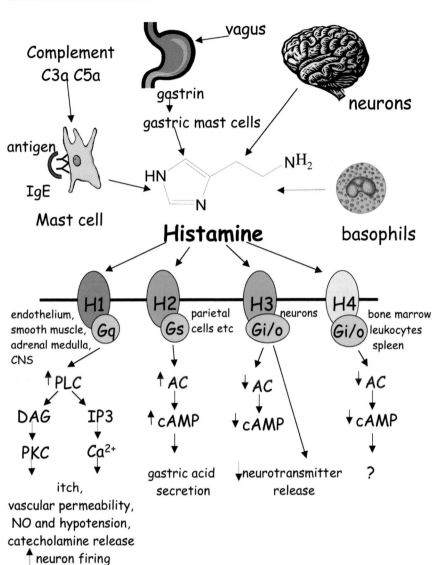

Fig. 1 Histaminergic System

senger cyclic AMP. In contrast, both the H_3- and H_4-receptors couple to the $G_{I/O}$-family of G-proteins that inhibit adenylyl cyclase activity and, in the case of the H_3-receptor, also inhibit neurotransmitter release in the central nervous system.

H_1-receptor. The human histamine H_1-receptor is a 487 amino acid protein that is widely distributed within the body. Histamine potently stimulates smooth muscle contraction via H_1-receptors in blood vessels, airways and in the gastrointestinal tract. In vascular endothelial cells, H_1-receptor activation increases vascular permeability and the synthesis and release of prostacyclin, platelet-acti-

vating factor, Von Willebrand factor and nitric oxide thus causing inflammation and the characteristic '▶ wheal' response observed in the skin. Circulating histamine in the bloodstream (from for example exposure to antigens or allergens) can, via the H_1-receptor, release sufficient nitric oxide from endothelial cells to cause a profound vasodilatation and drop in blood pressure (septic and anaphylactic shock). Activation of H_1-receptors in the adrenal medulla stimulates the release of the two catecholamines noradrenaline and adrenaline as well as enkephalins. In the heart, histamine produces negative inotropic effects via H_1-receptor stimulation, but these are normally

masked by the positive effects of H_2-receptor stimulation on heart rate and force of contraction. Histamine H_1-receptors are widely distributed in human brain and highest densities are found in neocortex, hippocampus, nucleus accumbens, thalamus and posterior hypothalamus, where they predominantly excite neuronal activity. Histamine H_1-receptor stimulation can also activate peripheral sensory nerve endings leading to itching and a surrounding vasodilatation ('▶ flare') due to an axonal reflex and the consequent release of peptide neurotransmitters from collateral nerve endings.

H_2-receptor. The histamine H_2-receptor (359 aminoacids) is best known for its effect on gastric acid secretion. Histamine H_2-receptor activation, in conjunction with gastrin and acetylcholine from the vagus, potently stimulates acid secretion from parietal cells. High concentrations of histamine are also present in cardiac tissues and can stimulate positive chronotropic and inotropic effects via H_2-receptor stimulation and activation of adenylyl cyclase. In smooth muscle, H_2-receptor stimulation leads to relaxation; this has been observed in airway, uterine and vascular smooth muscle. In the immune system, histamine H_2-receptors can inhibit a variety of functions. For example, H_2-receptors on lymphocytes can inhibit antibody synthesis, T-cell proliferation and cytokine production. In the CNS, H_2-receptor activation generally leads to inhibition of nerve cell activity, however in hippocampal neurones they produce a block of the long-lasting after-hyperpolarization and accommodation of firing, leading to potentiation of excitatory stimuli.

H_3- and H_4-receptors. The histamine H_3-receptor (445 aminocaids) was first identified as an ▶ autoreceptor, negatively regulating the synthesis and release of histamine from histaminergic neurons in the CNS. However, H_3-receptors have been identified on the terminals of many neurons in both the CNS, where they can inhibit the release of acetylcholine, serotonin, dopamine and noradrenaline, and on peripheral neurons where they inhibit the release of sympathetic neurotransmitters in human saphenous vein, heart, bronchi and trachea. Unlike the genes for H_1- and H_2-receptors, the H_3-gene contains ▶ introns (two

introns and three ▶ exons) thus, multiple H_3-receptor isoforms (▶ splice variants) can be produced from the single H_3-receptor gene. So far, several isoforms of the H_3-receptor have been detected in different species including six splice variants in the human CNS and in some of these cases, the subsequent signalling functions appear to be different. As several different H_3-splice variants exist with different signal transduction capabilities, this splicing mechanism offers a way for tightly regulating the biological actions of the H_3-receptor in different tissues. The H_3-receptor also appears to be expressed in a constitutively active form (▶ constitutive receptor activity) in the CNS providing a means for pharmacological intereference by ▶ inverse agonists as well as agonists and ▶ neutral antagonists.

The H_4-receptor (390 aminoacids) is the most recently identified and unlike the H_3-receptor appears to be exclusively expressed in the periphery. The H_4-receptor shows highest levels in bone marrow and leukocytes (mainly neutrophils and eosinophils), moderate levels in spleen and small intestine and has been detected on mast cells. It has a genomic structure consisting of two introns and three exons suggesting that splice variants may also occur.

Drugs

H_1-antagonists
A large number of histamine H_1-receptor antagonists drugs have been developed. These include mepyramine, chlorpheniramine, promethazine, triprolidine, diphenhydramine, cyclizine and cyproheptadine (although many of these are actually inverse agonists) and have proved to be very effective in the treatment of systemic and topical allergic and inflammatory disorders (hay fever, allergic rhinitis, insect bites, anaphylaxis etc). At therapeutic doses, many of the traditional antihistamines give rise to sedative effects because of blockade of the H_1-receptors in the brain. More recently, a second generation of H_1-antihistamines has been synthesised that have poor blood brain barrier penetration and therefore cause less central sedative effects. These include temelastine, acrivastine, astemizole, cetirizine and loratidine. Both chlorpheniramine and cetirizine exist as stereoisomers with markedly different affinities

for the human histamine H_1-receptor. In the case of cetirizine, the active levo-isomer is now available for clinical use. Many H_1-receptor antagonists also possess marked muscarinic receptor antagonist properties (e.g. promethazine, diphenhydramine, cyclizine) and this 'side effect' is exploited for the treatment of nausea and motion sickness. Several other classes of drugs, namely the antidepressants doxepin, amitriptyline and mianserin and the antipychotic drug chlorpromazine, are also potent H_1-antihistamines.

H_2-receptor Antagonists

The first H_2-antagonist that had selectivity for H_2- over H_1-receptors was burimamide. However, this compound is now known to be a more potent H_3-receptor antagonist. Cimetidine was developed directly from burimamide and proved to be an effective agent in the treatment of gastric and duodenal ulceration because of its ability to inhibit basal and gastrin-stimulated gastric acid secretion. A wide range of highly selective H_2-receptor antagonists are now available and are in regular clinical use including ranitidine, titotidine, nizatidine, famotidine and mifentidine. Most H_2-receptor antagonists penetrate poorly into the CNS, but zolantidine is an example of a selective brain-penetrating H_2-receptor antagonist. Studies in transfected cells overexpressing the H_2-receptor with constitutive receptor activity have shown that cimetidine and ranitidine are both inverse agonists at the H_2-receptors, while burimamide behaves as a neutral antagonist.

H_1- and H_2-receptor Agonists

Selective agonists, like selective antagonists, are useful for scientific characterization of receptors. Although not clinically used, a number of potent agonists are available that are able to selectively stimulate the histamine H_2-receptor. These include impromidine, arpromidine, sopromidine, dimaprit and amthamine. In the case of impromidine and apromidine, the compounds are 10–100 times more potent than histamine itself. However, whilst acting as agonists at the H_2-receptor, some of these compounds act as antagonists at other histamine receptors eg arpromidine is a potent H_1-receptor antagonist, and impromidine a potent H_3-receptor antagonist. Selective agonists for the H_1-

receptor (histaprodifen, N-methylhistaprodifen) have only become available recently.

Ligands for the Characterization of Histamine H_3- and H_4-receptors

Agonists with good selectivity for H_3-receptors (relative to H_1- and H_2-receptors) have been developed and these include R-α-methylhistamine, imetit and immepip. H_3-receptor antagonists include thioperamide, clobenpropit, iodoproxyfan, ciproxifan and impentamine and these all have substantially lower affinity for H_1- and H_2-receptors. The histamine H_4-receptor was discovered and cloned in 2000 and it is clear that there is considerable overlap in the pharmacology of the H_3- and H_4-receptors. High affinity H_3-agonists e.g. R-α-methylhistamine, imetit and immepip also have H_4-agonist properties although, their ▸ relative potency with respect to histamine is generally lower. For example, R-α-methylhistamine is several hundred-fold less effective as an H_4-receptor agonist than as a H_3-receptor agonist. The H_3-receptor antagonist clobenpropit also binds with high affinity to the H_4-receptor, but also possesses weak H_4-agonist activity. Thioperamide is an antagonist at both the H_3- and H_4-receptors but has 5–10 fold lower affinity for the H_4-receptor. Perhaps the most striking aspect of the pharmacology of the new H_4-receptor, however, is the fact that the atypical antipyschotic drug clozapine has agonist activity at the H_4-receptor but no agonist or antagonist activity at the H_3-receptor.

Drugs That Inhibit Histamine Synthesis, Metabolism and Release

Histamine synthesis from l-histidine can be selectively inhibited by α-fluoromethylhistidine. Metabolism by diamine oxidase is sensitive to aminoguanidine, while N-methylation of histamine by histamine methyltransferase can be inhibited by SKF 91488, tacrine and metoprine. Sodium cromoglicate and nedocromil are drugs that inhibit mediator release from mast cells (e.g. histamine) and are used in the prophylaxis of asthma (in children), allergic rhinitis and allergic conjunctivitis. Ketotifen is an H_1-receptor antagonist that has also been reported to inhibit mast cell degranulation.

References

1. Hill, S.J. (1990) Distribution, Properties and functional characteristics of three classes of histamine receptor. Pharmacol. Reviews 42:45–83
2. Hill, S.J., Ganellin, C.R., Timmerman, H., Schwartz, J.C., Shankley, N.P., Young, J.M., Schunack, W., Levi, R. & Haas, H.L. (1997) International Union of Pharmacology XIII Classification of histamine receptors. Pharmacol. Reviews 49:253–278
3. Hough, L.B. (2001) Genomics meets histamine receptors: New subtypes, new receptors. Molec. Pharmacol. 59:415–419
4. Schwartz, J.C., Arrang, J.M., Garbarg, M., Pollard, H & Ruat, M. (1991). Histaminergic transmission in the mammalian brain. Physiol. Rev. 71:1–51

Histone

A histone is a small, highly charged basic protein present in the eukaryotic nucleus, that helps to wrap up the genetic material into tightly packed chromosomes.

▶ Glucocorticoids

Histone Acetylation

The genetic material in the nucleus (genomic DNA) is highly organized. The organized structure (chromatin structure) regulates the transcriptional activity. DNA is wrapped around histone proteins forming so-called "nucleosomes". The post-translational modification of histone by methylation, phosphorylation or acetylation can alter the higher-order nucleosome structure. This regulated remodeling of the chromatin regulates the expression of genes. Aberrant transcription due to the altered expression or mutation of genes that encode enzymes, which are involved in histone-acetylation [histone acetyltransferases (HATs) and histone-deacetylases (HDACs)] or their binding partners, are key events in the onset and progression of cancer. Inhibitors of HDACs can reactivate gene expression and inhibit the growth and survival of tumor cells. Histone-deacetylase inhibitors are currently studied for their potential as new agents for the treatment of neoplastic diseases.

HIV

The human immunodeficiency virus (HIV) is the causative agent of the acquired immunodeficiency syndrome (AIDS). HIV is a retrovirus, whose replication includes the transcription of the single-stranded RNA genome into double stranded DNA (reverse transcription) and the covalent insertion of the DNA copy of the viral cDNA into the genome of the host cell (integration). Both steps are mediated by virus-encoded enzymes.

▶ Antiviral Drugs

HMG-CoA-reductase-inhibitors

ERIK BERG SCHMIDT, MOGENS LYTKEN LARSEN
Department of Preventive Cardiology, Aalborg Hospital, Denmark; Department of Cardiology, Aarhus University Hospital, Aarhus, Denmark
ebs@dadlnet.dk,
mogenslytkenlarsen@dadlnet.dk

Synonyms

Statins

Definition

A class of important pharmacological compounds that are the most effective drugs for lowering plasma levels of total cholesterol and in particular low-density-lipoprotein (LDL)-cholesterol.

Mechanism of Action

HMG-CoA-reductase-inhibitors (statins) inhibit the enzyme HMG-CoA-reductase that catalyzes the conversion of acetyl coenzyme A to meval-onate, which through several further biochemical steps is metabolized to cholesterol (Fig. 1). HMG-CoA-reductase is the rate-limiting enzyme for the endogenous formation of cholesterol in the human body, which takes place primarily in the liver. The reduced production of cholesterol leads to an increased formation (upregulation) of so-called ▶ LDL-receptors on the surface of hepatic cells that remove cholesterol from the circulating blood. By this the body ensures that its demand for cholesterol (cholesterol is a constituent of cell membranes, bile acids and various hormones) is met, and subsequently plasma cholesterol is low-ered. A second, although probably less important mechanism, by which statins reduce plasma cho-lesterol is by a reduction in hepatic synthesis of ▶ very-low-density-lipoprotein (VLDL) and LDL. Statins therefore markedly reduce plasma levels of ▶ atherogenic LDL-cholesterol and slightly reduce plasma ▶ triglycerides carried in VLDL's and in addition slightly increase plasma levels of antia-therogenic ▶ high-density-lipoprotein-choles-terol.

Furthermore, there is some evidence for pleio-trophic effects (for example effects on hemosta-sis, vascular function, antiinflammatory effects and stabilising effects on ▶ atherosclerotic plaques) of statins. The clinical relevance of this (and the potential difference between the various statins) is at present uncertain but subject to intense investigation.

Clinical Use

Statins are used to reduce plasma cholesterol in subjects believed to have too high levels of choles-terol in order to reduce their risk of cardiovascular and in particular coronary heart disease. They are used both in patients with established vascular disease and subjects considered at high risk for cardiovascular disease, including subjects with genetic disorders of lipid and lipoprotein metabo-lism. Statins are by far the most commonly used and the most effective class of drugs for pharma-cological lowering of plasma cholesterol. Statins were introduced as investigational drug com-pounds in the early 1980s and has been marketed since 1987.

Types of Statins

There are currently marketed three naturally derived statins (lovastatin, pravastatin and simv-astatin) and two synthetic statins (atorvastatin and fluvastatin). The structure of these statins is shown in Fig. 2. Other statins are in the process of being evaluated and will be launched within a short time.

Basic Pharmacology

The individual statins differ with respect to their pharmacological properties, but in general the clinical consequences of this are limited, but may occasionally be of importance with respect to side-effects and interactions with other pharmaceuti-cal drugs. Atorvastatin has the longest half-life and can be given at any time of the day, while the other statins are best administered in the evening (lovastatin with the evening meal), perhaps due to the fact that hepatic cholesterol biosynthesis is greatest during the night time. Despite this, all of the statins can be given in one daily dose. The stat-ins are mainly metabolized by the liver (approxi-mately 90%) apart from pravastatin, where 60% of the drug is excreted by the kidneys. Therapeuti-cally, much caution should be given if patients with liver or renal diseases are treated, and if stat-ins are used in such patients low doses should be administered under close control.

Statins should not be used in pregnant women. If women with child-bearing potential are treated with statins an efficient contraception should be secured. Statins should at present not be used in children unless they carry a very high risk of pre-mature vascular disease and in this case only by very experienced lipid specialists.

Effect on Plasma Lipids and Lipoproteins

Statins may reduce total cholesterol and LDL-cho-lesterol levels in plasma by 55%, reduce plasma triglycerides by up to 30% (best effect in individu-als with high triglycerides) and increase HDL-cho-lesterol by 5–10%. It should, however, be men-tioned that responsiveness to statins differ sub-stantially between individuals. The major effect of statins is to reduce the atherogenic LDL-choles-terol fraction and this effect is dose-dependent and typically increase by 6% for each doubling of the starting (lowest) approved dose of the drug. The effect on LDL-cholesterol vary between

H

Mechanism of Action of Statins Cholesterol Synthesis Pathway

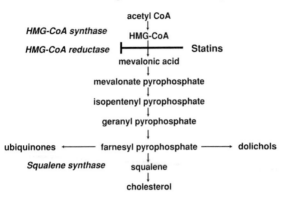

Fig. 1 Mechanism of Action of Statins – Cholesterol Synthesis Pathway. The conversion of acetyl Co-A to cholesterol in the liver. The step of cholesterol biosynthesis inhibited by HMG-CoA reductase inhibitors (statins) is shown.

preparations in maximal approved doses from 30% to 55% in the following order of efficacy: fluvastatin< pravastatin< lovastatin< simvastatin< atorvastatin. There is some evidence that atorvastatin may have the largest effect on triglycerides and that the best effect on HDL-cholesterol can be obtained by simvastatin.

The effect of statins on plasma lipids and lipoproteins is rapidly seen and fully achieved after 4–6 weeks of treatment. The effect persists unchanged during continued use for several years, but after stopping the drug, LDL-cholesterol rapidly increases to pretreatment levels. Treatment with statins is therefore usually continued indefinitely and not as a short-term cure. Finally, it is generally advisable to use the statins that have documented their efficacy in clinical trials (evidence based medicine).

Effect on Clinical Events

Five major well-conducted clinical trials have been published where subjects (4–10,000) have been treated with a statin or matching placebo for approximately 5 years: Three studies in patients with coronary heart disease (one study with simvastatin and two studies with pravastatin) and two studies in subjects without pre-existing heart dis-

ease (one study each with pravastatin and lovastatin, respectively). The results have been remarkably similar, with a reduction in deaths from vascular disease, heart attacks and the number of revascularisations (bypass surgery or baloon angioplasty) of roughly 30% in subjects given the statin compared to those receiving the placebo. The reduction in mortality from coronary heart disease has been achieved without any indication of adverse trends in non-coronary mortality. Moreover, the benefit has been observed in various age groups including old people, in both genders and in groups of patients with elevated plasma cholesterol as well as in patients with cholesterol values considered normal.

Side-Effects

Abdominal symptoms including changes in bowel function, rash and disturbances of sleep have been reported, but in general statins are remarkably free of side-effects. Thus, in the large clinical trials comprising several thousands of patients treated for approximately 5 years, side-effects and the rate of discontinuation due to suspected side-effects have been very similar in individuals receiving statins and placebo.

Two types of side-effects, however, need to be considered. Approximately 1% of subjects experience an increase in liver enzymes during statin treatment, and it is generally advised that a (repeatedly found) increase in liver enzymes to more than 2–3 times above normal levels should lead to discontinuation of the statin. This side-effect is asymptomatic to the patient, reversible and generally occurs shortly after institution of treatment and with high doses of the statin. Myositis which, during continued treatment may progress to ▶ rhabdomyolysis and acute renal failure, is a serious but very rare complication seen in less than 0.2% of patients. The risk of myositis is greatest when a statin is given together with certain other drugs including (but not exclusively) erythromycin (antibiotic), nicotinic acid and fibrates (other lipid-lowering drugs), ciclosporin (used in transplanted patients) and some drugs used for systemic treatment of fungal infections. A statin, cerivastatin, was recently (year 2001) withdrawn from the market due to an unacceptable high incidence of rhabdomyolysis, in particular when used in combination wirh gemfibrozil.

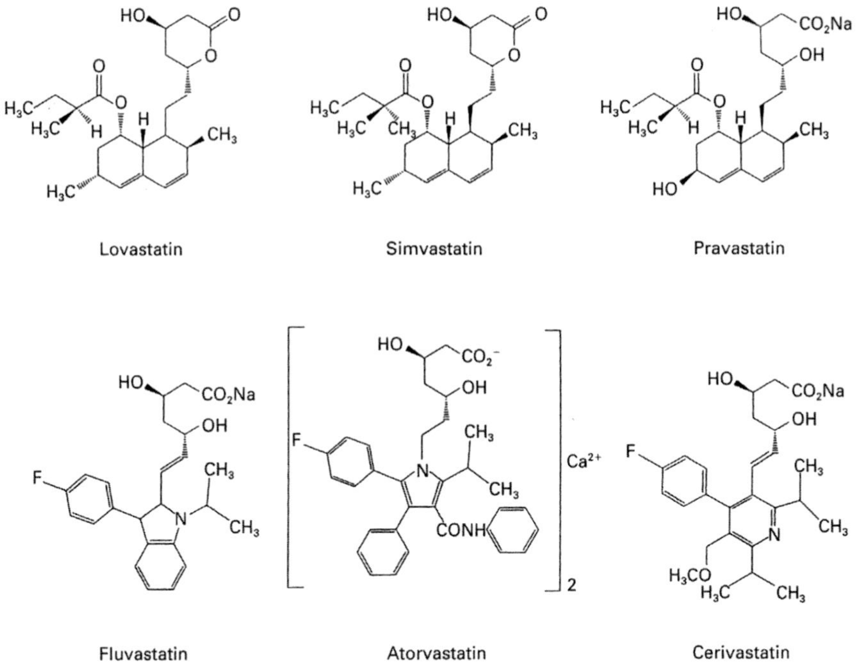

Lovastatin

Simvastatin

Pravastatin

Fluvastatin

Atorvastatin

Cerivastatin

H

Fig. 2 The chemical structure of the marketed HMG-CoA reductase inhibitors (statins) year 2001.

If side-effects occur on one statin a change to another statin may be tried under supervision, but commonly the same side-effect is encountered during treatment with the new statin. Statins (in particular simvastatin and lovastatin) that are metabolized via a hepatic enzyme system (C450) may interact with drugs metabolized by the same system (for example diltiazem and anticoagulant drugs) increasing plasma levels of the statin and/ or the simultanously used other drug. To date, however, few patient cases of clinically relevant drug interactions have been reported with the statins.

Treatment Control

The effect of a statin is usually determined by measuring fasting plasma lipids and lipoproteins after 4–6 weeks of treatment. Liver enzymes and eventually creatine kinase (in case of myositis liver enzymes are usually also elevated) are measured simultaneously to exclude side-effects related to liver and muscles. After the treatment goal has been reached, blood sampling is usually performed 2–3 times a year.

References

1. Law MR, Wald NJ, Thompson SG (1994) By how much and how quickly does reduction in serum cholesterol concentration lower risk of ischaemic heart disease. Br Med J 308:367–373
2. Wood D, de Backer G, Faergeman O, Graham I, Mancia G, Pyorala K (1998) Prevention of coronary heart disease in clinical practice. Eur Heart J 19:1434–1503
3. Knopp RH (1999) Drug treatment of lipid disorders. N Engl J Med 341:498–511
4. Vaughan CJ, Gotto AM, Basson CT (2000) The evolving role of statins in the management of atherosclerosis. J Am Coll Cardiol 35:1–10
5. Illingworth DR (2000) The management of hypercholesterolemia. Med Clin North Am 84:23–42

Homologous Desensitization

Homologous desensitization is a form of desensitization which is mediated by agonist-induced activation of the same receptor. G protein coupled receptor (GPCR) kinases (GRKs) and arrestins are involved in this process, which leads to an uncoupling of the receptor from its G protein.

► Desensitization

Homologous Proteins

Two proteins with related folds and related sequences are called homologous. Commonly, homologous proteins are further divided into orthologous and paralogous proteins. While orthologous proteins evolved from a common ancestral gene, paralogous proteins were created by gene duplication.

Homologous Recombination

Homologous recombination is a form of genetic alteration that occurs when DNA duplexes align at regions of sequence similarity and new DNA molecules are formed by the breakage and joining of homologous segments.

► Transgenic Animal Models

Homology

The similarity in base sequences of genes or amino acid sequences of proteins is called homology.

Hormone Replacement Therapy

Estrogens and progestins are diminished in menopausal or ovarectomized women. In hormone replacement therapy (HRT), these hormones are substituted to alleviate hot flushes, mood changes, sleep disorders and osteoporosis.

► Selective Sex-Steroid Receptor Modulators
► Sex Steroid Receptors

HPA Axis

► Hypothalamus-pituitary-adrenal Axis
► Glucocorticoids
► Gluco-/Mineralocorticoid Receptors

HRT

► Hormone Replacement Therapy
► Selective Sex-steroid Receptor Modulators
► Sex Steroid Receptors

HSP

► Heat Shock Protein
► Stress Proteins

Hsp70

Hsp70 is a molecular chaperone (relative molecular mass 70 kD) found in different compartments of eucaryotic cells. Hsp70 was originally described as heat shock protein 70.

► Stress Proteins
► Protein Trafficking and Quality Control

HSV (Herpes Simplex Virus)

Acute infection with Herpes simplex viruses (HSV) results in painful rashes on skin and mucous membranes. HSV-1 mainly causes cold sores around the mouth (herpes labialis) or eyes (keratitis), whereas infection by HSV-2 mostly results in sores in the genital or anal area. Less frequently, HSV also causes severe infections in newborns or a potentially fatal encephalitis. HSV remains latent and can be reactivated by stress, suppression of the immune system or other infections.

▶ Antiviral Drugs

Humanized Monoclonal Antibodies

TOM GELDART
Cancer Research UK Medical Oncology Unit,
Southampton General Hospital,
Southampton, UK
trg@soton.ac.uk

Definition

Monoclonal antibodies (mAb) are molecules that recognise and bind a specific foreign substance called an ▶ antigen. They are produced from a single clone of ▶ B lymphocytes. Conventionally, mouse mAbs have been generated for experimental and diagnostic use. Techniques have been developed to humanise mouse monoclonal antibodies to facilitate their therapeutic use in humans.

▶ Immune Defense

Mechanism of Action

Antibodies perform a key role in the vertebrate immune system recognising specific foreign antigens and directing a targeted, adaptive, immune response designed to protect the host from a wide variety of pathogens. Antibodies are also known as immunoglobulins. They are large, Y-shaped ▶ glycoproteins produced by specialised white blood cells known as B lymphocytes. Each B lymphocyte expresses immunoglobulin (mAb) on its cell surface where it acts as a receptor for one specific antigen. Following antigen recognition through surface immunoglobulin, B lymphocytes may differentiate and multiply into clones of antibody forming cells known as plasma cells. Plasma cells produce and secrete large quantities of antibody in soluble form. The antigen specificity is identical to the membrane-bound surface immunoglobulin receptor. Within the immune system, billions of antibodies with differing antigen specificities are produced. Individual B lymphocytes, however, may produce an antibody of a single specificity only. Antibodies produced from clones of an individual B lymphocyte will have identical antigen specificity and are known as monoclonal antibodies.

All antibodies possess the same basic Y-shaped structure comprised of two identical heavy and two identical light polypeptide chains linked together by a series of non-covalent and covalent disulphide bonds. Both light and heavy chains are folded into discrete regions called domains. Light chains exist in two different forms called κ and λ. Five distinct classes of antibody IgA, IgD, IgE, IgG and IgM are recognised in most vertebrates with antibody class being determined by heavy chain type, (α, δ, ϵ, γ or μ, respectively). Antibodies are bifunctional molecules: The arms at the top of the Y structure are primarily concerned with antigen binding and are known as Fab fragments. The amino acid sequences that make up part of each Fab fragment are characterised by sequence variability and are therefore referred to as variable regions. Within each variable region, three short polypeptide sequences show immense variability. These hypervariable regions together create the specific antigen binding site and as such are referred to as complementarity determining regions (CDRs). The intervening peptide fragments between the CDRs within the variable region act as a scaffold for the CDRs and are known as framework regions. The two Fab fragments are joined at an area of structural flexibility known as the hinge region. The remainder of the antibody molecule (the stem of the Y) is known as the Fc fragment and has a relatively constant structure. The Fc fragment is responsible for mediating immune effector functions such as complement activation or ▶ phagocyte binding following antigen recognition.

H

Antibodies are highly specific, binding only to a restricted part of a given antigen known as an epitope. Given the billions of antibody specificities that may be produced by the immune system, an antibody that recognises an epitope on virtually any molecule may be produced. It is this property that makes antibodies immensely powerful tools for experimental, diagnostic and therapeutic procedures.

In the laboratory, an antibody may be raised by injecting antigen into an animal and then collecting the resultant antibody rich serum. However, this antiserum will contain a variable, heterogeneous polyclonal mixture of antibodies produced by any number of different B lymphocytes that recognise a variety of epitopes present on the given antigen. In contrast, antibodies produced from identical copies or clones of a single B lymphocyte will have identical antigen epitope specificity and are known as monoclonal antibodies (mAbs). In 1975, Köhler and Milstein won the Nobel Prize for devising an experimental technique enabling stable and permanent production of mAb. Mice were injected with an antigen of interest thereby eliciting an antibody response. Antibody producing B lymphocytes (isolated from these animal's spleens) were then fused with cells previously derived from an immortal B lymphocyte tumour (myeloma). Hybrid cells (hybridomas) with the ability to make the specific antibody of interest and multiply indefinitely were then selected out, propagated and cloned, thereby providing a permanent and pure source of mAb from a single progenitor cell. Because mouse B lymphocytes are used to derive these hybridomas, the mAb produced by this system is of mouse origin (murine). Although murine mAbs have proven to be of immense importance in experimental and diagnostic techniques, their use in human therapy is problematic. Firstly, murine antibodies may be recognised by a patient's immune system as foreign, leading to the generation of a human anti-mouse antibody (HAMA) response. HAMA responses may adversely affect the clinical efficacy and half life of the antibody but also cause the clinical symptoms of ▶ serum sickness. Secondly, because the Fc fragment of the mAb is murine rather than human, it may fail to activate appropriate immune effector functions, and as such, prove ineffective.

It is clearly unacceptable to immunise humans to raise antibodies and technically it has proven difficult to produce fully human antibodies by cell fusion techniques. Therefore, in an attempt to overcome the HAMA response and improve the clinical efficacy of murine derived mAbs for therapy in humans, genetic engineering techniques have been developed to "humanize" murine antibodies. Chimeric antibodies with mouse variable regions and human constant regions may now be produced. This technique involves cloning the genes that encode for mouse antibody variable regions (specific to an antigen of interest) and inserting them into a vector along with the appropriate genes encoding for human immunoglobulin constant domains. This vector is then transfected into an appropriate cell line such as Chinese hamster ovary cells. These cells are then screened and cloned like conventional hybridomas. Colonies that secrete the resultant chimeric antibody can then be propagated, thereby providing a stable source of chimeric mAb. This humanization concept can be taken a step further to produce "CDR grafted" monoclonal antibodies. This approach requires the synthesis of a totally novel variable region using gene sequence information for the three epitope specific CDRs of interest from the variable regions of a mouse mAb, with compatible sequences from human variable framework regions. These humanized variable regions can then be linked to human constant region genes that, when expressed in an appropriate cell line, may produce an humanized mAb. In practice, the grafting of murine CDRs alone may result in some loss of antigen binding affinity, and a number of framework region amino acid residues may also need to be reintroduced alongside the CDRs to maintain antigen affinity. The result of both these approaches is to produce a mAb for human therapy that is specific to the antigen of interest, is less immunogenic, has a longer biological half-life and is more efficient at recruiting human Fc dependent immune effector functions.

An alternative technique for producing fully human monoclonal antibodies is the use of phage display libraries. Gene segments encoding for human variable domains of antibodies may be fused to genes that encode for ▶ bacteriophage coat proteins. Bacteria may then be infected with the bacteriophage and the resultant phage parti-

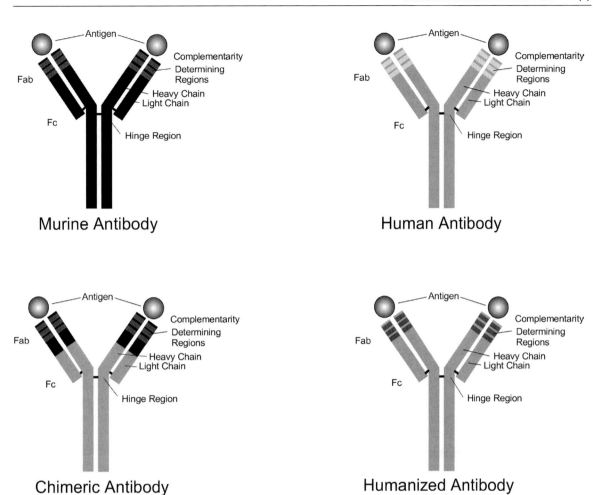

Fig. 1 Schematic representation of mouse, human, chimeric and humanized antibody.

cles that are produced will have coats that express the appropriate variable domain proteins. In this manner, phage display libraries may be built up consisting of a large collection of phages ($>10^{10}$), each expressing a different variable domain specific for a different antigen. Phage display libraries may then be challenged with an antigen of interest and phages that express appropriate antigen binding domains isolated and cloned. The gene encoding the variable region of interest may then be recovered from the isolated phage, joined to the remaining parts of an human immunoglobulin gene and transfected into an appropriate host cell capable of antibody secretion. The result is production of a fully monoclonal human antibody with appropriate antigen specificity. One final

approach to produce fully human monoclonal antibodies is to utilise transgenic animals. This technology requires deletion of an animals own immunoglobulin genes and the subsequent introduction of human immunoglobulin gene segments. Subsequent antigen immunisation then results in the generation of a fully human immunoglobulin.

Monoclonal antibodies are thought to exert their therapeutic effect through a variety of mechanisms: In the treatment of conditions such as cancer, mAbs may selectively bind to antigen on cells of interest, thereby targeting them for destruction through recruitment of the host's own immune system. Secondly, mAbs may act by blocking cellular communication, a mechanism thought to be important in the treatment of some autoimmune inflammatory conditions. At the molecular level, this effect might be achieved by binding and disabling cell surface receptors, or by binding and inactivating the signalling molecules themselves. Finally, mAbs may provide their own inhibitory or stimulatory signals on binding cell surface receptors, a mechanism also thought to be of importance in mAb cancer therapy.

Clinical Use (incl. side effects)

A number of chimerised or humanized mAbs have now been approved for therapeutic use in humans in the treatment of autoimmunity, malignancy, infection and cardiovascular disease. Some of the currently licensed mAbs will be discussed here. A much larger number of mAbs are currently being evaluated in Phase I, II and III trials. In general, chimeric or humanized mAbs are very well tolerated with few side effects. Chimeric or humanized mAbs still have the potential to evoke host immune response to the variable domains or CDRs of the antibody; so-called HACA (human anti chimeric antibody) or HAHA (human anti human antibody) responses, although these responses are uncommon. Short-lived and occasionally severe infusion-related acute hypersensitivity reactions such as fever, skin itching, shivering, respiratory compromise and low blood pressure sometimes occur. Such effects may be abrogated by slowing the infusion rate or by co-administration of antihistamines and steroids.

Infliximab, a chimeric mAb against tumour necrosis factor (TNF) α has proven beneficial in the treatment of inflammatory diseases such as Crohn's disease and rheumatoid arthritis. TNF is a ▶ cytokine with a broad spectrum of pro-inflammatory biological activities. Infliximab binds TNF thereby blocking its activity. Clinical trials have clearly demonstrated significant clinical efficacy compared to placebo or conventional therapy. TNF blockade by Infliximab has been associated with a number of specific side-effects, notably an increase in opportunistic infections and the development of other autoimmune syndromes. Delayed hypersensitivity manifested by joint and muscle aches, rash and facial swelling have been reported rarely in patients retreated with Infliximab after a considerable treatment-free interval. Basiliximab,

a chimeric mAb, and Daclizumab, a humanized IgG mAb, are two mAbs that are thought to exert at least some of their clinical effects through cell signal blockade. They are both licensed for the suppression of graft rejection following allogeneic organ transplantation. Both mAbs are specific for the interleukin-2 (IL-2) receptor (CD25) expressed on activated T lymphocytes, blocking IL2 receptor binding and its resultant T lymphocyte proliferative effect. Rituximab, another chimeric IgG monoclonal antibody, binds to CD20, a transmembrane protein present on normal and malignant B lymphocytes. It has proven efficacy in non-Hodgkin's lymphoma and has been shown to be effective both as a single agent and in combination with standard chemotherapy. Early clinical trials are also beginning to show impressive therapeutic activity in some autoimmune conditions. Rituximab probably works through a variety of mechanisms that include immune effector targeting and receptor signalling. Trastuzumab, a humanized IgG mAb directed against the extracellular domain of the HER2 (ErbB-2) epidermal growth factor, has proven efficacy in 25% of patients with metastatic breast cancer whose tumours overexpress the HER2 receptor. Its effect is likely to be mediated through a number of mechanisms that include signal blockade and immune effector recruitment. Again, the antibody is effective as a single agent and has been shown to provide significant additional benefit to cytotoxic chemotherapy. Of note, Trastuzumab, particularly in combination with certain chemotherapeutic agents, has been associated with longer term cardiac dysfunction. The basis for the observed cardiotoxicity is, as yet, not fully explained. Abciximab is the Fab fragment of a chimeric mAb against the platelet glycoprotein IIb/IIIa receptor. This receptor is involved in the final common pathway of platelet aggregation and thrombus formation, and Abciximab can successfully inhibit receptor function. Abciximab also binds to the vitronectin receptor found on platelets and endothelial cells inhibiting its pro-coagulant function. As an adjunct to aspirin and heparin, it has proven beneficial in the treatment of high risk patients undergoing percutaneous transluminal revascularisation procedures for coronary artery disease, reducing the need for subsequent revascularisation and the risk of myocardial infarction and death. Bleeding and a low platelet count are recognised complications of therapy. Finally, mAbs have been developed to treat infective diseases. One example, Palivizumab, is a humanized mAb directed against an epitope on the fusion glycoprotein of the respiratory syncitial virus (RSV). It has potent neutralising and fusion inhibitory activity against RSV. It is licensed for the prophylactic treatment of infants at high risk of infection with this virus and randomised trials have proven clinical benefit compared to placebo.

Monoclonal antibodies have revolutionised experimental and diagnostic laboratory techniques. The humanisation of murine monoclonal antibodies has allowed the development of a wide variety of generally safe, clinically useful, therapies. The humanization approach may well eventually be superseded by the production of fully human antibodies produced by phage display techniques or through the use of transgenic animals. Given the large number of mAbs currently undergoing pre-clinical development and being evaluated in clinical trials, the indications for mAb therapy are set to increase dramatically.

References

1. Kohler G, Milstein C (1975) Continuous cultures of fused cells secreting antibody of predefined specificity. Nature 256:495–497
2. Breedveld FC. (2000) Therapeutic monoclonal antibodies. Lancet 355:735–740
3. Glennie MJ, Johnson PWM (2000) Clinical trials of antibody therapy. Immunology today 21(8):403–410
4. Clark M (2000) Antibody humanization: a case of the "Emperor's new clothes"? Immunology today 21(8):397–402
5. Gavilondo J, Larrick J (2000) Antibody engineering at the millennium. Biotechniques 29(1):128–145

5-HT

5-HT is 5-Hydroxytryptamine (serotonin, enteramine).

▶ Serotoninergic System

Humoral Immunity

Humoral immunity depends on soluble, non-cellular effector mechanisms of the immune system. These include defensins and complement components (proteins of the innate immune system) and antibodies (products of the adaptive immune system). They are capable of reacting with foreign substances (e.g. bacteria and viruses) to produce detoxification and elimination.

▶ Immune Defense

Hybridization

Hybridization is the act of treating e.g. a DNA array with one or more labelled preparations under a specified set of conditions, in order to bind complementary pairs of DNA molecules.

Hydroxypyridones

▶ Antifungal Drugs

5-Hydroxytryptamine

▶ Serotonin
▶ Serotoninergic System

Hyoscine (scopolamine)

▶ Muscarinic Receptors

Hyperactivity Disorder

▶ Psychostimulants

Hyperaldosteronism

Hyperaldosteronism is a syndrome caused by excessive secretion of aldosterone. It is characterized by renal loss of potassium. Sodium reabsorption in the kidney is increased and accompanied by an increase in extracellular fluid. Clinically, an increased blood pressure (hypertension) is observed. Primary hyperaldosteronism is caused by aldosterone-producing, benign adrenal tumors (Conn's syndrome). Secondary hyperaldosteronism is caused by activation of the ▶ renin-angiotensin-aldosterone system. Various drugs, in particular ▶ diuretics, cause or exaggerate secondary aldosteronism.

Hyperalgesia

Increased responsiveness to noxious stimuli is termed hyperalgesia. It occurs following injury or disease and encompasses enhanced responses as well as reduced thresholds to a given noxious stimulus. "Primary" hyperalgesia occurs in the damaged area whereas 'secondary' hyperalgesia occurs in the area surrounding it.

▶ Nociception

Hypercholesterolaemia

▶ HMG-CoA-reductase Inhibitors

Hyperekplexia

Hyperekplexia (startle disease, stiff baby syndrome; OMIM databank: #138491) is a congenital human motor disorder that follows autosomal-recessive and dominant traits. Affected patients suffer from exaggerated startle responses to unexpected acoustic and tactile stimuli as well as episodic muscle stiffness. The startle response may trigger a sudden loss of postural control resulting in immediate and unprotected falling. In addition to profound startle responses, affected neonates exhibit a severe muscular hypertonia which may cause fatal apneic attacks. Muscle tone normalizes during infancy, while excessive startling persists throughout life. The clinical appearance varies considerably even within families with more than one afflicted member. A variety of mutant alleles of the glycine receptor subunit genes *GLRA1* and *GLRB* have been found to cause hyperekplexia. These mutations affect glycine receptor affinity and ion conductance, or represent null alleles.

▶ Glycine Receptors

Hyperglycaemia

▶ Diabetes Mellitus

Hyperkalaemia

Hyperkalemia is an excess of potassium in the blood. Clinical symptoms are muscle weakness and cardiac arrhythmias. It is caused by, e.g., ▶ hyperaldosteronism and angiotensin-converting enzyme (ACE) inhibitors.

▶ Renin-Angiotensin-Aldosterone System

Hyperlipidaemia/ Hyperlipoproteinaemia

▶ Dyslipidemia
▶ HMG-CoA-reductase-inhibitors

Hyperplasia

Hyperplasia is enlargement of an organ due to an increased number of cells.

Hyperpolarization-activated and Cyclic Nucleotide-gated (CNG) Channels

▶ Cyclic Nucleotide-Gated Channels

Hypersensitivity

Hypersensitivity (or allergy) describes an inappropriate immune response to foreign substances, allergens, giving rise to irritant or harmful reactions.

▶ Allergy

Hypertension

Hypertension is a chronic elevation of blood pressure which is a major modifiable risk factor for cardiovascular and renal disease. There is no specific level of blood pressure where clinical complications start to occur; thus the definition of hyper-

tension is arbitrary but needed in clinical practice for patient assessment and treatment. The diagnosis of hypertension in adults is made when the average of 2 or more diastolic blood pressure measurements on at least 2 separate visits is ≥90 mm Hg or when the average of multiple systolic blood pressure readings on 2 or more separate visits is consistently ≥140 mm Hg. Isolated systolic hypertension is defined as systolic blood pressure ≥ 140 mm Hg and diastolic blood pressure < 90 mm Hg. Essential, primary, or idiopathic hypertension is defined as high blood pressure in which causes of secondary hypertension or monogenic (mendelian) forms are not present. Essential hypertension accounts for 95% of all cases of hypertension. This condition is a heterogeneous disorder, with different patients having different causal factors that lead to high blood pressure and usually requires pharmacological treatment.

▶ Blood Pressure Control
▶ Antihypertensive Drugs

Hyperthyroidism

Hyperthyroidism (thyrotoxicosis), defined as excessive thyroid activity, causes a state of thyroid hormone excess (thyrotoxicosis) characterized by an increased metabolic rate, increase in body temperature, sweating, tachycardia, tremor, nervousness, increased appetite and loss of weight. Common causes of hyperthyroidism are toxic multinodular goiter, toxic adenoma or diffuse toxic goitre (▶ Graves' disease). ▶ Antithyroid drugs (methimazol, carbimazole, propylthiouracil) block thyroid hormone production and are hence suitable for the treatment of hyperthyroidism.

Hyperuricemia

Hyperuricemia is defined as serum uric acid concentration > 416 μmol/L or 7.0 mg/dL. With increasing serum uric acid concentration, the risk of acute gouty arthritis increases, but asympto-

H

matic hyperuricemia does not have to be treated pharmacologically.

▶ Anti-gout Drugs

Hypnotics

Hypnotics are a group of drugs, which facilitate the onset and maintenance of sleep.

▶ Benzodiazepines
▶ GABAergic System

Hypoaldosteronism

Hypoaldosteronism is defined as a deficiency of aldosterone. Renal secretion of potassium is decreased, causing ▶ hyperkalaemia. The treatment is replacement of a mineralocorticoid, e.g. fludrocortisone.

▶ Renin-Angiotensin-Aldosterone System

Hypocretin

▶ Orexins
▶ Appetite Control

Hypoglycaemia

Hypoglycaemia is a reduction of blood glucose concentration to below nomoglycaemia (euglycaemia). Severe hypoglycaemia will deprive the brain of adequate glucose (neuroglycopenia), which causes impaired neural function and can result in coma and death. Sulphonylureas, prandial insulin releasers and insulin can cause hypoglycaemia if administered in excess or if taken without appropriate food consumption.

▶ Oral Antidiabetic Drugs
▶ Insulin Receptor

Hypokalaemia

Hypokalaemia is a reduction of plasma potassium concentration below 3.5 mM. Hypokalaemia can result from a reduction in dietary K intake or from a shift of K into the intracellular space. The most common cause of hypokalaemia, however, is renal K loss.

▶ Hyperaldosteronism
▶ Diuretics

Hyposensitization

Hyposensitization is an empirically founded immunotherapy which is characterized by repeated exposure to the responsible (clearly defined) allergen. It can lead to a diminished Type I (IgE-dependent) allergic reaction.

▶ Allergy

Hypotension

Hypotension is defined as abnormally low blood pressure. In most cases, hypotension is adequately treated with general measures (e.g. physical exercise), drug treatment is rarely required. Drugs used for the treatment of hypotension include α-adrenoceptor agonists and compounds which activate both α and ß adrenoceptors.

Hypothalamus

The hypothalamus is a region of the brain which is critical for regulation of homeostatic processes such as feeding, thermoregulation, and reproduction. The hypothalamus senses neural, endocrine, and metabolic signals, integrates these inputs, and engages distinct effector pathways to exert its responses. The central role of the hypothalamus in appetite and satiety became obvious by lesion studies (▶ Appetite Control, ▶ Anti Obesity Drugs).

Hypothalamus-pituitary-adrenal Axis

The hypothalamus-pituitary-adrenal (HPA) axis is the regulatory circuit controlling glucocorticoid secretion and synthesis by the adrenal gland. In an endocrine cascade, corticotropin releasing hormone (CRH) in the hypothalamus stimulates adrenocorticotrope hormone (ACTH) production by the anterior pituitary, which then acts on the adrenal gland in order to release glucocorticoids. In a negative feedback loop, these hormones inhibit the HPA axis via binding to glucocorticoid receptors and mineralocorticoid receptors, thus ensuring homeostasis of glucocorticoid serum levels.

▶ Glucocorticoids
▶ Gluco-/Mineralocorticoid Receptors

Hypothyroidism

Decreased activity of the thyroid gland results in hypothyroidism and, in severe cases, myxoedema. It is often of immunological origin and the manifestations are low metabolic rate, slow speech, lethargy, bradycardia, increased sensitivity to cold, and mental impairment. Myxoedema includes a characteristic thickening of the skin. Therapy of thyroid tumours is another cause of hypothyroidism. Thyroid deficiency during development causes cretinism, characterized by retardation of growth and mental deficiency.

▶ Antithyroid Drugs

Hypoxia

Hypoxia is reduced or deficient oxygenation of the tissues by the blood.

I

IBS

▶ Irritable Bowel Syndrome (IBS)

IC$_{50}$ values

The IC50 value is that concentration of a drug that reduces the activity (or binding) of another drug to an enzyme by 50%. Under certain conditions it can used to express the affinity of the enzyme inhibitor.

▶ Drug Interactions
▶ Drug-Receptor Interaction

Idiosyncratic Reactions

An idiosyncratic reaction is a harmful, sometimes fatal reaction, that occurs in a small minority of individuals. The reaction may occur with low doses of drugs. Genetic factors may be responsible, e.g. glucose-6-phosphate dehydrogenase deficiency, although the cause is often poorly understood.

▶ Pharmacogenetics

IGF

▶ Insulin-like Growth Factor

IKr

Ikr is a rapidly activating component of the delayed rectifier K^+ current (IKr). Ikr stands for potassium (K) rectifier (r) current (I). Ikr is characterized by delayed activation and slow inactivation and contributes to the repolarization phase of the action potential.

▶ K^+ Channels
▶ Inward Rectifier K^+ Channels

Imidazoline Receptor

The imidazoline receptor is a hypothetical receptor for a subgroup of α_2 adrenergic agonists, which are characterized by their imidazoline structure (e.g. moxonidine). So far, there is no proof of the existence of imidazoline receptors.

▶ α-Adrenergic System

Immediate Early Genes

Immediate early genes, e.g., c-fos, c-jun, and c-myc, are the first genes whose expression is induced in cells after a growth stimulus. They encode transcription factors and induce the expression of other growth-related genes.

Immune Complexes

Immune complexes are aggregates of antibodies with their (foreign) antigens which physiologically initiate the clearance of the substance *via* ingestion and subsequent intracellular degradation by phagcoytic leukocytes. In type III allergic reactions immune complexes cause disease.

▶ Allergy

Immune Defense

MICHAEL U. MARTIN, KLAUS RESCH
Institute of Pharmacology, Hannover Medical School, Hannover, Germany
Martin.Michael@MH-Hannover.de,
Resch.Klaus@MH-Hannover.de

Synonyms

▶ Immunity

Definition

Immune defense is the ability of higher organisms to identify and combat potentially harmful microorganisms such as viruses, bacteria, fungi, protozoa and helminths by highly sophisticated mechanisms involving soluble factors (▶ Humoral Immunity) and immune competent cells (▶ Cellular Immunity). In humans two arms of the ▶ Immune System exist that comprise the innate immune response and the adaptive immune response. Mechanisms of immune defense are also utilized to identify and eliminate (neoplastic) tumor cells.

▶ Allergy
▶ Chemokine Receptors
▶ Cytokines
▶ Humanized Monoclonal Antibodies
▶ Immunosuppressive Agents
▶ Inflammation
▶ Interferons

Basic Characteristics

Acute Inflammation is the Immediate Response of Innate Immunity to Pathogens.

The task of ▶ innate immunity is to respond rapidly to challenges by pathogens by mounting an acute inflammatory response (▶ Inflammation) preferably at the site of infection in order to avoid a systemic spreading of pathogens (summarized in Fig. 1). Humoral components of innate immunity include the complement system, defensins, and antibacterial enzymes such as lysozyme. Cellular components of innate immunity comprise dendritic cells, monocytes/macrophages, mast cells, neutrophilic and eosinophilic granulocytes, basophils and natural killer cells. Tissue macrophages, dendritic cells and mast cells serve as sentinel cells at critical sites of pathogen entry such as skin and mucosa. They recognize structures from pathogens via pattern recognition receptors. Depending on the nature of the pathogen and its site of entry these sentinel cells release typical mediators including cytokines, chemokines, prostaglandins, leukotrienes, and in the case of mast cells, also histamine. Thus, dendritic cells and macrophages preferably recruit and activate neutrophilic granulocytes and mount an anti-bacterial response (left hand side of Fig. 1), whereas mast cells provide an environment enabling eosinophils to become activated with the aim to combat larger pathogens such as helminths (right hand side of Fig. 1). The activated infiltrating leukocytes support the resident phagocytic cells by effectively removing and/or killing the pathogens (neutrophilic granulocytes and monocytes/macrophages) or by killing (virus-) infected host cells (NK cells).

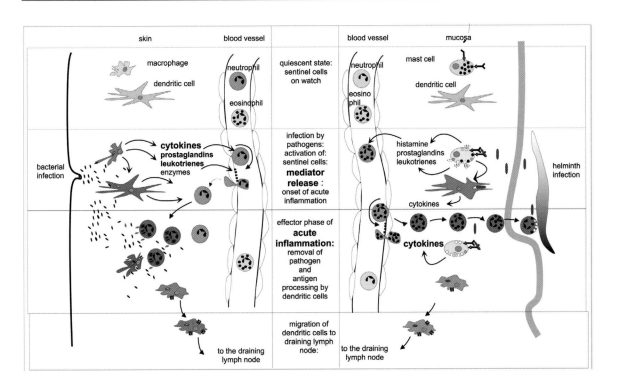

Fig. 1 Innate immune responses after challenge of skin or mucosa: Acute inflammation and priming of adaptive immunity.

In summary, critical steps in the activation of innate (and subsequently adaptive) immunity are the recognition of pathogens, the activation of sentinel cells and most importantly the synthesis and release of mediators such as cytokines. Inability to produce and release master cytokines largely abrogates immune defense mechanisms. It needs to be emphasized that innate and ▸ adaptive immunity closely interact and that the effector mechanisms of innate immunity are greatly enforced by products of lymphocytes, e.g. interferon-γ. On the other side, effectivity of complement factors is enhanced by the presence of antibodies, which are products of the adaptive immune system.

The Dendritic Cell is the Innate Link to Adaptive Immunity

Parallel to orchestrating acute inflammatory processes by providing an optimal milieu of cytokines, mediators and adhesion molecules in order to recruit and activate effector cells to the site of infection, dendritic cells also serve as professional antigen presenting cells (▸ Antigen Presentation, ▸ Antigen Receptors). After having ingested pathogens or pathogenic structures they move out of the (inflammed) tissue into the draining lymph node (bottom part of Fig. 1). During this migration they process antigens and present peptides from ingested particels on MHC class II molecules, which become upregulated.

Activation of the Adaptive Immune Response

In the specialized environment of the lymph nodes (or the spleen), dendritic cells provide the requirements for naive T lymphocytes to become activated and to proliferate. The professional antigen presenting cells present peptides in MHC II, they express ▸ co-stimulatory molecules, and release cytokines into the immunological synapse formed by the antigen presenting cell and the naive T-lymphocyte. Thus, cells of innate immunity initiate and facilitate the activation of naive lymphocytes, and it is easily conceivable that their repertoire of

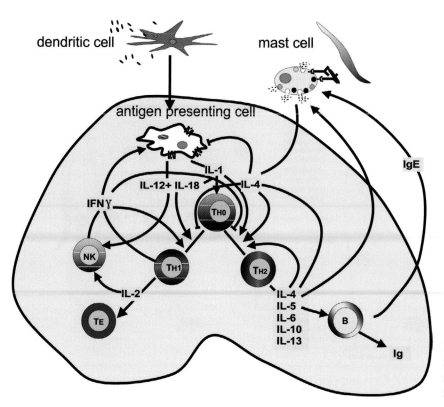

Fig. 2 Cytokines involved in the development of adaptive immune responses.

cytokines and adhesion molecules will instruct the naive T-lymphocyte during activation and differentiation to T-effector cells.

Cellular Components of Adaptive Immune Responses are T- and B-Lymphocytes whereas Humoral Components are Antibodies.

The hallmark of T- and B-lymphocytes is that each single lymphocyte expresses one specificity of antigen receptor that was created randomily during the development of only that lymphocyte. This is achieved by sequential genetic rearrangement of the gene segments coding for either the β- and α-chain of the T cell antigen receptor or the heavy and light chain of the surface immunoglobulin which serves as B cell antigen receptor. This process generates millions of individual mature naive T and B cells each carrying one type of antigen receptor with a single defined antigen specificity, thus creating a repertoire of millions of antigen specific lymphocytes. Upon encountering its specific antigen, one lymphocyte proliferates and expands to become an effector cell (▶ Clonal Selection). In strict contrast to T- and B- lym-

phocytes, cells of the innate immune system do not rearrange genes to create receptors recognizing pathogenic structures; innate immune receptors are always germ-line configurated.

T-Lymphocytes. This class of lymphocytes differentiates from immunologically incompetent stem cells of the bone marrow within the thymus – hence the name thymus-dependent (T-) lymphocytes. Two major subclasses develop simultaneously, T-helper lymphocytes (Th) and cytotoxic effector lymphocytes (Tc). The cytotoxic T-lymphocytes (carrying on the surface the differentiation marker CD8) destroy cells which carry their cognate antigen bound to MHC class I molecules on the surface by inducing apoptosis. Tc cells appear to have developed to cope with virus infections. As viruses can only replicate within cells, Tc eliminate them by destroying their "factories".

For an effective defense, antigen specific Tc have to proliferate, whereby up to a 10^7 fold increase in numbers may occur. This process is regulated by T helper lymphocytes, which recognize their specific antigen when it is presented on

MHC-class II molecules. A subpopulation, Th-1 cells, provides the central growth factor, interleukin-2 (IL-2). These cells also secrete interferon (IFN)γ, which represents the strongest activator of macrophages and thus recruits the innate immune system for adaptive immune responses, especially for the defense of bacteria or fungi.

A second population of Th-cells, Th-2, regulates B-cell responses (see below) by secreting a different set of cytokines including IL-4, IL-5, IL-6, IL-10, IL-13.

Th-1 and Th-2 cells develop during an immune response from a common ancestor, the Th-0 cells. Th-1 cells, once generated, promote their own differentiation and simultaneously block the development of Th-2 cells. Vice versa also Th-2 cells promote their own differentiation and inhibit that of their counterpart. In addition, Th-1 development is initiated by secretion of IL-12 and IL-18 from cells of the monocytic lineage, often stimulated by e.g. bacteria, and Th-2 by secretion of IL-4 from mast cells. Thus the balance between Th-1 and Th-2 cells is central for a physiological defense mechanism, which usually affects T- as well as B-cell responses (schematically depicted in Fig. 2). If it is skewed towards Th-1, chronic inflammatory situations may occur, if it is skewed towards Th-2, allergy can be the result.

B-lymphocytes. Also derived from the hemopoetic stem cells, B-lymphocytes differentiate in the bone marrow, which gave them the name. Upon binding of an antigen to its immunoglobulin receptor a B-cell starts to proliferate and differentiate into plasma cells synthesizing and secreting antigen-specific antibodies. Initially the high molecular weight IgM is secreted, upon continued or repeated antigen-binding the B-lymphocyte switches to other immunglobulin classes, IgG, IgA, or IgE, which preserve the original antigen specificity. These antibody classes fulfil different functions. IgM is very effective in activating complement that can kill bacteria and thus constitutes an early defense mechanisms against invading infectives. Because of its size, however, it does not penetrate into tissues. IgG, which is the most abundant immunoglobulin, can reach sites outside the circulation, it is less effective in complement activation, but additionally induces phagocytosis by interacting with immunglobulin Fc-receptors on

phagocytic cells. IgA is secreted into gut, mucosal membranes of the respiratory tract or tear ducts and constitutes an early barrier for invading infectives literally outside of the body. IgE has an important function in fighting infections that are too large to be ingested by cells, such as parasites. In highly industrialized countries, predominantly IgE is associated with allergy.

Effective antibody synthesis and switching from IgM to the other Ig-classes requires help by Th-cells, predominantly but not exclusive by Th-2 cells. The master cytokine responsible for a switch to IgE and thus development of an allergy is interleukin-4.

Drugs

Reasons to Intervene in Immune Defense Mechanisms
Immune defense mechanisms can become deleterious for an individual when they are not controlled properly. Then they can cause disease. In such situations therapy is aimed to dampen immune reactions. Important examples are septic shock, allergy, autoimmune diseases and chronic inflammatory diseases such as rheumatoid arthritis. Also, the success of organ transplantation depends on the inhibition of the immune response against the foreign organ.

But also several situations can be anticipated in which support of the immune system is required. These include congenital defects in the immune repertoire, acquired immune deficiencies, but also situations in which the immune system is compromised after treatment of patients, e.g. after radiation or chemotherapy.

Support of Immune Mechanisms

Vaccination. Probably the oldest and most efficient method of supporting immune defense mechanisms is vaccination. The principle is to induce an immune reaction towards a dead or denatured pathogen or parts of it in order to raise a high titre, high-affinity specific antibody response or to generate memory T effector cells. Upon re-exposure this will allow rapid and efficient clearance of the pathogen before it can cause harm. If such protective antibodies are generated by vaccination of the individual, one calls this active immunization. If the antibodies are raised

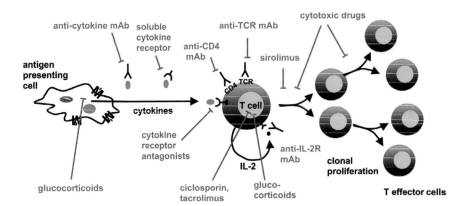

Fig. 3 Drugs involved in suppressing innate and adaptive immune response. Abbreviations: mAb: monoclonal antibody, TCR: T cell antigen receptor, IL-2 interleukin-2, R: receptor, CD: cluster of differentiation.

in other individuals or animals and injected into the recipient for immediate protection this is denominated passive immunization. Vaccination has proven to be an extremely powerful and successful tool to combat many viral infections, with increasing success also in bacterial infections.

Tumor Cell Vaccination. Tumor cells are recognized and killed by cytotoxic T cells. Unfortunately, frequently the cytotoxic response mounted against the tumor cells is not sufficient in patients to eliminate the tumor. The number and activation status of tumor-specific T cells can be increased by tumor cell vaccination. This technique uses dendritic cells derived from the patient that are loaded with tumor antigens by different methods. This results in the presentation of peptides of the tumor cells on the dendritic cell. These modified antigen-presenting cells are reintroduced into the tumor patient where they are capable of either mounting a non-existent anti-tumor response by T cells or by enhancing an existing but ineffcient T cell response to the tumor. This novel strategy is presently in an experimental stage with encouraging clinical results.

Use of Antibodies. Human immunoglobulin preparations from pools of a great number of people (>1000) with assumed antibodies against common viruses are used as a means of "passive immunization" in acute infections. More specific antibody preparations with high titers from patients who recovered recently from a viral disease or were immunized against toxins are also available in some countries. With the advent of monoclonal antibody technology a series of murine antibodies

were probed with respect to therapeutic intervention. To avoid rapid formation of human anti-mouse antibodies, often non-antigen binding parts of the antibody molecule are replaced by human homologues (humanized monoclonal antibodies). The use of therapeutic antibodies is rapidly increasing, including anti-tumor antibodies, antibodies that prevent blood clotting or inhibit immune reactions (see below).

Application of Recombinant Cytokines. Several cytokines are in clinical use that support immune responses, such as interleukin-2, interferons, colony stimulating factors etc. IL-2 supports the proliferation and effector function of T-lymphocytes in immune compromised patients such as after prolonged dialysis or HIV infection. Interferons support antiviral responses or antitumoral activites of phagoytes, NK cells and cytotixic T-lymphocytes. Colony stimulatory factors enforce the formation of mature blood cells from progenitor cells e.g. after chemo- or radiotherapy (G-CSF to generate neutrophils, TPO to generate platelets, EPO to generate erythrocytes).

Unspecific Stimulation of the Immune Response. Dead or live bacteria may be effective to stimulate inflammatory reactions of phagocytic cells against tumor cells. The best-characterized treatment is the use of Bacillus Calmette Guerin (BCG) in the case of bladder cancer where activation of the immune response is capable of controlling tumor growth.

Similar results may be obtained with muramyl dipetides and CpG oligonucleotides, most commonly used as adjuvants in the course of vaccination.

Inhibition of Immune Mechanisms. Two main strategies are presently used to suppress immune responses (summarized in Fig. 3). The first focuses on cytokines, the central mediators of the immune system. Effcient inhibition of cytokine production can be achieved by glucocorticoids. Specific anti-cytokine strategies include the use of monoclonal antibodies, soluble receptors or receptor constructs.

The second target is the T-lymphocyte as the central regulatory cell of specific or adaptive immunity. Inhibition of T cell activation can be achieved on different levels. Drugs like ciclosporin or tacrolimus (FK506) affect activation, whereas cytostatic drugs or sirolimus (rapamycin) inhibit proliferation. Specific elimination of T cells can be achieved by anti CD3 antibodies or anti CD4 antibodies, unspecific cell killing of proliferating T-cells by cytotoxic drugs. The aim is to impair immune reactions by removing the source of T-cell help (→ immunosuppression).

Glucocorticoids. At pharmacological concentrations glucocorticoids are the most efficient inhibitors of the synthesis of several cytokines, including those produced by T-lymphocytes, like IL-2, IL-4, or IFNγ, or by inflammatory cells e.g. IL-1, IL-6, IL-8, IL-12, IL-18, or TNFα (→ cytokines). The molecular mechanisms of the inhibition of cytokine protein synthesis – in contrast to their physiological action, i.e. the induction of metabolic enzymes (→ glucocorticoids) – is not completely understood. Contributing factors are the interaction of the cytosolic glucocorticoid receptors after they have bound glucocorticoids with transcription factors regulating cytokine synthesis, and thereby blocking their binding to DNA, as well as the induction of inhibitory proteins. Glucocorticoids are effective in severe forms of allergy, autoimmune diseases, and all forms of chronic inflammatory diseases.

Anti-cytokine Regimens (Treatments). In addition to inhibiting cytokine synthesis by glucocorticoids, cytokine effects can be prevented by scavenging the cytokine either with neutralizing antibodies or soluble receptors or by blocking the respective cytokine plasma membrane receptors with blocking antibodies or receptor antagonists.

Examples are:
▶ Anti-cytokine antibodies
Infliximab: Humanized monoclonal antibody against TNFα. Effective in the treatment of severe forms of rheumatoid arthritis where it can halt disease progression, or inflammatory bowel disease (IBD).
▶ Soluble receptor constructs
Etanercept: This genetically engineered drug consists of the extracellular part of the TNF receptor type I and the Fc portion of human IgG. Its application mirrors that of infliximab.
▶ Anti-cytokine receptor antibodies
Basiliximab, Dacluzimab: Both are humanized monoclonal antibodies against the IL-2 receptor that block T cell proliferation by inhibiting IL-2 and thus decrease the T-cell mediated frequency of rejection episodes in organ transplantation.

There are further anti-cytokine approaches that have shown to be effective in clinical trials, but are not yet approved. Those include IL-1 receptor antagonist, a naturally occurring complete antagonist (anakinra®) in chronic inflammatory diseases such as rheumatoid arthritis; IL-4 receptor antagonist, a mutated IL-4 (protein) with properties of a complete antagonist in bronchial asthma, Anti IgE monoclonal antibody which blocks IgE (→ allergy) in bronchial asthma, or other IgE dependent allergic diseases.

References

1. Janeway CA, Travers P, Walport M, Shlomchik M (2001) Immunobiology, 5th edition, Churchill Livingstone, St. Louis.
2. Abbas AK, Lichtmann AH, Pober JS (1997) Cellular and Molecular Immunology, 4th edition, W.B. Saunders Co, Philadelphia.
3. Gemsa D, Kalden JR, Resch K (1997) Immunologie, Georg Thieme Verlag Stuttgart.

Immune System

The immune system is a distinct organ in vertebrates, specialized to defend against invading infections or poisons in order to preserve the integrity of the organism. For this task it is disseminated throughout the body in primary and secondary lymphoid organs and the circulating blood. It contains the cells responsible for innate and adaptive immunity and humoral factors.

▶ Immune Defense

Immunity

Immunity is the innate or acquired ability of a higher organism to succesfully defend life against potentially harmful agents like infections or poisons.

▶ Immune Defense

Immunoglobulins (Immunoglobulin Superfamily)

▶ Immune System
▶ Antibodies
▶ Humanised Monoclonal Antibodies
▶ Allergy
▶ Table appendix: Adhesion Molecules

Immunomodulators

Immunomodulators are a group of mostly stimulatory effectors which act on cells of the immune system (e.g. cytokines, interferons).

▶ Cytokines
▶ Interferons

Immunophilin

Immunophilins are the intracellular binding proteins of several immunosuppressive drugs. Cyclosporin A exerts its action after binding to cyclophilin. Tacrolimus and sirolimus predominantly bind to the protein FKBP-12 (FK binding protein-12).

▶ Immunosuppressive Agents

Immunosuppressive Agents

VOLKHARD KAEVER, MARTA SZAMEL
Institute of Pharmacology, Medical School
Hannover, Hannover, Germany
kaever.volkhard@mh-hannover.de,
szamel.marta@mh-hannover.de

Synonyms

Immunosuppressants

Definition

Immunosuppressive agents (immunosuppressants) are drugs that attenuate immune reactions. An application is indicated in case our immune system reacts inadequately leading to serious diseases or normal immune reactions are unwanted e.g. following transplantations.

▶ Allergy
▶ Glucocorticoids
▶ Humanized Monoclonal Antibodies
▶ Immune Defense
▶ Inflammation

Mechanism of Action

Immunosuppressive drugs comprise a large spectrum of substances with different mechanisms of action where ▶ T-lymphocytes represent a major target (1,2). In general, immunosuppressants can be divided into those that

▶ inhibit T-lymphocyte proliferation in an unspecific manner
▶ decrease the pool of circulating lymphoytes
▶ more specifically attenuate the activation of T-lymphocytes and
▶ inhibit the interaction between antigen or antigen-presenting cells (APC) and T-lymphocytes.

Antiproliferative drugs

Cyclophosphamide. This drug belongs to the group of alkylating antineoplastic drugs. Alkylation finally results in covalent cross-linkage of DNA strands that interrupts the replication of all dividing cells including activated lymphocytes. Thus, both cellular and humoral immune reactions (antibody production) are inhibited.

Methotrexate including its polyglutamates. Metotrexate belongs to the class of antimetabolites. As a derivative of folic acid it inhibits the enzyme dihydrofolate reductase resulting in a decreased production of thymidine and purine bases. This interruption of the cellular metabolism and mitosis leads to cell death.

Inhibitors of de novo purine biosynthesis
Inosine monophosphate dehydrogenase (IMPDH) is a key enzyme of purine nucleotide biosynthesis. Purine synthesis in lymphocytes exclusively depends on the *de novo* synthesis, whereas other cells can generate purines via the so-called "salvage pathway". Therefore, IMPDH inhibitors preferentially suppress DNA synthesis in activated lymphocytes.

Azathioprine. *In vivo* azathioprine is rapidly converted into its active metabolite 6-mercaptopurine by the enzyme thiopurine methyltransfrase (TPMT). The active agent inhibits IMPDH function. Furthermore, it also acts as antimetabolite of the RNA and DNA synthesis particularly in T-lymphocytes leading to cell death. Due to genetic polymorphism of TPMT, therapy may fail, thus it is currently discussed whether individual patients should be monitored before use of azathioprine.

Mycophenolate mofetil. The active metabolite of this drug is mycophenolic acid (MPA), which inhibits IMPDH, too. MPA is metabolized *in vivo* by glucuronidation. It has to be noted that its acyl glucuronide inhibits IMPDH with similar potency compared to the parent compound.

Mizoribine. This immunosuppressive drug, which is only marketed in Japan, is a nucleoside analog. Its phosphorylated form, mizoribine-5-phosphate, is a potent inhibitor of IMPDH activity.

Inhibitors of the de novo pyrimidine biosynthesis

Leflunomide. The active metabolite of leflunomide, the ring-opened drug A771726, inhibits dihydroorotate dehydrogenase (DHOD) which is the key enzyme of the *de novo* pyrimidine synthesis. Inhibition of synthesis stops proliferation of activated lymphocytes.

Brequinar. This drug also inhibits DHOD activity but has not been approved yet.

Immunosuppressive drugs acting by lymphocyte depletion

Antilymphocyte globulin (ALG) and antithymocyte globulin (ATG). Both globulins exert their effect by depletion of circulating lymphocytes either by complement-dependent lysis or by phagocytosis after opsonization. However, ALG and ATG are non-human polyclonal antibodies. To prevent sensitization application is restricted to a time period of several days only.

Anti CD3 (muronomab-CD3). Muronomab CD3 is a murine monoclonal antibody directed against the CD3 complex of the T-lymphocyte antigen receptor. This drug selectively diminishes the T-lymphocyte pool resulting in a strong lymphopenia. Similar to other non-human antibodies the generation of human anti murine antibodies (HAMA) limits its long-term use.

I

Anti CD4 (OKT-4a). Murine monoclonal antibodies reacting with CD4, which is solely located on T-helper lymphocytes and monocytes/macrophages, may also be suited for immunosuppression.

Campath 1H (alemtuzumab). This is a humanized anti CD52 ► monoclonal antibody. At present it is in clinical use after bone marrow transplantation and for the treatment of refractory chronic lymphocytic leukemia.

Inhibitors of interleukin-2 induced T-lymphocyte proliferation

Anti interleukin-2 (IL-2) receptor (CD25) antibodies (basiliximab/ dacluzimab/ inolimomab). The chimeric human/murine (basiliximab and dacluzimab) or murine (inolimomab) monoclonal antibodies are specifically directed against a part (CD25) of the IL-2 receptor. Binding of one of these antibodies to CD25 thereby displaces physiological interleukin-2 and prevents proliferation of activated T-lymphocytes.

P70S6 kinase inhibitorsSirolimus (SRL). SRL (also termed rapamycin) is a macrolide lactone isolated from the ascomycete species *Streptomyces hygroscopicus*. After binding to its cytosolic receptor FKBP-12 the resulting complex inhibits the multifunctional serine-threonine kinase mTOR (mammalian target of rapamycin). Inhibition of mTOR prevents activation of the p70S6 kinase and successive G_1 to S phase cell-cycle transition. Transition is required for the onset of IL-2 induced T-cell proliferation. Additionally, SRL also attenuates growth factor induced proliferation of several non-immune cells and also inhibits metastatic tumor growth and angiogenesis.

Everolimus (RAD). This is the synthetic derivative (40-O-(2-hydroxyethyl)rapamycin) of sirolimus. Its molecular mode of action resembles that of SRL. It is still in clinical trials.

Inhibitors of IL-2 synthesis

► Glucocorticoids. After diffusion through the cell membrane, glucocorticoids bind to their specific receptor, which acts as hormone-dependent transcription factor. In the nucleus transcription of several genes is regulated after binding at specific glucocorticoid responsive elements of the DNA or by transactivation through interaction with other co-activators. In several cell types glucocorticoids induce transcription of the protein IκBα, which binds to the transcription factor NFκB thus preventing its activation and nuclear translocation. The important feature for the strong immunosuppressive action of glucocorticoids is inhibition of the synthesis of those cytokines that are involved in the activation of lymphocytes, i.e. interleukin-1 and -2. Therefore, especially cellular immune reactions are affected. In addition, a short-term reduction of circulating lymphocytes in the blood is observed after glucocorticoid treatment, due to a reversible sequestration in the bone marrow.

Calcineurin phosphatase inhibitors

Cyclosporine A (CsA). CsA is a water-insoluble cyclic peptide from a fungus composed of eleven amino acids. CsA binds to its cytosolic recector cyclophilin. The CsA/cyclophilin complex reduces the activity of the protein phosphatase calcineurin. Inhibition of this enzyme activity interrupts antigen receptor induced activation and translocation of the transcription factor ► NFAT to the nucleus which is essential for the induction of cytokine synthesis in T-lymphocytes.

Tacrolimus (TRL). TRL (in the past also named FK506) belongs to the group of macrolides and is produced by a special actinomycete species. TRL binds to its cytosolic receptor FKBP-12, however, it also blocks calcineurin activity and subsequently cytokine synthesis.

Pimecrolimus (ASM 981). ASM 981 is a ascomycin derivative that has been approved for topic application only.

Inhibitors of interaction between antigen or antigen-presenting cells (APC) and T-lymphocytes

15-Deoxy-sperguanilin (gusperimus). The exact molecular mode of action of this drug, which is so far only marketed in Japan, is not clear. Presumably, it interferes with antigen processing in antigen presenting cells.

CTLA4-Ig fusion protein. This is a immunoglobulin fusion protein with the cytotoxic lymphocyte antigen 4 (CTLA-4) receptor. By binding to CD80/86 on APCs it inhibits the CD28 costimulatory signal in lymphocytes. It is speculated that this can result in tolerance but up to now there is only experimental data (3).

Anti CD40 specific monoclonals. Such antibodies, which are still in an experimental status inhibit CD40 – CD40L (= CD154) interaction.

Vitamin D3 analogues. In addition to its classical role as regulator of calcium homeostasis, 1,25-dihydroxyvitamin D_3 (calcitriol) displays immunosuppressive properties. Inhibition of T-lymphocyte proliferation seems to be mediated via regulation of CD80/86 co-stimulatory molecule expression on antigen presenting cells. For clinical use as immunosuppressant, however, analogues of vitamin D_3 that do not influence calcium metabolism are needed.

Inhibitors of adhesion molecules and lymphocyte homing

CD2 antagonist (alefacept). Alefacept is a human recombinant integrin LFA3-IgG fusion protein that binds to the CD2 receptor thus blocking T-cell activation.

Anti CD11a antibody (antilfa). This is a murine anti-leukocyte functional antigen (LFA)-1α antibody that blocks LFA-1α (CD11a) - ICAM-1 (CD54) interaction.

Anti ICAM-1 antibody (enlimomab). This murine antibody also blocks LFA-1α - ICAM-1 interaction.

FTY720. This experimental drug is a derivative of myriocin. After phosphorylation FTY720 modulates chemotactic responses and lymphocyte trafficking, leading to reversible lymphocyte sequestration in secondary lymphoid tissues.

Clinical Use (incl. side effects)

Specific immunity is a highly sophisticated defense mechanism of higher organisms. A high level of specificity is given by immune responses directed against antigen epitopes of pathogenic microorganisms, foreign (transplant) or transformed cells (tumor) or even autologous cells (autoimmunity). Thus treatment with immunosuppressive agents is indicated for transplantations, systemic autoimmune diseases, chronic inflammatory diseases and certain types of allergic disease.

In any case, immunosuppressive therapy has to be carefully balanced in order to achieve a sufficient reduction of the unwantedimmune reactions and to avoid complete suppression of host defence that might result in bacterial, viral, fungal, and parasitary infections or increases in the incidence of various malignancies. Besides these unspecific adverse effects of all immunosuppressants drug-specific side effects, i.e. organ toxicity or metabolic alterations (hypertension, hyperglycaemia, hyperlipidaemia) are apparent (4). All antiproliferative immunosuppressive drugs can lead to hematologic disorders like leukopenia, thrombocytopenia, and anaemia indicating a continuous control of hematopoiesis.

Indications for the clinical use of immunosuppressive drugs are: transplantation, autoimmune diseases, chronic inflammatory diseases, allergic reactions.

Transplantation

The allogenic transplantation of solid organs, i.e. kidney, heart, liver, lung, small intestine, and pancreas, constitutes an absolute indication for a lifelong treatment with immunosuppressive agents. The major goal of the therapy is to prevent acute or chronic rejection of the donor organ. Patients transplanted with allogenic bone marrow have to be saved from non-desired immune reactions caused by transfered mature lymphocytes (graft-versus-host reaction).

Immunosuppressive therapy in allogenic transplantation consists of an induction phase (first four weeks) followed by the maintenance phase (normally lifelong). Because of the higher risk of acute organ rejection especially in the induction phase a combination of several immunosuppressants including antibodies with high dosages and blood target concentrations are utilized.

Treatment with specific antibodies (ALG, ATG, anti CD3, anti CD25) is indicated during the induction phase after transplantation and in the case of acute rejection for short time periods. Therapy with non-human antibodies may cause sensitization. Muromonab CD3 might initiate a cytokine release syndrome (fever, chills, headache).

During the maintenance phase dose reductions are aimed. However, in most cases a dual or triple combination therapy is still necessary. The use of drugs with different mechanisms of immunosuppressive action allow the application of lower doses additionally resulting in decreased toxicity.

Glucocorticoids belong to the oldest immunosuppressive agents given to transplant recipients and are part of most treatment regimens. However, due to their numerous side effects (see: glucocorticoids) particularly at high and continuous dosage, they are withdrawn or doses are largely reduced within months.

Current immunosuppressive regimens depend on a combination of a T-lymphocyte specific calcineurin phosphatase inhibitor (CsA or TRL) and a newer antiproliferative drug (MPA or SRL). Although CsA and TRL display a similar mechanism of action some differences in their side effect profiles are obvious. The most common unwanted effects of CsA comprise of nephrotoxicity, hepatotoxicity, neurotoxicity, hypertension, hyperlipidaemia, increased diabetogenic risk, hirsutism, and gingival hyperplasia. TRL appears equally nephrotoxic but hypertension and hyperlipidaemia occurs less ; hyperglycaemia is more frequent than after CsA treatment. Gingival hyperplasia is lacking but TRL may result in alopecia. In contrast, MPA and SRL are not nephrotoxic, however, myelosuppression is a common side effect of both drugs. The use of MPA is limited by dose-related gastrointestinal disorders. SRL, CsA, TRL and glucocorticoids induce hyperlipidaemic effects including increases in cholesterol as well as triglyceride serum levels that have to be treated with hydroxymethylglutaryl coenzym A (▶ HMG-CoA-reductase-inhibitors.

Most immunosuppressive drugs applied in the maintenance phase after transplantation are substrates of the efflux pump P-glycoprotein (MDR1)

and the cytochrome P450 3A4 (CYP3A4) metabolising enzyme system in the gastrointestinal tract and the liver. Both MDR1 and CYP 3A4 are focal points of numerous pharmacokinetic interactions. Thus, co-administered drugs can either induce (e.g. rifampicin, St John's wort) or inhibit (e.g. erythromycin, diltiazem, fluconazol) MDR1 and CYP3A4 expression or activity resulting in reduced or elevated blood concentrations of the immunosuppressants. For this reason it is also advised that the oral intake of CsA and SRL should be interrupted by a four hour interval.

Therapeutic Drug Monitoring (TDM)

Individualisation of treatment by TDM is indicated for most immunosuppressive agents exhibiting a narrow therapeutic index and broad interindividual pharmacokinetic variability. A careful monitoring of the respective target concentrations of MPA, CsA, TRL, SRL, and RAD can help to minimize their toxicity and to reduce the incidence of acute organ rejection. It is a matter of discussion whether trough or maximum blood levels should be determined in clinical practice (5).

Autoimmune diseases

Immunosuppressive agents are indicated for the therapy of systemic autoimmune diseases (e.g. systemic lupus erythematodes, myasthenia gravis) exhibiting severe organ-specific disorders which cannot be treated by other drugs. In general, immunosuppressive treatment of autoimmune disease is less successful as compared to organ transplantation, because of intra-individual variabilities.

Chronic inflammatory diseases

In the pathogenesis of many chronic inflammatory diseases (e.g. ▶ rheumatoid arthritis, glomerulonephritis, colitis ulcerosa, Morbus Crohn, atopic dermatitis, psoriasis) autoimmune processes play an important role, too. Although first of all nonsteroidal antiinflammatory agents or glucocorticoids should be applied, immunosuppressive agents may also be indicated.

Low-dose methotrexate is used for treatment of rheumatoid arthritis despite side effects such as disorders of the gastrointestinal tract and the liver. Leflunomide is also approved for this indication, however, hepatoxicity limits its use as first option.

For the topical treatment of some chronic inflammatory skin diseases (like atopic dermatitis) immunosuppressive macrolides (like TRL and pimecrolimus) that permeate the inflamed epidermis are of benefit for patients. Severe side effects comparable to those after systemic application of TRL in transplanted patients (see above) have not been observed so far. For the treatment of psoriasis vulgaris these drugs are less effective. The CD2 antagonist alefacept may be a suitable alternative.

Allergic reactions

Allergic reactions (especially those of type IV) can lead to disorders which resemble autoimmune or chronic inflammatory diseases. If an immediate elimination of the antigen is not feasible, immunosuppressive drugs can represent a reasonable addendum.

References

1. Allison AC (2000) Immunosuppressive drugs: the first 50 years and a glance forward. Immunopharmacology 47:63–83
2. Kilic M, Kahan BD (2000) New trends in immunosuppression. Drugs of Today 36:395–410
3. Goodnow CC (2001) Pathways for self-tolerance and the treatment of autoimmune diseases. Lancet 357:2115–2121
4. Paul LC (2001) Overview of side effects of immunosuppressive therapy. Transplantation Proceedings 33:2089–2091
5. Holt DW, Armstrong VW, Griesmacher A, Morris RG, Napoli KL, Shaw LM (2002) International federation of clinical chemistry/international association of therapeutic drug monitoring and clinical toxicology working group on immunosuppressive drug monitoring. Therapeutic Drug Monitoring 24:59–67

IMPDH

Inosine monophosphate dehydrogenase (IMPDH) is the key enzyme of purine nucleotide biosynthesis. Proliferation of activated lymphocytes depends on rapid *de novo* production of purine nucleotides for DNA synthesis.

▶ Immunosuppressive Agents

Importins

Importins are transport proteins at the nuclear pore complex, needed for the selective import of proteins into the nucleus. They recognize nuclear localization signal sequences of cargo proteins.

▶ Small GTPases

Inflammation

JOSEF PFEILSCHIFTER, ANDREA HUWILER
pharmazentrum frankfurt, Johann Wolfgang
Goethe-Universität Frankfurt am Main, Germany
pfeilschifter@em.uni-frankfurt.de,
huwiler@em.uni-frankfurt.de

Definition

Inflammation occurs when a living tissue is injured or infected by microorganisms. It is a beneficial, self limited response that requires phagocytic cells and elements of circulating plasma to enter the affected area. In principle it may achieve resolution and repair as the ideal outcome of inflammation. The persistent accumulation and activation of leukocytes is a hallmark of chronic inflammation.

▶ Allergy
▶ Glucocorticoids
▶ Immune Defense
▶ Immunosuppressive Agents
▶ Non-steroidal Anti-inflammatory Drugs

Basic Mechanisms

Introduction

The clinical characteristics of acute inflammation are familiar to anyone who has suffered from a burned or infected finger. The account comprises the cardinal symptoms of inflammation with heat, redness and painful swelling that were reported by the Roman encyclopedist Celsus as calor, rubor, tumor and dolor. Galen of Pergamon added a further sign of inflammation, the impaired function or functio laesa. Though unpleasant these signs are indicators of useful processes going on with the aim for limiting tissue damage and infection and initiating repair. Inflammation starts after an initial injury by mechanical trauma, infections, UV-irradiation, burns, ischemia and many others. It initially comprises the release of chemical mediators like histamine from a population of cells that are distributed throughout the connective tissue and are extremely sensitive to injury, the mast cells. The same is true for the blood basophil, which in many aspects resembles the mast cell. Histamine and secondary mediators like eicosanoids and nitric oxide cause vasodilatation and increase the calibre of arterioles, capillaries and venules, which results in increased blood flow to the injured area and consequently redness and heat. An increase in the vascular permeability causes the loss of solutes and proteins from the blood plasma, a process called exsudation, which leads to swelling and oedema formation (tumor). The local increase in tissue turgor and the activation of the kinin cascade with the generation of particularly bradykinin are major factors causing pain, the fourth cardinal symptom of inflammation. Besides these changes of the microcirculation the acute inflammatory response essentially requires the extravasation of leukocytes and phagocytosis of microorganism and cell or tissue debris.

Cells and Mediators of Acute Inflammation

The migration of phagocytic cells to the site of damage is one of the most fundamental components of the acute inflammatory response, and the key players in this process will be presented next.

The Endothelial Cell. The vascular endothelium plays an important role in regulation of vascular tone and permeability. Dilatation of arterioles to increase blood flow and constriction of endothelial cells of postcapillary venules causing exsudation of plasma constituents illustrates the complex nature of this cell type. Moreover, by expression of adhesion moledules and secretion of

▶ chemokines endothelial cells play an important role in the recruitment of leukocytes to the inflamed area. Endothelial cells express two basic types of adhesion molecules on their surface:
a) ▶ Selectins (E-Selectin, P-Selectin)
b) Members of the immunglobulin gene superfamily (VCAM-1, ICAM-1, ICAM-2)

Selectins are a family of glycoproteins that allow the initial attachment and rolling of leukocytes on endothelial cells. Selectins are not expressed on the surface of resting endothelial cells but are exposed upon activation with a number of mediators like ▶ interleukin 1 (IL-1), tumor necrosis factor α (▶ TNFα), lipopolysaccharide or thrombin. Two endothelial selectins have been reported. E-selectin is synthesized *de novo* and expressed on endothelial cell surface following stimulation. The specific ligand for E-selectin is stored in Weibel-Palade bodies of endothelial cells and in α-granules of platelets and is translocated within minutes to the plasma membrane following exposure to inflammatory mediators. The ligand for P-selectin is the so-called P-selectin glycoprotein ligand 1 (PSGL-1), which has the sugar lacto-n-fucopentose III in its core domain and is present on hematopoietic cells.

The second class of adhesion molecules expressed on endothelial cells belong to the immunglobulin gene superfamily. These transmembrane glycoproteins structurally resemble in certain parts the structure of immunglobulins. Whereas intercellular cell adhesion molucule 1 (ICAM-1) and ICAM-2 are constitutively expressed on endothelial cells, the third member vascular cell adhesion molecule 1 (VCAM-1) is not present on resting endothelial cells but is upregulated together with ICAM-1 in the course of acute inflammation by cytokines like IL-1 or TNFα within a few hours. The counterreceptor on the cell membrane of leukocytes that binds to ICAMs and VCAM-1 belong to the ▶ integrin family of adhesion molecules.

The Neutrophil. In the very early phases of the acute inflammatory response most of the cells invading the damaged area are polymorphonuclear neutrophils, also denoted as PMNs, which serve as initial line of defense and source of proinflammatory cytokines. These cells, which usually live for 4–5 days, circulate in the blood until they

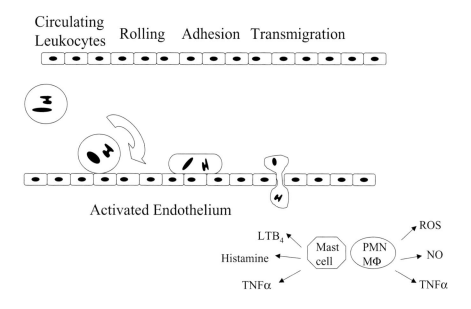

Fig. 1 Sequence of events in the recruitment of leukocytes in postcapillary venules adjacent to injured tissue.
At the site of lesion, diverse reactive substances stimulate the endothelium to produce inflammatory cytokines, chemoattractants and other inflammatory mediators. The cytokine-activated endothelium expresses adhesion molecules that lead to the low affinity interactions between leukocytes and endothelium, which is mediated by selectins and described as rolling. Subsequently integrins mediate the firm adhesion of leukocytes, which allows emigration of the cells from venules into the interstitial compartment. Activated mast cells, PMNs and macrophages secrete cytokines (TNFα), lipid mediators (LTB$_4$) and other inflammatory players (histamine, NO).

are attracted by ▶ chemokines into injured tissues. Whereas physical injury does not recruit many neutrophils, infections with bacteria or fungi elicit a striking neutrophil response. The characteristic pus of a bacterial abscess is composed mainly of ▶ apoptotic and necrotic PMNs. Emigration of neutrophils from the blood starts with a process denoted as margination where neutrophils come to lie at the periphery of flowing blood cells and adhere to endothelial cells (Fig. 1). L-Selectin is expressed constitutively on most leukocytes and interacts with ligands that are induced in endothelial cells exposed to inflammatory cytokines. The second class of surface molecules that mediate adhesion of neutrophils and monocytes to endothelial cells are the integrins. Leukocyte integrins are heterodimeric transmembrane proteins consisting of α and β chains with short cytoplasmic domains that are engaged in signal transduction. Many cells express integrins, and some of the known integrins are cell-type specific. Integrins mediate firm adhesion that follows the initial rolling of leukocytes along the endothelial cell lining. All the leukocyte integrins share a common small subunit, the β$_2$ subunit. There are at least four larger α subunits known that can associate with the β$_2$ subunit to form unique receptors. It is these β$_2$-integrins that adhere to the endothelial ICAMs in the course of acute inflammation. Once the neutrophils have made firm contact to the endothelial cells they protrude pseudopodia and leave the blood vessel by squeezing through the gap between adjacent endothelial cells and subsequently pass the basement membrane (Fig. 1). The whole process takes a few minutes.

The Monocyte/Macrophage. The very early peak of neutrophil invasion into an inflamed area is followed several hours later by a wave of a second class of phagocytic cells, the macrophages. This biphasic pattern of inflammatory cell movement and accumulation is observed in most acute

Tab. 1 Endogenously produced mediators of inflammation.

Category	Mediators
preformed mediators released from activated cells	histamine serotonin lysosomal enzymes
mediators derived from activated plasma protein cascades	complement system kinin cascade clotting pathway fibrinolytic system
de novo synthesized mediators	prostaglandins leukotrienes cytokines reactive oxygen species nitric oxide

inflammatory responses. The mononuclear phagocyte in the blood is known as the monocyte and differentiates into the macrophage upon entering into tissues. The differentiation process markedly increases the phagocytic and secretory capacities of the cell. Chemotactic factors that act on macrophages include complement cleavage products, membrane components of microorganisms and fibrin degradation products that also attract neutrophils. In addition, there are specific chemokines that act exclusively on macrophages. Macrophages in turn release large amounts of growth factors and cytokines.

Mediators of Inflammation. Many low weight compounds produced by microorganism-like formylated peptides as well as endogenous mediators are chemotactic for leukocytes and promote the inflammatory process. The main endogenous compounds are listed in Table 1 and are derived from activated plasma protein cascades that function as amplification mechanisms, are performed and released from activated cells or are *de novo* synthesized on demand by cells participating in or being affected by inflammatory events. The major modulators of leukocyte adhesion to endothelial cells are listed in Table 2.

Healing

The objectives of the inflammatory response can be viewed as a hierarchical ordered panel of events. The most successful consequence of an inflammatory response is the complete restoration of function and structure of the affected tissue, also denoted as resolution. If this is not possible, inflammation aims for healing by repair and replacement of lost tissue by scar tissue.

Central to resolution is the cessation of initiating stimuli, e.g. the killing of invading bacteria and microorganisms, and the complete removal of inflammatory exudate. Whereas neutrophils carry out the killing of invading microorganisms that subsequently die by apoptosis, macrophages are mainly responsible for clearing dead neutrophils and fluid phase debris by phagocytosis and extremely active pinocytosis. It should be emphasized that the clearing of apoptotic cells by phagocytes is extremely fast and efficient, and dying cells release chemokines to speed up their removal by attracting macrophages. Moreover, cytokines like interleukin 6 and antiinflammatory lipid mediators such as lipoxins or prostaglandines D_2 and E_2 play important roles in providing stop signals for acute inflammatory processes. Most macrophages emigrate from the inflamed site to reach draining lymph nodes. Subsequently tissue that has been lost must be replaced in an orderly fashion. The replacement of lost cells by compensatory proliferation and phenotypic change of surviving resident cells is part of the healing process. If the removal of inflammatory exudate fails, a process denoted as organization is triggered. The exsudate is invaded by macrophages and fibroblasts and the formation of new blood vessels (angiogenesis) is initiated. This series of events finally results in the formation of tissue scar, which may be considered as an essential component of wound healing not only in skin.

Chronic Inflammation

If the endogenous control mechanisms of inflammation fail and resolution or healing by repair cannot be achieved, the inflammatory process may persist for weeks, months or even years and is termed chronic. The inflammatory macrophage is not only a ringmaster for safe resolution and repair of inflammation but also for chronicity of the disease. Some of the products secreted by macrophages are relevant to chronic inflammation such as IL-1, TNFα, IL-6 or IL-10, just to name a few. A further characteristic feature is the presence

Tab. 2 Modulation of leukocyte adhesion to endothelial cells.

Target cell	Endothelial cell	Leukocyte
Anti-adhesive	Interleukin 4	Interleukin 4
	Interleukin 10	Interleukin 10
	Interleukin 13	Interleukin 13 Prostacyclin
	Adenosine	Adenosine
	Nitric oxide (NO) Glucocorticoids	Nitric oxide (NO)
Pro–adhesive	TNFα	TNFα
	IL-1	IL-1
	Interferon γ	Interferon γ Interleukin 8 MCP-1
	Leukotrien B_4	Leukotrien B_4
	PAF	PAF
	Endotoxin	Endotoxin C3b, C5a
	Histamine	Neuropeptides

of activated B and T lymphocytes, which represent a local immune response to antigens presented to them by macrophages or dendritic cells. B cells differentiate upon activation to plasma cells that release immunglobulins which in most cases is a good indicator of chronicity of inflammation. Further attempts to repair are clearly unsuccessful and tissue necrosis and inflammation continue as is the case in chronic ulcerative colitis or chronic pyelonephritis and other diseases. The mechanisms by which the inflammatory response resolves is under intense investigations and may provide new targets in the treatment of chronic inflammation.

References

1. Ley K (ed) (2001) Physiology of inflammation. Oxford University Press, Oxford, 1–546
2. Sherlian CN, Ward PA (eds) (1999) Molecular and Cellular Basis of Inflammation, Humana Press, Totowa New Jersey, 1–338
3. Woolf N (ed) (1998) Pathology, Basic and Systemic. WB Saunders Company Ltd., London, 35–91

Inflammatory Disorders

Inflammatory disorders are due to hyperactivity of leukocytes and over-expression of their associated integrins, cytokines, and chemokines, which leads to various disorders including arthritis, bowel diseases and other chronic inflammations.

▶ Inflammation

Influenza

Influenza is an acute viral disease caused by Influenza A (sporadic, epidemic and pandemic) or B (sporadic outbreaks) virus. Symptoms typically occur suddenly and include high fever, chills, headache, muscle aches, sore throat and malaise. Serious complications can be caused by bacterial superinfection of the respiratory tract.

▶ Antiviral Drugs

Infrared Spectroscopy

Infrared spectroscopy is an analytical technique which differentiates molecules on the basis of their vibrational states.

Innate Immunity

Innate immunity describes inborn effector mechanisms defending the organism against harmful foreign substances by humoral (defensins, complement) or cellular (phagocytic cells, natural killer cells) mechanisms. In innate immunnity, recognition of foreign substances is always by receptors such as pattern recognition receptors, which are germ-line configured and not rearranged like the T- and B-cell antigen receptors. From a phylogenetical point of view, the innate defense system developed much earlier than the adaptive immune system of lymphocytes; the innate system is found in many invertebrates.

▶ Immune Defense

Inorganic Phosphate Transporters

Type 1 Na^+-dependent inorganic phosphate transporters are a family of proteins isolated in a screen for genes that increase Na^+-dependent inorganic phosphate transport. Further characterization with heterologous expression of the rat kidney NaPi-1 isoform in particular, demonstrated that phosphate transport did not correlate with the level of messenger RNA (mRNA) expressed. However, expression did correlate with the saturable transport of inorganic anions such as penicillin

and probenecid. It has also been shown that NaPi-1 mediates an anion conductance that can be blocked by transport substrates. Sialin, VGLUT1 and VGLUT2 are closely related to the type INa^+-dependent inorganic phosphate transporters.

▶ Vesicular Transporters

Inositol

D-*myo*-inositol is a six carbon polyalcohol in a ring structure arranged in a chair configuration.

▶ Phospholipid Kinases

Inositol Trisphosphate

Inositol triphosphate is inositol that is phosphorylated at positions 1, 4 and 5. It is a product of the hydrolysis of phosphatidylinositol bisphosphate by phospholipase C and releases Ca^{2+} ions from stores in the endoplasmic reticulum.

▶ Phospholipases

INR

▶ International Normalized Ratio
▶ Anticoagulants

Insulin

▶ Diabetes Mellitus
▶ Insulin Receptor

Insulin-like Growth Factor

Insulin-like growth factor IGF1 (also called somatomedin C) and IGF2 are ubiquitously expressed peptides with sequence homology to insulin. Both factors bind to specific receptors. The IGF1 receptor is a receptor tyrosine kinase with similar structure ($\alpha_2\beta_2$) and molecular function to the insulin receptor (INSR). The receptor for IGF2 lacks a tyrosine kinase activity and is identical with the mannose-6-phosphate receptor. IGF1 also binds to the INSR, although with much lower affinity; IGF2 binds to the IGF1 receptor with high affinity.

▶ Insulin Receptor

Insulin Receptor

ANDREAS BARTHEL, #HANS-GEORG JOOST
Department of Endocrinology,
Heinrich-Heine-University, Düsseldorf and
#German Institute of Human Nutrition,
Potsdam-Rehbrücke, Germany
Andreas.Barthel@uni-duesseldorf.de,
joost@mail.dife.de

Synonyms

INSR (gene name)

Definition

The insulin receptor is a transmembrane ▶ receptor tyrosine kinase located in the plasma membrane of insulin-sensitive cells (e. g. adipocytes, myocytes, hepatocytes). It mediates the effect of insulin on specific cellular responses (e. g. glucose transport, glycogen synthesis, lipid synthesis, protein synthesis).

▶ Diabetes Mellitus

Basic Characteristics

Structure and Function

The INSR is a heterotetrameric protein consisting of two extracellular α-subunits (molecular weight 135 kD) and two membrane-spanning β-subunits (molecular weight 95 kD). These subunits are covalently linked by disulfide bonds ($\alpha_2\beta_2$-structure) (Fig. 1). The receptor is encoded by a single gene that is located on human chromosome 19 and consists of 22 exons (exon 1-11 = α-subunit, exon 12-22 = β-subunit). The single chain polypeptide precursor is posttranslationally cleaved in the endoplasmic reticulum into the α- and β-subunit which subsequently dimerize. Both subunits are glycosylated in the Golgi apparatus.

In addition to insulin, the INSR can also bind ▶ insulin-like growth factors (IGF1 and IGF2) albeit with considerably lower affinity (2 and 3 orders of magnitude, respectively).

The insulin-binding domain of the INSR is located within a cysteine-rich region of the α-subunits. Alternative splicing of exon 11 generates two isoforms of the α-subunit which differ in their C-terminus and in their tissue distribution (type A: leukocytes; type B: liver; type A and B: skeletal muscle and fat). The isoforms differ in their affinity to insulin (A>B), but their relevance for normal and impaired insulin action is not entirely clear (1,2).

Activation of the tyrosine kinase activity of the INSR is essential for receptor function. The tyrosine kinase domain of the INSR is localized in the cytoplasmic region of the β-subunit. In the absence of insulin, the α-subunits strongly repress the tyrosine kinase activity of the β-subunits. Binding of insulin releases this block through a conformational change and induces dimerization and/or oligomerization of β-subunits, resulting in receptor trans-autophosphorylation. While several phosphorylated tyrosine residues in the catalytic domain (Y1158, Y1162, Y1163 of human INSR) are essential for the kinase activity of the receptor, phosphorylation of two tyrosine residues in the juxtamembrane domain (Y965 and Y975 of human INSR) is critical for the interaction of the receptor with other signaling components of the insulin receptor signaling cascade (Fig. 1) (1).

Signaling through the INSR systems has evolved early and has been highly conserved dur-

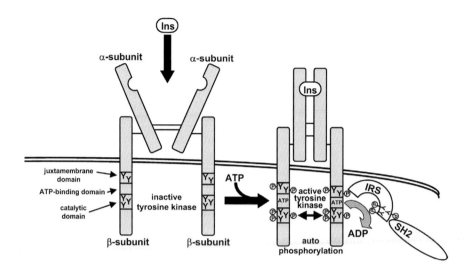

Fig. 1 Structure and function of the insulin receptor. Binding of insulin to the α-subunits leads to activation of the intracellular tyrosine kinase (β-subunit) by autophosphorylation. The insulin receptor substrates (IRS) bind via a phospho-tyrosine binding domain to phosphorylated tyrosine residues in the juxtamembrane domain of the β-subunit. The receptor tyrosine kinase then phosphorylates specific tyrosine motifs (YMxM) within the IRS. These tyrosine phosphorylated motifs serve as docking sites for some adaptor proteins with SRC homology 2 (SH2) domains like the regulatory subunit of PI 3-kinase.

ing evolution. Proteins related to the human INSR gene product have been found in *C. elegans* (DAF-2) as well as in *D. melanogaster* (DIR). Insulin-like signaling peptides (e. g. bombyxin) have been found in such distantly related organisms as the silkworm (1,3).

Structurally and functionally related receptors to the INSR in mammalian organisms are the insulin-like growth factor 1 receptor (IGF1R) and the insulin receptor-related receptor (INSRR). Although the function and signal transduction of the IGF1R and the INSRR resembles that of the INSR, major differences appear in the tissue distribution of the receptors. In contrast to the INSR, the IGF1R is expressed in adipocytes only at low levels and is almost absent in hepatocytes. The INSRR is an orphan receptor whose endogenous ligand is yet unknown. It has been found in few neuronal cell types e.g. in the dorsal root ganglion and trigeminal neurons.

Deletion of the INSR gene results in normal development but early postnatal lethality because of ketoacidosis. Organ specific INSR-knockout models (>95% reduction of the receptor protein content in the organ) exhibit less severe pheno-

types. Mice with a liver-specific insulin receptor knockout ('LIRKO') show severe insulin resistance and hyperglycemia due to an increased hepatic ▶ gluconeogenesis, whereas mice with a skeletal muscle-specific insulin receptor knockout ('MIRKO') have normal blood glucose and normal glucose tolerance but elevated serum free fatty acids and triglycerides. Mice with a neuron-specific INSR knockout develop an obese phenotype with mild insulin resistance and impaired fertility. These data emphasize the importance of insulin action in liver for glucose homeostasis, and indicate that the INSR plays an important role in the central regulation of body weight and reproduction (4).

There are two clinical syndromes with an impaired function of the INSR: Leprechaunism is a rare genetic disease characterized by growth retardation, hyperinsulinemia and insulin resistance due to mutations in the INSR gene. Acanthosis nigricans is a syndrome of hyperpigmentation and hyperandrogenism associated with hyperinsulinemia and ▶ diabetes mellitus. Insulin resistance in this syndrome is either due to mutations in the

Tab. 1 The effect of insulin on metabolism in some organs. Other, more general effects of insulin on cellular function include stimulation of cell growth (increase in DNA- and protein synthesis), inhibition of apoptosis and stimulation of potassium influx into the cell.

Organ	Effect	Mechanism	Comments
Liver	Activation of glycogen synthesis	Activation of glycogen synthase (GS)	Inactivation of glycogen synthase kinase 3 (GSK3) through phosphorylation by Akt.
	Inhibition of gluconeogenesis/ increased glycolysis	Inhibition of gluconeogenic gene expression/ activation of some glycolytic enzymes	Akt-dependent inhibition of phosphoenolpyruvate carboxykinase (PEPCK) and glucose-6-phosphatase (G6Pase) gene expression. Decrease of cAMP, the second messenger of glucagon. Induction of pyruvate kinase and glycerinaldehyde dehydrogenase.
Fat	Increased glucose transport	GLUT4-translocation	PI 3-kinase/Akt mediated translocation of GLUT4 into the plasma membrane. Potential involvement of atypical forms of protein kinase C (PKC ζ and λ).
	Increased lipid synthesis/ inhibition of lipolysis	Activation of lipoprotein lipase (LPL)/ induction of fatty acid synthase (FAS)/ inactivation of hormone sensitive lipase (HSL)	Facilitated uptake of fatty acids by LPL-dependent hydrolysis of triacylglycerol from circulating lipoproteins. Increased lipid synthesis through Akt-mediated FAS-expression. Inhibition of lipolysis by preventing cAMP-dependent activation of HSL (insulin-dependent activation of phosphodiesterases?)
Skeletal muscle	Increased glucose transport	GLUT4-translocation	See above (fat)
	Activation of glycogen synthesis	Activation of glycogen synthase	See above (liver)
	Increased protein synthesis	Increased amino acid uptake/ increased translation of mRNA	Akt-mediated stimulation of system A amino acid transporter and stimulation of mRNA-translation through activation of p70S6-Kinase and elongation initiation factor 4 (eIF4). Possible involvement of atypical PKCs.

insulin receptor gene (type A) or to autoantibodies to the INSR (type B).

Signal Transduction and Insulin Action

Stimulation of the insulin receptor results in the activation of two major pathways: a) the mitogen-activated protein (MAP) kinase cascade (▶ MAP kinase cascades) and b) the phosphatidylinositol 3-kinase (PI 3-kinase) pathway which has been extensively studied in the context of the metabolic responses to insulin (summarized in Table 1 and Fig. 2).

The major intracellular target molecules of the tyrosine kinase activity of the INSR β-subunit are the insulin receptor substrates (IRS). Interaction of phosphotyrosine-binding domains (PTB) within the N-terminal region of an IRS with the juxtamembrane phosphotyrosines of the INSR β-

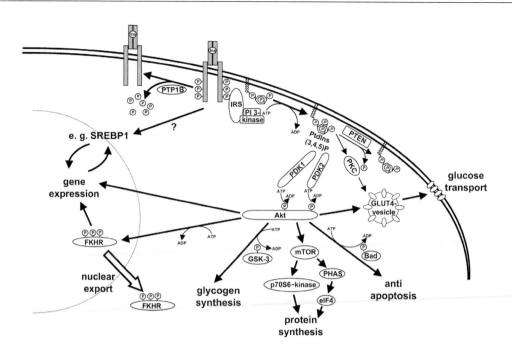

Fig. 2 Signal transduction of the insulin receptor. Activation of the insulin receptor leads to stimulation of the PI 3-kinase pathway. Generation of 3'-phosphorylated PI-phospholipids mediates the effect of insulin on glucose transport, cell survival, protein synthesis, glycogen synthesis and gene expression. The protein kinase Akt plays a central role in the regulation of these PI 3-kinase dependent processes.

subunit results in tyrosine phosphorylation of consensus motifs (YMXM) in the C-terminus of IRS (Fig. 1). Four different mammalian IRS isotypes have been identified (IRS1–4). IRS1 knockout mice develop a mild state of insulin resistance (impaired glucose intolerance) without diabetes, whereas knockout of the IRS2 gene causes a phenotype with severe insulin resistance (liver >muscle), diabetes and impaired pancreatic β-cell function. Both IRS1 and IRS2 knockout mice exhibit growth retardation (IRS1>IRS2). IRS3 knockout mice appear to be normal, whereas disruption of the IRS4 gene produces mild glucose intolerance and growth retardation in male animals. IRS1 and IRS2 are ubiquitously expressed. IRS3 is expressed only in adipocytes, β-cells and hepatocytes; IRS4 mRNA is detected in thymus, brain and kidney. Taken together, the data suggest that the major effects of insulin on metabolism are mediated via IRS1 and IRS2 (2).

Tyrosine phosphorylated IRS interacts with and activates ▶ phosphatidylinositol 3-kinase (PI 3-kinase). Binding takes place via the SRC homology 2 (SH2) domain of the PI 3-kinase regulatory subunit. The resulting complex consisting of INSR, IRS and PI 3-kinase facilitates interaction of the activated PI 3-kinase catalytic subunit with the phospholipid substrates in the plasma membrane. Generation of PI 3-phosphates in the plasma membrane recruits phospholipid dependent kinases (PDK1 and PDK2) that subsequently phosphorylate and activate the serine/threonine kinase ▶ Akt (synonym: protein kinase B, PKB). Three isotypes of Akt have been identified (Akt1, 2, 3). AKT1-knockout mice exhibit growth retardation and increased apoptosis, but no increased prevalence in diabetes. Disruption of the Akt2 gene produces diabetes due to insulin resistance of skeletal muscle and liver. There is solid evidence that activation of Akt is essential for the effect of insulin on glucose transport (▶ Glucose Transporters), glycogen synthesis, ▶ gluconeogenesis, protein synthesis and gene expression (1,3) (summarized in Table 1 and Fig. 2). ▶ Glycogen synthase kinase 3

(GSK3) and FKHR, a transcription factor regulating the expression of gluconeogenic enzymes, have been shown to be substrates of Akt. Recently, sterol regulatory-element binding protein 1 (SREBP1) knockout animals were found to have impaired insulin-dependent upregulation of lipogenesis related enzymes. Regulation of SREBP1 gene expression involves activation of Akt and other IRS-2 independent mechanisms.

Furthermore, some of the effects of insulin on cell proliferation and survival may be explained by an Akt-dependent inhibition of ▶ apoptosis through phosphorylation and inactivation of pro-apoptotic proteins (BAD, caspase 9).

INSR signaling is terminated by specific phosphotyrosine phosphatases (e.g. PTP1B), and mice lacking the PTP1B gene exhibit increased insulin sensitivity. Furthermore, it has been suggested that the lipid phosphatases PTEN and SHIP2, the ligand-induced endocytosis and degradation of the activated INSR, and the degradation of insulin by insulin-degrading enzyme (insulysin) are involved in the termination of insulin signaling.

Drugs

Agents Stimulating the Receptor or the Signaling Pathway

Insulin Analogs. At present, the only known ligands of the insulin receptors are insulin isotypes from different species and a number of synthetic analogs with insulin-like activity. Three analogs generated by site-directed DNA mutagenesis are used in clinical practice because of their pharmacokinetic characteristics: insulin lispro (generated by swap of prolin B28 and lysine B29) and insulin aspart (generated by exchange of proline B28 for aspartate) are rapid and short-acting insulins (see Chapter Diabetes Mellitus); insulin glargine is a long acting analog which carries two additional arginines at B31 and B32. It is soluble at low pH and precipitates after injection from its solution, thereby forming a stable, long-acting depot.

Thiazolidinediones. Thiazolidinediones (synonyms glitazones, insulin sensitizers) are a novel class of oral anti-diabetic drugs that activate the transcription factor peroxisome proliferator-activated receptor gamma (PPARγ). Thiazolidinediones have been found to decrease the level of insulin resistance in individuals with type-2-diabetes. Although the target genes of PPARγ and the precise mechanism of action of thiazolidinediones is largely unknown, recent evidence suggests that thiazolidinediones may increase the insulin dependent activation of the PI 3-kinase/Akt pathway, or stimulate differentiation of preadipocytes. The latter effect would lower serum triglycerides and free fatty acids which are thought to be involved in the pathogenesis of insulin resistance (see also Chapter Diabetes Mellitus).

Concanavalin A. Concanavalin A is a plant lectin from the jack bean (*Canavalia ensiformis*) that binds with high affinity to mannose residues of glycoproteins. Concanavalin A is known to stimulate the tyrosine kinase activity of the INSR β-subunit with consecutive activation of kinases downstream the insulin receptor (IRS, PI 3-kinase). It is believed that concanavalin A stimulates the activation and autophosphorylation of the INSR kinase through aggregation of the receptor, although the precise mechanism of action is unclear.

Vanadate. Vanadate (sodium orthovanadate or peroxovanadate) exhibits insulin-like effects *in vitro* (activation of insulin receptor tyrosine kinase, PI 3-kinase, Akt) and *in vivo* (diabetic rats, humans). These effects can be explained at least in part by the inhibition of phosphotyrosine phosphatases that deactivate the INSR tyrosine kinase.

Hydrogen peroxide. Hydrogen peroxide (H_2O_2) exhibits insulin-like activity in isolated cells. Like that of vanadate, this effect is thought to be mediated by inhibition of protein-tyrosine phosphatases. Interestingly, recent evidence suggests that stimulation of cells with insulin leads to a rapid intracellular generation of endogenous H_2O_2 *in vivo* with consecutive inhibition of protein-tyrosine phosphatase 1B, which inactivates the INSR tyrosine kinase.

Agents Inhibiting Insulin Receptor Signaling

Insulin Analogs. Interestingly, several covalently dimerized insulin analogs are partial agonists of the insulin receptor. The intrinsic activity of the dimers decreases with the length of the spacer, with B29-B29'-suberoyl-insulin exhibiting the highest antagonist efficacy at the receptor (5).

Wortmannin. Wortmannin is a fungus-derived inhibitor of PI 3-kinase. The agent binds and inhibits the enzyme covalently and irreversibly. It is very potent and considered to be highly specific (IC_{50} in most cells in the low nanomolar range).

LY294002. LY294002 is a synthetic drug which reversibly inhibits PI 3-kinases. It is less toxic and also less potent than wortmannin. The IC_{50} in most cells is in the micromolar range.

Rapamycin. Rapamycin is an immunosuppressive drug and an inhibitor of ▶ **p70S6-kinase** that phosphorylates ribosomal S6 protein. p70S6-kinase is activated in response to insulin via activation of Akt. Rapamycin binds to a specific target protein (mTOR=mammalian target of rapamycin) which is functionally located downstream of Akt, but upstream of p70S6 kinase. The IC_{50} in most cells is in the high nanomolar range.

References

1. Kido Y, Nakae J, Acilli D (2001) Clinical review 125: The insulin receptor and its cellular targets. J Clin Endocrinol Metab 86:972–979
2. Withers DJ, White M (2000) Perspective: the insulin signaling system- a common link in the pathogenesis of type 2 diabetes. Endocrinology 141:1917–1921
3. Le Roith D, Zick Y (2001). Recent advances in our understanding of insulin action and insulin resistance. Diabetes Care 24:588–597
4. Saltiel AR (2001) New perspectives into the molecular pathogenesis and treatment of type 2 diabetes. Cell 104:517–529
5. Weiland M, Brandenburg C, Brandenburg D, Joost HG (1990) Antagonistic effects of a covalently dimerized insulin derivative on insulin receptors in 3T3-L1 adipocytes. Proc Natl Acad Sci USA 87:1154–1158

Insulin Resistance

Insulin resistance is a condition in which the biological effectiveness of insulin is impaired. This is mostly due to defects in the cellular pathways of insulin action. Insulin resistance is typically an early feature in the pathogenesis of type 2 diabetes.

▶ Diabetes Mellitus

Integrase

Integrase is the enzyme of retroviruses that performs the incorporation of the viral DNA genome into the genome of the host cell. The enzyme is carried inside the viral particle and released into the host cell during infection. Upon back-transcription of the viral RNA genome into DNA by reverse transcriptase, integrase binds to the ends of this DNA product and removes two nucleotides. In a second step, integrase nicks the host cell genome and integrates the recessed viral nucleic acid into the cellular DNA.

▶ Viral Proteases

Integrins

Integrins constitute a large family of $\alpha\beta$ heterodimeric cell surface, transmembrane proteins that interact with a large number of extracellular matrix components through a metal ion-dependent interaction. The term "integrin" reflects their function in integrating cell adhesion and migration with the cystoskeleton.

▶ Anti-integrins, therapeutic and diagnostic implications
▶ Inflammation
▶ Table appendix: Adhesion Molecules

Integrin, αIIbβ3

αIIbβ3 Integrin is a selective platelet integrin that generally binds to the RGD domain within fibrinogen and vWF. It mediates platelet-platelet aggregation that is essential for thrombosis and haemostasis.

▶ Anti-integrins, therapeutic and diagnostic implications

Integrin, α4β1

The leukocyte integrin α4β1 (also known as VLA-4 and CD49d/CD29) is a cell adhesion receptor, which is predominantly expressed on lymphocytes, monocytes and eosinophils. VLA-4 is generally selective for the CS1 domain within fibronectin, with an essential requirement for LDV sequence for binding. VLA-4 also binds to VCAM-1 as a counter receptor.

▶ Anti-integrins, therapeutic and diagnostic implications

Integrin, α4β7

The integrin α4β7 is restricted to leukocytes and can bind not only to VCAM1 and fibronectin, but also to MAdCAM the mucosal addressin or homing receptor, which contains immunoglobulin-like domains related to VCAM-1.

▶ Anti-integrins, therapeutic and diagnostic implications

Integrin, αvβ5

αvβ5 integrin generally binds to soluble and, with a higher affinity, to immobilized vitronectin via an RGD binding domain. αvβ5 integrin is expressed on endothelial, epithelial, and other cells.

▶ Anti-integrins, therapeutic and diagnostic implications

Integrin, αvβ3

αvβ3 Integrin is generally binds via RGD domain within various matrix proteins including vitronectin, osteopontin, and fibrinogen. It is widely distributed on various cells.

▶ Anti-integrins, therapeutic and diagnostic implications

Interactions

▶ Drug Interaction

Interferons

R. ZAWATZKY
Deutsches Krebsforschungszentrum Heidelberg, Germany
r.zawatzky@dkfz.de

Synonyms

Antiviral cytokine

Definition

Interferons (IFNs) are a family of multifunctional secreted proteins in vertebrates. Their most prominent functions are their antiviral properties on homologous cells against a wide range of viruses. It is important to note that prior exposure to IFN is required to render cells resistant to viral infection and replication. In contrast to antibodies, IFNs have no direct neutralizing effect on viruses.

▶ Antiviral Drugs
▶ Immune Defense

Nomenclature

In mammals the type I IFN genes form a large multigene family comprising the species -α, -β, -ω and -τ. The best studied representatives are the IFN-α group, which comprise at least 14 genes in man, and the single IFN-β gene. These species are rapidly induced by viruses or ▶ double-stranded (ds) RNA molecules. IFN-β is produced in almost all cell types, whereas the most efficient IFN-α producing cells are lymphocytes and antigen-presenting cells of the monocyte/macrophage differentiation lineage (▶ Inflammation). IFN-ω constitute a minor species of type I IFN coinduced by viruses with α and β IFN in leucocyte cultures. IFN-τ, formerly called trophoblastin or ovine trophoblast protein, was isolated from sheep and bovine embryonic tissues. This IFN species is not virus-inducible but is released constitutively by ▶ trophoblast cells during the period immediately prior to implantation and therefore seems to play a key role in the establishment of maternal recognition and of pregnancy in ruminants. All typeI IFN species are encoded by intronless genes and bind to a common cell-surface receptor present on virtually all nucleated cells. Sequence homology of type I IFN species ranges from 50 to >90% with polypeptide chain lengths of 165–166 amino acids for most.

In contrast to the large group of type I IFN genes, type II IFN comprises only IFN-γ. The gene contains three ▶ introns, displays no homology to type I IFN and is expressed exclusively by T-lymphocytes following stimulation with certain interleukins (IL-2, IL-7, IL-12 and IL-18), ▶ mitogens or the specific antigen of sensitized T-lymphocytes. IFN-γ binds to its specific receptor as a homodimer. All natural type I and II IFNs are glycosylated, but non-glycosylated recombinant IFN shows the same spectrum of biological activities. Before the availability of specific antibodies, type I

and type II IFNs were distinguished by their differential sensitivity to acid treatment. The biological activity of IFN-α and -β is resistant to pH2 whereas IFN-γ is not. This essay focusses on IFN-α, -β and -γ.

Mechanism of Action

Regulation of IFN Gene Expression

Type I IFN. Type I IFNs are considered an integral part of the innate defense system (▶ Innate Immunity) against viral infection. Large amounts of IFN are produced in many cell types upon infection by various viruses, and production is controlled at the transcriptional level. Efficient inducers of type I IFN also include bacteria or bacteria-derived ▶ lipopolysaccharide. Initiation of transcription requires activation of the IFN-α and -β ▶ gene promoters located 110 to 40 base pairs upstream of the start codon.

The events leading to activation of the IFN-β promoter have been studied in detail. This promoter is composed of an overlapping set of four regulatory elements, two of which are target sequences for members of the Interferon-Regulatory-Factor (IRF) family of ▶ transcription factors. This family is comprised of nine members with remarkable homology in the DNA-binding domain, and IRF-3 and IRF-7 being crucial for inducing maximal type I IFN expression. The strong IFN-α/β response measured after viral infection is critical for survival of the host. As explained in Fig. 1, this response is due to a positive feedback regulation involving IRF-7, and is generated in a two-step process. IRF-7 has been shown to represent the key element of this two-step process since the gene carries a sequence named 'Interferon-Stimulated-Response-Element' (ISRE) – a conserved sequence in the regulatory region shared by most IFN-inducible genes – and also particiates in the induction process through binding to the IFN-β promoter. Due to the pronounced effects of IFNs on cell growth and immune functions, the duration of 'bulk' synthesis is generally limited. Two mechanisms are known to mediate rapid post-induction turnoff of IFN-β gene expression: First, virus-inducible competitive factors downregulate the IFN-β promoter activity; second, IFN-β mRNA has a rapid turno-

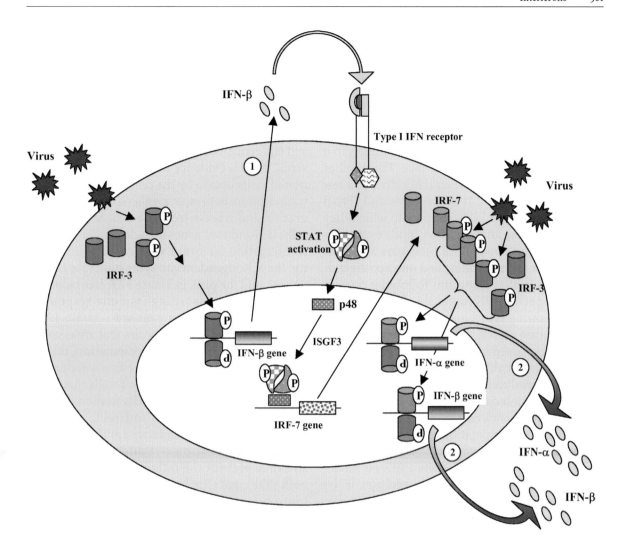

Fig. 1 Virus infection results in two-step induction of type I IFN. 1. In the first step IRF-3 is activated by phosphorylation during viral infection and translocates to the nucleus, a rapid process independent of protein synthesis due to the constitutive expression of IRF-3 with low to moderate yields of IFN–β. In a positive feedback regulation the secreted 'early' IFN–β then stimulates the type I IFN receptor and – via formation of ISGF3 – activates the IRF-7 gene through binding to its ISRE element (see also Fig. 2 for further details regarding the signal transduction). **2.** In concert with IRF-3 *de novo* produced IRF-7 is also phosphorylated in the cytoplasm during ongoing viral infection, and in the nucleus both IRF-3 and IRF-7 activate IFN–α and IFN–β gene promoters. This second step is highly efficient resulting in an amplified 'bulk' IFN response.

ver. In addition, in non-induced cells transcriptional repressors prevent transcriptional activation of the IFN-β promoter.

Type II IFN. In contrast to IFN-α/β, the expression of IFN-γ is strictly limited to T-cells and large granular lymphocytes, also often referred to as

▶ natural killer (NK) cells. This is probably due to a silencing effect by ▶ DNA methylation, since a CpG target region in the IFN-γ promoter near the ▶ TATA box was found to be methylated in cells that do not express IFN-γ but not in T_h1 lymphocytes (▶ Immune Defense). Hypomethylation *per se*, however, does not result in IFN-γ expression since continuous production of IFN-γ would be harmful to the host. It is therefore assumed that in unstimulated cells nuclear factors keep the gene in the 'off' position.

Signal Transduction and Biological Activity in Response to IFNs

Any IFN-mediated activity requires binding to a specific receptor on the cell surface. The number of receptors varies from several hundred to a few thousand per cell. All IFN-α species and IFN-β share the same type I IFN receptor to which they bind with similar affinity. IFN-γ binds to the distinct type II receptor. Both receptors are composed of one ligand-binding and one non-ligand-binding chain that associates following contact with the specific IFN molecule. The signaling events following type I and type II IFN receptor stimulation are depicted on a simplified scheme in Fig. 2 and explained in the legend. Crucial components of this signaling pathway are the so-called '▶ Signal-Transducer-and-Activator-of-Transcription' (STAT) molecules. Although IFN-γ specifically activates genes carrying a GAS element in their regulatory region, it can also indirectly activate genes harboring only an ISRE via binding of the transcription factor IRF-1, since IRF-1 is inducible by both IFN-α/β and IFN-γ. In addition, IFN-γ signaling is dependent on simultaneous or prior stimulation of the IFN-α/β receptor that results from a cross-talk between IFNAR1 and IFNGR1 receptor components. This is borne out by observations that on one hand a low constitutive IFN-β expression observed in some cell types, such as macrophages and embryonic fibroblasts, considerably enhances their sensitivity towards IFN-γ, whereas on the other hand the IFN-γ induced antiviral activity is strongly reduced in cells lacking the IFNAR1 chain.

Oligonucleotide arrays (▶ Microarray Technology) using cRNA prepared from IFN-α/β and IFN-γ treated cells have identified >300 inducible genes, displaying cell type specific variations. Of course, not all of them are inducible solely by IFNs, some of them being activated by virus infection, dsRNA, lipopolysaccharide or other cytokines. In turn, IFNs also act via stimulation or inhibition of other members belonging to the cytokine family, all of which constitute central regulators of immune responses. Some cellular genes,

in particular those involved in cell proliferation are inhibited by type I IFN. This all accounts for the pleiotropic effects of IFNs on cell growth, viral infection and the immune system. In particular, the antiviral properties against many viruses with different infection and replication strategies rely on the concerted action of many induced genes and still remain obscure. Depending on the type of virus, there is evidence for IFN-mediated inhibition of virus uptake by the cell, inhibition of viral transcription, of protein synthesis or of virus maturation and release from the cell. More specifically, IFN-induced genes include the IRF family of transcription factors, a wide range of enzymes, e.g. the 2′,5′oligoadenylate-synthetase (2′,5′OASE), RNaseL and the protein kinase PKR (see below) as well as factors governing immune responses. Among these are the ▶ proteasome subunits LMP2 and LMP7 and ▶ MHC molecules that are essential for antigen processing and presentation, respectively. Type I IFN also non-specifically induce the proliferation of CD8$^+$ memory T-cells that interact with antigen presenting cells to elicit immune responses. This effect is indirect, mediated through the secondary induction of IL-15. Interestingly, type I IFN also exert direct growth arrest and thus prevent the induction of apoptosis in both CD4$^+$ and CD8$^+$ memory T-cells. This fine-tuned balance seems to depend on the amount of IFN secreted from fibroblasts, stromal cells and monocytic cells and contributes to the long-lasting persistence of memory T-cells in the immune system. Dysregulation of its synthesis, however, may prevent elimination of autoreactive T- and B-cells and is associated with T-cell dependent chronic joint inflammation or the presence of autoreactive antibodies.

IFN-induced proteins are involved in cell growth inhibition, as for instance the transcription factor IRF-1, the cyclin-dependent kinase inhibitor p21/waf (▶ Cell-cycle Control), and members of the p200 family. The latter inhibit several transcriptional activators including the ▶ proto-oncogenes c-myc, c-fos and c-jun and bind to the retinoblastoma protein (Rb), which is a major player in cell-cycle regulation (▶ Cell-cycle Control). IFN-induced mediators of antiviral activity are the proteins of the Mx and GBP families with GTPase activities. Among the IRF group of transcription factors, 'Interferon-Consensus-

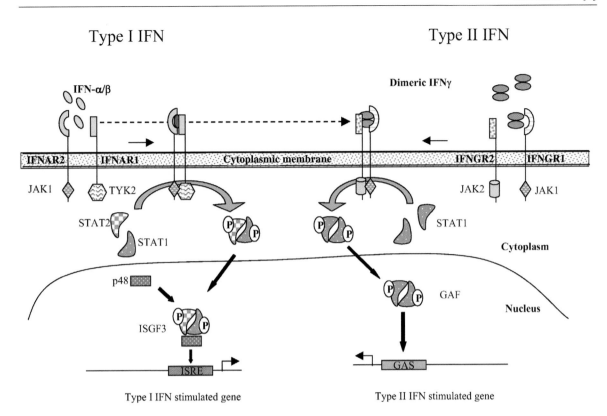

Fig. 2 Receptor stimulation and signal transduction by type I and type II IFN. *Type I IFN:* The receptor is composed of two chains, IFNAR1 and IFNAR2. Their cytoplasmic domains are associated with the tyrosine kinases Tyk2 and Jak1, respectively, which are essential for signaling. Upon IFN–α/β binding, the ligand-binding subunit IFNAR2 associates with IFNAR1, and bound IFN is internalized via receptor-mediated endocytosis. The receptor associated kinases Jak1 and Tyk2 get into closer contact and are activated by transphosphorylation. Subsequently, Tyk2 phosphorylates first a tyrosine residue of the IFNAR1 chain and then the STAT2 molecules that in turn have been attracted to this phosphorylated residue. STAT1 molecules will then be recruited to the phosphorylated STAT2 and become phosphorylated as well. The phosphorylated STAT1/STAT2 heterodimer thus formed finally dissociates from the IFNAR1 chain and translocates to the nucleus where it associates with the DNA-binding protein p48/IRF-9 to form the trimeric complex interferon-stimulated-gene-factor 3 (ISGF3). The ISGF3 complex binds to a conserved target sequence in the promoter of IFN-inducible genes. This interferon-stimulated-response-element (ISRE) is essential for activation by IFN–α/β. Interestingly, the ISRE shares significant homology with defined domains in the type I IFN promoter and can therefore also be stimulated by members of the IRF family. *Type II IFN:* Similar to the type I IFN receptor, the type II (IFN–γ) receptor is also composed of two chains, the ligand-binding IFNGR1 and the non-ligand binding IFNGR2 chain, which are associated with the kinases Jak1 and Jak2, respectively. IFNGR1 associates with IFNGR2 after binding of the dimeric IFN–γ. In contrast to type I IFN signaling pathway, the IFNGR associated kinases only recruit STAT1 molecules to a C-terminal IFNGR1 sequence containing several tyrosine residues phosphorylated previously. The STAT1 molecules are also phosphorylated and dissociate from the receptor to form a homodimer named γ-activated-factor (GAF), which in the nucleus interacts with defined elements of IFN–γ inducible genes named γ-activated-sequences (GAS). In cells constitutively secreting IFN–α/β – such as macrophages and embryonic fibroblasts – the IFNAR1 chain is constitutively phosphorylated. Through association with the non-ligand binding chain IFNGR2 – indicated by the dashed arrow – the phosphorylated IFNAR1 contributes to type II IFN signaling by providing phosphorylated STAT2 molecules that enables ISGF3 assembly and activation of the ISRE in type I IFN-inducible gene promoters.

Sequence-Binding-Protein' (ICSBP/IRF-8) is specifically induced by IFN–γ and its expression is limited to cells of monocytic and lymphoid origin. Cytogenetic analyses have provided evidence for tumor suppressor activities of both IRF-1 and ICSBP/IRF-8. Blood samples from patients with chronic myelogenous ▶ leukemia (CML) exhibited impaired ICSBP expression, whereas deletion of the *ICSBP* gene in mice led to a CML-like syndrome. Chromosomal deletions or point mutations within the *IRF-1* locus are among the most frequent cytogenetic abnormalities in myeloid leukemia and myelodysplastic syndromes, and experimental deletion of the IRF-1 gene facilitates oncogenic transformation *in vitro*.

From a certain size, tumor growth is dependent on blood vessel supply, a process defined as ▶ angiogenesis. Angiogenesis in turn is dependent on growth factors such as vascular endothelial growth factor (VEGF) and basic fibroblast growth factor (bFGF) and involves dissociation of endothelial cells and basement membranes of pre-existing vessels by way of matrix metaloproteinases (MMP). IFNs are known to mediate angiostatic effects and may thus contribute to inhibition of tumor spreading. Their angiostatic effects are caused by inhibition of bFGF and MMP-9 expression in tumor cells by type I IFN and of induction by IFN-γ of IP-10 (CXCL10) in macrophages. IP-10 belongs to the CXC family of ▶ chemokines and injection of the purified protein into experimental tumors exerted direct anti-angiogenic effects by an unknown mechanism.

A complicated interplay exists between both types of IFN and ▶ nitric oxide (NO), the details of which are still far from clear. NO generated by macrophages in response to IFN-γ plays an important role in host defense against viruses, bacteria and eukaryotic parasites but has also been implicated in the pathogenesis of chronic inflammatory syndromes.

The pathway leading to 2′5′OASE/RNaseL activation also contributes to the antiviral and antiproliferative effects of IFN-α/β. Both are induced by IFNs but require dsRNA or viral infection for activation. 2′5′OASE polymerizes ATP into 2′5′linked oligoadenylates (2-5A) of different lengths. In turn, these molecules bind to and activate the latent RNaseL, which is also involved in IFN-mediated apoptosis. Much attention has also

been attributed to the serine-threonine kinase PKR. In the presence of dsRNA, PKR undergoes autophosphorylation and phosphorylates selected cellular proteins of which the most well known is eIF2α, a translation initiation factor. Phosphorylation inactivates eIF2α leading to an arrest of cellular protein synthesis. Most importantly, PKR displays the properties of a tumor suppressor since its inactivation *in vitro* causes malignant transformation and prevents apoptosis of virus-infected cells. In addition to PKR and RNaseL, a variety of other proteins participate in the initiation of ▶ apoptosis; for instance IRF-1 and TNF-Related-Apoptosis-Inducing-Ligand (TRAIL) induced by type I and type II IFN. The selective induction of TRAIL in T-cells and fibroblasts may also represent an important component of host defense against virus-infected or tumor cells. Due to its rather specific action on malignant cells and few adverse effects *in vivo*, TRAIL is a promising antitumor agent for clinical trials. Finally, in a tumor line a heterogenous group of IFN-γ induced Death-Associated-Proteins (DAP) has been identified and characterized. Each of these findings reveals that programmed cell death is part of the IFN-mediated cellular defense and is an efficient means for an organism to combat virus infection.

Clinical Use (incl. side effects)

IFNs were the first therapeutic products resulting from recombinant DNA technology. In view of their pronounced antiproliferative effects, crude preparations of natural leucocyte IFN were already being used for the treatment of various tumors well before the availability of recombinant material. However, due to limited supply, the number of patients and duration of treatment did not allow for the evaluation of long lasting beneficial effects. Today, numerous clinical trials have been conducted for a variety of different human diseases. Based on the results approved indications have been formulated for the therapeutical application of IFNs (Table 1). As can be seen, most of the responding tumors are of hematopoietic origin and the response rates wthin this group of tumors were comparable to ▶ chemotherapy. Combination regimen mainly using recombinant IFN-α2 and chemotherapeutic drugs yielded promising results with even higher rates of complete hemato-

Tab. 1 Approved indications for interferon therapy eitheras adjuvant or for monotherapy.

Malignancy class	IFN-α	IFN-β
Hematological Malignancies	Hairy Cell Leukemia Chronic Myelogenous Leukemia Multiple Myeloma Low-Grade Non-Hodgkin-Lymphoma Adult T-cell Lymphoma Cutaneous T-cell Lymphoma	
Other Malignancies	Metatastatic Renal Cell Carcinoma Metatastatic Melanoma Kaposi Sarcoma	
Virus-associated Benign Tumors		Anogenital Warts Juvenile Laryngeal Papilloma
Viral Diseases	Hepatitis B Hepatitis C	
Diseases of unclear Etiology		Multiple Sclerosis

logic remissions and survival. For sufferers with hairy cell leukemia, a rare chronic lymphoproliferative disorder, IFN-α is the therapeutic agent of choice with overall response rates of 75%. Generally used treatment schedules consist of daily parenteral application of 3×10^6 IU/m^2 for six months followed by maintenance treatment three times weekly for one year. Fortunately, in patients with hematologic relapses, readministration of IFN-α is successful in most cases. Striking effects have also been obtained for IFN-α treatment of CML. This hematopoietic stem cell malignancy is characterized by a reciprocal translocation between chromosomes 9 and 22 giving rise to the constitutive expression of the chimeric BCR-ABL tyrosine kinase that is essential for malignant transformation. Cytogenetic responses to IFN-α therapy were seen in 30–40% of the treated patients with complete responses in about 10%. Long term survival can therefore be expected in these patients. Recently, the BCR-ABL tyrosine kinase inhibitor STI-571 has been introduced for CML therapy and in future will be used in combination with IFN-α to further improve response rates. In addition, IFN-α has therapeutic potentials for multiple myeloma, low-grade non-Hodgkin lymphoma, cutaneous T-cell lymphoma and adult T-cell lymphoma. Thus, IFN-α is one of the most useful and wide-ranging antitumor agents in hematological malignancies.

Metastatic renal cell carcinoma has a poor prognosis and resists conventional chemotherapy. Immunotherapy with IL-2 and/or IFN-α is currently regarded as the most effective therapy with, however, modest response rates of 15–20%. Similar results are also observed in patients with metastatic melanoma and the response to IFN-α and IL-2 correlates with the occurrence of tumour-infiltrating CD4$^+$ T-lymphocytes identified in aspirates from melanoma metastases. Determination of these cells therefore seems to be a method to predict responders prior to the initiation of cytokine therapy.

Kaposi sarcoma (KS) – an angiogenic-inflammatory neoplasm – is the most prevalent cancer in ► HIV-infected patients and its appearance is preceeded by infection with human Herpesvirus-8 (HHV-8). KS showed a 30% response rate to combined treatment with ► reverse transcriptase inhibitors and IFN-α. There is much clinical evidence for a role of HIV in the etiology of KS, it is therefore likely that the therapeutic response of KS is at least in part due to inhibition of HIV-1 replication. Whether or not the observed inhibition of HHV-8 by IFN-α also contributes to its activity against KS is unclear at present.

Although there has been substantial success using IFN for the treatment of some cancers, until this point, the great majority of tumors are resistant or show an initial moderate response soon followed by disease progression under treatment. One likely reason for resistance is the progredient loss of susceptibility to IFN, due for instance to down-regulation of IFN receptors, a phenomenon known from *in vitro* studies, or to *in vivo* selection of single therapy-resitant tumor cells.

Since their discovery in 1957, type I IFNs have been noted to have protective effects against human viral infections. This is why, apart from malignancies, diseases of viral etiology have also been successfully treated with IFNs. For anogenital warts, a commonly acquired sexually transmitted disease caused by Human Papilloma Viruses (HPV), the most effective response is obtained after intralesional administration of IFNs in contrast to systemic treatment that only prevents the development of new warts. Juvenile laryngeal papilloma is a rare but severe benign lesion also caused by HPV infection and mainly observed in childhood. Recurrence is a characteristic feature of this disease and calls for repeated surgical removal. Treatment with type I IFN has proven highly effective and, most importantly, prevents recurrence of lesions.

Successful treatment with IFN-α also includes patients with chronic ▶ Hepatitis B virus (HBV) infections. Despite the availability of an efficient vaccine, chronic Hepatitis B virus infection remains a major worldwide public health problem. The World Health Organization estimates that there are still 350 million chronic carriers of the virus who are at risk of developing chronic hepatitis, liver cirrhosis and hepatocellular carcinoma. The success of IFN-α treatment has been measured by the normalization of liver enzymes, loss of Hepatitis B e antigen and loss of detectable viral DNA in the serum of patients. It has been estimated from several clinical trials that as many as 40% of treated HBV patients would respond to therapy with IFN-α or combined treatment with nucleoside analogues and IFN-α.

Similar to HBV, infections with ▶ Hepatitis C virus (HCV) have a high rate of progression from an acute to a chronic state that frequently leads to cirrhosis or hepatocellular carcinoma. Monotherapy for HCV infection with IFN-α or combined therapy with ribavirin and IFN-α is associated with initial rates of response as high as 40%. The rates of sustained responses are, however, lower and also depend on the viral genotype. In patients infected with HCV genotype 2 or 3 the response was maximal after 24 weeks of treatment, whereas patients infected with genotype 1 – the most frequent in the US and Europe – required a minimum treatment course of 48 weeks for an optimal outcome.

Considerable success has been obtained with IFN-β monotherapy of multiple sclerosis (MS) although a definite cure seems unlikely even after treatment for years at highest tolerable doses 3 times weekly. The beneficial effects of IFN-β consist of significantly reduced clinical attack and relapse rates and delay of disability progression and are clearly dose-dependent with highest doses achieving maximal clinical response. This chronic inflammatory disease of the central nervous system (CNS) is assumed to result from autoaggressive T cell-mediated immune responses to self antigens such as myelin basic protein (MBP). Stimulated by proinflammatory cytokines like IL-1, TNF-α and IFN-γ, and cellular adhesion molecules these T-cells and also macrophages cross the ▶ blood-brain barrier and gain access to the CNS. This transendothelial migration process involves the release of MMPs, which cleave type IV collagen, a component of the blood-brain barrier. ▶ Astrocytes and microglia in the CNS are activated by the infiltrating immune cells resulting in a chronic inflammatory process with irreversible axonal damage. The mechanism of the favorable response of MS to IFN-β treatment most likely resides within its immunregulatory effects on the autoreactive T-cells. In this context the most important effects are repression of IL-2 receptor expression and of IL-2 dependent release of MMP-2 and MMP-9 in a dose-dependent manner resulting in inhibition of T-cell migration across the blood-brain barrier. In addition, IFN-β reduces the induction by inflammatory cytokines of ▶ adhesion molecules and of ▶ MHC class I and II complex on endothelial cells, a process preceeding attachment and transendothelial migration of T-cells. These antiinflammatory effects of IFN-β exemplify antagonistic actions of type I and type II IFN. There is, indeed, much clinical evidence for the involvement of IFN-γ in inflammatory processes – through activation of iNOS and subsequent secretion of NO – leading to the establishment of ▶ autoimmune diseases as for instance in rheumatoid arthritis.

On the other hand, IFN-α may also be involved in the activation of autoreactive T-cells as has been proposed for type I diabetes. An IFN-α inducible ▶ superantigen encoded by the truncated envelope gene of a human endogenous retrovirus and specifically activating Vβ7 T-cells has been detected in pancreatic lesions from type I diabetes patients infiltrated by Vβ7 T-cells. Since IFN-α expression could be detected in pancreatic β cells in concert with persistent viral infections, there is a clear link between viral infections and autoimmunity via IFN-α stimulated ▶ superantigen expression.

Side Effects of IFN Therapy

During clinical trials aimed at defining the optimal IFN dose for therapy, various side effects became manifest with increasing doses. The most common side effects that develop independently of the IFN preparation used are transient nausea, skin reactions, chills and fever; the latter two often being managed by prophylaxis with ibuprofen and paracetamol. In addition, however, therapeutic effectiveness is compromised by more severe secondary effects such as myelosuppression, cardiomyopathy and impaired renal function requiring limitation of IFN therapy. Thyroid dysfunction resulting in ▶ hypothyroidism is also a known complication during IFN therapy in 10 to 20% of patients and may be caused by an autoimmune reaction. Fatigue is a common symptom of hypothyroidism and accounts for the most frequent side effect, reported in up to 50% of treated patients. IFN-mediated fatigue is recognized as a complex neurophysiologic phenomenon that is not transient but worsens with ongoing IFN therapy and may finally result in cognitive slowing, general lethargy and depression. Finally, a substantial number of patients develop neutralizing antibodies during IFN treatment and their presence is associated with a poor therapeutic response. Most of these antibodies are specific for non-glycosylated, recombinant type I IFN.

Second Generation IFNs

Improvements in therapy are expected through the development of 'second generation' IFN.

Reduced immunogenicity and enhanced stability have been reported for pegylated IFN-α, a conjugate of recombinant IFN-α and monomethyl-polyethylenglycol. Pharmakokinetic studies comparing pegylated and non-pegylated IFN-α preparations have revealed an increase of biological half life from 4 h to 30 h and a seven-fold delay in the mean elimination time. For IFN-β, a complex with the soluble portion of the ligand-binding receptor chain IFNAR2 was tested in preclinical studies and showed a prolonged clearance and potentiated biological effects.

References

1. Sen GC (2001) Viruses and interferons. Ann. Rev. Microbiol. 55:255–281
2. Taniguchi T, Takaoka A (2001) A weak signal for strong responses: interferon-alpha/beta revisited. Nat Rev Mol Cell Biol. 2:378–386
3. Lauer GM, Walker BD (2001) Hepatitis C virus infection. N Engl J Med. 345:41–52
4. Pitha PM et al. (2000) Introduction: interferon's connection to cancer. Semin.Cancer Biol. 10:69–72 (whole issue dedicated to IFN)
5. Goodbourn S, Didcock L, Randall RE (2000) Interferons: cell signalling, immune modulation, antiviral response and virus countermeasures. J.Gen.Virol.81:2341–2364

Interleukin-1

The interleukin-1 (IL-1) family of proteins currently comprises IL-1α, IL-1β and the IL-1 receptor antagonist (IL-1RA). The biological activities of IL-1 are shared by IL-1α and IL-1β, whereas IL-1RA is a true receptor antagonist. IL-1 is a key player in acute and chronic inflammatory diseases. Whether IL-1 has a role in normal physiology is still unresolved. IL-1 can activate a wide range of cells important in both immunity and inflammation and is a promising novel target of anti-inflammatory therapy.

▶ Inflammation
▶ Cytokines

Interleukin-2

The cytokine interleukin-2 (IL-2) represents the ultimate growth factor of activated T-lymphocytes.

▶ Immune Defense
▶ Cytokines

Intermediate Filaments

Intermediate filaments are present in most animal cells. They are composed of more than 50 proteins which are expressed in a cell-type specific manner. Their diameter is about 10 nm and thus between those of the larger microtubules and the smaller F-actin. They form scaffolds and networks in the cyto- and nucleoplasm.

▶ Cytoskeleton
▶ Cytokeratin

Internalization

Internalization is an agonist-induced endocytosis of membranous receptors which occurs in seconds to minutes. It involves the formation of receptor containing vesicles (e.g. clathrin-coated pits) and is followed by an endosomal acidification permitting dephosphorylation of the receptor and dissociation of the agonist. Internalized receptors are recycled to the cell surface or degraded in lysosomes.

▶ Tolerance and Desensitization

International Normalized Ratio (INR)

The international normalized ratio (INR) is a method to standardize reporting of the prothrombin time, using the formula, $INR = (PT_{patient}/PT_{control})^{ISI}$, where PT indicates the prothrombin times (for the patient and the laboratory control), and ISI indicates the "international sensitivity index", a value that varies depending upon the thromboplastin reagent and laboratory instrument used to initiate and detect clot formation respectively.

▶ Anticoagulants

Intracellular Transport

CONSTANZE REINHARD, FELIX T. WIELAND
Biochemie-Zentrum Heidelberg,
University Heidelberg, Heidelberg, Germany
reinhard@sun0urz.uni-heidelberg.de,
felix.wieland@urz.uni-heidelberg.de

Definition

In this review the term intracellular transport comprises both the correct targeting and the mechanism of transport of newly synthesized proteins and lipids to their destination and their retrieval from organelles and the plasma membrane to maintain the structural and functional organization of a eukaryotic cell.

▶ Protein Trafficking and Quality Control
▶ Exocytosis

Basic Mechanisms

At any given time, a typical eukaryotic cell carries out a multitude of different chemical reactions, many of them mutually incompatible. Therefore, cells have developed strategies for segregating and organizing their chemical reactions. Thus e.g.,

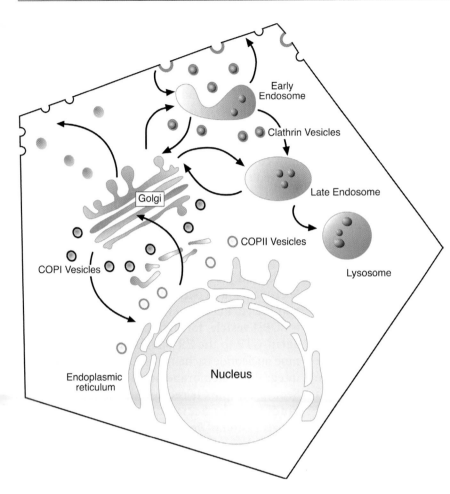

Fig. 1 Model of intracellular transport within a mammalian cell: Export from the ER to the IC occurs in COPII vesicles. Anterograde transport from the *cis-* to the *trans-*side of the Golgi is mediated by COPI vesicles. COPI vesicles are also involved in retrograde traffic from the Golgi to the ER. Sorting and transport at the exit side of the Golgi to organelles of the endocytic pathway and to the plasma membrane is mediated by clathrin vesicles. Additionally, other types of vesicles may be involved in sorting at the Golgi-exit.

multi-enzyme complexes have evolved. Of particular importance in this respect are the membrane-bounded compartments, like the nucleus, endoplasmic reticulum (ER), Golgi apparatus, lysosomes, endosomes, peroxisomes and mitochondria. The specialized functions of each organelle require distinct protein and lipid compositions. Since a cell cannot usually make these organelles from *de novo*, information is required in the organelle itself. Thus, most of the organelles are formed from pre-existing ones, which are divided during the cell-division cycle and distributed between the two daughter cells. Thereafter, organelle growth needs a supply of new lipids and proteins. Even in resting cells, lipids and proteins must be continuously delivered to organelles; some for eventual secretion from the cell, and some to replace molecules that have been degraded due to their physiological turnover.

Therefore, the problem of how to make and maintain organelles is largely one of how to direct newly synthesized lipids and proteins to their correct destinations.

The synthesis of virtually all proteins in a cell begins on ribosomes in the cytosol (except a few mitochondrial, and in the case of plants, a few chloroplast proteins that are synthesized on ribosomes inside these organelles). The fate of a protein molecule depends on its amino acid sequence, which can contain sorting signals that direct it to its corresponding organelle. Whereas proteins of mitochondria, peroxisomes, chloroplasts and of the interior of the nucleus are delivered directly from the cytosol, all other organelles receive their set of proteins indirectly via the ER. These proteins enter the so-called ▶ secretory pathway (Fig.1).

Stations of the Secretory Pathway

The journey along the secretory pathway begins with the targeting of the nascent polypeptide-chain to the ER by a hydrophobic signal sequence. This signal sequence interacts with the signal recognition particle complex and the growing polypeptide chain is translocated across the ER membrane to the ER lumen or inserted into the ER membrane via a translocation pore. On the luminal side of the ER, various chaperones associate with the polypeptide chain in order to mediate translocation and to control and support correct folding. In addition, the newly synthesized protein undergoes co- and post-translational modifications, i.e. glycosylation, disulfide bond formation and oligomerization. Once the protein is properly matured, it passes the quality control of the ER and exits the compartment via transport ▶ vesicles. Protein transport from the ER to the Golgi complex involves the ER-Golgi intermediate compartment (IC), also termed 15°C compartment or vesicular tubular clusters. Although the nature as a stable compartment of the IC is discussed controversially, it is generally accepted that the IC plays a role as a sorting station of anterograde and retrograde membrane flow. Subsequently, en route through the secretory pathway secretory proteins next enter the Golgi apparatus at the *cis*-Golgi network (CGN). They continue their passage through the several subcompartments of the Golgi (CGN, *cis*-, *medial*-, *trans*-Golgi and *trans*-Golgi network (TGN)), where proteins are subjected to various kinds of post-translational processing, e.g. remodeling of *N*- and *O*-linked oligosaccharide side chains, sialylation and tyrosine sulfatation. Once a protein has reached the exit side of the Golgi, the *trans*-Golgi network, it has to be sorted to its final destination.

Transport Through the Secretory Pathway

The various transport steps between the stations of the secretory pathway are linked by a membrane flow that is mediated by transport vesicles. In general, vesicles are formed from their donor membrane upon recruitment of coat proteins. Thereafter, the vesicles move to their target membranes where they dock. After uncoating they fuse with the target membranes. Export from the ER is the first step in the vectorial movement of cargo through the secretory pathway. The generation of vesicles from the ER is driven by the recruitment of a set of soluble proteins from the cytoplasm to the ER membrane that form a coat structure, termed COPII. Components of the COPII coat have initially been identified as Sec (Sec for secretion) mutants of the yeast *S. cerevisiae* causing defects at distinct steps of intracellular transport. This led to the identification of three soluble protein components that make up the coat of ER-derived transport vesicles: Sar1p, Sec23p complex and Sec13p complex. Sar1p is a small GTP-binding protein with a molecular mass of 21 kD that shares primary structure identity with GTPases of the Ras family. The Sec23p complex is composed of two proteins: Sec23p, a 85 kD protein and a tightly associated protein of 105 kD called Sec24p. The Sec13p complex contains the 34 kD subunit Sec13p and the 150 kD protein Sec31p. The initial step of ▶ COPII vesicle formation is the recruitment of Sar1p-GTP to the ER membrane through a guanine nucleotide exchange reaction catalyzed by the integral ER-membrane protein Sec12p. Next, the Sec23p complex is recruited, a prerequisite for binding of the Sec13p complex. As mentioned above, fusion of vesicles requires prior dissociation of the coat. Uncoating of COPII vesicles is achieved by hydrolysis of Sar1p-bound GTP, a reaction catalyzed by Sec23p, part of the coat complex. GTP hydrolysis results in the dissociation of Sar1p from the vesicle membrane followed by the removal of the coat.

Anterograde transport of material from the *cis*- to the *trans*-side of the Golgi and also retrograde transport back from the Golgi to the ER is mediated via COPI coated vesicles. *In vitro* generation of ▶ COPI vesicles from isolated Golgi membranes has allowed their biochemical characterization. Components that make up the coat of COPI vesicles are the cytosolic proteins ADP-rybosylation factor 1 (ARF1) and ▶ coatomer, a stable heteroheptameric protein complex. ARF1, like Sar1p, belongs to the family of Ras GTP-binding proteins. The coatomer complex consists of seven different subunits termed α-, β-, β'-, γ-, δ-, ε-, and ζ-COP (COP for coat protein), present in a one by one stoichiometry in both the cytosolic and the membrane-associated form of the coatomer complex. Similar to COPII, the formation of COPI-coated vesicles is initiated by recruitment from the cytoplasm to the membrane of the GTP-binding protein ARF1. Membrane binding and activation of ARF1 is triggered by the exchange of GDP for GTP, a reaction that requires catalysis by a nucleotide exchange factor. Several exchange factors for ARF1 have been characterized to date, all of them are soluble proteins found in the cytoplasm. An important difference between COPI and COPII is the GTP hydrolysis reaction needed for uncoating. While for COPII disassembly Sar1p-mediated GTP hydrolysis is activated by the coat protein Sec23p, acceleration of GTP hydrolysis in ARF1 needs the activation by ARF-specific GAPs (GTPase activating proteins) that are recruited from the cytoplasm to the membranes.

Along their route through the Golgi, secretory and membrane proteins destined for the various post-Golgi pathways are intermixed. Thus, proteins of distinct routes, i.e. the endosomal and the secretory route, are sorted into individual types of transport vesicles at the TGN. Among the best-characterized types of TGN-derived vesicles are ▶ clathrin-coated vesicles. In addition, several types of non-clathrin-coated vesicles have been identified but their specific functions remain to be characterized.

Biochemical characterization of clathrin-coated vesicles revealed that their major coat components are ▶ clathrin and various types of adaptor complexes. Clathrin assembles in triskelions that consist of three heavy chains of approximately 190 kD and three light chains of 30–40 kD. Four types of adaptor complexes have been identified to date, AP-1, AP-2, AP-3 and AP-4 (AP for adaptor protein). Whereas AP-1, AP-3 and AP-4 mediate sorting events at the TGN and/or endosomes, AP-2 is involved in endocytosis at the plasma membrane. Each adaptor complex is a heterotetrameric protein complex, and the term "adaptin" was extended to all subunits of these complexes. One complex is composed of two large adaptins (one each of $\gamma/\alpha/\delta/\epsilon$ and β1–4, respectively, 90–130 kD), one medium adaptin (μ1–4, ~50 kD), and one small adaptin (σ1–4, ~20 kD). In contrast to AP-1, AP-2 and AP-3, which interact directly with clathrin and are part of the clathrin-coated vesicles, AP-4 seems to be involved in budding of a certain type of non-clathrin-coated vesicles at the TGN.

A prerequisite for clathrin coat assembly is the recruitment to the membrane of an adaptor complex. Similar to what has been observed for the recruitment of coatomer to Golgi membranes, adaptor binding is dependent on the presence of ARF-GTP. But in contrast to COPI vesicle formation, ARF-GTP is suggested to act in a process before budding and not as a stoichiometric coat component. Other differences between COP-coated and clathrin-coated vesicles concern their uncoating mechanism. Disassembly of clathrin-coated vesicles is believed to depend on the chaperone hsc70 and on auxilin.

Membrane Proteins in Vesicle Formation and Cargo Selection

Formation of vesicles is likely to require interaction with the soluble coat components of cytoplasmic domains of certain integral membrane proteins that may serve as coat receptors. Likewise, interaction of cytoplasmic domains of membrane cargo proteins with coat components may result in their selective packaging in a certain type of transport vesicle. Sorting of soluble cargo requires involvement of transmembrane receptors which may couple sorting in the lumen of an organelle to coat assembly at the cytoplasmic surface. The expected properties of a transmembrane cargo receptor include one or more transmembrane domains, a luminal domain able to interact with cargo species, and a cytoplasmic domain that interacts with coat subunits. Further, such proteins must cycle between the donor and the acceptor organelle. Coupling of coat assembly and cargo selection is best understood for clathrin-coated vesicles. The best known example for a cargo/coat receptor is the ▶ mannose 6-phosphate receptor of TGN-derived clathrin-coated vesicles. On the luminal side, the receptor recognizes a mannose 6-phosphate signal of lysosomal hydrolases. On the cytoplasmic face, the receptor tail interacts with AP-1, thus initiating coat assembly. Sorting of membrane proteins into TGN-derived clathrin-coated vesicles has been shown to depend on a tyrosine-based motif (YXXF, where F can be replaced by a bulky hydrophobic amino acid) similar to the signal established for internalization via AP-2 at the plasma membrane. Sorting of membrane cargo into COPII pre-budding complexes was described for several proteins, and is believed to be mediated via an interaction with the Sec23p complex. For sorting of soluble cargo into retrograde COPI-coated vesicles, two types of membrane proteins are known to date that fulfil the criteria for cargo/coat receptors. One is the ▶ KDEL receptor, a multi-spanning membrane protein that mainly localizes to the Golgi and recognizes a carboxy-terminal tetrapeptide (KDEL) of soluble luminal proteins. The KDEL-sequence has been shown to serve as a retrieval signal of soluble proteins that have escaped from the ER. Another type of vesicular transmembrane proteins is referred as to the p24 family, some members of which have been found in both COPII- and COPI-coated vesicles. These type I membrane proteins share a common structural organization: a large luminal domain with the tendency to form coiled-coil structures, one membrane spanning domain, and a short cytoplasmic domain with two conserved motifs: a di-phenylalanine motif and a di-basic motif at the extreme C-terminus. p23 and p24, two members of the p24 family, were the first transmembrane proteins to be identified in COPI-coated vesicles. Both proteins are abundant in Golgi membranes and are concentrated into Golgi-derived COPI-coated vesicles where they are present in approximately stoichiometric amounts relative to ARF1 and coatomer. p23 and p24 bind directly to coatomer and cycle within the early secretory pathway. It was also shown that both proteins interact with COPII *in vitro* and that they form heterooligomeric complexes with various members of the ▶ p24-family (p25, p26 and p27). Reconstitution of COPI-coated vesicles from chemically defined liposomes revealed that p23 is part of the minimal machinery for budding of COPI-coated vesicles. The data presently available make the p24 proteins strong candidates for coat receptors.

Mechanism of Vesicle Fusion

Once a coated vesicle is formed, delivery of its cargo to the correct destination depends on the accurate and specific recognition of the target membrane and subsequent fusion. A conceptual framework for explaining how transport vesicles dock to an acceptor membrane was formulated in the ▶ SNARE hypothesis. This hypothesis states that the specificity of vesicle targeting is generated by highly specific complexes that form between membrane proteins of the vesicle (v-SNAREs) and membrane proteins of the acceptor membrane (t-SNAREs). Structural and biophysical studies have shown that the cytoplasmic domains of v- and t-SNAREs form α-helical bundles with high thermal stability. During pairing of cognate v- and t-SNAREs the cytoplasmic core domains build a rod-shaped coiled-coil complex that is composed of four α-helices. Formation of this stable complex pulls the vesicle and the target membrane in close proximity, thus providing the driving force for fusion. Thus, the SNARE-complex represents the minimal machinery needed for the fusion process, as has been shown by reconstitution in liposomes with defined proteins. In addition, specificity of SNARE-pairing is controlled by so-called tethering proteins and another class of GTP-binding proteins, the Rabs.

Pharmacological Intervention

Progress during the last few years to understanding the mechanisms that underlie transport of proteins and lipids within the secretory pathway, as well as the sequencing of the human genome revealed that many human diseases are due to defects in intracellular trafficking, like e.g. I-cell disease and familial hypercholesterolaemia. Obviously, a better understanding at the molecular level of intracellular transport within the secretory pathway, combined with increasing knowledge of the molecular basis of "transport diseases" will open ways to therapeutic interventions.

References

1. Rothman, JE, and Wieland, FT (1996) Protein sorting by transport vesicles. Science 272:227–234
2. Harter C, Reinhard C (2000) The secretory pathway: from history to the state of the art. Subcell. Biochem. 34:1–38
3. Robinson MS, Bonifacino JS (2001) Adaptor-related proteins. Curr. Opinion Cell Biol. 13:444–453
4. Rothmann JE (1994) Mechanisms of intracellular protein transport. Nature 372:55–63
5. Mellman I, Warren G (2000) The road taken: past and future foundations of membrane traffic. Cell 100:99–112
6. Nichols BJ, Pelham HR (1998) SNAREs and membrane fusion in the Golgi apparatus. Biochim. Biophys. Acta 1404:9–31

Intrathecal Space

The intrathecal space is located between the arachnoid and the pia mater of the spinal cord. It contains the cerebrospinal fluid, spinal nerves and blood vessels.

Intrinsic Efficacy

Efficacy in drug receptor theory was originally defined by R.P. Stephenson (1956) as a dimensionless quantity of excitation given to a receptor to induce a response. Furchgott (1966) refined the definition to intrinsic efficacy as the quantal unit of stimulus given to a single receptor by an agonist. Subsequent research indicates that receptors mediate behaviors in addition to physiological response (some independent of ligands such as ▶ constitutive activity). Hence a more encompassing definition of intrinsic efficacy is the property of a ligand that causes the receptor to change its behavior toward the host cell.

▶ Drug-Receptor-Interaction

Intron

An intron is a non-coding region only found in eucaryotic genes. During transcription in the nucleus, RNA is generated from both introns and exons - the coding regions - but the introns are exised by RNA splicing when mRNA is produced. During this process, the splicing machinery recognizes defined splice sites in the RNA sequence.

▶ Exon

Inverse Agonist

An inverse agonist binds with higher affinity to the inactive state of a receptor and thus alters the equilibrium in favour of there being more inactive receptors than active receptors present. This has the effect of turning off a receptor which demonstrates constitutive activity, leading to a decrease in the basal activity of the cell. An inverse agonist will block an agonist response by physically preventing the agonist from binding to the receptor, as well as turning off the basal cellular response. A lot of 'antagonists' in clinical use are in fact inverse agonists. A neutral antagonist binds equally to both states of the receptor, regardless of activation state, and therefore blocks the actions of agonists and inverse agonists alike.

▶ Drug-Receptor Interaction
▶ G-protein-coupled Receptors
▶ Transmembrane Signalling
▶ Histaminergic System

Inward Rectification

Inward rectification refers to decreased conductance upon depolarization. In classical inward rectifier potassium channels, rectification is "strong" and currents rapidly decline at membrane potentials positive to the reversal potential. In contrast, in other potassium channels rectification is "weak" and currents decline only gradually at potentials positive to the reversal potential.

▶ Inward Rectifier K^+ Channels

Inward Rectifier K$^+$ Channels

ANATOLI N. LOPATIN, COLIN G. NICHOLS
Department of Physiology, University of
Michigan, Ann Arbor andWashington University
School of Medicine, St. Louis, USA
alopatin@umich.edu, cnichols@cellbio.wustl.edu

Synonyms

Inwardly rectifying potassium channels, anomalous rectifiers, ▶ Kir channels

Definitions

Inward rectifier potassium channels, or Kir Channels: a class of potassium channels generated by the tetrameric arrangement of one-pore/two-transmembrane helix (1P/2TM) protein subunits, often associated with additional β subunits. As potassium channels, they serve to modulate cell ▶ excitability, being involved in ▶ repolarization of ▶ action potentials [see Fig. 1], setting the ▶ resting potential [Fig. 1] of the cell, and contributing to ▶ K$^+$ homeostasis.

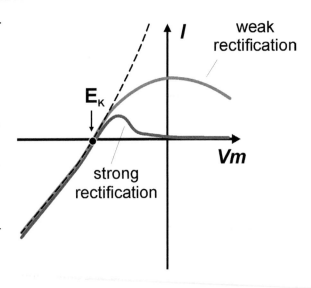

Fig. 2 High [K$^+$] inside cells relative to outside results in 'normal' rectification, whereby outward (positive by convention) potassium currents (I) when cells are depolarized (Vm = positive) are bigger than inward (negative) currents at hyperpolarized (negative) voltages. Inward or anomalous rectifiers show 'strong' or 'weak' inward rectification whereby outward currents are smaller than inward currents.

▶ Inward Rectification: decreased conductance upon depolarization. In classical inward rectifiers, rectification is "strong" and currents rapidly decline at voltages positive to the reversal potential. [Fig. 2]. In other Kir channels, rectification is "weak" and currents decline only gradually at voltages positive to the reversal potential. [Fig. 2].

▶ ATP-dependent K$^+$ Channel
▶ K$^+$ Channels
▶ Voltage-gated K$^+$ Channels

Molecular Basis and Functional Diversity of Kir Channels

Seven sub-families of Kir channels are known each sharing ~60% amino acid identity between individual members within each subfamily and ~40% identity between subfamilies [3].

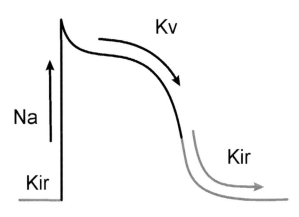

Fig. 1 The role of inward rectifier (Kir) channels in cardiac action potentials. Depolarization is generated and maintained by Na and Ca currents (iNa, iCa). Voltage-gated K currents (Kv) and Kir channels contribute to repolarization and maintenance of a negative resting potential.

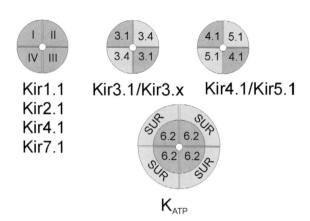

Fig. 3 Kir channels may be homo- or hetero-tetra-meric complexes, in some cases in tight association with β-subunits (e.g. the K$_{ATP}$ channel). SUR – sulfonylurea receptor.

Kir1 Subfamily

Kir1.1 (ROMK1, gene *KCNJ1*) [1] encodes a "weak" (see below) inward rectifier and is expressed predominantly in the kidney. Alternate splicing at the 5' end also generates multiple Kir1.1 splice variants, Kir1.1a (ROMK2) through Kir1.1f (ROMK6), some of which are ubiquitously expressed in various tissues, including kidney, brain, heart, liver, pancreas and skeletal muscle. In the kidney the renal Kir1.1 channels control salt reabsorption.

Kir2 Subfamily

Four distinct Kir2 subfamily members (Kir2.1-Kir2.4; *KCNJ2, KCNJ12, KCNJ4, KCNJ14*) have been cloned to date [2,3], all encoding classical "strong" inward rectifiers that differ in single channel conductance and in sensitivity to phosphorylation and other second messengers. Kir2 subfamily members are highly expressed in the heart, skeletal muscle and nervous system. The time- and voltage-dependent rectification (see below) of the expressed Kir2.x channels is virtually indistinguishable from native I$_{K1}$ channels in the heart. Kir2.1 subunits are probably the key players in classical inward rectifier current I$_{K1}$ present in atrial and ventricular myocytes while Kir2.2 and 2.3 may also contribute.

Kir3 Subfamily

Four members of the Kir3 subfamily (Kir3.1-Kir3.4: *KCNJ3, KCNJ6, KCNJ9, KCNJ5*) express G-protein activated "strong" inward rectifier ▶ K$^+$ Channels (GIRK channels) underlying G-protein coupled receptor activated currents in heart, brain, and endocrine tissues. Functional channels require co-assembly of two different subunits (Kir3.1 and Kir3.4). Several studies have provided evidence for a promiscuous coupling between the various members of the Kir3 subfamily.

Kir4 and 5 Subfamilies

These subfamilies of Kir channels (Kir4.1 and Kir4.2, *KCNJ10, KCNJ15*, Kir5.1, *KCNJ16*) are abundantly expressed in brain and kidney. Kir4.1 forms "weak" inward rectifier K channels when expressed alone, while Kir5.1 does not form homomeric channels. Co-expression of Kir4.1 and Kir5.1 subunits results in formation of channels with properties significantly different from those of homomeric Kir4.1 channels. Little is known about the physiological role of channels derived from Kir4 and Kir5 subfamilies. However, the activity of the Kir5.1/Kir4.1 heteromeric channels is very sensitive to intracellular pH and this property is conferred predominantly by the Kir5.1 subunits.

Kir6 Subfamily

Two members (Kir6.1, Kir6.2, *KCNJ8, KCNJ11*) of this subfamily encode ATP-sensitive K$^+$ channels (K$_{ATP}$) that are inhibited by intracellular ATP and activated by ADP, thereby coupling cell metabolism to excitability. K$_{ATP}$ channels are found in many tissues including ventricular and atrial cells (Kir6.2 in the cell membrane, Kir6.1 potentially in mitochondrial membranes). Functional expression of active channels requires co-expression of Kir6.x subunits with a sulfonylurea receptor (SUR1 or SUR2). K$_{ATP}$ channels display "weak" rectification, allowing substantial outward current to flow at positive potentials, and thus causing action potential shortening, or inexcitability, when activated.

Kir7 Subfamily

The only known member (Kir7.1, *KCNJ13*) is primarily expressed in brain, retinal pigment epithelium, but it is also found in a variety of other tissues, including kidney and intestine. This weakly

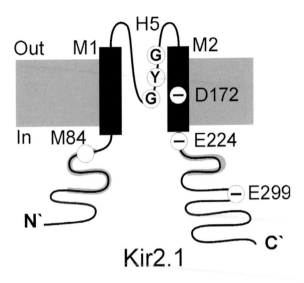

Fig. 4 Kir channel subunits consist of two transmembrane domains (M1, M2) separated by a pore loop (P-loop) that contains the signature K$^+$-selectivity sequence (-GYG-) as well as extended cytoplasmic N- and C- termini. Several residues (indicated) have been implicated in causing rectification (see text).

rectifying channel has an apparently low single channel conductance, shallow dependence on external K$^+$ and is virtually insensitive to intracellular Mg^{2+}. The exact physiological role of this channel is obscure although suggestions are made that Kir7.1 may contribute to K$^+$ recycling processes.

Molecular Structure of Kir Channels

All Kir channels are tetrameric proteins [Fig. 3] of one-pore/two-transmembrane (1P/2TM) domain subunits that equally contribute to the formation of highly selective K$^+$ channels. Most Kir channels can be assembled in functional homo tetramers while some require heteromeric assembly [Fig. 3]. For example, functional GIR K channels underlying IK$_{ACh}$ current in atria are heteromultimers of two members of Kir3 subfamily: Kir3.1 and Kir3.4. It should be noted though that only some of Kir channels rectify strongly enough to fit the definition based on the property of rectification. A feature of all K$^+$ selective channels is the signature G-Y-G sequence within the P-loop [Fig. 4] that acts

as a filter to confer high selectivity to K$^+$ ions and also contributes to single channel conductance and kinetics. Two transmembrane domains with N'- and C'-termini facing the cytoplasm flank the P-loop [Fig. 4]. It has been shown that the selectivity filter of Kir2.1 channels is stabilized by interaction of negatively charged E138 and positively charged R148 residues, which probably interact electrostatically and/or through formation of a salt bridge. These, and probably other, residues beyond the selectivity filter also play an essential role in conduction and stabilization of the pore. The assembly of the Kir2.1 channel is supported by the presence of intrasubunit disulfide bonds between highly conserved cysteine residues (at positions 122 and 154) which are absolutely required for proper channel folding, although disruption of the bond with reducing agents does not disrupt channel activity once the channel is already assembled. Scanning cysteine mutagenesis studies of relatively large stretches of N- and C-termini of Kir2.1 reveal that nearly half of them are water accessible, and potentially facing the pore, in addition to residues in the second transmembrane region. There is accumulating evidence that the overall structure of the core region of all Kir channels is very similar to that of the recently crystallized bacterial K$^+$ channel KcsA [4].

The Mechanism of Strong Inward Rectification

Inward, or 'anomalous', rectification of potassium permeability refers to increases of potassium conductance under hyperpolarization and decreases under depolarization, the effect opposite to that of 'normal' outward or delayed rectification that is seen in voltage gated potassium channels [Fig. 2]. Classical inward rectification is so strong that only small currents can be measured in the outward direction at voltages positive to the K$^+$ reversal potential (E$_K$) while large inward currents can be easily observed negative to it. This strongly voltage-dependent rectification also strongly depends on the concentration of external K$^+$ ([K$_{OUT}$]), such that increasing K$_{OUT}$ relieves the rectification, so that the mid-point voltage of rectification shifts nearly perfectly with corresponding change in E$_K$. It is now established that strong inward rectification results primarily from voltage-dependent block by intracellular organic cations called ▶ **polyamines** [3]. Of the polyamines, spermine

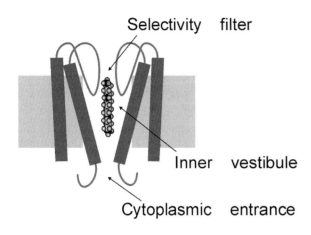

Selectivity filter

Inner vestibule

Cytoplasmic entrance

Fig. 5 Proposed 3-dimensional arrangement of the transmembrane region of inward rectifiers. Two of four subunits are indicated. The pore consists of an external selectivity filter, a central inner vestibule, and a cytoplasmic entrance. Spermine may block in the inner cavity or in the selectivity filter.

[Figs. 5, 6] and spermidine (▶ Spermine/Spermidine) are the most potent inducers of rectification although contributions of putrescine and of Mg^{2+} ions are also important. Both the steady state and the kinetic properties of rectification result from the combined action of polyamines and Mg^{2+} ions. Micromolar concentrations of spermine and spermidine are required to reproduce the degree of rectification seen in native cells. With exogenously expressed Kir channels at physiologically relevant membrane potentials, total cellular polyamine levels (10–10,000 μM) are clearly sufficient [3].

The degree of rectification varies greatly among members of the Kir superfamily and is fundamental to their respective functional roles. Kir2 and Kir3 encode classical "strong" inward rectifier channels, while other members encode channels with variably "milder" or "weaker" rectification [Fig. 2]. For example, because of mild rectification of the K_{ATP} channel its activation causes considerable shortening of cardiac action potential, thus reducing entry of Ca^{2+} through voltage-dependent Ca^{2+} channels and hence conserving ATP under conditions of metabolic stress. Conversely, the strong inward rectification of Kir2.1 channels underlying I_{K1} current in the heart

results in very small currents flowing through these channels during depolarization phase of action potential while increased conductance around ▶ resting potential leads to its stabilization [5].

Structural Elements of Inward Rectification

Each Kir subunit consists of two transmembrane helices (M1, M2), with a pore-forming selectivity filter linking them, and cytoplasmic N' and C'-termini [Fig. 4]. Based on the crystal structure of a distantly related bacterial K channel [4], the channel is proposed to be formed as a tetrameric arrangement of these subunits, surrounding an external selectivity filter, an inner vestibule and a cytoplasmic entrance to the pore [Fig. 5]. Aspartate 172 located in the M2 region of Kir2.1 was the first residue implicated in the classical rectification of these channels and is sometimes referred to as the 'rectification controller'. Later, E224, residing in the C terminus of Kir2.1, was also shown to contribute to polyamine-induced ▶ rectification [3]. Neutralization of both of these charges transforms the strongly rectifying Kir2.1 channel into one that is nearly insensitive to blockage by polyamines and Mg^{2+}. Other cytoplasmic residues were also shown to be important for channel blockage by intracellular cations. For example, M84 and E299 in Kir2.1 situated beyond the TM domains are also involved in controlling rectification. At present the question about the location(s) of the binding sites for polyamines remains unanswered. While one spermine molecule is probably required to completely block the channel, either within the inner vestibule or perhaps within the selectivity filter itself, there have been reports that the Kir pore region may be 'unprecedentedly wide' allowing simultaneous binding of three Mg^{2+} ions or 3 polyamine molecules. Reconciliation of conflicting interpretations can probably be achieved by assuming that gating of Kir channels may involve substantial conformational changes including helix rotations and translational movements similar to those observed in the related bacterial KcsA channel [4]. The selectivity filter of Kir2.1 is probably the best candidate for binding of polyamines. Despite the relatively large size of the spermine molecule (~20 Å long) [Fig. 3], its diameter is close to that of a dehydrated K$^+$ion, thus potentially allowing its head

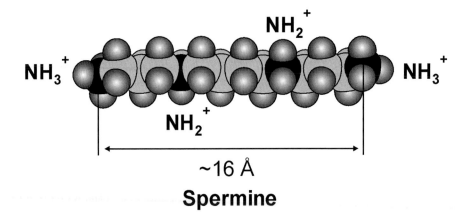

~ 16 Å

Spermine

Fig. 6 Spermine (amino-propyl-amino-butyl-amino-propyl amine) is a long linear naturally occurring polyamine containing four spaced positively charged (at normal pH) amines. Although 16 Å long, the molecule is only about 3 Å wide, similar to a dehydrated potassium ion.

amine group to 'squeeze' into the selectivity filter and block ion flow [Fig. 6]. Spermine may also permeate Kir channels and can clearly permeate as well as block other non-selective cationic channels, consistent with such an interpretation.

Pharmacology of Kir Channels

Voltage-dependent block by external Ba^{2+} and Cs$^+$ ions, and insensitivity to the Kv channel blocker tetraethyl ammonium (TEA) have been the classical tools to examine Kir channel activity. Recently, the honeybee venom tertiapin has been found to be an effective blocker of certain (Kir1, Kir3) inward rectifier subfamily members. The tight association of Kir6 family members with SUR subunits endows K$_{ATP}$ channels with a rich pharmacology: Channel activity is very specifically inhibited by sulfonylurea drugs such as tolbutamide and glibenclamide, and is activated by a broad class of 'potassium channel opening' (KCO) drugs such as pinacidil and diazoxide.

A potent antiarrhythmic drug RP58866 has been shown to block IKACh (encoded by Kir3.x members) and I_{K_1} (encoded by Kir2.x members) currents in the heart in low micromolar range. Unfortunately, RP58866 does not discriminate well between Kir and other K channels (for example, underlying ▶ Ito and ▶ Ikr) and thus did not get

much attention as a selective blocker for Kir channels.

Known Diseases (Channelopathies) Resulting from Kir Channel Mutations

Several ▶ chanelopathies resulting from mutations in Kir channels are known.

Kir1.1. ▶ Bartter syndrome. Several mutations in the core region as well as in the N' and C' terminus of Kir1.1 are found in patients with hyperprostaglandin E syndrome (HPS; renal disorder resulting from impairment of tubular reabsorption), an antenatal form of Bartter syndrome. Some of these mutations result in the loss of function of Kir1.1 channels causing impaired renal K$^+$ secretion and NaCl reabsorption.

Kir2.1. Andersen syndrome. Dominantly inherited LQT syndrome, a disorder of cardiac action potential ▶ repolarization is usually assigned to mutations in cardiac Na$^+$ or voltage-gated K$^+$channels. Recently, it has been found that mutations in Kir2.1 cause Andersen's syndrome, a rare disease characterized by periodic paralysis, cardiac arrhythmias and dysmorphic features. Two mutations in Kir2.1 associated with Andersen syndrome were found to cause dominant negative suppression of the wild type Kir2.1 channels when expressed in *Xenopus* oocytes thus mimicking the effects of the Kir2.1 gene knock-out which is characterized by prolonged QT interval.

Kir3.2 Weaver mouse. The Weaver mouse is a mutant mouse with cerebellar degeneration and motor dysfunction resulting from a serine for glycine substitution in the -GYG- sequence of the K selectivity filter of Kir3.2. G-protein activated K conductances are abolished in the cerebellar neurons, leading to Ca^{2+} overload and cell death.

Kir6.2/SUR Persistent Hyperinsulinemic Hypoglycemia of Infancy (PHHI) (▶ ATP-dependent K^+ Channel). Lowered blood glucose normally causes decreased ATP/ADP ratios in the pancreatic islet β-cells, causing the opening of K_{ATP} channels, hyperpolarization, inhibition of Ca^{2+} entry and cessation of insulin secretion. In PHHI, K_{ATP} channel mutations lead to abolition of activity and hence maintained depolarization and maintained Ca^{2+} entry and insulin secretion. Many mutations in the SUR subunit abolish ADP activation of channels, but point mutations in Kir6.2 are implicated in abolition of channel activity in some cases.

References

1. Ho K, Nichols CG, Lederer WJ, Lytton J, Vassilev PM, Kanazirska MV and Hebert SC (1993) Cloning and expression of an inwardly-rectifying, ATP-regulated potassium channel. Nature 362:31–38
2. Kubo Y, Baldwin TJ, Jan YN, Jan LY (1993) Primary structure and functional expression of a mouse inward rectifier potassium channel. Nature 362:127–33
3. Nichols CG and Lopatin AN (1997) Inward rectifier potassium channels: Review of Physiology 59:171–191
4. Doyle DA, Morais CJ, Pfuetzner RA, Kuo A, Gulbis JM, Cohen SL, Chait BT, MacKinnon R (1998) The structure of the potassium channel: molecular basis of K+ conduction and selectivityy 280(5360):69–77
5. Lopatin AN and Nichols CG (2001) Inward Rectifiers in the Heart: An update on IK1. Journal of Molecular and Cellular Cardiology 33:625–638

Inwardly Rectifying K^+ Channel Family

There are seven subfamilies of the inwardly rectifying potassium (Kir) channel family (Kir1.0, Kir2.0, Kir3.0, Kir4.0, Kir5.0, Kir6.0, Kir7.0) with two transmembrane domains, M1 and M2, linked by a pore loop (the H5 region) which is critical for K^+ ion selectivity. The asparagine residue in M2 is critical for the rectification property.

▶ ATP-dependent Potassium Channels
▶ Inward Rectifier Potassium Channels

Iodide

▶ Antithyroid Drugs

Iodine

▶ Antithyroid Drugs

Ion Channels

Ion channels are proteins which span the plasma membrane and can be opened by transmembrane voltage changes (voltage-dependent ion currents) or by binding of a neurotransmitter. Ion channels which are selective for Na^+ or Ca^{2+} ions cause excitation, ion channels with selectivity for Cl^- or K^+ usually cause inhibition of cells.

Ion channels are often multimeric and are regulated by a wide variety of mechanisms (e.g. ligand binding, voltage changes, phosphorylation).

Ionic Contrast Media

Ionic contrast media are triiodobenzene derivatives carrying a negative electrical charge, water soluble only as sodium or meglumine (an organic cation similar to glucosamine) salts.

▶ Radiocontrast Agents

Ionotropic (channel-linked) Receptors

Ionotropic (channel-linked) receptors are membrane receptors which are directly coupled to an ion channel, e.g. receptors on which fast neurotransmitters act such as the nicotinic acetylcholine receptor, γ-aminobutyric acid$_A$ (GABA$_A$) receptor, N-methyl-D-aspartate (NMDA) receptors, α-amino-3-hydroxy-5-methyl-4-isoxazole propionic acid (AMPA) receptors and P2X-receptors.

▶ Ionotropic Glutamate Receptors
▶ Transmembrane Signalling

Ionotropic Glutamate Receptors

AXEL H. MEYER, ELKE C. FUCHS, HANNAH MONYER
Interdisziplinäres Zentrum für
Neurowissenschaften (IZN),
Heidelberg, Germany
axmeyer@urz.uni-hd.de,
E.Fuchs@urz.uni-heidelberg.de,
monyer@urz-hd.de

Definition

Most neurons in the central nervous system are stimulated by L-▶ glutamate, the major excitatory amino acid in the brain. The postsynaptic actions of this neurotransmitter are mediated by two categories of glutamate receptors: the ionotropic gluta-mate receptors that directly gate channels and the metabotropic glutamate receptors that indirectly gate channels via second messengers. The ionotropic glutamate receptors can be further subdivided into N-methyl-D-aspartate (NMDA) receptors (▶ NMDA receptor) and non-NMDA receptors, with AMPA (L-α-amino-3-hydroxy-5-methyl-4-isoxazolepropionic acid) and ▶ kainate receptors constituting the latter group (1,2). These three major subtypes of ionotropic glutamate receptors are named according to their selective agonists NMDA, AMPA and kainate. These receptors mediate most of the fast excitatory neurotransmission in the brain.

NMDA- and AMPA receptors (▶ AMPA receptor) are co-localized in the postsynaptic membrane of excitatory synapses. Glutamate released from presynaptic terminals binds to both types of receptors. Upon activation by glutamate, AMPA receptors generate the large early component of an excitatory postsynaptic current (EPSC) because of their rapid ▶ gating kinetics. This synaptic current is mainly generated by Na$^+$ and K$^+$, but not Ca^{2+} ions, since AMPA receptors in excitatory neurons are usually impermeable to Ca^{2+}. In contrast to this, NMDA receptors have relatively slow gating kinetics and contribute to the late component of the EPSC. The NMDA receptors are permeable for Na$^+$ and K$^+$ as well as Ca^{2+} ions and require extracellular glycine as a cofactor for activation. Most importantly, this activation is not only dependent on the presence of the agonist, but also depends on the membrane voltage. Therefore, the receptor is not involved in generation of the early component of the EPSC after the binding of glutamate. The channel gets activated only when the binding of glutamate plus the co-agonist glycine and depolarization of the membrane occur at the same time. This voltage dependence is due to extracellular Mg^{2+}. At resting membrane potential extracellular Mg^{2+} binds tightly to a site in the pore and blocks the channel. Only at depolarized membrane potentials, which are generated by the AMPA receptors, Mg^{2+} is expelled from the pore by electrostatic repulsion, thereby lifting the Mg^{2+} block and Na$^+$, K$^+$ and Ca^{2+} cations can cross the channel. Most neurons express both NMDA and AMPA receptors. However, the EPSC generated at resting membrane potential is mainly generated by activation of AMPA receptors. NMDA receptors do not contribute significantly to the EPSC since at membrane resting potential Mg^{2+} is blocking the channel. Only with increasing membrane depolarization NMDA receptors contribute to the EPSC, since Mg^{2+} is removed and ions flow through the channel.

Whereas the role of AMPA and NMDA receptors in fast synaptic transmission is well characterized, only few examples demonstrating synaptic responses due to kainate receptor activation are known so far.

▶ Table appendix: Receptor Proteins
▶ Metabotropic Glutamate Receptors

Basic Characteristics

Sequence homologies and sometimes similarity in gene structure suggest a common evolutionary origin for all ionotropic glutamate receptors. The cloning of the ionotropic glutamate receptor genes revealed that NMDA, AMPA and kainate receptor subunits are encoded by at least six gene families (a single family for AMPA receptors, two for kainate, and two for NMDA receptors).

The primary structure of the cloned receptor subunit genes revealed prominent structural similarities between NMDA, AMPA and kainate receptors (Fig. 1). The transmembrane topology of these receptors is very different from that of other ionotropic channels. Members of other ionotropic receptor families, which are activated by acetylcholine, GABA (γ-aminobutyric acid) or glycine, contain four transmembrane segments. In contrast to these, the ionotropic glutamate receptor subunits contain three transmembrane domains (M1, M3 and M4) and a cytoplasm-facing membrane loop (M2), which connects the transmembrane domains M1 and M3 and forms the channel pore. Key amino acids in the M2 segment are responsible for the differences in ion selectivity displayed by the various receptor subunits. Two regions of the glutamate receptors are extracellularly located: the amino-terminus and the region between M3 and M4, which are involved in building the ligand-binding site. The carboxy-terminal part after M4 reaches into the cytoplasm of the cell and is important for intracellular modifications like phosporylation or interaction with cytoplasmic proteins.

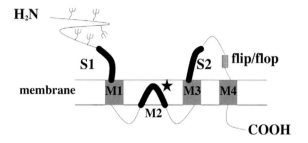

Fig. 1 Schematic structure of a ionotropic glutamate receptor subunit. The three transmembrane domains M1, M3 and M4 are shown as grey boxes, the membrane loop M2 forms the channel pore. The star indicates the position of key amino acids regulating the ion selectivity, e.g. the Q/R for AMPA, N for NMDA receptors. S1 and S2 designate the two ligand-binding domains. The alternatively spliced flip/flop exon occurs in AMPA receptors and is located extracellulary. Potential glycosilation sites are shown as trees in the N-terminal region.

Both AMPA and NMDA receptors are multimeric, probably tetrameric, assemblies of various molecularly distinct subunits, giving rise to large receptor diversity. For AMPA receptors this is achieved by assembling the receptor from four types of subunits, termed GluR (glutamate receptor)-A, -B, -C and –D (in an alternative nomenclature GluR1, GluR2, GluR3 and GluR4), with additional molecular diversity generated by ▶ RNA editing at the glutamine/ arginine (Q/R) and arginine/ glycine (R/G) site as well as alternative splicing of the flip-flop module. NMDA receptors are assembled from NR1 subunits and NR2A, B, C or D subunits. Several splice variants have been identified for the NR1 subunits, and the NR3 subunit, that has been identified recently, appears to be part of a glycine-gated channel. Kainate receptors are formed by subunits that can be divided into two subfamilies: the first subfamily contains the subunits GluR5, GluR6 and GluR7, whereas the second subfamily comprises KA1 and KA2. All subunits of the first group can form functional channels, whereas the subunits of the second group do not form homomeric channels. Several splice variants have been identified for the GluR5 and GluR7 subunits. This large number of combinatorial possibilities accounts for a considerable molecular diversity of glutamate receptor channels.

Recombinant expression of the AMPA receptor subunits has shown that homomeric AMPA receptors assembled from different subunits are different in a number of characteristics. These are mostly determined by the GluR-B subunit. Receptors formed from GluR-B subunits show low Ca^{2+} permeability whereas receptors assembled from GluR-A, -C and -D subunits are highly Ca^{2+} permeable. A single amino acid difference in the pore-forming segment M2 has been identified as the molecular determinant of the subunit-specific difference in Ca^{2+} permeability. Whereas the GluR-B subunit contains a positively charged arginine (R), the GluR-A, -C and -D subunits contain a neutral glutamine residue (Q) at this position. This amino acid exchange at the Q/R site is sufficient to abolish the permeability to Ca^{2+}, possibly through electrostatic repulsion, indicating that the Q/R site is the main determinant of the Ca^{2+} permeability in recombinant AMPA receptors. In native AMPA receptors, which are heteromeric assemblies, the Ca^{2+} permeability of recombinant receptors is determined by the GluR-B(R) subunits. Therefore strong differences in Ca^{2+} permeability can be observed between different cell types (1). Excitatory neurons strongly express GluR-B(R), which leads to the formation of Ca^{2+} impermeable AMPA receptors. In contrast, inhibitory neurons express the GluR-B(R) subunit to a low extent and therefore contain AMPA receptors that are highly permeable to Ca^{2+} ions.

Interestingly, the genomic sequences of all AMPA receptor subunits contain a Q codon for this position and the R codon is selectively introduced into the GluR-B pre-mRNA by RNA editing (3). Additionally, the Q/R site is a critical determinant of current ▶ rectification and single-channel conductance. In recombinant AMPA receptors, GluR-B(R)-containing channels show a linear current-voltage relation (I-V), whereas it is inwardly or doubly rectifying in AMPA receptors that only contain GluR-A, -C or -D subunits. It has been shown that this current rectification is due to a voltage-dependent block by intracellular ▶ polyamines, such as spermine or spermidine, which block GluR-B(R)-free but not GluR-B(R)-containing AMPA receptors. The physiological significance of this block is unknown, but it may act

similar to the extracellular Mg^{2+} block of NMDA receptor channels. But whereas a single GluR-B(R) subunit per channel is possibly sufficient to abolish Ca^{2+} permeability, several GluR-B(R) subunits are necessary to suppress polyamine sensitivity. Another basic property of the AMPA receptor that is determined by the Q/R site is the single-channel conductance. If the receptor contains a GluR-B(R) subunit, it has a two- to three-fold lower single-channel conductance. Each AMPA receptor subunit exists as either a flip or a flop variant, which is determined by mutually exclusive splicing of an exon encoding a domain of 38 amino acids. Alternative splicing and editing of the GluR-B, -C and –D subunit at the R/G site influences receptor deactivation, desensitization and recovery from ▶ desensitization. The flip-flop module as well as the R/G site is probably located in the extracellular loop between M3 and M4, which is thought to be part of the agonist-binding site. This suggests relationships between agonist binding and gating properties of the receptor.

Functional NMDA receptors are heteromeric channels, which are composed of a principal NR1 subunit and modulatory NR2 subunits (NR2A, -B, -C and D). They differ from AMPA receptors in several properties. Some of the most important properties are requirement for glycine for activation, the very high permeability for Ca^{2+}, the voltage-dependent block by extracellular Mg^{2+} and the slow gating kinetics. NMDA receptors require not only glutamate for activation, but also glycine as a co-agonist. In the receptor the binding site for glutamate is generated by the NR2 subunit whereas the binding site for glycine is supplied by the NR1 subunit.

In contrast to AMPA receptors, NMDA receptor channels display a prominent Ca^{2+} permeability, which is largely independent of the subunit composition. It has been shown by mutational analysis that the Ca^{2+} permeability of recombinant NMDA receptors is dependent on a residue at a position equivalent to the Q/R site of AMPA subunits. Both NR1 and NR2 subunits contain an asparagine (N) residue at this position. Replacing this N with an R within the NR1 subunit led to the formation of NMDA receptors with a strongly reduced Ca^{2+} permeability, whereas exchanging N for Q in the NR2 subunit had only a small effect, indicating that the N site of the NR1 subunit is the main determinant of the Ca^{2+} permeability of recombinant NMDA receptors. The situation is more complex for the other important property of the NMDA receptor, the extracellular Mg^{2+} block. Mutational analysis has revealed that the two residues downstream of the Q/R/N site are important for the control of the Mg^{2+} block. Furthermore, differences in Mg^{2+} sensitivity in the different NR1-NR2 combinations are generated at multiple locations throughout the subunit, including M1, the M1/M2 linker and the M4 segment.

Another characteristic distinguishing NMDA from AMPA receptors is the slow gating kinetics. Whereas recombinant AMPA receptors display deactivation time constants in the range of a few milliseconds, deactivation time constants for recombinant NMDA receptors are in the range of hundreds of milliseconds up to seconds, depending on which NR2 subunit is used to form the receptor. Desensitization of NMDA receptors is more complex than of AMPA receptors. At least three different forms have been described, all of which are mediated by the NR2 subunit.

The two kainate receptor subunits GluR5 and GluR6 undergo post-transcriptional modification similar to AMPA receptors. These two subunits also contain a Q/R site that is modified by RNA editing (3). The Q/R site seems to have a strong influence on the functional properties of kainate receptors, similar to what has been observed in AMPA receptors. The GluR6(Q) subunit shows strong inward rectification whereas GluR6(R) does not rectify. And, like in AMPA receptors, the inward rectification of GluR6(Q) channels is most likely due to blocking of the channel by intracellular polyamines. But in contrast to AMPA receptors, where the GluR-B subunit is almost completely Q/R site-edited, significant proportions of the kainate subunits remain unedited. No editing occurs on the KA1 and KA2 subunit mRNAs, which carry a Q at the Q/R site. Editing of the Q/R site has a strong influence on single-channel conductance. Homomeric channels formed by edited subunits have a smaller single-channel conductance than homomeric channels formed by unedited subunits or heteromeric channels containing unedited subunites. Such a larger single-channel conductance for unedited receptors compared to edited receptors has also been observed for AMPA receptors. Desensitization and recovery from desensiti-

zation are different compared to other glutamate receptors. Whereas desensitization of kainate receptors is very fast, recovery from desensitization is very slow.

Drugs

Changes in the physiological function of glutamate are thought to contribute to the pathogenesis of neurological diseases. Derivatives of quinoxaline-2,3-diones have long been shown to have an antagonistic effect on AMPA, kainate and NMDA receptor channels (4). Representative examples of this group acting on AMPA receptors are 6-cyano-7-nitroquinoxaline-2,3-dione (CNQX) and 2,3-dihydroxy-6-nitro-7-sulfamoylbenzo(f)quinoxinaline (NBQX). In addition to being glycine-site antagonists for NMDA receptors they have also been shown to be competitive antagonists for AMPA and kainate receptors, with a much higher affinity for AMPA and kainate receptors than for the glycine binding-site of the NMDA receptors. The advent of these compounds allowed the study of the mechanism of fast synaptic transmission by AMPA receptors as well as of their potential in neuroprotection. But due to their nephrotoxic side effects and their poor solubility in water they are of limited therapeutic importance.

NMDA receptors play key roles not only in synaptic plasticity, but also in neurological diseases such as epilepsy and neurodegeneration. Their ability to participate in excitotoxic events is due to the high Ca^{2+} permeability, their high affinity for glutamate and their relative lack of desensitization. This has prompted extensive research for selective NMDA receptor antagonists (4). Different types of antagonists have been developed, in part acting on different parts of the receptor. Compounds such as dizocilpine (MK-801), aptiganel, phencyclidine and ketamine are activity-dependent channel blockers. They need channel opening in order to bind to and block the receptor. Therefore, they are noncompetitive antagonists. Antagonists of the glutamate- and glycine-recognition site have also been developed. Antagonists against the glycine-recognition site such as kynurenic acid are of special interest because glycine is a co-agonist at the NMDA receptor, but glutamate acts as the neurotransmitter. In contrast, glycine plays a more modulatory role, since it is always present in the extracellular fluid. Therefore, these antagonists would limit the level of NMDA receptor activation, but still allow for a certain physiological activation. Another approach taken is the development of subunit-selective compounds. One compound of this group of antagonists is ifenprodil. It is selective for the NR2B subunit and has a much lower affinity on receptors containing NR2A, C or D subunits. The action of ifenprodil is not only subunit-specific, but also state-dependent. It binds to the activated and desensitized receptor with a higher affinity than to a receptor without a bound ligand, in this way exerting a stronger blockade on receptors continuously activated in a disease state whereas leaving normal fast synaptic transmission largely unaffected.

Antagonists selective for kainate receptors are not available yet. The non-NMDA receptor antagonist 6-cyano-7-nitroquinoxaline-2,3-dione (CNQX) blocks AMPA as well as kainate receptors. Nevertheless, compounds like GYKI 53655, which acts as a non-competitive antagonist of AMPA receptors and completely blocks AMPA receptor function at certain concentrations at which no antagonistic effect on kainate receptors is discernible, has been used to demonstrate the kainate receptor-mediated currents in neurons.

References

1. Monyer, H., Jonas, P., Rossier, J. (1999) Molecular determinants controlling functional properties of AMPARs and NMDARs in the mammalian CNS. Chapter 9; Ionotropic glutamate receptors in the CNS. Springer Verlag
2. Lerma, J. (1999) Kainate receptors. Chapter 8; Ionotropic glutamate receptors in the CNS. Springer Verlag
3. Seeburg, P.H., Higuchi, M., Sprengel, R. (1998) RNA editing of glutamate receptor channels: Mechanism and physiology. Brain Res. Brain Res. Rev. 26:217–219
4. Kemp, J.A., Kew, J.N.C., Gill, R. (1999) NMDA receptor antagonists and their potential as neuroprotective agents. Chapter 16; Ionotropic glutamate receptors in the CNS. Springer Verlag

IPC

▶ Ischemic Preconditioning

IPSP

An inhibitory postsynaptic potential is a local hyperpolarizing potential at a postsynaptic membrane, which is elicited by the release of an inhibitory neurotransmitter via an inhibitory postsynaptic current.

▶ GABAergic System

IRAG

IRAG is an inositol 1,4,5-triphosphate (IP_3) receptor-associated cGMP kinase substrate of 130 kD, that is present in all smooth muscles and platelets. Its phosphorylation decreases calcium release from intracellular IP_3-sensitive stores.

▶ Smooth Muscle Tone Regulation

Irreversible Antagonists

According to ▶ Michaelis-Menten kinetics, ligands have affinity for receptors determined by their rate of offset from the binding domain divided by their rate of onset to the binding domain. Reversible ligands occupy different proportions of receptor sites according to this ratio and the concentration present in the receptor compartment. Irreversible ligands have negligible rates of offset (i.e. once the ligand binds to the receptor it essentially stays there) therefore receptor occupancy does not achieve a steady-state but rather increases with increasing time of exposure of the receptors to the ligand. Thus, once a receptor is occupied by an irreversible antagonist, it remains inactivated throughout the course of the experiment.

▶ Affinity
▶ Drug-Receptor-Interaction

Irritable Bowel Syndrome

Irritable bowel syndrome (IBS) is an exceedingly common condition in all societies, characterized by abdominal discomfort or pain in association with altered bowel habit or incomplete stool evacuation, bloating and constipation or diarrhoea. easily go undetected and do not show up with common tests such as blood tests or x-rays.. The estimated prevalence in the community is about 10%. Irritable bowel syndrome and its variants, collectively called functional gastrointestinal disorders, constitute 40-50% of all the patients seen by gastroenterologists in Western countries.

▶ Serotoninergic System

Ischemic Preconditioning

IPC is the endogenous cellular protective mechanism in the heart by which brief periods of ischemia induce protection against infarction due to subsequent longer periods of ischemia.

▶ ATP-dependent Potassium Channels

Islet Amyolid Peptide

Amylin

Isoform

Multiple forms of a protein, that may be encoded by different genes or by a single gene whose transcript is alternatively spliced, are called isoforms.

Isoprenoid

Isoprenoids are intermediates and products of the biosynthetic pathway that starts with mevalonate and ends with cholesterol and other sterols.

Ito

Ito is a component of the outward potassium current in cardiac myocytes. Ito stands for transient (t) outward (o) current (I). Ito is characterized by relatively fast activation and inactivation and contributes to a fast phase of action potential repolarization.

▶ Inward Rectifier K^+ Channels

JAK-STAT Pathway

Thomas Meyer, Uwe Vinkemeier
Forschungsinstitut für Molekulare
Pharmakologie, Berlin-Buch, Germany
meyer@fmp-berlin.de,
vinkemeier@fmp-berlin.de

Definition

The Janus kinase-signal transducer and activator of transcription (JAK-STAT) signaling pathway is activated in response to a large number of ▶ cytokines, hormones, and growth factors. As their name implies, the STAT proteins exhibit the dual function of transducing signals from the cell surface into the nucleus as well as activating transcription of target genes, thus converting extracellular stimuli to a wide range of appropriate cellular responses. STATs have been identified as important regulators of a multitude of cellular processes, such as immune response, antiviral protection, and proliferation.

▶ Cytokines
▶ Tyrosine Kinases
▶ MAP Kinase Cascades

Basic Characteristics

The JAK-STAT pathway is widely used by members of the cytokine receptor superfamily. Upon ligand binding and oligomerization of the cognate receptor chains, the receptor-associated JAKs themselves become tyrosine phosphorylated and consecutively phosphorylate critical tyrosine residues on the cytoplasmic domain of the receptors, thereby generating docking sites for STAT proteins and other intracellular signaling molecules. The STATs are recruited to specific phospho-tyrosine-containing motifs located in the cytoplasmic part of the receptor via their Src-homology-2 (SH2) domain and in turn are phosphorylated by activated JAKs at a single tyrosine residue in their C-terminus. Tyrosine ▶ phosphorylation causes the homo- or heterodimerization of STAT molecules by virtue of reciprocal SH2-phospho-tyrosine interactions. The dimeric STATs are capable of binding to nonameric palindromes with relaxed sequence specificity in the promoter regions of cytokine-inducible genes, termed GAS sites, to regulate gene expression. An unidentified ▶ tyrosine phosphatase located in the nucleus dephosphorylates STAT molecules.

Physiological Functions of JAKs

The mammalian JAK family of protein tyrosine kinases consists of 4 members (JAK1, JAK2, JAK3 and TYK2), which are characterized by the possession of a kinase and an adjacent pseudokinase domain. JAKs have a molecular mass of approximately 130 kD and are composed of seven JAK homology domains. The essential role of JAKs in mediating signal transduction via members of the cytokine receptor superfamily became apparent from studies of knockout mice. Targeted disruption of the mouse JAK1 gene results in perinatal lethality, obviously caused by defective neural function and altered lymphoid development. JAK2-deficient mice exhibit an embryonic lethal phenotype caused by a block in definite erythropoiesis but show intact lymphoid development, demonstrating the obligatory and nonredundant roles of JAKs in cytokine-induced biological

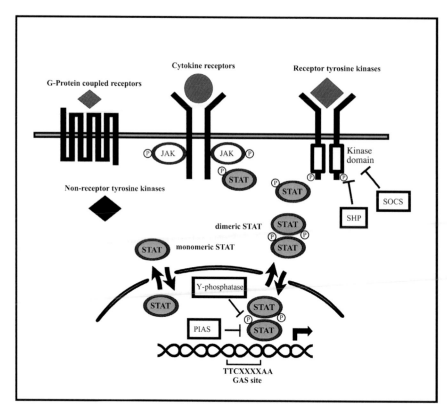

Fig. 1 Activating and inhibitory mechanisms of the JAK-STAT-pathway.

responses. Mutant mice lacking JAK3 are viable but display severe defects in both cellular and humoral immune responses with profound reduction in mature B and T cells, resembling the clinical symptoms of patients suffering from an autosomal-recessive form of severe combined immunodeficiency in which inactivating mutations in the JAK3 gene have been identified.

Roles of STAT Proteins in Cytokine-inducible and Constitutive Gene Induction

In mammals, seven different members encoded by distinct genes have been identified, all of which are activated by a distinct set of cytokines. Diversity in signaling is provided by variants of STAT proteins derived from either alternative splicing of RNA transcripts or proteolytic processing (e.g. STATs 1, 3, 4, and 5) and the ability of certain STATs to form both homodimers and heterodimers with each other. In response to ▶ interferon-γ monomeric STAT1 dimerizes, while upon interferon-α stimulation a heterotrimeric complex consisting of STAT1 and STAT2 with associated p48 is formed, known as the ISGF3 ▶ transcription factor. Major

structural features in STAT proteins are the N-terminal region involved in cooperative DNA binding of multiple STAT dimers, the central DNA-binding domain, the dimerization region containing the SH2 domain and the site of tyrosine phosphorylation, and the C-terminal transcriptional transactivation domain. Phosphorylation of a critical serine residue within the transactivation domain is necessary for maximal transcriptional activity of some STAT family members.

STAT1 knockout mice exhibit selective signaling defects in their response to interferon, including an impaired expression of MHC class II, complement protein C3, the MHC class II transactivating protein CIITA, interferon regulatory factor-1, and guanylate-binding protein 1. STAT3 activated through binding of IL-6, leptin, EGF, PDGF, LIF, or other ligands to their cognate receptors appears to have important roles in preventing apoptosis and promoting proliferative processes. A deficiency in STAT3 causes embryonic lethality in mice, indicating the essential role of STAT3 in growth regulation, embryonic development and organogenesis. STAT4 is activated in T cells in response to IL-12 and stimulates the development of T_H1 cells. The two ubiquitously expressed STAT5 proteins (STAT5a and 5b) are encoded by distinct genes and share more than 90% sequence identity. They are activated by many growth stimulatory ▶ cytokines, including interleukins, ▶ GM-CSF, ▶ GH, ▶ prolactin, ▶ EGF, as well as ▶ erythropoietin, and exert critical roles in antiapoptosis and proliferation. STAT6 functions in response to IL-4 and IL-13 signaling to induce T_H2 cell development, CD23 and MHC class II expression, immunoglobulin class switching, and B- and T-cell proliferation.

Originally discovered as DNA-binding proteins that mediate interferon signaling, recent data demonstrated that STAT1 can also exert constitutive functions in the nucleus, which do not require STAT activation with tyrosine phosphorylation. Cells lacking STAT1 are resistant to apoptotic cell death induced by tumor necrosis factor due to an inefficient expression of caspase genes, while reintroduction of STAT1 in these cells restores protease expression and sensitivity to apoptosis. For the transcription of certain target genes a phosphorylation of the critical tyrosine residue 701 is not necessary, suggesting that unphosphorylated STAT1 can also bind to DNA. Recent data indicate that unphosphorylated STAT1 can either positively or negatively regulate the constitutive expression of a wide range of different genes. It was shown that tyrosine phosphorylated and unphosphorylated STAT1 molecules shuttle between the cytoplasm and the nucleus via independent pathways to distinct sets of target genes.

Besides the cytokine receptors that lack intrinsic kinase activity but have associated JAK kinases, STAT proteins can be activated by a variety of G-protein coupled receptors and growth factor receptors with intrinsic tyrosine kinase activity (for example EGF, PDGF, CSF-1, and angiotensin receptor). Increasing evidence suggests a critical role for STAT family members in oncogenesis and aberrant cell proliferation. Constitutively activated STATs have been found in many transformed cell lines and a wide variety of human tumor entities. Numerous non-receptor tyrosine kinases and viral oncoproteins, such as v-Src, v-Abl, v-Sis, and v-Eyk, have been identified to induce DNA-binding activity of STAT proteins.

Mechanisms negatively regulating the JAK-STAT pathway have been identified. Besides the dominant-negative effects of naturally occurring STAT variants lacking the transactivation domain, ▶ PIAS proteins (protein inhibitor of activated STAT) have been shown to interact with STATs and to suppress their DNA-binding activity. The ▶ SOCS proteins (suppressor of cytokine signaling), also named as CIS (cytokine inducible src homology 2-domain containing protein), JAB (JAK-binding protein) or SSI (STAT-induced STAT inhibitor), are induced by cytokine signaling and act in a negative feedback loop to inhibit JAK kinase activity. Another important negative regulatory mechanism involves the recruitment of tyrosine phosphatases containing tandem SH2 domains (SHP-1 and SHP-2) to the intracytoplasmic portion of receptor complexes, where they dephosphorylate and thus inhibit JAK activity.

Pharmacological Implications

Components of the JAK-STAT signaling pathway represent novel targets for pharmacological interventions. Antagonists of cytokines and growth factor receptors may have therapeutic potentials in selectively inhibiting this pathway. Pharmacological inhibitors that specifically interrupt tyrosine kinase signaling including JAK kinases (e.g. tyrphostin AG490) are currently under clinical investigation. Because of the high levels of STAT activation in tumor cells, drugs specifically blocking dimeric STAT molecules are of promising value in the treatment of cancer. Structural targets for the development of novel therapeutics within the STAT molecule include the SH2 domain responsible for dimerization and recruitment to the receptor, the DNA-binding domain as well as the recently discovered nuclear import signal for activated STAT1.

References

1. Akira S. (1999) Functional roles of STAT family proteins: lessons from knockout mice. Stem Cells 17:138–146
2. Catlett-Falcone R, Dalton WS, Jove R. (1999) STAT proteins as novel targets for cancer therapy. Signal transducer an activator of transcription. Curr Opin Oncol. 11:490–496

3. Darnell JE. (1997) STATs and gene regulation. Science 277:1630–1635
4. Horvath CM. (2000) STAT proteins and transcriptional responses to extracellular signals. Trends Biochem Sci. 25:496–502
5. Ward AC, Touw I, Yoshimura A. (2000) The Jak-Stat pathway in normal and perturbed hematopoiesis. Blood 95:19–29

K⁺ Channels

CHAR-CHANG SHIEH
Abbott Laboratories, Abbot Park, USA
char-chang.shieh@abbott.com

Synonyms

Potassium channels

Definition

Potassium channels are a diverse and ubiquitous family of membrane proteins present in both excitable and non-excitable cells that selectively conduct K^+ ions across the cell membrane along its electrochemical gradient at a rate of 10^6–10^8 ions/sec.

▶ Table appendix: Membrane Transport Proteins (K^+ Channels)
▶ ATP-dependent K^+ Channel
▶ Inward Rectifier K^+ Channels
▶ Voltage-gated K^+ Channels

Basic Characteristics

In normal physiological conditions, the concentration of K^+ ions inside the cell is around 25-fold greater than that outside the cell membrane. An outward current is generated due to the efflux of K^+ ions by the opening of K^+ channels that brings membrane potential to close to the resting state (repolarization) of the cells. K^+ channels set the resting membrane potential, shorten the action potential, terminate periods of intense activity, and determine the interspike intervals during repetitive firing (1). Activators of K^+ channels tend to stabilize cellular excitability or dampen the effectiveness of excitatory inputs whereas blockers have the opposite effects. In addition to controlling cellular excitability, K^+ channels can also regulate fluid and electrolyte transport and cell proliferation.

More than 78 human genes, encoding a variety of K^+ channels and auxiliary subunits, have been identified (Fig. 1 and Table 1). While the K^+ channels are diverse, they share a salient feature: a conducting pore highly selective for K^+ ions. The K^+ channels are tetramers composed of four α subunits that form the conducting pore. On the basis of primary amino acid sequence of α subunit, K^+ channels can be classified into three major families (Fig. 2).

A. Six Transmembrane One-Pore Channels

Recent molecular biology studies have identified a loop containing 20–25 amino acid residues between S5 and S6 (or M1 and M2, Fig. 2) forming the pore. The G(Y/F)G motif located in the pore represents the K^+-selectivity signature that is common to all K^+ channels. The external entry to the channel pore and its adjacent residues constitute binding sites for toxins and blockers. The internal vestibule of the pore and the adjacent residues in S5 and S6 contribute to binding sites for compounds such as 4-aminopyridine and quinidine. The S4–S5 linker lies close to the permeation pathway and forms part of the receptor for the inactivation. The S4 segment, containing 5–7 positive charges at approximately every third position, serves as a voltage-sensor governing the channel opening.

Name	Gene	Chromosome	Disorders	Tissue expression	Type
Kv1.5	KCNA5	12p13		B, H, K, L, Sk m	Voltage-gated K⁺ channel (*Shaker*)
Kv1.6	KCNA6	12p13		B	"
Kv1.7	KCNA7	19q13.3		H, Panc, Sk m	"
Kv1.4	KCNA4	11q13.4-14.1		B, H, Panc	"
Kv1.3	KCNA3	1p21-p13.3		Lym, B, L, Th, S	"
Kv1.2	KCNA2	1		B, H, Panc	"
Kv1.1	KCNA1	12p13	EA	B, H, R, Panc	"
Kv4.1	KCND1	Xp11.23-11.3		H, B, L, K, Li, Pl	Voltage-gated K⁺ channel (*Shal*)
Kv4.3	KCND3	1p13.2		H, B	"
Kv4.2	KCND2	7q31-32		B	"
Kv3.2	KCNC2	19q13.3-13.4		B	Voltage-gated K⁺ channel (*Shaw*)
Kv3.3	KCNC3	19q13.3-13.4		B, L	"
Kv3.4	KCNC4	1p21		B, Sk m	"
Kv3.1	KCNC1	11p15		B, M, Lym	"
Kv5.1 (KH1)	KCNF1	2p25		B	Voltage-gated K⁺ channel
Kv8.1		8q22.3-24.1		B	"
Kv2.1 - Kv2.2	KCNB1	20q13.2		B, H, K, Sk m, R	Voltage-gated K⁺ channel (*Shab*)
Kv9.1	KCNS1			B	Voltage-gated K⁺ channel
Kv9.3	KCNS3	2p24		L, B, artery	"
Kv9.2	KCNS2	8q22		B	"
Kv6.2	KCNF2	18q22-23		H	"
Kv6.1 (KH2)	KCNG1	20q13		B	"
KvLQT1	KCNQ1	11p15.5	LQT1 (JLNS)	H, Co, K, L, Pl	"
KvLQT3	KCNQ3	8q24	BFNC	B, neuron	"
KvLQT2	KCNQ2	20q13.3	BFNC	B, neuron	"
KvLQT5	KCNQ5	6q14		B, Sk m	"
KvLQT4	KCNQ4	1p34	Deafness	Hair cell, inner ear	"
TASK2	KCNK5	6p21		B, L	Two-pore K⁺ channel
TALK1	KCNK16	6p21		Panc	"
TALK2	KCNK17	6p21		Panc, Pl, L, H, Li	"
TRAAK	KCNK4	11q13		B, Spin, R	"
TREK2	KCNK10	14q31		B	"
TREK1	KCNK2	1q41		B	"
KCNK7	KCNK7	11q13		B	"
TWIK1	KCNK1	1q42-q43		B, K, H	"
TWIK2	KCNK6	19q13.1		K	"
TASK5	KCNK15	20q12		Adr g, Panc	"
TASK1	KCNK3	2pP23		H, B, Panc, Pl	"
TASK3	KCNK9	8		B, K, Li, L	"
THIK1	KCNK13	14q24.1-24.3		ubiquitous	"
THIK2	KCNK12	2p22-2p23		B, K	"
BK_Ca	KCNMA1	10q23.1		B, Sm, Panc	Ca²⁺-activated K⁺ channel
IK_Ca1	KCNN4	19q13.2		Lym, Col, Pros, Pl	"
SK_Ca1	KCNN1	19p13.1		B, H	"
SK_Ca3	KCNN3	1q21.3		B, Adr g, T cells	"
SK_Ca2	KCNN2	5q21.2-q22.1		B, H, L	"
Kir7.1	KCNJ13	2q37		GI, K, B	Inward rectifier K⁺ channel
Kir5.1	KCNJ16	17q25		B, periphery	"
Kir3.1	KCNJ3	2q24.1		H, cerebellum	"
Kir3.3	KCNJ9	1q21-23		H, B, Sk m	"
Kir3.2	KCNJ6	21q22.1-22.2		Panc, cerebellum	"
Kir3.4	KCNJ5	11q24		H, Panc	"
Kir2.4	KCNJ14	19q13		B, R	"
Kir2.3	KCNJ4	22q13.1		H, B, Sk m	"
Kir2.1	KCNJ2	17q23	Andersen's	H, B, Sm, Sk m, K	"
Kir2.2	KCNJ12	17p11.1-11.2		H	"
Kir6.1	KCNJ8	12p11.23	PHHI	ubiquitous	"
Kir6.2	KCNJ11	11p15.1		ubiquitous	"
Kir1.1	KCNJ1	11q24	Bartter's	K, Panc	"
Kir4.1 (Kir1.3)	KCNJ10	1q		Glia	"
Kir4.2 (Kir1.2)	KCNJ15	21q22.2		K, L, B	"
HERG	KCNH2	7q35-36	LQT2	B, H	Voltage-gated K⁺ channel
EAG	KCNH1	1q32-41		B	"
BEC1	KCNH3	12q13		B	"
BEC2	KCNH4			B	"

◀ **Fig. 1 Human potassium channel genes: localization and diseases.** Human K⁺ channel genes are sorted by similarity of amino acid sequence. The dendrogram was generated using Pileup program of the Wisconsin Sequence Analysis Package (Genetics Computer Group (GCG), Madison, Wisconsin). Abbreviations: Adr g, adrenal gland; Andersen's, Andersen's syndrome; B, brain; Bartter's, Bartter's syndrome; BEC, brain-specific eag-like channel; BFNC, Benign familial neonatal convulsions; BK_{Ca}, large-conductance Ca^{2+}-activated K⁺ channel; Co, cochlea; EA, Episodic ataxia/myokymia syndrome; EAG, *ether-a-go-go* gene encoded K⁺ channel; H, heart; HEAG, human *ether-a-go-go*; hSK, human small-conductance Ca^{2+}-activated; IK_{Ca}, intermediate-conductance Ca^{2+}-activated; JLNS, Jervell and Lange-Nielsen syndrome; K, kidney; Kv, voltage-gated; Kir, inward-rectifier K⁺ channel; L, lung; Li, liver; LQT, long-QT syndrome; Lym, lymphocyte; M, muscle; Pan, pancreatic islet; PHHI, persistent hyperinsulinemic hypoglycemia of infancy; Pl, placenta; Pros, prostate; R, retina; Sk m, skeletal muscle; Sm, smooth muscle; Spin, spinal cord; TASK, TWIK-related acid-sensitive K⁺ channel; TASK, TWIK-related acid-sensitive K⁺ channel; TRAAK, TWIK-related arachidonic acid-stimulated K⁺ channel; TWIK, two-pore weak inward rectifier.

B. Two Transmembrane One-Pore Channels

The inward rectifier K⁺ channels (Kir) represent this class of channels that conduct K⁺ ions more in the inward direction than outward and regulate resting membrane potential. The occlusion of internal vestibule of the pore by Mg^{2+} and ▶ polyamines contribute to this inward rectification. These channels are tetrameric, although a more complex octameric arrangement has been described for a ATP-sensitive K⁺ channel. This channel is composed of four inward rectifiers, contributing to ion conducting pore, and four sulfonylurea receptors as regulatory subunits.

C. Four Transmembrane Two-Pore Channels

This class of K⁺ channel subunits contains four putative transmembrane and two pore domains. They represent a class of K⁺ channel with >50 distinct gene members. The G(Y/F)G motif is preserved in the first pore loop but this motif is replaced by GFG or GLG in the second pore loop. The two-pore K⁺ channel family plays important role in conducting K⁺ leak currents that regulate cellular excitability by shaping the duration, frequency and amplitude of action potentials through their influence over the resting membrane potential (2).

K⁺ Channelopathies

A. Genetically Linked Diseases. Genetic linkage analyses have identified inherited human disorders due to abnormal function of K⁺ channels. These naturally occurring mutations result in loss or changes in K⁺ channel function (3).

Cardiac diseases: In heart, multiple K⁺ channels regulate cardiac excitability and determine cardiac action potential duration. Both KvLQT1 and ▶ MinK have wide distribution in different tissues; these two subunits coassemble to form a slowly activating delayed rectifier K⁺ channel (IK_S) that plays role in repolarization of cardiac action potential in heart and regulates transepithelial K⁺ ion secretion in the inner ear. Mutations in either KvLQT1 or MinK have been linked to cardiac arrhythmia in the dominant ▶ Long-QT syndromes (LQT) or to recessive LQT, in which cardiac arrhythmia is associated with congenital deafness. Another cardiac rapid delayed rectifier K⁺ channel (IK_R), in contrast to IK_S, is composed of ▶ HERG and MiRP1, and is responsible for repolarization of cardiac action potential. Aberrant function of HERG/MiRP1 resulting from mutations in either subunit has been identified in families associated with LQT. Mutations in *KCNJ2*, encoding Kir2.1, lead to Andersen's syndrome.

CNS diseases: In CNS, mutations in *KCNA1* (Kv1.1) impair the capacity of the affected neurons to repolarize effectively following an action potential and are linked to the type 1 ▶ Episodic ataxia/myokymia (EA1). KCNQ3 and KCNQ2 or KCNQ5 constitute diverse ▶ M-channels that play important roles in determining the excitability threshold, firing properties and responsiveness of neurons to synaptic inputs. Mutations in both KCNQ2 and KCNQ3 that render the function of M-channels have been identified in the family associated with ▶ benign familial neonatal convulsions (4).

Deafness: KCNQ4 is highly expressed in vestibular system, brain and cochlea sensory hair cells.

Tab. 1 Human K⁺ channel auxiliary subunits: genes, localization, function and disorders.

Name	Gene	Chromosome	Tissue Expression	Association with α subunits	Functions	Disorders
Kvβ1	KCNAB1	3q26.1	Brain, heart	Kv1.4; Kv1.5	Inactivation	
Kvβ2	KCNAB2	1p36.3	Brain, heart	Kv1.4	Inactivation	
Kvβ3	KCNAB3	17p13.1	Brain	Kv1.5	Inactivation	
MINK	KCNE1	21q22.1-22.2	Heart, kidney, uterus	KvLQT1	Coassemble to form the cardiac IK_S channel.	LQT5
MiRP1	KCNE2	21q22.1	Heart, skeletal muscle	HERG	Coassemble with HERG to form the cardiac IK_R channel.	LQT6
MiRP2	KCNE3	11q13-q14	Small intestine, colon, kidney	KvLQT1; KvLQT4; HERG	1. Coassemble with KvLQT1 to from cAMP-activated K⁺ channel in intestine. 2. Suppress KvLQT4 currents. 3. Suppress HERG currents.	
SUR1	SUR1	11p15.1	Pancreas, neurons, skeletal muscle	Kir6.2	Coassemble to from K_{ATP} channels.	PHHI
SUR2A/ SUR2B	SUR2	12p12.1	SUR2A: Heart, skeletal muscle SUR2B: Brain, smooth muscle, liver	Kir6.2 or Kir6.1	Coassemble to from K_{ATP} channels.	
BK$_{Ca}$-β1	KCNMB1	5q34	Smooth muscle, cochlea, pancreas	BK$_{Ca}$	Alter Ca^{2+} and voltage-dependency.	
BK$_{Ca}$-β2	KCNMB2	3q26.2-q27	Kidney, heart, uterus	BK$_{Ca}$	Inactivation; iberiotoxin-resistant	
BK$_{Ca}$-β3	KCNMB3	3q26.3-q27.1	Spleen, testis, placenta, pancreas	BK$_{Ca}$		
BK$_{Ca}$-β4	KCNMB4	12q14.1-q15	Brain, heart, kidney	BK$_{Ca}$	Iberiotoxin-, charybdotoxin-resistant	

KCNQ4 has been mapped to human chromosome 1p34 in which *DFNA2* is located. Loss of KCNQ4 function due to deletion or mutation contributes to progressive hearing loss (4).

Renal diseases: In kidney, mutations in *KCNJ1* disrupt the function of Kir1.1 in apical renal outer medullar. The loss of tubular K⁺ channel function and impaired K⁺ flux probably prevent apical membrane potassium recycling and lead to antenatal ▶ Bartter's syndrome.

Metabolic diseases: In the pancreatic β-cells, multiple ion channels regulate insulin secretion. These include the ATP-sensitive K⁺ (K_{ATP}) channel (composed of four SUR1 and four Kir6.2 subunits) which link cellular metabolism to electrical activity. Mutations in SUR1 and Kir6.2 that leads to loss of K_{ATP} channel function have been identified in families with ▶ familial persistent hyperinsulinemic hypoglycemia of infancy (PHHI).

B. Acquired Aberrant K⁺ Channel Function. In addition to naturally occurring mutations in K⁺ channels leading to various human disorders, acquired dysfunction of K⁺ channels induced by drugs or diseases can also occur (3). Blockade of HERG channel by certain H1 antagoinsts, antipsychotics, tricyclic antidepressants, antibiotics and antiemetic agents contributes to the drug-induced LQT leading to polymorphic ventricular dysrhythmia, the torsade de pointes. H1 receptor antagonists such as loratadine and rupatadine can also induce cardiac arrhythmia by blocking Kv1.5. Upor down-regulation of K⁺ channel gene expression has been shown to be involved in cardiac hypertrophy, atrial fibrillation, apoptosis, oncogenesis and Alzheimer's disease. In neuromuscular junctions, inhibition of delayed rectifier K⁺ channels (Kv1.1 and Kv1.6) by autoantibodies is the underlying mechanism leading to muscle twitching observed in Isaacs' syndrome, an acquired neuromyotonia.

Therapeutic Indications and Drug Developments

Concurrent with the progress in our understanding of molecular diversity, structure and function of K⁺ channels, genetically linked and acquired diseases involved in alterations in the K⁺ channel, the interests in discovery and development of

A. Six transmembrane one-pore

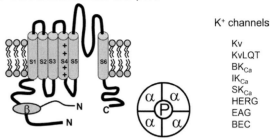

K⁺ channels

Kv
KvLQT
BK_{Ca}
IK_{Ca}
SK_{Ca}
HERG
EAG
BEC

B. Two transmembrane one-pore

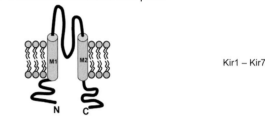

Kir1 – Kir7

C. Four transmembrane one-pore

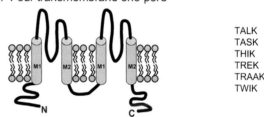

TALK
TASK
THIK
TREK
TRAAK
TWIK

Fig. 2 Schematic representation of the structural classification of K⁺ channel subunits. A, Six transmembrane one-pore subunits. This represents a class of the K⁺ channels composed of four subunits each containing six transmembrane segments (S1–S6) and a conducting pore (P) between S5 and S6 with a voltage sensor (positive charge of amino acid) located at S4. Some of the voltage-gated K⁺ channels include an auxiliary β-subunit (Kvβ), which is a cytoplasmic protein with binding site located at the N-terminus of the α-subunit. The inset shows the general assembly of K⁺ channels. The homotetrameric K⁺ channel consists of four identical subunits while different α-subunits form heterotetrameric K⁺ channels. **B, Two-transmembrane one-pore subunits.** The inward rectifier K⁺ channel belongs to a superfamily of channels with four subunits each containing two transmembrane segments (M1 and M2) with a P-loop in between. **C, Four transmembrane two-pore subunits.** This represents a class of K⁺ channel that has four transmembranes with two P-loops. This figure is adapted from (3).

selective modulators of various classes of K^+ channels are evolving (5).

A. Voltage-Gated K^+ Channels

Kv1.3. The Kv1.3 channel plays a critical role in controlling Ca^{2+} influx that regulates proliferation in human T lymphocytes. Blocking Kv1.3 inhibits activated-T cell proliferation, thereby making this channel an attractive target for immunosuppressant agents. Recent studies have identified correolide as a Kv1.3 blocker. Other emerging Kv1.3 blockers that could be used as potential immunosuppressants include H-37, WIN-17317-3, CP-339818 and UK-78282 (Table 2).

Kv1.5. In human atria, the Kv1.5 represents the ultra-rapid delayed rectifier that contributes to the repolarization in early phase of cardiac action potential. Selective blockers of Kv1.5 channels could potentially be beneficial in the treatment of atrial fibrillation since blocking Kv1.5 could delay repolarization and prolong refractoriness selectively in cardiac myocytes.

HERG. HERG/MiRP is the major target for the class III antiarrhythmic agents. Novel and selective agents include dofetilide, ibutilide and azimilide that block HERG, prolong cardiac action potential and represent useful agents for the treatment of arrhythmias (Table 2).

KvLQT1. KvLQT1/MinK has been suggested as a promising avenue for the class III antiarrhythmic approach. As noted above, most known class III antiarrhythmic drugs block HERG/MiRP and lead to prolongation of cardiac action potentials. However, HERG/MiRP blockade typically causes excessive prolongation of action potentials at slow heart rates, whereas at higher rates blockade is much less effective. This so-called reverse use-dependent action can lead to life-threatening arrhythmias. Thus, selective KvLQT1/MinK blocker might be more promising with less pro-arrhythmic potential. Recent developments have identified chromanol 293B as a prototypical inhibitor of KvLQT1/MinK. Other blockers include HMR-1556 and L-73582.

Other KCNQ-Derived Channels. The M-channel is emerging as an attractive target to enhance cognition; this is encouraged by the observation that neurotransmitter release enhancers for Alzheimer's disease such as linopirdine, DMP-543, and XE-991 are M-channel blockers. Mutations in KCNQ2 and KCNQ3 linking to benign familial neonatal convulsions suggest M-channel openers as potential antiepileptic agents. The antiepileptic agent retigabine has been shown to activate KCNQ2/KCNQ3 channels, indicating that M-channel activation may be a new mode of action for anticonvulsant drugs.

B. ATP-Sensitive K^+ Channels (KATP Channels)

As noted previously, SUR1/Kir6.2 constitutes the pancreatic K_{ATP} channel. The molecular composition of the cardiac/skeletal muscle K_{ATP} channel is SUR2A/Kir6.2, whereas SUR2B/Kir6.2 is thought to form the major K_{ATP} channel in smooth muscle cells. Like sarcolemmal K_{ATP} channel, mitochondria K_{ATP} channel also couples the energy metabolism to cellular activities, although its molecular composition remains to be elucidated.

SUR1/Kir6.2. Glibenclamide and glipizide, which block pancreatic K_{ATP} channels, have been used for the treatment of type II diabetes. New classes of insulin secretagogues includes repaglinide and nateglinide, which improve insulin secretion, action and reduce carbohydrate absorption.

Mitochondria KATP Channels. Cardiac K_{ATP} channel opening has a role in myocardial preconditioning, a paradoxical form of cardioprotection wherein brief ischemic episodes can protect the heart from subsequent lethal ischemic injury. Recent developments have shown that BMS-180448 and BMS-191095 have cardioprotective over vasorelaxant effects by activating mitochondria K_{ATP} channels.

SUR2B/Kir6.2. Recent efforts have been focused on the development of selective K_{ATP} channel openers for vascular and nonvascular indications including angina, airway hyperactivity, bladder over-activity and erectile dysfunction (Table 3).

Ca^{2+}-Activated K^+ Channels. This subfamily includes the large- (BK_{Ca}), intermediate- (IK_{Ca})

Tab. 2 Potassium channel openers*.

Channel family	Therapeutic Indications	Compounds
Voltage-gated K$^+$ channels		
Kv1.3	Immunosuppressant	Correolide, WIN-17317-3, CP-339318, UK-78,282, H-37
Kv1.5 (IK$_{UR}$)	Atrial fibrillation	NIP-142
Kv4.2 (IK$_{TO}$)	Arrhythmia	Flecainide, Clofilium
Kv (other)	Multiple sclerosis	Fampridine (4-aminopyridine)
	Epilepsy	BIIA 0388
HERG/MiRP (IK$_R$)	Arrhythmia	Dofetilide, Ibutilide
	Atrial fibrillation/flutter	Almokalant, E4031, MK499, Sematilide, Azimilide (NE 10064), D-Sotalol
KvLQT1/MinK (IK$_S$)	Arrhythmia	Chromanol 293B, HMR1556, E-047/1, L768673, L735821, L364373
Kv1.5, HERG/MiRP, KvLQT1/MinK	Arrhythmia, angina	Ambasilide (LU 47710), Tedisamil
ATP-sensitive K$^+$ channels (K$_{ATP}$)		
SUR1/Kir6.2	Type II diabetes	Tolbutamide, Chlorpropamide, Glibenclamide, Glipzide, Nateglinide, Repaglinide
SUR2A/Kir6.2	Ventricular arrhythmia, sudden cardiac death	HMR-1883 (Clamikalant), HMR-1098
SUR2B/Kir6.2 (?)	Arrhythmia, diuretics	PNU-37883A, PNU-99963, IMID-4F
Ca^{2+}-activated K$^+$ channels		
Intermediate-conductance (IK$_{Ca}$)	Sickle cell anemia, diarrhea	Clotrimazole, ICA-15451
	Immunosuppressant	TRAM-34
	Rheumatoid arthritis	
Small-conductance (SK$_{Ca}$)	Sleep apnea	Dequalinium, Tubocurarine
	Neuromuscular disorders	UCL-1684, UCL-1530
M-channels		
KCNQ2/KCNQ3	Cognition enhancer	Linopirdine (DUP 996)
	Alzheimer's diseases	DMP-543, XE-991

* Adapted from (3).

K

Tab. 3 Potassium channel blockers*.

Channel family	Therapeutic Indications	Compounds
ATP-sensitive K$^+$ channels (K$_{ATP}$)		
Cardiac Mitochondria K$_{ATP}$ (SUR2A/Kir6.2)	Myocardial Ischemia	BMS-180448, BMS-191095, Diazoxide
SUR2B/Kir6.2	Angina	Nicorandil, JTV-506
(SUR2B/Kir6.1?)	Hypertension	Pinacidil
(SUR2B splice variant/Kir6.2)		Aprikalim (RP 52891), Bimakalim (EMD52692), Cromakalim, Celikalim, Emakalim, NIP121 RO 316930, RWJ 29009, SDZ PCO 400, Rimakalim (HOE234), Symakalim (EMD 57283), YM-099, YM-934
	Airway hyperactivity	SDZ-217-744
	Alopecia	P1075, Minoxidil
	Bladder overactivity	ZM244085, ZD6169, WAY233537, WAY151616, ZD0947
	Erectile dysfunction	PNU83757
Ca^{2+}-activated K$^+$ channels (K$_{Ca}$)		
Large-conductance (BK$_{Ca}$)	Cerebral ischemia	BMS-204352
	Vascular/nonvascular disorders, Antipsychotic	NS-1608, NS-4, NS-1619 (also Ca^{2+} channel blocker)
	Urinary incontinence, Pollakisuria	NS-8
Intermediate (IK$_{Ca}$)-, Small-conductance (SK$_{Ca}$)	Vascular disorder, Cystic fibrosis	1-EBIO, Chlorzoxazone, Zoxazolamine
M-channels		
KCNQ2/KCNQ3	Epilepsy	Retigabine (also GABA$_A$ agonist), BMS-204352

* Adapted from (3).

and small-conductance (SK$_{Ca}$) Ca^{2+}-activated K$^+$ channels that are activated by increases in intracellular free Ca^{2+} concentration. The opening of IK$_{Ca}$ and SK$_{Ca}$ channels are less voltage-dependent, whereas the activation of BK$_{Ca}$ channel has steep voltage sensitivity.

BKCa. The diversity of BK$_{Ca}$ channels can be attributed to the assembly of pore-forming α subunit together with four different auxiliary subunits (β1–β4). BMS-204352 has been identified as a BK$_{Ca}$ channel opener for the treatment of acute ischemic stroke although it has also been shown to be a M-channel activator. Therapeutic applications for channel openers include epilepsy, bladder over-activity, asthma, hypertension and psychosis. Other known BK$_{Ca}$ channel openers include NS-8, NS-1619 and NS-4 (Table 3).

IKCa. The IK$_{Ca}$ channel has been known as a Gardos channel in red blood cells. Blockers of IK$_{Ca}$ channels have been suggested for the treatment of sickle cell anemia, diarrhea and rheumatoid arthritis. Blockers of IK$_{Ca}$ channels may be used as immunosuppressive agents because these channels are up-regulated following antigenic or mitogenic stimulation in T-cells. IK$_{Ca}$ channel blockers include clotrimazole, ICA-15451 and TRAM-34. Openers of IK$_{Ca}$ channels may be therapeutically beneficial in cystic fibrosis and peripheral vascular diseases. Although not highly specific, 1-EBIO (1-ethyl-2-benzimidazolinone) and benzoxazoles have been shown to activate IK$_{Ca}$ channels.

SKCa. The SK$_{Ca}$ channels are responsible for the slow after-hyperpolarization and play important roles in determining the firing frequency. Distinct genes are known to encode SK$_{Ca}$1, SK$_{Ca}$2 and SK$_{Ca}$3, in which SK$_{Ca}$2 and SK$_{Ca}$3 are highly apamin-sensitive. Over expression of SK$_{Ca}$3 can induce abnormal respiratory responses to hypoxic challenge and compromised parturition, suggesting SK$_{Ca}$3 as a potential target for sleep apnea and for regulating uterine contractions during labor. Other indications for SK$_{Ca}$ channel modulators include myotonic muscular dystrophy, gastrointestinal dismotilities, memory disorders and epilepsy. The SK$_{Ca}$ channel blockers include dequalinium analogs and more potent agents such as UCL-1684 and UCL-1530.

D Two-Pore K$^+$ Channels
The newly identified two-pore K$^+$ channels are thought to function as background channels involved in the regulation of resting membrane potential. Recent studies have shown that neuroprotective agents such as riluzole and volatile general anesthetics can activate two-pore K$^+$ channels, suggesting these channels might be attractive targets for novel neuroprotective and anesthetic agents.

Conclusions
K$^+$ channels have emerged as underlying molecular targets in a number of diseases. Recent cloning and the knowledge of structure and function, genetic- and disease-induced regulation of K$^+$ channels could undoubtedly improve diagnosis and offer specific candidate genes for the development of appropriate therapies. Technology to improve high throughput assays for K$^+$ channel modulators such as planar patch should be helpful to identify potent and selective drug candidates.

References
1. Hille B (2001) Ion channels of excitable membranes. 3rd ed, Sinauer, Sunderland, MA.
2. Goldstein SA, Bockenhauer D, O'Kelly I, Zilberberg N (2001) Potassium leak channels and the KCNK family of two-P-domain subunits. Nat Rev Neurosci 2:175–184
3. Shieh CC, Coghlan M, Sullivan JP, Gopalakrishnan M (2000) Potassium channels: molecular defects, diseases, and therapeutic opportunities. Pharmacol Rev 52:557–594
4. Jentsch TJ (2000) Neuronal KCNQ potassium channels: physiology and role in disease. Nat Rev Neurosci 1:21–30
5. Coghlan MJ, Carroll WA, Gopalakrishnan M (2001) Recent developments in the biology and medicinal chemistry of potassium channel modulators: update from a decade of progress. J Med Chem 44:1627–1653

K$^+$ Channel Openers

Typical KCO members are diazoxide, pinacidil, cromakalim, and nicorandil. KCOs activate K$_{ATP}$ channels by binding to SUR subunits. Diazoxide and nicorandil are clinically used in treatment of PHHI and angina pectoris, respectively.

▶ ATP-dependent Potassium Channels

K⁺ Homeostasis

Potassium homeostasis refers to the maintaining and regulating of a relatively stable and mostly internal (intracellular) potassium balance (concentration), although more generally it refers to the maintenance of potassium balance in any compartment (e.g. in the blood).

K⁺-sparing Diuretics

▶ Diuretics

Kainate Receptor

Kainite receptors are a subtype of ionotropic glutamate receptors that are permeable to Na^+, K^+ and Ca^{2+} ions.

▶ Ionotropic Glutamate Receptors

Kallidin

▶ Kinins

Kallikrein

▶ Kinins

K$_{ATP}$ Channels

▶ ATP-dependent Potassium Channels

KCNQ-channels

KCNQ-channels are assembled from KCNQ α-subunits. Mutations in the KCNQ1 gene are associated with heart arrhythmia and deafness (LQT1 syndrome, Romano-Ward Syndrome, Jervyll-Lange-Nielsen Syndrome). Mutations in KCNQ2 and KCNQ3 genes are associated with a benign form of juvenile epilepsy (BFNC). Mutations in the KCNQ4 gene are associated with deafness.

▶ Antiepileptic Drugs
▶ K⁺ Channels
▶ KvLQT1-channels
▶ Long-QT Syndromes
▶ M-channels
▶ MinK subunits
▶ Voltage-gated K⁺ Channels

KCOs

▶ K⁺ Channel Openers

K$_D$

K_D is the dissociation constant for a drug-receptor complex. It is a measurement of the affinity of a drug for a receptor. The lower the value, the higher the affinity.

KDEL Receptor

Interaction of the KDEL-receptor with soluble luminal proteins bearing the tetrapeptide KDEL at their carboxy-terminus retrieves these proteins back from the Golgi to the endoplasmic reticulum.

▶ Intracellular Transport

KELL Blood Group Antigen

KELL blood group antigen is a plasma membrane protein isolated from red cells homologous to zinc-binding glycoproteins with neutral endopeptidase activity.

K_i Values

The K_i value is the dissociation constant of an enzyme-inhibitor complex. If $[E]$ and $[I]$ are the concentrations of enzyme and its inhibitor and $[EI]$ is the concentration of the enzyme-inhibitor complex, there is an equilibrium of complex formation and detachment as follows:

$$[E][I] \rightleftharpoons [EI]$$

Under these circumstances, K_i can be defined as:

$$K_i = \frac{[E][I]}{[EI]}$$

Kinase

A kinase is an enzyme that catalyzes the transfer of the terminal phosphate of a nucleotide to suitable substrates. Protein and lipid kinases play important roles in signaling. The kinase domain is a two lobed structure with an ATP binding site and a substrate-binding site. Protein kinases can be tyrosine kinases (e.g. receptor tyrosine kinases (RTKs)), serine/threonine kinases (e.g. protein kinase C (PKC)) or dual specificity kinases (e.g. MEK). Kinases that can phosphorylate histidine and arginine residues have been identified in lower organisms.

Kinase Domain

▶ Kinase

Kinetochore

Kinetochores are the attachment sites on the condensed chromosomes. During mitosis, microtubules attach and segregate the two sets of chromosomes.

Kinins

HEIKO HERWALD, WERNER MÜLLER-ESTERL
Lund University, Lund, Sweden; University of Frankfurt Medical School, Frankfurt, Germany
Heiko.Herwald@medkem.lu.se,
wme@biochem2.de

Synonyms

Bradykinin, kallidin (lysyl-bradykinin), desArg^9-bradykinin, desArg^{10}-kallidin (Lys^0, desArg^9-bradykinin), T-kinin (Ile-Ser-bradykinin)

Definition

Kinins are a group of oligopeptides of 8 to 11 residues that act locally as proinflammatory agents, often through the release of powerful downstream effectors such as nitric oxide and/or prostaglandins.

▶ Inflammation
▶ Nociception

K

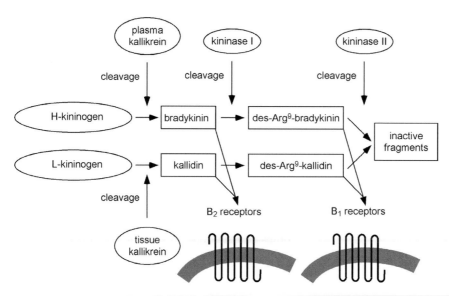

Fig. 1 Scheme of kinin liberation, turnover and action.

Basic Characteristics

Liberation of Kinins

Typically, kinins are produced at injured or inflamed tissue sites where they act through a combined endocrine/paracrine mode. In a first step, the large kinin precursor proteins, i.e. kininogens, are targeted to the inflamed site where the kinins are eventually liberated from the kininogens by specific kininogenases, i.e. kallikreins. In humans, two types of kininogens exist, termed high-molecular-weight (H-)kininogen (H-kininogen) and low-molecular-weight (L-)kininogen (Fig. 1). Both types of kininogens are encoded by distinct mRNAs generated by alternative splicing from a single kininogen gene. A third type of kininogen, T-kininogen, appears to be unique for the rat and is not found in humans or other mammalian species. Kininogens are primarily synthesized by hepatocytes and secreted into the human plasma via constitutive routes. Kidney and secretory glands are among the prominent extrahepatic sites of kininogen production.

The most common kinin-releasing enzymes are kallikreins, a group of serine proteases that are found in glandular cells, ▶ neutrophils and biological fluids such as plasma and urine. Kallikreins fall into two distinct groups, i.e. tissue kallikrein and plasma kallikrein, that differ by their struc-tural, immunological and functional characteristics (2). In some mammalian species, tissue kallikrein preferentially utilizes L-kininogen as the substrate to produce kallidin, whereas plasma kallikrein acts on H-kininogen to generate bradykinin (Table 1). Kinins can also be released by common proteases such as trypsin, elastase or cathepsin D. Apart from human kininogenases, a large number of proteases derived from pathogenic microorganisms has been found to liberate kinins from kininogens.

Kinins are extremely short-lived peptide hormones (<15 s) that are prone to rapid conversion and inactivation. For instance, bradykinin and kallidin are cleaved at their carboxy-terminal ends by carboxypeptidases of the N and M type, collectively referred to as kininases type I, to form desArg^9-bradykinin and desArg^{10}-kallidin, respectively (Table 1). Because bradykinin and kallidin act on B_2 receptors, and desArg^9-bradykinin and desArg^{10}-kallidin bind exclusively to B_1 receptors, the proteolytic conversion of the kinins results in a receptor "switch" (Fig. 1). Both types of agonists are rapidly degraded and inactivated by the action of the dipeptidylpeptidase angiotensin-converting enzyme, also known as kininase type II, and neutral endopeptidase that inactivate kinins by trimming the kinin peptides at their carboxy-terminal ends (Table 1).

Tab. 1 Enzymes involved in the generation and degradation of kinins.

Substrate	Processing Enzyme	Product	Kinin Receptor
H-kininogen	plasma kallikrein tissue kallikrein	bradykinin (RPPGFSPFR) kallidin	B_2 receptor
L-kininogen	tissue kallikrein plasma kallikrein	kallidin (KRPPGFSPFR) bradykinin	B_2 receptor
bradykinin	carboxypeptidase N carboxypeptidase M neutral endopeptidase (NEP) angiotensin converting enzyme (ACE)	$desArg^9$-bradykinin (RPPGFSPF) bradykinin 1-7 (RPPGFSP) bradykinin 1-7 (RPPGFSP) 1-5 (RPPGF)	B_1 receptor inactive inactive inactive
kallidin	carboxypeptidase N carboxypeptidase M neutral endopeptidase (NEP) angiotensin converting enzyme (ACE)	$desArg^{10}$-kallidin (KRPPGFSPF) kallidin 1-8 (KRPPGFSP) kallidin 1-8 (KRPPGFSP) 1-6 (KRPPGF)	B_1 receptor inactive inactive inactive
$desArg^9$-bradykinin (RPPGFSPF)	neutral endopeptidase (NEP) angiotensin converting enzyme (ACE)	bradykinin 1-7 (RPPGFS), 1-4 (RPPG) bradykinin 1-5 (RPPGF)	inactive inactive
$desArg^{10}$-kallidin (KRPPGFSPF)	neutral endopeptidase (NEP) angiotensin converting enzyme (ACE)	kallidin 1-5 (KRPPG) kallidin 1-6 (KRPPGF)	inactive inactive

K

In humans as well as in other but not all mammalian species, kininogens are modified by post-translational hydroxylation of a single proline residue of their kinin sequence, i.e. position 3 in bradykinin or position 4 in kallidin. Hydroxylation does not affect the specificity, affinity or intrinsic efficacy of the kinins.

Kinins in Biological Fluids

The determination of kinins in humans has been limited due to the inherent difficulties in accurately measuring the concentration of ephemeral peptides. Thus, strict measurements have to be taken to prevent rapid degradation of the kinins *in vitro*. Kinins and their degradation products have been studied in various biological milieus such as plasma/serum, urine, joint fluids, kidney, lung and skeletal muscle (1). Under normal conditions, the concentration of kinins in these compartments is extremely low; for instance kinin levels in human plasma are in the femtomolar and lower picomolar range. Because plasma concentration of kininogens is in the micromolar range, i.e. the ratio of

effector to precursor concentrations is maintained at an extremely low level of 10^{-6} to 10^{-9}, and therefore kinin release must be extremely tightly controlled. Kinin levels, however, can considerably rise in patients with underlying diseases such as hereditary angioedema or in more severe complications such as ▶ sepsis and ▶ septic shock.

Receptors

The physiological functions executed by kinins are mediated by their interaction with specific receptors. In humans, two types of kinin receptor have been identified, namely B_1 and B_2 receptors (2). The two receptor types are products of distinct genes on two closely apposed loci of human chromosome 14q32 that likely arose from a common progenitor, though their sequence identity is limited. The two proteins belong to the large family of G protein-coupled receptors characterized by seven transmembrane-spanning helices. Unlike B_2 receptors that are constitutively expressed in many cell types and tissues, the expression levels of B_1 receptors are very low under non-stimulated con-

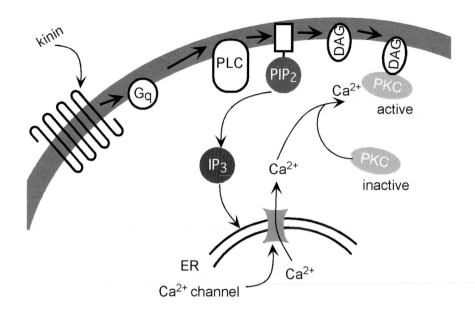

Fig. 2 Intracellular signaling cascades triggered by kinins. Following binding of kinins to the receptor the associated heterotrimeric G protein complex dissociates. The α subunit stimulates phospholipase C (PLC) which in turn catalyses the breakdown of phosphatidylinositol-4,5-bisphosphate (PIP_2) into 1,2-diacylglycerol (DAG) and inositol-1,4,5-trisphosphate (IP_3). IP_3 reacts with Ca^{2+} channels in the endoplasmatic reticulum (ER) releasing Ca^{2+} into the cytosol. The increase in intracellular Ca^{2+} levels activates protein kinase C (PKC), which translocates to the plasma membrane, anchoring to DAG and phosphatidylserine.

ditions. However, inflammatory or noxious stimuli boost the biosynthesis of the B_1 receptor. Several ▶ cytokines such as interleukin IL-1β, as well as ▶ growth factors and bacterial ▶ lipopolysaccharides can up-regulate the transcription of the B_1 gene. B_1 and B_2 receptors are predominantly coupled to the ▶ pertussis toxin-insensitive G_q type of G protein leading to phospholipase C activation, mobilization of intracellular calcium by inositol-1,4,5-trisphosphate (IP_3) and activation of ▶ protein kinase C (Fig. 2). Kinin receptors are vigorous stimulators of the biosynthesis of potent downstream effectors such as ▶ prostaglandins and ▶ leukotrienes due to ▶ phospholipase A_2 activation, and of ▶ nitric oxide via stimulation of the endothelial isoform of ▶ nitric oxide synthase (eNOS).

Kinin Receptor-Deficient Mice
Mice that are homozygous for a disrupted B_1 or B_2 receptor gene are healthy, fertile and normotensive. In B_1-deficient mice, bacterial lipopolysac-charide-induced ▶ hypotension is diminished and the recruitment of polymorphonuclear leukocytes to the sites of tissue injury is impaired and the animals show signs of hypoalgesia. Deletion of the B_2 gene in mice leads to salt-sensitive ▶ hypertension and altered ▶ nociception. B_2 knockout embryos subjected to salt stress *in utero* show suppressed renin expression and an abnormal kidney phenotype and develop early postnatal hypertension.

Biological Functions and Clinical Implications
Kinins are implicated in many physiological and pathological processes including the induction of pain and hypotension, contraction of smooth muscles, regulation of local blood flow, stimulation of electrolyte fluxes, activation of sensory neurons and increase of vascular permeability. Many of these effects are triggered at least in part via the major downstream effectors ▶ prostaglandins, ▶ leukotrienes and ▶ nitric oxide.

In rare cases of a systemic release, kinins have the potential to cause severe hypotension. Uncontrolled activation of the contact system (Fig. 3) is thought to trigger a massive formation of kinins under certain pathological conditions (3). For instance, this situation is seen in patients with underlying diseases such as systemic inflammatory response syndrome (SIRS) due to sepsis or trauma. During the progression of the disease, depletion of contact system factors may occur and low levels of H-kininogen and plasma kallikrein are indicative of a fatal outcome (4). Other diseases associated with a massive, often systemic release of kinins are hereditary angioedema and pancreatitis. Kinins are also generated during allergic and non-allergic rhinitis and ▶ asthma. Notably, kinins are important endogenous mediators exerting acute protective effects in the ischemic myocardium via ▶ nitric oxide-dependent mechanisms.

Drugs

Aprotinin (Trasylol®) was the first drug to be used in the clinic to prevent the formation of kinins. More recently this potent serine protease inhibitor has received much attention in cardiac surgical practice as a pharmacologic intervention to improve the hemostatic derangement associated with cardiopulmonary bypass. Interestingly, aprotinin isolated from bovine lung not only inhibits contact activation but also impinges on a number of interrelated pathways, thereby providing an antifibrinolytic effect, attenuating platelet dysfunction and down-regulating inflammatory responses. As a drug, aprotinin is also used to reduce blood loss and transfusion requirements in patients with a risk of hemorrhage, though the underlying molecular mechanisms responsible for the beneficial effects of aprotinin are still obscure.

A large number of specific B_1 and B_2 receptor antagonists have been developed. Some of them are orally available and are resistant to proteolytic degradation. Kinin antagonists have been tested in clinical trials and it appears that they have some effects on the survival in patients with severe systemic inflammatory response syndrome and sepsis and in patients suffering from severe traumatic brain injury. Kinin antagonists are drug candidates for diseases such hyperalgesia and

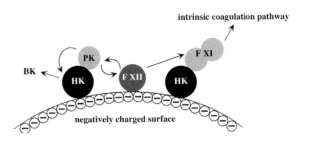

Fig. 3 Activation of the contact system on negatively charged surfaces. Upon perturbation or damage, endothelial cells change their properties from a non-thrombogenic to a thrombogenic state, thereby initiating different pro-coagulative and pro-inflammatory cascades. The contact system contributing to this conversion comprises 4 factors, i.e. three inactive proteinases, factor XII (F XII), factor XI (F XI), plasma kallikrein (PK), and a single non-enzymatic co-factor, H-kininogen (HK). Under physiological conditions, these proteinases circulate as zymogens. The contact system associates with the surface of many cell types, e.g. platelets and endothelial cells. Negatively charged artificial surfaces such as kaolin are also capable to assemble and subsequently activate the contact system; the initial step of this process is FXII activation, and active F XIIa converts plasma kallikrein and factor XI to their active proteolytic forms. Activated factor XI triggers the endogenous coagulation cascade, whereas activated plasma kallikrein cleaves H-kininogen and releases bradykinin (BK). The mechanisms of activation of the contact system on cellular surfaces is less clear and may well differ from that on artificial surfaces.

angioedema, and the use of kinin agonists in the treatment of brain tumors is anticipated.

Angiotensin-converting enzyme (ACE) inhibitors represent a class of drugs that have proven anti-hypertensive and anti-proteinuric effects. They delay the progression of renal disease in conjunction with the ability to reduce systemic blood pressure. Furthermore they have been shown to reduce mortality and morbidity in myocardial infarction associated with chronic heart failure. The cardioprotective effect of ACE inhibitors is a combined result of the diminished conversion of angiotensin I and of the attenuated kinin breakdown leading to kinin accumulation in ischemic myo-cardia. Given their pleiotropic effects, ACE inhibi-tors may well use alternative mechanism(s) to exert their beneficial roles, e.g. through the resen-sitization of kinin receptors, however, the precise modes of action remain to be determined.

References

1. Blais, C Jr., Marceau F, Rouleau JL, and Adam A (2000) The kallikrein-kininogen-kinin system: les-sons from the quantification of endogenous kinins. Peptides 21:1903–1940
2. Mahabeer R, Bhoola, KD (2000) Kallikrein and ki-nin receptor genes. Pharmacol. Ther. 88:77–89
3. Colman RW,Schmaier A H (1997) Contact system: a vascular biology modulator with anticoagulant, profibrinolytic, antiadhesive, and proinflammatory attributes. Blood 90:3819–3843
4. Pixley RA, Colman RW (1997) The kallikrein-kinin system in sepsis syndrome. Handbook of Immu-nopharmacology - The Kinin System. Farmer SG, ed. New York: Academic Press 173–186

Kir Channels

Kir (inwardly rectifying K^+) channels are a class of potassium channels generated by the tetrameric arrangement of one-pore/two-transmembrane helix (1P/2TM) protein subunits, often associated with additional beta subunits. Kir Channels serve to modulate cell excitability, being involved in repolarization of action potentials, setting the resting potential of the cell and contributing to potassium homeostasis.

▶ Inwardly Rectifying K^+ Channel Family

K_{NDP} Channel

▶ NDP-dependent K^+ Channels

Knockout Mice

Knockout mice are mice carrying a mutation lead-ing to the disruption of a certain gene. Using a molecular genetic technique called "gene target-ing", a gene is rendered non-functional in totipo-tent embryonal stem cells in culture. These mutant cells are then used to generate mice carrying the mutation in the germ line, thus leading to the establishment of an animal colony with a loss of function of the desired gene.

▶ Transgenic Animal Models

k_{off}

K_{off}, or the dissociation constant of a drug, refers to the rate at which the drug-receptor complex dis-sociates into separate drug and receptor units.

Korsakoff Psychosis

Korsakoff psychosis is an advanced and irreversi-ble stage of the so called Wernicke encephalopa-thy, caused, e.g., by alcohol abuse. Typical symp-toms include confabulation, disorientation and reduced memory.

Kvβ-subunits

Kvβ-subunits are auxiliary subunits of *Shaker*-related Kv-channels, which belong to the Kv1 sub-family of voltage-gated potassium channels. Kvβ-subunits may function as chaperones in Kvα-sub-unit assembly and may modulate the gating prop-erties of Kv-channels. In particular, some Kvβ-subunits may confer a rapid inactivation to other-wise non-inactivating Kv-channels.

Kv-channels

Kv-channels is an abbreviation of voltage-gated potassium channels. K stands for potassium and v for voltage.

KvLQT1-channels

The subunits of KvLQT1-channels were cloned by positional cloning from mutant human DNA obtained from patients suffering from a hereditary LQT1 (long QT) syndrome associated with heart arrhythmia and deafness. The corresponding gene is abbreviated as KCNQ1. KCN stands for K-channel, Q for the K-channel subfamily, and 1 indicates it as the first member of the KCNQ subfamily. Relatives of this channel (KCNQ2-KCNQ5) underlie the M-channels in the nervous system.

▶ M-channels

▶ K^+ Channels

Kynurenine Pathway

The kynurenine pathway accounts for most of the non-protein tryptophan metabolism in most tissues. Several metabolites produced by this pathway have been shown to be biologically active. Kynurenic acid produced *via* kynurenine has been shown to be an antagonist at N-methyl D-aspartate (NMDA), kainate and α-amino-5-methyl-3-hydroxy-4-isoxazole propionic acid (AMPA) receptors. It can block glutamate receptors in various species in distinguish subpopulations of kainate receptors. 3-hydroxykynurenine can produce neuronal damage by generating radicals. Quinolinic acid, another metabolite produced by the kynurenine pathway, functions as an agonist at NMDA receptors.

▶ Ionotropic Glutamate Receptors

K

L

L-Arginine

▶ NO-synthases

Lasofoxifene

Lasofoxifene is a second generation selective estrogen receptor modulator (SERM) that displays estrogenic effects in bone and the cardiovascular system, but functions as an antiestrogen in the breast and uterus.

Lateral Hypothalamic Area

The lateral hypothalamic area has been identified as a feeding center by studies involving electric stimulation and discrete lesions. Neurons in the lateral hypothalamic area and the neighbouring perifornical area express neuropeptides that stimulate feeding when injected into cerebral ventricles (orexins 1 and 2, melanin-concentrating hormone (MCH)).

Laxatives

Laxatives, also called purgatives or cathartics, are substances used to hasten the transit of food through the intestine. Laxatives function by differ-
ent mechanisms. Bulk laxatives, like methylcellulose or bran, contain agents like polysaccharide polymers, which are not fermented by the normal processes of digestion. They retain water in the gut lumen and promote bowel movements. Osmotic laxatives consist of poorly absorbable solutes such as salines containing magnesium cations or phosphate anions or non-digestable sugars and alcohols (glycerin, lactulose, sorbitol or mannitol). Osmotic laxatives retain an increased volume of fluid in the lumen of the bowel by osmosis, which accelerates the transfer of the bowel contents. Faecal softeners alter the consistency of the faeces. They are also called emollients and contain surface-active compounds similar to detergents, like docusate salts. Stimulant laxatives/purgatives increase the motility of the gut (peristalsis) and stimulate water and electrolyte secretion by the mucosa. Stimulant laxatives, which can cause abdominal cramps and deterioration of intestinal function, include diphenylmethane derivatives (bisacodyl, phenolphthalein), anthraquinone laxatives (derivatives of plants such as aloe, cascara or senna) and ricinoleic acid.

LD$_{50}$

▶ Lethal Dose

L-dihydroxyphenylalanine

▶ L-DOPA / Levodopa

LDL-receptors

LDL-receptors are receptors on the cell surface that remove LDL (and some other forms of) lipoproteins from the plasma into the cell.

▶ HMG-CoA-Reductase Inhibitors

L-DOPA / Levodopa

The immediate metabolic precursor to dopamine, L-DOPA (L-dihydroxphenylalanine) is converted to the active neurotransmitter ▶ dopamine by the action of the enzyme aromatic amine acid decarboxylase (AADC). L-DOPA (INN name Levodopa) is the main drug used to treat ▶ Parkinson's disease.

Lead

A lead is a hit compound that displays specificity and potency against a target in a library screen and continues to show the initial positive dose-dependent response in more complex models such as cells and animals.

Leptin

The cytokine leptin is secreted by adipocytes (fat cells) in proportion to the size of the adipose depot and circulates via the bloodstream to the brain, where it ultimately affects feeding behaviour, endocrine systems including reproductive function and, at least in rodents, energy expenditure. Leptin exerts its effects *via* binding to the leptin receptor in the brain (specifically in the hypothalamus), which activates the ▶ JAK-STAT Pathway.

▶ Appetite Control

Lethal Dose

The lethal dose (LD_{50}) is a measure of the toxicity of a compound. In an LD_{50} toxicity test, various doses of a drug are administered to groups of animals, and the mortality in each group is determined. The lethal dose 50 is the dose, which is lethal for 50% of a group of animals.

Leucin Zipper

A leucine zipper is a structural motif present in a large class of transcription factors. These dimeric proteins contain two extended alpha helices that "grip" the DNA molecule much like a pair of scissors at adjacent major grooves. The coiled-coil dimerization domain contains precisely spaced leucine residues which are required for the interaction of the two monomers. Some DNA-binding proteins with this general motif contain other hydrophobic amino acids in these positions; hence, this structural motif is generally called a basic zipper.

Leukemia

Leukemia is a progressive, malignant disease of the blood-forming organs, characterized by distorted proliferation and development of leukocytes and their precursors in the blood and bone marrow. It is classified according to the degree of cell differentiation as acute or chronic (terms no longer referring to the duration of disease) and according to predominant type of cell involved as myelogenous or lymphocytic.

▶ Bone Metabolism

Leukopoiesis

Leukopoiesis denotes the formation of leukocytes (white blood cells, a general term for granulocytes and lymphocytes) from precursor cells.

Leukotriene Receptor Antagonists

Leukotriene receptor antagonists are agents that inhibit the cysLT receptor and prevent the actions of the leukotrienes LTC_4, LTD_4, and LTE_4.

▶ Leukotrienes

Leukotrienes

ALAN R. LEFF
Deptartment of Medicine, MC6076,
University of Chicago, Chicago, IL, USA
aleff@medicine.bsd.uchicago.edu

Synonyms

▶ Cysteinyl leukotriene, B-leukotrienes

Definition

Leukotrienes are the last stage synthetic products resulting from hydrolysis of phospholipid by the ubiquitous 85 kD enzyme, $cPLA_2$. This results in the production of arachidonic acid (AA) from which platelet activating factor is also synthesized as a by-product of lipid hydrolysis. Arachidonic acid is subseqeuntly converted by the enzyme, ▶ 5-lipoxygenase (5-LO), into two bioactive classes of leutotriene (LT): 1) LTB_4, which is chemotactic for neutrophils and minimally chemotactic for human ▶ eosinophils, and 2) the ▶ cysteinyl leukotrienes (cysLT), LTC_4, D_4 and E_4. There is no known physiological function of the cysLTs. These com-pounds play a significant role in allergic responses and contribute variably to the bronchoconstrictor response in human ▶ bronchial asthma.

▶ Inflammation
▶ Prostanoids

Basic Characteristics

Synthesis and Metabolism

The site of synthesis of leukotrienes within cells remains incompletely defined. Increases in intracellular Ca^{2+} concentration triggered by inflammatory stimuli including chemokines and cytokines cause migration of $cPLA_2$ to the nuclear envelope of inflammatory cells and, possibly, to cytosolic lipid bodies (see below). AA produced by hydrolysis of the associated membranes is converted by 5-LO into 5-hydroperoxy-6,8,11-eicosatetraneoic acid (5-HPETE). 5-LO then further converts 5-HPETE into LTA_4 in the presence of 5-lipoxygenase activating protein, which serves as a substrate-concentrating rather than enzyme-activating function. LTA_4 [5(s)-trans-5,6-oxido-7,9-trans11,14-cis-eicosatetranonic acid] is an unstable intermediate that undergoes attack by water, nucleophiles and alcohols. LTA_4 thus is converted by a hydrolase into LTB_4 in neutrophils, eosinophils, mast cell, alveolar macrophages and airway epithelial cells (Fig. 1). Eosinophils, mast cells and alveolar macrophages also possess a LTC_4 synthase, which converts LTA_4 into LTC_4. LTC_4 is transported rapidly out of the cell where it is quickly converted by γ-glutamyltranspeptidase into LTD_4. LTD_4 is converted more slowly into LTE_4, which is secreted into the urine and is sometimes used (controversially) as a marker for cysLT synthesis. Leukotriene B_4 binds to its own BLT receptor. The cysLTs are characterized by a side chain containing 3, 2 or 1 amino acids (cysteine is always present); there are two or more specific cysLT receptors in tissues at various sites including airway smooth muscle, vascular smooth muscle and inflammatory cells themselves. The high affinity cysLT receptor recently has been cloned. All cysLTs bind to this receptor.

Recent investigations have suggested that cysLT may also be synthesized in the cytosol in lipid bodies that are formed during cellular activation in eosinophils. It has been suggested that all

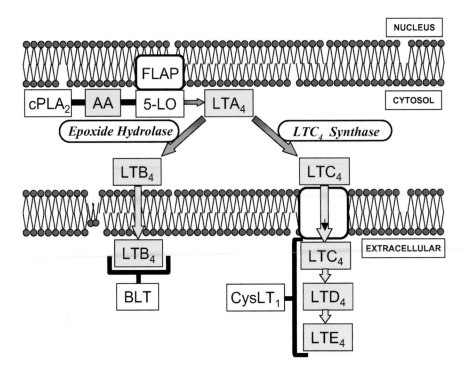

Fig. 1 Schema representing synthesis of cysteinyl leukotreine (cysLT) and BLT at the nuclear membrane. In this schema, cPLA$_2$ has migrated from the cytosol to the nuclear envelope and 5-LO is secreted from the nucleus to produce the unstable metabolite, LTA$_4$, which catalyzed by 5-LO from the 5-HPETE (not shown). Upon synthesis, catalyzed by LTC$_4$ synthase, there is active secretion of LTC$_4$, which is converted rapidly to LTD$_4$ outside of the inflammatory cell. Note that a specific hydrolase catalyzes the formation of LTB$_4$, a non-cysLT, which has its own receptor. See text for details. Reprinted with permission from reference 6.

enzyme and transport systems essential to cysLT synthesis exist in these lipid bodies, and hence synthesis could occur with translocation of cPLA$_2$ to the nuclear envelope. Likewise, it has been suggested that 5-LO is not stored within the nucleus, but rather is an enzyme dispersed throughout the cytosol, which migrates to the nuclear membrane and cytosolic lipid bodies upon activation. The role of secretory PLA$_2$ in leukotriene synthesis also is not completely defined. Recent studies in cell free systems indicates that group V sPLA$_2$, a 14 kD protein with a high predilection for phosphatidylcholine on the plasma membrane of granulocytes, is capable of causing AA synthesis through hydrolysis of the outer plasma membrane. This is presumed to be followed by subsequent internalization of AA, 5-LO activation and cysLT synthesis by a mechanism that does not involve cPLA$_2$ or metabolites/ isoforms of the mitogen-activated

protein kinase (MAPK) pathway. Reports of this novel pathway are still unverified, but the role of sPLA$_2$ isoforms in leukotriene sythesis remains an area of considerable interest. sPLA$_2$s have been identified in the bronchoalveolar lavage fluid of asthmatic subjects.

Role of Leukotrienes in Inflammatory Diseases

LTB$_4$, a B-leukotriene, is a potent chemotaxin for neutrophils and a weak chemotaxin for human eosinophils. There is no indication that it is an essential chemotactic receptor, and eosinophil migration progresses *in vivo* even in the presence of LTB$_4$-receptor blockade. In human neutrophils, LTB$_4$ causes translocation of intracellular calcium that initiates an autocrine pattern of stimulated cellular activity. Some studies have shown that LTB$_4$ may cause contraction of both human bronchus and guinea pig parenchymal strips *in vitro*;

Tab. 1 **Pharmacologic actions of the leukotrienes**[1]. Reprinted with permission from reference 5.

LTB_4	Cysteinyl LTs (LTC_4, LTD_4, LTE_4)
PMN aggregration	Airway smooth muscle contraction
PMN chemotaxis	Constriction of conducting airways
	Contraction of guinea pig parenchyma
Exudation of plasma	Secretion of mucus
Translocation of calcium	Fluid leakage from venules
Stimulation of PLA_2 (guinea pig)	Edema formation
Contraction of human bronchus (?)	Chemoattraction of eosinophils
Contraction of guinea pig parenchyma (?)	Autocrine activation of PLA_2 (guinea pig)
No effect with LTRA	Blocked by LTRA

[1]Adapted from Leff AR Discovery of leukotrienes and development of antileukotriene agents. (2001) Annals of Allergy, Asthma and Immunol 8(supp):864–868.

however, blockade of LTB_4 has little or no therapeutic action in human asthma.

The cysLTs were formerly known as SRS-A (slow reacting substance of anaphylaxis) because of the slow, sustained contraction of airway smooth muscle that resulted from the secretion of this substance(s) upon mast cell activation. Although originally identified in tissue mast cells, eosinophils and mast cells both have substantial cysLT synthetic capacity. Because the eosinophil is ubiquitous in asthma and allergic disease and because it is capable of cysLT synthesis, this cell has generally been regarded as the primary mechanism for sustained cysLT secretion in allergic states (Table 1).

Asthmatic exacerbations are associated with chemotaxis of eosinophils from the peripheral blood across endothelial membranes into the parenchyma and lumen of the conducting airways of the lung. This process is facilitated by the upregulation of β_1- and β_2-integrin, which bind to counterligands of the immunoglobulin supergene family on the endothelial surface. Diapedesis is facilitated by the presence of these ligands on both sides of the endothelium (lumenal and parencymal). The migration of eosinophils from the peripheral blood to human airways provides a continuous reservoir for leukotriene synthesis in allergic and asthma reactions. The 85 kD phospholipase $cPLA_2$ that catalyzes the first steps of leukotriene synthesis also serves as a messenger protein for cellular adhesion, likely from the synthesis of lysophospholipid, which is the by-product of membrane hydrolysis in which AA is also synthesized.

Leukotrienes may play a more important role in allergy than asthma. While cysLTs are highly efficacious bronchoconstricting agents when administered exogenously to human asthmatics (Fig. 2) (1,000-fold the potency of histamine), a critical role for cystLT in asthmatic bronchoconstriction has not been established. Amelioration of inflammatory response by corticosteroids in both asthma and allergic reactions is highly efficacious and does not appear to result from blockade of leukotriene synthesis. No other chronic inflammatory disease has been linked directly to cysLT secretion despite the capacity for these compounds to cause edema and inflammatory cell migration.

Drugs

The effects of leukotrienes can be blocked at several levels. Inhibitors of 5-lipoxygenase activating protein (FLAP) or 5-lipoxygenase inhibit LT synthesis at all levels. However, FLAP antagonists developed to date have been too hepatotoxic for human use. Zileuton, a 5-LO inhibiting drug, also demonstrated some hepatotoxicity in a small per-

L

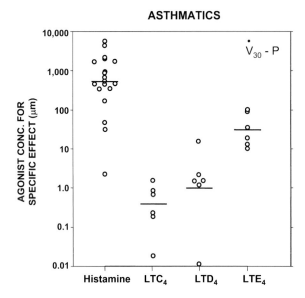

ASTHMATICS

Fig. 2 **Relative airway responsives of asthmatic patients to inhaled cysteinyl leukotrines versus histamine.** CysLTs have up to 1000-fold greater potency in causing bronchoconstriction than histamine.
Reprinted from (2), by permission of the publisher.

centage of patients, which was nonetheless entirely reversible. However, the short half-life of this compound requires 4-times daily administration in, and, accordingly, this compound is rarely prescribed. The most widely used anti-LT drugs are the ▶ leukotriene receptor antagonists, which were synthesized before the cloning of the cysLT receptor. These include pranlukast, which is widely used in Japan, and zafirlukast and montelukast, which are used in the United States, Europe and Asia. In controlled studies in human asthmatics, these compounds causes 5–8% improvement in bronchoconstriction as measured by the forced expiratory volume in 1 second (FEV_1). LTRAs have been shown to reduce the need for inhaled corticosteroids (ICS) and β-adrenoceptor agonists in human asthma. Additional studies have suggested that addition of an LTRA to loratadine, an antihistamine, or to ICS or β-adrenoceptor agonists augments the improvement in FEV_1. Nonetheless, LTRAs are fairly expensive and substantially less efficacious than either long acting β-adrenergic agonists (LABA) or ICS, particularly when LABA and ICS are used in combination. Accordingly, the use of LTRAs is often relegated to either mild asthma or as supplemental therapy for patients failing to respond to other drugs.

There arefew definitive data to substantiate the efficacy of LTRA therapy in refractory asthma, except for patients with "aspirin-sensitive asthma". This is a fairly uncommon form of asthma that occurs generally in adults who often have no prior (i.e. childhood) history of asthma or ▶ atopy, may have nasal polyposis, and who often are dependent upon oral corticosteroids for control of their asthma. This syndrome is not specific to aspirin but is provoked by any inhibitors of the cycloxygenase-1 (COX-1) pathway. These patients have been shown to have a genetic defect that causes overexpression of the enzyme LTC_4 synthase. However, the mechanism by which this bronchoconstriction is provoked by COX-1 inhibition remains unexplained. In such patients, LTRAs are specifically indicated. There is limited evidence suggesting that patients with aspirin-sensitive asthma can use selective COX-2 inhibitors safely; however, COX-2-specific analgesics still are not recommended for use in aspirin-sensitive asthma by the FDA in the United States.

Although some studies have shown no change in the excretion of LTE_4 in the urine of patients treated with corticosteroids, other investigations indicated that corticosteroids inhibit $cPLA_2$ translocation to the nuclear nuclear membrane in inflammatory cells, thus attenuating stimulated synthesis of cysLTs. This would suggest that oral and possibly inhaled corticosteroids may also inhibit production of cysLTs both directly (see above) and indirectly by causing necrosis and apoptosis of eosinophils, which are the predominant leukotriene-sythesizing cells in asthmatic airways (see above).

In the United States, LTRAs have largely replaced theophylline as the incremental drug for the treatment of moderate and severe asthma, where LABA and ICS do not effect adequate control. For patients with mild persistent asthma, LTRAs have been designated as a suitable substitute for low dose ICS by the National Asthma Education Panel Program (NAEPP) of the National Heart and Lung Institute (National Institutes of Health).

Therapeutic Response to Anti-leukotriene Drugs

When given acutely to patients who have no prior exposure to LTRA therapy, FEV_1 increases measureably within 30 min and results in a maximal improvement of about 10% in 1 hr. For short acting drugs, e.g. zileuton, this response returns rapidly to baseline, and the drug must initially be administered in 4 doses daily. In this regard, the initial effects of 5-LO inhibition are more like bronchodilators than disease modifying agents. However, with prolonged use (>60 days) there is little difference between peak and trough response in FEV_1, even if zileuton administration is decreased to twice daily. This acquired, longer acting effect has been suggested to imply a disease modifying effect of anti-leukotriene therapy. In some studies, even acute administration of LTRAs has caused a modest decrease in eosinophil migration into asthmatic airways, and the presence of the cysLT receptor, which has been recently identified on eosinophils, suggests a possible mechanism for this action. Other recent studies indicate that the LTRA, montelukast, if infused intravenously causes rapid incremental increase in FEV_1 in patients seeking treatment for acute asthma. The reason for the improved efficacy by intravenous infusion is unclear, but further investigations are examining the future role of LTRAs as potential rescue drugs in acute asthma.

LTRAs are extremely safe for patient use. However, the present generation of LTRAs is only modestly efficacious. Many patients show no clinically meaningful response, and current recommendations suggest a one month trial period to determine if patients will benefit from these drugs. With the exception of aspirin-sensitive asthmatics, there is currently no means for predicting which patients or under what circumstances anti-leukotrine therapies will be effective.

References

1. Samuelsson B (1983) Leukotrienes: mediators of immediate hypersensitivity reactions and inflammation. Science 220:568
2. Drazen JM (1988) Comparative contractile responses to sulfidopeptidyl leukotrienes in normal and asthmatic human subjects. NY Acad. Sci. 524:289–295
3. Expert Panel Report 2 (1997) Guidelines for the Diagnosis and Management of Asthma. NIH publication 97-4051, 86 pp.
4. Leff AR (2001) Regulation of leukotrienes in the management of asthma: biology and clinical therapy. Annu. Rev. Med. 52:1–14
5. Leff AR. (2001). Annals of Allergy and Immunology 86 (supp):4-8.
6. Fisher AR, Drazen JM (1997). Leukotrienes. In Asthma, ed. P. Barnes, MM Grunstein, AR Leff and A. Woolcock. Vol 1, pp. 547-58. Philadelphia, Lippincott-Raven

Levodopa

▶ L-DOPA / Levodopa

Lewy Bodies

Lewy bodies are typical in neuronal degeneration, which is accompanied by the presence of these eosinophilic intracellular inclusions of 5–25 μm in diameter in a proportion of still surviving neurons. Lewy bodies contain neurofilament, tubulin, microtubule-associated proteins 1 and 2, and gelsolin, an actin-modulating protein.

Liddle's Syndrome

Liddle's syndrome is an autosomal dominant disorder that is caused by persistent hyperactivity of the epithelial Na channel. Its symptoms mimic aldosterone excess, but plasma aldosterone levels are actually reduced (pseudoaldosteronism). The disease is characterized by early onset arterial hypertension, hypokalemia, and metabolic alkalosis.

Disease-causing mutations are found in the cytoplasmic regulatory region of the β and γ subunits of the epithrlial sodium channel (ENaC) genes. In general, patients with Liddle's syndrome

L

can be treated successfully with the ENaC inhibitor amiloride.

▶ Epithelial Sodium Channels

Ligand

A ligand can be an antagonist or agonist that binds to a receptor.

Ligand-gated Ion Channels

Ion channels that are opened by binding of a neurotransmitter (or drug) to a receptor domain on extracellular sites of the channel protein(s) are defined as ligand-gated. Nicotinic acetylcholine, ▶ glutamate, γ-aminobutyric acid$_A$ (GABA$_A$) and ▶ glycine receptors are examples of this type of receptor-linked ion channel.

▶ Benzodiazepines
▶ Cyclic Nucleotide-gated Channels
▶ Ca^{2+} Channels
▶ Ionotropic Glutamate Receptors
▶ Nicotinic Receptors
▶ K$^+$ Channels
▶ Serotoninergic System
▶ Purinergic System
▶ Tolerance and Desensitization
▶ Table appendix: Receptor Proteins

Limbic System

The limbic system is part of the brain, consisting of the amygdala, the hippocampus and evolutionarily old regions of the cortex, takes part in the representation of emotions in the brain.

Lipid Modifications

PATRICK J. CASEY
Duke University Medical Center, Durham, USA
Casey006@mc.duke.edu

Synonyms

Lipidation, S-acylation, N-myristoylation, myristoylation, S-prenylation, prenylation, palmitoylation, isoprenylation, ▶ GPI anchors, glypiation

Definition

Covalent attachment of lipid moieties to proteins plays important roles in the cellular localization and function of a broad spectrum of proteins in all eukaryotic cells. Such proteins, commonly referred to as lipidated proteins, are classified based on the identity of the attached lipid (Fig. 1). Each specific type of lipid has unique properties that confer distinct functional attributes to its protein host. S-acylated proteins, commonly referred to as palmitoylated proteins, generally contain the 16-carbon saturated acyl group palmitoyl attached via a labile thioester bond to cysteine residue(s), although other fatty acyl chains may substitute for palmitoyl group. N-myristoylated proteins contain the saturated 14-carbon myristoyl group attached via amide bond formation to amino-terminal glycine residues. S-prenylated proteins contain one of two ▶ isoprenoid lipids, either the 15-carbon farnesyl or 20-carbon geranylgeranyl. The fourth major class of lipidated proteins is those containing the glycosylphosphatidylinositol (GPI) moiety, a large and complex structure of which the lipid component is an entire phospholipid.

Basic Mechanisms

S-acylated proteins include many GTP-binding regulatory proteins (G-proteins), including most α subunits of ▶ heterotrimeric G-proteins and also many members of the Ras superfamily of monomeric G proteins, a number of ▶ G protein-coupled receptors, several nonreceptor ▶ tyrosine kinases, and a number of other signaling molecules. S-acylation is post-translational and reversi-

Lipid	Structure	Position of Modification
N-myristoyl	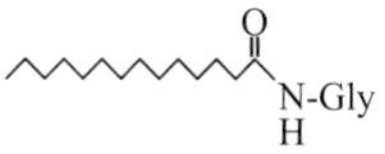 (structure) N-Gly	Amino-terminal glycine
S-acyl (S-palmitoyl)	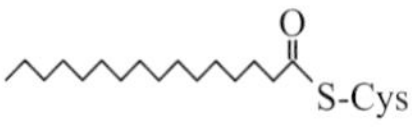 (structure) S-Cys	Cysteine, no defined consensus
S-prenyl (farnesyl)	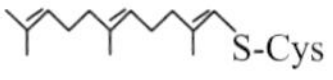 (structure) S-Cys	Cysteine at/near carboxyl-terminus
S-prenyl (geranylgeranyl)	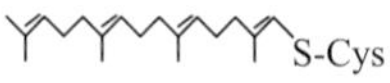 (structure) S-Cys	Cysteine at/near carboxyl-terminus
GPI anchor	Complex structure includes phosphatidylinositol and sugars	Carboxyl-terminus

Fig. 1 Major classes of lipid-modified proteins.

ble, a property that allows the cell to control the modification state, and hence the localization and biological activity, of the protein. The lipid substrates for S-acylation are ▶ Acyl-CoA molecules. The molecular mechanism of S-acylation is only recently being elucidated; the first identified acyltransferase specifically involved in the process being the product of the *Skinny Hedgehog (Ski)* gene in Drosophila (1). *Ski* orthologs have also been identified in mammalian genomes. This acyltransferase appears to specifically process secreted proteins, in particular a molecule important in development termed Hedgehog. Hedgehog proteins undergo two lipid modifications during their maturation involving covalently modification by cholesterol at their carboxyl-terminus (a modification that has not been characterized for any other protein to date) and the S-acylation catalyzed by Ski on a conserved amino-terminal cysteine residue. Since the acylation of Hedgehog is apparently coupled to passage through the secretory pathway, there are most likely other unidentified enzymes that handle the numerous intracellular S-acylated proteins. In addition, nonenzymatic acylation of cysteine thiols on proteins incubated in the presence of acyl-CoA has been described, although the biological importance of this process is still unclear.

N-myristoylated proteins include select α subunits of heterotrimeric G proteins, a number of nonreceptor tyrosine kinases, a few monomeric G-

proteins, and several other proteins important in biological regulation. There is some overlap between S-acylated and N-myristoylated proteins such that many contain both lipid modifications. Such "dual lipidation" can have important consequences, most notably the localization of the dually modified species to distinct membrane subdomains termed ▶ lipid rafts or ▶ caveolae (2). N-myristoylation is a stable modification of proteins. The myristoyl moiety is attached to the protein cotranslationally by the enzyme myristoyl CoA: protein N-myristoyltransferase (NMT); the lipid substrate is myristoyl-CoA. NMT has been extensively studied in regard to substrate utilization and kinetic properties, and crystal structures of fungal enzymes are available (3). There are two distinct but closely related genes encoding NMTs in mammalian cells, *NMT1* and *NMT2*, although differences between the two isoforms have not yet been described.

S-prenylation is the most recent of the four major types of lipid modifications to be described. As with S-acylation, S-prenylation is posttranslational. The lipid substrates for these modifications are farnesyl diphosphate and geranylgeranyl diphosphate. The mechanism involves attachment of the isoprenoid lipid to cysteine residues at or near the carboxyl terminus through a stable thioether bond (4). Two distinct classes of S-prenylated proteins exist in eukaryotic organisms. Proteins containing a cysteine residue fourth from the carboxyl terminus (the so-called CaaX-motif) can be modified by either the 15-carbon farnesyl or 20-carbon geranylgeranyl isoprenoid by one of two closely-related termed protein farnesyltransferase (FTase) and protein geranylgeranyltransferase type 1 (GGTase-1); these enzymes are collectively referred to as CaaX prenyltransferases. FTase and GGTase-1 are $\alpha\beta$ heterodimers; the α subunits of the enzymes are identical while the β subunits are the products of distinct, but related, genes. The identity of the "X" residue of the CaaX motif dictates which of the two enzymes recognize the substrate protein. Following prenylation, most CaaX-type proteins are further processed by proteolytic removal of the three carboxyl-terminal residues (i.e. the –aaX) by the Rce1 CaaX protease and methylation of the now-exposed carboxyl group of the prenylcysteine by the Icmt methyltransferase. A number of S-prenylated proteins are also subject to S-acylation at a nearby cysteine residue to produce a dually lipidated molecule, although this type of dual modification does not apparently target the protein to the same type of membrane subdomain as the dual acylation noted above.

The second class of S-prenylated proteins is members of the Rab family of proteins, which are involved in membrane trafficking in cells. These proteins are geranylgeranylated at two cysteine residues at or very near to their carboxyl-terminus by protein geranylgeranyltransferase type 2 (GGTase-2), also known as Rab GGTase. GGTase-2 is also a $\alpha\beta$ heterodimer and its subunits show significant sequence similarity to the corresponding subunits of the CaaX prenyltransferases. However, unlike the CaaX prenyltransferases, monomeric Rab proteins are not substrates for GGTase-2. In order to be processed by the enzyme, newly synthesized Rab proteins first bind and form a stable complex with a protein termed Rep, and it is the Rab-Rep complex that is recognized by GGTase-II. The enzyme acts in a processive fashion, attaching both geranylgeranyl groups to closely spaced cysteine residues at or near the carboxyl-terminus of the Rab proteins. All three of the protein prenyltransferases (FTase, GGTase-1, GGTase-2) have been extensively characterized in regard to substrate recognition, mechanism and structure.

GPI-anchored proteins constitute a quite diverse family of cell-surface molecules that participate in such processes as nutrient uptake, cell adhesion and membrane signaling events. All GPI-linked proteins are destined for the cell surface via trafficking through the secretory pathway, where they acquire the pre-assembled GPI moiety. The entire procedure, which involves assembly of the GPI moiety from ▸ phosphatidylinositol and sugars and proteolytic processing of the target protein to expose the GPI addition site at the carboxyl-terminus of the protein, involves a number of gene products. Many of the genes associated with GPI biosynthesis have been cloned by complementation of GPI-deficient mammalian cell lines and temperature-sensitive yeast GPI mutants. The precise mechanisms through which these enzymes work in concert to produce a GPI-anchored protein are just now begining to be elucidated.

Pharmacological Intervention

Since the mechanisms of protein S-acylation are so poorly understood, there is little in the way of good pharmacological agents that target this process. One compound that has been used with modest success is cerulenin, which apparently mimics the acyl-CoA substrate in the reaction catalyzed by the putative S-acyltransferase that acts on intracellular proteins. In contrast, there has been substantial effort to identify and characterize specific inhibitors of N-myristoylation. Genetic and biochemical studies have established NMT as a target for development of anti-fungal drugs. The enzyme is also a potential target for the development of antiviral and antineoplastic agents. Both peptidic and nonpeptidic inhibitors of NMTs, particularly fungal NMTs, have been described.

There has been enormous effort in the past 10 years to develop pharmacological agents targeting the S-prenylation by CaaX prenyltransferases, especially FTase. This is primarily due to the interest in one subset of S-prenylated proteins, the Ras proteins, due to the importance role of Ras in ▸ oncogenesis. Ras proteins are modified by the 15-carbon farnesyl isoprenoid, and farnesylation of these proteins is indispensable for both normal biological acitvity and oncogenic transformation. Selective inhibitors of FTase, termed FTIs, can reverse Ras-mediated oncogenic transformation of cells, and several are in clinical development as anti-cancer therapeutics. Literally hundreds of potent inhibitors of FTase, and many of GGTase-1, have been identified using several strategies, including design of analogs of the CaaX peptide and isoprenoid substrates and by high-throughput screening of natural product and compound libraries. These compounds can be placed into four distinct categories: mimics of CaaX tetrapeptides, mimics of FPP, ▶ bisubstrate analogs, and organic compounds selected from natural product and chemical libraries. There has been relatively little development of pharmacological agents targeting GGTase-2. It is likely, however, that some of the isoprenoid analogs that show activity against GGTase-1 will also have inhibitory activity on GGTase-2 given that both enzymes use the same isoprenoid substrate.

There is also increasing interest in developing pharmacological agents targeting the biosynthesis of GPI-anchored proteins (5). Such proteins are particularly abundant on the surface of a number of protozoan organisms. Several devastating tropical diseases such as African sleeping sickness and Chagas disease are caused by protozoan parasites that rely heavily on cell-surface GPI-anchored proteins for both inhabiting their host and escaping immune detection. In studies primarily involving gene disruption approaches, several of the enzymes involved in GPI biosynthesis have been identified as attractive targets for development of anti-parasitics. To date, there is very little publically available information on specific inhibitors of the enzymes involved in GPI biosynthesis and attachment, but it is likely that such information will be forthcoming.

References

1. Ingham PW. (2001) Hedgehog signaling: a tale of two lipids. Science 29:1879–1881
2. Simons K, Toomre D (2000) Lipid rafts and signal transduction. Nat Rev Mol Cell Biol 1:31–39
3. Bhatnagar RS, Futterer K, Waksman G, Gordon JI (1999) The structure of myristoyl-CoA: protein N-myristoyltransferase. Biochim Biophys Acta 1441:162–172
4. Fu, HW, Casey, PJ (1999). Enzymology and biology of CaaX protein prenylation. Recent Progress Hormone Res 54:315–343
5. Ferguson, MAJ (2000) Glycosylphosphatidylinositol biosynthesis validated as a drug target for African sleeping sickness. Proc. Natl. Acad. Sci. (USA) 97:10673–10675

Lipid Phosphate Phosphohydrolases

Lipid phosphate phosphohydrolases (LPPs), formerly called type 2 phosphatidate phosphohydrolases (PAP-2), catalyse the dephosphorylation of bioactive phospholipids (phosphatidic acid, ceramide-1-phosphate) and ▶ lysophospholipids (lyso-phosphatidic acid, sphingosine-1-phosphate). The substrate selectivity of individual LPPs is broad in contrast to the related sphingosine-1-phosphate phosphatase. LPPs are characterized by a lack of requirement for Mg^{2+} and insensitivity to N-ethylmaleimide. Three subtypes (LPP-1, LPP-2, LPP-3) have been identified in mammals. These enzymes have six putative transmembrane domains and three highly conserved domains that are characteristic of a phosphatase superfamily. Whether LPPs cleave extracellular mediators or rather have an influence on intracellular lipid phosphate concentrations is still a matter of debate.

Lipid Rafts

Lipd rafts are specific subdomains of the plasma membrane that are enriched in cholesterol and sphingolipids; many signaling molecules are apparently concentrated in these subdomains.

▶ Lipid Modifications

Lipid-lowering Drugs

Lipid-lowering drugs are drugs that affect the lipoprotein metabolism and that used in therapy to lower plasma lipids (cholesterol, triglycerides). The main classes of drugs used clinically are statins (HMG-CoA reductase inhibitors), anion exchange resins (e.g. cholestyramine and cholestipol), fibrates (bezafibrate, gemfibrozil or clofibrate) and other drugs like nicotinic acid.

▶ HMG-CoA-reductase-inhibitors
▶ Fibrates
▶ Anion Exchange Resins

Lipopolysaccharide

A lipopolysaccharide (LPS) is any compound consisting of covalently linked lipids and polysaccharides. The term is used more frequently to denote a cell wall component from Gram-negative bacteria. LPS has endotoxin activities and is a polyclonal stimulator of B-lymphocytes.

Lipoprotein

▶ HMG-CoA-reductase Inhibitors

5-lipoxygenase

5-lipoxygenase is the enzyme causing catalysis of arachidonic acid into leukotriene A4.
▶ Leukotrienes

Lipoxygenases

▶ Leukotrienes

Lithocholic Acid

Lithocholic acid is a 3α-hydroxy-5β-cholanoic acid, a hepatotoxic and cholestatic secondary bile acid, which is formed by bacterial dehydroxylation of primary bile acids in the intestine.

L-NAME

L-NAME (N-nitro-L-arginine methyl ester), like L-NMMA, is a structural analogue of L-arginine and competes with L-arginine for NO-synthase, which uses L-arginine as a substrate for the formation of NO. L-NMMA and L-NAME are very effective NO-synthesis inhibitors, both *in vitro* and *in vivo*.

▶ NO Synthase

Local Anaesthetics

MICHAEL BRÄU
Universitätsklinikum, Justus-Liebig-Universität, Gießen, Germany
meb@anesthesiologie.de

Definition

Local anaesthetics are drugs that reversibly interrupt impulse propagation in peripheral nerves thus leading to autonomic nervous system blockade, analgesia, anaesthesia and motor blockade in a desired area of the organism.

▶ General Anaesthetics
▶ Voltage-dependent Na$^+$ Channels

Mechanism of Action

Impulse propagation in the ▶ peripheral nervous system depends on the interplay between ion channels selective to potassium and sodium. Briefly, few voltage insensitive potassium chan-

lipophilic moiety   bond   termi

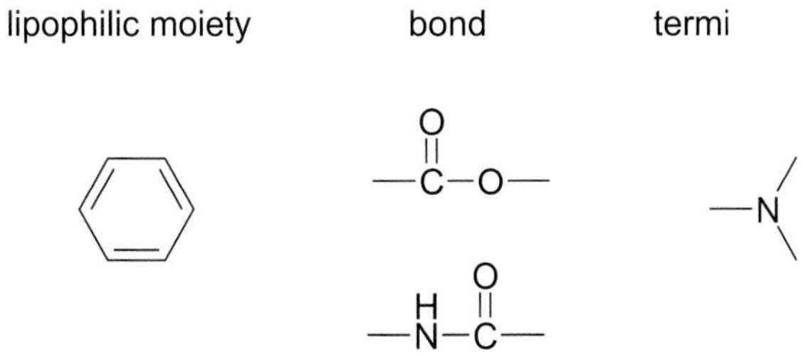

Fig. 1 Common structure of local anaesthetics. A
lipophilic moiety on the left, an aliphatic spacer containing an ester or amide bond in the middle and an
amine group on the right are the typical structural elements for local anaesthetic drugs.

nels allow diffusion of positively charged potassium ions from the internal side of the axon to the
exterior. This leaves a negative charge at the internal side that is called resting potential and
amounts to approximately -80 mV over the
▶ axonal membrane. Upon a small depolarisation
of the membrane, ▶ voltage gated sodium channels open (activate) and conduct positively
charged sodium ions from the exterior to the interior of the axon that depolarises the membrane to
about $+60$ mV (action potential). After a few milliseconds the channels close spontaneously (inactivation) terminating the action potential and thus
giving it an impulse like character. The action
potential spreads electrotonically to neighbouring
sodium channels that also open to produce an
action potential. In this way, the impulse is propagated along the nerve to (afferent) or from (efferent) the central nervous system. Local anaesthetics
inhibit ionic current through voltage gated sodium
channels in a concentration dependent and reversible manner therefore directly blocking the
impulse propagation process in either direction
(1). The interaction between the local anaesthetic
molecule and the sodium channel is complex. The
binding affinity is low for resting channels, but
dramatically increases when the channel is activated. Thus, at high stimulus frequency sodium
current block increases (use-dependent block).
Use-dependent block is not important for conduction block during local anaesthesia since very high
concentrations are reached locally producing complete and sufficient block. However, when local

anaesthetics such as lidocaine are applied intravenously, lower systemic concentrations may already
induce use-dependent block and thus reduce
excitability in electrically active cells. This mechanism is important for the successful use of lidocaine as an antiarrhythmic or analgesic drug.

The putative binding site for local anaesthetic
molecules at the sodium channel has been identified as two amino acids in the sixth membrane-
spanning segment of domain IV (2). This binding
site is located directly underneath the channel
pore and can only be reached from the internal
side of the membrane. Because local anaesthetics
are applied exterior to the nerve fibre, they have to
penetrate the axonal membrane before they can
bind to the channel.

Besides sodium channels, other ion channels
such calcium- and potassium channels as well as
certain ligand-gated channels are affected by local
anaesthetics. However, this plays only a minor role
for nerve block but may have more impact on
adverse effects induced by systemical concentrations of these drugs.

Structure Activity Relation
Local anaesthetics comprise a lipophilic and a
hydrophilic portion separated by a connecting
hydrocarbon chain (Fig. 1). The hydrophilic group
is mostly a tertiary amine such as diethylamine;
the lipophilic group is usually an unsaturated aromatic ring such as xylidine or para-aminobenzoic
acid. The lipophilic portion is essential for anaesthetic potency whereas the hydrophilic portion is
required for water solubility. Both groups are
important for binding the drug molecule to the
sodium channel. The connecting hydrocarbon
chain usually contains an ester or an amide, in
rare cases also an ether, and separates the
lipophilic and hydrophilic portions of the molecule in an ideal distance for binding to the channel. Local anaesthetics are classified by the nature
of this bond into ester or amide local anaesthetics.
This bond is also important for metabolism of the
drugs and to adverse reactions such as allergic
reactions. Clinically relevant local anaesthetics
have an efficacy of 100%, i.e. at high concentrations they completely abolish the sodium current.
Their blocking potencies range from a few micromolar to millimolar half-maximal blocking concentration and are highly dependent on lipid solu-

Tab. 1 Examples of clinically used local anaesthetics. The ending 'caine' stems from cocaine, the first clinically employed local anaesthetic. Procaine and tetracaine are ester-linked substances, the others are amides. Amide bonded local anaesthetics usually contain two i's in their name, ester-bonded only one. In the structure drawings, the lipophilic portion of the molecule is depicted at the left, the amine at the right. The asterisk marks the chiral centre of the stereoisomeric drugs. Lipid solubility is given as the logarithm of the water:octanol partition coefficient, log(P).

Name	Structure	Relative potency	Mean blocking duration [h]	Lipid solubility log[P]	Molwt. [g/mol]	pKa
procaine	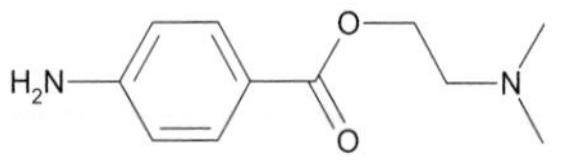 (chemical structure)	1	0.5–1	1.92	236	9.1
tetracaine	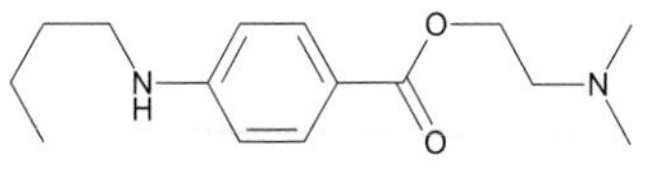 (chemical structure)	8	2–3	3.73	264	8.6
lidocaine	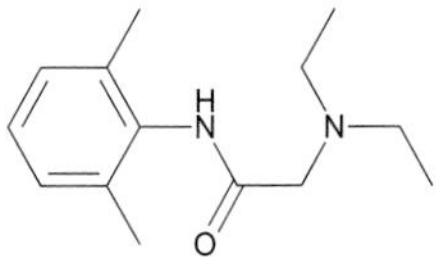 (chemical structure)	2	1–2	2.26	234	8.2
prilocaine	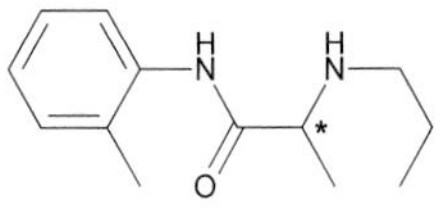 (chemical structure)	2	1–2	2.11	220	7.9
mepivacaine	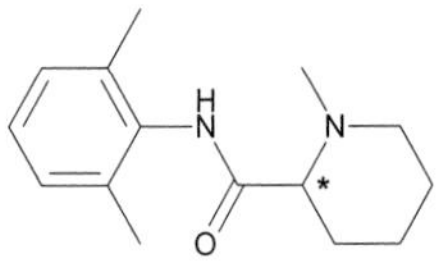 (chemical structure)	2	1,5–2	1.95	246	7.9
ropivacaine	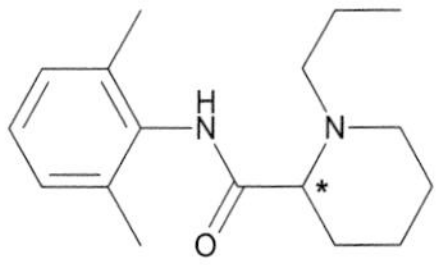 (chemical structure)	6	3–5	2.90	274	8.2
bupivacaine	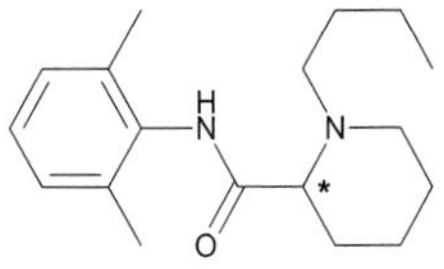 (chemical structure)	8	4–6	3.41	288	8.2

bility. To a smaller amount potency also depends on the structure of the molecule and on the type of bonding (Table 1). Further determinants of blocking potency are the membrane potential and the state in which the sodium channel is in (resting, activated, inactivated). The tertiary amine group can be protonated giving most local anaesthetics a pK_a of about eight so that a larger amount of the drug is in the hydrophilic form when injected into tissue with physiological pH. However, only the unprotonated lipophilic form is able to penetrate the axonal membrane, which is required before binding to the sodium channel can occur. In a very acidic environment, like inflamed tissue, local anaesthetics are highly protonated, therefore cannot penetrate the axonal membrane and have little effect.

Toxicity

Local anaesthetics interfere with all voltage-gated sodium channel isoforms in an organism and thus with all electrically excitable cells in organs such as brain, heart and muscle. The major unwanted effects of local anaesthetics are thus disturbances of brain and heart function occurring during systemically high concentrations after overdosing or after accidental intra-vascular injection. Cerebral convulsions, general anaesthesia as well as dysrhythmias up to asystolic heart failure or ventricular fibrillation are feared as rare but most harmful complications. Other adverse effects can be allergic reactions. This occurs especially with ester-bonded local anaesthetics because their metabolism produces para-aminobenzoic acid that may serve as a hapten. As a special case, the local anaesthetic prilocaine is metabolised to o-toluidine, which may induce methemoglobinemia, especially in patients that have a glucose-6-phosphatase deficiency. The ▶ S-stereoisomers of the piperidine local anaesthetics bupivacaine and ropivacaine have now been introduced into clinical practise to reduce side effects. Their blocking potencies are minimally lower compared to their R-counterparts but their therapeutic index is wider.

Clinical Use

Local anaesthetics are mainly employed to induce regional anaesthesia and analgesia to allow surgical procedures in a desired region of the organism. Nerve block result in autonomic nervous system blockade, analgesia, anaesthesia and motor blockade. The patient normally stays awake during surgical procedures under regional anaesthesia, but regional anaesthesia can also be combined with general anaesthesia to reduce the requirement of narcotics and analgesic drugs. Local anaesthetics have to be injected locally into the circumference of a peripheral nerve, which gives sufficiently high concentrations to achieve conduction block. Certain injection techniques and procedures such as single nerve block as well as spinal, ▶ epidural, or intravenous regional anaesthesia have evolved to achieve the desired nerve block. It is also possible to place a catheter adjacent to a nerve and continuously apply local anaesthetics to receive long-term analgesia. Low concentrations of lipophilic local anaesthetics may be used for differential nerve block, i.e. only block of sympathetic and nociceptive fibres whereas somatosensory and motor fibres are less affected. Differential nerve

block for example is useful in labour analgesia or for analgesia after surgical procedures of the extremities.

After local anaesthetic injection, onset of nerve block and duration depends mainly on lipid solubility and on the region in where the drug is injected. In some formulations adrenaline is added to prolong the blocking action by inducing regional vasoconstriction and hereby reduce absorption and metabolisation.

The amide local anaesthetic lidocaine may also be used as an antiarrhythmic for ventricular tachycardia and exrasystoles after injection into the blood circulation. Drugs with high lipid solubility such as bupivacaine cannot be used for these purposes because their prolonged binding to the channel may induce dysrhythmias or asystolic heart failure (3). Systemically applied lidocaine has also been used successfully in some cases of ▶ neuropathic pain syndromes (4). Here, electrical activity in the peripheral nervous system is reduced by used-dependent but incomplete sodium channel blockade.

References

1. Butterworth JF, Strichartz GR. (1990) Molecular mechanisms of local anesthesia: A review. Anesthesiology 72:722–734
2. Ragsdale DS, McPhee JC, Scheuer T, Catterall WA (1994) Molecular determinants of state-dependent block of Na+ channels by local anesthetics. Science 265:1724–1728
3. Clarkson CW, Hondeghem LM. (1985) Mechanism for bupivacaine depression of cardiac conduction: Fast block of sodium channels during the action potential with slow recovery from block during diastole. Anesthesiology 62:396–405
4. Tanelian DL, Brose WG (1991) Neuropathic pain can be relieved by drugs that are use-dependent sodium channel blockers: lidocaine, carbamazepine, and mexiletine. Anesthesiology 74:949–951

Locus Ceruleus

The locus ceruleus is a structure located on the floor of the fourth ventricle in the rostral pons. It

L

contains more than 50% of all noradrenergic neurons in the brain, and projects to almost all areas of the central nervous system. The locus ceruleus is important for the regulation of attentional states and autonomic nervous system activity. It has also been implicated in the autonomic and stress-like effects of opiate withdrawal. A noradrenergic pathway originating from the locus ceruleus which descends into the spinal cord is part of the descending inhibitory control system, which has an inhibitory effect on nociceptive transmission in the dorsal horn.

Long-QT Syndromes

Long-QT syndromes (LQTS) are potentially fatal inherited cardiac arrhythmias characterized by prolonged or delayed ventricular repolarization, manifested on the electrocardiogram as a prolongation of the QT interval. LQTS can be caused by mutations of at least six genes including *KCNQ1* for LQT1, *KCNH2* for LQT2, *SCN5A* encoding a cardiac sodium channel for LQT3, *KCNE1* for LQT5 and *MiRP1* for LQT6. LQT4 is linked to the mutations located in chromosome 4q25-27. Blockade of HERG channels is the most commonly identified drug-induced LQT.

▶ K^+ Channels
▶ Voltage-dependent Na^+ Channels

Long-term Depression

Long-term depression (LTD) is a synaptic plasticity phenomenon that corresponds to a decrease in the synaptic strength (decrease in the post-synaptic response observed for the same stimulation of the presynaptic terminals) observed after a specific stimulation of the afferent fibers. This decreased response is still observed hours after its induction.

Long-term Potentiation

Long-term potentiation (LTP) is a synaptic plasticity phenomenon that corresponds to an increase in the synaptic strength (increase in the post-synaptic response observed for the same stimulation of the presynaptic terminals) observed after a high frequency stimulation (tetanus) of the afferent fibers. This increased response is still observed hours and even days after the tetanus. The phenomenon is often observed at glutamatergic synapses and involves, in most cases, the activation of the N-methyl D-aspartate (NMDA) subtype of ▶ ionotropic glutamate receptors.

Loop Diuretics

▶ Diuretics

Low-density-lipoprotein (LDL)-cholesterol

LDL is the major carrier of cholesterol to the periphery and supplies the cholesterol essential for the integrity of nerve tissue, steroid hormone synthesis, and cell membranes. The association between elevated plasma cholesterol carried in LDL and the risk of coronary heart disease has been well established. LDL is also sometimes called the "bad" cholesterol.

Low-dose Oral Contraceptives

All formulations of combination oral contraceptives which contain less than 50 μg ethinyl estradiol per pill are called low-dose oral contraceptives.

► Contraceptives

LPS

► Lipopolysaccharide

LTD

► Long Term Depression

3′,5′,3,5-L-tetraiodothyronine

► Thyroxine

LTP

► Long Term Potentiation

3′,5,3-L-triiodothyronine

► Triiodothyronine

L-type Ca^{2+} Channel

The L-type calcium channel is the dihydropyridine-sensitive $Ca_v1.2$ calcium channel, that is essential for smooth muscle contraction and the target for the calcium channel blocker/calcium antagonists.

Luteinizing Hormone

► Contraceptives

Lymphangiogenesis

Lymphangiogenesis is the growth of lymphatic vessels, which is critically controlled by the interaction of VEGF-C and VEGF-D with the receptor VEGF-R3 on lymphatic endothelial cells.

► Angiogenesis and Vascular Morphogenesis

Lymphocytes

Lymphocytes are specialized white blood cells that play a crucial role in an immune response. They can be T lymphocytes, which can directly target and destroy defective cells, or B lymphocytes, which produce antibodies directed against specific antigens. Both T and B lymphocytes produce a variety of cytokines to augment and amplify the immune response.

► Immune Defense

Lysophosphatidic Acid

Lysophosphatidic acid (LPA) is the prototype of a group of bioactive lysophospholipids that act on specific G protein-coupled receptors to mediate a wide variety of cellular functions.

► Lysophospholipids

Lysophospholipids

DAGMAR MEYER ZU HERINGDORF
Universitätsklinikum Essen, Essen, Germany
meyer-heringdorf@uni-essen.de

Synonyms

Lysolipid mediators; phospholipid growth factors; lyso-glycerophospholipids and lyso-sphingolipids

Definition

The term "lysophospholipids" comprises a number of small bioactive lipid molecules that share some common features regarding structure and biological activity. The lysolipid structure renders these lipids more hydrophilic and versatile than their complex membrane bound precursors. Chemically, two subgroups can be distinguished: molecules containing the sphingoid base backbone (lyso-sphingolipids) and molecules containing the glycerol backbone (lyso-glycerophospholipids). Biologically, these lipids act as extracellular mediators activating specific G protein-coupled receptors (GPCRs), although some of them additionally play a role in intracellular signal transduction. The best characterized lysophospholipids are ▶ sphingosine-1-phosphate (S1P) and ▶ lysophosphatidic acid (LPA), and the concept of lysophospholipids as a group of mediators is supported by the high homology between S1P- and LPA-specific GPCRs. However, more candidate lipids are emerging that share the lysolipid structure and for which specific GPCRs have been identified, such as sphingosylphosphorylcholine (SPC) and lysophosphatidylcholine (LPC); some of them do not contain a phosphate, such as psychosine and glucopsychosine. Lysophospholipids play a functional role in many tissues, e.g. in the cardiovascular system, immune system and brain. In general, they appear to be auto- or paracrine regulators of cell growth, migration, differentiation and thus morphogenesis and regeneration. Relatives of the lysophospholipid family are platelet-activating factor and the endocannabinoids arachidonyl ethanolamide and 2-arachidonyl glycerol.

▶ Phospholipases

Basic Characteristics

Metabolism and Occurrence

S1P (Fig. 1) is formed from sphingosine by ▶ sphingosine kinase and degraded by S1P lyase or S1P phosphatase; in addition it can be cleaved by the non-specific ▶ lipid phosphate phosphohydrolases (LPPs), which also cleave LPA. S1P is stored in platelets and released upon platelet activation. Accordingly, it has been found in serum in higher concentrations (~0.5–0.8 µM) than in plasma (~0.2–0.4 µM). S1P in plasma is bound to albumin and lipoproteins, mainly high-density lipoproteins. The lipoproteins may regulate the bioavailability of plasma S1P. A constitutive release of S1P is found in several types of differentiated cells as well as in tumor cells. In addition to its role as extracellular mediator, S1P also plays a role as intracellular second messenger. Accordingly, production of intracellular S1P by sphingosine kinase is highly regulated by plasma membrane receptors. Regulation of extracellular S1P levels is less well understood.

LPA, i.e. monoacyl-glycerol-3-phosphate, can be formed and degraded by multiple metabolic pathways (Fig. 1). Depending on the precursor molecule and respective pathway, the fatty acid chain in LPA differs in length, degree of saturation and position (sn-1 or sn-2), which has an influence on biological activity. LPA analogs with ether-bound alkyl or alkenyl chains are quantitatively less abundant than those with ester-bound acyl chains. LPA may be produced intracellularly as well as extracellularly. Extracellular production of LPA from phosphatidic acid probably requires rearrangement of membrane phospholipid polarity as found in shed microvesicles, since most of phosphatidic acid is located in the inner plasma membrane leaflet. Alternatively, extracellular LPA may be formed from other lyso-glycerophospholipids by lyso-phospholipase D. In degradation of LPA, LPPs play a predominant role.

Like S1P, LPA is a constituent of plasma, formed during coagulation and present in serum in micromolar concentrations where it is bound to albumin. Recently, interesting differences in the fatty acid composition of plasma- versus serum-LPA

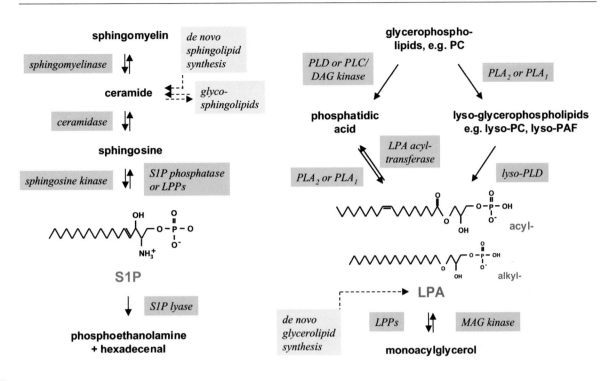

Fig. 1 Formation and degradation of S1P and LPA. DAG, diacylglycerol; LPPs, lipid phosphate phosphohydrolases; MAG, monoacylglycerol; PAF, platelet-activating factor; PC, phosphatidylcholine; PLA, phospholipase A; PLC, phospholipase C; PLD, phospholipase D.

were found, suggesting that the sources of these LPA pools were different. LPA is produced by many cell types, e.g. fibroblasts, adipocytes and tumor cells. It is found in aqueous humor after corneal injury, corresponding to its role in wound healing. Furthermore, LPA occurs in malignant ascites in substantially high concentrations, acting as an autocrine tumor cell growth factor.

Biological Actions

Cellular responses to S1P and LPA can be classified as growth-related (stimulation of cell proliferation and survival, protection from apoptosis), cytoskeleton-dependent (shape change, migration, adhesion, chemotaxis) and Ca^{2+}-dependent (contraction, secretion). In addition to the strong growth-promoting and antiapoptotic actions of S1P and LPA in many cell types, they occasionally inhibit proliferation or induce apoptosis. Cell migration likewise can be stimulated or inhibited. In cells of neural origin, S1P and LPA usually cause cell rounding and neurite retraction, while in

other cell types differentiation is induced. Both lysophospholipid mediators cause a mobilization of intracellular Ca^{2+} ($[Ca^{2+}]_i$) in many cell types and also have an influence on various ion channels.

S1P is a major stimulus of vascular endothelium (Fig. 2), inducing proliferation and migration of macro- and microvascular endothelial cells; the magnitude of its effects is comparable to that of vascular endothelial growth factor. In endothelial cells, S1P furthermore activates NO synthase (via protein kinase B (Akt)) and induces formation of adherens junction assembly, decrease in monolayer permeability and differentiation into capillary-like networks. LPA has a rather weak influence on migration of endothelial cells, but, like S1P, promotes surface expression of leukocyte adhesion molecules. Of the two platelet-derived lysophospholipids, LPA but not S1P induces platelet aggregation. Both S1P and LPA stimulate fibroblast proliferation and migration and LPA

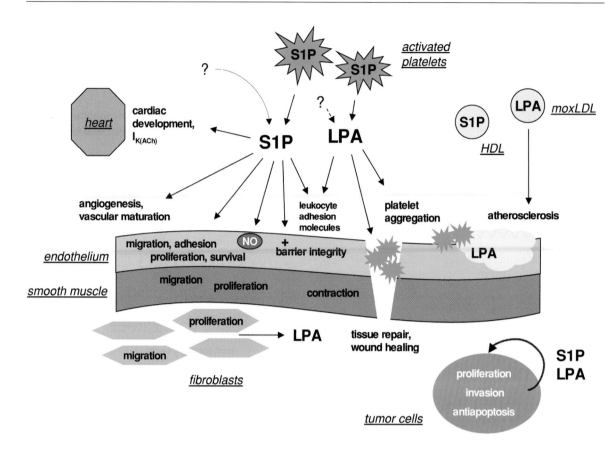

Fig. 2 Putative roles of S1P and LPA in the cardiovascular system, in wound healing and in tumor cell growth. HDL, high-density lipoproteins; moxLDL, mildly oxidized low-density lipoproteins.

promotes wound healing *in vivo* (Fig. 2). Thus, S1P and LPA interact in vessel formation and tissue repair.

S1P and LPA induce smooth muscle cell contraction, e.g., they cause vasoconstriction. Another action of S1P is activation of $I_{K(ACh)}$ in atrial myocytes. However, systemic cardiovascular parameters such as blood pressure or heart rate are marginally affected by intravenous S1P, consistent with a role of S1P as a local rather than systemic mediator. With regard to LPA, considerable species differences have been observed in blood pressure alterations. Other tissues that are responsive to S1P or LPA include the respiratory tract (activation of airway smooth muscle cells and cytokine release induced by S1P), kidney (diuresis caused by S1P), adipose tissue (preadipocyte proliferation induced by autocrine LPA), Schwann

cells (morphology, adhesion and survival regulated by LPA) and many others.

S1P, LPA and other lysolipids have been detected in lipoproteins and probably play a role in atherosclerosis. The major part of lipoprotein-bound S1P is associated with high-density lipoproteins (HDL), and the ability of HDL to protect endothelial cells from apoptosis has been attributed to HDL-bound S1P, SPC, and lysosulfatide. In contrast, LPA is produced during mild oxidation of low-density lipoproteins (LDL) and accumulates in atherosclerotic plaques where it acts proinflammatory and promotes thrombus formation. Another pathophysiological role of S1P and LPA is the promotion of tumor cell growth and metastasis. The two mediators are produced by several tumor cells and stimulate proliferation and survival of these cells in an autocrine manner. The

Tab. 1   G protein-coupled receptors that are activated by lysophospholipids and lysosphingolipids.

Receptors	Synonyms	Ligands
S1P$_1$	EDG-1; LP$_{B1}$	
S1P$_2$	EDG-5; LP$_{B2}$; AGR16; H218	SPP (nM)
S1P$_3$	EDG-3; LP$_{B3}$	Dihydro-S1P (nM)
S1P$_4$	EDG-6; LP$_{C1}$	SPC (low µM)
S1P$_5$	EDG-8; LP$_{B4}$; NRG-1	
LPA$_1$	EDG-2; LP$_{A1}$; VZG-1; MREC1.3	
LPA$_2$	EDG-4; LP$_{A2}$	LPA (nM)
LPA$_3$	EDG-7; LP$_{A3}$	
SPC$_1$	OGR1; GPR68	SPC (nM)
SPC$_2$	GPR4	SPC (nM) LPC (nM)
LPC$_1$	G2A	LPC (nM) SPC (nM-µM)
PSY$_1$	TDAG8	Psychosine (low µM) Glucopsychosine Lysosulfatide

antiapoptotic action of S1P and LPA may protect the cells from chemotherapy or radiation. Furthermore, S1P and LPA stimulate tumor cell motility and invasiveness. However, it has to be noted that motility of certain cancer cells (e.g., melanoma or breast cancer cells) is inhibited by S1P. Finally, S1P might play a role in tumor angiogenesis.

G Protein-coupled Receptors

S1P and LPA activate two groups of GPCRs, termed S1P$_{1-5}$ and LPA$_{1-3}$, respectively (Table 1). Amino acid identity is ~50% within these groups and ~35% between the two groups. Since the first member was cloned as an orphan receptor from differentiating vascular endothelial cells, the receptors were first named EDG (endothelial differentiation gene) receptors. According to an IUPHAR commitee, they are now named after the primary natural ligand and numbered in order of identification. Usually, several S1P or LPA receptors are co-expressed within a single cell type, rendering investigation of individual endogenous receptors difficult. Overexpression studies revealed that S1P and LPA receptors in general

couple to $G_{i/o}$, $G_{q/11}$ and $G_{12/13}$ proteins and thereby inhibit or stimulate adenylyl cyclase, stimulate phospholipase C, increase $[Ca^{2+}]_i$, stimulate or inhibit cell growth via ERK, JNK and p38, and modulate the cytoskeleton via Rho and Rac. The S1P$_1$ receptor appears to be unique since it exclusively couples to $G_{i/o}$, has little effect on $[Ca^{2+}]_i$ but a strong impact on cytoarchitecture and contains a phosphorylation consensus site for protein kinase B (Akt). In endothelial cells, S1P$_1$ activates Akt, which in turn phosphorylates S1P$_1$ and thereby enables Rac activation and endothelial cell migration.

S1P$_1$, S1P$_2$ and S1P$_3$ are widely expressed, however, most information is available about their role in the cardiovascular system. Both S1P$_1$ and S1P$_3$ collaborate to mediate the effects of S1P on endothelial cell growth and survival, migration and morphogenesis. Knockout of the S1P$_1$ receptor in mice results in hemorrhage and death during embryogenesis caused by a defect in blood vessel maturation. Furthermore, deletion of S1P$_1$ in fibroblasts impairs chemotaxis towards platelet-derived growth factor (PDGF), implicating a role for autocrine S1P secretion in PDGF signalling. In contrast, S1P$_3$ knockout mice have no obvious phenotypic abnormality. Evidence for a role of S1P$_2$ in heart development is derived from the zebrafish, in which a mutation of a S1P$_2$-like receptor (called "miles apart") causes formation of two separate hearts due to a defect in migration of the cardiomyoblasts. Expression of S1P$_4$ is limited to lymphoid and hematopoetic tissues; this receptor has a relatively low homology to the other S1P receptors. S1P$_5$ is mainly expressed in brain, predominantly in white matter (it has to be noted that S1P$_1$, S1P$_2$ and S1P$_3$ are also found in the brain), and in skin. The physiological roles of these latter receptors remain to be elucidated.

With regard to LPA receptors, most information is available about their role in the nervous system. The LPA$_1$ receptor was originally cloned from cerebral cortical neuroblasts and is highly expressed in the neurogenic ventricular zone of the embryonic cerebral cortex. In the adult nervous system, it is predominantly found in myelinating cells, i.e. oligodendrocytes and Schwann cells. LPA$_1$ is also widely expressed outside the nervous system, while expression of LPA$_2$ and LPA$_3$ is more limited. All three receptors are found in several cancer cells. Functional comparison of overexpressed LPA$_1$, LPA$_2$ and LPA$_3$ in a neuroblastoma cell line which is not responsive to LPA revealed that all three receptors mediated inhibition of adenylyl cyclase and activation of phospholipase C, mitogen-activated protein kinase and arachidonic acid release induced by LPA, but only LPA$_1$ and LPA$_2$ mediated LPA-induced cell rounding. Overexpression of LPA$_3$ even increased the length and number of neurites. In a cortical neuroblast cell line, overexpressed LPA$_3$ counteracted LPA-induced cell rounding which was most likely mediated by endogenous LPA$_1$ and LPA$_2$ receptors. Interestingly, overexpression of S1P$_1$, S1P$_2$ and S1P$_3$ in PC12 cells promoted S1P-induced cell rounding and neurite retraction, indicating that this is a more common response to S1P/LPA receptors. Deletion of LPA$_1$ in mice resulted in ~50% neonatal lethality, the survivors showing reduced size, craniofacial dysmorphism and impaired suckling behavior. The defect in suckling behavior caused malnutrition of the pups, leading to growth retardation and death and was attributed to a defective olfaction.

Functional data suggest that other LPA receptors remain to be discovered. A putative LPA-GPCR, PSP24, with no specific homology to the above mentioned S1P and LPA receptors, has been cloned from Xenopus oocytes. Overexpression of xPSP24 in the oocyte clearly augmented the maximum Cl$^-$ current elicited by LPA, while antisense oligonucleotides inhibited the response. However, the mammalian PSP24 isoforms failed to mediate LPA-induced activation of G proteins or of a serum response element-driven reporter gene and thus the role of these receptors remains unclear.

Recently, a number of GPCRs have been identified that are activated by lysolipids other than S1P or LPA. OGR1, GPR4, G2A and TDAG8 were activated by SPC, LPC and psychosine as shown in Table 1. SPC and LPC are the phosphocholine-containing analogs of S1P and LPA, respectively. SPC (lyso-sphingomyelin) may be derived from sphingomyelin by sphingomyelin-deacylase; it accumulates in Niemann-Pick disease (deficiency of acid sphingomyelinase) but is also a normal constituent of plasma and serum. SPC is a low-affinity or partial agonist at S1P receptors, but a high-affinity agonist at OGR1 and GPR4. Psychosine (1-galactosyl-sphingosine) and glucopsychosine (1-glucosyl-sphingosine) likewise were suspected to act via GPCRs according to functional data; this assumption was confirmed recently by detection that the T cell death-associated gene, TDAG8, is a GPCR which is activated by psychosine, glucospychosine and lysosulfatide.

Drugs

The development of drugs acting on the lysolipid mediator system is difficult because receptor binding studies are hampered by high non-specific binding of the lipophilic ligands. However, it is known from homology modeling and mutational analysis of the S1P$_1$ receptor that the hydrophilic headgroup plays a major role in ligand recognition. In S1P$_1$, two arginines bind the phosphate and a glutamic acid associates with the ammonium ion of S1P. While the glutamic acid is conserved among S1P receptors, all known LPA receptors contain glutamine in the respective position, corresponding to the lack of an amino group in LPA. Interestingly, if the glutamic acid in S1P$_1$ is exchanged for glutamine, the receptor is activated by LPA and not S1P. The lipophilic part in natural LPA is variable as described above and also plays an important role in receptor binding, e.g., the LPA_3 receptor prefers sn-2 linked unsaturated fatty acids. In contrast, LPA_1 and LPA_2 are less selective and are activated by LPA containing sn-1 linked fatty acids as well.

Drug development in LPA signalling has largely made use of compounds in which the glycerol backbone was replaced by serine, tyrosine or ethanolamine, with the fatty acid linked to the amino group. N-palmitoyl-serine-phosphoric acid (NPSerPA) and N-palmitoyl-tyrosine-phosphoric acid (NPTyrPA) inhibited LPA-induced Cl^- currents in Xenopus oocytes in a competitive manner with an IC_{50} in the nanomolar range, while Cl^- currents induced by other agonists remained unaffected. Furthermore, NPSerPA and NPTyrPA inhibited responses to LPA in platelets and human vascular endothelial cells. However, NPSerPA was a weak agonist at heterologously expressed LPA_1 and LPA_2 receptors. N-acyl-ethanolamine-phosphoric acid (NAEPA) was as efficient as LPA at LPA_1 and LPA_2 receptors, and less active at LPA_3. Recent work shows that 2-substituted NAEPA derivatives can be agonists or antagonists dependent on size and position of the substituent. Compounds with small substituents such as methyl, methylene hydroxy or methylene amino groups stimulated G protein activation by LPA receptors in the order $LPA_1 > LPA_2 > LPA_3$ and acted like LPA on cardiovascular parameters in the anesthetized rat. In contrast, a compound with a large hydrophobic substituent (benzyl-4-oxybenzyl) acted as competitive antagonist at LPA_1 (K_i ~130 nM) and LPA_3 (K_i ~430 nM) receptors, with no effect on LPA_2. Interestingly, the 2-substituted NAEPA derivatives acted in a stereoselective manner, which is not observed with LPA itself. Another recently described subtype-selective LPA receptor antagonist, dioctylglycerol pyrophosphate (DGPP), was principally obtained by the same strategy of introducing a second large hydrophobic group into a LPA-like molecule. DGPP competitively inhibited the LPA_3 (K_i ~100 nM) and LPA_1 (K_i ~6.6 μM) receptors but, like the above mentioned NAEPA derivative, was inactive at LPA_2.

Less drugs are available for modulation of S1P signalling. The polyanionic compound suramin, which interferes with ligand binding of many receptors, blocked the activation of heterologously expressed $S1P_3$, but not $S1P_1$ or $S1P_2$, with an IC_{50} of ~20 μM. Interestingly, suramin inhibited S1P-induced activation of $I_{K(ACh)}$ in human atrial myocytes with high potency, the IC_{50} being ~0.2 nM. However, suramin also inhibits LPA-induced mitogenesis (IC_{50} ~70 μM). S1P homophosphonate strongly inhibited S1P binding to $S1P_1$, had a slight effect on $S1P_3$ and no effect on $S1P_2$, however, it is not known whether it is an agonist or antagonist. Another approach is the development of sphingosine kinase inhibitors.

References

1. Fukushima N, Ishii I, Contos JA, Weiner JA, Chun J (2001) Lysophospholipid receptors. Annu. Rev. Pharmacol. Toxicol. 41:507–534
2. Moolenaar WH (1999) Bioactive lysophospholipids and their G protein-coupled receptors. Exp. Cell Res. 253:230–238
3. Pagès C, Simon M-F, Valet P, Saulnier-Blache JS (2001) Lysophosphatidic acid synthesis and release. Prostaglandins & other Lipid Mediators 64:1–10
4. Pyne S, Pyne N (2000) Sphingosine-1-phosphate signalling in mammalian cells. Biochem. J. 349:385–402
5. Spiegel S, Milstien S (2000) Functions of a new family of sphingosine-1-phosphate receptors. Biochim. Biophys. Acta 1484:107–116
6. Tigyi G (2001) Selective ligands for lysophosphatidic acid receptor subtypes: gaining control over the endothelial differentiation gene family. Mol. Pharmacol. 60:1161–1164

M

Macrolides

Macrolides are a group of antibiotics, produced in nature by many actinomycetes strains, that are composed of a 12- to 16-membered lactone ring, to which one or more sugar substituents is attached. They target the peptidyl transferase center on the 50S ribosomal subunit and function primarily by interfering with movement of the nascent peptide away from the active site and into the exit tunnel.

▶ Ribosomal Protein Sythesis Inhibitors

Macrophage

A macrophage is a white blood cell, preferentially located near potential entry sites for microbial pathogens and specialized for the uptake of particulate material by phagocytosis. Most macrophages originate from peripheral blood monocytes and are able to leave the circulation following stimulation by chemotactic agents.

▶ Inflammation

Macula Densa

The macula densa is a dense aggregation of cells in the distal tubule of nephrons facing the glomerular tuft of capillaries. These cells sense the salt content of the distal tubular fluid and adjust glomerular perfusion and renin secretion accordingly.

▶ Renin-Angiotensin-Aldosteron System

Major Histocompatibility Complex

The major histocompatibility complex (MHC) is a complex of genes coding for a large familiy of cell surface proteins. MHC molecules bind peptide fragments of foreign proteins and present them to T-lymphocytes. MHC-I molecules are required for a cytolytic T-cell response, MHC-II molecules are recognized by T-helper cells. The human MHC is also known as 'HLA', the murine MHC as 'H-2'complex.

▶ Immune Defense

Malaria

Malaria remains a major public health problem in many parts of the world, including Southeast Asia, sub-Saharan Africa and Latin America where an estimated 300–500 million people are infected. 1–3 million die of malaria every year. The etiologic agents of malaria are protozoan parasites of the genus Plasmodium. Of the four pathogens that can cause malaria in humans (*Plasmodium falci-*

parum, P. vivax, P. ovale, P. malariae), P. falci-parum is responsible for the most severe form. At particular risk of developing severe malaria-associated pathology are the non-immune, including tourists and, in endemic areas, children and pregnant women during first pregnancy.

Malarial parasites feature a complex life cycle alternating between vertebrate and invertebrate hosts. The life cycle begins with the bite of an infected *Anopheles* mosquito and the injection of sporozoites into the blood stream. Sporozoites enter the liver and infect hepatocytes where they replicate and produce merozoites. Upon rupture of an infected hepatocyte, merozoites are released. The merozoites infect erythrocytes to establish the erythrocytic developmental cycle. The clinical symptoms of malaria are largely associated with the intraerythrocytic stages and include intermittent fever followed by shaking chills, headache, muscle pain, nausea, vomiting and diarrhoea. Infections with *P. falciparum* can cause life-threatening complications including cerebral malaria and multi-organ failure.

▶ Antiprotozoal Drugs

MALDI-MS

▶ Matrix-assisted Laser Desorption/Ionization Mass Spectrometry

Malignant Hyperthermia

Human individuals with the genetic trait malignant hyperthermia show characteristic signs and symptoms including tachycardiac arrhythmia, cyanosis, acidosis, muscle contracture and high fever when they are exposed to an inhalation general anesthetic, particularly halothane. Use of a depolarizing muscle relaxant is precipitating. The trait is linked with human chromosome 19 q 13.1 in many cases where a single amino acid in ryanodine receptor (RyR1) is mutated. The mutated sites are classified generally into three regions: region 1

(residues 36 - 614), region 2 (residues 2162 - 2458) and region 3 (residues 4637 - 4898). In some cases, other disorders such as central core disease (CCD) are complications with this. Similar abnormality is observed in other mammals, particularly in pigs (porcine stress syndrome, PSS), where psychic stress can be a critical trigger.

Mannose 6-phosphate Receptor

The mannose 6-phosphate receptor is the cargo/coat-receptor for trans-Golgi network (TGN)-derived clathrin vesicles. The receptor recognizes the mannose 6-phosphate tag of lysosomal hydrolases on the luminal side and the adaptor-1 complex of clathrin on the cytoplasmic face.

▶ Intracellular Transport

MAO

▶ Monoamine Oxidase

MAP

MAP is the acronym for both, ▶ Microtubule Associated Protein Mitogen Activated Protein

MAPK

Mitogen activated protein kinase.

▶ MAP Kinase Cascade

MAP Kinase Cascades

AMY N. ABELL, MARK T. UHLIK, BRUCE D. CUEVAS,
GARY L. JOHNSON
University of Colorado Health Sciences Center,
Denver, Colorado, USA
amy.abell@uchsc.edu, mark.uhlik@uchsc.edu,
bruce.cuevas@uchsc.edu,
Gary.Johnson@uchsc.edu

Synonyms

Serine/threonine protein kinase phosphorelay
modules.

Definition

Mitogen activated protein ▶ kinase (MAPK) cascades are three kinase modules activated by
▶ phosphorylation. The three kinase modules are
composed of a MAPK, a MAPKK, and a MAP-
KKK. There are multiple members of each component of the MAPK cascade that are conserved from
yeast to human. Activation of selective MAPK
modules by specific stimuli regulates cell functions such as gene expression and migration.

Basic Characteristics

Characteristics of MAPK Cascades

MAPK cascades are signaling modules that serve
as important mediators of signal transduction
from the cell surface to the nucleus (1–4). MAPK
modules are activated by diverse stimuli including
growth factors, hormones, ▶ cytokines, bacterial
products such as lipopolysaccharide (LPS), and
stresses to the cell including γ and ultraviolet irradiation, heat and cold shock, hyperosmolarity, and
oxidative stress. Activation of MAPK signaling by
these stimuli contributes to the regulation of many
different cell functions including growth, differentiation, survival, ▶ apoptosis, cytokine production, migration and adhesion (2).

MAPK cascades are composed of three cyto-
plasmic kinases, the MAPKKK, MAPKK, and
MAPK, that are regulated by phosphorylation
(Fig. 1) (1–3). The MAPKKK, also called MEKK for
MEK kinase, is a serine/threonine kinase. Selective

activation of MAPKKKs by upstream cellular
stimuli results in the phosphorylation of MAPKK,
also called MEK for MAP/ERK kinase by the MAP-
KKK. MAPKKK members are structurally diverse
and are differentially regulated by specific
upstream stimuli. MAPKK is phosphorylated by
MAPKKK on two specific serine/threonine residues in its activation loop. The MAPKK family
members are dual specificity kinases capable of
phosphorylating critical threonine and tyrosine
residues in the activation loop of MAPKs. MAP-
KKs have the fewest members in the MAPK signaling module. MAPKs are a family of serine/threo-
nine kinases that upon activation by their respective MAPKKs are capable of phosphorylating
cytoplasmic substrates as well as translocating to
the nucleus where they phosphorylate transcription factors and thus regulate gene expression.
MAPKs are divided into four main subfamilies
including the extracellular signal-regulated
kinases (ERKs), Jun amino-terminal kinases
(JNKs), and p38 kinase members. This review will
focus on four of best characterized MAPK cascades including ERK1/2, ERK5, JNK, and p38
kinase.

M

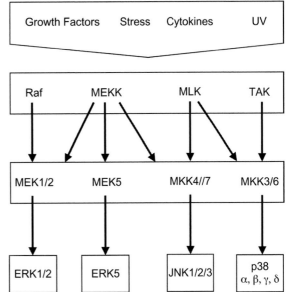

Fig. 1 Organization of MAPK cascades (see text for
details).

Characteristics of the ERK1/2 Pathway

Extracellular signal-regulated kinase (ERK) 1 and ERK2, also called p44 MAPK and p42 MAPK respectively, are nearly 85% identical. ERK1 and 2 are involved in the regulation of cell growth, differentiation, survival, and cell cycle progression. While these factors are ubiquitously expressed in mammalian tissues, the majority of their functions and biological properties have been characterized in the context of fibroblasts (2). Similar to other MAPKs, ERK1 and ERK2 are terminal components of a three kinase signaling module. Extracellular stimuli (such as growth factors, cytokines and serum) or events (such as cell adhesion) promote the activation of Raf kinases (MAPKKKs), which proceed to phosphorylate MAPK/ERK kinase (MEK) 1 and MEK2 (MAPKKs). Activation of ERK1/2 is accomplished by the MEK1- or MEK2-mediated dual phosphorylation of threonine and tyrosine of the conserved threonine-glutamate-tyrosine (TEY) motif present in the catalytic domains of ERK1/2 (3). Once activated, ERK1/2 phosphorylate cytosolic substrates, including ribosomal S6 kinase (p90^{rsk}), phospholipase A$_2$ (PLA$_2$), and microtubule associated proteins (MAPs). Additionally, activated ERK1 and ERK2 are capable of translocating to the nucleus where they phosphorylate a number of transcription factors (Elk1, Ets1, Sap1a, and c-Myc) and, thereby, increase their transcriptional activities (2). Downregulation of ERK1/2 is achieved chiefly through the dephosphorylation of their TEY motifs by a family of MAPK ▶ phosphatases (MKPs)(3).

The biological functions of ERK1 and ERK2 have been further defined by mouse models in which the genes coding for these proteins have been knocked out. ERK1 knockout mice appear to be grossly phenotypically normal and fertile but have defects in thymocyte proliferation and maturation. However, ERK2 knockouts are not viable and die early in embryogenesis (day E7.5) as a result of defects in placental development. Raf-1, an upstream activator of ERK1/2, has also been knocked out in mice and displays similar placental defects leading to embryonic mortality. Knockouts of other upstream activators of ERK1/2, including the MAPKKK B-Raf and the MAPKK MEK1, are also embryonic lethal and have vascular and angiogenic defects (2). Thus, from these studies important roles for ERK1/2 in cell prolifer-ation, cell migration, cell differentiation, and angiogenesis can be inferred.

Characteristics of the ERK5 Pathway

The MEK5/ERK5 pathway is a more recently identified MAPK signaling module (1,2). The MAPK ERK5, also known as Big MAP kinase (BMK1) possesses a TEY activation motif similar to ERK1/2 and is activated by growth factor stimulation, albeit with slightly different kinetics than ERK1/2. Stimulation of cells with epidermal growth factor (EGF) promotes ERK5 dependent cell proliferation and cell-cycle progression. In addition to being responsive to growth factors, ERK5 is also activated by cell stress stimuli including oxidative stress and hypersosmolarity similar to the MAPK members JNK and p38 kinase. Although ERK5 is stimulated by activators common to other MAPK members, ERK5 is activated by unique upstream MAPKK termed MEK5 that is not utilized by other MAPKs (1,2). Additionally, the structure of ERK5 is significantly different from other MAPK members. ERK5 possesses a unique, long C-terminal tail containing a nuclear localization signal and a distinct N-terminal domain that binds MEK5. ERK5 is an important regulator of serum-induced immediate early gene expression. Active ERK5 has been shown to phosphorylate MEF2c, a member of the MEF2 transcription factor family, resulting in an increase in c-jun transcription, a gene required for cell proliferation. Thus, ERK5 plays an important biological role in the coordination of cell response to different stimuli and promotes cell growth.

Characteristics of the JNK Pathway

The MAPKs termed Jun amino-terminal kinases (JNKs) are a subgroup comprised of three known members, JNK1, 2, and 3. This group of kinases is thus named due to their specific phosphorylation of the transcription factor c-Jun, a component of the AP-1 transcription complex. JNK pathway regulation of AP-1 activity is critical for transcriptional control of a number of gene products resulting from a variety of stimuli, ranging from growth factor receptor ligation to cytoskeletal alteration and other cellular stresses. Indeed, JNKs were originally identified as stress-activated protein kinases (SAPKs) (2,3). Through the regulation of AP-1, JNKs influence the expression of genes as diverse as cytokines, growth factors, inflammatory mediators and matrix ▶ metalloproteinases. Thus, JNK signaling is expected to play a key role in cellular survival and disease processes stemming from inflammation and cell death. JNKs 1 and 2 are widely expressed, whereas JNK3 expression is limited to neuronal tissue and cardiac myocytes (2,5).

As with other MAPKs, JNK is phosphorylated and activated by upstream MAPKKs of which the dual-specificity kinases MKK4 and MKK7 have been identified as JNK activators. MKK4/7 are, in turn, phosphorylated by a number of upstream MAPKKKs, including MEKK1/2/3/4, and MLKs (1). Several JNK pathway component knockouts have been produced by ▶ homologous recombination, and these tools are helping to define the biological function of JNK signaling. These studies have thus far shown JNK1 and 2 as having a role in immune cell function, and a simultaneous deletion of both JNK1 and 2 is embryonic lethal. All JNKs seem to regulate cell survival. For example JNK1/2 double knockout fibroblasts show increased resistance to radiation (3,5).

Characteristics of the p38 Kinase Pathway

p38 kinases are members of the mitogen-activated protein kinase (MAPK) family of serine/threonine kinases that phosphorylate and regulate both cytoplasmic proteins and transcription factors, thus regulating gene transcription (1,3). Several investigators have independently identified p38 kinase during experiments designed to isolate kinases involved in cell responses to cellular stresses. Four isoforms of p38 kinase have been isolated: α, β, γ, and δ. These isoforms have been classified as p38 kinases based on both the presence of a conserved threonine-glycine-tyrosine (TGY) sequence in their activation loop and a high amino acid identity. For example, p38α and β are 60% identical to p38γ and δ, further suggesting p38 kinases as a subfamily of MAPKs (2). Stimuli including heat and cold shock, osmotic shock, irradiation, LPS, and cytokines have been shown to activate p38. However, the MEKKs activated upstream of p38 in response to these stimuli remain unclear. These stimuli have been shown to activate the MKKs MKK3/MKK6 that phosphorylate p38 kinase on highly conserved tyrosine and threonine residues. Phosphorylation of p38 kinase

results in the nuclear translocation of this kinase where it can phosphorylate and activate transcription factors such as ATF-2 and ELK1. However, not all targets of p38 kinase are nuclear. p38 kinase also phosphorylates cytoplasmic proteins such as tau protein, MAPKAP3 and 5 and Mnk1/2. Activation of p38 has been shown to affect multiple cell functions including growth, apoptosis, spreading, adhesion, cytokine production and cell-cycle progression (4). For example, γ irradiation activates MKK6, stimulating p38γ and blocking G2-M transition. Similarly, UV irradiation activates p38 α and β that may serve as an early sensor of DNA damage. Finally, stimulation of cells with LPS activates p38 kinase, resulting in the production of the cytokines IL-1 and TNFα and leading to increased inflammation. Disruption of the p38 pathway would therefore be useful clinically in the arrest of the inflammatory response and in the treatment of inflammatory diseases (5).

Drugs

To date, no compounds have been identified that directly and specifically inhibit either ERK1 or ERK2. However, a number of inhibitors have been developed that affect the activities of the kinases upstream of ERK1/2. The most useful compounds for the inhibition of ERK1/2 activity have been the MEK1/2 inhibitors PD98059 and UO126 (Table 1). These compounds have high specificity for MEK1 and MEK2, and at low concentrations, do not cause appreciable inhibition of MAPK pathways other than ERK1 and ERK2. Both PD98059 and UO126 bind to MEK1 and MEK2 at sites distinct from the ATP-binding pocket, but cause allosteric changes in the proteins that render them unable to activate ERK1/2. More recently a second-generation compound, PD184352, has been developed and been found to successfully reduce elevated levels of ERK1/2 activity in colon carcinoma cells and reduce tumor growth in mice (Table 1) (5). As a result of this preliminary efficacy for controlling cancer cell proliferation, PD184352 is currently in Phase I oncology trials. Additionally, a Raf-1 inhibitor, Bay439006, has shown promise as an inhibitor of ERK1/2-mediated cancer cell growth and ▶ metastasis and is also in Phase I trials (5).

Selective inhibitors of ERK5 have not been described. However, studies of MEK1/2 inhibitors

M

Tab. 1 Pharmacological inhibitors of MAPK cascades.

Kinase	Inhibitors	Mechanism of Action	Biological Consequences
Raf	Bay 439006	unknown	reduces MEK1/2 activity and tumor growth
MEK1/2	PD98059 U0126 PD184352	binds to MEK1/2 at a site distinct from the ATP binding pocket	reduces ERK1/2 activity and cancer cell growth
MEK5	PD98059 U0126 PD184352	unknown	reduces ERK5 activity by partial blocking of MEK5
JNK1/2	SP600125	binds the ATP binding pocket of JNK	blocks LPS-induction of TNFα expression; blocks TCR mediated apoptosis
p38 kinase α/β	SB203580 SB202190 VK19911 Vertex 745 SB235699	binds the ATP binding pocket of p38 kinase	blocks p38 stimulation of production of pro-inflammatory cytokines

have detected effects on MEK5, the upstream activator of ERK5. In addition to inhibition of MEK1/2 activation of ERK1/2, both PD98059 and U0126 have been shown to partially reduce EGF and hydrogen peroxide activation of the ERK5 pathway in mammalian cell lines (Table 1). Inhibition of the ERK5 pathway occurs at the level of MEK5, however the precise mechanism is unknown. Similarly, the MEK1/2 inhbitor PD184352 also inhibited EGF-stimulation of the MEK5/ERK5 pathway, but a 10-fold higher concentration of inhibitor was required relative to that required for MEK1/2 inhibition (Table 1). Addtionally, low doses ($2\,\mu M$) of PD184352 that completely block ERK1/2 activity were shown to prolong activation of ERK5 in response to EGF and hydrogen peroxide. The additional effects of MEK1/2 inhibitors on MEK5/ERK5 signaling alters the interpretation of results related to studies of these inhibitors on ERK1/2 signaling (5). Although selective inhibitors of MEK5/ERK5 are yet to be identified, the ability of ERK5 signaling to promote cell proliferation makes it a potentially useful clinical target for inhibitors.

The recent development of the JNK-specific inhibitor SP600125 will likely aid efforts to define the biological significance of JNK signaling (Table 1). SP600125 is an anthrapyrazolone that competes with ATP for the nucleotide-binding site in the JNK catalytic domain (5). Importantly, as JNK activity is necessary for expression of some extracellular proteinases linked to invasiveness, JNK inhibition may represent an avenue by which to affect tumorigenesis, cancer metastasis and inflammatory immune response. Further, manipulation of JNK activity may potentially allow alleviation of cell death-mediated pathologies, such as ischemic injury and myocardial infarction.

The most extensive development of pharmacological inhibitors of MAPK members has been for p38 (Table 1) (5). Small-molecule inhibitors have been developed for two p38 isoforms (α and β). Pyridinyl imidazole compounds have been known to block inflammation since the early 1970s. Structural analyses have revealed that p38 kinase inhibitors bind to the ATP binding pocket of p38 thereby acting as competitive inhibitors. The p38 kinase inhibitor SB202190 is able to bind both the low activity nonphosphorylated form and the high activity phosphorylated form of p38 suggesting that the inhibitor is able to disrupt the activation of p38 (Table 1) (5). Several p38 inhibitors such as Vertex 45 and SB235699(HEP689) are in clinical trials (Table 1). Vertex 45 is in clinical trials for rheumatoid arthritis and SB235699 is in trials as a topical treatment for psoriasis.

References

1. Garrington TP, Johnson GL (1999) Organization and regulation of mitogen-activated protein kinase signaling pathways. Current Opinion in Cell Biology 11:211–218
2. Pearson G, Robinson F, Gibson TB, Xu B, Karandikar M, Berman K, Cobb MH (2001) Mitogen-activated protein (MAP) kinase pathways: regulation and physiological functions. Endocrine Reviews 22:153–183
3. Widmann C, Gibson S, Jarpe MB, Johnson GL (1999) Mitogen-activated protein kinase: conservation of a three-kinase module from yeast to human. Physiological Reviews 79:143–179
4. Pearce AK, Humphrey TC (2001) Integrating stress-response and cell-cycle checkpoint pathways. Trends in Cell Biology 11:426–433
5. English JM, Cobb MH (2002) Pharmacological inhibitors of MAPK pathways. Trends in Pharmacological Sciences 23:40–45

Marijuana

Marijuana is the name given to the dried leaves and flower heads of the hemp plant, *Cannabis sativa*, prepared as a smoking mixture.
Cannabinoid System

Marimastat

▶ Matrix Metalloprote(in)ases

Mast Cells

Mast cells are connective tissue cells that can release histamine under certain conditions.

▶ Allergy
▶ Histaminergic System

Matrix Metalloprote(in)ase 2

MMP-2 (also known as gelatinase A) is a secreted metalloproteinase homologous with interstitial collagenase, with the exception of an additional fibronectin-like domain. It degrades collagen types I, II and III.

Matrix Metalloprote(in)ase 9

MMP-9 (also known as gelatinase B) is a secreted metalloproteinase structurally similar to MMP-2 (gelatinase A). It degrades gelatin types I and V and collagen types IV and V.

Matrix Metalloprote(in)ases

Matrix metalloproteinases (MMP), are a family of extracellular proteinases, which depend on metal ions (zinc) for catalytic activity (▶ metalloprote(in)ase), and which are very potent in degrading structural proteins of their extracellular matrix. MMPs influence a wide variety of physiological and pathological processes, including aspects of embryonic development, tissue morphogenesis, wound repair, inflammatory diseases and cancer. In vertebrates about 25 MMPs have been identified. Inhibitors of MMPs (e.g. marimastat, prinomastat) are currently being tested for their potential therapeutic use in treating various disease states, such as chronic inflammatory diseases or cancer (to prevent tumor invasion, metastases and tumor angiogenesis).

▶ Angiogenesis and Vascular Morphogenesis
▶ Endothelins
▶ Non-viral Proteases

M

Matrix Proteins

▶ Fibrinogen

Matrix-assisted Laser Desorption/Ionization Mass Spectrometry

Matrix-assisted laser desorption mass spectrometry (MALDI-MS) is, after electrospray ionization (ESI), the second most commonly used method for ionization of biomolecules in mass spectrometry. Samples are mixed with a UV-absorbing matrix substance and are air-dried on a metal target. Ionization and desorption of intact molecular ions are performed using a UV laser pulse.

▶ Proteomics

MCH

▶ Melanin-concentrating Hormone

M-channels

M-channels (M for Muscarine) are voltage-gated potassium channels, assembled from KCNQ-subunits. They are expressed in the peripheral sympathetic neurons and CNS. In the absence of acetylcholine, the M channel opens at resting membrane potential and dampens neuronal responsiveness to synaptic inputs. Acetylcholine inhibits M channel activity by activation of the muscarinic M1 receptor.

▶ K$^+$ Channels

MDMA

▶ 3,4-Methylenedioxymethamphetamine
▶ Psychostimulants

Mechanism-based Enzyme Inhibition

Mechanism-based inhibition is irreversible metabolic inhibition caused by covalent binding of the inhibitor to the enzyme after being metabolized by the same enzyme. The inhibitory effect remains after elimination of the inhibitor from the body.

▶ Viral Proteases

Mechano-sensory Transduction

The process whereby mechanical stimulation leads to stimulation of sensory nerve terminals.

Meglitinide

▶ ATP-dependent Potassium Channels
▶ Oral Antidiabetic Drugs

Meglitinide-related Compounds

Meglitinide contains a benzamide group. Meglitinide-relatedcompounds such as nateglinide are non-sulfonylurea oral hypoglycemic drugs used in the treatment of type 2 (non-insulin dependent) diabetes mellitus.

► ATP-dependent Potassium Channels
► Oral Antidiabetic Drugs

Melanin-concentrating Hormone

Melanin-concenttrating hormone (MCH) is a cyclic neuropeptide of 19 amino acids. It is involved in the modulation of feeding behavior. Its actions are mediated by G-protein coupled receptors (MCH1 and MCH2).

► Appetite Control

Melanocortins

Melanocortins are a group of peptides consisting of corticotropin (ACTH), α-melanocyte-stimulating hormone (α-MSH), β-MSH and γ-MSH, which are derived from a common larger precursor protein termed prepro-opio-melanocortin (POMC). While ACTH, which is produced in the anterior pituitary, stimulates the adrenal cortex to secrete glucocorticoids, the melanocyte-stimulating hormones have a wide variety of functions. Besides their effects on melanocytes, they have multiple functions in the regulation of various behaviors, most notably the control of body weight homeostasis by inhibition of food intake. In addition, they regulate the immune system, having anti-inflammatory and anti-pyretic actions. The effects of melanocortins are mediated by at least five melanocortin receptors (MC_{1-5}). While the MC_2 receptor mediates the action of ACTH, the other melanocorticoid receptors bind MSHs. MSH peptides are detectable in many central and peripheral locations, including the hypothalamus, the adrenal medulla, neurons of the intestine and the skin. Two mediators, the agouti and the agouti-related protein show a wide distribution and function as competitive antagonists at melanocortin receptors, especially MC_1, MC_3 and MC_4.

► Appetite Control

Melanocyte-stimulating Hormone

Melanocyte-stimulating hormones (αMSH, βMSH, γMSH; also called melanocortins or melanotropins) are generated by proteolytic cleavage of proopiomelanocortin. MSH isoforms increase the synthesis of eumelanin by melanocytes and regulate body weight by activating anorexigenic pathways in the hypothalamus.

► Appetite Control

Melatonin

Melatonin is synthesized from serotonin in the pineal gland via *N*-acetyl-serotonin. The synthesis of melatonin is highly regulated by environmental lighting, melatonin synthesis and release is stimulated in the dark and inhibited in the light. This effect is mediated by the suprachiasmatic nucleus of the hypothalamus, the major circadian pacemaker in the brain. Melatonin released from the pineal gland binds to receptors in a variety of organs. Three melatonin receptors, MT_1, MT_2 and MT_3, have been described. The function of melatonin in humans remains elusive. Because it is believed to promote sleep and based on its ability to reset the circadian clock, it has been proposed as a treatment for jet lag and other sleep disorders.

Membrane Transport Protein

► Table appendix: Membrane Transport Proteins

M

Ménière's Disease

Ménière's disease is a condition in which there is an increased volume of endolymph with dilatation of the membranous labyrinth. It is brought about by excessive production of endolymph or impaired outflow from the labyrinth. It is characterised by attacks of vertigo, tinnitus, nausea and vomiting.

Mesangial Cells

Mesangial cells are the smooth muscle-like cells of the capillaries in the glomerulus of the kidney.

Mesolimbic System / Reward System

In 1954 experiments by Olds and Milner revealed that the brain has specialized "centers" for reward functions. In these studies, electrical stimulation of certain brain sites was found to be highly rewarding in the sense that rats operantly responded to electrical stimulation of these sites, often to the exclusion of any other activity. A neurotransmitter system that is particularly sensitive to electrical self-stimulation is the mesolimbic dopamine projection that originates in the ventral tegmental area and projects to structures closely associated with the limbic system, most prominently the nucleus accumbens shell region and the prefrontal cortex. Because of its ubiquitous involvement in the regulation of reward-related behavior this system has been characterized as a neurochemical system of reward.

Metabolic Syndrome

A syndrome consisting of obesity, insulin resistance, hypertension, dyslipidemia (elevated very low density lipoprotein (VLDL)-triglycerides and low high density lipoprotein (HDL)-cholesterol levels), and impaired glucose tolerance. The main component of the syndrome is obesity which is believed to cause insulin resistance, hypertension and dyslipidemia. The syndrome is frequently associated with type 2 diabetes mellitus which is a consequence of insulin resistance and a defect in insulin secretion. Sedentary lifestyle and high-fat and high-sucrose diets are responsible for the continuous increase of its prevalence in Western countries.

▶ Diabetes Mellitus

Metabotropic Glutamate Receptors

JEAN-PHILIPPE PIN
CNRS, Mécanismes Moléculaires des Communications Cellulaires, Montpellier, France
pin@montp.inserm.fr

Synonyms

▶ G-protein coupled ▶ glutamate receptors

Definition

▶ Glutamate is the transmitter of most fast excitatory synapses in the central nervous system. To excite (depolarize) the post-synaptic neuron, glutamate activates various types of receptor channels (the ▶ ionotropic glutamate (iGlu) receptors) known as the NMDA, AMPA and kainate receptors (Fig. 1). Glutamate also acts on receptors called the ▶ metabotropic glutamate (mGlu) receptors that are coupled to heterotrimeric G-proteins to activate intracellular pathways. Eight mGlu receptors have been identified in mammals and all play important roles in the fine-tuning of most glutamatergic as well as other synapses (1).

▶ Ionotropic Glutamate Receptors

Basic Characteristics

The mGlu receptor family

The mGlu receptors were first identified as receptors responsible for the glutamate stimulation of phospholipase C (PLC) in neurons. Latter, other mGlu receptors were shown to inhibit ▶ adenylyl cyclase (AC). Molecular cloning and the sequencing of mammalian genomes identified eight genes encoding mGlu receptors (1). Additional mGlu receptors subtypes exist due to alternative splicing of the mRNA encoding mGlu1 (splice variants a, b and d are the best characterized), mGlu5 (a and b), mGlu7 (a and b) and mGlu8 (a and b). All these splice variants differ in the sequence of their carboxy-terminal intracellular tail. These receptors can be classified into three groups based on their sequence similarity, their pharmacology (see bellow) and their transduction mechanism (1). The sequence similarity is around 60–70% between members of a given group, and drops to 40% between receptors of two distinct groups. The group-I is composed of mGlu1 and mGlu5 receptors, which are both coupled to the stimulation of PLC. The mGlu2 and mGlu3 receptors form the group-II, whereas the mGlu4, mGlu6, mGlu7 and mGlu8 constitute the group-III. Both group-II and group-III mGlu receptors can inhibit AC in transfected cells.

Transduction Mechanism and Function of mGlu Receptors

Group-I mGlu receptors are mainly found on the side of the post-synaptic element (Fig. 1). By activating PLC, they stimulate the formation of inositol triphosphate leading to the release of Ca^{2+} from intracellular stores. This Ca^{2+} signal can then regulate the activity of enzymes such as protein kinase C and phopholipase A2. Group-I mGlu receptors can also regulate the activity of various channels, including Ca^{2+}-channels. They also inhibit or activate K^+-channels leading either to a decrease or to an increase in neuronal excitability. Group-I mGlu receptors also modulate (mainly

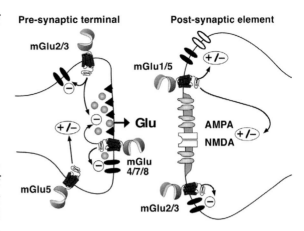

Fig. 1 The mGlu receptors and the fine tuning of glutamatergic synapses. Release of glutamate from nerve terminals activates the iGlu receptors (the NMDA and AMPA subtypes) in the post-synaptic element, leading to neuronal excitation. The group-I mGlu receptors (mGlu1 or mGlu5) located on the side of the post-synaptic element regulates the activity of Ca^{2+} (in black) and K^+-channels (in white) as well as iGlu receptors via intracellular pathways. The group-II mGlu2 and mGlu3 receptors regulate either the release of glutamate when located on the pre-synaptic terminal, but can also participate in the glutamate response when located in the post-synaptic element. Most group-III mGlu receptors (4, 7 and 8) are located in the pre-synaptic release zone where they inhibit glutamate release.

positively) the activity of the iGlu receptors of the AMPA and NMDA types, and can therefore modulate the excitatory effect of glutamate. NMDA receptors are known to be responsible for the ▶ excitotoxic effect of ▶ glutamate and to play an important role in synaptic plasticity including ▶ long-term potentiation (LTP) and ▶ long-term depression (LTD). It is therefore not surprising that antagonists of group-I mGlu receptors have neuroprotective effects and can inhibit synaptic plasticity such as LTP and LTD. Although they have never been directly observed in nerve terminals, electrophysiological experiments also suggest a pre-synaptic localization of mGlu5 receptors that can either facilitate or inhibit the release of glutamate.

The mGlu1 receptors are expressed at high density in the Purkinje neurons in the cerebellum where they are involved in a synaptic plasticity phenomenon important for the control of eye movements. These receptors are also found in the thalamus, the olfactory bulb and in some neurons of the hippocampus. The mGlu5 receptors are highly expressed in the pyramidal neurons of the hippocampus where they regulate a LTP phenomenon important for spatial memory. The mGlu5 receptors are also found in glial cells, but their function in these cells is still not yet fully elucidated. Both group-I mGlu receptors are expressed in many other brain regions and as such are involved in many processes such as the central response to pain, the control of movements via the extrapyramidal motor circuit. Group-I mGlu receptors are also found outside the central nervous system, such as in the sensory terminals in the skin where they can be at the origin of the inflammatory pain sensation. These various observations help understand the anxiolytic, anti-Parkinsonian and analgesic effects, as well as the decrease in the development of cocaine dependence observed with a mGlu5 receptor antagonist (▶ MPEP) (2). In addition neuroprotective and antiepileptic effects have been observed with a mGlu1 receptor antagonist (BAY367620).

Group-II mGlu receptors have been observed in pre-synaptic as well as post-synaptic elements. These receptors can inhibit AC activity, but their main action in neurons is to regulate the activity of various types of channels, including inhibition of Ca^{2+} channels (and as such they can inhibit the release process at the pre-synaptic level).

In the brain, mGlu2 receptors are highly expressed in Golgi cells in the cerebellum and in the dentate granule neurons of the hippocampal formation where they are involved in a LTD phenomenon. The other group-II mGlu receptor, mGlu3, is found not only in neurons, but also in astrocytes where its role is not yet elucidated. The mGlu3 receptor is mainly expressed in the reticular nucleus of the thalamus. Group-II mGlu receptors are also expressed in many other brain areas, and the recent development of selective and systematically active group-II mGlu receptor agonists (such as LY354740) reveal the potential use of such compounds for the treatment of anxiety, Parkinson's disease, schizophrenia and drug dependence, and for neuroprotection (3).

Group-III mGlu receptors are mostly found in the pre-synaptic element within the synaptic release site (Fig. 1), except the mGlu6 receptor, which is responsible for the post-synaptic action of glutamate on the ON bipolar cells in the retina. These receptors are therefore considered as autoreceptors controlling the glutamate release process. The mGlu7 and 4 receptors are also found in GABA-ergic terminals where they inhibit the release of the inhibitory transmitter GABA. Like group-II receptors, group-III mGlu receptors can inhibit AC activity, but their main action is the inhibition of Ca^{2+} channels leading to the inhibition of the release process. Due to their localization at the synaptic vesicle release site, it is likely that group-III mGlu receptors can directly control the release machinery.

The mGlu7 receptor type is widely expressed in the brain and is activated by high concentration of glutamate (100–1000 µM). It may serve to prevent over-activity of glutamatergic synapses, and accordingly, the deletion of its gene in mice leads to the rapid development of general epilepsy and death. The mGlu4 receptor is mostly expressed in the cerebellum and the olfactory bulb, but also in other areas. It has been shown to play a role in certain types of absence epilepsy. The mGlu8 receptor is expressed in some restricted areas in the brain and its physiological function is not yet elucidated.

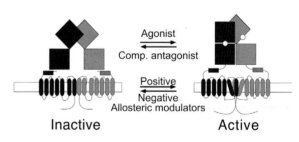

Fig. 2 The original structure of mGlu receptors. These receptor proteins are composed of a Venus Flytrap (VFT) module connected to an heptahelical domain via a cystein-rich region. The mGlu receptors are homodimers (one subunit in black, the other in grey) and this appears to play a crucial role in receptor activation. Binding of agonist in at least one VFT module induces a change in conformation of the dimer of VFTs, and leads to the activation of the dimer of heptahelical domains.

Original Structure and Activation Mechanism of mGlu Receptors

Like any other G-protein coupled receptors (GPCRs), mGlu receptors have 7 transmembrane helices, also known as the ▶ heptahelical domain (Fig. 2). As observed for all GPCRs, the intracellular loops 2 and 3 as well as the C-terminal tail are the key determinants for the interaction with and activation of G-proteins. However, sequence similarity analysis as well as specific structural features make these mGlu receptors different from many other GPCRs, and were the first members of the family 3 GPCRs. The main structural originality of these receptors is their large extracellular domain (Fig. 2) that contains the glutamate binding site (4). The structure of this extracellular domain has been solved recently (4). It is composed of two lobes that are separated by a wide cleft in the absence of glutamate. Upon binding of the agonist within this cleft, the two lobes close like a Venus Flytrap trapping an insect. This domain is therefore often called the "Venus Flytrap (VFT) module", and is connected to the first transmembrane segment of the ▶ heptahelical domain by a cysteine-rich domain (Fig. 2).

The second original feature of the mGlu receptors compared to other GPCRs is that they are always found as dimers in the brain. A disulfide-bond linking the two ▶ VFT modules stabilizes this dimeric structure. Today, only homodimers have been identified. This dimeric structure of mGlu receptors is probably critical for glutamate to activate the receptor. Indeed, the resolution of the structure of the extracellular domain of mGlu1 revealed a dimer of VFT modules, and a large change in the general conformation of the dimer is seen in the presence of glutamate. This change is such that the C-terminal ends of the two VFT modules become closer in the presence of agonists (Fig. 2). Because the C-terminal ends on the VFT modules are linked to the heptahelical domain via the cysteine-rich region, such a change of conformation is likely to induce a change of the conformation of the dimeric heptahelical domain leading to G-protein activation.

As we will see below, this original and complex structure of the mGlu receptors offers multiple possibilities to develop drugs modulating their activity.

Drugs

All compounds identified so far acting at the glutamate binding site share a glutamate-like structure. Such compounds are either agonists or competitive antagonists (Fig. 2). Within the last ten years a number of group-selective compounds have been characterized. However, due to the high conservation of the glutamate binding site between receptors of the same group, very few subtype selective compounds have been characterized (3). More recently, ▶ allosteric modulators of group-I mGlu receptors have been identified (2,5). Such molecules have a structure very different from glutamate and do not bind to the VFT module but rather in the heptahelical domain (Fig. 2). These can be either non-competitive antagonists (2), or positive ▶ allosteric modulators (5) and are subtype selective. Such compounds offer new possibilities to modulate mGlu receptor activity in the brain. Although no such compounds have been described for group-II and group-III mGlu receptors, these are expected and would likely be the first really subtype selective compounds. Most importantly, because compounds activating group-II and group-III receptors are expected to have multiple therapeutic application (see above), positive allosteric modulators may be more efficacious than pure agonists since they are less likely to induce receptor desensitization.

Group-I mGlu Receptor Compounds

Quisqualate was the first compound shown to activate group-I mGlu receptors. Although it is also active on the AMPA type of iGlu receptors, it remains the most potent group-I agonist. 1S,3R-▶ ACPD was the first selective mGlu receptor agonist identified, but it activates group-I, group-II and some group-III mGlu receptors. 3,5-DHPG remains the best characterized selective group-I agonist, though it has a low potency (10 μM). So far, CHPG is the only group-I subtype selective agonist that is active only at mGlu5, but its low affinity (1 mM) limits its usefulness. A few competitive group-I antagonists have been identified (the first was MCPG which is also active on group-II receptors) such as LY367366 and LY393675 which are acting on both mGlu1 and mGlu5, and LY367385 which is mGlu1 selective.

M

As mentioned above, non-competitive antagonists have been identified for group-I mGlu receptors that bind within the heptahelical domain. These are ▶ MPEP, selective for mGlu5, and BAY367620, selective for mGlu1. These highly selective and potent compounds have helped identify the important physiological roles of group-I mGlu receptors mentioned above.

Other molecules also acting within the heptahelical domain of mGlu1 have been shown to potentiate the action of glutamate and are therefore positive allosteric modulators. Such compounds have no effect on their own but increase both the efficacy and potency of agonists. No behavioral effect has already been reported for these molecules but according to the known function of group-I mGlu receptors, positive action on cognition are expected.

Group-II mGlu Receptor Compounds

Potent and selective compounds have been identified for group-II receptors. The first one was DCG-IV but this compound also antagonizes group-III mGlu receptors and activates NMDA receptors limiting its usefulness. LY354740 and its analog LY379268 are actually the best group-II agonists, and, most interestingly, they are systemically active and have unraveled the various possible applications of group-II agonists described above. However, no subtype selective group-II compounds have so-far been identified.

MCPG was the first described antagonist acting at group-II mGlu receptors but it is not selective, being also an antagonist of group-I and some group-III receptors. Today, the commonly used group-II competitive antagonists are derivatives of the non-selective mGlu agonist L-CCG-I: LY341495 > XE-CCG-I > PCCG4 > MCCG-I. However, LY341495 is active at all mGlu receptors, being more potent at group-II but also at most group-III receptors (mGlu6, 7 and 8). Moreover, the activity of the other compounds on group-III receptors remains to be characterized.

Group-III mGlu Receptor Compounds

L-AP4 and the natural compound, L-SOP, were the first identified group-III agonists. More recently, Z-CPrAP4, (+)ACPT-III, (+)-PPG and DCPG were shown to be additional group-III agonists. DCPG, being 50–100 times more potent on mGlu8 than on the other group-III receptors, is proposed as a selective mGlu8 agonist. Today, the number of group-III antagonists is rather limited. The only selective compounds are MAP4, MSOP and CPPG.

Currently, more group-selective and subtype-selective compounds remain to be discovered. The recent demonstration of a possible action of new subtype selective group-I modulators opens a new route for the discovery of such molecules for either group-II or group-III receptors. These will certainly be useful for the identification of the physiological roles of these different receptors and for the discovery of new therapeutic drugs.

References

1. Conn P, Pin J-P (1997) Pharmacology and functions of metabotropic glutamate receptors. Ann. Rev. Pharmacol. Toxicol. 37:205–237
2. Spooren WP, Gasparini F, Salt TE, Kuhn R (2001) Novel allosteric antagonists shed light on mGlu5 receptors and CNS disorders. Trends Pharmacol. Sci. 22:331–337
3. Schoepp DD, Jane DE, Monn JA (1999) Pharmacological agents acting at subtypes of metabotropic glutamate receptors. Neuropharmacology 38:1431–1476
4. Kunishima N, Shimada Y, Tsuji Y, Sato T, Yamamoto M, Kumasaka T, Nakanishi S, Jingami H, Morikawa K (2000) Structural basis of glutamate recognition by a dimeric metabotropic glutamate receptor. Nature 407:971–977
5. Knoflach F, Mutel V, Jolidon S, Kew JN, Malherbe P, Vieira E, Wichmann J, Kemp JA (2001) Positive allosteric modulators of metabotropic glutamate 1 receptor: Characterization, mechanism of action, and binding site. Proc. Natl. Acad. Sci. U S A 98:13402–13407

Metabotropic Receptors

For differentiation of G-protein-coupled receptor subtypes from subtypes permanently linked to ion channels (ligand-gated ion channels) the terms metabotropic *versus* ionotropic receptors, respectively, are used.

▶ Transmembrane Signalling

Metalloprote(in)ase

A family of proteinase depending on metal ions.
▶ Matrix metalloprote(in)ases are a subfamily of metalloprote(in)ases.

▶ Non-viral Proteases

Metastasis

Metastasis is the process by which tumor cells disconnect from the primary tumor and disseminate to distant sites to establish secondary colonies. Metastasis is a complex pro-cess, which requires a phenotypical change in the tumor cell as it has to lose its attachment to neighboring cells, gain motility, become resistant to apoptosis and be able to attach to cells of the blood vessels. A variety of proteins have been found to be involved in metastasis, including adhesion molecules (e.g. E-cadherin), proteases (e.g. plasminogen activator, matrix metalloproteinases) or growth factors (e.g. epidermal growth factor (EGF)).

Methicillin-resistant Staphylococci

Methicillin-resistent staphylococci are strains of staphylococci, which show resistance to a wide variety of antibiotics.They are named for their resistance to methicillin, a β-lactamase-resistant penicillin. Methicillin-resistante *Staphylococcus aureus* (MRSA) has become a serious problem particularly in hospitals.

3,4-Methylenedioxymeth-amphetamine

3,4-Methylenedioxymethamphetamine (MDMA; ecstasy) is a synthetic analog of amphetamine that produces hallucinations, an elevation in mood, and a feeling of "emotional closeness". This latter property has led to Ecstasy being referred to as the "hug drug". The unique properties of Ecstasy as compared to the parent compound amphetamine are believed to be due to the more selective effects of Ecstasy in promoting transporter-mediated release of serotonin. The use of Ecstasy has become a part of the culture associated with "rave" style dance parties.

▶ Psychostimulants

2-Methyl-6-(phenylethynyl) Pyridine

MPEP (2-methyl-6-(phenylethynyl) pyridine) is the best characterized mGlu5 selective non-competitive antagonist. This compound was one of the first of the allosteric regulators of the mGlu receptor identified as a non-competitive antagonist. MPEP is systemaically active and has been very helpful in identifying the role of the mGlu5 receptor subtype, including its involvement in inflamatory pain, anxiety and the development of cocaine addiction.

▶ Metabotropic Glutamate Receptors

1-Methyl-4-Phenylpyridium

1-methyl-4-phenylpyridinium (MPP$^+$), a permeant organic cation, is an excellent substrate for all organic cation transporters, but also for vesicular (VMAT) and some neuronal (e.g. DAT, NET) monoamine transporters. It is a potent neurotoxin and produces Parkinson's disease-like symptoms. It is generated *in vivo* from MPTP (1-methyl-4-phenyl-tetrahydropyridinium).

▶ Organic Cation Transporters

1-Methyl-4-phenyl-1,2,3,6-tetrahydropyridine

1-methyl-4-phenyl-1,2,3,6-tetrahydropyridine (MPTP) is a toxic agent which selectively destroys nigrostriatal neurons, but does not effect dopaminergic neurons elsewhere. MPTP is converted to its toxic metabolite, MPP^+, by the enzyme monoamine oxidase. MPP^+ is taken up via dopamine transporters and acts selectively on dopaminergic neurons by inhibiting mitochondrial oxidation reactions, which eventually results in the destruction of the cell. MTPT produces a severe form of Parkinson disease in primates.

▶ Nigrostriatal tract/pathway

Methylxanthines

Mehtylxanthines are naturally occurring drugs, including theophylline, theobromine and caffeine. Methylxanthines at relatively high doses inhibit phosphodiesterases, which results in an increase in intracellular cAMP levels. Inhibition of phosphodiesterase may be responsible for the tachycardia and relaxation of smooth muscles observed in response to methylxanthines. Already at lower doses, methylxanthines act as antagonists on adenosine receptors. The latter effect is believed to be responsible for the psychomotor stimulant effects of methylxanthines. Theophylline is used clinically as an anti-asthmatic drug, due to its strong bronchodilator effects.

▶ Phosphodiesterase
▶ Adenosine Receptors

MHC

▶ Major Histocompatibility Complex

MIC

▶ Minimal Inhibitory Concentration

Michaelis-Menten Kinetics

In 1913 L. Michaelis and M.L. Menten realized that the kinetics of enzyme reactions differed significantly from the kinetics of conventional chemical reactions. They put the reaction of substrate plus enzyme yielding enzyme plus substrate into the form of the equation: reaction velocity = (maximal velocity of the reaction x substrate concentration)/ (concentration of substrate + a fitting constant K_m). This latter constant characterized the tightness of the binding of the reaction between substrate and enzyme or the concentration at which the reaction was half the maximal value. This equation is formally identical to the Langmuir adsorption isotherm that relates the binding of a chemical to a surface. Both of these models form the basis of drug receptor interaction, thus the kinetics involved are referred to as 'Michaelian', or 'Langmuirian' in form.

▶ Drug-receptor Interaction

Microarray Hybridization

Microarray hybridization is a process by which nucleic acids are detected by hybridizing with complementary sequences bound to wafers at specific array coordinates. Hundreds to thousands of gene products may be measured in a single experiment.

▶ Microarray Technology
▶ Gene Expression Analysis

Microarray Technology

FRANCESCO FALCIANI, MARIA LIOUMI
University of Birmingham, Birmingham and
Lorantis Ltd, Cambridge, UK
f.falciani@bham.ac.uk,
maria.lioumi@lorantis.com

Synonyms

Biochip, gene ▶ array, gene chip

Definition

Microarray technology is a method to study the
activity of a large numbers of genes simultaneously. This method uses high speed robotics to
precisely apply tiny droplets containing biologically active material (DNA, proteins, chemicals) to
glass slides. In Functional Genomics, DNA microarrays are used to monitor ▶ gene expression at
the RNA level to identify genetic mutations and to
discover novel regulatory regions in genomic
sequences. Protein or chemical arrays are used to
monitor protein expression and to identify protein-protein or drug-protein interactions. Typically tens of thousands of genes or interactions can
be monitored in a single experiment.

▶ Combinatorial Chemistry
▶ Gene Expression Analysis

Description

Gene Expression Profiling

The most common application of microarray technology is in monitoring gene expression (gene
expression profiling).

The Principle. The technique is based on a classic
molecular biology procedure called reverse Northern blot. ▶ mRNA is extracted from a biological
sample and reverse transcribed in the presence of

a radioactive or fluorescent precursor. The reaction produces a pool of labeled complementary
DNA copies (cDNAs) representative of the original mRNA pool (defined as the target). The
expression of an individual gene is quantified by
hybridizing the target to the gene specific cDNA
(defined as the probe) which has been previously
spotted on a solid surface. The amount of radioactive or fluorescent signal associated to the spot is
proportional to the amount of gene specific RNA
originally present in the cell. Multiple cDNAs can
be spotted in an ordered pattern (array) allowing
the quantification of multiple genes. Before the
advent of microarray technology researchers were
employing low complexity nylon-based arrays
manufactured using manual devices. The technology subsequently evolved with the introduction of
robotics which made possible to generate repro-
ducible high density nylon filters (50 spots per
square centimeter). This technology employed
large membranes with up to 50,000 DNA spots,
required several milliliters of ▶ hybridization
solution and furthermore was relatively time consuming. The introduction of high precision and
high speed robotics brought to a further miniaturization of the technology with the production of
microarrays (up to 10,000 DNA spots per square
centimeter).

Because of the high density of signals in the
processed arrays the conversion of the radioactive
or fluorescent emissions in a numeric value is performed by sophisticated image analysis software
that identifies the position of every spot in the
array, determines the spot and the local background intensities and derives a number representing a spot-specific signal (Fig. 1H). Spot coordinates are then associated to gene identities
within the image analysis program or in a specific
gene expression profiling database (Fig. 1I). Differentially expressed genes are identified by comparing two or more arrays derived from different biological samples. When a gene is represented by
multiple spots in an array and/or replicated
hybridizations are available, statistical tests can be
used to assess the significance of the observed differences. Furthermore, data-mining techniques
are used to identify groups of genes with similar
expression profiles across different samples (Fig.
1J).

M

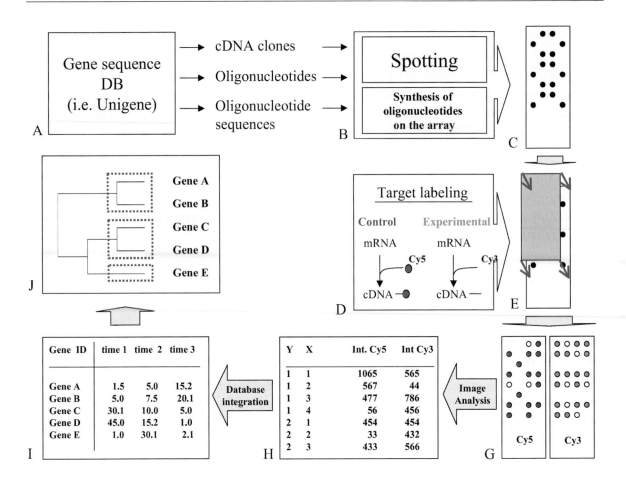

Fig. 1 Microarray technology applied to gene expression profiling. The figure summarises the process from the construction of the microarray to data analysis. **(A) This panel describes the first step in manufacturing a microarray for gene expression profiling:** the choice of the cDNA clones or the oligonucleotide sequences to represent the genes of interest. Clones or sequences are selected from sequence databases such as Unigene. **(B) cDNA clones are PCR amplified and spotted on a slide whereas oligonucleotides can be synthesised and spotted or synthesized *in situ*. (C) The result is an array of DNA samples representing several thousands of genes.** Thousands of arrays can be manufactured from micrograms of DNA. **(D) This panel represents the basic protocol to synthesize a labelled target.** In this example, mRNAs derived from experimental and control samples are differentially labelled, mixed and **(E) hybridised on an array.** Typically the hybridisation reaction is performed under a coverslip (marked in pink). **(G) After hybridisation the array is washed and scanned.** Two images are produced for each array. **(H) An image analysis program identifies the spots and derive a numerical value representing the intensity of the signal subtracted by the local background.** The panel represents the output of a typical image analysis software. X and Y are spot coordinates. Int. Cy5 and Int. Cy3 are the signal intensities for each spot in the two channels. **(I) Database integration associate a gene identity to each spot and integrate data from different arrays within the experiment.** The example refers to a timecourse. Gene expression intensities for genes A–E are reported for time 1, time 2 and time 3 of an hypothetical experiment using three arrays. Each value is expressed as a ratio between the experimental and the control sample. **(J) Result of cluster analysis applied to the data schematised in panel I.** Profile of expression of genes A and B are similar and therefore are grouped together. Similarly, genes C and D are grouped.

Array Types. There are two main type of arrays: a) ► oligonucleotide and b) cDNA arrays. In the first type short 20–25 mers are synthesized on a silica chip using photolithography (Affymetrix arrays, www.affymetrix.com) or using an ink-jet based technology (Rosetta Inpharmatics, www.rii.com). Alternatively, pre-synthesized oligonucleotides can be printed onto glass slides. In the second type, nucleic acids (usually in the form of PCR products) are robotically printed on glass slides as spots in defined locations. The first glass based high density cDNA arrays were developed in Pat Brown's laboratory at Stanford University, USA (1). cDNA arrays are now a very common choice in academic institutions because they offer a great degree of flexibility in the choice of the arrayed elements. Manufacturing them, however, requires a considerable infrastructure. The process needs liquid handling workstations to work with large collection of cDNA clones and to support the production of the purified probes and, of course, it requires robotics for the production of the proper microarrays.

The first step in designing a microarray is the choice of the cDNA clones or the determination of the oligonucleotide sequence that will represent the genes of interest. In both cases it is essential to use highly specific sequences in order to minimize cross-hybridization with related genes. An excellent source of gene information to design microarray probes are public domain expressed sequence databases such as Unigene, Genebank, db ► EST. The Unigene database (www.ncbi.nlm. nih.gov/UniGene/) is a collection of sequence clusters that represents the large majority of transcribed genes in a variety of species. It is also an excellent source of general information since it provides links to functional and genetics data, to scientific literature and indicates the source of the physical cDNA clones (Fig. 1A–C).

Because of the high gene coverage achievable with this technology it is possible to design arrays that cover the entire transcriptional capacity of an organism. For some species genome-wide arrays are already available. These are mainly bacteria and yeast open reading frame (ORF) based arrays. Human arrays covering the majority of the expressed genes are also available but it is still not practical to design human arrays that cover all the possible splicing variants encoded in the genome.

With the amount of effort dedicated to the annotation of the human genome it is expected that more comprehensive arrays will be soon available.

The Target. In the last few years more methods to synthesize a labeled target have been introduced. The new methods are still based on a ► reverse transcription reaction but diverge in the way the fluorescent dye is incorporated in the target. For example, Genechip^{TM} technology developed by Affymetrix uses a reverse transcription step followed by an RNA *in vitro* transcription reaction to produce a biotinylated target. The detection of the target, after hybridization, is achieved with a streptavidin-bound single fluorescent dye. Targets derived from different biological samples are always hybridized to multiple arrays. In the case of spotted arrays, two or more samples (typically experimental and control sample) can be compared on a single array. This is possible because the targets are labeled by direct incorporation of different fluorescent dyes (eg. Cy3 and Cy5). After labeling, the targets are mixed and hybridized to the same array, resulting in competitive binding of the target to the sequences on the array (Fig. 1D,E). With both methods, after hybridization and washing, the slides are scanned using one (Affymetrix) or multiple (spotted arrays) wavelengths corresponding to the dyes used (Fig. 1F).

A relatively large amount of RNA needs to be labeled with fluorescent dyes in order to obtain satisfactory results (20–100 µg of total RNA or 1–2 µg of mRNA). These requirements could make microarrays incompatible with the very limited RNA yields obtained from some types of biopsy or microdissected samples. To bypass these limitations several amplification methods have been developed. PCR-based amplification methods are quite straightforward but they introduce a bias in the gene representation due to the exponential amplification of the original mRNA molecules. Slightly more complex protocols are based on linear *in vitro* transcription. Although more reliable than PCR-based methods they also introduce some bias. An alternative strategy to amplification methods has been developed by Genisphere Inc. (www.genisphere.com). The target is synthesized using a reverse transcriptase reaction that introduces a sequence tag at the 3' end of every cDNA. A large agglomerate of oligonucleotides containing several hundreds of fluorescent dyes (dendromere) and containing a tag complementary to the cDNA tag is hybridized to the target to form a labeled cDNA that can be hybridized to the microarray. The large number of fluorophores attached to each cDNA molecule results in a two hundred fold signal enhancement.

Amplification based methods can be used with as little as nanograms of total RNA (corresponding to <1000 cells), whereas the dendromer-based methods require at least a microgram of total RNA.

Data Analysis. The rapid spread of microarray gene expression profiling has created an unprecedented situation in biology: An incredibly large amount of genome-wide gene expression data has been rapidly produced creating the need of appropriate data analysis tools. Many applications have been produced in academic groups and many others are available through commercial providers. Briefly, there are three levels of analysis that have been applied to gene expression profiling. The first uses statistical tests to identify genes differentially expressed between two or more samples. The second utilizes data reduction techniques to simplify the complexity of the dataset by identifying clusters of genes with similar expression profiles across different experimental conditions. One of the most common data reduction methods is called Cluster analysis. This method is based on a correlation measure that assigns a high score to genes that have very similar expression profiles. Using this matrix a roadmap displaying the degree of similarity between the genes in the array is built and visualized in a form of a hierarchical tree. The most correlated genes being on very close branches. Even the simple visual inspection of the tree is usually sufficient to identify meaningful associations. The third level uses reverse engineering algorithms to reveal the structure of transcriptional pathways within the cell. Although in principal very powerful, this approach still uses highly experimental algorithms that are in the process of experimental verification in a number of laboratories (for an extensive overview of data analysis methods see (2)).

Other Applications

Genotyping of Human Single Nucleotide Polymorphism (SNPs). The human genome project has produced large amounts of genome sequence and polymorphism data that is extremely useful to investigate the genetic bases of human diseases. Among these, ▶ single nucleotide polymorphisms (SNPs) are the most frequent variant in the human genome and they occur once every 1kb of genomic DNA. Identification of disease genes, however, require linkage and association analysis of thousands of SNPs in thousands of individuals. This is an impossible task without a high throughput genotyping method. Microarray based sequencing have been successfully used to genotype SNPs in human populations (3).

Protein Arrays. The amount of steady state RNA in a cell does not always reflect the biological activity of an expressed gene. It is the protein, translated from the RNA pool, that exerts the function, and it has been shown that mRNA and protein abundance are often not correlated. It follows that information about protein levels and their interactions are essential to understand the biological mechanisms. Microarray technology has been used to increase the throughput of classical protein detection methods and recently to study protein-protein interactions. Protein arrays are more complex than DNA arrays. The major issue is that proteins must bound to the slide while retaining their correct folding. In spite of these difficulties the field is rapidly expanding. Many companies are investing in developing and improving the technology. An excellent example of protein arrays and their applications is described by MacBeath et al. (4). The authors have deposited 10,000 protein spots on a glass microscope slide and demonstrated that their arrays could detect protein-protein interactions, reveal interactions between enzymes and their substrates, and detect small molecules-protein interactions. Protein microarrays consisting of either printed antibodies or printed protein antigens are used to monitor protein levels or antibody levels, respectively. With the effort now being concentrated in developing antibodies for the whole of the human proteome, the broad use of protein microarrays is not far off in the future.

Pharmacological Relevance

The ability of microarray technology to describe the behavior of thousands of molecular markers is well suited to identify and characterize the effect of a drug in complex biological systems and provide insights in the drug mechanism of action, its toxicity and the molecular basis of drug resistance. Below are some examples of the use of microarray technology in the pharmacology/drug discovery area.

Sensitivity to Drugs

It is known that the expression of certain genes can influence the response to drugs. Mis-expression or mutations in these genes can sometimes be responsible for treatment failure. This problem is particularly severe in anti-cancer therapy where resistant cell clones can expand very rapidly and generate secondary tumors that are completely unresponsive to therapy. A general method for the rapid identification of genes influencing drug sensitivity is therefore crucial for the development of future therapies. Uwe Scherf at the National Cancer Institute (NCI) in Bethesda (USA) has used a gene expression profiling based approach to identify genes responsible for influencing the response of a panel of sixty human cancer cell lines (NCI-60 panel) to a number of anti-cancer drugs. The data were analyzed using a clustering-based method that relate gene expression in the tumor cell before drug treatment to its capacity to respond to the drug (5). Interestingly, the authors identified a large number of significant correlations, many of them related to known mechanisms of drug resistance.

Drug Mode of Action Studies (MOA)

Conventional molecular and biochemical approaches to MOA studies are usually time consuming and resource demanding. A group of researchers from Rosetta Inpharmatica has recently developed a gene expression profiling-based method to identify drug targets that may significantly speed up investigation in this area.

The principle is simple; the expression fingerprint of yeast cells treated with a compound with unknown MOA is compared with a reference set of transcriptional profiles representing three hundred *S. cerevisiae* gene knock out mutants. The mutant with the closest expression fingerprint to the compound treated cells will most likely be mutated in a gene related to the drug target. Sequence homology to the identified yeast gene may then reveal the potential drug target in more broadly pharmaceutically relevant species (i.g. mouse, rat and man). Interestingly, the analysis of the expression profiles of yeast cells treated with the anesthetic drug dyclonine identified the human neuroactive σ factor as a potential target. Although there are potential complications in a broader application of gene expression profiling to the analysis of a drug mode of action directly in mammalian cells, several more studies have been reported (5).

Toxicology

Many companies are known to use gene expression profiling to assess the potential toxicity of lead compounds. This approach may require a database of reference compounds with known pharmacological and toxicological properties. Lead compounds can be compared to the database to predict compound-related or mechanism-related toxicity (5).

Pharmacogenomics

This rapidly expanding field examines the genetic basis for individual variations in response to therapeutics. Mutations in certain genes involved in drug metabolism make some populations unresponsive to a certain drug. Microarray technology can be used to genotype patients and predict their response to therapy. In this contest pharmacogenetics promises to increase the success of pharmaceutical research by developing individualized medicines tailored to patients' genotypes (5).

References

1. Schena M, Shalon D, Davis RW, Brown PO. (1995) Quantitative monitoring of gene expression patterns with a complementary DNA microarray. Science 20:467–470
2. J. Dopazo, E. Zanders, I. Dragoni, G. Amphlett and F. Falciani (2001) Methods and approaches in the analysis of gene expression data. Journal of Immunological Methods 250:93–112
3. Tilib SV, Mirzabekov AD (2001) Advances in the analysis of DNA sequence variations using oligonu-

cleotide microchip technology. Current Opinion in Biotechnology 12:53–58

4. MacBeath G, Schreiber SL. (2000) Printing proteins as microarrays for high throughput function determination. Science 289:1760–1763

5. Clarke PA, te Poele R, Wooster R, Workman P. (2001) Gene expression microarray analysis in cancer biology, pharmacology, and drug development: progress and potential. Biochemical Pharmacology 62:1311–1336

Microbial Resistance to Drugs

IRITH WIEGAND, BERND WIEDEMANN
Rheinische Friedrich-Wilhelms-Universität,
Bonn, Germany
unc30002@uni-bonn.de
B.Wiedemann@uni-bonn.de

Synonyms

Antibiotic resistance

Definition

A bacterial strain is called resistant if it grows in a relatively high concentration of a specific antibacterial drug. Thus, it is insensitive. The sensitivity is measured with standardized methods as the ▶ minimal inhibitory concentration (MIC). Guidelines from institutions like NCCLS (National Committee for Clinical Laboratory Standards) and DIN (Deutsches Institut für Normung e.V.) define specific breakpoints above which MIC a strain is regarded as resistant. This breakpoint usually is derived from microbiological and clinical experience. Resistant strains are regarded as non responding in an antibiotic therapy (Fig. 1).

▶ β-lactam Antibiotics
▶ Quinolones
▶ Ribosomal Protein Synthesis Inhibitors

Basic Mechanisms

Bacteria can develop resistance to antimicrobial agents as a result of mutational changes in the chromosome or via the acquisition of genetic material (resistance genes carried on ▶ plasmids or ▶ transposons or the recombination of foreign DNA into the chromosome) (Fig. 2).

The basic biochemical mechanisms leading to bacterial resistance can be classified into three different categories.

Antibiotic Inactivation

A common means that causes resistance is the inactivation of the antibiotic before it reaches the target site. Antibiotics can be either enzymatically cleaved or modified. In both cases the antibiotic loses its capacity to bind to its target.

Enzymatic Cleavage. β-Lactamases are enzymes that hydrolyse the β-lactam ring of β-lactamantibiotics (penicillins, cephalosporins, monobactams and carbapenems). They are the most common cause of β-lactam resistance. Most enzymes use a serine residue in the active site that attacks the β-lactam-amid carbonyl group. The covalently formed acylester is then hydrolysed to reactivate the β-lactamase and liberates the inactivated antibiotic. Metallo-β-lactamases use Zn(II) bound water for hydrolysis of the β-lactam bond.

β-Lactamases constitute a heterogeneous group of enzymes with differences in molecular structures, in substrate preferences and in the genetic localistions of the encoding gene (Table 1).

Another group of antibiotics that can be inactivated by hydrolysis are 14- and 15- membered macrolides (2). Esterases cleave the lactone ring. The plasmid encoded *ere* genes are found in members of the Enterobacteriaceae and increase the intrinsic resistance to a clinically important level. Furthermore, these esterases can also be found in some strains of erythromycin resistant staphylococci.

Resistance to streptogramin type B antibiotics can be mediated in staphylococci and enterococci by plasmids carrying a *vgb* gene (2). The Vgb enzyme is a lyase that linearizes the cyclic hexadepsipeptide by cleavage of the ester bond via an elimination reaction.

Chemical Modification. Several bacterial enzymes can modify antibiotics to inactive derivatives (Table 2).

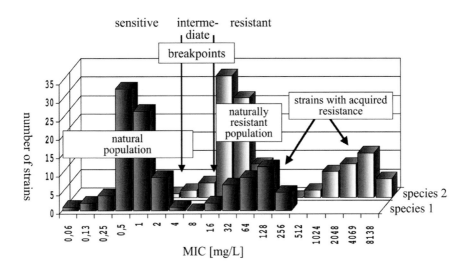

Fig. 1 MIC-Distribution showing the number of strains of one species with a certain MIC. The breakpoints are usually derived from microbiological and clinical experience as resistant strains are regarded as non-responding in an antibiotic therapy. Some bacterial species are naturally resistant (intrinsic resistance) to drugs because their natural MIC is above the breakpoint. Naturally sensitive strains as well as naturally resistant ones can acquire resistance and with that increase their MIC (acquired or secondary resistance).

Enzymatic modification is the most important mechanism of aminoglycoside resistance in gram-positive and gram-negative bacteria. There are three different types of enzymatic activity. N-acetyltransferases (AAC) use acetyl-CoA as a donor to modify aminogroups in the aminoglycoside. ATP dependent O-adenyltransferases (ANT) and ATP dependent O-phosphoryltransferases (APH) modify hydroxyl-residues. Numerous enzymes have been described. The nomenclature includes the regiospecifity of the group transfer (e.g. 3″), a roman numbering distinguishes between substrate specificities and an alphabetic prefix differentiates different genes. The localisation of the genes can be chromosomal but is usually plasmidic and can often be found on transposable elements (3).

Acetyl-CoA is also utilized as a cofactor to modify chloramphenicol by O-acetyltranferases (CATs). These enzymes have been found in many different bacterial genera and are usually plasmid encoded in clinical isolates. Furthermore, streptogramin type A antibiotics are acetylated by Vat enzymes that occur on plasmids in staphylococci and enterococci.

Nucleotidylation – the addition of adenylate-residues by Lnu enzymes – can also be the cause of resistance to lincosamid antibiotics in staphylococci and enterococci.

O-phosphotransferases that modify macrolides are produced by highly macrolide resistant *E. coli* strains. However, these enzymes have no clinical importance for macrolide resistance in gram-positive bacteria, and gram-negative ones are regarded as naturally resistant (2).

A minor percentage of fosfomycin resistance in gram-positive and gram-negative species is due to plasmids carrying a *fos* gene. The Fos protein, a glutathione-S-transferase, catalyzes the opening of fosfomycin followed by the addition of the tripeptide glutathione to the antibiotic.

Prevention of Access to the Target

The second general mechanism to cause resistance to antibacterial agents is to prevent the drug from reaching its target site. This is either achieved by altered rates of entry (reduced uptake) or by the active removal of the drug (active efflux) (4).

Reduced Uptake. The outer membrane of gram-negative bacteria is a permeability barrier that

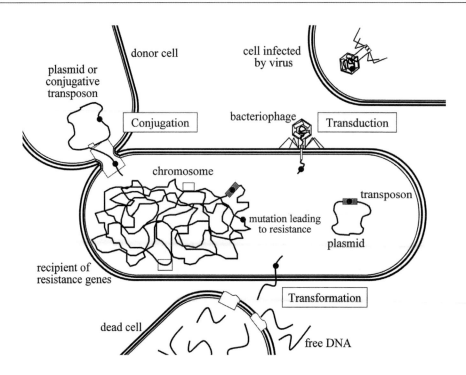

Fig. 2 Bacterial cells can obtain resistance genes in three ways: 1. Bacteria receive a plasmid or a conjugative transposon carrying resistance genes by a mechanism that involves direct cell-to-cell contact between donor and recipient cell (conjugation). 2. A bacteriophage infects a bacterium carrying a resistance gene and transfers the gene to the recipient cell where it can be incorporated into the genome (transduction). 3. Free DNA from dead cells in the vicinity of the recipient cell is taken up and integrated into the chromosome (transformation).

allows the passive diffusion of small hydrophilic antibiotics only through aqueus channels, the porins. Drugs larger than 800 Da are excluded. Mutational changes that lead to a reduction in the number of porins or the size of their diameter slow down the penetration process. In combination with a second contributor, e.g. a β-lactamase, porin changes can have a pronounced effect on the MIC. Accordingly, carbapenem resistance has been described in clinical *Enterobacter* and *Citrobacter* strains due to the loss of a major porin protein combined with a high-level production of an AmpC β-lactamase that is normally not able to confer resistance to carbapenems.

Furthermore, if the antibiotic passes membranes through a specific port of entry, its mutational loss leads to resistance. The lack of the outer membrane protein OprD in *Pseudomonas aeruginosa* causes resistance to the β-lactam antibiotic imipenem. Fosfomycin passes the cytoplasmic

membrane via a L-α-glycerolphosphate permease. This transport system is not essential for bacterial growth and therefore mutants with a reduced expression are frequently selected under therapy.

Active Efflux. Bacterial resistance can be caused by actively pumping antibiotics out of the cell and therefore decreasing the concentration at the target site. Drug efflux systems in bacteria are classified into four major groups based on their sequence homologies and functional similarities (Table 3).

ABC (ATP-binding cassette) transporters are efflux pumps that derive the energy needed for drug extrusion from the hydrolysis of ATP. Bacterial ABC antibiotic efflux transporter encoded on plasmids are a significant contributor to the aquired resistance of staphlyococci to macrolide and streptogramin antibiotics. The energy for the efflux mediated by the other three groups of bacte-

Tab. 1 **The most recent classification scheme according to Bush, Jacoby and Medeiros (BJM-scheme) divides the enzymes into four different classes according to their substrate and inhibitor profile (1).**

Functional group	Major subgroups	Molecular class*	Attributes	Example
1		C	chromosomal enzymes in gram-negative bacteria, may be also plasmid encoded; confer resistance to all classes of β-lactams except carbapenems; not inhibited by clavulanic acid	AmpC
2		A, D	most enzymes are inhibited by clavulanic acid	
	2a	A	confer high resistance to penicillins	Staphylococcal penicillinase
	2b	A	broad-spectrum β-lactamases [OSBL] (hydrolyse penicillins, broad-spectrum cephalosporins)	TEM-1, SHV-1
	2be	A	extended-spectrum β-lactamases [ESBL] conferring resistance to oxyimino-cephalosporins and monobactams	TEM-3 to TEM-20, SHV-2
	2br	A	broad-spectrum β-lactamases resistant to β-lactamase-inhibitors	TEM-30 to TEM-40
	2c	A	carbenicillinases	PSE-1, PSE-3
	2d	D	cloxacillin (oxacillin) hydrolysing enzymes	OXA-1 to OXA-10, PSE-2
	2e	A	cephalosporinases inhibited by clavulanic acid	FPM-1
	2f	A	serine-carbapenemases inhibited by clavulanic acid	MNC-A, Sme-1
3	3a 3b 3c	B	metallo-enzymes conferring resistance to all β-lactams except monobactams; not inhibited by clavulanic acid	IMP-1, L1 CphA
4		unknown	miscellaneous unsequenced enzymes not fitting into other groups	

older classification according to Ambler (similarities of the active site at aminoacid level)

rial transporters is provided by the proton-motive-force. Transporters of the SMR family (*Staphylococcus* multi drug resistance) are plasmid-encoded small cytoplasmic-membrane proteins. The Smr transporter of *S. aureus* pumps out quarternary ammonium compounds (e.g. benzalkonium chloride) and therefore confers resistance to these disinfectants. Within the MFS (major facilitator superfamily) group there are several pumps acting on different classes of antibiotics (see Table 3). The respective genes are found on conjugative and non-▸ conjugative plasmids or within the chromosome. They can be part of ▸ conjugative transposons as seen with the *mef* genes. Transporters of the RND (resistance/nodulation/division) family are chromosomally encoded. These systems are typically tripartite. A pump protein is located in the cytoplasmic membrane and an "outer membrane protein" forms a transperiplasmic tunnel and a channel through the outer membrane. The contact between them is established by a "membrane fusion protein". The efflux pumps of *P. aeruginosa* contribute significantly to the natural resistance of this species to a wide range of antibiotics. Furthermore, they can

Tab. 2 Antibiotic modifying enzymes (2,3).

Enzymes	Substrates	Host	Gene localisation
Acetyltransferases			
AAC	aminoglycosides	gram-negative and gram-positive bacteria	plasmid, transposon, chromosome
Vat	streptogramin A	staphylococci, enterococci	plasmid
CAT	chloramphenicol	gram-negative and gram-positive bacteria	plasmid, chromosome, transposon
Adenyltransferases			
ANT	aminoglycosides	gram-negative and gram-positive bacteria	plasmid, transposon
Lnu	lincomycin	staphylococci, E. faecium	plasmid
Phosphotransferases			
APH	aminoglycosides	gram-negative and gram-positive bacteria	plasmid, transposon
Mph	macrolides	E. coli, S. aureus	plasmid
Glutathionetransferase			
Fos	fosfomycin	gram-negative and gram-positive bacteria	plasmid

confer high levels of resistance when overexpressed as a result of mutations within regulatory genes.

Altered Target

A third general mechanism of bacterial resistance is to obtain an unsusceptible target. The affinity of the antibiotic to the target is diminished without impairing the physiological function of the target considerably. This can be either achieved by altering the usual target or by the acquisition of a new unsusceptible target (5).

Alteration of the Usual Target. One general mechanism is to exchange residues within the target molecule.

Resistance to fluoroquinolones is frequently mediated by amino acid changes within specific domains of the target proteins gyrase and topoisomerase IV. Mutations occur at hotspots in a qui-

nolone resistance-determinig region (QRDR) of the genes *gyrA* (coding for subunit A of gyrase) and *parC/grlA* coding for subunit A of topoisomerase IV.

One amino acid substitution within a specific region in the β-subunit of the RNA-polymerase, the target molecule of rifampicin, is necessary to establish high-level resistance to this antibiotic.

Macrolide, lincosamide and streptogramin B resistance (MLS_B phenotype) can be linked to specific nucleotide changes within the 23S rRNA of the large ribosomal subunit, mainly at position A2058 or neighbouring bases (*E. coli* numbering). This is the major mechanism of macrolide resistance in *Helicobacter pylori*, a species that does not possess multiple but only two *rrn* operons.

The acquisition of a *van*A gene cluster carried on a transposon is the major mechanism to confer glycopeptide resistance in enterococci. A coordinated expression of several *van* genes leads to the

Tab. 3 Examples of frequent bacterial efflux systems.

System	Substrates	Species	Gene Location
ABC			
MsrA	14-,15- membered macrolides, streptogramin type B	staphylococci	plasmid
Vga, Vga(B)	streptogramin type A	S. aureus	plasmid
SMR			
Smr(QacC)	quarternary ammonium compounds	S. aureus	plasmid
MFS			
NorA	fluoroquinolones	S. aureus	chromosome
TetK	tetracycline	S. aureus	plasmid
QacA	quarternary ammonium compounds	S. aureus	plasmid
TetA	tetracycline	E. coli	plasmid
MefA	14-,15- membered macrolides	S. pyogenes	chromosome
MefE	14-,15- membered macrolides	S. pneumoniae	chromosome
RND			
AcrAB-TolC	tetracycline, fluoroquinolones, chloramphenicol, β-lactams except imipenem, novobiocin, erythromycin, fusidic acid, rifampicin	E. coli	chromosome
MexAB-OprM	tetracycline, fluoroquinolones, chloramphenicol, β-lactams except imipenem, novobiocin, erythromycin, fusidic acid, rifampicin, trimethoprim, sulfamethoxazol	P. aeruginosa	chromosome

M

synthesis of modified peptidoglycan precursors: The D-alanyl-D-alanine moiety, the target of glycopeptides, is replaced by D-alanyl-D-lactate, which has a decreased affinity for vancomycin and teicoplanin.

A similar complex mechanism is responsible for the penicillin resistance of pathogenic *Neisseria* and *Streptococcus pneumoniae*. These bacteria are naturally competent, meaning they are able to take up free DNA. They alter the targets for penicillin, the penicillin binding proteins (PBPs), by recombining parts of their PBP genes with homologous DNA from related species. The resulting mosaic genes then encode PBPs with low affinity to penicillin.

A second mechanism that can be grouped into the category of alteration of the usual target is the overproduction of the target.

The enterococcal penicillin-binding-protein PBP5 binds penicillin with low affinity. The overproduction of this PBP is able compensate the loss of the others which are inhibited by the drug.

Overproduction of the chromosomal genes for the dehydrofolate reductase (DHFR) and the dihydropteroate synthase (DHPS) leads to a decreased susceptibility to trimethoprim and sulfamethoxazol, respectively. This is thought to be the effect of titrating out the antibiotics. However, clinically significant resistance is always associated with amino acid changes within the target enzymes leading to a decreased affinity of the antibiotics.

A third common means to alter the target is its modification. A widespread mechanism, with high clinical relevance in staphylococci and streptococci, leading to a MLS$_B$ phenotype is encoded by *erm* genes, mainly found on conjugative and non-conjugative transposons. The Erm enzymes mono- or dimethylate the adenine residue A2058 of the 23S ribosomal RNA. This phenotype is either constitutive or inducible by macrolide antibiotics via a translational attenuation mechanism.

Resistance to tetracyclines is often caused by the acquisition of genes (e.g. *tetO* and *tetM*) coding for so-called ribosome protection proteins. These proteins bind to the ribosome and protect them from tetracycline action.

Acquisition of New Unsusceptible Targets. Methicillin resistant *Staphylococcus aureus* strains (MRSA) produce an acquired new PBP with low affinity to almost all β-lactam antibiotics. It allows functional cell wall synthesis even if the normally occuring PBPs are inhibited. This PBP2a (or PBP2′) is encoded by the *mecA* gene that is part of a region of foreign DNA (*mec* region) that has been integrated into the staphyloccocal chromosome. MRSA are a major problem as these strains also tend to display a multi-resistance phenotype to other classes of antibiotics.

Resistance to trimethoprim can be due to the acquisition of plasmid encoded non-allelic variants of the chromosomal DHFR enzyme that are antibiotic unsuspectible. The genes may be part of transposons that then insert into the chromosome. For instance, in gram-negative bacteria the most widespread gene is *dhfrI* on transposon Tn7.

Accessory DHPS enzymes confer resistance to sulfonamides. Two different types encoded by the genes *sulI* (located on transposons) and *sulII* (located on plasmids) have been described. These resistance determinants are often genetically linked to trimethoprim resistance genes. Therefore, the combination of sulfonamide antibiotics with trimethoprim does not prevent resistance selection.

Drug resistance in the defined sense, however, is not always the reason for treatment failures. The formation of biofilms may be as well regarded as a resistance mechanism. Cells within such a film withstand the antibiotic treatment. Some antibiotics (e.g. the aminoglycoside tobramycin) penetrate only slowly into the film. A further explanation is the existence of cells living in a non-growing, protected phenotypic state .

Formation of spheroblasts, which are not attacked by antibiotics interfering with the peptidoglycan metabolism, is another example how bacteria could circumvent the antibiotic action.

Furthermore, the inability of the drug to reach the focus of the infection or to reach bacteria with intracellular location may be a common reason for the failure of antibiotic treatment.

Pharmacological Relevance

The presence of a specific resistance mechanism in a bacterial strain does not necessarily implicate that this strain is resistant in clinical terms. However, a strain expressing a resistance mechanism will be eliminated less easily as compared to a susceptible one. In clinical practice, only rarely resistance mechanisms will be identified. Usually the sensitivity of strains will be determined and reported to the clinician by using the interpretive criteria sensitive, intermediate or resistant. Some bacteria, however, harbouring resistance mechanisms may show up as sensitive in the standard test, although therapy will probably fail.

References

1. Bush K (2001) New β-Lactamases in Gram-negative Bacteria: Diversity and Impact on the Selection of Antimicrobial Therapy. Clinical Infectious Diseases 32:1085–1089
2. Roberts MC, Sutcliffe J, Courvalin P, Jensen LB, Rood J, Seppala H (1999) Nomenclature for Macrolide and Macrolide-Lincosamide-Streptogramin B Resistance Determinats, Antimicrob. Agents Chemother. 43:2823–2830
3. Mingeot-Leclerq M-P, Glupczynski Y, Tulkens PM (1999) Aminoglycosides: Activity and Resistance.
4. Hiroshi N (1994) Prevention of Drug Acces to Bacterial Targets: Permeabilty Barriers and Active Efflux. Science 264:382–387
5. Spratt BG (1994) Resistance to Antibiotics Mediated by Target Alterations. Science 264:388–393

Microtubule

A microtubule is a hollow tube of 25 nm diameter formed by 13 protofilaments. Each protofilament consists of polymerised α and ß tubulin heterodimers. Microtubules are polarized and have a plus and a minus end.

▶ Cytoskeleton

Microtubule Associated Proteins

Microtubule associated proteins (MAPs) are attached to microtubules *in vivo* and play a role in their nucleation, growth, shrinkage, stabilization and motion.

▶ Cytoskeleton

Mineralcorticoids

The main endogenous mineralocorticoid is aldosterone, which is mainly produced by the outer layer of the adrenal medulla, the *zona glomerulosa*. Aldostorone, like other steroids, binds to a specific intracellular (nuclear) receptor, the mineralocorticoid receptor (MR). Its main action is to increase sodium reabsorption by an action on the distal tubules in the kidney, which is accompanied by an increased excretion of potassium and hydrogen ions.

▶ Gluco-/Mineralocorticoid Receptor

Minimal Inhibitory Concentration

The minimal inhibitory concentration (MIC) is the concentration which is able to prevent 10^5 cells/ml from growing up to a visable density (~10^8 cells/ml) under standardized conditions.

MinK Subunits

MinK stands for minimal K-channel. In fact, MinK are auxiliary subunits. They do not form K-channels by themselves. They are associated with KvLQT1 subunits and are important for the properties of native KvLQT1 (I_{KR})-channels in cardiac tissue. Mutations in the MinK (KCNE1)-gene are associated with the same type of long QT syndrome (Romano-Ward syndrome; Jervyll-Lange-Nielson syndrome) as mutations in the KvLQT1 (KCNQ1)-gene.

▶ K^+ Channels

MirP Subunits

MirP subunits are relatives of MinK subunits. The abbreviation means MinK related Protein. So far, four MirP subunits are known. The corresponding human genes are KCNE2 to KCNE5. MirP1 (KCNE2) may associate with ▶ HERG channels. Mutations in MirP1 have been associated with certain forms of the long QT syndrome.

▶ K^+ Channels

M

Mitochondrial Permeability Transition Pore

Mitochondrial permeability transition involves the opening of a larger channel in the inner mitochondrial membrane leading to free radical generation, release of calcium into the cytosol and caspase activation. These alterations in mitochondrial permeability lead eventually to disruption of the respiratory chain and depletion of ATP. This in turn leads to release of soluble intramitochondrial membrane proteins such as cytochrome C and apoptosis-inducing factor, which results in apoptosis.

▶ Apoptosis

Mitogen

Mitogens are substances that cause cells, particularly lymphocytes, to undergo cell division. Mitogens are also referred to as polyclonal activators, since they stimulate proliferation of lymphocytes irrespective of their clonal origin. The best known mitogens are phytohemagglutinins isolated from certain plants.

Mitogen-activated Protein Kinase

MAPK

▶ MAP Kinase Cascades
▶ Glucocorticoids

Mitosis

Mitosis is the phase of the cell cycle in which the sister chromatids are separated and distributed into two daughter nuclei. First, upon entry into mitosis, the chromosomes are condensed, followed by the breakdown of the nuclear envelope (prophase). The two centrosomes are separated and induce the formation of the mitotic spindle. Then, the chromosomes are captured by the spindle and aligned on the metaphase plate (metaphase). The sister chromatids are separated and pulled to the poles of the spindle (anaphase). In telophase two new nuclei are formed around the separated chromatids.

Mixed Function Oxygenase

▶ P450 Mono-oxygenase System

MLCK

▶ Myosin Light Chain Kinase

MLCP

▶ Myosin Phosphatase

MMP-2

▶ Matrix Metalloprote(in)ase 2

MMP-9

▶ Matrix Metalloprote(in)ase 9

Molecular Chaperones

Molecular chaperones are a family of proteins that mediate the correct folding of other proteins, and, in some cases, their assembly into oligomeric structures. Chaperones assist protein folding by inhibiting alternative folding pathways that lead to nonfunctional structures. Chaperones are also part of the quality control system and play a role in the retention of misfolded proteins.

▶ Protein Trafficking and Quality Control

Molecular Dynamics Simulation

The principle of the molecular dynamics simulation approach is the movement of atoms under the action of a force field.

This approach starts with an initial low-energy structure and the integrated Newton's equation of motion is solved for all atoms simultaneously. Often the protein is placed in a box, which is filled up with solute molecules, e.g. water. To avoid effects at the edges a trick is used, the so-called periodic boundary condition. At the beginning, a starting velocity is assigned to every atom. The velocities are selected to couple the system on a certain temperature bath e.g. 310 K. For every atom, the force which is acting on this particle by the surrounding atoms is calculated. With a given step, usually 1 femtosecond, the next position is calculated over time to obtain classical atomic trajectories, which define conformational motions.

▶ Molecular Modelling

Molecular Modelling

GERD KRAUSE
Forschungsinstitut für Molekulare
Pharmakologie, Berlin-Buch, Germany
gkrause@fmp-berlin.de

Synonyms

Bio-computing, molecular simulation, molecular dynamics, structural ▶ bioinformatics

Definition

Molecular modelling itself can be simply described as the computer assisted calculation, modulation and visualisation of realistic three-dimensional molecular structures and their physical-chemical properties using molecular mechanics/▶ force fields.

Moreover, molecular modelling is one key method of a wide range of computer-assisted methods to analyse and predict relationships between protein sequence, three-dimensional molecular structure and biological function (sequence-structure-function relationships). In molecular pharmacology these methods focus predominantly on analysis of interactions between different proteins and between ligands (hormones, drugs) and proteins as well gaining information at the amino acid and even to atomic level.

▶ Bioinformatics
▶ NMR-based Ligand Screening

Description

The constantly increasing amount of data coming from high throughput experimental methods, genome sequences, and functional- and ▶ structural genomics has given a rise to a need for computer assisted methods to elucidate sequence-structure and function relationships.

Sequence Similarity
Protein sequences encoded by genome sequences encode biological functions.

There are two different dimensions, breadth and depth, used to reveal sequence-structure-functional relationships by computational methods (1). The aim of the first dimension breadth is to reveal sequence-function relationships by comparing protein sequences by sequence similarity. Simple bioinformatic algorithms can be used to compare a pair of related proteins or for sequence similarity searches e.g. BLAST (Basic Local Alignment Search Tool). Improved algorithms allow multiple alignments of larger number of proteins and extraction of consensus sequence pattern and sequence profiles or structural templates that can be related to some functions, see e.g. underhttp://www.expasy.ch/tools/#similarity.

The aim of the second dimension depth is to consider protein three-dimensional structures to uncover structure-function relationships. Starting from the protein sequences, the steps in the depth dimension are structure prediction, homology modelling of protein structures and the simulation of protein-protein interactions and ligand-complexes.

Protein Structure Predictions

Starting from the protein sequence (primary structure) several algorithms can be used to analyse the primary structure and to predict secondary structural elements like β-strands, turns and helices. The first algorithms from Chou and Fasman occurred in 1978. The latest algorithms, e.g. under http://dodo.cpmc.columbia.edu, are able to make predictions of transmembrane and coiled coil regions just from the primary sequence.

Approaches of *de novo* predictions, which try to calculate how the structural elements are folded into the three-dimensional structure (tertiary structure) of complete proteins are nowadays far away from reliable large-scale applications. On the other hand, this topic is under strong development indicated by recent successful results at the contest for structural prediction methods CASP4. With the fast growing number of experimentally solved 3D-structures of protein and new promising approaches like threading tools combined with experimental structural constraints, one can expect more reliable *denovo* predictions for 3D-protein structures in the future.

Homology Models of Protein Structures

The primary sequence of proteins with identical function varies within different species by natural mutations of amino acids. With increasing distance in the evolutionary process the number of variations between the sequences of proteins increase.

In the protein structure database PDB (http://www.rcsb.org/pdb) all by X-ray crystallography and NMR spectroscopy experimentally solved three-dimensional protein structures are available to the public. Homology model building for a query sequence uses protein portions of known three-dimensional structures as structural templates for proteins with high sequence similarity.

If the sequence of a protein has more than 90% identity to a protein with known experimental three-dimensional structure, than it is an optimal case to build a homologous structural model based on that structural template. The margins of error for the model and for the experimental method are in similar ranges. The different amino acids have to be mutated virtually. The conformations of the new side chains can be derived either from residues of structurally characterized amino acids in a similar spatial environment or from side chain rotamer libraries for each amino acid type which are stored for different structural environments like β-strands or α-helices.

The discrepancies between homologous protein sequences occur predominantly at the surfaces and in the so-called loop regions. With decreasing sequence identities, insertions and deletions of loop chains modelling of completely different loop chains are necessary. Segmentation of the loop in overlapping sequence fragments (3–10 residues) and searching for sequence similarity using BLAST or FASTA in the PDB database has proven to be most successful in loop modelling. Those fragments occurring several times in different protein structures with a common backbone conformation have a high probability of adopting the same backbone conformation also in the query sequence. The overlap almost allows knowledge-based assembly of the fragments to a new loop conformation. This segmentation strategy is also part of the successful algorithm, Rosetta (http://depts.washington.edu/bakerpg/) for predicting complete folds for new proteins.

Similar residues in the cores of protein structures especially hydrophobic residues at the same positions are responsible for common folds of homologous proteins. Certain sequence profiles of conserved residue successions have been identified which give rise to a common fold of protein domains. They are organized in the smart database (simple modular architecture research tool) http://smart.embel-heidelberg.de

Natural mutation of amino acids in the core of a protein can stabilize the same fold with different complementary amino acid types, but they can also cause a different fold of that particular portion. If the sequence identity is lower than 30% it is much more difficult to identify a homologous structure. Other strategies like secondary structure predictions combined with knowledge based rules about reciprocal exchange of residues are necessary. If there is a reliable assumption for common fold then it is possible to identify interacting residues by search for correlated complementary mutations of residues by correlated mutation analysis, CMA.

Predicting a likely conformation or fold of a particular region of a protein with less or no sequence similarity to protein structures recoded

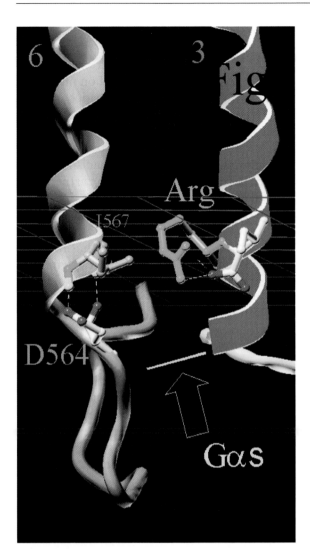

Fig. 1 Structural detail of the glycoprotein LH receptor model in its inactive state at the intracellular portion between TM6 and TM3. An N-terminal helix capping conformation of the side chain of Asp 564 formed by a hydrogen bond towards the main chain stabilises an extended helical portion of TM6 into the intracellular phase. The extended TM6 seals the cleft between TM6 and TM3 at the intracellular site hindering the infiltration of the G-protein Gαs. Release of the TM6 extension or movement of TM6 allows the infiltration of G-protein between TM6 and TM3. Instead of stabilising the inactive state via a salt-bridge between TM6 and TM3 (conserved arginine) like in rhodopsin, a new stabilising mechanism for constraining the inactive, basal receptor state was identified for glycoprotein receptors.

in the PDB is the main challenges for homology modelling of proteins.

Sequence conservation is, in general much, weaker than structural conservation. There are proteins, which are clearly not related in sequence but are closely related in 3D-structure and fold, like heamoglobin and myoglobin, which have similar functions. In many proteins, fold elements like 4-helical bundles are repeated. Classifications of known structural folds of proteins are organized in the SCOP or CATH database see e.g.http://scop.mrc-lmb.cam.ac.uk/scop/.

Taken together the procedure to build a starting protein structural model for a protein combines similarity searches by sequences and by folds in different 3D structure databases and filling in remaining unknown conformations by information resulting from bioinformatic, knowledge based approaches and overlapping segmentation of sequence fragments.

After the construction phase of a model follows the optimisation of the geometrical structure by force fields.

Molecular Simulation

Simulation in general describes calculations with models where different options and combinations of variables can be quickly played through. Molecular simulations allow the characterization of molecular properties during the motions of the molecular models over time.

Force field or molecular mechanics calculations of molecular models are energy minimisations. Starting with energy for an unfavourable molecular geometry, the algorithm searches for the next local energy minimum at the energy hyper-surface. Starting with different unfavourable geometries can lead to different conformations at other local energy minima. For larger molecular structures and especially for structural models built on templates with lower sequence identity, it is necessary to evaluate the geometrical stability.

Importantly, all biological procedures operate at a temperature of 310 Kelvin, not at 0 Kelvin, as the potential energy is calculated by the force fields. The kinetic energy must also be considered. Molecules and proteins at room temperature change the conformation at least at the surface and in loop region. ▶ Molecular dynamics simulation

(MD) is an approach to tackle these kinetic and stability problems.

An approach to overcome the multi minima problem of proteins is ▶ simulated annealing (SA) run. Besides global molecular properties such as structural and thermal motions, functional properties of fast biological reactions are studied by MD.

Accuracy and Limitations

Molecular models are only an approximation to reality, but good models can often closely approach reality.

The margin of error of a final structural model depends on the sequence or fold similarity to the starting structural template.

An important measure for quality is the verification by MD or SA of the stability of a molecular model. Other programs (e.g. PROCHECK) can also be used to check the globular geometrical quality of a structure to avoid serious defects in the geometry of proteins. Even the most elaborate models are worthless if there is no experimental examination at all.

Functional insights based on structural relationships can only rise to the level of hypotheses, and these hypotheses must be tested by direct functional experiments.

The strongest verification for a 3D protein model comes from the experimental 3D structure. This is objective of the contest for protein structure predictions CASP4 etc., where the structural models are made in advance of the experimental structure of a particular protein.

In molecular pharmacology research an indirect proof of a structural model is possible by functional examinations e.g. by molecular biological experiments. Well selected site directed mutageneses and their functional characterization allows confirmation or rejection of a molecular protein model. The process is organized as an iterative procedure, where the biological answer of suggested mutations is used to refine the model. The iteration continues until the model is consistent with the biological experiments and the functional predictions of mutations are confirmed.

Pharmacological Relevance

In general the relevance of predictions of structure-function relationships based on molecular modelling and structural bioinformatics are three fold. First they can be used to answer the question of which partners (proteins) might interact. Second, predictions generate new hypotheses about binding site, about molecular mechanisms of activation and interaction between two partners, and can lead to new ideas for pharmacological intervention. The third aim is to use the predictions for structure based drug design.

Common to all three aims is, that *in silico* derived predictions can rationalize experimental efforts either by specific molecular biological experiments like site directed mutations or e.g. by reducing the number of compounds to screen experimentally for drug design.

Structure–Function Prediction

From the human genome project it is known, that roughly 30,000 proteins exist in humans. Currently only the 3D structures of few thousand human proteins or protein domains are known. Structures of membrane-bound proteins are several magnitudes more rare. Beside efforts to solve further structures like structural genomics, there is a challenge for computational approaches to predict structures and function for homologous proteins.

This is eminently necessary for large protein classes with important functions, e.g. the ▶ G-protein coupled receptors (GPCR), where several hundred different human GPCR are known. Out of this large family of seven transmembrane–helix proteins, there is only one structure known - rhodopsin. The rhodopsin structure is used as a template for homologous receptor models. Incorporation of further experimental results like scanning accessible cysteines, cross linking, spin labelling, ligand binding and site directed mutations allow molecular modelling to predict successfully ligand binding sites and local activation mechanisms of diverse GPCR. Although all GPCR contain the seven transmembrane helix pattern it seems to be that rather small structural differences cause diverse activation mechanisms even within one family of GPCR. Such differences can be revealed by molecular simulations and characterized by molecular experiments. For example, in general, the inactive conformation of GPCR is constrained by the interaction of complementary residues in the interior side of the receptor. At the intracellular phase the only structural template, rhodopsin, is constrained via a very highly conserved arginine at transmembrane (TM) helix 3 by forming a salt-bridge to a glutamate at the opposite TM6. Although in the group of glycoprotein receptors at the same positions an arginine in TM3 and an aspartate in TM6 occur, site-directed mutagenesis could not confirm the mechanism of rhodopsin. Instead of a salt-bridge as constrain of the inactive basal state for the glycoprotein receptors, an intracellular extension of TM6 could be identified by molecular modelling (Fig. 1). The helical extension is stabilized by helix capping via

the aspartate side chain of TM6 and was confirmed by site-directed mutagenesis and NMR studies of corresponding peptides (2).

Structural similarity can sometimes be a strong indicator of similar function but does not necessarily mean having similar function. More important structural similarity can show evolutionary links between proteins whose ancestors may have had similar functions.

Several different types of protein domains are known to function in binding to phosphotyrosine, including ▶ src homology-2 domain (SH2 domain) and ▶ PTB domain. For example, the crystal structure of the amino-terminal domain from the human signalling protein Cbl revealed the presence of a cryptic SH2 domain followed by a C3HC4 ring finger domain. The sequence of this

M

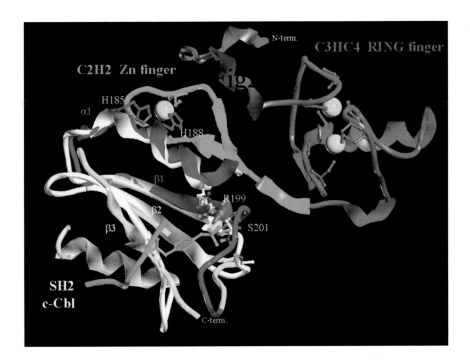

Fig. 2 Molecular model of Hakai based on structural bioinformatics, molecular modelling and biochemical experiments. Comparison of the structural model of Hakai, incomplete SH2 domain (magenta) with the SH2 domain X-ray structure of Cbl (white). The missing beta-strand fold β2, β3 at the incomplete SH2 sequence is exactly replaced by a beta sheet fold found in Fibronectin (yellow) with similar sequence to Hakai in that portion. The SH2 like fold of Hakai is assembled by sequence similarity and fold similarity. An incomplete C2H2 Zn finger domain (blue) is completed by merging with helix α1 of the SH2 domain. Side chains H 185, H188 of the merged Zn finger domain and R199 and S201 of the P-tyrosine binding site showed strong sensitive functional influences on mutations and confirm indirectly the proposed model at that region.
red: the preceding ring finger domain; green: putative phosphotyrosine peptide of E-cadherin.

SH2 domain was so divergent that its existence had not been previously suspected. The conservation of unique and important structural elements in the X-ray structure however identified it clearly as a member of the SH2 family. A recently isolated E-cadherin binding protein called Hakai contained, according to sequence similarity, a C3H4 ring-finger domain and a small portion of an incomplete SH2 domain. These are similar domains as in Cbl but with inverse order, and the sequences around the incomplete SH2 domain were even more divergent from canonical SH2 domain and also from that of Cbl. Combination of sequence and fold similarity with structural alignments and functional investigation showed that Hakai is a Cbl-like protein where the SH2 domain and ring-finger domain are in the same spatial arrangement. A two stranded β-sheet identified in the fibronectin structure by sequence similarity to Hakai replaced the missing part in the incomplete SH2 fold. Although divergent to SH2 sequences the particular portion resembles the corresponding SH2 fold. Moreover, an additional incomplete C2H2 Zn finger domain between the ring-finger and SH2 domain could be assigned to a complete Zn finger by its structural merging with the first helix of the SH2 domain carrying the two missing histidines (Fig. 2). Mutations and functional characterization of the two histidines participating in Zn finger formation as well as the suspected arginine and serine for phosphotyrosine binding of SH2 confirmed the structural model of Hakai (3).

Simulation of Functional Properties

With growing computer power, the abilities to simulate functional properties and dynamics of fast biological reactions are increasing. Today molecular dynamics can be traced over a time range of about 1 millisecond. Relevant dynamics of fast biological processes (vision and photosynthesis) like electron transfer reactions, proton translocation (bacteriorhodopsin) and ion transport (potassium channels) in proteins have been studied. MD simulations can provide a realistic description of the actual reactive event.

Recently the dynamics and mechanisms of water permeation through biological membranes via pore proteins were studied using aquaporin 1 (AQP1) and the homologous glycerol facilitator (GlpF). The selective pattern for transport of water at AQP1 and glycerol at GlpF could be identified. Also a fine-tuned water dipole rotation during the passage through the pores could be simulated by MD (4). Critical examinations of dynamic effects showed that they are rather unlikely to contribute to processes with significant activation barriers. Even in cases of ion channels it is found that the most important effects are associated with energies rather than dynamics (5).

The resulting insight of MD is crucial in studies of fast photo biological reactions and instructive in cases of slower processes. Very slow processes like protein folding cannot be traced by MD, since folding takes a time range between 20 milliseconds and one hour.

References

1. Luscombe NM, Greenbaum D, Gerstein (2001) What is Bioinformatics? A proposed definition and overview of the field. Method Infom Med 40:346–358
2. Schulz A, Bruns K, Henklein P, Krause G, Schubert M, Gudermann T, Wray V, Schultz G, Schöneberg T. (2000) Requirement of specific intrahelical interactions for stabilizing the inactive conformation of glycoprotein hormone receptors. J Biol Chem. 275(48):37860–37869
3. Fujita Y, Krause G, Scheffner M, Zechner D, Leddy HEM, Behrens J, Sommer T, Birchmeyer W. (2002) Hakai, a c-Cbl-like protein, ubiquitinates and induces endocytosis of the E-cadherin complex. Nature Cell Biology 4(3):222–231
4. Groot BL de, Grubmüller H. (2001) Water permeation across biological membranes: mechanism and dynamics of aquaporin-1 and GlpF. Science 294:2353–2357
5. Warshel A. (2002) Molecular dynamics simulations of biological reactions. Acc Chem Res. 35(6):385–395

Monoamine Oxidase

Two related but distinct enzymes, MAO A and MAO B, are major neurotransmitter-degrading enzymes in the central nervous system (CNS) and periphery. Both enzymes require the cofactor FAD (flavin adenine dinucleotide) but each has a unique substrate specificity. MAO A has a higher affinity for the substrates serotonin, norepinephrine and dopamine, while MAO B prefers phenylethylamine and benzylamine. Despite this, MAO B appears to be the form that catalyzes the oxidation of dopamine to DOPAC (3,4-dihydroxyphenylacetic acid) in humans. Selective MAO B inhibitors have therefore been used as an adjuvant to L-DOPA therapy in Parkinson's disease (PD) patients.

Monoclonal Antibodies

▶ Humanized Monoclonal Antibodies

Monocytes

▶ Inflammation

Monophasic Preparations

In monophasic preparations a fixed estrogen/progestin combination is present in each contraceptive pill.

▶ Contraceptives

Mood Disorders

▶ Affective Disorders

Mood-stabilising Drugs

In contrast to antidepressants (mood-elevating agents), mood-stabilizing drugs are not only effective in treating a state of depression, but can also control the manic phase of a manic-depressive (bipolar) illness. Mood-stabilizing drugs are often used prophylactically in bipolar depression. The most important mood-stabilizing agents are lithium salts which are able to prevent swings of mood in bipolar depression. In the acute phase, lithium is effective only in reducing mania, but not depression. It is currently not clear how lithium exerts its mood-stabilizing effects. Two main molecular mechanisms have been preposed. Lithium has been shown to inhibit inositol phosphatases. This results in a reduced formation of free inositol, which is required for the formation of phosphatidyl inositols, serving as substrates for phospholipases (e.g. phospholipase-β). Lithium, thus, blocks the phosphatidyl inositol (PI) pathway resulting in the inhibition of agonist-stimulated inositol 1,4,5-triphosphate (IP_3) formation by a variety of receptors. Recently lithium has been shown to inhibit glycogen synthesis kinase-3β (GSK-3β), which is involved in various neuronal regulatory processes, including the Wnt-pathway.

Morpholines

Morpholines are a chemical class of organic compounds with the six-membered ring tetrahydro-1,4-oxazine, as their basic structure.

Motilin

Motilin is a 22-amino acid peptide hormone, secreted by the enterochromaffin cells of the small intestine, which exerts a profound effect on gastric motility by inducing contractions of the antrum and duodenum. Motilin acts on a G-protein cou-

M

pled receptor, which is expressed in a subset of interstitial cells of the human duodenum, jejunum and colon. Macrolide antibiotics like erythromycin and roxithromycin act as agonists on the motilin receptor.

▶ Macrolides

Motion Sickness

▶ Emesis

Motor Proteins

Motor proteins move along microtubules or F-actin. The respective motor domains are linked to their cargoes *via* adaptor proteins. Kinesin motors move only to the plus and dynein motors only to the minus ends of microtubules. Myosin motors move along F-actin. When motors are immobilized at their cargo binding area, they can move microtubules or F-actin respectively.

▶ Cytoskeleton

MPEP

▶ 2-Methyl-6-(Phenylethynyl) Pyridine

MPP$^+$

▶ 1-Methyl-4-Phenylpyridinium

MPTP

1-Methyl-4-phenyl-1,2,3,6-tetrahydropyridine

▶ 1-Methyl-4-Phenylpyridinium
▶ Organic Cation Transporters

mRNA

Messenger RNA (mRNA) is the intermediate template between DNA and proteins. The information from a particular gene is transferred from a strand of DNA by the construction of a complementary strand of RNA through a process known as transcription. The amount of any particular type of mRNA in a cell reflects the extend to which a gene has been 'expressed'.

MS/MS

▶ Tandem Mass Spectrometry

Mucolipin

Mucolipin, also known as mucolipin 1 or mucolipidin (encoded by the *MCOLN1* gene), is a TRP-channel-related membrane protein, most probably residing in intracellular membranes. Is defective in mucolipidosis type IV disease, a developmental neurodegenerative disorder characterized by lysosomal storage disorder and abnormal endocytosis of lipids. The function of mucolipin is unknown.

▶ TRP Channels

Multidrug Resistance

Multidrug resistance is the simultaneous resistance of a cell to a broad spectrum of structurally and functionally unrelated chemotherapeutic drugs. Resistance may be present before exposure to a drug (intrinsic resistance) or may occur following initial exposure (acquired resistance).

▶ Multidrug Transporter

Multidrug Resistance Gene

▶ Multidrug Transporter

Multidrug Transporter

MELISSA J. PEART, ASTRID A. RUEFLI,
RICKY W. JOHNSTONE
Cancer Immunology Division, The Peter
MaccCallum Cancer Institute, Trescowthick
Research Laboratories, Smorgon Family
Building, St Andrews Place, East Melbourne 3002
Victoria, Australia
r.johnstone@pmci.unimelb.edu.au

Synonyms

P-glycoprotein

Definition

P-glycoprotein (P-gp) is an energy-dependent efflux pump that can transport a wide variety of compounds including anti-cancer drugs, conferring multidrug resistance to tumors. Recently, other functions have been assigned to P-gp that may affect cell development and survival and additionally protect cells from drug-induced death.

▶ Tolerance and Desensitization

Basic Characteristics

The phenomenon of multidrug resistance (MDR) was first described in 1970 by Biedler and Riehm (1), who noted that cells selected for resistance to a single cytotoxic drug simultaneously acquired resistance to other structurally and functionally unrelated drugs. While we now know that there are multiple mechanisms by which tumor cells are able to resist the cytotoxic effects of ▶ chemotherapy, one of the first identified mechanisms was overexpression of the multidrug transporter, P-glycoprotein (P-gp). Over the last two decades, the genetic, biochemical and molecular characteristics of P-gp have been extensively studied (see ref 2 for review). However, although more effective drugs and chemotherapeutic strategies are continually being developed, MDR remains a major obstacle to successful cancer chemotherapy. In addition, it is becoming increasingly apparent that P-gp is much more than a simple drug efflux pump. This chapter summarises the current knowledge and proposed functions of the multidrug transporter, P-glycoprotein.

P-gp is a 170–180 kD cell surface molecule and a member of the ATP-binding cassette (ABC) superfamily. ▶ ABC transporters are conserved throughout evolution and include many bacterial transporters as well as eukaryotic proteins such as Ste6p, a yeast mating-factor transporter, the cystic fibrosis transmembrane regulator (CFTR) and the human multidrug resistance related protein (MRP). They transport a wide variety of substrates such as drugs, ions, sugars, lipids and peptides across cellular membranes in an energy-dependent manner. P-gp is encoded by the multidrug resistance-1 gene (*MDR1*) in humans and in mice is encoded by two genes, *mdr1a* and *mdr1b*. *MDR1* expression can be induced after several rounds of chemotherapy (acquired resistance) and by a number of stress stimuli including hypoxia, growth factor withdrawal, heat shock, UV- and γ-irradiation, activated oncogenes and HIV-1.

As well as being overexpressed in a wide range of human tumors, P-gp is present in many normal tissues including the surface of cells found in the gut, liver, kidney tubules and at blood-tissue barriers. P-gp has a proposed physiological function in protecting vital organs from xenotoxins by active transport of these compounds into bile,

M

urine and the lumen of the intestine. P-gp is also expressed in the adrenal gland, on various cells of the immune system including hemopoietic stem cells, natural killer cells, monocytes, antigen presenting dendritic cells and T- and B- ▸ lymphocytes, and in the developing embryo and placenta. This wide distribution of P-gp in normal human cells provides cancers derived from these tissues with an intrinsic resistance to chemotherapeutic drugs and suggests that additional physiological functions for P-gp exist.

P-gp is composed of two homologous halves separated by a linker region. Each half contains 6 predicted transmembrane (TM) domains that are thought to recognize and transport substances across the bilayer, and an intracellular nucleotide binding domain (NBD), or ATP-binding site, which couples ATP hydrolysis to drug transport. The precise number of substrate binding sites is still uncertain. Photoaffinity labeling with P-gp substrate analogs and mutational data have identified two drug binding sites, but suggest that additional regions are also involved. Unlike other ▸ ABC transporters, each of which is relatively specific for its substrate, P-gp transports a wide variety of structurally diverse compounds including steroid hormones and ▸ cytokines, in addition to drugs. Original models of drug efflux by P-gp hypothesized that drugs were transported from the cytosol to the outside of the cell through a pore formed by P-gp. Further structural and functional studies have led to a revised model of transport, where P-gp acts as a drug 'flippase'. This 'flippase' model proposes that P-gp intercepts the drug as it moves through the lipid membrane and flips it from the inner to the outer leaflet of the membrane into the extracellular media. During this transport cycle, P-gp undergoes significant conformational changes in response to ATP binding and hydrolysis and the two NBDs are thought to interact. There is a lack of understanding of this series of conformational changes however, and in the absence of a high resolution three-dimensional structure, it remains unclear how a single molecule can recognize and transport such a broad range of compounds across the lipid bilayer.

The mechanism by which P-gp mediates MDR appears more complex than originally thought. It is clear that P-gp acts as a drug efflux pump, reducing intracellular drug accumulation and as a consequence, drug toxicity. This has been confirmed in *mdr1a/1b* knock-out mice, which have an increased sensitivity to toxins and altered drug distribution especially in the brain, highlighting the importance of P-gp as a component of the blood-brain barrier. The expression of P-gp often alters the biophysical properties of the cell, such as increasing intracellular pH and altering membrane potential and ion transport, which may contribute to MDR in some cells. Recent evidence however, has suggested that drug efflux may not be the only mechanism of resistance mediated by P-gp, as discussed below.

Additional Physiological Functions for P-gp
In addition to drug transport, P-gp has been implicated in the regulation of chloride channel activity, lipid transport, ▸ cholesterol esterification, cytotoxic effector cell function, dendritic cell migration, ▸ cytokine export, ▸ alloimmunity, viral infection and cell death (Fig. 1). However the physiological significance of P-gp for each of these functions remains poorly understood.

Chloride Channel Activity.
Several ABC transporters, such as CFTR, which functions as a cAMP-activated chloride channel, have been shown to act as ▸ ion channel regulators. It is now clear that P-gp itself is not an ion channel but that it regulates the rate of activation of an as yet unidentified volume-activated chloride channel. Human *MDR1* and murine *mdr1a* possess this regulatory activity, however *mdr1b* does not. The ability of P-gp to act as a chloride channel regulator is separate to its drug efflux function as defined by mutation studies, and can be inhibited by protein kinase C-induced phosphorylation. The mechanism by which P-gp regulates this chloride channel activity is unknown and is unlikely to be elucidated until the channel being regulated is identified.

Lipid Transport and Cholesterol Esterification.
Many ABC transporters have been associated with the trafficking of lipids and sterols. *In vitro* studies have shown that *MDR1* and *mdr1a* can transport a wide variety of short chain phospholipids, such as platelet-activating factor and native phosphatidylcholine and sphingomyelin (SM), across the plasma membrane. *In vitro* expression of P-gp correlates with increased esterification of plasma

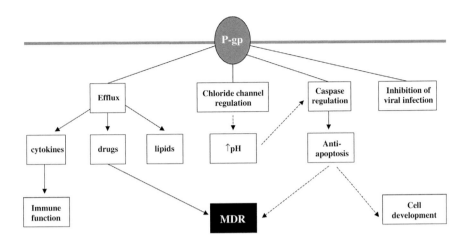

Fig. 1 Proposed functions of P-glycoprotein (P-gp). P-gp may mediate multidrug resistance (MDR) via 2 distinct, yet interrelated, mechanisms; firstly through its efflux function to decrease the intracellular accumulation of drug, and secondly by inhibiting the apoptotic pathways required for drug action. In addition, the proposed ability of P-gp to efflux cytokines and lipids may be responsible for regulating a range of different physiological functions, including effector cell function, alloimmunity, cell migration and cholesterol esterification. An increase in intracellular pH (pHi) resulting from functional expression of P-gp may affect drug efflux and caspase activation, which in turn impacts on cell development and survival. Separate to its efflux and anti-apoptotic functions, P-gp regulates chloride channel activity. P-gp may also inhibit viral infection by an as yet unidentified mechanism.

M

membrane ▶ cholesterol, and in *mdr1a/1b* knock-out mice the kinetics of cholesterol accumulation and esterification are affected in the liver. Depletion of SM can induce cholesterol esterification, thus these two functions may be interrelated, however this is speculative and the mechanism through which P-gp affects cholesterol trafficking remains unknown.

Immune Functions. P-gp is expressed on a wide variety of cells of the human immune system, thus a potential role for P-gp in a number of immune functions has been intensely investigated. P-gp has been reported to play a role in the cytotoxic effector function of NK cells and T ▶ lymphocytes, in the migration of antigen presenting dendritic cells and T cells during immune/inflammatory responses, and to facilitate the secretion of ▶ cytokines such as IL-1β, IL-2, IL-4 and IFN-γ. Recently a novel role for P-gp in ▶ alloimmunity was defined, as anti-P-gp antibodies were shown to inhibit alloantigen-dependent T cell proliferation by blocking IL-2, IFN-γ and TNF-α release in stimulated lymphocytes. However, these studies were in contrast to others showing T cells from *mdr1a-/-* mice exhibited normal proliferation, cytokine secretion and cytotoxic effector function when compared to wild-type T cells, although ▶ alloimmune T cell responses were not investigated in this particular study. The development of more specific P-gp inhibitors will help in determining whether these responses are directly mediated by P-gp, and further studies using the *mdr1a/1b* knock-out mice will help to clarify any immune regulatory role that P-gp may have.

A recent report found that *mdr1a-/-* mice spontaneously develop ▶ colitis characterised by destruction of the epithelial tissue and lymphocyte infiltration. This phenotype could be reversed using broad spectrum antibiotics. Subsequently, it was shown that these mice had altered development and function of intraepithelial lymphocytes (IEL), which are associated with the skin epithelium and mucosal surfaces and are important in the host immune response against pathogens. Taken together, these studies suggest a role for P-gp in the maintenance of the intestinal epithelial barrier and it is possible that the lack of functional IELs results in the colitis phenotype.

Viral Infection. Recent studies have demonstrated that P-gp overexpressing MDR cells and stem cells that express P-gp are resistant to infection by enveloped viruses such as the influenza virus and HIV-1, which enter the cell via fusion with the plasma membrane. P-gp is proposed to provide protection by blocking insertion of the viral fusion protein into the membrane, although an indirect effect of P-gp expression on membrane structure cannot be excluded. In addition, in cells directly transfected with HIV-1 to bypass the fusion step, P-gp inhibited virus production independent of its efflux function. Collectively, these studies suggest that P-gp may play an important role in protecting cells from viral infection. Further studies are required to dissect the mechanism of this inhibition and its physiological significance. To date, there have been no published reports on the susceptibility of *mdr1* knock-out mice to viral challenge.

Cell Death. Although chemotherapeutic drugs have diverse intracellular targets, most kill tumor cells primarily by activating ▶ apoptosis pathways. Hence the susceptibility of a cell to undergo apoptosis may determine its drug sensitivity. A role for P-gp in regulating apoptosis has been postulated based on the fact that P-gp can confer cross-resistance to non-drug death stimuli such as radiation. In addition, although P-gp is an efficient efflux pump, it only serves to lower the intracellular accumulation of cytotoxic agents, but does not completely inhibit entry and accumulation. Despite the fact that drug influx often surpasses drug efflux, P-gp^{+ve} cells are still protected from cell death. Studies by several groups have suggested that in addition to drug efflux, *MDR1* protects against drug-induced cell death by inhibiting the apoptotic program (3).

While somewhat controversial, functional P-gp has been shown to confer resistance to a range of cell death stimuli, including UV- and γ-irradiation, serum starvation and ligation of the cell surface ▶ death receptors Fas and tumor necrosis factor (TNF) receptor. The apoptotic pathways induced by these stimuli are mediated by ▶ caspases, and

P-gp has been shown to inhibit caspase activation. This inhibition can be reversed by anti-P-gp monoclonal antibodies or pharmacological blockers of P-gp function. While there is an increasing amount of data demonstrating P-gp-mediated protection against caspase-dependent death stimuli, it appears that P-gp does not protect cells against stimuli that induce death independent of caspase activation. For example, caspase-independent stimuli including the pore-forming proteins perforin and complement, and chemotherapeutic drugs such as staurosporine, hexamethylene bisacetamide (HMBA) and the histone deacetylase inhibitor suberoylanilide hydroxamic acid (SAHA) induce equivalent death in P-gp^{+ve} and P-gp^{-ve} cells. Thus, P-gp can inhibit caspase-dependent cell death, possibly by inhibiting caspase activation, but does not inhibit caspase-independent cell death. This suggests that P-gp may protect cells on two levels, both through its efflux function and by inhibiting apoptotic pathways activated by drugs to induce cell death. Despite the large volume of work demonstrating that P-gp can confer resistance to non-drug induced death stimuli, the mechanism by which P-gp mediates this protection remains unknown.

P-gp may also provide protection against death induced through the SM-ceramide apoptotic pathway. Stimulation of sphingomyelinase following cell stress generates ceramide, a pro-apoptotic molecule that can induce cell death. P-gp expression has been found to correlate with a significant decrease in inner leaflet-associated SM and inhibition of TNF-induced ceramide production and apoptosis. Since P-gp is able to transport phospholipids, it has been proposed that P-gp may inhibit ceramide production by reducing intracellular pools of SM. However, the importance of ceramide in apoptosis induction is still controversial, thus it is not clear whether the effect of P-gp on TNF-mediated cell death occurs due to decreased intracellular SM levels or by inhibiting caspase activation by another, as yet unidentified, manner.

A role for P-gp in regulating primary cell survival and/or growth has recently been proposed. P-gp is expressed in hemopoietic stem cells, and the most primitive cells contain the highest amount of P-gp. Overexpression of *MDR1* facilitates stem cell expansion in culture and results in the development of a myeloproliferative syndrome in transplanted mice, suggesting that P-gp may influence self-renewal decisions in repopulating stem cells. Interestingly, treatment of activated primary human mononuclear cells with anti-P-gp antibodies induces apoptosis induced by the Fas death receptor pathway, suggesting that P-gp may regulate the survival of activated lymphocytes.

Future Directions

In principle, P-gp mediated MDR can be circumvented by treatment regimes that either exclude P-gp substrate drugs and those that require the activation of caspases to induce cell death, or include P-gp inhibitory agents. Efforts in the clinic to overcome MDR have explored the therapeutic benefit of P-gp inhibitors, such as the calcium channel blocker verapamil and the cyclosporin A analog PSC-833, to sensitise resistant cells to the action of cytotoxic drugs. Unfortunately, there has been limited success with these compounds to date due to their toxic side effects and the complexity and multiplicity of cellular resistance, although new compounds are currently being tested in clinical trials with renewed optimism. Interestingly, a new class of small molecules was recently discovered that are able to modulate the substrate specificity of P-gp, dramatically changing the MDR phenotype by making P-gp more active against some classes of drugs and inactive against others. Further insights into the structure and function of P-gp will lead to an improved understanding of its mechanism of action as an efflux pump, which should in turn lead to the development of novel drugs and more specific P-gp inhibitors to use both in the clinic and as a research tool. In addition, as the molecular basis for drug sensitivity and initiation of resistance is defined, better treatment strategies will be designed in order to circumvent resistance associated with P-gp, or more ideally to prevent initiation of MDR.

While the ability of P-gp to efflux xenotoxins has been firmly established, it appears that additional functions of P-gp may enhance cell survival. However, the question regarding the true physiological function of P-gp remains unanswered. There is a need for better controlled experiments using non-drug selected cells and more specific P-gp inhibitors. In addition, further studies involving the *mdr1a/mdr1b* "knock-out"

mice to assess the role of P-gp in hemopoietic cell development, immune cell function and viral infection are required.

References

1. Biedler JL, Riehm H (1970) Cellular resistance to actinomycin D in Chinese hamster cells in vitro: cross-resistance, radioautographic and cytogenetic studies. Cancer Res. 30(4):1174-84.
2. Ambudkar SV, Dey S, Hrycyna CA, Ramachandra M, Pastan I and Gottesman MM (1999). Biochemical, cellular, and pharmacological aspects of the multidrug transporter. Annu Rev Pharmacol Toxicol 39:361–98
3. Johnstone RW, Ruefli AA, Tainton KM and Smyth MJ (2000). A role for P-glycoprotein in regulating cell death. Leuk Lymphoma 38(1-2):1–11

Multiple Sclerosis

Multiple scelerosis is an autoimmune disease mediated by T and B lymphocytes and macrophages. Which is chracterized by extensive inflammation and demyelination of the myelin sheath that surrounds the nerve fibre. The death of the nerve fibre results in a variety of symptoms that can lead to impairment of movement, paralysis and death.

M

Muscarinic Receptors

JÜRGEN WESS
National Institutes of Health (NIDDK),
Bethseda, USA
jwess@helix.nih.gov

Synonyms

Muscarinic acetylcholine receptors

Definition

Muscarinic acetylcholine receptors (mAChRs) form a class of cell surface receptors that are acti-

Tab. 1 Summary of key features of the five human mAChRs (M$_1$–M$_5$).

Receptor subtype	M1	M2	M3	M4	M5
Amino acids	460	466	590	479	532
Chromosomal localization	11q12	7q35-36	1q43-44	11p12-11.2	15q26
GenBank/EMBL accession number	X15263	X15264 M16404	X15266	X15265 M16405	M80333
G protein coupling selectivity	G$_{q/11}$	G$_{i/o}$	G$_{q/11}$	G$_{i/o}$	G$_{q/11}$

vated upon binding of the neurotransmitter, ace-tylcholine. Structurally and functionally, mAChRs are prototypical members of the superfamily of G protein-coupled receptors. Following acetylcholine binding, the activated mAChRs interact with distinct classes of heterotrimeric G proteins resulting in the activation or inhibition of distinct downstream signaling cascades.

▶ Nicotinic Receptors

Basic Characteristics

The neurotransmitter acetylcholine (ACh) exerts its diverse pharmacological actions via binding to and subsequent activation of two general classes of cell surface receptors, the nicotinic and the muscarinic acetylcholine receptors (mAChRs). These two classes of ACh receptors have distinct structural and functional properties. The ▶ nicotinic receptors, which can be selectively activated by the alkaloid, nicotine, represent ACh-gated ion channels. In contrast, the mAChRs, which can be selectively activated by the alkaloid, muscarine, are members of the ▶ G protein-coupled receptor (GPCR) superfamily.

General Structural Features
Molecular cloning studies have revealed the existence of five molecularly distinct mammalian mAChRs (M$_1$–M$_5$; Table 1; Fig. 1) (1,2). All five receptor subtypes are members of the so-called class I GPCR subfamily (rhodopsin-like receptors) with which they share about twenty highly conserved amino acids (Fig. 1). These highly conserved residues play important roles in proper receptor folding and receptor activation (2,3). The structural hallmark of mAChRs (and GPCRs in

general) is the presence of seven α-helically arranged transmembrane domains (TMI–VII; Fig. 1) that form a tightly packed transmembrane core. The N-terminal portion of the receptor protein is located extracellularly, whereas the C-terminal segment protrudes into the cytoplasm. The seven transmembrane helices are linked by three intracellular (i1–i3) and three extracellular loops (o2–o4; Fig. 1). A characteristic structural feature of mAChRs is the presence of a rather large third intracellular loop (i3 loop; 157–240 amino acids in length), which, except for the N- and C-terminal segments, displays virtually no sequence homology among the different subtypes. The N- and C-terminal portions of the i3 loop play important roles in receptor/G protein coupling (2), whereas the central portion of the i3 loop is involved in the regulation of receptor activity (see below). The five receptor subtypes share the highest degree of sequence homology with the seven membrane-spanning domains (Fig. 1), which are known to be involved in ACh binding (2,3).

Distribution and Physiological Functions of mAChRs
mAChRs are found in virtually all organs, tissues and cell types (4). All five mAChRs are expressed in both the central nervous system (CNS) and the body periphery. Whereas the M$_2$ and M$_3$ receptor subtypes are the predominant mAChRs found in peripheral tissues, the M$_1$ and M$_4$ mAChRs are abundantly expressed in the CNS, specifically in higher brain regions. The M$_5$ mAChR is expressed at rather low levels in various central and peripheral tissues. Characteristically, most tissues or organs express multiple mAChR subtypes (4).

Peripheral mAChRs are known to mediate the well-documented actions of ACh at parasympathetically innervated effector tissues (organs)

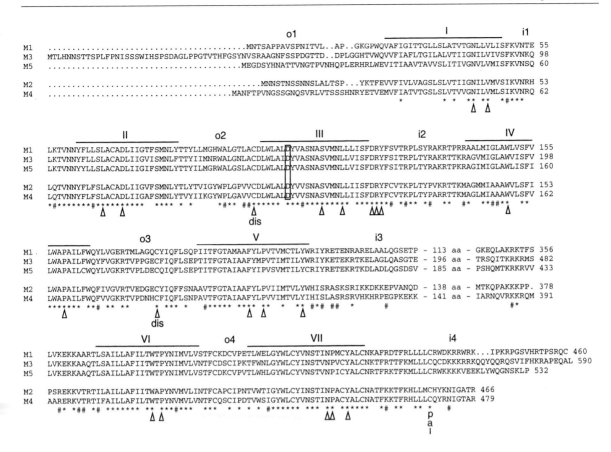

Fig. 1 Alignment of the amino acid sequences of the human M₁–M₅ mAChRs. The predicted positions of the seven transmembrane helices (I–VII) and the four extracellular (o1–o4) and four intracellular (i1–i4) domains are indicated above the sequences. The central portions of the i3 loop sequences, which show very little homology among the five receptors, have been omitted. The o1 regions contain two or more consensus sites (N-X-S/T) for N-linked glycosylation (not shown). Arrowheads indicate amino acids that are highly conserved among class I GPCRs (rhodopsin family). *, amino acids identical among all five receptor subtypes. #, amino acids identical in the M₁, M₃, and M₅ mAChRs, which are replaced with different (identical) residues in the M₂ and M₄ mAChRs. The boxed TM III aspartate residue plays a key role in the binding of muscarinic ligands (see text for details). *pal*, predicted site of receptor palmitoylation. *dis*, Cys residues predicted to link the 'top' of TM III and the second extracellular loop (o3 region) via formation of a disulfide bridge.

including heart, endocrine and exocrine glands, and smooth muscle tissues (1). The most prominent peripheral actions mediated by activation of these receptors are reduced heart rate and cardiac contractility, contraction of smooth muscle tissues (e.g. smooth muscles of the eye, gastrointestinal system, lung or urinary bladder), and stimulation of glandular secretion (e.g. lachrymal, salivary and gastrointestinal glands). Whereas the cardiac muscarinic actions of ACh are mediated by M₂ receptors, the M₃ receptor subtype plays a major role in mediating ACh-dependent stimulation of glandular secretion and smooth muscle contraction (1).

Central mAChRs are involved in modulating a very large number of behavioral, autonomic, sensory and motor functions. For example, central muscarinic mechanisms play important roles in the control of body temperature, cardiovascular and pulmonary functions, learning and memory, emotional responses, arousal, attention, rapid eye movement (REM) sleep and stress modulation.

Moreover, increased or decreased muscarinic cholinergic neurotransmission has been implicated in the pathophysiology of several important disorders of the brain, including ▶ Alzheimer's and ▶ Parkinson's disease, depression, schizophrenia and epilepsy. The roles of the individual mAChRs in mediating the diverse central muscarinic functions of ACh are not well understood at present, primarily due to the lack of muscarinic ligands with a high degree of receptor subtype selectivity (see below).

Ligands and Mechanisms Involved in Ligand Binding

Various lines of evidence indicate that ACh binds to the M_1–M_5 receptors within a cleft enclosed by the ring-like arrangement of TMI–VII, about 10–15 Å away from the membrane surface (2,3). ACh binding induces as yet poorly understood changes in the arrangement of individual transmembrane helices. These conformational changes are then transmitted to the intracellular surface of the receptor protein, enabling the receptor to productively interact with specific classes of ▶ heterotrimeric G proteins. The amino acids involved in ACh binding are located on different TM helices, primarily TMIII, V, VI and VII (2,3). Importantly, the positively charged ammonium head group of ACh (or the amino/ammonium head group of other classical muscarinic agonists or antagonists) is engaged in an ion-ion interaction with a TMIII aspartate residue (shown boxed in Fig. 1) that is conserved among all ▶ biogenic amine GPCRs. This ion pair is surrounded by a cluster of aromatic amino acids, thus creating a charge-stabilized aromatic cage (2,3).

The ACh binding pocket partially overlaps with that of competitive muscarinic antagonists such as atropine, scopolamine or quinuclidinyl benzilate. However, antagonists usually form additional strong interactions with hydrophobic receptor residues, thus stabilizing the inactive state of the receptor (2,3).

The amino acids lining the ligand-binding cavity are highly conserved among the M_1–M_5 mAChRs. For this reason, the development of agonist or antagonist ligands able to interact with individual mAChR subtypes with a high degree of selectivity has proven to be difficult. At present, agonists that display a high degree of selectivity for a particular mAChR subtype are not available

(2,5). Moreover, the degree of receptor subtype selectivity of so-called 'selective' muscarinic antagonists that are currently used to distinguish pharmacologically between different mAChR subtypes is generally rather modest (5). Such compounds include, for example, pirenzepine (M_1 receptor-preferring), tripitramine (M_2 receptor-preferring), darifenacin (M_3 receptor-preferring), or PD 102807 (M_4 receptor-preferring) (5). Antagonists that preferentially bind to M_5 receptors are not available at present.

Recently, several snake toxins have been identified that display an unprecedented degree of mAChR subtype selectivity. For example, MT7 and MT3 toxins are highly selective antagonists for M_1 and M_4 mAChRs, respectively (5). The binding of these polypeptide ligands appears to involve interactions with less well conserved amino acids present on the extracellular surface of the mAChRs.

The binding of muscarinic ligands to the primary recognition site can be modulated by so-called allosteric ligands that interact with a secondary (allosteric) site (5). The best-known ligands of this class are certain neuromuscular blocking agents including gallamine. Most allosteric ligands exhibit negative cooperativity with classical muscarinic agonists and antagonists. However, allosteric agents that display positive cooperativity with ACh or certain muscarinic antagonists at specific mAChR subtypes have also been recently identified (5). The receptor-binding site for allosteric muscarinic ligands is thought to be located just "above" the classical ligand-binding pocket.

G Protein-Coupling Properties of mAChRs

Based on their G protein coupling properties, the M_1–M_5 mAChRs can been subdivided into two major functional subclasses (1,2). The M_1, M_3 and M_5 mAChRs are preferentially coupled to G proteins of the $G_{q/11}$ family, which mediate the activation of different isoforms of phospholipase Cβ, resulting in the breakdown of phosphatidyl inositol and the generation of the second messengers, inositol 1,4,5-trisphosphate (IP_3) and diacylglycerol. In contrast, the M_2 and M_4 mAChRs are selectively linked to G proteins of the $G_{i/o}$ class, which, at a biochemical level, inhibit the accumulation of intracellular cAMP via inhibition of

▶ adenylyl cyclase. However, the G protein coupling selectivity of the individual mAChRs is relative rather than absolute, as has been observed with most other GPCRs. Mutagenesis studies have shown that amino acids located within the i2 loop and the membrane-proximal portions of the i3 loop play key roles in determining the G protein coupling profile of the individual mAChRs (2).

Signaling Pathways Activated by mAChR Subtypes

At a cellular level, the activation of mAChRs leads to a wide spectrum of biochemical and electrophysiological responses (1,5). The precise pattern of responses that can be observed does not only depend on the nature of the activated G proteins (receptor subtypes) but also on which specific components of different signaling cascades (e.g. effector enzymes or ion channels) are actually expressed in the studied cell type or tissue. The observed effects can be caused by direct interactions of the activated G protein(s) with effector enzymes or ion channels, or may be mediated by second messengers (Ca^{2+}, IP_3, etc.) generated upon mAChR stimulation. Activation of M_1, M_3 and M_5 mAChRs not only leads to the generation of IP_3 followed by the mobilization of intracellular Ca^{2+}, but also results in the stimulation of phospholipase A2, phospholipase D, and various tyrosine kinases. Similarly, M_2 and M_4 receptor activation not only mediates inhibition of adenylyl cyclase, but also induces other biochemical responses including augmentation of phospholipase A2 activity. Moreover, the stimulation of different mAChR subtypes is also linked to the activation of different classes of mitogen-activated protein kinases (MAP kinases), resulting in specific effects on gene expression and cell growth or differentiation.

Stimulation of mAChRs also results in the activation or inhibition of a large number of ion channels (1). For example, stimulation of M_1 receptors leads to the suppression of the so-called M current, a voltage-dependent K^+ current found in various neuronal tissues. M_2 receptors, on the other hand, mediate the opening of cardiac $I_{K(ACh)}$ channels, and both M_2 and M_4 receptors are linked to the inhibition of voltage-sensitive calcium channels (1).

Regulation of mAChR Activity

Like most other GPCRs, mAChRs are subject to desensitization, which is defined as diminished responsiveness of the receptor/effector signaling pathway upon prolonged exposure of the receptor to an activating ligand. The phenomenon of GPCR desensitization involves a complex series of events, including G protein uncoupling, receptor sequestration/internalization (removal of receptors from the cell surface), and receptor down-regulation associated with the net loss of receptor protein (2). Many of these processes are regulated by receptor phosphorylation catalyzed by various protein kinases including different members of the family of GPCR kinases (GRKs), casein kinase 1α, or second messenger-dependent protein kinases. Phosphorylation occurs on threonine and serine residues located within the i3 loop and the C-terminal tail of the mAChRs. The individual mAChR subtypes differ in their ability to serve as substrates for phosphorylation by these various kinases. The rapid removal of mAChRs from the cell surface following agonist stimulation (referred to as receptor internalization/sequestration) occurs through multiple pathways, one of which involves the targeting of receptors to clathrin-coated pits.

Drugs

Current Clinical Uses of Muscarinic Drugs

Muscarinic agonists and antagonists are used for the treatment of a variety of pathophysiological conditions. For example, muscarinic agonists (pilocarpine, carbachol or aceclidine) reduce intraocular pressure when applied locally to the eye and are therefore widely used for the treatment of glaucoma. Moreover, muscarinic agonists (carbachol or bethanechol) are employed in certain cases of atonia of the stomach, bowel, or urinary bladder. The agonist pilocarpine is used to stimulate salivation under conditions where the function of the salivary glands is impaired. The antagonist, scopolamine, is highly effective in preventing motion sickness. Centrally-acting muscarinic antagonists (e.g. trihexyphenidyl, procyclidine, or biperiden) are useful for the treatment of Parkinson's disease or Parkinson-like symptoms caused by the administration of antipsychotic drugs, probably due to their ability to reduce excessive striatal muscarinic neurotransmission

M

resulting from the lack of striatal dopamine. Muscarinic antagonists are also of considerable value in the treatment of clinical disorders characterized by an increased tone or motility of the gastrointestinal and urogenital tract, and in the local therapy of obstructive pulmonary diseases including chronic bronchitis and bronchial asthma. Antimuscarinic agents are widely used in ophthalmology to produce mydriasis and/or cycloplegia, are effective in the treatment of peptic ulcer disease (e.g. pirenzepine) and certain forms of cardiac arrhythmias, and can be used as part of routine preoperative medication, primarily to reduce reflex bradycardia and excessive bronchial secretion.

Potential Clinical Uses of Muscarinic Drugs

A major problem associated with the use of classical muscarinic drugs is the rather common occurrence of side effects, primarily due to the stimulation or blockage of cardiac, glandular, smooth muscle or central mAChRs. It is likely that the development of muscarinic agonists and antagonists that can interact with individual mAChRs with a high degree of selectivity will lead to novel muscarinic drugs with reduced side effects and increased efficacy. For example, it has been proposed that selective activation of central M_1 receptors or selective blockage of presynaptic M_2 receptors mediating autoinhibition of ACh release may represent potentially useful strategies for the treatment of Alzheimer's disease. Such agents could offer therapeutic benefits by facilitating signaling through cortical and hippocampal M_1 mAChRs that lack proper cholinergic innervation in patients with Alzheimer's disease. Selective M_3 receptor antagonists are likely to produce fewer side effects in the treatment of smooth muscle disorders including urinary urge incontinence, irritable bowel syndrome and chronic obstructive pulmonary disease. The application of subtype-selective muscarinic drugs may also be beneficial in the management of pain (centrally active muscarinic agonists are potent analgesics) and in the treatment of schizophrenia.

References

1. Caulfield MP (1993) Muscarinic receptors - characterization, coupling and function. Pharmacol. Ther. 58:319–379
2. Wess J (1996) Molecular biology of muscarinic acetylcholine receptors. Crit. Rev. Neurobiol. 10:69–99
3. Lu ZL, Saldanha JW, Hulme EC (2002) Seven-transmembrane receptors: crystals clarify. Trends Pharmacol. Sci. 23:140–146
4. Levey AI (1993) Immunological localization of M1–M5 muscarinic acetylcholine receptors in peripheral tissues and brain. Life Sci. 52:441–448
5. Caulfield MP, Birdsall NJM (1998) International Union of Pharmacology. XVII. Classification of muscarinic acetylcholine receptors. Pharmacol. Rev. 50:279–290

Muscle Relaxants

Muscle relaxants reduce the tone of the voluntary muscles. Centrally acting muscle relaxants like benzodiazepines or baclofen reduce the background tone of the muscle without seriously affecting its ability to contract transiently under voluntary control. Baclofen is a selective agonist of presynaptic γ-aminobutyric acid$_B$ (GABA$_B$)-receptors. Its antispastic action is due to the inhibition of the activation of motor neurons in the spinal cord. Peripherally acting muscle relaxants block neuro-muscular transmission. They either inhibit the synthesis of acetylcholine (e.g. hemicholinium) or inhibit acetylcholine release (e.g. botulinum toxin) or act postsynaptically as antagonists of the muscular nicotinic acetylcholine receptor (non-depolarising blocking agents; e.g. tubocurarine, pancuronium, vecuronium, atracurium, gallamine) or as agonists of the receptor (depolarizing blocking agents; e.g. suxamethonium). The peripherally acting relaxants are also called "neuromuscular blocking agents".

Muscle Type Nicotinic Receptors

Nicotinic receptors (nicotinic acetylcholine receptors, nACHR) exist not only in the membrane of vertebrate skeletal muscle at the synapse between nerve and muscle (muscle-type nAChR) but also at various synapses throughout the brain, mainly at presynaptic positions (neuronal-type nAChR). Whereas the muscle-type nAChR is precisely composed of two α1-subunits, one β-subunit, one γ-subunit and one γ-subunit (adult) or one ε-subunit (embryonic), the neuronal receptors exist as homopentamers (e.g. $[\alpha 7]_5$) or heteropentamers comprising various combinations of α2- to α6- with β2- to β4-subunits or α9- with α10-subunits.

▶ Nicotinic Receptors

Mutation

A mutation is a change in the DNA sequence, typically arising from DNA damage or errors during DNA replication.

▶ Pharmacogenetics

Myasthenia Gravis

Myasthenia gravis is an autoimmune disorder caused by antibodies to nicotinic receptors of the skeletal muscle endplate. The antibodies block the receptors directly, for example by occupying the acetylcholine binding site. They also increase the rate of degradation of the receptors. Symptoms are muscle weakness and fatigue. Cholinesterase inhibitors such as physostigmine improve muscle strength by preservation of released acetylcholine, so that a greater number of still intact receptors is exposed to effective concentrations of the transmitter.

▶ Nicotinic Receptors
▶ Muscle Relaxants

Myelin Basic Protein

Myelin basic protein is a component of the myelin sheath surrounding the axons of nerve cells. Additional compounds of the myelin sheath are phospholipids, cholesterol, cerebrosides and specific keratins. The myelin sheath constitutes an isolating barrier during electrophysiological axonal signaling.

Myelosuppression

Myelosuppression is suppression of the production of blood cells by the bone marrow.

▶ Hematopoietic Growth Factors

M

Myosin Light Chain Kinase

Myosin light chain kinase (MLCK) specifically phosphorylates the regulatory light chain of myosin after activation by calcium-calmodulin. Several isozymes of approximately 135 kD exist.

▶ Smooth Muscle Tone Regulation

Myosin Phosphatase

Smooth muscle myosin phosphatase (MLCP) contains three subunits, a 110 - 130 kD myosin phosphatase targeting and regulatory subunit (MYPT1), a 37 kD catalytic subunit (PP-1C) and a 20 kD subunit of unknown function.

▶ Smooth Muscle Tone Regulation

Myotonia

Myotonia is muscle stiffness, in which muscle relaxation after voluntary contraction is impaired. Mutations in several ion channel genes (Cl, Na, Ca, K channels) can cause myotonias, which can sometimes be differentiated clinically (e.g. paramyotonia is cold-sensitive). ClC-1 mutations cause 'pure' myotonia congenita which is not sensitive to temperature. Channel myotonia comes in a recessive (Becker type) form and a dominant (Thomsen type) form. In myotonic dystrophy (due to mutations in a kinase gene), myotonia is one of the symptoms. In contrast to myotonic dystrophy, myotonia congenita is a non-dystrophic, rather benign disorder in which the skeletal muscle is not dystrophic, but rather shows hypertrophy secondary to 'exercise' by prolonged contractions.

▶ Cl⁻ Channels
▶ Voltage-dependent Na⁺ Channels

Myristoylation

Myristoylation is the post-translational addition of the 14-carbon fatty acid myristate to the N-terminal glycine of proteins *via* an amide link. Myristoylation of proteins helps to anchor them to membranes.

▶ Lipid Modifications

N

Na$^+$ Channels

▶ Voltage-dependent Na$^+$ Channels

nAChR

Nicotinic Acetylcholine Receptor.

▶ Nicotinic receptors
▶ Table appendix: Receptor Proteins

Na$^+$-dependent Glucose Cotransporter

Sodium-dependent glucose cotransporters (SGLT) transport glucose into the cell against its concentration gradient. These transporters catalyze intestinal glucose adsorption and renal re-absorption. SGLT1 is a high-affinity transporter present in both intestinal brush border membranes and renal proximal tubules. The Na$^+$/sugar stoichiometry of SGLT1 is 2:1. SGLT2 is a low-affinity transporter expressed in the S1 segment of the early proximal tubules of the kidney. SGLT2 exhibits a Na$^+$/glucose stoichiometry of 1:1. SGLT3 is a low-affinity transporter expressed in both kidney and intestine. The Na$^+$/glucose stoichiometry of SLGT3 is 2:1.

▶ Glucose Transporters

Na$^+$Cl$^-$ Cotransporter

The thiazide-sensitive NaCl cotransporter (NCC) is the major pathway of NaCl entry in the distal convoluted tubule of the kidney. Seven percent of the sodium that is filtered by renal glomeruli is reabsorbed by Na/Cl cotransport in the distal convoluted tubule of the nephron. Na/Cl cotransport is a target of thiazide and related diuretics. Like the Na$^+$,K$^+$,2Cl$^-$cotransporter 2 (NKCC2), NCC contains 12 putative transmembrane domains and long intracellular amino- and carboxy-tails. NCC and NKCC, as well as the KCl cotransporter KCC, are members of the same gene family, and have considerable homology.

▶ Antihypertensive Drugs

Na$^+$/H$^+$ Exchanger

The apical Na$^+$/H$^+$ exchanger (NHE) is a member of a family of 5 membrane proteins (NHE1 through NHE5) that mediate electroneutral countertransport of Na and H and are involved in the regulation of cellular pH, cellular volume and Na and H transport. NHE proteins consist of two functional domains, a membrane-spanning transport domain and a cytosolic regulatory domain. The tissue distribution of NHE proteins ranges from ubiquitous expression in the case of NHE1 to more specific expression in kidney, stomach, intestine, testes, ovaries, and brain.

Na$^+$K$^+$ 2Cl$^-$ Cotransporter

The bumetanide-sensitive Na$^+$, K$^+$, 2Cl$^-$ cotransporter (NKCC) mediates the electroneutral uptake of chloride across epithelial cell membranes and is found in both absorptive and secretory epithelia (airways, salivary gland). NKCC exists in two isoforms, the secretory isoform NKCC1, and the absorptive isoform NKCC2. NKCC is a heavily glycosylated protein with 12 putative membrane-spanning regions. Thirty percent of the sodium that is filtered by renal glomeruli is reabsorbed by Na-K-2Cl cotransport in the ascending limb of Henle in the nephron. Na-K-2Cl cotransport is a target of all loop diuretics.

▶ Antihypertensive Drugs
▶ Diuretics

Na$^+$K$^+$-ATPase

The Na$^+$K$^+$-ATPase transports 3 Na$^+$ ions out of and 2 K$^+$ ions into the cell, using the energy of ATP hydrolysis (electrogenic transport). It maintains the high sodium and potassium gradient across the cell membrane. The Na$^+$K$^+$-ATPase (also called the "cellular sodium pump") is selectively inhibited by cardiac glycosides.

▶ Epithelial Na$^+$ Channel

N-Acetyltransferases

N-Acetyltransferases (NATs) catalyze the conjugation of an acetyl group from acetyl-CoA on to an amine, hydrazine or hydroxylamine moiety of an aromatic compound. NATs are involved in a variety of phase II-drug metabolizing processes. There are two isozymes NAT I and NAT II, which possess different substrate specificity profiles. The genes encoding NAT I and NAT II are both multi-allelic. Especially for NAT II, genetic polymor-phisms have been shown to result in different phenotypes (e.g. fast and slow acetylators).

▶ Pharmacokinetics

NADPH-diaphorase

NADPH-diaphorase activity is the ability of an enzyme to reduce soluble tetrazolium salts to an insoluble, visible formazan. This activity is being used by many laboratories to localize NO synthase histochemically.

▶ NO Synthases

NANC Transmission/Mediators

▶ Non-adrenergic Non-cholinergic transmission/ mediators

Narcolepsy

Narcolepsy is a sleep disorder - affecting 0.06–0.5% of the population - characterized by excessive daytime sleepiness, sleep fragmentation and the intrusion of rapid eye movement (REM) sleep behaviors into wakefulness. Other typical symptoms are kataplexy, hypnagogic hallucinations and sleep paralysis. Defects in the orexinergic system have recently been found to cause some forms of narcolepsy.

Narcotics

▶ General Anaesthetics

Natriuretic Drugs

▶ Diuretics

Natriuretic Peptides

Natriuretic peptides are a family of peptide hormones. All of them contain a 17-amino acid long ring that is closed by a disulfide bond between two cysteine residues. ANP (atrial natriuretic peptide) is mainly expressed in the atria of the heart, whereas BNP (B-type natriuretic peptide) is synthesized in the ventricular myocardium. CNP occurs mainly in the endothelium and is thought to have a paracrine function. ANF and BNF lower blood pressure by a direct effect on smooth muscle and on the salt retention in the kidney. Natriuretic peptides bind and activate particulate guanylyl cyclases.

▶ Guanylyl Cyclase

Natural Killer Cells

Natural killer (NK) cells are large granular lymphocytes, not belonging to either the T- or B-cell lineages. NK cells are considered as part of the innate defense system since, in contrast to cytotoxic T-cells, they are able to kill certain tumor cells *in vitro* without prior sensitization. The basal activity of NK cells increases dramatically following stimulation with type I interferons. In addition, NK cells display Fc-receptors for IgG and are important mediators of antibody-dependent-cell-mediated-cytotoxicity (ADCC).

▶ Immune Defense
▶ Interferons

Nausea

▶ Emesis

NDP-dependent K$^+$ Channel

The NDP-dependent potassium (K_{NDP}) channel is activated by nucleoside diphosphates (NDPs) in the presence of Mg^{2+} and is relatively insensitive to inhibition by ATP. K_{NDP} channels are present in vascular smooth muscle.

▶ ATP-dependent K$^+$ Channels

Necrosis

Necrosis is a form of cell death, which involves multiple cells at the same time, all of which share a similar susceptibility. For example, blockage of an artery to an organ leads to anoxia to all of the cells of the tissue and leads to the death of these cells, which is called necrosis. Necrosis can also be seen in response to pharmacologic agents at very high doses, such as suicidal doses of acetaminophen. The process of cell death by necrosis can share some mechanisms with that of single cell death or apoptosis. For example, when similar cytotoxic drugs are given at much lower doses, single cells die by apoptosis rather than by necrosis. Another example is when the cell death process leads to depletion of ATP as it does with apoptosis and then extends to a secondary aggravation of the mitochondrial lesions leading to more extensive ATP depletion, which causes multiple cells to die synchronously; this is called necrosis.

▶ Apoptosis

N

N-end Rule

The N-end rule relates the *in vivo* half-life of a protein to the identity of its N-terminal residue. Proteins with destabilizing N-terminal residues such as arginine and leucine are recognized by a RING-type ubiquitin ligase (termed N-recognin or E3-α) that, together with a specific ubiquitin c, mediates poly-ubiquitylation.

▶ Ubiquitin/Proteasome System

NEP

▶ Neutral Endopeptidase

Nephrogenic Diabetes Insipidus

In nephrogenic diabetes insipidus (NDI), the kidney's ability to respond to antidiuretic hormone (ADH) is impaired by different causes, such as drugs (e.g. lithium), chronic disorders (e.g. sickle cell disease, kidney failure) or inherited genetic disorders (X-linked or autosomal NDI). This type of ▶ diabetes insipidus cannot be treated by exogenous administration of arginine vasopressin (AVP) or AVP analogues. Instead, diuretics (hydrochlorothiazide, combined or not with amiloride) and non-steroidal antiinflammatory drugs (NSAIDs) (indomethacin) are administrated to ameliorate polyuria.

Neprilysin

▶ Neutral Endopeptidase

Nerve Growth Factor

NGF

▶ Neurotrophic Factors

Neural Network

A neural network is a computer algorithm to solve non-linear optimisation problems. The algorithm was derived by analogy to the way in which the densely interconnected, parallel structure of the brain processes information.

Neuraminidase

▶ Antiviral Drugs

Neuraxis

The neuraxis is the rostro-caudal extension of the nervous system including forebrain, midbrain, brainstem, spinal cord and peripheral nerves.

Neuregulin

Neuregulins are a complex family of factors consisting of neuregulins-1, -2, -3 and -4, that perform many functions during morphogenesis of various organs. Neuregulins exert their effects by activating the ErbB-family of receptor tyrosine kinases. While neuregulin-1 and -2 bind both ErbB3 and ErbB4, neuregulin -3 and -4 bind only ErbB4. Neuregulin-1 is also known as "neu differentiation factor" or "heregulin".

Neurodegeneration

ALVIN V. TERRY JR.
Program in Clinical and Experimental
Therapeutics, University of Georgia,
College of Pharmacy, Augusta, Georgia, USA
aterry@mail.mcg.edu

Synonyms

Neuronal cell deterioration, neuronal cell death

Definition

Neurodegeneration refers to the processes whereby damaged neuronal cells deteriorate or degenerate and eventually die.

Since the body's ability to replace lost neurons (i.e., such as via neurogenesis) is quite limited when compared to many non-neuronal cells, degenerative processes affecting neurons can be quite devastating.

Basic Mechanisms

The basic mechanisms underlying the neuronal cell degeneration and death observed in the neurologic disorders as diverse as Alzheimer's Disease and stroke have not been fully elucidated. However, a number of distinct factors and processes clearly contribute to neurodegeneration including increased oxidative stress and free radical damage, impaired mitochondrial function, excitotoxicity, immunologic and inflammatory mechanisms, impaired trophic factor support and altered cell signaling. In the process of neuronal degeneration, cells eventually die as a result of one of two processes, ▶ apoptosis or ▶ necrosis.

Necrosis

Necrosis occurs as a pathological response to cell injury, most commonly resulting from trauma, ischemia, hypoxia, neurotoxins or infection. Necrosis occurs when a cell is too severely damaged for the orderly energy-dependent process of apoptosis (see below) to occur. Following one or more of the insults listed above, neuronal degeneration or death occurs in groups of contiguous cells in a localized region and the initiation of inflammatory processes can be clearly observed in tissue sections[1]. In the process of necrosis, an initial swelling of the cell occurs (see Fig. 1 and Table 1), little or no chromatin condensation is evident, mitochondria and other organelles swell and rupture, the plasma membrane lyses, and spillage of the cellular contents into the extracellular space follows. A general inflammatory response is then triggered and macrophages attack and phagocytize the cellular debris.

Apoptosis

Neuronal apoptosis is triggered by a number of factors including lipid peroxidation (and membrane damage) induced by reactive oxygen species, genetic mutation, or DNA damage (or degradation) resulting from radiation or other destructive agents. A loss of trophic factor support, as well as some of the same factors that induce necrosis (see above) can also initiate apoptotic processes. The processes involved in apoptosis differ from necrosis (see Table 1) in several important details; most notably, neuronal death with apoptosis usually involves individual cells that are phagocytized before they can release their cytoplasmic contents and induce an inflammatory response in adjacent tissues, and phagocytes are able to recognize dying or degenerating cells by their expression of death related cell surface epitopes. Furthermore, mitochondria are preserved until the late stages of apoptosis, whereas they swell and disintegrate early in necrosis. The apoptotic sequence begins (see Fig. 2) with shrinkage of the cell, chromatin becomes pyknotic and condenses then migrates to the nuclear membrane. DNA fragmentation and degradation occurs, the Golgi apparatus disappears, and loss of the endoplasmic reticulum becomes evident. Afterwards, blebbing of the plasma membrane occurs and the cell then fragments into small apoptotic bodies that are subsequently phagocytosed and digested without triggering inflammation. The key execution process is now known to result from activation of a set of specific proteases (e.g. ▶ caspases).

Neuronal apoptosis serves a number of important roles in normal brain development and is a key mechanism by which defective or damaged neurons are removed from the brain. However, in a number of brain disorders including Alzhe-

N

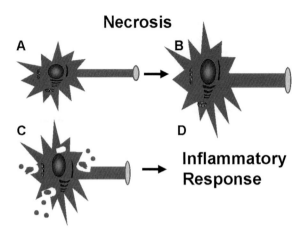

Fig. 1 Illustration of the major cellular changes observed in neuronal necrosis. A normal neuronal cell (A) when exposed to an insult (e.g., trauma, ischemia, hypoxia, neurotoxins, infection, etc.) initially swells (B), mitochondria and other organelles swell and rupture, the plasma membrane lyses (C), and spillage of the cellular contents into the extracellular space follows. A general inflammatory response (D) is then triggered and macrophages attack and phagocytose the cellular debris.

imer's disease, dementia with Lewy bodies and Parkinson's disease, inappropriate apoptosis may occur leading to accelerated neuronal loss and progressive disease symptoms. Apoptosis may be accelerated or retarded by a variety of hormones, metabolic byproducts, electrolytes and other endogenous substances. For example, altered serum levels of thyroid hormone or ammonia, altered plasma or extracellular levels of excitatory amino acids such as glutamate and aspartate, imbalances of calcium and other electrolytes, and lactic acidosis are all known to initiate or modify apoptotic processes.

Apoptosis is also influenced by synaptic communication in both the central and peripheral nervous systems. For example, in transsynaptic degeneration, neurons deteriorate and often undergo apoptosis if they fail to be innervated (from the afferent side) due to the loss of presynaptic neurons. This process has been observed in the lateral geniculate body after optic nerve lesions and in the inferior olivary nucleus after destruction of the central tegmental tract. Efferent, motor neurons degenerate if they fail to match with target muscle fibers or their muscle targets are lost, such as after amputation of a limb.

There is an increasing body of evidence that supports an apoptosis-necrosis cell death continuum. In this continuum, neuronal death can result from varying contributions of coexisting apoptotic and necrotic mechanisms[2]. Therefore the distinct designations above (necrosis versus apoptosis) are beginning to blur.

Important mediators of Neurodegeneration

Oxidative Stress. A variety of metabolic pathways generate highly reactive by-products known as free radicals including hydrogen peroxide, superoxide anions and hydroxyradicals. These substances can be used by various cells as part of the immune response to serve useful functions such as to combat infectious organisms and neoplastic cells, and to execute cells programmed for death during the normal course of development. In abnormal circumstances, such as associated with traumatic and ischemic injury or neurodegenerative diseases such as Alzheimer's and Parkinson's disease, free radicals may be excessively produced, aberrantly controlled or inadequately scavenged. In such cases, free radicals cause injury as a result of membrane lipid peroxidation, DNA damage, iron accumulation and protein nitrosylation. Excess free radicals are normally scavenged and inactivated by several endogenous substances such as vitamin E (α-tocopherol), which can quench lipid peroxidation, superoxide dismutase that scavenges superoxide radicals, and glutathione peroxidase that removes hydrogen peroxide and lipid peroxides. Therefore alterations or deficits in any of these endogenous substances can contribute to and/or initiate neurodegeneration.

Excitotoxic Amino Acids. Excitotoxic amino acids play a deleterious role in a number of neurologic diseases and are known to contribute to neurodegeneration. These compounds are released in response to a wide variety of insults to the CNS and include glutamate, aspartate and several oxidation products of cysteine and homocysteine. For example in stroke, excitatory amino acids are released in the penumbra of ischemic lesions and further released when perfusion is restored, and

Tab. 1 Comparison of necrosis and apoptosis.

Necrosis	Apoptosis
Cellular swelling	Cellular shrinkage
	Nuclear and cellular pyknosis
Little or no chromatin condensation	Chromatin condensation
Rupture of organelles and plasma membrane	Organelles and plasma membrane not usually ruptured
Release of cytoplasmic contents and inflammation	Release of cytoplasmic contents and inflammation not usually present
Random DNA degradation	DNA fragmentation
Caspases not involved	Activation of caspases
	Cytoplasmic blebbing
	Formation of apoptotic bodies which are engulfed and cleared by phagocytes

thus are believed to contribute significantly to reperfusion injury. These compounds are also released following traumatic brain injury, during prolonged seizures, and are thought to contribute to the neurotoxicity associated with the amyloid plaques observed in Alzheimer's disease. Overactivation of N-methyl-D-asparate (NMDA) receptors (a subtype of glutamate receptor) by glutamate leads to alterations in a number of signal systems and ion channels activating apoptosis.

Energy Failure and Ion Dysregulation. Neuronal degeneration may result as a consequence of energy failure within mitochondria precipitated by ischemia, free radical damage and several acquired and genetic disorders of metabolism. For example, mitochondrial energy disruption and neurodegeneration occur in Wernicke's encephalopathy, an acquired metabolic disorder resulting from ethanol abuse and/or thiamine deficiency. Similar neuropathology can be observed in Leigh's syndrome, an inherited neurometabolic disorder in which point mutations in mitochondrial DNA are evident. Friedrich's ataxia, the most common inherited ataxia, is an autosomal recessive disease in which protein aggregates appear to disrupt mitochondrial iron metabolism, leading to abnormal free radical formation and altered energy metabolism. In the cases highlighted above, specific irreversible processes lead to a decrease in high energy phosphates (e.g., ATP, creatine phosphate), possibly leading further to elevated acyl CoA levels that inhibit multiple metabolic processes. Local electrolyte (ion) imbalances and/or ion channel dysfunction are also thought to contribute significantly to neurodegenerative processes. Ion changes are commonly among the early events in apoptosis; in fact, alterations in calcium homeostasis are among the best-documented factors in neurodegeneration. Direct evidence of the importance of ion channels in neurodegeneration comes from genetic disorders that affect specific ion channels (i.e., channelopathies). Channelopathies may underlie certain forms of migraine, episodic ataxias and epilepsy. Indirect evidence that ion dysregulation plays an important role in some forms of neurodegeneration comes from preclinical studies (i.e, stroke models in animals) in which calcium and sodium channel blockers reduce infarct size.

Inflammation. Several lines of evidence indicate that inflammatory processes contribute to the neurodegeneration found in a number of disease states. A common feature in neurodegenerative diseases is microgliosis. Microglia, in addition to releasing oxygen free radicals, also secrete a variety of compounds and substances known to stimulate local inflammation such as inflammatory cytokines, complement and coagulation proteins, as well as binding proteins. As an example, inflammatory factors found in degenerating sites in Alzheimer's disease brains include activated microglia, the cytokines interleukin Il-1 and Il-6, an early component of the complement cascade, Clq, as well as ▶ acute phase reactants such as C-reactive protein.

Neurotrophin Support and Altered Cell Signaling. A continuous supply of a variety of polypeptide molecules known as neurotrophic factors (or neuro-

Apoptosis

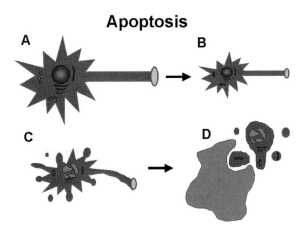

Fig. 2 Illustration of the major cellular changes observed in neuronal apoptosis. A normal neuronal cell (A) when exposed to specific triggers (e.g., lipid peroxidation, genetic mutation, DNA damage, excitotoxic injury, etc.) initially shrinks, chromatin becomes pyknotic and condenses, then migrates to the nuclear membrane, DNA fragmentation and degradation occurs, and several organelles disappear. Afterwards, blebbing of the plasma membrane occurs (C), the cell then fragments into small apoptotic bodies that are subsequently phagocytosed and digested (D) without triggering inflammation.

trophins) is essential to the nervous systems of all vertebrates throughout development as well as in adult life[3]. These important molecules interact with specific receptors and initiate a variety of cellular signaling systems. During the period of target innervation, limiting amounts of neurotrophic factors regulate neuronal numbers by allowing survival of only some of the innervating neurons; the remaining being eliminated by apoptosis. Increasing evidence indicates that several neurotrophic factors also influence the proliferation, survival and differentiation of precursors of a number of neuronal lineages. In the adult, neurons continue to be dependent on trophic factor support, which may be provided by the target or by the neurons themselves. Altered trophic factor support and cell signaling as a result of excess free radicals or peroxynitrites has been implicated in the neurodegenerative processes associated with several neurologic diseases. Furthermore, the ability of neurotrophins to promote survival of

peripheral and central neurons during development and after neuronal damage has stimulated the interest in these molecules as potential therapeutic agents for the treatment of nerve injuries and neurodegenerative diseases.

Pharmacological Intervention

There are multiple mechanisms known to underlie neuronal cell damage associated with injury or disease that at least theoretically could be targeted for pharmaceutical intervention. Currently, however, there is no clinically available therapeutic agent that can reliably protect the brain from progressive neurodegenerative processes for sustained periods. Due to the extensive amount of preclinical research that has been conducted in recent years, there is a basis for optimism. It appears likely that some of these approaches will result in clinically effective therapeutic modalities in the near future. A short overview of some of the investigational approaches to combat neurodegeneration appears below.

Inhibitors of Inflammatory Processes

Inflammatory processes associated with neurodegenerative disease suggest a number of therapeutic targets, including inhibitors of complement activation or cytokines, free radical scavengers and inhibitors of microglial activation. In retrospective studies, the use of non-steroidal anti-inflammatory drugs (NSAIDS) has been associated with a reduced incidence or slowed progression of Alzheimer disease, indicating a potential for therapeutic use of this class of agent.

Inhibitors of Apoptosis and Growth Factor-like Molecules

While all cells have the genetic programs for apoptosis, the process is inhibited by certain genes, such as *bcl-2* and *bcl-x*. In contrast, the proto-oncogenes *bax* and ▶ p53 have been shown to enhance the onset of apoptosis. Accordingly, drugs that have the ability to enhance the expression of *bcl-2* and *bcl-x* or to inhibit the expression *bax* and p53 could theoretically have the potential to reduce neurodegeneration[4]. Drugs that inhibit apoptosis-inducing enzymes including caspases may also have a role. *Bcl-2* and other genes in this family are also modulated by trophic factors such as nerve growth factor (NGF) and basic fibroblast growth factor (FGF), endogenous neurotrophins that have been shown to block cell death and preserve the phenotype of various cells in the nervous system. NGF is well known to support basal forebrain cholinergic neurons, cells reproducibly ravaged in Alzheimer's disease and known to be critically important for many cognitive processes. Accordingly, there has been interest in using NGF as a therapeutic modality for Alzheimer's disease and potentially other conditions in which cholinergic deficits may be present (e.g., dementia with Lewy bodies). In other investigations, the potential role of trophic molecules in stroke has been evaluated. For example, in animal models of stroke, ischemia is reduced following treatment with FGF. Unfortunately, NGF, FGF, as well as most other peptide molecules fail to adequately penetrate the brain from peripheral administration and are thus considerably limited from a therapeutic standpoint. Recent interest has thus focused on low molecular weight growth factor-like molecules or small organic molecules that increase the release of growth factors in the brain or increase the expression of growth factor receptors.

Inhibitors of Oxidative Stress

Human trials have evaluated vitamin E, selegeline and other antioxidant molecules for their ability to prevent or slow the progressive neurodegeneration associated with several neurologic diseases. To date, the data have provided conflicting or equivocal results with some studies showing slightly positive effects and others showing little or no effect. A number of issues require further attention such as the identification of optimal doses of the various antioxidant compounds as well as the evaluation of selected combinations of these agents. These issues are important since specific compounds are known to scavenge or inactivate specific oxidative agents, and thus a single compound would not intuitively be expected to combat free radicals originating from several sources.

Modulators of Glutamate Transmission

Several glutamate antagonists have been or are in the process of being evaluated both preclinically and clinically as neuroprotective agents. For example, MK-801 is an NMDA antagonist that reduces the detrimental effects of excess glutamate (as well as other insults to neurons) in a variety of animal models. Unfortunately the compound is too toxic for use in humans. Other antiglutamatergic agents such as citicoline, riluzole and aminoadamantanes are being investigated in human trials. Riluzole, in fact, became available clinically for the treatment of amyotrophic lateral sclerosis after it was shown to be somewhat effective in slowing progression in patients with the disease. Riluzole has also been shown to reduce infarct size in stroke and brain injury after trauma in animal models, and accordingly human studies are anticipated in the near future. Citicoline was beneficial in several human stroke treatment protocols and is also being evaluated further. Other agents that modulate glutamate receptors, such as AMPA antagonists and compounds that interact allosterically at the polyamine and glycine receptor sites, are also being evaluated.

Other Investigational Approaches

Other pharmaceutical and molecular therapies are currently being developed to antagonize neurodegenerative processes. For example, compounds designed to prevent toxic reactions of free radicals, such as nitric oxide (NO) and reactive oxygen species (ROS), new calcium channel antagonists, as well as compounds that stimulate the expression of antioxidant enzymes such as superoxide dismutase, are being developed. Further, the low incidence of cardiovascular disease in those who consume large amounts of omega-3 fatty acids and their known ability to protect cell membranes from a variety of insults has provided the impetus to evaluate these agents as potential neuroprotectants.

In conclusion, the steadily increasing size of geriatric populations in developed countries and the resultant increases in age-related diseases of the brain have provided the impetus for intensive study of the processes underlying neurodegeneration. A better understanding of these process will likely lead to better methods of treatment not only for progressive memory disorders such as Alzheimer disease, but also for motor disorders such as amyotrophic lateral sclerosis and cerebrovascular disorders such as stroke.

N

References

1. Schwartz LM, and Osborne BA, eds (1995) Methods in Cell Biology, Vol 46. Academic Press, San Diego, CA.
2. Martin LJ. (2001) Neuronal cell death in nervous system development, disease, and injury (Review). Int J Mol Med 7:455–478
3. Huang EJ, Reichardt LF. (2001) Neurotrophins: roles in neuronal development and function. Annu Rev Neurosci 24:677–736
4. Michel PP, Lambeng N, Ruberg M. (1999) Neuropharmacologic aspects of apoptosis: significance for neurodegenerative diseases. Clin Neuropharmacol 22:137–50

Neurokinin A

Substance K.

▶ Tachykinins
▶ Neuroleptics

Neuroleptic-like Malignant Syndrome

Neuroleptic-like malignant syndrome is a serious but very rare adverse effect of some drugs, of e.g., neuroleptics, some anaesthetics and apparently tolcapone. Symptoms include hyperthermia, muscle deterioration, even dissolution.

▶ Neuroleptics

Neuroleptics

Neuroleptics or antipsychotics suppress the "positive symptoms" of schizophrenia such as combativeness, hallucinations and formal thought disorder. Some also alleviate the 'negative symptoms'

such as affective blunting, withdrawal and seclusiveness. Neuroleptics also produce a state of apathy and emotional indifference. Most neuroleptics block dopamine D_2-receptors but some, like clozapine, also block dopamine D_4-receptors or serotonin 5-hydroxytryptamine$_{2A}$-receptors.

▶ Antipsychotic Drugs
▶ Dopamine System

Neuromedin B

▶ Bombesin-like Peptides

Neuromedin U

Neuromedin U is a neuropeptide which is widely distributed in the gut and central nervous system. Peripheral activities of neuromedin U include stimulation of smooth muscle, increase in blood pressure, alteration of ion transport in the gut, control of local blood flow and regulation of adrenocortical function. The actions of neuromedin U are mediated by G-protein coupled receptors (NMU1, NMU2) which are coupled to $G_{q/11}$.

Neuromuscular Blocking Agents

▶ Muscle Relaxants

Neuropathic Pain

Neuropathic pain is initiated or caused by a primary lesion in the peripheral or central nervous system. The causative agent may be trauma, nerve-invading cancer, herpes zoster, HIV, stroke, diabetes, alcohol or other toxic substances. Neuropathic pain is refractory to most analgesic drugs. Altered sodium channel activity is characteristics of neuropathic pain states.

- ▶ Analgesics
- ▶ Local Anaesthetics
- ▶ Voltage-dependent Na$^+$ Channels

Neuropeptide FF

The octa-peptide neuropeptide FF is generated together with a related octa-peptide (neuropeptide AF) from a common precursor protein. It is involved in nociception and in the modulation of opiate-induced analgesia, morphine intolerance and morphine abstinence. The effects of neuropeptide FF are mediated by G-protein coupled receptors (NPFF1, NPFF2).

Neuropeptide Y

MARTIN C. MICHEL
Academisch Medisch Centrum,
Amsterdam, The Netherlands
m.c.michel@amc.uva.nl

Synonym

NPY

Definition

Neuropeptide Y (NPY) is a 36 amino acid polypeptide with tyrosine residues at both ends of the molecule. It is characterised structurally by a "PP-fold" consisting of an extended polyproline helix and an α-helix connected by a β-turn. Based on structural and evolutionary criteria, NPY is closely related to ▶ peptide YY (PYY) and ▶ pancreatic polypeptide (PP).

- ▶ Appetite Control

Basic Characteristics

NPY is primarily (but not exclusively) synthesized and released by neurons, which in the peripheral nervous system are predominantly sympathetic neurons. In most cases, NPY acts as a co-transmitter that is preferentially released upon high frequency nerve stimulation.

As to be expected from a peptide that has been highly conserved during evolution, NPY has many effects e.g. in the central and peripheral nervous system, in the cardiovascular, metabolic and reproductive system. Central effects include a potent stimulation of food intake, anxiolytic effects, anti-seizure activity and various forms of neuroendocrine modulation. In the central and peripheral nervous system NPY receptors (mostly Y_2 subtype) mediate prejunctional inhibition of neurotransmitter release. In the periphery NPY is a potent direct vasoconstrictor, and it potentiates vasoconstriction by other agents (mostly via Y_1 receptors); despite reductions of renal blood flow, NPY enhances diuresis and natriuresis. NPY can inhibit pancreatic insulin release and inhibit lipolysis in adipocytes. It also can regulate gut motility and gastrointestinal and renal epithelial secretion. In some cell types, e.g. in vascular smooth muscle cells, NPY appears to enhance cell growth.

NPY, PYY and PP act upon the same family of receptors, which are classified together as NPY receptors. Based on IUPHAR recommendations, the NPY receptors are designated by a capital Y and the various receptors within the family are designated by subscript numbers. At present five mammalian subtypes of NPY receptors have been cloned and are designated Y_1, Y_2, Y_4, Y_5 and y_6. Among the cloned receptors the Y_1, Y_2, Y_4 and Y_5 receptors represent fully defined subtypes, but no functional correlate of the cloned y_6 receptor has been reported to date. The Y_4 receptor preferentially binds PP, whereas NPY (and PYY) are much less potent at the Y_4 receptor than at the other subtypes; hence this PP-preferring subtype will not be discussed here. The y_6 receptor represents a non-functional pseudo-gene in humans and primates, is absent from the rat genome, and its pharmacological recognition profile remains controversial; hence, it will also not be discussed here.

Sequence comparisons show that receptors Y_1, Y_4 and y_6 are more closely related to each other

N

than to the receptors Y_2 and Y_5. This is apparent not only from sequence identity but also from other features, such as cysteines believed to form disulfide bonds and the size of the third cytoplasmic loop, which is large in Y_5. The receptors Y_2 and Y_5 are equally distantly related to one another as to the $Y_1/Y_4/y_6$ group. In fact the $Y_1/Y_4/y_6$ group, the Y_2 and the Y_5 receptor are more distantly related to one another than any other G-protein-coupled receptors that bind the same endogenous ligand, despite the fact that Y_1, Y_2 and Y_5 each bind two distinct endogenous ligands, namely NPY and PYY. However, based on pharmacological recognition profiles, the receptors Y_1 and Y_5 are more similar to one another than to the receptor Y_4 (see below). Therefore, at present no formal division of NPY receptors into subfamilies is recommended.

▸ Y1 receptors have been cloned from rats, mice, humans and from non-mammals such as Xenopus laevis. The genomic organization of the Y1 subtype gene has been determined in humans and mice, and the human gene has been located on chromosome 4q(31.3–32). Three splice variants in the 5' region of the human Y1 receptor yield multiple promoters with tissue-specific expression patterns. Two splice variants of the murine Y1 receptor have been described. While both variants bind NPY, the form with a shortened seventh transmembrane-spanning region and a lacking C-terminal tail does not appear to couple to signal transduction as efficiently as the full length form. Messenger RNA for the Y1 receptor has been detected in a variety of human, rat and murine tissues including brain, heart, kidney and gastrointestinal tract.

▸ Y2 receptors were originally cloned from human SMS-KAN cells. Later cloning studies in rats demonstrated that the cloned Y2 receptor is also the molecular correlate of a previously proposed PYY-preferring receptor in the gastrointestinal tract. Messenger RNA for the Y2 receptor has been detected in various parts of the CNS, while apparently low levels of Y2 mRNA were found in human peripheral tissues.

▸ Y5 receptors were cloned from rats and humans. Interestingly, the corresponding gene resides on human chromosome 4q in the same location as the human Y1 receptor gene, but apparently in opposite orientation. Messenger RNA for Y5 receptors was detected by Northern blotting and in situ hybridization in several rat brain areas, including those believed to be important for the regulation of food intake, as well as in testis.

All known NPY receptors belong to the large superfamily of G-protein-coupled, heptahelical receptors. They appear to use similar signal transduction pathways, and no clear and consistent alignment of a specific receptor type with a distinct transduction pathway has been identified. In almost every cell type studied (with the possible exception of some prejunctional receptors), NPY receptors act via pertussis toxin-sensitive G-proteins, i.e. members of the G_i and G_o family. The typical signalling responses of NPY receptors are similar to those of other G_i/G_o-coupled receptors. Thus, inhibition of adenylyl cyclase is found in almost every tissue and cell type investigated and also with all cloned NPY receptor subtypes upon heterologous expression. Additional signalling responses that are restricted to certain cell types include inhibition of Ca^{2+} channels, e.g. in neurons, and activation and inhibition of K^+ channels, e.g. in cardiomyocytes and vascular smooth muscle cells, respectively. Based on experiments with Ca^{2+} entry blockers, it has been postulated that NPY stimulates Ca^{2+} channels in the vasculature. In some cell types, members of the NPY family can mobilize Ca^{2+} from intracellular stores. While this appears to involve inositol phosphates in some cells, inositol phosphate-independent Ca^{2+} mobilization has been postulated in other cell types. A sensitivity of certain responses to NPY to the cyclooxygenase inhibitor, indomethacin, indicates possible activation of a phospholipase A_2 by NPY receptors, but this has yet to be demonstrated definitively. Activation of a phospholipase D or of a tyrosine kinase, which can occur with some G_i/G_o-coupled receptors has also not clearly been demonstrated. Thus, in general, Y receptors demonstrate a preferential coupling to pertussis toxin-sensitive G-proteins, i.e. the G_i and G_o family, which is followed by the responses typically under the control of these G-proteins.

Drugs

NPY receptors and NPY-induced responses were originally classified based on agonist orders of potency, but the advent of several subtype-selective antagonists has at least partly superseded the use of agonists classification purposes. In some cases, however, particularly *in vivo*, agonists may still be required for receptor characterisation. This is based on the use of NPY, PYY, [Pro^{34}]-substituted analogues (which may or may not contain an additional [Leu^{31}] substitution) and on C-terminal fragments of NPY and PYY (including the endogenous NPY$_{3-36}$ and PYY$_{3-36}$).

Y_1 receptors are characterised by an agonist order of potency of NPY ≥ PYY ≥ [Pro^{34}]-substituted analogue >> C-terminal fragment > PP. C-Terminal fragments may act as partial agonists at Y_1 receptors and in some cell lines even as antagonists; whether such partial antagonism also occurs with intact tissues or *in vivo* remains to be determined. Y_1-selective antagonists include BIBO 3304 ((R)-N-[[4-(aminocarbonylaminomethyl)-penyl]methyl]-N2-(diphenylacetyl)-argininamide trifluoroacetate, K_i or K_B 0.2–1 nM), and BIBP 3226 ((R)-N^2-diphenylacetyl)-N-[(4-hydroxyphenyl)methyl]-arginine amide, K_i or K_B 1–10 nM), with BIBP 3435 ((S)-N^2-(diphenylacetyl)-N-[(4-hydroxyphenyl)methyl]-argininamide) being a much less active stereo-isomer which can be used as an inactive control for the latter one. Other Y_1 receptor antagonists include SR 120819A ((R,R)-1-(2-[2-{2-naphthylsulphamoyl}-3-phenyl-propionamido]-3-[4[N-(4-[dimethylaminomethyl]-cis-cyclohexylmethyl)amidino}phenyl]propionyl)-pyrrolidine) or the polypeptide GR 231118 (also known as 1229U91 or GW1229, homodimeric Ile-Glu-Pro-Dpr-Tyr-Arg-Leu-Arg-Tyr-CONH$_2$), but the latter has also been reported to be an agonist at Y_4 receptors in some cases.

Y_2 receptors are characterised by an order of potency of NPY ≈ PYY ≥ C-terminal fragment >> [Pro^{34}]-substituted analogue > PP. BIIE 0246 ((S)-N^2-[[1-[2-[4-[(R,S)-5,11-dihydro-6(6h)-oxodibenz[b,e]azepin-11-yl]-1-piperazinyl]-2-oxoethyl]cyclopentyl]acetyl]-N-[2-[1,2-di-hydro-3,5-(4H)-dioxo-1,2-diphenyl-3H-1,2,4-triazol-4-yl]ethyl]-argininamide) is a Y_2-selective antagonist with an affinity of 3 nM.

Y_5 receptors are characterised by an order of potency of NPY ≥ PYY ≈ [Pro^{34}]-substituted analogue ≈ NPY$_{2-36}$ ≈ PYY$_{3-36}$ >> NPY$_{13-36}$; rat PP had very low potency at the rat and human Y_5 receptor, while human and bovine PP had affinities similar to those of NPY and PYY. Y_5-selective antagonists include CGP 71683A (trans-naphthalene-1-sulfonic acid {4-[4-amino-quinazolin-2-ylamino)methyl]-cyclohexylmethyl}amide hydrochloride) with an affinity of 1 nM.

As additional tools, transgenic mice overexpressing NPY and knockout mice lacking NPY, Y_1 receptors or Y_5 receptors have been published.

References

1. Cerda-Reverter JM, Larhammar D (2000) Neuropeptide Y family of peptides: structure, anatomical expression, function, and molecular evolution. Biochem Cell Biol 78:371–392
2. Michel MC, Beck-Sickinger AG, Cox H, Doods HN, Herzog H, Larhammar D, Quirion R, Schwartz TW, Westfall TC (1998) XVI. International Union of Pharmacology recommendations for the nomenclature of neuropeptide Y, peptide YY and pancreatic polypeptide receptors. Pharmacol Rev 50:143–150
3. Wieland HA, Hamilton BS, Krist B, Doods HN (2000) The role of NPY in metabolic homeostasis: implications for obesity therapy. Expert Opin Investig Drugs 9:1327–1346

Neuropeptides

The neuropeptides are peptides acting as neurotransmitters. Some form families such as the tachykinin family with substance P, neurokinin A and neurokinin B, which consist of 11 or 12 amino acids and possess the common carboxy-terminal sequence Phe-X-Gly-Leu-Met-CONH$_2$. Substance P is a transmitter of primary afferent nociceptive neurones. The opioid peptide family is characterized by the C-terminal sequence Tyr-Gly-Gly-Phe-X. Its numerous members are transmitters in many brain neurones. Neuropeptide Y (NPY), with 36 amino acids, is a transmitter (with noradrenaline and ATP) of postganglionic sympathetic neurones.

▶ Neuropeptide Y
▶ Opioid Systems
▶ Synaptic Transmission

Neurosteroids

Neurosteroids are neuroactive steroids, which are synthesized in the brain. Neurosteroids can bind to and modulate the activity of γ–aminobutyric $acid_A(GABA_A)$ receptors.

▶ GABAergic System

Neurotensin

Neurotensin is a 13-amino acid peptide synthesized as part of a larger precursor, which also contains neuromedin N, a 6-amino acid neurotensin-like peptide. Neurotensin functions as a neurotransmitter or neuromodulator in the nervous system and as a local hormone in the periphery. It has been shown to modulate dopamine transmission and anterior pituitary hormone secretion. It exerts potent hypothermic and analgesic effects in the brain. In the periphery, neurotensin is a paracrine and endocrine modulator of the digestive tract and of the cardiovasular system. It also acts as a growth factor on a variety of normal or tumor cells. The effects of neurotensin are mediated by G-protein coupled receptors (NTS1 and NTS2).

Neurotransmitters

Neurotransmitters are molecules that convey a signal from one nerve cell to the other. Neurotransmitters can be biogenic amines (e.g. norepinephrine, serotonin), amino acids (e.g. γ-aminobutyric acid, glutamate) or neuropeptides (e.g. corticotropin releasing hormone, substance P).

▶ Synaptic Transmission

Neurotransmitter Transporters

ERIC L. BARKER
Purdue University School of Pharmacy
and Pharmacal Sciences, West Lafayette, USA
ericb@pharmacy.purdue.edu

Synonyms

Uptake pumps, reuptake system, neurotransmitter carriers

Definition

There are two major types of neurotransmitter transporters: Vesicular transporters and plasma membrane transporters. Vesicular transporters (Table 1) are located intracellularly on ▶ synaptic vesicles and are responsible for packaging cytoplasmic neurotransmitter into vesicles in preparation for exocytotic release events. By controlling the amount of neurotransmitter in ▶ synaptic vesicles, these vesicular uptake systems in many ways control the magnitude of neurotransmitter response (1). Plasma membrane transporters (Table 2) are responsible for removing neurotransmitter from the synaptic space after release, thus limiting the spatial and temporal action of neurotransmitters (1).

▶ Organic Cation Transporters
▶ Vesicular Transporters
▶ Antidepressant Drugs

Basic Characteristics

Vesicular Neurotransmitter Transporters

Vesicular Amine Transporters. A small gene family of 12 transmembrane spanning domain (TMD) antiporters have been identified that mediate the vesicular uptake of amine-containing neurotransmitters such as dopamine, norepinephrine, serotonin (5-hydroxytryptamine; 5-HT) and acetylcholine. This family of proteins is also sometimes referred to as the toxin-extruding proton-translocating antiporter (TEXAN) family due to their ability remove various toxins from the cytoplasm

Tab. 1 Summary of vesicular transporters.

	Amines			Inhibitory Amino Acids	Excitatory Amino Acids
Structure	12 TMDs			11 TMDs	6–8 TMDs
Bioenergetics	Outward H^+ gradient (ΔpH)			Outward H^+ gradient ($\Delta\psi$, ΔpH)	Outward H^+ gradient ($\Delta\psi$), Cl^-(?)
Subtypes	VMAT1	VMAT2	VAChT	VGAT	VGLUT
Substrates	Norepinephrine Dopamine Serotonin	Norepinephrine Dopamine Serotonin	Acetylcholine	GABA Glycine	Glutamate Inorganic Phosphate (Na^+-dependent)
Drugs	Reserpine	Reserpine Tetrabenazine		Vigabatrin	

Tab. 2 Summary of plasma membrane transporters.

	Excitatory Amino Acid Transporters (EAATs)					Amine Neurotransmitter Transporters				
Structure	8 TMDs					12 TMDS				
Bioenergetics	3 Na^+, 1 H^+ in: 1 K^+ out					1 Na^+, 1 Cl^- in				
Subtypes	EAAT1	EAAT2	EAAT3	EAAT4	EAAT5	DAT	NET	SERT	GAT1-3	GlyT1-2
Substrate(s)	Glutamate Aspartate	Glutamate Aspartate	Glutamate Aspartate	Glutamate Aspartate	Glutamate Aspartate	Dopamine	Norepinephrine, Dopamine	Serotonin	GABA	Glycine
Drugs	Trans-2,4-PDC	Trans-2,4-PDC, TBOA, Kainite	Trans-2,4-PDC	Trans-2,4-PDC	Trans-2,4-PDC	Cocaine, Amphetamine	Cocaine, Desipramine, Amphetamine	Cocaine, Fluoxetine, MDMA	Tiagabine	

N

and thus protect cellular constituents from reactive species. Indeed, this "toxin-extruding" property was exploited in the original cloning strategy where protection from the neurotoxin, 1-methyl-4-phenylpyridinium (MPP^+) was used to identify the first vesicular monoamine transporter (VMAT-1). Sequence similarities allowed the identification of additional members of the gene family that include VMAT-2 as well as the vesicular acetylcholine transporter (VAChT). This family of transporters relies upon the H^+ electrochemical gradient to drive accumulation of cytoplasmic neurotransmitter into ▶ synaptic vesicles. The acidic pH of the vesicle lumen is maintained by a H^+-adenosine triphosphatase (ATPase) that transports cytoplasmic protons into the vesicles. The vesicular uptake of amine neurotransmitters is mediated by the outward transport of a lumenal H^+ and the countertransport of neurotransmitter into the vesicle. VMAT1 and VMAT2 demonstrate broad substrate recognition transporting dopamine, norepinephrine and 5-HT. The major difference between these two transporters is their tissue localization, where VMAT1 is found in endocrine cells and VMAT2 is expressed in neuronal and some neuroendocrine tissues.

Vesicular Inhibitory Amino Acid Transporters.

Vesicular uptake of the inhibitory neurotransmitters γ-aminobutyric acid (GABA) and glycine is mediated by a proton-dependent transporter that resides in a distinct gene family from VMATs and VAChT. Unlike the VMATs that rely heavily upon the proton chemical gradient for driving transport, the vesicular GABA transporter (VGAT) is dependent upon both the electrical and chemical components created by the H^+ gradient. This protein is predicted to possess eleven TMDs and is a member of the gene family of transporters classically defined by biochemical studies as Systems N and A.

Vesicular Glutamate Transporters.

The vesicular glutamate transporter (VGLUT) was originally identified as a brain-specific sodium-dependent inorganic phosphate transporter (BNPI). Localization studies suggested that BNPI was found in glutamatergic neurons which eventually led to the identification of the glutamate transporting properties of this protein. Hydropathy plots suggest a proposed topology for VGLUT of 6–8 TMDs. The bioenergetics of this protein are somewhat unique in comparison to other vesicular neurotransmitter transporters. Whereas the uptake of inorganic phosphate is Na^+-dependent, the uptake of glutamate into vesicles is Na^+-independent. Similar to other vesicular transporters, the accumulation of glutamate into ▶ synaptic vesicles is dependent upon the proton gradient maintained by the H^+/ATPase. Whereas the vesicular amine transporters also rely upon the proton electrochemical gradient to drive vesicular accumulation of neurotransmitter, VGLUTs appear to be more dependent upon the electrical component of the H^+ gradient than VMATs. Interestingly, a complex biphasic Cl^--dependence for vesicular uptake of glutamate has been described. In addition, VGLUTs exhibit a channel-like Cl^- conductance that is blocked by the presence of the substrate glutamate.

Because VGLUT also transports inorganic phosphate, a role in promoting biosynthesis of glutamate has been proposed for this transporter. Glutaminase, which converts glutamine to glutamate, is activated by inorganic phosphate. Thus, VGLUT-mediated influx of inorganic phosphate could stimulate glutamate biosynthesis. The role of VGLUT in regulating glutamate synthesis is not yet fully understood.

Plasma Membrane Transporters

Excitatory Amino Acid Transporters (EAATs).

Three related proteins from non-human species were cloned that when heterologously expressed in mammalian cells imparted high-affinity uptake of the excitatory amino acids glutamate and aspartate. These proteins named GLAST-1 (Glutamate/Aspartate Transporter), GLT-1 (Glutamate Transporter) and EAAC1 (Excitatory Amino Acid Carrier) define a gene family of neurotransmitter transporters that exhibit ~50% shared sequence identity. Human homologs of these three transporters have been identified and named EAAT1, EAAT2 and EAAT3, respectively. EAAT1 and EAAT2 are mainly found in the glial cells of the CNS, whereas EAAT3 has been found in both neurons and glial cells as well as in several peripheral tissues. Two additional human EAATs have been cloned, EAAT 4 and EAAT5, with EAAT 4 primarily localized to the cerebellum and EAAT5 expressed in the retina (2).

EAATs are electrogenic transporters that couple the co-transport of three Na^+ ions, a proton, and the countertransport of one K^+ ion to the uptake of glutamate. These transporters also possess a thermodynamically uncoupled ion channel activity for Cl^- that is gated by both Na^+ and substrate (glutamate). A series of studies have been performed seeking to elucidate the membrane topology of the EAAT family of carriers. In general these studies have used accessibility of engineered cysteine residues to modifying reagents to define the intracellular and extracellular domains of the protein. Results from these studies suggest that the topology consists of an intracellular amino terminus followed by six α-helical TMDs, a membrane-inserted re-entrant loop, a seventh TMD, an extracellular facing membrane-inserted re-entrant loop, an outwardly accessible hydrophobic linker to the eighth TMD, and an intracellular carboxy tail. Evidence from cross-linking studies as well as freeze-fracture electron microscopy experiments suggest that EAATs exist as oligomeric structures with the strongest evidence pointing toward pentameric assembly.

Amine Neurotransmitter Transporters. The molecular cloning of the GABA and norepinephrine transporters (GAT and NET, respectively) in the early 1990s led to the identification of a large gene family of Na^+-dependent transport proteins now referred to as the GAT/NET gene family. Members of this gene family include transporters for serotonin (5-HT), dopamine, glycine, proline, creatine and taurine (3). These transporters are predicted to possess a twelve TMD topology, intracellular amino and carboxy terminal tails, a large extracellular loop between TMDs III and IV with sites for N-linked glycosylation, and multiple intracellular phosphorylation sites. These transporters have complex activity and can be considered as multifunctional proteins. The transporter must first bind substrate and the co-transported ions and then move the substrates across the membrane in a translocation step. In addition to the transport processes, members of the GAT/NET gene family have a conducting state that is dependent upon the transport cycle, yet in many gene family members appears electrogenically uncoupled to the trans-

port process. Once neurotransmitter has been transported back into the presynaptic terminal, the transmitter either, 1) undergoes metabolism by intracellular enzymes or 2) is recycled into vesicles for subsequent release events. Thus, reuptake of neurotransmitters by Na^+-dependent transporters not only contributes to clearance and termination of neurotransmitter action, but also in the conservation of neurotransmitter molecules. In addition to participating in the clearance of neurotransmitter, evidence suggests that under certain conditions members of this transporter family can engage in reverse transport or efflux of neurotransmitter. In such situations, the transporters would promote non-vesicular release of neurotransmitter, thus implicating the transporters in the initiation of signaling as well as the termination of exocytotically released neurotransmitter action (4).

Early biochemical studies of transporters in this gene family identified the inward movement of substrates as being coupled to the energetically favorable influx of Na^+ down its concentration gradient (3). Additional studies on bioenergetics of these transporters led to the development of a model whereby 1 Na^+, 1 Cl^- and 1 substrate molecule are transported into the cell, and 1 K^+ is countertransported per translocation cycle. Interestingly, the absolute requirement of Na^+ for transport is preserved throughout the Na^+-dependent transporter family, whereas the requirements for Cl^- and K^+ appear much less rigid for many members of this gene family. The precise molecular events surrounding the interactions of ions with transporters or the mechanism by which they facilitate the transport process is not known. The studies of transporter ion dependence eventually led to the development of the "alternating access" model for transport whereby ions and substrate bind in an ordered sequence to the external face of the transporter, the binding event promotes a conformational change in the protein occluding access to the extracellular environment so that the substrate and ions now have access to the cytoplasmic environment, dissociation of the ionic species in an ordered sequence promotes dissociation of bound substrate into the cytoplasm, and binding of K^+ or some other countertransported ion to the "empty" transporter promotes reorientation to the external side where K^+ dissociates generating an "available" transporter for another cycle. In general, much of the work leading to this model has been verified using cloned transporters; however, biophysical studies of these transporters have revealed discrepancies in this model suggesting that substrate translocation is a more complex event than described by the "alternating access" model.

Clear evidence exists that the amine neurotransmitter transporters exist as hetero- and homo-oligomers. Interactions with other cellular proteins such as the syntaxins and phosphatases have been demonstrated and appear to play an important role in the trafficking of transporters in and out of the plasma membrane (5). Protein kinase C-dependent phosphorylation of many of these transporters appears to stimulate transporter internalization, an effect that may be modulated by the presence of substrate. Homo-oligomeric structures for members of this gene family have been described, but the functional consequences of such multimeric structures is not known.

Drugs

Vesicular Neurotransmitter Transporter Pharmacology

Historically, drugs that block the uptake of biogenic amines (norepinephrine, dopamine and 5-HT) were some of the first highly efficacious antihypertensive agents. The *Rauwolfia serpentina* alkaloid Reserpine is the prototype in this drug class. Reserpine is highly effective in depleting vesicular stores of biogenic amines by inhibiting both VMAT1 and VMAT2. The non-selective action of Reserpine most likely accounts for many of the serious side effects including depression and ▶ Parkinsonism associated with clinical use of the drug. Tetrabenazine is a more selective inhibitor of the neuronal VMAT2 than the peripherally localized VMAT1. Vigabatrin is an anti-epileptic drug that inhibits VGAT. Drugs targeted toward VChAT and VGLUT have yet to be developed for clinical use.

EAAT Pharmacology

L-*trans*-Pyrrolidine-2,4-dicarboxylic acid (*trans*-2,4-PDC) is a non-selective inhibitor of all members of the EAAT family. EAAT2 is more selectively inhibited by compounds such as dihydrokainate,

kainate and threo-β-benzyloxyaspartate (TBOA). Development of selective EAAT inhibitors has been hampered by concerns that such compounds would potentiate the neurotoxic effects of glutamate. However, there is substantial interest in modulators of EAATs since evidence suggests that reduced EAAT activity may form the molecular basis of several neurodegenerative and psychiatric disorders.

Amine Transporter Pharmacology

The biogenic amine transporters (NET, DAT, SERT) have generated the most clinical interest as molecular targets for antidepressants and psychostimulants. The older antidepressant drugs such as imipramine and amitriptyline inhibit both NET and SERT. New antidepressants have been generated that are more seletive for SERT and have been marketed as ▶ selective serotonin reuptake inhibitors or SSRIs. The ▶ SSRI class of drugs include fluoxetine, paroxetine, citalopram and sertraline. ▶ Psychostimulants such as cocaine inhibit all three biogenic amine transporters. The ability of cocaine to inhibit DAT and thus elevate synaptic dopamine levels has been implicated as the major activity leading to the potent reinforcing and addictive properties of cocaine. The ▶ amphetamines including ▶ 3,4-methylenedioxymethamphetamine (MDMA, "Ecstasy") are substrates for the biogenic amine transporters and induce efflux of neurotransmitter through the transporter proteins. This non-vesicular transporter-mediated release of neurotransmitter is responsible for the stimulant action of these drugs.

The three subtypes of the GATs (GAT1-3) are non-selectively inhibited by nipecotic acid. Tiagabine is a more selective inhibitor of GAT1 and is used therapeutically as an anticonvulsant. Inhibitors of the glycine transporters (GlyT1-2) have yet to be marketed, but such compounds have been implicated as having therapeutic potential in the treatment of schizophrenia and pain conditions.

References

1. Fon EA, Edwards RH (2001) Molecular mechanisms of neurotransmitter release. Muscle & Nerve 24:581–601
2. Kanner BI, Kavanaugh MP, Bendahan A (2001) Molecular characterization of substrate-binding sites

in the glutamate transporter family. Biochemical Society Transactions. 29:711–716

3. Rudnick G (1998) Ion-coupled neurotransmitter transport: Thermodynamic vs. kinetic determinations of stoichiometry. In: Amara SG (ed) Methods in Enzymology: Neurotransmitter Transporters. Academic Press, Inc., San Diego, 296:233–247
4. Falkenburger BH, Barstow KL, Mintz IM (2001) Dendrodendritic inhibition through reversal of dopamine transport. Science 293:2465–2470
5. Blakely RD, Bauman AL (2000) Biogenic amine transporters: regulation in flux. Current Opinion in Neurobiology 10:328–336

Neurotrophic Factors

KERSTIN KRIEGLSTEIN
Universität Göttingen, Göttingen, Germany
kkriegl@gwdg.de

Synonyms

Neurotrophins

Definition

Neurotrophic factors are operationally defined as molecules that support neuron survival during development and subsequent to lesions. During development a significant portion of neurons undergoes apoptosis, the extent of which is widely believed to be controlled by limiting amounts of trophic factors provided by target tissues. Neurotrophic factors considered here include members of the nerve growth factor (NGF) family, the glial cell line-derived neurotrophic factor (GDNF) family, the ciliary neurotrophic factor (CNTF) family, as well as some members of the fibroblast growth factor (FGF) and transforming growth factor β (TGF-β) families.

▶ Growth Factors
▶ Hematopoietic Growth Factors

Mechanism of Action

NGF Family (neurotrophins)

Neurotrophins (NGF, brain-derived neurotrophic factor, BDNF; neurotrophin-3, NT-3; NT-4, NT-6) are important regulators of neural survival, development, function and plasticity of the vertebrate nervous system. Neurotrophins generally function as noncovalently associated homodimers. They activate two different classes of receptors, through which signalling pathways can be activated, including those mediated by ras and members of the cdc42/rac/rho G protein families, MAP kinase, PI-3 kinase and Jun kinase cascades.

NGF binds to the transmembrane receptor tyrosine kinase (trk, or p140^{trk}), now referred to as TrkA. BDNF binds to TrkB, whereas NT-3 can bind to all three Trk (A,B,C) receptors, with a preference to TrkC, and NT-4/5 can bind both TrkA and TrkB. Furthermore, all neurotrophins also bind with equal affnity to a 75 kD transmembrane glycoprotein, p75^{NTR} (also referred to as low affinity receptor). The p75^{NTR} appears to be essential for certain biological responses, such as ▶ apoptosis, and can modulate the response of Trk activation at the biological level.

Neurotrophin binding leads to autophosphorylation of the cytoplasmic tyrosine kinase domain of trk, containing 10 conserved tyrosine residues. Three of them (Y670, Y674, Y675) are present in the autophosphorylatory loop that controls kinase activity, whereas the others create docking sites for adaptor proteins containing phosphotyrosine-binding (PTB) or src-homology-2 (SH-2) motifs. These adaptor proteins couple Trk receptors to intracellular signaling cascades, which include the Ras/ERK protein kinase pathway, the phosphatidylinositol-3-kinase (PI-3 kinase)/Akt kinase pathway, and phospholipase C (PLC)-γ1. Neurotrophins induce rapid ruffling and cytoskeletal rearrangements involving small G proteins of the Cdc-42/Rac/Rho family, which regulate the polymerization and turnover of F-actin. The ability of Trk receptors to activate specific signaling pathways is regulated by membrane trafficking. Transmission of the signals from the nerve terminal to neuronal cell bodies requires retrograde transport of e.g. NGF together with the activated Trk receptors in endocytotic vesicles, whereby membrane sorting is thought to determine which pathways

N

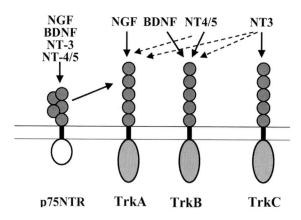

Fig. 1 Neurotrophic Factors

are activated by Trk receptors. Tyrosine kinase-mediated signaling by endogenous Trk receptors has been shown to promote survival and differentiation of all respective neuron populations.

Several signaling pathways are also activated via the p75^{NTR} receptor. Intracellulary, p75^{NTR} interacts with proteins including TRAF6, RhoA, NRAGE and NRIF and regulates gene expression, cell cycle, apoptosis, mitogenic responses and growth cone motility. An important pathway promoting cell survival of many cell populations involves activation of NFκB. All neurotrophins have been shown to promote association of p75^{NTR} with the adaptor protein TRAF-6, whereas only NGF seems to be able to induce nuclear translocation of NFκB. Binding of neurotrophins to p75^{NTR} has also been shown to activate the Jun kinase pathway.

GDNF Family
GDNF is described as a survival promoting and neuroprotective activity for mesencephalic dopaminergic neurons *in vitro* and *in vivo*, as well as for spinal motoneurons. Gene targeting has revealed that GDNF signaling is also required for the development of the enteric nervous system and kidney morphogenesis. GDNF utilizes a receptor system comprised of a signaling component encoded by the c-ret protooncogene and a glycosylphosphatidylinositol (GPI)-anchored co-receptor, GDNF family receptor α1 (GFRα1), which is required for ligand binding. The GDNF family

comprises four members, all of which utilize Ret as signaling receptor wih the aid of different members of the GPI-linked co-receptor: neurturin - GFRα2, artemin - GFRα3, and persephin - GFRα4, although promiscuity between the different receptors is also possible.

The current model of GDNF signaling proposes a rather stringent devision in the functions of Ret and the GFRα receptor, whereby Ret is regarded as the signaling receptor and GFRα as the ligand-binding receptor. Signaling is initiated upon formation of the heterodimeric RET/GFRα receptor complex. In this context, GDNF-induced signaling leads to autophosphorylation of the intracellular tyrosine kinase of RET, the involvement of Grb2 adaptor and Shc docking proteins resulting in activation of the Ras/ERK, PI-3 kinase/Akt pathways as well as PLC-γ.

Recent studies have shown that GFRα receptors are localized in lipid rafts of the plasma membrane. The binding of GDNF to GFRα1 also recruits Ret to the lipid rafts and triggers an association with Src, which is required for effective downstream signalling. Furthermore, GDNF has been shown to activate intracellular signaling in the absence of Ret via GFRα1-associated Src-like kinase activity.

CNTF Family
CNTF is expressed in glial cells within the central and peripheral nervous system. CNTF lacks a signal sequence and is not secreted by the classical secretory pathway, but is thought to convey its cytoprotective effects after release from adult glial cells by some mechanism induced by injury.

CNTF supports survival and differentiation of selected neuron populations incuding sensory, sympathetic and motoneurons. Also, nonneuronal cells, such as oligodendrocytes, microglial cells, liver cells and skeletal muscle cells, respond to exogenous CNTF. Mice lacking CNTF develop normally and only in adulthood do they exhibit a mild loss in motoneurons, suggesting that CNTF acts on the maintenance of these cells.

The CNTF receptor complex is most closely related to, and shares subunits with, the receptor complex for interleukin-6 (IL-6) and leukemia inhibitory factor (LIF). The specificity conferring α subunit of the CNTF receptor complex (CNT-FRα) is a GPI-anchored membrane protein lack-

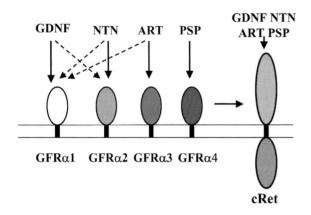

Fig. 2 Neurotrophic Factors

ing a conventional transmembrane domain. Mice lacking CNTFRα die perinatally, suggesting a developmentally important CNTF-like ligand. CNTF binding to CNTFRα results in the formation of a heteromeric tripartite receptor complex upon recruitment of pg130 and LIFRβ. IL-6 requires IL6Rα and a homodimer of gp130 for activity, and LIF requires gp130 and LIFRβ. Signal transduction is mediated via tyrosine phosphorylation through constitutively associated Janus kinases (JAK) and signal transducers and activators of transcription (STAT). Activated STATs dimerize, translocate to the nucleus to bind specific DNA sequences and resulting in enhanced transcription of responsive genes.

FGF-Family

FGFs have been demonstrated to influence the growth and function of cells of the vascular, muscular, epithelial and nervous systems. They are now thought to be involved in processes ranging from morphogenesis, tissue maintenance and repair to oncogenesis. To date, 20 distinct FGFs have been discovered, numbered consecutively from 1 to 20. Particulary FGF2, FGF5, FGF9 and FGF20 have been discussed in the context of regulating neuron survival of e.g. motoneurons, mesencephalic dopaminergic neurons, cholinergic neurons. FGFs are small polypeptide growth factors, many of which contain signal peptides for secretion. FGFs have a strong affinity for heparin and heparan-like glycosaminoglycans (HLGAG) of

the extracellular matrix. There are four FGF receptors, FGFR-1 to FGFR-4, known, containing two intracellular tyrosine kinase domains. FGFR diversity is additionally increased by alternative splicing of the individual FGFR genes. FGF signaling is propagated via PLCγ, src, Crk-mediated and SNT-1/FRS2 signalling pathways.

TGF-β Family

TGF-βs are a growing superfamily of cytokines with widespread distribution and diverse biological functions. TGF-β has been described to control neuronal performances including the regulation of proliferation of neuronal precursors, survival/death decisions and neuronal differentiation. TGF-βs fall into several subfamilies including the TGF-βs 1, 2 and 3, the bone morphogenetic proteins (BMPs), the growth/differentiaton factors (GDFs), activins and inhibins. TGF-β signal through heteromeric complexes of type II and type I serine-threonine kinase receptors (▶ Receptor Serine/Threonine Kinases), which activate the downstream Smad signal transduction pathway. Three classes of Smads have been defined: receptor-regulated Smads (R-Smads), common-mediator Smads (co-smads) and inhibitory Smads (I-Smads). TGF-β binding results in the phosphorylation of Smad2 (R-Smad), its dissociation from the receptor and assembly of heteromeric complexes with Smad4 (co-Smad), which finally translocates to the nucleus where it modulates gene expression.

Clinical Use (incl. side effects)

Over the past 15 years neurotrophic factors have generated considerable excitement because of their therapeutic potential for a wide variety of currently uncurable degenerative neurological disorders. Attempts to replicate the success of animal studies in demonstrating the therapeutic efficacy in clinical trials has been less successful. CNTF, BDNF and IGF-I have been tested in clinical trials for the treatment of ▶ amyotrophic lateral sclerosis, NGF in clinical trials for ▶ peripheral neuropathies and GDNF in trials for ▶ Parkinson's disease. However, many issues with regard to technical and pharmacological parameters, such as drug delivery to the site of action, and mode of application, remain to be solved before a final

N

judgement on the use of neurotrophic factor therapy can be drawn.

References

1. Huang EJ, Reichardt LF (2001) Neurotrophins: Roles in neuronal development and function. Ann Rev Neurosci 24:677–736
2. Unsicker K, Suter-Crazzolara C, Krieglstein K (1999) Neurotrophic roles of GDNF and related factors. Handbook of Exp Pharmacol 134:189–224
3. Sleeman MW, Anderson KD, Lambert PD, Yancopoulos GD (2000) The ciliary neurotrophic factor and its receptor, CNTFRα. Pharm Acta Helv 74:265–272
4. Böttner M, Krieglstein K, Unsicker K (2000) The transforming growth factor-βs: structure, signaling, and roles in nervous system development and functions. J Neurochem 75:2227–2240
5. Sendtner M (1999) Neurotrophic factors and amyotrophic lateral sclerosis. Handbook of Exp Pharmacol 134: 81–117

Neutral Antagonist

A neutral antagonist binds equally to both active and inactive states of a G-protein-coupled receptor, regardless of activation state, and therefore blocks the actions of ▶ agonists and ▶ inverse agonists alike.

▶ Drug-Receptor Interaction
▶ Histaminergic System

Neutral Endopeptidase

Neutral endopeptidase (NEP, nephrilysin) is an enzyme that preferentially catalyzes cleavage at the amino group of hydrophobic residues of the B-chain of insulin as well as opioid peptides and other biologically active peptides. The enzyme is inhibited primarily by EDTA, phosphoramidon, and thiorphan and is reactivated by zinc. NEP is identical to common acute lymphoblastic leukemia antigen (CALLA), a marker protein of human acute lymphocytic leukaemia.

▶ Endothelins

Neutropenia

Neutropenia is a drop in the number of circulating leukocytes, especially neutrophils. It can be induced by a variety of drugs. Treatment with cytotoxic antineoplastic drugs usually results in severe neutropenia, which can be treated with colony-stimulating factors (G-CSF, GM-CSF).

Neutrophils

▶ Inflammation

NFAT

The nuclear factor of activated T-lymphocytes (NFAT) is a transcription factor responsible for the regulation of cytokine gene transcription (e.g. IL-2) in activated T-cells.

▶ Immune Defense
▶ Immunosuppressive Agents

NF-IL6

NF-IL6 is a nuclear factor for interleukin-6, a transcription factor which is activated by IL-6 and other cytokines and stimulates stress protein gene expression.

▶ Cytokines

NF-κB

▶ Nuclear Factor–κB

NGF

Nerve Growth Factor.

▶ Neurotrophic Factors

NHE

Na^+/H^+ Exchanger

Niacin

▶ Vitamins, watersoluble

Nicotinic Acetylcholine Receptor

nAChR

▶ Nicotinic receptors
▶ Table appendix: Receptor Proteins

Nicotinic Receptors

FERDINAND HUCHO
Freie Universität Berlin,
Institut für Chemie/Biochemie, Berlin, Germany
hucho@chemie.fu-berlin.de

Synonyms

Nicotinic acetylcholine receptors; cholinergic receptors, nicotinic; ▶ nAChR

Definition

Nicotinic receptors are membrane proteins that convert extracellular signals into intracellular effects. They are members of the group of ▶ Ligand-Gated Ion Channels (LGIC) (1,2). Together with the glycine, GABA_A, serotonin (5HT_3) and P2X receptors, they belong to a superfamily of ▶ ionotropic receptors. In contrast to the other family of cholinergic receptors, the ▶ muscarinic receptors, they are activated by nicotine, not by muscarine, and antagonized e.g. by α-bungarotoxin and other snake venom α-neurotoxins (for subtype specificity see below) and not by atropine.

▶ Table appendix: Receptor Proteins
▶ Muscarinic Receptors

Basic Characteristics

Function and Occurence
Nicotinic acetylcholine receptors (nAChR) are neurotransmitter receptors. They occur in the central nervous system, in peripheral ganglia and at the neuromuscular endplate. Their physiological function is to participate in nerve impulse transmission at nicotinic cholinergic synapses. At striated muscles nAChRs are key molecules in the development and function of neuromuscular synapses. Not all functions of nAChRs in the CNS are understood: From knockout mouse mutants (3) it is known that for example the α4 subunit seems to be involved in nicotine-elicited anti ▶ nociception. A similar effect can be observed with β2 knockout mutants. In addition, β2 deficient mice show

N

impairment in spatial learning, especially with aged animals, and reduced protection against age-related neocortical and hippocampal alterations. nAChRs in the CNS may therefore participate in addictive drug behavior, in learning and aging. Presently they are a target for ▶ Alzheimer drug development.

Structure and Mechanism of Function

nAChRs (4,5) are composed of five membrane spanning polypeptide chains. Each chain is characteristically folded as shown in Fig. 1: The extracellular N-terminal domain is glycosylated. It contains a 17 amino acids–long loop formed by a disulfide bridge. This loop is considered to be a "signature" characterizing nAChR resembling members of the superfamily of LGICs. Other characteristic features are the four membrane spanning sequences M1–M4 and the large cytoplasmatic loop connecting M3 and M4. nAChRs represent either homo- or hetero-pentameric protein complexes comprising at least three functional domains: "R", the signal recognition (ligand binding) domain, "E", the effector (a cation selective ion channel) and "T", the transducer coupling "R" with "E". These functional domains are not separable molecules, rather they are integral parts of the pentamer. "T" is represented by the allosteric properties of the receptor protein.

Within the superfamily of LGICs, nAChRs form a family of iso-receptors: there are five different subunits composing the muscle-type peripheral nAChRs, named $\alpha 1$, $\beta 1$, $(\gamma)\epsilon$, δ. ϵ replaces the embryonic γ polypeptide chain in the adult muscle. Furthermore, there are twelve subunits expressed in neuronal tissue: $\alpha 2$–10 and $\beta 2$–4 (these neuronal "β-subunits" are frequently called "non-α" subunits, because they have little resemblance to the muscle β-subunits). The physiology (ion channel properties, rate of gating and desensitization) and pharmacology of the various pentamers formed by these polypeptide chains are different; the physiological significance of these differences is largely unknown. The ion channels formed by these subunits (see below) are permeable to monovalent cations, predominantly Na^+ and K^+, to a lesser extent also to divalent cations. The homo-pentameric channel formed in the CNS by five $\alpha 7$ subunits is a calcium channel.

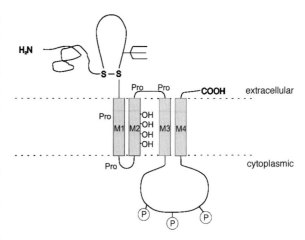

Fig. 1 Nicotinic Receptors

The primary structures of all nAChR subunits from a large variety of organisms have been deduced from the cloned and sequenced cDNAs obtained by reverse transcription of the respective mRNAs. They are similar in sequence, indicating that they may have derived early in evolution from a common ancestor. The primary structures are supplemented by several posttranslational modifications (glycosylation, acylation, phosphorylation). They add up to a total of about 15% of the relative molecular mass of the receptor complex (total M_r ca. 290 kD). The function of these modifications is largely unknown.

As to the secondary structure β strands and β pleated sheets prevail (36–42%; nAChR from the electric tissue of *Torpedo californica*, the model organism for much nAChR research). α helical structures (32–33%) are largely located in the transmembrane part of the molecule.

Due to fundamental problems with the crystallization of membrane proteins, the tertiary structure of nAChRs is unknown. Information as to the folding of the receptor's polypeptide chains is indirect and rather fragmentary. Especially scarce is our knowledge of the three dimensional structure of the functional domains. It derives from mutational analysis in combination with patch clamp electrophysiology and from photo-affinity labeling in combination with microsequencing techniques, including mass spectrometry. A gross picture is obtained by cryo-electron microscopy, yielding at present images at 4.6 Angstrom resolution. It shows the overall dimensions (120 Angstroms perpendicular to the membrane plane with about 65% of the protein's mass extending to the extracellular and cytoplasmic side of the membrane; 65 Angstrom diameter as seen from the synaptic side, with a 25 Angstrom "hole" in the center, surrounded by the five subunits, probably forming the entrance to the channel (see below).

Briefly, detailed here are some prominent features of the nAChR's three-dimensional structure: "R", the receptor's agonist and competitive antagonist binding sites, is located at the interfaces between the α/γ and the α/δ subunits. It is formed by three loops of the α- and one or more of the δ polypeptide chain. Most of the crucial amino acid residues participating in the binding of cholinergic ligands are aromatic. Downstream (C-terminal) from this domain the five polypeptide chains are folded each four times through the membrane (4TM receptor, Fig. 1, see above). The four (largely α-helical) transmembrane helices of each subunit form a hydrophobic helix bundle, in the center of which is located the effector "E", the ion channel. The wall of this channel is formed by the five transmembrane helices M2, one contributed by each of the five subunits (Helix M2 Model, Fig. 2). The five helices form a funnel; the channel's selectivity filter is located at the narrowest part of it. At the upper (extracellular) end it widens to the 25 Angstrom 'hole', visualized by the electron microscope. This upper part, which admits cations in their hydrated form, is called the channel's vestibule.

The third functional domain of the RTE three-partite receptor model is "T", the transducer, coupling R with E (converting the agonist binding signal into channel gating). As mentioned above, T is not a separate protein, like the G protein in a G-protein coupled receptor (▶ GPCR) it cannot be separated from "R" and "E". Rather it is an intrinsic property of the pentameric protein complex. This is defined as the receptor's allosterism. In terms of the three-dimensional structure discussed here there are two facts to be considered: Allosterism is a regulatory property based on the quaternary structure of a protein. And the allosteric site (s) is (are) a ligand-binding site different from the agonist and competitive antagonist sites. As to the latter, a major group of allosterically act-

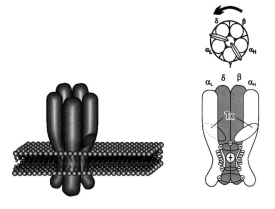

Fig. 2 Nicotinic Receptors

ing ligands are the non-competitive antagonists (NCIs). They have been shown by affinity labeling and by mutational analysis to bind to the 'upper' part of the funnel-shaped channel. As to the importance of the quaternary structure for nAChR's allosterism there is experimental proof that the subunit interface (like with the allosteric model protein hemoglobin) is involved; preventing quaternary structure changes by cross-linking the subunit interfaces abolishes allosteric regulation of nAChR.

The mechanism of function can best be described on the basis of the Induced-fit Model as follows: The receptor can exist in at least three functional states: resting (channel closed), active (channel open), desensitized (channel closed, high affinity for agonists). Two agonist molecules bind to the two α-subunits and their neighboring polypeptide chains. The binding energy is used for conformational changes in the protein complex, resulting in transient opening (gating) of the channel. Removal, and in the case of the natural agonist acetylcholine, hydrolytic cleavage of the agonist converts the receptor back to its resting state. After prolonged presence of the agonist the receptor desensitizes, i.e. the channel closes, and the affinity for the agonist increases by two orders of magnitude. The three functional domains R, T, and E are located closely together near to and within the membrane and form an active center only a few Angstroms across (2).

N

In addition to allosteric regulation there seems to be regulation through phosphorylation catalysed by protein kinases. nAChRs contain consensus phosphorylation sites and are phosphorylated by PKA, PKC and tyrosine kinase. The physiological functions of these covalent modifications are poorly understood.

The most interesting part of the nAChR is "E", the pore representing the receptor's effector, the ion channel. The lipid bilayer poses a huge energy barrier for charged entities like cations; the receptor's channel serves the purpose to decrease this energy barrier in postsynaptic membranes in a regulated manner. Photo-affinity labeling experiments using the non-permeant organic cation triphenymethylphosphonium (TPMP$^+$) identified the structure of the channel ("Helix M2-model", Fig. 2): The membrane spanning helix M2 contributed by each of the five receptor subunits forms the wall of the channel. Its hydrophilic serine side chains facilitate the permeation of cations and three rings of negative charges formed by glutamate side chains on the luminal surface of M2 seem to represent the channel's selectivity filter.

Drugs

Three types of drugs can be discriminated: agonists, competitive antagonists, non-competitive antagonists (NCIs, channel blockers).

Besides the physiological agonist acetylcholine, a variety of natural and synthetic agonists are available: e.g. nicotine (the "signature agonist" used to discriminate nicotinic cholinergic nAChRs from muscarinic mAchRs), phenyltrimethylammonium and the persisting 'partial' agonists decamethonium and succinylcholine. Agonists specific for neuronal AchRs of the autonomic ganglia and the CNS are the natural compounds cytisine and epibatidine.

Competitive antagonists include the natural alkaloid tubocurarine, synthetic compounds like the bis-quaternary hexamethonium, and the Elapid snake venom α-neurotoxins (α-Bungarotoxin).

Characteristic non-competitive antagonists are the natural alkaloid histrionicotoxin, local anesthetics like tetracaine, certain neuroleptics (chlorpromazine) and synthetic compounds like triphenylmethylphosphonium (TPMP$^+$).

References

1. Le Novére N, Changeux J-P (2002) http://www.pasteur.fr/LGIC/LGIC.html.
2. Hucho F, Tsetlin V, Machold J (1996) The emerging three-dimensional structure of a receptor. The nicotinic acetylcholine receptor. Eur. J. Biochem. 239:539–555
3. Cordero-Erausqui M, Marubio L.M. Klink R. Changeux J.-P. (2000) Nicotinic receptor function: new perspectives from knockout mice. TIPS 21:211–217
4. Hucho F, Weise C (2001) Ligand-gated ion channels. Angew. Chem. Int. Ed. 40: 3100–3116
5. Unwin N (1998) The nicotinic acetylcholine receptor of the Torpedo electric ray. J. Struct. Biol. 121:181–190

Nigrostriatal Tract/Pathway

The nigrostriatal tract is one of the four main dopaminergic pathways in the central nervous system. About 75% of the dopamine in the brain occurs in the nigrostriatal pathway with its cell bodies in the substantia nigra, whose axons project in the corpus striatum. Degeneration of the dopaminergic neurons in the nigrostriatal system results in Parkinsons disease.

▶ Dopamine System

Nitrates

▶ Guanylyl Cyclases

Nitrergic Transmission

Nitrergic transmission is synaptic transmission by nitric oxide. In contrast to other transmitters, NO is not preformed and stored in synaptic vesicles. When an action potential arrives at a nitrergic terminal, the Ca^{2+} entered through the presynaptic Ca^{2+} channels activates neuronal NO synthase and NO is then produced *ad hoc* from arginine. It is released not by exocytosis but by diffusion through the plasma membrane. In further contrast to other transmitters, the postsynaptic receptor is not a membrane protein but the cytosolic enzyme soluble guanylyl cyclase which catalyzes formation of the second messenger cyclic GMP. Finally, NO is not inactivated by enzymatic degradation or cellular uptake but by spontaneous oxidation. NO is a transmitter in the enteric nervous system and in some blood vessels where it causes vasodilation.

▶ Synaptic Transmission

Nitric Oxide

▶ NO
▶ NO Synthase
▶ Guanylyl Cyclase

Nitric Oxide Synthase

NOS

▶ NO Synthase

Nitrovasodilators

▶ Nitrates

NK Cells

▶ Natural Killer Cells

NK Receptors (Neurokinins Receptors)

▶ Tachykinins

NMDA

NMDA (N-methyl-D-aspartic acid) is a synthetic deriviative of aspartic acid and represents the prototypical agonist at the ▶ NMDA receptors for which the latter were named.

NMDA Receptor

NMDA receptors are subtypes of ionotropic glutamate receptors activated by ▶ NMDA forming heteromers containing NRI (isoform 1-4) and NR2 (NR2A-NR2D) and in some cases NR3 subunits. They are permeable to Na^+, K^+ and Ca^{2+} ions. Inward ionic current through the receptor is voltage-dependent due to Mg^{2+} block at negative membrane potentials. Other families of ionotropic glutamate receptors are AMPA (α-amino-5-methyl-3-hydroxy-4-isoxazole propionic acid) and kainate receptors.

▶ Ionotropic Glutamate Receptors

N-Methyl D-aspartate Receptors

▶ Ionotropic Glutamate Receptors

N

NMR

NMR, nuclear magnetic resonance, is an analytical technique based on the energy differences of nuclear spin systems in a strong magnetic field. It is a powerful technique for structural elucidation of complex molecules.

▶ NMR-based Ligand Screening

NMR-based Ligand Screening

HARTMUT OSCHKINAT
Forschungsinstitut für Molekulare
Pharmakologie, Berlin, Germany
oschkinat@fmp-berlin.de

Synonyms

Sequence-Activity-Relationship (SAR)-by-NMR, lead discovery by NMR, NMR-screening.

Definition

SAR-by-NMR is a method for generating systematically lead compounds in the early stages of a drug finding process. NMR is used as a method for detecting protein-ligand interactions site-specifically through the application of correlation spectroscopy (1). The inherent parameter of NMR signals, the chemical shift, is dependent on the chemical environment of the respective nucleus that gives rise to the signal. Binding of a ligand close to this nucleus changes the chemical environment and therefore also the chemical shifts. The monitoring of chemical shift changes through correlation spectroscopy thus indicates the binding site. This information can be used to either i) search for two compounds that bind close to each other in the active center of a protein, and that can be linked chemically to one compound that supposedly binds tighter (1), or ii) to detect the binding of so-called molecular frameworks (small organic compounds) as a basis for the design of focussed compound libraries and improvement of the binding affinity of these frameworks by addition of further substitutions to them through the library approach (2).

In its original form (version i), SAR-by-NMR involved the following steps:

▶ Screening of a compound library to detect compounds that bind to the active site of the protein by correlation spectroscopy
▶ Screening of derivatives of these compounds, optional synthesis of a focussed library yielding such derivatives to obtain compounds with improved affinity
▶ Screening for a second compound that binds in the vicinity of the first one using the same procedure
▶ Determination of a three-dimensional structure of the protein with both ligands
▶ Design of a linker for both ligands and synthesis of this compound
▶ Detection of the affinity of the new compound and further improvement by synthesis of focussed library on the basis of the design.

Typically, between 1,000 and 10,000 substances are screened to find weakly binding ligands.

The linking of two weaker binding compounds may lead to a strong binding one, primarily due to the saving of one entropical factor if both original compounds are chemically connected:

$$\Delta G_{AB} = \Delta G_A + \Delta G_B + \Delta G_{link}$$

The binding constant increases then:

$$K_d(AB) = K_d(A) * K_d(B) * L,$$

where L is the linking coefficient derived from ΔG link.

In its modified form (ii), the first three steps of the original procedure as outlined above are applied to obtain a good starting point for the chemists to synthesize new compounds in a more focused manner.

▶ Bioinformatics
▶ Combinatorial Chemistry
▶ Molecular Modelling

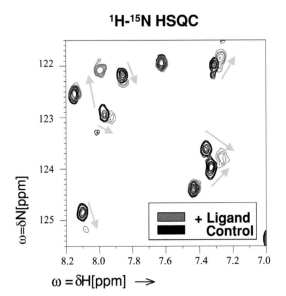

¹H-¹⁵N HSQC

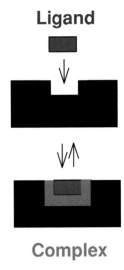

Ligand

Complex

Fig. 1 Overlay of regions from ¹H-¹⁵N correlation spectra of a protein without (black) and with (red) bound ligand (left). In case of ligand binding, only signals in the vicinity of the binding sites show chemical shift changes (red, right).

Description

The NMR screening technology in general is a tool to detect interactions between ligands and proteins in the milli- to picomolar range, using a direct binding assay that detects binding in a site-specific manner.

In both variants of the approach, i) and ii), the ligands detected in a NMR screen would be subjected to further modifications, and become larger during the design process. The properties of the compound library therefore need to fulfill a number of NMR-specific requirements. The compounds need to be soluble in water and their molecular weight should be around 250-300. hydrogen bond donors and acceptors. The latter allows for generation of still pharmacologically relevant molecules at the end of the design process.

Most commonly, protein-ligand interactions are monitored by ¹H-¹⁵N correlation spectroscopy (Fig. 1), requiring ¹⁵N-labeled protein and approximately 10 min of measurement time for each spectrum. These correlation spectra are particularly well suited for the detection of the binding site, as each amino acid in the protein leads to exactly one cross-peak caused by its backbone amid moiety in a usually well-resolved spectrum. Only few amino acids, like arginine, asparagine, glutamine and lycine show additional NH correlation peaks due to the presence of such moieties in the side chain. The correlation signals in ¹H-¹⁵N correlation spectra are the so-called fingerprint of a protein, since the ¹H and ¹⁵N chemical shifts depend on the protein sequence and structure, and therefore occur on individual positions, whereby the secondary structure has a systematical influence on peak position. Due to the occurrence of only a few signals, such spectra are usually also well resolved. Upon binding of a ligand (Fig. 1, right) only those signals in the spectrum of the undistorted protein (black) show chemical shift changes, which are in the direct neighbourhood of the ligand in the complex (red). Chemical shift changes are usually quantified as a linear combination of δ^1H and $\delta^{15}N$, e.g.

$$\Delta\delta(^1H,^{15}N)=\Delta\delta(^1H)+\Delta\delta(^{15}N)/5.$$

In principle, any type of NMR spectroscopy may be used to detect the chemical shift changes upon ligand-binding. For very small proteins, 1D-NMR might even be sufficient. Other two-dimensional techniques, such as ¹H-¹³C correlation spectroscopy or 2D-Total Correlation Spectroscopy (TOCSY) might be useful in individual cases.

Screening of compound libraries with medium throughput is only possible if the spectra can be recorded in a short period of time, and if one measurement simultaneously gives a number of

N

answers. In practice, several ligands are usually measured in one protein sample, depending on the problem[3]. Mostly 10–20 ligands are combined to multiplexes, which need to be deconvoluted if a positive answer is obtained, as shown in Fig. 1. The hits obtained may be analyzed automatically or by hand through manual inspection of the spectra.

Several ligands are often found to interact with the protein but showing different binding modes. An analysis concerning the binding modes of groups of ligands is possible through a principle component analysis that is used to cluster the results according to concerted chemical shift changes in the respective correlation spectra [4].

The chemical shift changes observed in correlation spectra may be used for measuring binding constants. The position of the protein signal in the absence of a ligand is the concentration of the free protein, whereas an excess of ligand shifts the signal to the position of the one in the complex. The result is a binding curve that may be evaluated by applying standard methods. The data are conveniently fitted with the following equation:

$$K_D = \frac{([P]_0 - x)([L]_0 - x)}{x}$$

$[P]_0$ is the total molar concentration of the protein and $[L]_0$ is the total molar concentration of ligand. X is the molar concentration of the bound species determined according to the chemical shift change:

$$x = \frac{\delta_{obs} - \delta_{free}}{\Delta}$$

δ_{obs} and δ_{free} are the chemical shift values for the target molecule determined at each concentration of ligand and for the protein in the absence of ligand, respectively. Δ is the difference between the chemical shift at saturating amounts of ligand and δ_{free}.

In the case of tighter binding (nanomolar range), the signal of the free protein would not start to change its position upon addition of a ligand, but rather decrease in intensity, and at the position of the chemical shift of the respective resonance in the complex, a signal would appear and its intensity rise with increasing ligand concentration. This may also be plotted as a binding curve.

Examples of the application of SAR-by-NMR include the design of stromeolysin and human papillomavirus E2 protein inhibitors[5,6].

A detailed analysis of designed inhibitors for stromeolysin by thermodynamical methods [5] showed that the combination of two ligands, a biphenyl derivitive and acetohydroxamic acid, yields an increase in the enthalpic contributions to the binding energy, whereas the entropical factor remained constant. In the application of the method to the design of the virus E2 protein, the potential of NMR to detect low affinity binding was exploited by starting a ligand refinement from compounds that bound in the millimolar range, and combining features of two compounds to one which finally showed an IC 50 of 10 micromolar in the applied test.

References

1. Shuker SB, Hajduk PJ, Meadows RP, Fesik SW (1996) Discovering High-Affinity Ligands for Proteins: SAR by NMR. Science 274:1531–1534.
2. Fejzo J, Lepre CA, Peng JW, Bemis GW, Ajay, Murcko MA, Moore JM (1999) The SHAPES strategy: an NMR-based approach for lead generation in drug discovery. Chem. Biol. 6(10):755–769.
3. Hajduk PJ, Gerfin T, Boehlen JM, Häberli M, Marek D, Fesik SW (1999) High-Throughput Nuclear Magnetic Resonance-Based Screening. J. Med. Chem. 42:2315–2317.
4. Ross A, Schlotterbeck G, Klaus W, Senn H (2000) Automation of NMR measurements and data evaluation for systematically screening interactions of small molecules with target proteins. J. Biomol. NMR 16:139–146.
5. Olejniczak ET, Hajduk PJ, Marcotte PA, Nettesheim DG, Meadows RP, Edalji R, Holzman TF, Fesik SW (1997) Stromelysin Inhibitors Designed from Weakly Bound Fragments: Effects of Linking and Cooperativity. J. Am. Chem. Soc. 119:5828–5832.
6. Hajduk PJ, Dinges J, Miknis GF, Merlock M, Middleton T, Kempf DJ, Egan DA, Walter KA, Tobins TS, Shuker SB, Holzman TF, Fesik SW (1997) NMR-Based Discovery of Lead Inhibitors that Block DNA binding of the Human Papillomavirus E2 Protein. J. Med. Chem. 40:3144–3150.

N-nitro-L-arginine Methyl Ester

▶ L-NAME

NO

Nitric oxide (NO) is produced in most cells by one of three isozymes (▶ NO synthases) and has many modulatory effects on all kinds of cells and organs. It is used therapeutically as a gas or in the form of nitrates. NO activates soluble guanylyl cyclase, but also has effects independent of cGMP through nitrosylation of regulatory cysteines.

▶ Guanylyl Cyclases
▶ NO Sythases

NO Donator

NO donators are a group of drugs, which are able to release NO. They include organic nitrates, sodium nitroprusside and molsidomine.

▶ Guanylyl Cyclases

NO Synthases

ULRICH FÖRSTERMANN
Johannes Gutenberg University, Mainz, Germany
ulrich.forstermann@uni-mainz.de

Synonyms

Nitric oxide synthase

Definition

NO synthases (NOS) represent a family of enzymes (EC 1.14.13.39) that catalyze the formation of nitric oxide (NO) from the amino acid L-arginine. In mammals, three isoforms of NOS have been identified. They are termed neuronal NOS (nNOS, NOS I, NOS1), inducible NOS (iNOS, NOS II, NOS2), and endothelial NOS (eNOS, NOS III, NOS3). Classically, nNOS and eNOS were considered "constitutive" enzymes, whereas iNOS is cytokine-induced. Recent evidence suggests, that also nNOS and eNOS are subject to important regulation of expression (1). Within the human species, amino acid sequences of the three NOS isoforms share 52–58% identity. Each isoform is well conserved across mammalian species (>90% amino acid identity for nNOS and eNOS, >80% for iNOS). NOS enzymes exist in organisms as low as nematodes, protozoa, and even in plants.

▶ Guanylyl Cyclase
▶ Smooth Muscle Tone Regulation

Basic Characteristics

All NOS isoforms utilize L-arginine as the substrate, and molecular oxygen and reduced nicotinamide adenine dinucleotide phosphate (NADPH) as cosubstrates. Flavin adenine dinucleotide (FMN), flavin mononucleotide (FAD) and (6R)-5,6,7,8-tetrahydro-L-biopterin (BH_4) are cofactors of the enzyme. All NOS isoforms contain heme and bind calmodulin. In nNOS and eNOS, calmodulin binding is brought about by an increase in intracellular Ca^{2+} (half-maximal activity between 200 and 400 nM). In iNOS, calmodulin already binds at low intracellular Ca^{2+} concentrations (below 40 nM) due to a different amino acid structure of the calmodulin binding site. The flow of electrons requires dimerization of the enzymes. In nNOS and eNOS, a zinc ion is coordinated tetrahedrally to pairs of cysteine motifs (CXXXXC), one motif being contributed by each NOS monomer. The zinc in NOS seems to be structural rather than catalytic and is important for optimal function of constitutive NOS. The C-terminal portion of all three NOS isozymes conveys ▶ NADPH-diaphorase activity. The NO formed by NOS can act on a number of target enzymes and proteins. The most important target of signal transduction quantities of NO is the soluble guanylyl cyclase.

N

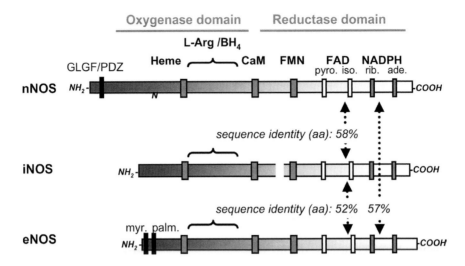

Fig. 1 Schematic diagram displaying the spatial relationships between the three cloned isoforms of NOS. Alignment of the deduced amino acid sequences of the three isoforms revealed 50–60% sequence identity between the enzymes. The reductase domain shows about 35% sequence identity with cytochrome P_{450} reductase, and this enzyme shares the cofactor binding regions of the NOS for reduced nicotinamide adenine dinucleotide phosphate (NADPH), flavin adenine dinucleotide (FAD) and flavin mononucleotide (FMN). Consensus sequences for the binding of the cosubstrate NADPH (adenine and ribose), FAD (isoalloxazine and pyrophosphate), FMN and calmodulin (CaM) are indicated. The proximal part of the N-terminal oxygenase domain (braces) shows 65–71% sequence identity between the three NOS isoforms and contains the binding region for L-arginine and (6R)-5,6,7,8-tetrahydro-L-biopterin (BH_4). The C-terminal portion of the isozymes (reductase domain) is responsible for the NADPH diaphorase activity that is common to all three isozymes. nNOS contains an N-terminal tail that includes a GLGF (glycine, leucine, glycine, phenylalanine)-motif or PDZ (*postsynaptic density protein 95/discs large/ZO-1* homology)-domain. This motif targets nNOS to other cytoskeletal proteins in brain and skeletal muscle. eNOS contains N-terminal myristoylation (myr.) and palmitoylation (palm.) sites. These lipid anchors contribute to the membrane localization of this isozyme.

Neuronal NO Synthase (nNOS)

nNOS is constitutively expressed in neurons of the brain. Its activity is regulated by Ca^{2+} and calmodulin. Half-saturating L-arginine concentrations are around $2\,\mu M$. cDNAs encoding nNOS have been cloned from rat and human brain. The open reading frame of human nNOS consists of 4299 bp, corresponding to 1433 aa. This predicts a protein of 160 kD, which is in accordance with the molecular mass of the purified protein.

nNOS is not only found in brain. Immunochemical studies identified the enzyme in the spinal cord, in sympathetic ganglia and adrenal glands, in peripheral nitrergic nerves, in epithelial cells of lung, uterus and stomach, in kidney macula densa cells, in pancreatic islet cells and in vascular smooth muscle. In terms of tissue mass, the largest source of nNOS in mammalians is skeletal muscle.

The gene for human nNOS is located in the 12q24.2-24.31 region of chromosome 12. The nNOS gene is by far the largest of the three NOS genes, spanning over 150 kb of genomic DNA. The mRNA is encoded by 29 exons with translation start and stop sites in exons 2 and 29, respectively. More than 10 different exons 1 have been identified, that are mostly spliced to a common exon 2. Moreover, skeletal muscle and some other tissues express an elongated protein (nNOSμ), containing a 102 bp cassette exon insertion between exons 16 and 17 of the human nNOS gene. There is no evidence for a difference in function between "brain-type" nNOS and "muscle type" nNOSμ.

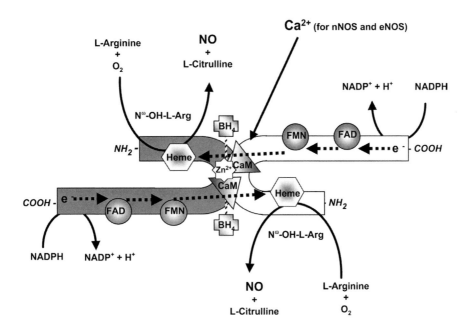

Fig. 2 Scheme of catalysis by dimeric NOS. NOS transfers electrons from reduced nicotinamide-adenine-dinucleotide phosphate (NADPH), via flavin-adenine-dinucleotide (FAD) and flavin- mononucleotide (FMN) in the carboxy-terminal reductase domain, to the heme in the amino-terminal oxygenase domain, where the substrate L-arginine is oxidized to L-citrulline and NO. Electrons for catalysis flow in a calmodulin-dependent manner from the reductase domain of one subunit to the heme of the other subunit (the two monomers are shown in white and dark, respectively). Due to differences in the CaM-binding domain, elevated Ca^{2+} is required for CaM binding (and thus catalytic activity) in nNOS and eNOS, whereas CaM binds to iNOS with high affinity even in the absence of Ca^{2+}. The normal flow of electrons requires dimerization of the enzymes, the presence of the substrate L-arginine, and the cofactor (6R)-5,6,7,8-tetrahydro-L-biopterin (BH_4). In nNOS and eNOS a zinc ion is coordinated tetrahedrally to pairs of cysteines at the dimer interface. This zinc sulfur center probably stabilizes the dimer and is important for maintaining enzymatic activity in constitutive NOS.

Functions of nNOS include long-term regulation of synaptic transmission in the CNS (long-term potentiation, long-term depression), whereas there is no evidence for an involvement of nNOS-derived NO in acute neurotransmission. Retrograde communication across synaptic junctions is presumed to be involved in memory formation, and there is evidence that inhibitors of NOS impair learning and can produce amnesia in animal models. Evidence is also accumulating that NO formed in the CNS by nNOS is involved in the central regulation of blood pressure. In the periphery, many smooth muscle tissues are innervated by nitrergic nerves, i.e. nerves that contain nNOS and generate and release NO. NO produced by nNOS in nitrergic nerves can be viewed as an unorthodox neurotransmitter that decreases the tone of various types of smooth muscle. By mediating the relaxation of corpus cavernosum smooth muscle, nNOS is responsible for penile erection. This represents the basis of the effect of the ▶ phosphodiesterase 5 inhibitor sildenafil (Viagra®).

On the pathophysiological side, hyperactive nNOS has been implicated in N-methyl-D-aspartate (NMDA)-receptor-mediated neuronal death in cerebrovascular stroke. Some disturbances of smooth muscle tone within the gastrointestinal tract (e.g. gastro-esophageal reflux disease) may also be related to an overproduction of NO by nNOS in peripheral nitrergic nerves.

Inducible NO Synthase (iNOS):

iNOS is usually not constitutively expressed, but can be induced in macrophages by bacterial lipopolysaccharide (LPS), cytokines and other agents. Although primarily identified in macrophages, expression of the enzyme can be stimulated in virtually any cell or tissue, provided the appropriate inducing agents have been identified (for review see 1;3).

Once expressed, iNOS is active independently from the intracellular Ca^{2+} concentration. Half-saturating L-arginine concentrations for iNOS have been reported between 3 and 30 µM. cDNAs encoding iNOS have been cloned from murine, rat and human cells and tissues. The open reading frame of human iNOS is 3459 bp, corresponding to 1153 aa and predicting a protein of 131 kD, which is in agreement with data obtained for purified iNOS. The human gene for iNOS has been localized to the 17p11-17q11 region of chromosome 17. The gene contains 26 exons and spans 37 kb of DNA.

When induced in macrophages, iNOS produces large amounts of NO which represents a major cytotoxic principle of those cells. Due to its affinity to protein-bound iron, NO can inhibit a number of key enzymes that contain iron in their catalytic centers. These include ribonucleotide reductase (rate-limiting in DNA replication), iron-sulfur cluster-dependent enzymes (complex I and II) involved in mitochondrial electron transport and cis-aconitase in the citric acid cycle. In addition, higher concentrations of NO, as produced by induced macrophages, can directly interfere with the DNA of target cells and cause strand breaks and fragmentation. A combination of these effects is likely to form the basis of the cytostatic and cytotoxic effects of NO on parasitic microorganisms and tumor cells.

However, the high levels of NO produced by activated macrophages (and probably neutrophils and other cells) may not only be toxic to undesired microbes, parasites or tumor cells, but, when released at the wrong site, may also harm healthy cells. *In vivo*, cell and tissue damage can be related to the NO radical (·NO) itself or an interaction of NO with superoxide leading to the formation of peroxynitrite ($ONOO^-$). The large majority of inflammatory- and autoimmune lesions are characterized by an abundance of activated macrophages and neutrophils. High levels of NO can be secreted by those cells, leading to damage of the surrounding tissue. Interestingly, non-immune cells can also be induced with cytokines to release amounts of NO large enough to affect neighboring cells. Cytokine-activated endothelial cells have been shown to lyse tumor cells, pancreatic islet endothelial cells can be induced to destroy adjacent β-cells, and induced hepatocytes can use NO to kill malaria sporozoites. iNOS activity is likely to be responsible for all of these effects. Also, tissue damage produced in animal models of immune complex alveolitis and dermal vasculitis is likely to depend on the presence of excess NO. iNOS-derived NO seems to be involved also in non-specific allograft rejection. Finally, iNOS is likely to play an important role in septic shock. This disease is characterized by massive arteriolar vasodilatation, hypotension and microvascular damage. Bacterial endotoxins initiate the symptoms. A number of mediators such as platelet-activating factor, thromboxane A_2, prostanoids, and cytokines such as interleukin-1, tumor necrosis factor-α and interferon-γ are elevated in septic shock and have been implicated in its pathophysiology. However, the fall in blood pressure is largely due to excess NO production by iNOS induced in the vascular wall. Similarly, interleukin-2 therapy is complicated by hypotension, and iNOS induction in response to cytokines may also take place in the vascular system of these patients.

Endothelial NO Synthase (eNOS)

eNOS expression is relatively specific for endothelial cells. However, the isozyme has also been detected in certain neurons of the brain, in syncytiotrophoblasts of human placenta and in LLC-PK_1 kidney tubular epithelial cells.

The cDNAs encoding eNOS have been cloned from bovine and human endothelial cells. The open reading frame of human eNOS encompasses 3609 bp, corresponding to 1203 aa and predicting a protein of 133 kD, which is in good agreement with the molecular mass determined for the purified protein. Its activity is regulated by Ca^{2+} and calmodulin. Half-saturating concentrations for L-arginine are around 3 µM. The human endothelial NOS gene has been localized to the 7q35-7q36 region of chromosome 7. The gene contains 26 exons spanning about 22 kb of genomic DNA.

Similar to nNOS, Ca^{2+}-activated calmodulin is important for the regulation of eNOS activity. However, several other proteins interact with eNOS and regulate its activity. Heat shock protein 90 (hsp90) is found associated with eNOS and probably acts as an allosteric modulator that activates the enzyme. Caveolin-1 binds eNOS and directs it to caveolae. Caveolin-1 is viewed as an inhibitor of eNOS activity, that is being replaced by CaM upon activation of endothelial cells (2). In addition, eNOS is subject to protein phosphorylation. The enzyme can be phosphorylated at Ser-1177 by protein kinase B/Akt, which increases enzyme activity. Factors activating eNOS through this signaling pathway include shear stress, vascular endothelial growth factor (VEGF), insulin-like growth factor 1 (IGF-1) and estrogens. In contrast, phosphorylation at Thr-497 reduces eNOS activity. Recent work has demonstrated that protein kinase A signaling leads to phosphorylation at Ser-1177 and dephosphorylation at Thr-497, thereby increasing eNOS catalytic activity. Protein kinase C, on the other hand, promotes dephosphorylation at Ser-1177 and phosphorylation at Thr-497, leading to a reduction of eNOS activity. Other kinases that have been shown to phosphorylate Ser-1177 and activate eNOS are the protein kinases A and G, as well as the AMP-activated kinase (that phosphorylates Ser-1177 in addition to Thr-497) (for review see 2).

In addition to its vasodilator properties, eNOS-derived NO can convey vasoprotection in several ways. NO released towards the vascular lumen is a potent inhibitor of platelet aggregation and adhesion to the vascular wall. Besides protection from thrombosis, this also prevents the release of platelet-derived growth factors that stimulate smooth muscle proliferation and its production of matrix molecules. Endothelial NO also controls the expression of genes involved in atherogenesis. NO decreases the expression of chemoattractant protein MCP-1 and of a number of surface adhesion molecules thereby preventing leukocyte adhesion to vascular endothelium and leukocyte migration into the vascular wall. This offers protection against an early phase of atherogenesis. Also, the decreased endothelial permeability, the reduced influx of lipoproteins into the vascular wall and the inhibition of low density lipoprotein (LDL) oxidation may contribute to the anti-atherogenic properties of eNOS-derived NO. Furthermore, NO has been shown to inhibit DNA synthesis, mitogenesis and proliferation of vascular smooth muscle cells as well as smooth muscle cell migration, thereby protecting against a later phase of atherogenesis. Based on the combination of those effects, NO produced in endothelial cells can be considered an anti-atherosclerotic principle (for review see 4).

Impaired NO-mediated vasodilatation has been seen in hypercholesterolemia and atherosclerosis. Arteries, especially human coronary arteries, may thereby be predisposed to vasoconstriction and vasospasm. Indeed, the paradoxical vasoconstriction in response to the endothelium-dependent vasodilator acetylcholine can be used as a diagnostic indicator of beginning coronary atherosclerosis during coronary catheterization. Reduced eNOS-mediated vasodilatation has also been found in arteries from hypertensive and diabetic animals, and impaired responses to endothelium-dependent vasodilators has been demonstrated in the forearm of hypertensive patients. In isolated blood vessels from animals with pathophysiological conditions such as hypertension, diabetes or nitroglycerin tolerance, evidence has been obtained for eNOS uncoupling. Under these conditions, superoxide is generated from the oxygenase domain instead of NO. Concomitant addition of L-arginine and BH_4 restores NO production and abolishes superoxide generation by eNOS. Administration of BH_4 also restored endothelial function in animal models of experimental diabetes and insulin resistance, as well as in patients with hypercholesterolemia and in smokers. Oxidative stress occurs in pathological conditions such as hypercholesterolemia, diabetes, aging and smoking, and oxidation of BH_4 may be the common cause of eNOS dysfunction in these situations (for review see 5).

N

References

1. Förstermann U (2000) Regulation of nitric oxide synthase expression and activity. In: Mayer B (ed.) Handbook of Experimental Pharmacology - Nitric Oxide. vol. 143. Springer, Berlin, 71–91
2. Fulton D, Gratton JP, Sessa WC (2001) Post-translational control of endothelial nitric oxide synthase:

why isn't calcium/calmodulin enough? J Pharmacol Exp Ther 299: 818–824

3. Kleinert H, Boissel J-P, Schwarz PM, Förstermann U (2000) Regulation of the expression of nitric oxide synthases. In: Ignarro LJ (ed.) Nitric Oxide, Biology and Pathobiology. Academic Press, San Diego, 105–128

4. Li H, Förstermann U (2000) Nitric oxide in the pathogenesis of vascular disease. J. Pathol. 190: 244–254

5. Li H, Wallerath T, Münzel T, Förstermann U (2002) Regulation of endothelial-type NO synthase expression in pathophysiology and in response to drugs. Nitric Oxide Biol Chem 7: 149-164.

Nociceptin/Orphanin FQ

Nociceptin is an opioid peptide, which is the endogenous ligand for the opioid receptor-like protein (ORL).

▶ Opioid System

Nociception

ROHINI KUNER
Pharmakologisches Institut,
Universität Heidelberg, Heidelberg, Germany
Rohini.kuner@urz.uni-heidelberg.de

Definition

Pain is a combination of sensory (discriminative) and affective (emotional) components. The sensory component of pain is defined as nociception.

Physiological pain constitutes a protective function as it warns the body against potentially damaging stimuli. Under certain circumstances, pain becomes pathological and manifests itself clinically as nociceptive hypersensitivity (▶ hyperalgesia and ▶ allodynia) or spontaneous pain. Pathological pain syndromes include ▶ neuropathic pain, chronic inflammatory pain (e.g. rheumatic pain, Morbus Crohn), neuralgias, ▶ causalgias, phantom limb syndrome and chronic ischemic pain (e.g. cardiac, cancer pain).

▶ Analgesics
▶ Kinins
▶ Non-steroidal Anti-inflammatory Drugs
▶ Opioid Systems

Basic Mechanisms

Physiology of pain and analgesia

The table illustrates the anatomical components of nociceptive systems and their physiological functions. Harmful stimuli applied to the body activate the peripheral endings of primary sensory neurons, called ▶ nociceptors, whose cell bodies lie in the dorsal root ganglia (DRG) or the trigeminal ganglia. Distinct classes of nociceptors encode discrete intensities and modalities of pain. Receptor molecules that impart their signalling mechanisms constitute a novel area of intense investigation in pain research. One important molecule amongst them is the Vanilloid receptor 1 (VR1), which serves as a transducer of noxious thermal and chemical (protons) stimuli and can be activated by capsaicin, the active ingredient of hot chilli peppers.

Nociceptive input is conveyed from the peripheral endorgans to the central nervous system predominantly by two classes of primary afferent fibers (Fig. 1). Of these the slowly conducting, thinly myelinated Aδ-fibers mediate thermal and mechanical nociception whereas the unmyelinated, polymodal C-fibers are activated by a variety of high intensity mechanical, chemical, hot and cold stimuli. Conduction of nociceptive signals in nociceptors is mediated via activation of voltage-gated sodium channels. A newly described family of sensory neuron-specific TTX-r sodium channels further modulates the excitability of nociceptive afferents, and likely mediates pathophysiological alterations thereof (see Table).

The terminals of C-fibers and Aδ-fibers synapse with and activate numerous second order neurons located in the superficial laminae of the spinal dorsal horn (Fig. 1). The functioning of the primary afferent-second order neuron synapses is of arch significance in context of the physiology as well as the pathophysiology of pain (see below). The amino acid neurotransmitter, glutamate,

Tab. 1 Physiology and pathophysiology of the nociceptive system.

Anatomical component	Nociceptor	Afferent	Spinal cord	Brain
Normal function	Transduction	Conduction	Processing, mono- and poly-synaptic reflexes	Processing, perception, polysynaptic reflexes
Pathological change	Sensitization, Desensitization, Changes in activation thresholds	Aberrent conduction, ectopic activity, sprouting	Hypersensitivity, hyposensitivity, changes in activation thresholds, expansion or reduction of receptive fields, deafferentation, spontaneous activity	
Etiology	Trauma, ischemia, inflammation, genetic defects	Neuropathy, genetic defects	Peripheral inflammation, peripheral neuropathy, trauma, viral infections (e. g. Herpes Zoster), genetic defects	
Clinical manifestation	Primary hyperalgesia, allodynia, spontaneous pain		Secondary hyperalgesia, allodynia, spontaneous pain, aberrently-referred pain	
Pharmacological intervention	NSAIDs, local anesthetics		Opioid analgesics	

serves as the primary nociceptive neurotransmitter at these synapses by activating several types of ▶ glutamate receptors such as α-amino-3-hydroxy-5-methyl-4-isoxazolepropionic acid (AMPA) receptors, N-methyl-D-aspartate (NMDA) receptors and metabotropic glutamate receptors (mGluRs). Neurotransmission at primary afferent-second order neuron synapses is further modulated and/or mediated by other agents that are released synaptically from primary afferent terminals upon peripheral nociceptive stimulation. These include peptide neurotransmitters, such as ▶ substance P (Fig. 1), calcitonin gene related peptide, somatostatin, and ▶ neurotrophins such as brain-derived neurotrophic factor (BDNF). It is believed that AMPA receptors mediate transmission of basal (physiological) pain whereas mGluRs and substance P-, NMDA- and BDNF-receptors play a key role in induction and maintenance of pathological central pain.

Afferent input from cutaneous and visceral nociceptors is known to converge on spinal neurons, which accounts for the referral of pain between visceral and cutaneous structures (e.g. cardiac pain gets referred to the chest and left upper arm in patients suffering from angina pectoris). Projection neurons in the spinal dorsal horn project to cell nuclei in supraspinal areas such as the thalamus, brainstem and midbrain. Of these, the synaptic junctions in the thalamus play a very important role in the integration and modulation of spinal nociceptive and non-nociceptive inputs. Nociceptive inputs are finally conducted to the cortex where the sensation of pain is perceived (Fig. 1). The mechanisms via which the cortex processes nociceptive inputs are poorly understood.

Nociceptive activity can be modulated at several peripheral and central relay points in pain pathways. For example, activation of myelinated primary fibers that conduct non-nociceptive input reduces the activity of spinal nociceptive projection neurons and thereby reduces the perception of pain. Local interneurons exert excitatory or inhibitory influences on projection neurons in the spinal cord (Fig. 1) and thalamus. Furthermore, spinal nociceptive output is strongly modulated by descending inhibitory systems that originate at supraspinal sites such as the periaqueductal gray, rostroventromedulla and pons. Stimulation of these brain regions, either electrically or chemically, e.g. by morphine and other opiates, produces

N

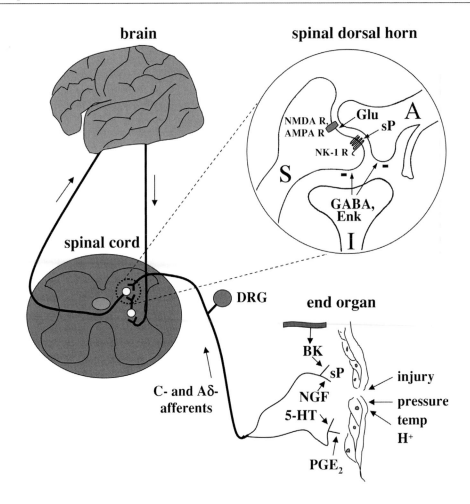

Fig. 1 Schematic Representation of Nociceptive Pathways: Noxious stimuli such as protons (H+), temperature (temp) etc. applied to endorgans activate nociceptors. Injury leads to the release of prostaglandins such as pros-taglandin E2 (PGE2), serotonin (5-HT), nerve growth factor (NGF) from damaged cells, Bradykinin (BK) from blood vessels and substance P (sP) from nociceptors. These agents either activate nociceptors directly or sensi-tize them to subsequent stimuli by parallel activation of intracellular kinases by G-protein coupled receptors and tyrosine kinase receptors. Primary nociceptive afferents (C-fibers, Ad-fibers) of dorsal root ganglion (DRG) neurons synapse on second order neurons (S) in the spinal dorsal horn (magnified in inset). Here, gluta-mate (Glu) and sP released from primary afferent terminals (A) activate glutamate receptors (NMDA R, AMPA R, mGluRs) and neurokinin-1 (NK-1) receptors, respectively, located post-synaptically on spinal neurons. These synapses are negatively modulated by spinal inhibitory interneurons (I), which employ enkephalins (Enk) or γ-amino-butyric acid (GABA) as neurotransmitters. Spinal neurons convey nociceptive information to the brain and brainstem. Activation of descending noradrenergic and/or serotonergic systems, which originate in the brain and brainstem, leads to the activation of spinal inhibitory interneurons (I) thereby resulting in anti-nociception.

analgesia in humans. These inhibitory pathways utilise monoamines such as noradrenaline and serotonin as neurotransmitters and terminate on nociceptive neurons in the spinal cord as well as on spinal inhibitory interneurons that store and release opioids (Fig. 1). The latter exert both pre-synaptic and post-synaptic inhibitory actions at primary afferent synapses in the spinal dorsal horn by activating specific opioid receptors. Thus, supraspinal pathways and local spinal circuits co-ordinately modulate incoming nociceptive signals.

Processes underlying pathological pain

Common pathological alterations in nociceptive pathways and their underlying etiological factors are listed in Table. Damaging stimuli such as trauma, viral infections, noxious temperature or noxious pressure (e.g. by tumor outgrowth) can elicit both short-term and long-term changes in the activity of nociceptors and/or central nociceptive neurons. Peripheral effects include the release of chemoactive substances from damaged cells, blood vessels or from nociceptors themselves (see Fig. 1 for details) which either activate or sensitize nociceptors. These peripheral mechanisms are typically short-term in nature and are predominantly manifest as primary hyperalgesia. Chronic nociceptor activity can also produce long-lasting sensitization of nociceptors by transcriptional regulation of genes encoding important nociceptive molecules in dorsal root or trigeminal ganglia neurons, thereby leading to the up- or down-regulation of receptors, enzymes or other signalling molecules on primary afferent terminals. Such molecular events lead to alterations in transduction as well as conduction properties of primary afferents.

Nociceptive neurons in the spinal cord as well as in higher centers such as the thalamus can also undergo alterations in activity following chronic peripheral changes and trauma. (Table). These changes are typically long-term in nature and lead to the clinical syndromes of centrally-maintained pain (secondary hyperalgesia, allodynia, spontaneous pain). Alterations in the synaptic efficacy of primary afferent-first order neuron synapses constitute the prime underlying mechanism. At the molecular level, these are brought about by long-term changes in the expression and signalling mechanisms of receptors for nociceptive neurotransmitters and neuromodulators at pre-synaptic terminals and post-synaptic cells in the spinal cord.

Pharmacological Intervention

Avenues targeted by contemporary analgesics

Synthesis pathways for peripheral chemoactive agents. Prime examples for this class of analgesics are Non-steroidal Anti-inflammatory Drugs (NSAIDs, e.g. aspirin, ibuprofen), which act by blocking cyclooxygenases (COX-1 and /or COX-2), the enzymes responsible for synthesis of prostaglandins, mainly prostaglandin E_2 (PGE_2), in peripheral tissues and thereby preventing or terminating the sensitization of nociceptors by PGE_2 (Fig. 1). A central component to NSAID-produced analgesia has been described, the mechanisms underlying it being complex (5, 6). NSAIDs are particularly effective against pain in the extremities, headache, migraine and dental pain, and are generally unsuitable for treating chronic central pain.

Nociceptive conduction by primary afferents. Anesthetics such as lidocaine and tetracaine reversibly block the generation and conduction of action potentials in primary afferent fibers without inducing systemic effects when applied locally to dermatomes. Their main action is to block voltage-dependent sodium channels by physically plugging the transmembrane pore. The degree of blockade is inversely proportional to the extent of myelination on the nerve fibers. Therefore the nociceptive C-fibers and Aδ-fibers are blocked preferentially in comparison with thickly myelinated, non-nociceptive primary afferents.

Opioid receptors. Similarly to the endogenous opioids, opiates like Morphine and other synthetic opioids activate G-protein-coupled receptors which couple to G-proteins of the $G_i/_0$ family. They act as analgesics by depressing nociceptive transmission at central synapses. This is achieved at the spinal level by inhibiting release of nociceptive neurotransmitters from primary afferent terminals as well as by depressing post-synaptic potentials on second order neurons. Thus, opiates and opioids basically mimic the effect of endogenous opioids released in the spinal cord upon activation by the descending anti-nociceptive systems (see above). Moreover, activation of opioid receptors at supraspinal sites leads to the activation of

N

descending inhibitory systems (see above). Although opioid receptors are present on some (in particular visceral) nociceptors, the contribution of peripheral mechanisms in opioid-produced analgesia is being investigated. Opioid analgesics are used in the treatment of various central pain syndromes, cancer pain and pain associated with labour. Although they are capable of causing side effects on the functioning of the central nervous system, such as euphoria, dysphoria, sedation, respiratory depression and lead to tolerance and dependence upon chronic use, opioid analgesics currently constitute prime therapeutics used in the treatment of severe chronic pain.

Anticonvulsants. Anticonvulsants have been empirically found to be effective in symptomatic management of neuropathic pain, probably owing to the similarities between the pathophysiological phenomena underlying epilepsy and neuropathic pain. Recent clinical trials support the use of carbamezapine and gabapentin in the treatment of neuropathic pain syndromes such as painful diabetic mononeuropathy, post-herpetic neuralgia and trigeminal neuralgia.

Novel drug targets

NMDA receptors and mGluRs. The NMDA subtype of glutamate receptors are key mediators of chronic nociceptive phenomena in the spinal cord and the thalamus. NMDA receptor antagonists like MK-801; d, 1-2-amino-5-phosphonovaleric acid etc. effectively inhibit several kinds of chronic pain, such as neuropathic and inflammatory pain, in corresponding animal models. In clinical trials, NMDA receptor antagonists effectively inhibited chronic pain in humans but produced side effects on the central nervous system including psychotomimetic effects, which limit their therapeutic application. Clinically used agents which block NMDA receptors weakly include ketamine and dextromethorphan. The newly developed subtype-specific NMDA receptor antagonists offer new hope for achieving analgesic effects specifically. Furthermore, drugs acting on specific mGluR subtypes involved in nociception are currently being developed as potential analgesics.

GABA receptors. GABA is the most prominent inhibitory neurotransmitter in the mammalian nervous system (▶ GABA Receptors). Activation of $GABA_B$ receptors by GABA released from local spinal interneurons (Fig. 1) negatively modulates nociceptive transmission in the spinal cord. Agonists at $GABA_B$ receptors (e.g. baclofen) inhibit pain in animal models and in humans, but also produce motor effects such as flaccidity and paralysis. The recent cloning of $GABA_B$ receptor subtypes with site specific expression therefore provides scope for finding drugs affecting $GABA_B$ receptors on nociceptive neurons without affecting motor neurons.

Novel nociceptive transducers. (▶ Nocicptive Transducers) These molecules largely include membrane bound cation channels such as VR1, acid-sensing ion channels etc., several splice variants of acid-sensing ion channels are selectively expressed in nociceptors. Pharmacological intervention at these channels therefore holds promise for producing analgesics with fewer side effects on other organs.

Neurotrophin receptors. Neurotrophins such as nerve growth factor (NGF) and brain-derived neurotrophic factor (▶ BDNF) are now emerging as important modulators of nociceptor activity in adult life. Receptors and signalling mechanisms involved in neurotrophin-produced modulation of nociception are areas of intensive current research and represent novel avenues for pharmacological intervention in chronic pain states. Furthermore, because of their trophic effects on injured nerves, neurotrophins may be useful in arresting and reversing disease processes underlying peripheral neuropathies and the neuropathic pain syndromes associated with them.

References

1. Caterina MJ, Julius D (1999) Sense and specificity: a molecular identity for nociceptors. Curr Opin Neurobiol (5):525–30
2. Woolf CJ, Salter MW (2000) Neuronal plasticity: Increasing the gain in pain. Science 288:1765–1768
3. Wood JN (2000) Genetic approaches to pain therapy. Am J Physiol Gastrointest Liver Physiol. 278(4):G507–12

4. Attal N. (2000) Chronic neuropathic pain: mechanisms and treatment. Clin J Pain 16(3 Suppl):S118–30

5. Svensson CI, Yaksh TL. The spinal phospholipase-cyclooxygenase-prostanoid cascade in nociceptive processing. Annu Rev Pharmacol Toxicol 2002;42:553-83

6. Vanegas H, Schaible HG. Prostaglandins and cyclooxygenases in the spinal cord. Prog Neurobiol 2001 64(4):327-63

Nociceptive Transducers

Nociceptive transducers are ion-channel complexes which generate depolarizing currents in ▶ nociceptors in response to specific noxious stimuli. Transducer proteins for irritant and chemical stimuli include the vanilloid receptors VR1 and VRL1 (cation-channels gated by protons, capsaicin and noxious heat i.e. 46° C) , the purinergic receptor P2X3 (ATP-gated ion channel) and acid-sensing ion channels such as ASIC-α, ASIC-β and DRASIC (proton-gated ion-channels). The molecular identity of the transducers for noxious mechanical stimuli is as yet unknown. Expression of nociceptive transducers is altered following tissue injury or disease, which contributes to long-term sensitization of nociceptors.

▶ Nociception

Nociceptors

Nociceptors are a specific subset of peripheral sensory organs which respond to noxious stimuli. Aδ mechanoreceptors and C-polymodal nociceptors are the two main classes of cutaneous nociceptors. The sensory quality of pain evoked by activation of Aδ-fibers is generally described as 'pricking', whereas that evoked by activation of C-fibers is generally described as 'burning'.

▶ Local Anaesthetics
▶ Nociception

Nodes of Ranvier

The nodes of Ranvier are the gaps formed between myelin sheath cells along the axons. The sodium channels are densely localized at the nodes of Ranvier.

Non-adrenergic Non-cholinergic (NANC) Transmission/Mediators

Non-adrenergic non-cholinergic (NANC) transmission/mediators describes a part of the autonomic nervous system which does not use acetylcholine or noradrenaline as transmitters. NANC-transmitters often function as co-transmitters, which are released together with acetylcholine or noradrenaline. Substances believed to function as NANC transmitters include ATP, which is found e.g. in postganglionic sympathetic neurons of blood vessels and may contribute to the fast contraction of smooth muscle cells, γ-aminobutyric acid (GABA) and serotonin which are found in enteric neurons and are involved in peristaltic reflexes, dopamine, found in some sympathetic neurons (e.g. kidney) and involved in vasodilatation and NO which is released from pelvic or gastric nerves and plays a role in penile erection or gastric emptying. A variety of peptides have also been described to function as NANC transmitters, e.g. neuropeptide Y (postganglionic sympathetic neurons), vasoactive intestinal peptide (parasymphathetic nerves to salivary glands), substance P (sympathetic ganglia, enteric neurons) or calcitonin gene-related peptide (CGRP) (non-myelinated sensory neurons).

▶ Synaptic Transmission

N

Non-competitive Antagonism

If an antagonist binds to the receptor and precludes agonist activation of that receptor by its occupancy, then no amount of agonist present in the receptor compartment can overcome this antagonism and it is termed non-competitive. This can occur either by binding to the same binding domain of the agonist or another (allosteric) domain. Therefore, this definition is operational in that it does not necessarily imply a molecular mechanism, only a cause and effect relationship. The characteristic of non-competitive antagonism is eventual depression of the maximal response, however, parallel displacement of agonist dose-response curves, with no diminution of maximal response, can occur in systems with ▶ receptor reserve for the agonist.

▶ Drug-receptor-interaction

Non-ionic Contrast Media

Non-ionic contrast media are neutral water-soluble triiodobenzene derivatives; the solubility is provided by hydrophilic groups in the side chains, preferentially hydroxy groups.

▶ Radiocontrast Agents

Non-neuronal Monoamine Transporters

Non-neuronal monoamine transporters is the collective designation for OCT1, OCT2, and EMT; the term indicates that these three carriers share some substrates with the neuronal monoamine transporters (such as DAT, NET, SERT) and the vesicular monoamine transporters (VMAT), but they are expressed (at least predominantly) in non-neuro-nal cells (e.g. in glia cells, hepatocytes or in the proximal tubule).

▶ Organic Cation Transporters
▶ Vesicular Transporters

Non-opioid Analgesics

Non-opioid analgesics can be divided into two groups. The first group contains substances having anti-inflammatory effects in addition to their analgesic and antipyretic activity and are called ▶ non-steroidal anti-inflammatory drugs (NSAIDs). The second group of non-opioid analgesics, which are not classified as NSAIDs, consists of substances that lack anti-inflammatory properties, such as phenazones, metamizole (=dipyrone) and paracetamol.

Non-selective Cation Channels

VEIT FLOCKERZI
Universität des Saarlandes, Homburg, Germany
veit.flockerzi@uniklinik-saarland.de

Definition

Non-selective cation channels are macromolecular pores in the cell membrane that form an aequous pathway. These enable cations such as Na^+, K^+ or Ca^{++} to flow rapidly, as determined by their ▶ electrochemical driving force, at roughly equal rates ($>10^7$ cations per channel pore and per second).

▶ TRP Channels

Basic Characteristics

In general, ion channels are multi protein complexes residing in cellular membranes and allowing ions, mainly Na^+, K^+, Ca^{++} and Cl^-, to flow rapidly as determined by their electrochemical driving force in a thermodynamically downhill

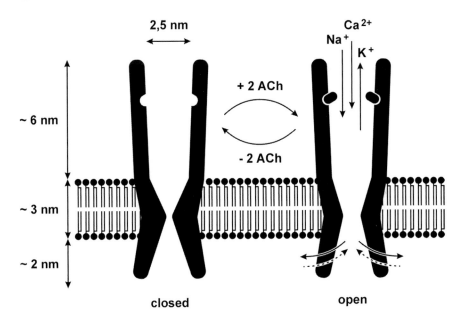

2,5 nm

~ 6 nm

~ 3 nm

~ 2 nm

+ 2 ACh

- 2 ACh

Ca^{2+}
Na^+
K^+

closed

open

Fig. 1 The nicotinic acetylcholine receptor (nAChR) is localized within the cell membrane; above the cell membrane is the synaptic cleft, below the cytoplasm. Drawing of the closed (left) and open (right) nAChR showing acetylcholine (ACh) binding and cation movement. Dimensions of the receptor were taken from references 2 and 3.

direction. The channel proteins are dynamic structures; they form channels that can exist in at least two conformational states, open and closed. In the closed state the channel can be inactive and/ or is reluctant to be activated. Fast shifts in the submillisecond range between these states can be regulated by the membrane potential (▶ voltage gated channels), by ligands or agonist (▶ ligand- or agonist-gated channels). In many cases these shifts can be modulated on a longer time scale (milliseconds to minutes) by hormones, neuro-transmitters, drugs and toxins.

The open channel has in most cases a selective permeability, allowing a restricted class of ions to flow, for example Na^+, K^+, Ca^{++} or Cl^- and, accordingly, these channels are called Na^+-chan-nels, K^+-channels, Ca^{++}-channels and Cl^{--}-chan-nels. In contrast, cation-permeable channels with little selectivity reject all anions but discriminate little among small cations. Little is known about the structures and functions of these non-selec-tive cation channels (1), and so far only one of them, the ▶ nicotinic acetylcholine receptor (nAChR, see Nicotinic Receptors), has been char-acterized in depth (2,3). The nAChR is a ligand-gated channel (see below) that does not select well among cations; the channel is even permeable to choline, glycine ethylester and tris buffer cations. A number of other plasma membrane cation chan-nels including certain ▶ ionotropic glutamate

receptors, the ▶ capsaicin receptor and ▶ cyclic nucleotide-gated (CNG) channels are also some-times called non-selective; they favour the flow of Ca^{++} over Na^+ with relative permeabilities of ~4 (▶ glutamate receptors of the NMDA-type), ~10 (capsaicin receptor) and ~90 (CNG channels). Others, like ▶ hyperpolarization-activated and cyclic nucleotide-gated (HCN) channels conduct both K^+ and Na^+, but are impermeable to divalent cations. Yet another group of channels, which belong to the superfamily of ▶ TRP channels (4), have been implicated to represent non-selective cation channels. However, their mode of gating and, most importantly, their pore regions have not been determined and characterized as yet. There are two exceptions: The capsaicin receptor, which is mentioned above as slightly Ca^{++} selective channel and the ▶ epithelial Ca^{++} channel 1 or ECaC1 (synonym TRPV5). The latter channel is highly selective for Ca^{++} compared to Na^+ with a relative permeability above 100. Finally, a subset of channels activated by stretch have been impli-cated to be non-selective cation channels (1). These channels appear to be ubiquitous, but their structures are unknown.

Acetylcholine-activated channels are found in the membrane of vertebrate skeletal muscle at the synapse between nerve and muscle, also called the neuromuscular junction (muscle type nAChR). Their function is to depolarize the postsynaptic

N

muscle membrane when the presynaptic nerve terminal releases its chemical neurotransmitter, acetylcholine. The channel is composed of four protein subunits that are assembled in a predetermined arrangement and stoichiometry ($\alpha_2\beta\gamma\delta$) around a central, cation-selective pathway. Transmembrane segments of the AChR subunits like those of other channels are mainly formed by 19 to 21 amino acid residues that are folded into a α helix. The α helix is a rod-like structure, the tightly coiled polypeptide main chain of which forms the inner part of the rod, and the side chains extend outward in a helical array (5). Each residue is related to the next one by a rise of 0.15 nanometer along the helix axis and a rotation of 100°, which gives 3.6 amino acid residues per turn of helix. Accordingly, one turn of the helix is 0.54 nanometer, which is equal to 0.15 times the number of residues per turn. The hydrocarbon core of cellular membranes is typically 3 nanometers wide, which accordingly, can be traversed by a α helix consisting of 19 to 21 residues.

The nAChR is cylindrical with a mean diameter of about 6.5 nanometers (Fig. 1). All five rod-shaped subunits span the membrane. The receptor protrudes by ~6 nanometers on the synaptic side of the membrane and by ~2 nanometer on the cytosolic side (2). The pore of the channel is along its symmetry axis and includes an extracellular entrance domain, a transmembrane domain and a cytosolic entrance domain. The diameter of the extracellular entrance domain is ~2.5 nanometer and it becomes narrower at the transmembrane domain. The pore is lined by five α-helices, one from each subunit, and adjacent extended loop regions (3). If two ACh molecules bind to the receptor sites at the extracellular surface of the receptor, far from each other and from the pore, this pathway opens, allowing permeation of Na^+ (crystal radius 0.095 nanometer) K^+ (crystal radius 0.133 nanometer) and Ca^{++} (crystal radius 0.099 nanometer), and initiates depolarization.

Monovalent or divalent cations, but not anions, readily flow through the open form of the AChR channel. What makes the channel cation selective? The amino acid sequences of the pore-forming helices and the adjacent loop components contain three rings of negatively charged residues. One of them is located within the transmembrane region of the pore, and the other two flank the cytosolic entrance to the pore. Apparently, the upper part of the channel, namely the α-helical components act as a water pore, whereas the lower loop components contribute to the selectivity filter of the channel (3). Anions, such as Cl^- cannot enter the pore because they are repelled by the negatively charged rings. Studies on the permeability of a series of organic cations differing in size, such as alkylammonium ions, triaminoguanidinium, histidine and choline, indicate that the narrowest part of the pore has the dimension of ~0.65 nanometers by 0.65 nanometers.

At the level of a ▶ single channel, addition of ACh is followed by transient openings of the channel. The current i flowing through an open channel is 4 picoamperes (pA) at a membrane potential V of –100 mV. Since one ampere (A) represents the flow of 6.24×10^{18} charges per second, 2.5×10^7 Na^+ ions per second flow through an open channel. The conductance g of a plasma membrane channel is the measure of the ease of flow of current between the extracellular space and the cytosol or *vice versa* and is equal to $i/(V-Er)$, where Er is the reversal potential at which there is no ionic net flux; g is expressed in units of siemens (the reciprocal of an ohm), i in amperes, and V in volts. Er equals 0 mV for non-selective cation channels, thus, a current of 4 pA at a potential of 100 mV corresponds to a conductance of 40 picosiemens.

References

1. Hille B (2001) Ionic Channels of Excitable Membranes. 3rd Ed. Sinauer Associates, Sunderland, Massachusetts USA
2. Miyazawa A, Fujiyoshi Y, Stowell M, Unwin N (1999) Nicotinic acetylcholine receptor at 4.6 A resolution: Transverse tunnels in the channel wall. J Mol Biol 288:765–786
3. Corringer P-J, LeNovère N, Changeux J-P (2000) Nicotinic receptors at the amino acid level. Annu Rev Pharmacol Toxicol 40:431–458
4. Montell C, Birnbaumer L, Flockerzi V (2002) The TRP channels, a remarkable functional family. Cell 108:595–598
5. Stryer, L. 1995. Biochemistry, 4th Ed. W.H.Freemann and Company, New York USA

Non-selective Monoamine Reuptake Inhibitor

Non-selective monoamine reuptake inhibitors (NSMRI) are a group of antidepressants, which function by inhibiting the reuptake of noradrenaline and serotonin from the synaptic cleft by blockade of the neurotransmitter transporters specific for noradrenaline and serotonin. Most tricyclic antidepressants are non-selective monoamine reuptake inhibitors (e.g. imipramine, amitriptyline, desipramine).

► Antidepressants
► Synaptic Transmission

Non-steroidal Anti-inflammatory Drugs

G. Geisslinger, J. Lötsch
pharmazentrum frankfurt, Institut für Klinische Pharmakologie, Klinikum der Johann Wolfgang Goethe-Universität Frankfurt am Main, Frankfurt, Germany
geisslinger@em.uni-frankfurt.de,
j.loetsch@em.uni-frankfurt-de

Synonyms

NSAIDs, non-steroidal anti-rheumatic drugs, NSAR; (► aspirin-like drugs, ► Inflammation).

Definition

► Non-opioid analgesic agents can be divided into two groups. The first group contains substances having anti-inflammatory effects in addition to their analgesic and antipyretic activity and are called non-steroidal anti-inflammatory drugs (NSAIDs). The members of this group, with the exception of the selective inhibitors of cyclooxygenase 2 (► COX-2), are acids. Acidic NSAIDs, which include salicylates, derivatives of acetic acid and propionic acid and oxicams among others, comprise molecules containing a lipophilic and a hydrophilic region and are more than 99% bound to plasma proteins.

The second group of non-opioid analgesics, which are not classified as NSAIDs, consists of substances that lack anti-inflammatory properties, such as phenazones, metamizole (=dipyrone) and paracetamol. Their molecules are neutral or weakly basic, have no hydrophilic polarity, and are much less strongly bound to plasma proteins than NSAIDs.

► Analgesics
► Inflammation
► Nociception
► Opioid Systems

Mechanism of Action

In the 1970s, NSAIDs were shown to interfere with the biosynthesis of ► prostaglandins (4). NSAIDs block cyclooxygenases (COX) that catalyze the formation of cyclic endoperoxides from arachidonic acid (Fig. 1). Cyclic endoperoxides are precursors of the prostaglandins, thromboxane A2 and prostacyclin. Prostaglandins have a major role in the pathogenesis of pain, fever and inflammation. Inhibition of their biosynthesis would therefore be expected to result in analgesic, antipyretic and anti-inflammatory activity. However, since prostaglandins are synthesized in most tissues and have a variety of physiological functions, inhibition of their biosynthesis also causes unwanted effects. The clinically most important of these are gastrointestinal erosion and ulceration with bleeding and perforation and kidney disorders with retention of sodium ions and water.

Moreover, there are cyclooxygenase independent effects of NSAIDs potentially contributing to the activity of NSAIDs [for review: (3)].

The identification of two distinct types of cyclooxygenases in 1990 (2) encouraged the search for NSAIDs devoid of the side effects associated with ► COX-1 inhibition. The cyclooxygenase isoform COX-1 is physiologically expressed in the stomach, platelets and the kidney and is there responsible for the synthesis of prostaglandins needed for normal organ function (Fig. 2). Its inhibition by conventional NSAIDs causes side

N

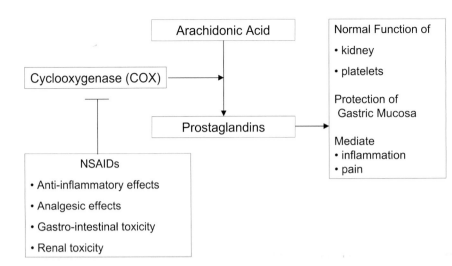

Fig. 1 Non-steroidal anti-inflammatory drugs (NSAIDs) block cyclooxygenase, an enzyme catalysing the production of prostaglandins. When fewer prostaglandins are produced, their physiological and pathophysiolgical effects are decreased, resulting in therapeutic as well as the unwanted effects of the NSAIDs.

effects e.g. inhibition of prostaglandin synthesis in the gastrointestinal tract results in a loss of protection in the gastrointestinal mucosa and ulcerations. The cyclooxygenase isoform, COX-2 is rapidly induced by various factors including cytokines, and its expression is triggered by inflammation, pain or tissue damage. It is clear from this division of cyclooxygenases into COX-1 and an inducible COX-2 that the anti-inflammatory, analgesic and antipyretic effects of the NSAIDs are mainly attributable to inhibition of COX-2 whereas inhibition of COX-1 is associated with most of the unwanted effects of the NSAIDs (Fig. 2).

It follows that drugs that selectively inhibit COX-2 should cause fewer side effects than those that inhibit both COX-1 and COX-2. At therapeutic doses, all currently available NSAIDs, with the exception of celecoxib and rofecoxib, are nonselective and inhibit both COX isoforms.

Newer research has shown that the assignment of physiological activity exclusively to COX-1 and pathophysiological activity exclusively to COX-2 is not strictly valid since COX-2 is expressed constitutively in organs such as spinal cord, kidney or uterus (Fig. 2). Furthermore, COX-2 is formed during various physiological adaptation processes such as the healing of wounds and ulcers.

Clinical Use (incl. side effects)

NSAIDs are indicated in the treatment of:
▶ various pain states (e.g. headache, toothache and migraine), primarily pathophysiological pain involving nociceptors e.g. rheumatic pain and pain caused by bone metastases,
▶ defects of the Ductus arteriosus Botalli (short circuit connection between arteria pulmonalis and aorta; non-closure after birth)
▶ fever.

Unwanted reactions of NSAIDs include:
▶ gastrointestinal disorders (e.g. dyspepsia) , gastrointestinal erosion with bleeding, ulceration and perforation,
▶ kidney malfunctions with retention of sodium and water,
▶ inhibition of platelet aggregation,
▶ central nervous symptoms such as dizziness and headache,
▶ disturbance of uterine motility,
▶ skin reactions,
▶ triggering of asthma attacks in asthmatics. This side effect is a pseudo-allergic reaction where COX-inhibition increases the availability of substrates for lipoxygenase which are converted to broncho-constrictive leukotriens.

Non-selective inhibitors of prostaglandin synthesis are contraindicated:
▶ in gastric and duodenal ulcer,
▶ in asthma,
▶ in bleeding disorders,
▶ during the last few weeks of pregnancy because of the danger in the early seal of the Ductus Botalli.

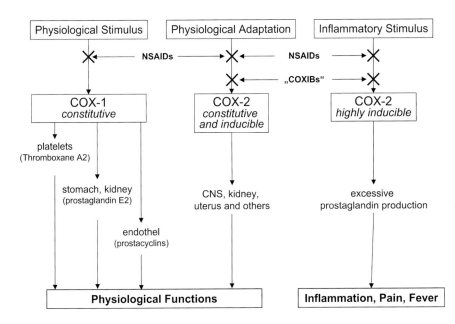

Fig. 2 **Physiological and pathophysiological functions of the cyclooxygenase isoenzymes COX-1 and COX-2,** and the consequences of their inhibition by either unselective conventional NSAIDs or COX-2 selective "COX-IBs".

Glucocorticoids increase the risk of gastrointestinal complications. Considerable caution is necessary when using NSAIDs in patients with severe liver and kidney damage and they should not be combined with coumarines. Owing to the limited experience obtained, these precautions and contraindications also apply to COX-2 selective inhibitors.

The following drug interactions are the most important that can occur when conventional NSAIDs are co-administered with other agents:

▸ the uricosuric effect of probenecid is reduced
▸ the diuretic effect of saluretics is weakened,
▸ the blood glucose-lowering effect of oral antidiabetics is increased,
▸ the elimination of methotrexate is delayed and its toxicity is increased,
▸ the elimination of lithium ions is delayed,
▸ the anti-coagulation effect of coumarin derivatives is enhanced and
▸ the antihypertensive effect of ACE-inhibitors is reduced.

Due to the short period of clinical use, the interaction profile of COX-2-selective inhibitors cannot be described at the present time.

Derivatives of Salicylic Acid

Salicylic acid for systemic use has been replaced by acetylsalicylic acid, amides of salicylic acid (sal-

icylamide, ethenzamide, salacetamide), salsalate and diflunisal.

Acetylsalicylic Acid (Aspirin). The esterification of the phenolic hydroxyl group in salicylic acid with acetic acid results not only in an agent with improved local tolerability but also greater antipyretic and anti-inflammatory activity and, in particular, more marked inhibitory effects on platelet aggregation (inhibition of thromboxane-A2 synthesis). Because of these qualities, acetylsalicylic acid is one of the most frequently used non-opioid analgesics, and the most important inhibitor of platelet aggregation.

Acetylsalicylic acid irreversibly inhibits both COX-1 and COX-2 by acetylating the enzymes. Since mature platelets lack a nucleus, they are unable to synthesize new enzyme. The anti-platelet effects of acetylsalicylic acid persist therefore throughout the lifetime of the platelet and the half-life of this effect is thus being much longer than the elimination half-life of acetylsalicylic acid (15 min). Since new platelets are continously launched into the circulation, the clinically relevant anti-platelet effect of aspirin lasts for up to five days. This is the reason why low doses of acetylsalicylic acid (ca. 100 mg per day) are sufficient in the prophylaxis of heart attacks.

After oral administration, acetylsalicylic acid is rapidly and almost completely absorbed but in the intestinal mucosa it is partly deacetylated to salicylic acid, which also exhibits analgesic activity. The plasma half-life of acetylsalicylic acid is approximately 15 min whereas that of salicylic acid, at low dosages of acetylsalicylic acid, is 2–3 h. Salicylic acid is eliminated more slowly when acetylsalicylic acid is administered at high dose rates because of saturation of the liver enzymes. The metabolites are mainly excreted via the kidney.

The dosage of acetylsalicylic acid in the treatment of pain and fever is 1.5–3 g daily and in the prophylaxis of heart attacks 30–100 mg daily.

Side effects of acetylsalicylic acid administration include buzzing in the ears, loss of hearing, dizziness, nausea, vomiting, and most importantly gastrointestinal bleeding, gastrointestinal ulcerations including gastric perforation. The administration of acetylsalicylic acid in children with viral infections can, in rare cases, produce ▶ Reye's syndrome involving liver damage, encephalopathy and a mortality rate exceeding 50%. Acute salicylate poisoning results in hyperventilation, marked sweating and irritability followed by respiratory paralysis, unconsciousness, hyperthermia and dehydration.

Derivatives of Acetic Acid

Indomethacin. Indomethacin is a strong inhibitor of both cyclooxygenase isoforms with a slight stronger effect in the case of COX-1. It is rapidly and almost completely absorbed from the gastrointestinal tract and has high plasma protein binding (>95%). The plasma half-life of indomethacin varies from 3 to 11 h due to intense enterohepatic cycling. Only about 15% of the substance is eliminated unchanged in the urine, the remainder being eliminated in urine and bile as inactive metabolites (O-demethylation, glucuronidation, N-desacylation).

The daily oral dose of indomethacin is 50–150 mg (up to 200 mg).

Indomethacin treatment is associated with a high incidence (30%) of side effects typical for those seen with other NSAIDs (see above). Gastrointestinal side effects, in particular, are more frequently observed after indomethacin than after administration of other NSAIDs. The market share of indomethacin (approximately 5%) is therefore low compared to that for other non-steroidal antirheumatic agents.

Diclofenac. Diclofenac is an exceedingly potent cyclooxygenase inhibitor slightly more efficacious (approximately 10-fold) against COX-2 than COX-1. Its absorption from the gastrointestinal tract varies according to the type of pharmaceutical formulation used. The oral bioavailability is only 30–80% due to a first-pass effect. Diclofenac is rapidly metabolised (hydroxylation and conjugation) and has a plasma half-life of 1.5 h. The metabolites are excreted renally and via the bile.

Epidemiological studies have demonstrated that diclofenac causes less serious gastrointestinal complications than indomethacin. However, a rise in plasma liver enzymes occurs more frequently with diclofenac than with other NSAIDs.

The daily oral dose of diclofenac is 50–150 mg. Diclofenac is also available as eye-drops for the treatment of non-specific inflammation of the eye and for the local therapy of eye pain.

Derivatives of Arylpropionic Acids

2-arylpropionic acid derivatives possess an asymmetrical carbon atom giving rise to S- and R-enantiomers. The S-enantiomer inhibits cyclooxygenases 2 to 3 times more strongly than the corresponding R-enantiomer. This finding has lead to the marketing of pure S-enantiomers (e.g. S-ibuprofen and S-ketoprofen) in some countries in addition to the racemates where the R-enantiomer is considered as "ballast". However, it is not yet proven whether 2-arylpropionic acids are better tolerated when given as S-enantiomer than as the racemate. Naproxen, for example, which is clinically available only as the S-enantiomer, does not cause less serious gastrointestinal side effects then, e.g., ibuprofen racemate.

Ibuprofen is the most thoroughly researched 2-arylpropionic acid. It is a relatively weak, nonselective inhibitor of COX. In epidemiological studies, ibuprofen compared to all other conventional NSAIDs, has the lowest relative risk of causing severe gastrointestinal side effects. Because of this, ibuprofen is the most frequently used OTC ("over the counter", sale available without prescription) analgesic. Ibuprofen is highly bound to plasma proteins and has a relatively short elimination half-life (approximately 2 h). It is mainly glucuronidated to inactive metabolites that are eliminated via the kidney.

The typical single oral dose of ibuprofen as an OTC analgesic is 200–400 mg and 400–800 mg when used in anti-rheumatic therapy. The corresponding maximum daily doses are 1200 or 2400 mg, respectively but the dose in anti-rheumatic therapy in some countries can be as high as 3200 mg daily.

Other arylpropionic acids include naproxen, ketoprofen and flurbiprofen. They share most of the properties of ibuprofen. The daily oral dose of ketoprofen is 50–150 mg, 150–200 mg for flurbiprofen, and 250–1000 mg for naproxen. Whereas the plasma elimination half-life of ketoprofen and flurbiprofen are similar to that of ibuprofen (1.5–2.5 h and 2.4–4 h, respectively), naproxen is eliminated much more slowly with a half-life of 13–15 h.

Oxicams

Oxicams e.g. piroxicam, tenoxicam, meloxicam and lornoxicam are non-specific inhibitors of cyclooxygenases. Like diclofenac, meloxicam inhibits COX-2 10 times more potently than COX-1. This property can be exploited clinically with doses up to 7.5 mg per day, but at higher doses COX-1 inhibition becomes clinically relevant. Since the dose of meloxicam commonly used is 15 mg daily, this agent cannot be regarded as a COX-2 selective NSAID and considerable caution needs to be exercised when making comparisons between the actions of meloxicam and those of other conventional NSAIDs. The average daily dose in anti-rheumatic therapy is 20 mg for piroxicam and tenoxicam, 7.5–15 mg for meloxicam, and 12–16 mg for lornoxicam. Oxicams have a long elimination half-lives (lornoxicam 3–5 h, meloxicam approximately 20 h, piroxicam approximately 40 h and tenoxicam approximately 70 h).

COX-2-selective NSAIDs (COXIBs)

The development of the COXIBs has been based on the hypothesis COX-1 is the physiological COX and COX-2 the pathophysiological isoenzyme. Inhibition of the pathophysiological COX-2 only is assumed to result in fewer side effects compared to non-selective inhibition of both COX isoenzymes (Fig. 2).

Rofecoxib and celecoxib were the first substances approved that at therapeutic doses inhibit only COX-2. Substances with higher COX-2-selectivity than rofecoxib and celecoxib have been recently approved or will shortly be approved (e.g., etoricoxib, parecoxib, valdecoxib).

Unlike conventional NSAIDs, the "COXIBs" marketed so far have no functional acidic group. The indications for these agents are in principle identical to those of the non-selective NSAIDs although celecoxib and rofecoxib have not yet received approval for the whole spectrum of indications of the conventional NSAIDs. Because they lack COX-1-inhibiting properties, COX-2-selective inhibitors show less side effects than conventional NSAIDs. However, they are not free of side effects because COX-2 has physiological functions that are blocked by the COX-2-inhibitors. The most frequently observed side effects are infections of the upper respiratory tract, diarrhoea, dyspepsia, abdominal discomfort and headache. Peripheral oedema is as frequent as with conventional NSAIDs. The frequency of gastrointestinal complications is approximately half that observed with conventional NSAIDs. The precise side effect profile of the selective COX-2-inhibitors however, will only be known after several years of clinical use.

References

1. Fereira S.H., Moncada, S. and Vane, J.R. (1971) Indomethacin and aspirin abolish prostaglandin release from the spleen. Nature New Biol. 231:237–239
2. Fu, J.Y., Masferrer, J.L., Seibert, K., Raz, A. and Needleman, P. (1990) The induction and suppression of prostaglandin H2 synthase (cyclooxygenase) in human monocytes. J Biol Chem. 265:16737–16740
3. Tegeder, I., Pfeilschifter, J. and Geisslinger, G (2001) Cyclooxygenase-independent actions of cyclooxygenase inhibitors. FASEB J. 15:2057–2072
4. Vane, J.R. (1971) Inhibition of prostaglandin synthesis as a mechanism of action for aspirin-like drugs. Nature New Biol. 231:232–235

N

Non-viral Proteases

JOHN C. CHERONIS
Source Precision Medicine, Boulder, CO, USA
jcheroni@SourceMedicine.com

Synonyms

Protease, proteinase, endopepetidase, exopeptidase, protein hydrolyase, peptide hydroloase, proteolytic enzymes.

Definition

Enzymes capable of peptide bond cleavage either within a polypeptide (endopeptidases) or at the amino or carboxy termini of a polypeptide chain (exopeptidase), together, ► proteinases, proteases or proteolytic enzymes, are among the most numerous and important general classes of enzymes found in mammalian systems. Furthermore, while these enzymes were originally thought to be solely metabolic or degradative in function, they are now understood to have important regulatory functions, as well. For example, they are directly involved in such diverse physiologic processes as fertility and reproduction, cell proliferation, apoptosis, tissue remodeling, wound healing, clotting, clot dissolution, blood pressure regulation, digestion and protein turnover. There has also been a rapid appreciation of the roles proteinases play in pathophysiologic processes such as cancer invasion and metastasis, the inflammatory response, antigen processing and presentation and degenerative diseases (Alzheimer's, atherosclerosis, emphesyma and osteo and rheumatoid arthritis, for example). It is not surprising, then, that proteinase inhibition has become a highly competitive area of research and development for the biopharmaceutical industry.

This chapter is intended to give the reader a basic overview of the mechanisms of proteolysis and the design of proteinase inhibitors as well as a general understanding of proteinase biology and the importance of proteinases as targets of drug development. For a thorough and encyclopedic review of both human as well as other proteolytic enzymes the reader should consult (1). A more complete discussion of the clinical potential of proteinase-directed therapies can be found in (2).

► Norepinephrine/Noradrenalin
► Proteinase-activated Receptors
► Ubiquitin/Proteasome System
► Viral Proteases

Basic Characteristics

Proteinase and proteinase inhibitor biochemistry

The terminology used to describe the physical interaction between the proteolytic enzyme and its preferred substrate is based on a model in which the catalytic site is flanked on either side by subsites that confer specificity for its substrate(s) based upon the interaction of these subsites with the side chains of the peptide residues making up the substrate. The substrate residues are numbered sequentially from P1 to Pn from the scissile bond towards the amino terminus of the substrate and P1' to Pn' towards the carboxy terminus of the substrate. The enzyme substies that flank the catalytic site and that interact with these residues are designated, correspondingly, S1...Sn and S1'...Sn' (see Fig. 1):

Mammalian proteinases fall into five general classes (serine, cysteine, threonine, aspartyl, and ► metalloproteinases) based upon the mechanism of peptide bond cleavage and the amino acid(s) or metal atom used to catalyze this cleavage. In each case, peptide bond cleavage is accomplished by nucleophilic attack on the carbonyl carbon of the scissile peptide bond resulting in the hydrolysis of that bond and the formation of new carboxy and amino termini for the two peptide fragments produced. Inhibition of proteinase activity by small molecules (as opposed to macromolecular, naturally occurring anti-proteinases) generally derives from either chemical modification (reversible or irreversible) of the active nucleophile (the

					Scissile Bond					
Substrate:	...P3	–	P2	–	P1	–	P1'	–	P2'	–	P3' ...
Enzyme:	...S3	–	S2	–	S1	–	S1'	–	S2'	–	S3' ...
					Catalytic Site					

Fig. 1 Non-viral Proteases

hydroxyl or sulfhydral moieties) of the active site serine, cysteine or threonine residues or complexation/chelation of the critical metal atom (usually zinc) found at the active sites of metalloproteinases. Inhibition of ▶ aspartyl proteinases is usually accomplished by tight binding "pseudo-substrates" that present a non-cleavable peptide bond mimetic to the active catalytic site. In simple terms, the portion of an inhibitor that interferes with the chemistry of peptide bond cleavage is called the "message" or "warhead" and the portion of the molecule that allows the warhead to interact with the enzyme in an effective way (in a sense, delivering the message) is defined as the "address". In general, any pharmacologically acceptable inhibitor will have both a message and an address.

Inhibitor specificity can be defined on the basis of the class(es) of proteinase(s) that can be inhibited by the chemistry of the warhead. For example, warheads such as aldehydes, halomethylketones, or α-keto heterocycles will inhibit serine, cysteine and threonine proteinases but will be ineffective against metallo- and aspartyl proteinases. Vinylsulfone-based inhibitors are potent irreversible inhibitors of ▶ cysteine proteinases but are devoid of activity against the other classes of proteolytic enzymes. Hydroxamic and carboxylic acids can be used as warheads for metalloproteinases but are ineffective against serine, cysteine, threonine and aspartyl proteinases. Finally, tight-binding pseudosubstrates are generally the only synthetic inhibitors that have been developed for aspartyl proteinases. However, pseudosubstrates have not been found to be of substantial utility in the development of inhibitors for the other classes of proteinases.

Inhibitor selectivity can be defined as the ability of a compound to discriminate between proteinases within a specific class of enzyme. Selectivity usually derives from inhibitor moieties that are not involved in the inhibition of the chemistry of catalysis. In other words, inhibitor specificity derives from the message (or warhead) and selectivity derives from the address. As a general principle, a proteinase inhibitor should have high specificity and a well-circumscribed spectrum of selectivity in order to avoid potential toxicity problems or side-effects. Potency is dependent on both the address and the message and is a measure

of how tightly the inhibitor binds to the enzyme and interacts with the active site nucleophile or metal atom.

Drugs

Structure/substrate-based Drug Design

An example of how these interactions can be used to design and develop highly potent and selective inhibitors is the ability to discriminate between two different types of ▶ serine proteinases using substrate-based chloromethylketones. Trypsin-like serine proteinases (trypsin, thrombin, plasmin, Factor Xa, tissue and plasma kallikrein, etc.) prefer positively charged amino acid side chains (arginine or lysine) in the P1 position, while ▶ elastase-like serine proteinases (pancreatic elastase, neutrophil elastase, proteinase-3, etc.) prefer aliphatic amino acid side chains (alanine, valine, leucine and isoleucine). A commonly used synthetic fluorgenic non-selective substrate for ▶ trypsin-like proteinases which is based on the known sequence specificities of many trypsin-like enzymes is NH_2-alanyl-prolyl-arginyl-paranitroanaline. Similarly, a general-purpose substrate for elasatase-like enzymes is NH_2-alanyl-prolyl-valyl-paranitroanaline.

In most cases, prototype small molecule inhibitors for serine proteinases can be easily generated from known small molecule substrates by substituting a "warhead" (cholormethylketone, trifluormethylketone, α-keto heterocycle, etc.) for the fluorphore moiety, in these cases, p-nitroanaline. Therefore, on the basis of the interaction between the peptide residue occupying the P1 position of the molecule, compounds such as NH_2-alanyl-prolyl-valyl-chloromethylketone will have more than 5 orders of magnitude greater potency and selectivity for human neutrophil elastase over trypsin or thrombin. Substituting an arginyl residue for the valyl residue will produce an inhibitor of trypsin-like serine proteinases with more than 5 orders of magnitude greater potency and selectivity for these enzymes over elastase-like enzymes.

Once a substrate-based inhibitor is developed, a variety of approaches can then be taken to generate a true drug candidate. Perhaps the most productive of these approaches is the combination of structure based design using x-ray crystallographic techniques to observe specific inhibitor-

Tab. 1 Non-viral Proteases – Potential clinical applications of and the target enzymes for non-viral protease inhibitors.

Clinical Indication	Proteinase Target(s)	Locus of Action	Class
Allergy and Autoimmunity	Cathepsin S	Intracellular	Cysteine
	Proteasome	Intracellular	Threonine
	Mast Cell Tryptase and Chymase	Extracellular	Serine
	Caspase-1 (Interleukin-1 Converting Enzyme)	Intracellular	Cysteine
	Granzyme B	Intracellular	Serine
General Inflammatory Diseases	Neutrophil Elastase and Proteinase 3	Extracellular	Serine
	Caspase-1	Intracellular	Cysteine
	TNFα Converting Enzyme	Extracellular	Metallo
	MMP-8, -9 and -12 (neutrophil collagenase, gelatinase B and metalloelastase)	Extracellular	Metallo
	Plasma and Tissue Kallikrein	Extracellular	Serine
	Proteasome	Intracellular	
Bone and Joint Diseases	Cathepsin K	Extracellular	Cysteine
	MMP-1, -8, -13 and -12 (collagenase 1, 2 and 3 and metalloelastase)	Extracellular	Metallo
	MT1-MMP	Extracellular	Metallo
Cancer	MMP-2 and -9 (gelatinase A and B)	Extracelllar	Metallo
	MT-MMPs 1-4	Extracellular	Metallo
	MMP-3, -10 and -11 (Stomelsyin 1, 2 and 3)	Extracellular	Metallo
	Urokinase plasminogen activator	Extracellular	Serine
	Guanadinobenzotase	Extracellular	Serine
Cardiovascular	Thrombin and Factor Xa	Extracellular	Serine
	Renin	Extracellular	Aspartyl
	Angiotensin Converting Enzyme	Extracelllular	Metallo
	Endothelin Converting Enzyme	Extracellular	Metallo

enzyme interactions with selected peptde-based inhibitors of interest and crystallography-directed medicinal chemistry to screen for substitute chemmical subunits that can provide similar binding motifs to those of the peptide-based inhibitors, thereby retaining and even improving selectivity and potency. Multiple iterations of crystallography-directed synthesis, then, can generate numerous drug candidates that have pharmacologically desirable characteristics such as oral bioavailability, prolonged serum or plasma half-lives, intracellular penetration (if needed), etc. This approach has been used with considerable success for th edevelopment of inhibitors fpr each of the classes of proteinases identified.

As a result of this understanding of how enzyme structure and inhibitor activity relate to each other, it is not surprising, then, that one of the most successful applications of structure-based drug design has been the design and development of proteinase inhibitors. The power of this approach is best exemplified by the extraordinarily short development time required for the introduction of HIV proteinase inhibitors into clinical use (see reference 2). In addition, inhibitors for angiotensin converting enzyme, which were also developed using these same techniques, have been a mainstay of therapy for hypertension and congestive hear failure for two decades (2). Drug candidates for other non-viral proteinases that have been generated using this approach that are in various stages of preclinical and clinical development include inhibitors for: serine proteinases (thrombin, Factor Xa, mast cell tryptase, urokinase, neutrophil elastase and proteinase-3), metalloproteinases (MMP-2, MMP-9, MMP-13, MT1-MMP, endothelin converting enzyme and TNFα converting enzyme) and cysteine proteinases (caspase-1, cathepsin K and cathepsin S).

Despite the obvious power of a structure-based approach, it is important to recognize that not all proteinase-proteinase inhibitor interactions can be predicted *a priori*. Directed combinatorial chemistry approaches also have utility, particularly in developing novel synthetic lead candidates that can be improved upon by structure-based modifications. Since combinatorial methods can be designed to limit inherent bias, they can survey idiosyncratic compound-induced conformational changes in the enzyme that could not have been predicted in advance. Many, if not most, programs will utilize both methodologies to enhance the potential for successful clinical candicdate compound identification.

Locus of Action

In addition to the type of proteolytic enzyme being considered as a potential therapeutic target, an additional consideration is the locus of action. Many important proteinase-dependent processes (thrombosis, thrombolysis, leukocyte migration, tumor cell invasion and metastasis, angiotensin conversion, to name a few) are extracellularly accessible even though the actual proteolytic events occur at the cell membrane. Other processes (apoptosis, antigen processing, cytokine, chemokine and hormone processing) are predominantly intracellular events that require significant intracellular penetration if an inhibitor is to be effective. Furthermore, the different proteinase classes tend to have different loci of action. Although specific exceptions to each general case can be found, extracellular proteolysis is generally a function of serine and metalloproteinases, while aspartyl, cysteine and threonine proteinase activities are generally restricted to the intracellular milieu. In fact, the only known threonine proteinases found in mammalian systems are the subunits of the 20S subcomplex of the 26S ▶ proteasome. Understanding the locus of action of different proteinases is a significant factor in selecting a target for drug development. As a result, many initial proteinase targets for drug development (thrombin, Factor Xa, angiotensin converting enzyme, neutrophil elastase and mast cell tryptase, for example) have been those enzymes that are accessible extracellularly.

Summary

Listed in Table 1 is a selected set of potential clinical indications that have been considered for treatment with inhibitors of endogenous proteinases. This table is by no means exhaustive and is only intended to give the reader a general understanding of the potential that proteinase inhibitors have for use in the treatment of human diseases. It is clear, however, that non-viral proteinase inhibitors have significant potential for the treatment of a wide variety of clinical conditions. Furthermore, given the well-understood relationships between the enzymes of interest and their substrates along with well-established chemistry for warhead design and synthesis, proteinase inhibition should quickly become a mainstay of human therapy.

References

1. Handbook of Proteolytic Enzymes (1998), Barrett, AJ, Rawlings, ND and Woessner, JF (eds), Academic Press, London/San Diego.

2. Handbook of Experimental Pharmacology, Vol.140, Proteases as Targets for Therapy, von der Helm, K, Korant, BD, and Cheronis, JC (eds), Springer-Verlag, Berlin.

Noradrenaline Transporter

Noradrenaline transporters (NAT) are localized in the presynaptic plasma membrane of adrenergic nerve terminals. They belong to a family of proteins with 12 putative transmembrane proteins which are responsible for recycling of released neurotransmitters (noradrenaline/adrenaline, dopamine, serotonin, amino acid transmitters) back into the presynaptic nerve ending. Noradrenaline transporters can be blocked by a number of different antidepressant drugs, including tricyclic antidepressants (e.g. desipramine) and selective noradrenaline reuptake inhibitors (e.g. reboxetine).

▶ Antidepressants
▶ Synaptic Transmission

Norepinephrine/Noradrenalin

Norepinephrine is a biogenic amine synthesized from tyrosine. It is generated in the brain, mostly by cells of the locus coeruleus located in the brainstem.

▶ α-Adrenergic System
▶ β-Adrenergic System

Normoglycaemia

Euglycaemia, blood glucose concentration within the normal range e.g. fasting blood glucose 3.5 – 6.5 mmol/l; postprandial blood glucose 5 – 11 mmol/l.

▶ Diabetes Mellitus

NOS

▶ NO Synthases

NSAIDs

▶ Non-steroidal Anti-inflammatory Drugs

NSF

NSF, the acronym for NEM-sensitive fusion protein, was originally discovered as an essential factor in intracellular membrane transport steps. NSF is now known to catalyze the disassembly of all SNARE complexes. NSF requires the binding of ▶ SNAPs to exert its action. NSF is an evolutionarily conserved protein that forms hexameric double-ring structures. During its catalytic cycle, ATP is cleaved and the N-terminal region undergoes massive conformational changes. Recently, NSF has been shown to interact with other proteins such as glutamate receptors, but the significance of these interactions is still controversial.

▶ Exocytosis

NSMRI

▶ Non-selective Monoamine Reuptake Inhibitors

Nuclear Factor-κB

Nuclear factor-κB (NF-κB) is a widely expressed transcription factor, which is involved in a wide variety of cellular functions, including communication between cells, embryonic development, response to stress, inflammation, viral infection apoptosis and the maintenance of cell-type specific expression of genes. NF-kappa B is activated by a variety of stimuli including cytokines, growth factors, cellular stress and others.

▶ Glucocorticoids

Nuclear Pore Complex

The nuclear pore complex, located in the nuclear envelope, contains more than 50 proteins. It allows diffusion of small proteins between cytoplasm and nucleoplasm. Larger molecules (>50kD) are selectively transported by an energy-dependent mechanism.

Nuclear Receptor Superfamily

▶ Gluco-/Mineralocorticoid Receptors
▶ Sex Steroid Receptors
▶ Nuclear Receptor Regulation of Drug-metabolizing P450 Enzymes
▶ Selective Sex-steroid Receptor Modulators
▶ Glucocorticoids
▶ Contraceptives
▶ Table appendix: Receptor Proteins

Nuclear Receptor Regulation of Drug-metabolizing P450 Enzymes

DAVID J. WAXMAN
Division of Cell and Molecular Biology,
Department of Biology, Boston University,
Boston, MA, USA
djw@bu.edu

Synonyms

None/Not Applicable

Definition

P450 induction is the process whereby cellular or tissue levels of one or more ▶ cytochrome P450 (CYP) enzymes is increased in response to treatment with certain drugs (e.g., phenobarbital (PB)) or environmental chemicals, which are designated P450 inducers. This leads to an increase in the cell's capacity for P450-catalyzed oxidative metabolism of xenochemicals and endogenous lipophilic substrates. Many phase II drug conjugation enzymes, e.g., glutathione S-transferases and UDP-glucuronyl transferases, are also subject to induction by classic P450 inducers.

▶ P450 Mono-oxygenase System
▶ Pharmacogenetics

Basic Characteristics

P450 induction can occur in many cell types and tissues, but is most prominent in liver, a major organ for metabolism of steroids, drugs and environmental chemicals. Many of the drug-inducible P450s are active catalysts of drug metabolism, and P450 induction typically leads to an enhanced capacity for foreign chemical biotransformation. P450 induction can have a major impact on: P450-dependent drug metabolism, pharmacokinetics and drug-drug interactions; the toxicity and carcinogenicity of foreign chemicals; and the activity and disposition of endogenous steroids and cer-

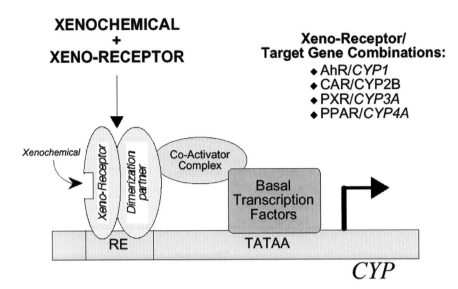

Fig. 1 General mechanism for transcriptional activation of CYP genes by xenochemicals (P450 inducers) that activate their cognate xeno-receptor proteins. In the case of Ah receptor, the receptor's heterodimerization partner is Arnt, whereas in the case of the nuclear receptors CAR, PXR and PPARα the heterodimerization partner is RXR. The coactivator and basal transcription factor complexes shown are each comprised of a large number of protein factors.

tain other hormones. Although some P450 substrates are also P450 inducers, there is not necessarily a correlation between the ability of a chemical to induce a particular P450 enzyme and its ability to serve as a substrate of that same P450.

Of the ~57 known human P450s, at least ten are subject to induction by xenochemicals. In most, but not all cases, the induction of P450 protein and enzyme activity occurs by a mechanism that involves increased transcription of the corresponding P450 gene. Members of four P450 gene families, CYP families 1, 2, 3 and 4, are induced by receptor-dependent transcriptional mechanisms (Fig. 1). P450 genes belonging to the *CYP1* gene family are induced *via* the Ah receptor, a PAS (Per-Arnt-Sim) family transcription factor (1), whereas individual members of the *CYP2, CYP3* and *CYP4* P450 gene families are respectively induced via the nuclear receptor superfamily members designated ▶ CAR (2,3), ▶ PXR and ▶ PPARα (3–5).

CAR, or constitutive androstane receptor, is an ▶ orphan nuclear receptor that mediates the widely studied induction of *CYP2B* genes by PB and many other 'PB-like' lipophilic chemicals. The pregnane X receptor (PXR) activates *CYP3A* genes

in response to diverse chemicals, including certain natural and synthetic steroids. The peroxisome proliferator-activated receptor PPARα mediates the induction of fatty acid hydroxylases of the CYP4A family by many acidic chemicals classified as non-genotoxic carcinogens and peroxisome proliferators. These three xenochemical receptors are most abundant in liver, where they may be responsive to endogenous ligands. The discovery of endogenous ligands for CAR (adrostanes, which inhibit receptor activity), PXR (certain pregnenolone derivatives, bile acids and other steroids) and PPAR (specific prostaglandins and other fatty acid metabolites) suggests that these three nuclear receptors play an important role in modulating liver gene expression in response to endogenous metabolic or hormonal stimuli in addition to their more obvious role in modulating liver drug and xenochemical metabolism by induction of cytochrome P450 and other enzymes of foreign compound metabolism.

CYP1 Induction via Ah Receptor

In contrast to the three nuclear superfamily receptors that activate *CYP2, CYP3,* and *CYP4* genes, the activation of *CYP1* genes is mediated by the Ah receptor (Aryl hydrocarbon receptor), a helix-loop-helix DNA-binding protein that belongs to the PAS family of transcription factors (1). The Ah receptor is activated by binding to an aromatic hydrocarbon ligand in the cytosol. The activated receptor then translocates to the nucleus where it can heterodimerize with the nuclear factor Arnt, bind to DNA enhancer sequences ('dioxin-response elements' or DREs) found upstream of *CYP1* and other Ah receptor-inducible genes, and stimulate target gene transcription. The overall pathway is conserved in many cell types and across species and accounts for the induction of *CYP1* genes by a large number of polycyclic aromatic hydrocarbons, including several important environmental carcinogens found in auto emissions and cigarette smoke.

Role of CAR in CYP2B Induction and Other PB Responses

Certain liver P450 enzymes are highly inducible *in vivo* following PB administration, with levels of specific P450s and their associated mRNAs and gene transcription rates increasing up to 50-fold (e.g., rat liver CYP2B1). The striking tissue specificity of the PB induction response (liver >> other tissues), the saturable dose response curves for induction, and the structure-activity relationships reported for certain classes of PB-like inducers (e.g., PCB congeners) all point to a receptor-dependent induction mechanism. The fact that diverse chemicals, with no obvious structural relationship other than their general lipophilicity, can each serve as PB-like inducers further suggests that these inducers bind with a 'sloppy fit' or an elastic recognition site to a common receptor; this has now been identified as the liver-enriched orphan nuclear receptor CAR. A similar paradigm of structurally diverse inducer ligands applies to the nuclear receptors that mediate induction of other classes of drug-metabolizing P450 enzymes, i.e., PXR and PPARα.

CAR is the key regulated transcription factor that mediates the effects of PB and PB-like inducers on liver P450 genes (2, 3). Mechanistically, P450 gene induction by CAR involves at least two distinct regulated steps. First, CAR is translocated from the cytosol to the nucleus. The mechanism whereby PB induces this nuclear translocation, which is essential for the PB induction response, is not well understood. It may reflect PB-stimulated nuclear import or, alternatively, PB-dependent blocking of a constitutive CAR nuclear export event. CAR nuclear translocation is followed by a second step, CAR binding to specific DNA response elements (PBREs) found upstream of *CYP2B* and other PB-inducible genes. This event is associated with recruitment to the promoter of co-activator complexes (Fig. 1) and leads to an increase in the rate of transcription of CAR target genes. CAR binds to these PBREs as a heterodimer with the nuclear receptor ▶ retinoid X receptor, RXR, which serves as a common heterodimerization partner for many orphan nuclear receptors, including PXR and PPARα. CAR nuclear translocation and (CAR-RXR)-PBRE binding are both strongly enhanced in liver *in vivo* following administration of PB. In the case of the potent PB-like inducer and pesticide contaminant TCPOBOP, but not in the case of PB, direct binding to CAR's COOH-terminal ligand-binding domain as an agonist ligand has been described.

Mouse *CAR* gene knockout studies confirm the importance of CAR in the PB induction response, and demonstrate that CAR is essential, not only for induction of the highly inducible *CYP2B* genes, but for multiple pleiotropic responses to PB-like inducing agents. These include the induction of many other genes involved in xenobiotic metabolism and repression of the expression of certain genes involved in energy metabolism. CAR is also required for various whole liver physiologic effects (e.g., hepatomegaly and enhanced hepatocyte proliferation) and pharmacologic responses that are characteristic of PB-treated liver (e.g., cocaine-induced hepatotoxicity).

Important unanswered questions regarding the role of CAR in PB-induction of P450 gene expression include the following: 1) By which mechanism is CAR retained in the cytoplasm in the absence of PB? 2) What contributions do phosphorylation/dephosphorylation reactions make to CAR nuclear localization, DNA binding or transcriptional activity? Modulation of the activity of other nuclear receptors through receptor phosphorylation reactions is well established. Finally, 3) do interindividual differences or species differences in the levels of CAR, in the ligand specificity of CAR, or in the synthesis or metabolism of CAR inhibitory lig-

N

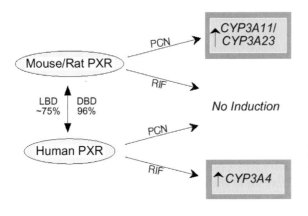

Fig. 2 Species-specificity of PXR's CYP3A induction response. Shown are the approximate amino acid sequence identities of the COOH terminal-ligand-binding domain (LBD) and the central DNA-binding domain (DBD) of rodent and human PXR. *CYP3A11* and *CYP3A23* are, respectively, mouse and rat P450 3A genes, whereas *CYP3A4* is a human P450 3A gene. PCN, pregnenolone 16α-carbonitrile; RIF, rifampicin.

ands (e.g., androstanediol) contribute to interindividual or interspecies differences in CAR-dependent liver induction responses?

PXR: A Novel Nuclear Receptor Involved in CYP3A Induction

CYP3A4, the single most abundant P450 enzyme in human liver, is highly expressed in liver and intestine, where it metabolizes structurally diverse drugs, environmental chemicals, endogenous steroid hormones and lipophilic bile acids. The high level expression, broad substrate specificity and widespread inducibility of this P450 enzyme in response to steroids, antibiotics and other pharmacological agents gives rise to many CYP3A-based drug interactions.

CYP3A enzyme induction can be stimulated by classic glucocorticoids, such as dexamethasone, and by certain anti-glucocorticoids (e.g., pregnenolone 16α-carbonitrile, PCN), indicating that CYP3A induction is not mediated by the classical glucocorticoid receptor. Important species differences in CYP3A induction have been observed. For example, the anti-glucocorticoid PCN is an efficacious CYP3A inducer in rat but not in humans or rabbits, whereas the antibiotic rifampicin is an

excellent CYP3A inducer in humans and rabbits, but not in rat. These species-specific responses are a function of intrinsic differences in the ligand specificity of the PXR protein in each species (3–5). For example, human PXR but not mouse PXR is activated by xenochemicals that preferentially induce *CYP3A* genes in human cells and tissues (e.g., rifampicin), whereas mouse PXR but not human PXR mediates the strong response to PCN that characterizes mouse *CYP3A* gene induction (Fig. 2). This conclusion is strongly supported by mouse *PXR* gene knockout studies, which establish PXR as the major mediator of CYP3A induction in response to various xenochemicals, and furthermore, demonstrate that a human pattern of *CYP3A* inducibility is achieved when the endogenous mouse *PXR* gene is replaced by its human *PXR* counterpart. Mouse and human PXR exhibit an uncharacteristically low amino acid conservation within the ligand-binding domain (~75% sequence identity), suggesting that these rodent and human PXRs are unusually divergent orthologs whose evolution reflects receptor adaptation to each species unique diet and distinct endogenous steroid profile.

PXR may serve as a broadly-based 'steroid and xenobiotic sensor' whose intrinsic physiologic function is to stimulate synthesis of CYP3A enzymes that catabolize endogenous steroidal substrates. This possibility is supported by the striking responsiveness of PXR to endogenous steroids belonging to several distinct classes (pregnanes, estrogens and corticoids) and by the catalysis by many CYP3A enzymes of 6β-hydroxylation reactions using diverse steroidal substrates, including androgens, corticoids, progestins and bile acids. More specifically, PXR plays a key role in bile acid homeostasis, as shown by the decreased production and increased hepatic uptake and detoxification of cholestatic bile acids, such as ► lithocholic acid, that is mediated by PXR. Thus, the activation of PXR by bile acids in liver leads to: 1) decreased expression of *CYP7*, cholesterol 7α-hydroxylase, which catalyzes a key rate-limiting reaction of bile acid biosynthesis; 2) increased expression of the transporter *Oatp2*, which increases hepatic uptake of bile acids from the sinusoidal blood; and 3) induction of CYP3A enzymes that detoxify lithocholic acid by catalyzing its 6β-hydroxylation.

PPARα: Xenochemical Induction of CYP4A Enzymes and Role in Rodent Hepatocarcinogenesis

CYP4A enzymes catalyze the oxygenation of biologically important fatty acids, including arachidonic acid and other eicosanoids. *CYP4A* gene transcription can be activated in both liver and kidney by a range of acidic drugs and other xenochemicals, including hypolipidemic fibrate drugs, ▶ phthalate ester plasticizers used in the medical and chemical industries, and other environmental chemicals. These CYP4A inducers are classified as ▶ peroxisome proliferator chemicals (PPCs) since they markedly induce liver peroxisomal enzymes, which in turn leads to a dramatic increase in both the size and the number of liver cell peroxisomes. PPARα is the nuclear receptor responsible for *CYP4A* induction, peroxisomal enzyme induction and hepatic peroxisome proliferation (3–5). The tissue distribution of PPARα (liver >kidney >heart >other tissues) mirrors the PPC responsiveness of these tissues. *CYP4A* induction in liver and kidney and hepatic peroxisome proliferation are both abolished in *PPAR* gene knockout mice, demonstrating the essential role of PPARα for these responses *in vivo*. This finding is consistent with the presence in the 5'-flank of *CYP4A* genes of functional DNA response elements (PPREs) that bind PPARα as a heterodimer with RXR and serve as functional enhancers with respect to the stimulation of *CYP4A* gene transcription. PPARα-RXR complexes bound to PPREs are permissive, in that they can be synergistically activated by the combination of a PPARα ligand with the RXR ligand 9-cis-retinoic acid.

Persistent activation of PPARα can induce the development of hepatocellular carcinoma in susceptible rodent species by a non-genotoxic mechanism, i.e., one that does not involve direct DNA damage caused by PPCs or their metabolites. This hepatocarcinogenic response is abolished in mice deficient in PPARα, underscoring the central role of PPARα, as opposed to the two other mammalian PPARs (PPARγ and PPARδ), in PPC-induced hepatocarcinogenesis. Other toxic responses to PPCs, such as kidney and testicular toxicities caused by certain phthalate di-ester plasticizers, are not abolished in PPARα-deficient mice, raising the possibility that PPARγ or PPARδ may mediate these PPC toxicities.

While many of the molecular details regarding PPARα and its transcriptional activation of *CYP4A* and other target genes have been elucidated, several important questions regarding the physiological role and toxicological impact of PPAR receptors remain: 1) What precise role does PPARα play in lipid metabolism and homeostasis? 2) What structural features enable PPARα to bind a broad range of xenochemicals, in addition to its structurally diverse endogenous fatty acids ligands? Crystallographic analysis of the ligand-binding domains of PPARγ and PPARδ has revealed ligand-binding pockets that are large in comparison to other nuclear receptors. This finding may have direct relevance for our understanding of the structural basis for the broad ligand specificity of PPARα, and perhaps that of CAR and PXR as well. Finally, 3) to what extent are PPARα-dependent responses (e.g., *CYP4A* gene induction, hepatocarcinogenesis) modulated *in vivo* through cross-talk with other nuclear receptors and other signaling molecules, e.g., thyroid hormone, which suppresses hepatic peroxisome proliferative responses, and growth hormone, which activates JAK/STAT signal transduction pathways that can inhibit PPAR transcriptional activity?

Importance of Nuclear Receptors for Drug Metabolism and Drug Development

The identification of specific nuclear receptors as molecular targets of P450 inducers impacts the fields of drug metabolism and drug development in two important ways:

1) Drug interactions, often associated with individual differences in drug metabolism, are a major contributor to idiosyncratic drug responses, which can sometimes be fatal. P450 induction, especially induction PXR and CYP3A enzymes, is likely to contribute significantly to interpatient differences in drug metabolism. Cell-based high throughput screens for P450 inducers that activate Ah receptor, CAR, PXR or PPARα have been developed and can readily be applied to characterize the P450 induction potential of drugs currently used in the clinic, as well as investigational drugs and lead compounds under development. These efforts may help to predict and thereby avoid idiosyncratic drug interactions associated with P450 metabolism and P450 induction. Further elucida-

tion of the factors that regulate cellular nuclear receptor levels (e.g., glucocorticoids, which increase expression of PXR in human hepatocytes) and the identification of any genetic polymorphisms that impact on receptor expression, ligand binding specificity or transcriptional activity are also likely to be important.

2) Receptor proteins involved in the induction of cytochromes P450 and other enzymes of drug metabolism may serve as novel drug targets. Examples of established nuclear receptor drug targets include PPARα, which is a target of hypolipidemic fibrate drugs, and PPARγ, which is targeted by anti-type II diabetes drugs of the thiazolidinedione class. Conceivably, potent activators of PXR could be useful for the relief of cholestasis associated with hepatotoxic bile acids, while PXR antagonists may be used to block CYP3A auto-induction responses, which can substantially shorten the plasma half-life of a drug that simultaneously serves as a CYP3A inducer and a CYP3A substrate, a characteristic of several AIDS protease inhibitors. The finding that genes encoding liver and intestinal drug transporters are also targets for PXR regulation presents additional opportunities and additional challenges as well.

Supported by NIH 5 P42 ES07381.

References

1. Whitlock JP Jr (1999) Induction of cytochrome P4501A1. Annu Rev Pharmacol Toxicol 39:103–125
2. Sueyoshi T, Negishi M (2001) Phenobarbital response elements of cytochrome P450 genes and nuclear receptors. Annu Rev Pharmacol Toxicol 41:123–143
3. Waxman DJ (1999) P450 gene induction by structurally diverse xenochemicals: central role of nuclear receptors CAR, PXR, and PPAR. Arch Biochem Biophys 369:11–23
4. Kliewer SA, Lehmann JM, Milburn MV, Wilson TM (1999) The PPARs and PXRs: nuclear xenobiotic receptors that define novel hormone signaling pathways. Recent Prog Horm Res 54:345–367
5. Savas U, Griffin KJ, Johnson, EF (1999). Molecular mechanisms of cytochrome P-450 induction by xenobiotics: An expanded role for nuclear hormone receptors. Mol Pharmacol 56:851–857

Nuclear Receptors

Nuclear receptors constitute a superfamily of intracellularly located proteins which share a common modular structure and act as transcription factors. At present 65 family members have been identified from nematodes to man. Specific to these transcription factors is their ability to bind small hydrophobic molecules such as steroids. This causes a change in the transcriptional activity of the respective receptor thereby leading to altered gene expression.

▶ Nuclear Receptor Regulation of Drug-metabolizing P450 Enzymes

Nucleic Acid Vaccination

▶ Genetic Vaccination

Nucleus Accumbens

The nucleus accumbens is part of the limbic system. It receives dopaminergic input through the mesolimbic system that originates from cell bodies in the ventral segmental area (A10 cell group). This mesolimbic dopaminergic pathway is part of the reward pathways. Drugs of abuse (cocaine, amphetamine, opiates or nicotine) have been shown to increase the level of dopamine release in these neurons.

▶ Drug Addiction/Dependence

O

Obesity

▶ Anti-obesity Drugs

OCT

▶ Organic Cation Transporters

Oestrogens

▶ Sex Steroid Receptors

Oedema

Oedema refers to an accumulation of interstitial fluid to a point where it is palpable or visible. In general this point is reached with a fluid volume of 2-3 liters. Oedema formation is the result of a shift of fluid into the interstitial space due to primary disturbances in the hydraulic forces governing transcapillary fluid transport and of subsequent excessive fluid reabsorption by the kidneys. Deranged capillary hydraulic pressures initiate oedema formation in congestive heart failure, and liver cirrhosis whereas a deranged plasma oncotic pressure leads to oedema in nephrotic syndrome

and malnutrition. Increased capillary permeability is responsible for oedema in inflammation and burns.

▶ Diuretics

Off-resin Analysis

Off-resin analysis is analysis of a compound cleaved off a polymeric carrier material, usually in solution.

▶ Combinatorial Chemistry

Oligonucleotide

An oligonucleotide is a short (typically up to 80 nucleotides) single stranded DNA molecule.

▶ Antisense Oligonucletides

Oncogenes

Oncogenes are genes, which confer malignancy on a cell. Proto-oncogenes are genes, that normally control cell division and differentiation, but which can be converted to oncogenes. Oncogenes often affect one or more signal transduction mechanisms, which impact on the cell division machinery.

▶ Proto-oncogenes

Oncogenesis

Oncogenesis is the process of cancer initiation; the term is essentially synonomous with carcinogenesis.

▶ Cancer (molecular mechanisms of therapy)

On-resin Analysis

On-resin analysis is analysis of compound attached to a poly-meric carrier material.

▶ Combinatorial Chemistry

Opiates

In the strict sense, opiates are drugs which are derived from opium and include the natural products morphine, codeine, thebaine and many semi-synthetic congeners derived from them. In the wider sense, opiates are morphine-like drugs with non-peptidic structures. The old term opiates is now more and more replaced by the term opioids which applies to any substance, whether endogenous or synthetic, peptidic or non-peptidic, that produces morphine-like effects through an action on opioid receptors.

▶ Opioid System

Opioid Systems

VOLKER HÖLLT
Otto-von-Guericke-Universität Magdeburg,
Magdeburg, Germany
Volker.Hoellt@medizin.uni-magdeburg.de

Synonyms

Opioid receptors, endogenous opioid peptides, nociceptin/orphanin FQ, ORL-1

Definition

Opioid systems comprise opiate alkaloids and the families of ▶ endogenous opioid peptides (β-endorphins, enkephalins and dynorphins) interacting with the three opioid receptor subtypes (μ, δ, κ). Pharmacological conventions define "opioid" when the action is produced by a prototypic opiate drug such as morphine and is antagonised by the antagonist naloxone. The classification of the three opioid receptors was confirmed by cloning of the three opioid receptor genes based on the fact that they share a homology of more than 60%. Interestingly, ▶ ORL1 an orphan receptor exhibits the same high degree of similarity to the opioid receptors. However, classical opioids do not binding to this receptor, and the endogenous ligand discovered for ORL-1 the peptide nociceptin or orphanin FQ (OFQ) causes actions which are different from that of the classical opioid peptides and which are not antagonized by naloxone. Nevertheless, based on the high degree of structural similarity nociceptin/ OFQ and the corresponding ORL-1 receptor are regarded to belong to the opioid systems.

▶ Analgesics
▶ Nociception
▶ Non-steroidal Anti-inflammatory Drugs

Basic Characteristics

During the last 25 years it became clear that there are three types of pharmacologically well-defined opioid receptors (μ, δ, κ) that belong to the hepta-helical group of G-protein-coupled receptors. The

Tab. 1   Opioid receptors and ligands.

Receptor subtype	μ (MOP)	δ (DOP)	κ (KOP)	ORL-1 (NOP)
Prototypic ligands	Morphine	Met/leu-enkephalin	Ethylketocyclacozine	Nociceptin/OFQ
Endogenous ligand	Endomorphin-1,-2	Met/leu-enkephalin	Dynorphin A	Nociceptin/OFQ
Selective agonists	DAMGO	DPDPE, D-ala^2-deltorphin II	Enadoline, U-50488	
Selective antagonists	(naloxone) CTAP	Naltrindole	Nor-binaltorphimine	J-113 397

genes of these receptors show a more than 60% homology to each other. A further "orphan" receptor sharing a similarly high degree of homology to the classical opioid receptors was recently identified and named ORL-1 ("opioid receptor like") (1; Table 1). The NC-IUPHAR Subcommittee on Opioid Receptors suggested the terms MOP for μ opioid, DOP for δ opioid, KOP for κ opioid and NOP for ORL-1 receptors (2).

The opioid receptors are targets of a large variety of exogenous (drugs) and endogenous ligands. Beginning with the discovery of the enkephalins in 1975, several endogenous opioid peptides have been isolated that derive from three precursor genes pro-opiomelanocortin (POMC), pro-enkephalin and prodynorphin (Table 2). β-endorphin derives from POMC. Besides in the pentapeptides met-enkephalin (ME) and leu-enkephalins (LE), proenkephalin is processed in the heptapeptide met-enkephalin-arg^6-phe^7 (MERF) and the octapeptide met-enkephalin-arg^6-gly^7-leu^8(MERGL). Prodynorphin is processed into dynorphin A, dynorphin A (1–8), dynorphin B, α-, β-neoendorphin (3). In addition, two endogenous pentapeptides have been isolated that exhibit a high selectivity for μ-opioid receptors and have been called endomorphin-1 and endomorphin-2. Attempts to clone the genes for the corresponding precursor molecules have not been successful.

The μ-opioid receptor (MOP) is the classical target for morphine and mediates the analgesic and addictive affects of the drug (3). Therefore, in MOP-deficient mice morphine does not exhibit analgesic and positive reinforcing properties (4). The human MOP gene encodes a heptahelical protein of about 400 amino acids and is localized on chromosome 6q24-25. Of the endogenous peptides, β-endorphin and to a lesser extent also the enkephalins and dynorphins have affinities for MOP. Endomorphin-1 and –2 are two pentapeptides that show the highest selectivity for this receptor. Another selective agonist is the synthetic peptide DAMGO (D-Ala^2, nMe-Phe^4, Gly^5-ol) enkephalin). The action of MOP agonists are competitively blocked by the antagonist naloxone, which is not absolutely specific for μ-opioid receptors. The somatostatin analogue CTAP (D-Phe-Cys-Thr-D-Trp-Arg-Thr-Pen-Thr-NH$_2$) has been found to be a more selective MOP antagonist. β-FNA (β-funaltrexamine) and naloxonazine are irreversible antagonists.

Several splice variants of MOP have been cloned (including MOP-A, -B, -C, -D, -E, -F) that differ in their amino acid sequence at the C-terminal end (5). These receptor variants differ in the rate of internalisation and desensitisation upon agonist exposure but have similar binding and coupling properties.

The existence of further alternative transcripts of MOP was postulated by the observation that in knockout mice with disrupted exon 1, heroin but not morphine was still analgesically active. Based on earlier observations that the antagonist naloxazone blocked morphine-induced antinociception but not morphine-induced respiratory depression, a subdivision of the μ-opioid receptor in μ_1 and $\mu_2$was proposed. However, no discrete mRNA for each of these μ-opioid receptor subtypes have been found. Highest concentrations of MOPs are found in the thalamus, caudate, neocortex in the brain, but the receptors are also present in gastrointestinal tract, immune cells and other peripheral tissues.

The δ opioid receptor (DOP) is the primary target for met- and leu-enkephalin which also exhibits affinities for μ and κ receptors (3). DPDPE

Tab. 2 Endogenous opioid peptides.

Proopiomelanocortin	Proenkephalin	Prodynorphin	Pronociceptin/OFQ	(Proendomorphin)
β-endorphin	Metenkephalin, leuenkephalin, MERF, MERGL	Dynorphin A, dynorphin A(1–8), dynorphin B, α-neoendorphin, β-neoendorphin	Nociceptin/OFQ	endomorphin-1, endomorphin-2

(D-Pen^2, D-Pen^5) enkephalin is a selective agonist, and naltrindole a selective antagonist on DOP. Only one DOP gene has been cloned to date. The human DOP is comprised of 372 amino acids and is localized on chromosome 1p34.3-36.1. Pharmacological experiments in rodents indicate the subdivision into δ_1 and δ_2 receptors (1). However, currently no genes encoding these δ receptor isoforms have been cloned. In addition, there is no evidence for the existence of splice variants of this receptor. A DOP that lacks the third intracellular loop was generated by atypical mRNA processing in human melanoma tissues. This atypically processed receptor did not couple to G-proteins.

A high concentration of DOPs are found in the olfactory bulb, the neocortex, caudate putamen and in the spinal cord, but they are also present in the gastrointestinal tract and other peripheral tissues. The functional roles of DOP are less clearly established than for MOP; they may have a role in analgesia, gastrointestinal motility, mood and behaviour as well as in cardiovascular regulation (3).

The κ opioid (KOP) receptor is the natural target for prodynorphin-derived peptides, such as dynorphin A, dynorphin B, α- neoendorphin etc. The prototypical ligand is ethylketocyclazocine. Enadoline and U-50488 are selective agonists and norbinaltorphimine is an irreversible selective antagonist (3). The human KOP gene encodes a protein of 380 amino acids which is localized on chromosome 8q11.12. From the binding characteristics of the prototypical ligand ethylketocyclazocine (EKC), evidence for the subdivisions in κ_1, κ_2 and κ_3 has been provided. However, there are no functional pharmacological data supporting this subdivisions. Moreover, no mRNAs coding for these receptor isoforms have been identified. Furthermore, in mice deficient in μ, δ and κ opioid receptors ("triple knockouts") no evidence for κ_2 binding sites could be found. A KOP with an alternative start site and with no known functional significance has been identified. High concentrations of KOP have been found in the cerebral cortex and hypothalamus; KOP is also present in the gastrointestinal tract, in immune cells as well as in other peripheral tissues. KOPs have been implicated in the regulation of nociception, diuresis, feeding, neuroendocrine and immune system functions (3).

The ORL-1 receptor was identified by its high homology to the other opioid receptor subtypes and termed "opioid receptor like" (1). However, none of the endogenous opioid peptides or the opiate drugs show a high affinity for this receptor. An endogenous ligand that binds to ORL-1 with high affinity has been identified and termed nociceptin or orphanin FQ (N/OFQ). Recently, J-113397, a drug with potent and selective antagonist activity at ORL-1 receptors, has been characterized.

According to the NC-IUPHAR Subcommittee on Opioid Receptors it was proposed to term ORL-1 receptor NOP receptor (2). The human NOP receptor gene encodes a protein of 370 peptide. Splice variants have been found in the human and mouse NOP receptor with no known functional significance. NOP receptors are widely distributed throughout the brain and in the spinal cord. They are also present in immune cells. A functional role for N/OFQ has been proposed in nociception, locomotoric activity, reward, stress and immunomodulation.

The OP group of receptors share common effector mechanisms. All receptors couple via pertussis toxin-sensitive Go and Gi proteins leading to: (1) inhibition of adenylate cyclase; (2) reduction of Ca^{2+} currents via diverse Ca^{2+} channels; (3) activation of inward rectifying K^+ channels. In

Tab. 3 Cellular responses to opioids.

Inhibition of adenylate cyclase	Activation of PLA$_2$
Inhibition of voltage operated potassium channels	Activation of PLCβ
	Activation of PLD$_2$
Activation of inwardly rectifying potassium channels	Activation of MAP kinase

addition, the majority of these receptors cause the activation of phospholipase A$_2$ (PLA$_2$), phospholipase Cβ (PLCβ), phospholipase D$_2$ and of MAP (mitogen-activated protein) kinase (Table 3).

In response to agonists, receptor desensitisation by phosphorylation leading to uncoupling as well as internalisation and recycling has been demonstrated for each receptor. β-Arrestin appears to play an important role in the development of morphine tolerance. Chronic administration of μ opioids has been shown to cause a superactivation of certain subtypes of adenylate cyclase. Long-term changes in adenylate cyclase activity results in activation of cAMP response element binding protein (CREB). This may result in changes in the expression of genes involved in opioid addiction.

In addition to the MOP, DOP, KOP and NOP receptors the existence of several other opioid receptors have been proposed. The σ receptor, originally classified as an opioid receptor, is no longer regarded as such, since naloxone does not act as an antagonist at this receptor. The σ receptor rather appears to be the target of phencyclidine and related drugs. A σ receptor that does not have the heptahelical structure of G protein coupled receptor has been recently cloned. A receptor with selective avidity for β-endorphin has been pro-

posed and termed ε receptor. In addition, a so-called λ receptor was postulated on the basis of binding experiments. Recently, a ζ opioid receptor was cloned that binds Met-enkephalin in a naloxone displaceable manner and is proposed to regulate cell growth. The relationship of the ζ receptor, which shares no sequence homology to the OP receptors, awaits elucidation.

There has been an extensive search for additional opioid receptor genes with homology to the μ, δ and κ receptors which was, however, unsuccessful. It is likely, therefore, that the functional properties of the subdivision of μ, δ and κ receptors as well as that of the ε and λ receptors results form alternate mRNA processing, post-translational modification of the receptor and/or from the formation of homo- and heterodimeric receptor complexes.

Drugs

Of the μ agonists (Table 3) morphine is the classical opioid alkaloid clinically used for treatment of pain. Undesirable effects of morphine such as respiratory depression, development of tolerance/dependence led to search for analogues. A first morphine derivative was diacetyl morphine (heroin) which, however, was soon shown to exhibit a higher addictive liability than morphine. Modification and simplification of the morphine structure lead to the development of drugs such as pethidine, methadone and piperidine derivates fentanyl (sufentanil, alfentanil). These opiates differ in their potencies and/or pharmakokinetics, but exhibit similar side effects than morphine. The long-acting methadone is a substitute for heroin in addicted patients. The short-acting and potent fentanyl derivatives are generally used during anesthesia. Other structural modifications lead to the development of the oripavine derivatives (e. g. etorphine and buprenorphine). Etorphine is much more potent than

Tab. 4 Opioid drugs

Agonists	Partial agonists	Antagonists
Alfentanil, dihydromorphine, etorphine, fentanyl, heroin, hydromorphone, levomethadone, morphine, oxymorphone, pethidine, piritramide, remifentanil, sufentanil, tilidine, tramadol	Buprenorphine, pentazocine	Naloxone, naltrexone

morphine and its catatonic action is used for sedating large animals. Buprenorphine is a long-acting partial agonist at μ opioid receptors which shows a ceiling effect. As compared to pure agonists partial agonists posses a lower addiction liability. The μ opioid antagonists (naloxone and naltrexone) are clinically used for treatment of heroin overdose.

κ receptor agonists produce a powerful antinociceptive effect and do not substitute for morphine in dependent animals. In addition, κ receptor agonists have neuroprotective effects in animal models of cerebral ischemia and traumatic head injury. However, clinical trials using κ agonists such as enadoline unmasked the dysphoric and psychotropic side effects of these drugs in humans. Clinical trials are presently being carried out to explore whether κ agonists that do not readily penetrate the blood brain barrier are useful in producing a peripheral analgesic effect in inflammatory pain.

Although preclinical studies suggest that δ agonists are potent analgesics with less side effects than μ agonists, none of the non-peptide agonists or antagonists have been introduced into clinical investigations. Similarly, the clinical perspectives of the use of agonists and antagonists on the ORL-1 (NOP) receptor have to wait the outcome of clinical trials. The recently discovered nonpeptide antagonist J-113397 is a promising candidate.

References

1. Corbett A, McKnight S, Henderson G (2000) Opioid receptors. (www.tocris.com).
2. Cox BM et al. (2000) Opioid receptors. NC-Iuphar Subcommittee on Opioid Receptors.
3. Herz A (1993) Opioids I, II. Handbook of Experimental Pharmacology, Springer, Heidelberg.
4. Kieffer BL (1999) Opioids; first lessons from knock-out mice. Trends in Pharmacol Sci 20:19–26
5. Pasternak GW (2001) Incomplete cross tolerance and multiple μ opioid peptide receptors. Trends in Pharmacol Sci 22:67–70

Opium

Opium is an extract of the juice of the poppy *Papaver somniferum*, which contains more than 20 distinct alkaloids, including morphine, codeine and papaverine.

▶ Opioid System

Oral Anticoagulants

▶ Anticoagulants

Oral Antidiabetic Drugs

CLIFFORD J BAILEY
Aston University, Birmingham, UK
c.j.bailey@aston.ac.uk

Synonyms

Oral hypoglycaemic agents; oral blood glucose-lowering drugs; insulin secretagogues; antihyperglycaemics.

Definition

Oral antidiabetic drugs are used to treat hyperglycaemia in type 2 (non-insulin-dependent) diabetes mellitus. They are used in conjunction with non-pharmacological interventions involving diet, exercise and health education. The classes of oral antidiabetic drugs are sulphonylureas, prandial insulin releasers (also termed meglitinides), the biguanide metformin, thiazolidinediones and α-glucosidase inhibitors (Table 1).

▶ ATP-dependent K$^+$ Channel
▶ Diabetes Mellitus

Mechanism of Action

Type 2 diabetes is a heterogeneous and progressive endocrine disorder associated with insulin resistance (impaired insulin action) and defective function of the insulin-secreting β-cells in the pancreatic islets of Langerhans. These endocrine disorders give rise to widespread metabolic

Tab. 1   Classes of oral antidiabetic drugs and their main mechanisms of action.

Class	Examples[a]	Main Mechanism of Action
Sulphonylureas	Chlorpropamide, glibenclamide[b], gliclazide, glimepiride, glipizide, gliquidone, tolazamide, tolbutamide	Stimulate insulin secretion (typically 6–24 h)
Prandial insulin releasers (meglitinides)	Repaglinide, nateglinide	Stimulate insulin secretion (rapid and short acting < 6 h)
Biguanide	Metformin	Improve insulin action
Thiazolidinediones	Pioglitazone, rosiglitazone	Improve insulin action (PPARγ agonists)
Alpha-glucosidase inhibitors	Acarbose, miglitol, voglibose	Slow rate of carbohydrate digestion

[a]Availability of agents and prescribing instructions vary between countries
[b]Glibenclamide is called glyburide in some countries

disturbances epitomized by hyperglycaemia. The five classes of oral antidiabetic agents act to either increase insulin secretion, improve insulin action or slow the rate of intestinal carbohydrate digestion.

Sulphonylureas

The first sulphonylureas were introduced in the 1950s. They stimulate insulin secretion by a direct effect on pancreatic β-cells. Sulphonylureas enter the β-cell and bind to a site at the cytosolic face of the sulphonylurea receptor (SUR). The SUR-1 isoform is expressed by the β-cell. It forms part of a transmembranal complex that includes ATP-sensitive Kir6.2 potassium efflux channels (K-ATP channels). The binding of a sulphonylurea to SUR-1 produces a conformational change that closes K-ATP channels, favouring local depolarisation of the plasma membrane. This opens voltage-dependent L-type calcium channels, increasing calcium influx and raising the cytosolic free calcium concentration. In turn, this activates calcium-dependent signalling proteins controlling the contractile activities of microtubules and microfilaments that mediate exocytosis of insulin granules. Pre-formed insulin granules adjacent to the plasma membrane are released first (first-phase insulin release). Newly formed granules contribute to the secretory pool within one hour of continued stimulation. Increased insulin release is sustained as long as drug stimulation is maintained, provided the β-cells are functionally competent (Fig. 1).

The SUR-Kir6.2 complex is a non-covalently bonded octamer (4 x SUR/4 x Kir6.2), with the pore-forming Kir6.2 channels located at the centre (Fig. 2). SUR molecules are members of the ATP binding cassette proteins (ABC proteins). Each SUR-1 molecule comprises 17 transmembrane domains, 2 cytosolic nucleotide binding domains and cytosolic binding domains for sulphonylurea, benzamido and other ligands. The Kir6.2 channel also has cytosolic binding regions, including one for ADP/ATP. Sulphonylureas bind to the sulphonylurea site with high affinity (eg. Ki for glibenclamide in low nanomolar range), being dependent on a 'U' shape to the ligand with 5.5 Å between the hydrophobic rings.

By closing K-ATP channels, sulphonylureas induce insulin release by activating a step along the normal pathway of glucose-induced insulin secretion. Activation of insulin secretion is therefore independent of glucose, provided there is sufficient glucose metabolism to stimulate proinsulin biosynthesis and service the energy requirements for the cellular processing and exocytosis of insulin. Hence sulphonylureas can stimulate insulin secretion at low glucose concentrations, creating the risk of hypoglycaemia. Sulphonylureas will also increase the amount of insulin secreted at any level of stimulation by glucose, subject to adequate β-cell function. Additionally, sulphonylureas may potentiate insulin release that is stimulated by glucose and other nutrients. This may involve SUR

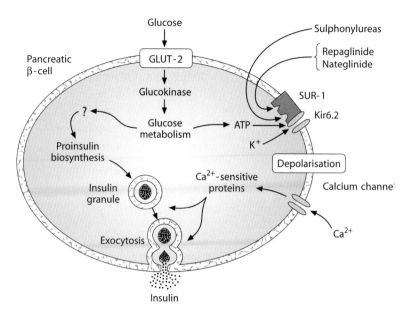

Fig. 1 Sulphonylureas stimulate insulin release by pancreatic β-cells. They bind to the sulphonylurea receptor (SUR-1), which closes Kir6.2 (ATP-sensitive) potassium channels. This promotes depolarisation, voltage-dependent calcium influx, and activation of calcium-sensitive proteins that control exocytotic release of insulin.

molecules located within the membranes of insulin granules and activation of certain isoforms of protein kinase C.

Although the main therapeutic effect of sulphonylureas is increased insulin secretion, there is evidence that these drugs exert weak extra-pancreatic effects. The latter effects include suppression of hepatic gluconeogenesis, possibly by suppression of a kinase which leads to increased formation of fructose-2, 6-bisphosphate. This stimulates phosphofructokinase and suppresses fructose-1, 6-bisphosphatase, thereby increasing glycolytic flux and suppressing gluconeogenic flux. Sulphonylureas might also enhance insulin-stimulated glucose transport by increasing translocation of GLUT-4 glucose transporters to the plasma membrane in adipocytes and muscle. However, these effects appear to require supra-therapeutic concentrations of sulphonylureas and are probably not therapeutically relevant. Sulphonylureas have been reported to reduce the hepatic extraction of insulin and to act on pancreatic A-cells to transiently stimulate and then suppress glucagon secretion.

The increase in insulin concentrations produced by sulphonylureas lowers blood glucose concentrations through decreased hepatic glucose output and increased glucose utilization, mostly by muscle (▶ insulin, ▶ insulin receptor).

Prandial Insulin Releasers (Meglitinides)

This class comprises the meglitinide analogue repaglinide and the structurally related D-phenylalanine analogue nateglinide. These recently introduced agents have a benzamido group that binds to a site on SUR-1 that is distinct from the sulphonylurea site, but probably in close proximity and capable of binding interference. Some sulphonylureas also have a benzamido moiety (eg. glibenclamide, glimepiride, glipizide) but the binding affinity for the sulphonylurea site has a higher affinity. Binding of repaglinide or nateglinide to the benzamido site closes the K-ATP channels and induces insulin secretion via the same pathway described for sulphonylureas.

Repaglinide and nateglinide are rapidly absorbed; their binding durations to SUR-1 are much shorter than sulphonylurea binding, and their hepatic metabolism and subsequent elimina-

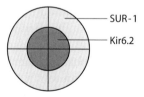

Fig. 2 Octameric structure (4 x SUR/4 x Kir6.2) of the SUR-Kir6.2 complex.

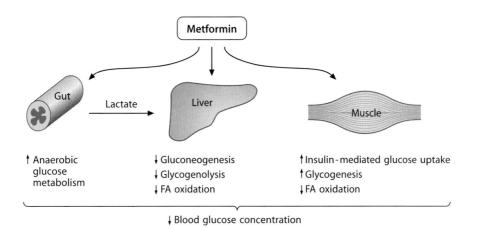

Fig. 3 The antihyperglycaemic effect of metformin involves enhanced insulin-mediated suppression of hepatic glucose production and muscle glucose uptake. Metformin also exerts non-insulin dependent effects on these tissues, including reduced fatty acid oxidation and increased anaerobic glucose metabolism by the intestine. FA, fatty acid; ↑, increase; ↓ decrease.

tion are faster. Consequently, repaglinide and nateglinide are faster-acting and shorter-acting insulin releasers than sulphonylureas. They can be taken immediately before a meal, and quickly stimulate insulin secretion to coincide approximately with the period of meal digestion, hence the categorization of 'prandial insulin releasers'.

Biguanide
Metformin is the main compound in this class, introduced in the late 1950s. Other biguanides, namely phenformin and buformin have been widely discontinued. The antihyperglycaemic effect of metformin results partly from a direct improvement of insulin action and partly from actions that are not directly insulin dependent. A presence of insulin is required for the therapeutic efficacy of metformin, but the drug does not stimulate insulin release and is often associated with a small decrease in basal insulin concentrations in hyperinsulinaemic patients. Metformin has a variety of metabolic effects: The main antihyperglycaemic actions involve a reduction of excess hepatic glucose production, increased insulin-mediated glucose utilization predominantly by muscle, decreased fatty acid oxidation and increased splanchnic glucose turnover.

Metformin restrains hepatic glucose production principally by suppression of gluconeogene-sis. The mechanisms involve potentiation of insulin action and decreased hepatic extraction of certain gluconeogenic substrates such as lactate. In addition, metformin reduces the rate of hepatic glycogenolysis and decreases the activity of hepatic glucose-6-phosphatase. Insulin-stimulated glucose uptake and glycogenesis by skeletal muscle is increased by metformin mainly by increased movement of insulin-sensitive glucose transporters (GLUT-4) into the plasma membrane. Metformin also appears to increase the transport function of glucose transporters and increases the activity of glycogen synthase. Further actions of metformin include insulin-independent suppression of fatty acid oxidation in liver and muscle, and insulin-independent increase in anaerobic glucose metabolism by the intestine. Lactate produced in this way is recycled to glucose by the liver. Thus metformin acts to a modest extent via several different effects to lower blood glucose concentrations (Fig. 3).

At a cellular level metformin improves insulin sensitivity by increasing insulin-stimulated tyrosine kinase activity of the β-subunit of the insulin receptor. Metformin also increases insulin signalling at more distal steps in the post-receptor cascades. Although metformin can increase insulin receptor binding when insulin receptor numbers are depleted, this does not appear to have a signifi-

O

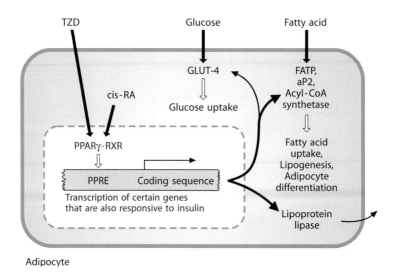

Adipocyte

Fig. 4 Thiazolidinediones stimulate the PPARγ moiety of the PPARγ-RXR nuclear receptor complex, which then binds to a response element, leading to transcription of certain genes that are also responsive to insulin. These facilitate increased uptake of fatty acids, lipogenesis and adipogenesis. PPARγ, peroxisome proliferator-activated receptor-γ; RXR, retinoid X receptor; PPRE, p,eroxisome proliferator response element; TZD, thiazolidinedione; *cis*-RA, *cis*-retinoic acid; GLUT-4, glucose transporter isoform-4; FATP, fatty acid transporter protein; aP2, adipocyte fatty acid binding protein.

cant impact on insulin action. The mediating steps that enable metformin to interface with insulin signalling pathways are not resolved. Metformin has been shown to alter membrane fluidity in hyperglycaemic states and to alter the activities of some metabolic enzymes (listed above), apparently independently of insulin. Very high concentrations of metformin that occur in the intestine could increase anaerobic glucose metabolism by suppression of the respiratory chain at complex I.

Thiazolidinediones

Two thiazolidinediones (TZDs) introduced in 1999 are presently available, pioglitazone and rosiglitazone. Another TZD, troglitazone has been withdrawn. TZDs improve insulin sensitivity and their principal mechanism of action is stimulation of the nuclear receptor peroxisome proliferator-activated receptor-γ (PPARγ). PPARγ is a member of the nuclear receptor superfamily for retinoid, steroid and thyroid hormones. PPARγ exists as a heterodimer with the retinoid X receptor (RXR). Binding of a TZD to PPARγ together with binding of *cis*-retinoic acid to the RXR moiety produces a

conformational change that prompts dissociation of co-repressors. The activated heterodimer then binds to the peroxisome proliferator response element (PPRE), which is a sequence (AGGTCAXAG-GTCA) located in the promoter region of the responsive genes. Recruitment of co-activators including PGC-1 and assembly of the RNA polymerase complex follows, initiating transcription (Fig. 4). Many of the responsive genes are also activated by insulin, hence the ability of TZDs to improve insulin sensitivity.

PPARγ is strongly expressed in adipocytes, and stimulation by TZDs promotes adipogenesis, predominantly in pre-adipocytes from subcutaneous depots. Increased transcription of transporters and enzymes involved in fatty acid uptake and lipogenesis increases the deposition of lipid in the adipocytes (Table 2). This appears to facilitate a reduction in hyperglycaemia by reducing circulating concentrations of non-esterified (free) fatty acids and triglycerides. The consequent effect on the glucose-fatty acid (Randle) cycle is to reduce the availability of fatty acids as an energy source, thereby favouring the utilization of glucose. Addi-

Tab. 2 Tissue expression, ligands, genes activated, and biological actions of the peroxisome proliferator-activated receptor-γ (PPARγ).

Tissue expression	Mainly white and brown adipose tissue; weak expression in liver, muscle, gut, macrophages, pancreatic β-cells and haemopoietic tissues
Natural ligands	Certain unsaturated fatty acids and prostaglandin metabolites
Synthetic ligands	Thiazolidinediones and some non-steroidal anti-inflammatory drugs
Gene activated	Lipoprotein lipase; fatty acid transporter protein; adipocyte fatty acid binding protein; acyl-CoA synthetase; malic enzyme; GLUT-4 glucose transporter; phosphoenolpyruvate carboxykinase
Biological actions	Adipocyte differentiation; fatty acid uptake; lipogenesis; glucose uptake; other effects on nutrient metabolism which lower hepatic glucose production

tionally, TZDs increase transcription of GLUT-4 glucose transporters that directly facilitates glucose uptake. Reducing free fatty acid concentrations also reduces the production of lipid metabolites, which suppress early postreceptor steps in the insulin-signalling pathway. TZDs may further improve insulin signalling by decreasing production of the adipocyte cytokine tumour necrosis factor-α (TNFα) and the adipocyte hormone resistin (and possibly leptin), which have been implicated in the pathogenesis of insulin resistance.

There is weak expression of PPARγ in muscle, liver and other tissues, enabling TZDs to support the effects of insulin in these tissues, notably increased glucose uptake in muscle and reduced glucose production in liver. TZDs may also affect nutrient metabolism by skeletal muscle through a direct mitochondrial action that is independent of PPARγ.

α-Glucosidase Inhibitors

The first member of this class, acarbose, was introduced in the early 1990s. α-Glucosidase inhibitors slow the intestinal process of carbohydrate digestion by competitive inhibition of the activity of α-glucosidase enzymes located in the brush border of the enterocytes (Fig. 5). Acarbose also causes a modest inhibition of pancreatic α-amylase activity. The principal α-glucosidase enzymes are glucoamylase, sucrase, maltase and dextrinase. The inhibitors bind to these enzymes with much higher affinity than their natural disaccharide and oligosaccharide substrates. Hence, when bound to the inhibitor, the enzyme fails to cleave the disaccharides and oligosaccharides into their absorbable monosaccharides. The available α-glucosidase inhibitors, acarbose, miglitol and voglibose, show different binding affinities for the enzymes, giving them different activity profiles. For example, the affinity profile of acarbose is glycoamylase > sucrase > maltase > dextrinase. Miglitol is a more potent inhibitor of sucrase, and voglibose of other α-glucosidases.

When α-glucosidase activity is inhibited, carbohydrate digestion is prolonged and takes place further along the intestinal tract. This in turn delays and spreads the period of glucose absorption, which reduces the extent of the postprandial rise in blood glucose concentrations. The effectiveness of α-glucosidase inhibitors is dependent on the consumption of a meal rich in complex carbohydrate.

Clinical Use

Type 2 (non-insulin-dependent) diabetes typically emerges in middle or later life. Unlike type 1 diabetes in which there is total loss of pancreatic β-cells and a critical need for exogenous insulin administration, type 2 diabetes is associated with a continued presence of β-cells and continued insulin production. However insulin resistance usually develops as a prelude to type 2 diabetes and creates a demand for a compensatory increase in insulin secretion. Eventually, the β-cells are unable to produce sufficient extra insulin to overcome the insulin resistance. This results in impaired insulin-

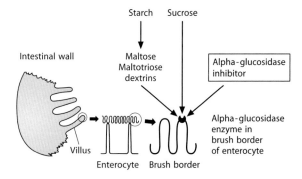

Fig. 5 α-Glucosidase inhibitors slow the rate of intestinal carbohydrate digestion by competitive inhibition of α-glucosidase enzymes in the brush border of enterocytes. The α-glucosidase inhibitors have a higher affinity for the α-glucosidase enzymes than the natural disaccharide and oligosaccharide substrates.

mediated glucose uptake by muscle, failure of insulin to suppress hepatic glucose production and consequently hyperglycaemia. Pancreatic β-cells of type 2 diabetic patients become increasingly sluggish in their responsiveness to raised glucose concentrations, and eventually β-cell function becomes severely impaired, leading to a state of hypoinsulinaemia and greater hyperglycaemia. The toxic effects of hyperglycaemia on the permeability of small blood vessels and nerve function result in the long-term microvascular and neuropathic complications of diabetes (retinopathy, nephropathy and neuropathy). The additional effects of other metabolic disturbances associated with insulin resistance (the so-called metabolic syndrome) are largely responsible for the long-term cardiovascular complications of type 2 diabetes.

Achieving and maintaining blood glucose concentrations as close to normal as possible reduces the morbidity and premature mortality of the long-term complications of type 2 diabetes. All treatments begin with non-pharmacological measures (diet, exercise and healthy living), but compliance is limited, and lasting glycaemic control occurs in only a small minority of patients. Patients are usually started on one oral antidiabetic drug. Recent studies suggest that metformin offers additional advantages beyond glycaemic control to reduce long-term cardiovascular complications. Thus, this is often the first oral agent to be used. The mecha-

nisms of action of metformin also prevent weight gain and avoid overswings into hypoglycaemia. Alternatively, a sulphonylurea or prandial insulin releaser may be favoured as the first oral antidiabetic agent if substantial β-cell failure is suspected. The prandial insulin releaser would be preferred for individuals with either mainly postprandial hyperglycaemia or irregular meal patterns which predispose to interprandial hypoglycaemia when taking a sulphonylurea. An α-glucosidase inhibitor can be used if the hyperglycaemia is modest and predominantly restricted to postprandial periods. The newly available thiazolidinediones are slower to take effect than other agents, presumably due to their largely genomic mode of action. At this time they are used a first-line therapy outside of Europe. However, in Europe the thiazolidinediones and nateglinide are presently recommended as second-line agents to be used in combination with another differently acting agent, when that agent alone does not achieve glycaemic control.

Type 2 diabetes is a progressive disease with continued insulin resistance and gradually declining β-cell function. Thus, hyperglycaemia increases with disease duration and glycaemic control becomes ever more difficult to maintain. If two or possibly three differently acting oral antidiabetic agents do not achieve glycaemic control then it is apposite to switch to insulin therapy (insulin, insulin receptor).

The main limitations and precautions for the use of oral antidiabetic drugs are listed in Table 3.

Hb, haemoglobin; Vit B12, vitamin B12; LFT, liver function test.

a) The dosage of each antidiabetic drug should be increased until either the target level of glycaemia is achieved or the last dosage increment produces no additional effect.

b) Appropriate monitoring of glycaemic control using fasting or random blood glucose, glycated haemoglobin (HbA1c) or fructosamine (glycated albumin) should be undertaken for all patients receiving oral antidiabetic drugs.

c) Depending upon pathways of metabolism and elimination of individual members of the class.

d) Prandial insulin releasers are less likely to produce severe or prolonged episodes of hypoglycaemia than sulphonylureas.

e) Liver function should be checked in patients on high dose acarbose.

Tab. 3 Main exclusions, adverse events and precautionary monitoring required for clinical use of oral anti-diabetic drugs.

Class[a]	Main exclusions	Main adverse events	Monitoring[b]
Sulphonylureas	Severe liver or renal disease[c]	Hypoglycaemia	--[b]
Prandial insulin releasers	Severe liver or renal disease[c]	Hypoglycaemia[d]	--[b]
Metformin	Renal or liver disease; any predisposition to hypoxia	Gastro intestinal upsets; risk of lactic acidosis if wrongly prescribed	Creatinine, Hb or Vit B12[b]
Thiazolidinediones	Cardiac failure; liver disease	Oedema, anaemia	LFT[b]
α-glucosidase inhibitors	Chronic intestinal disease	Gastrointestinal upsets	LFT[b, e]

Hb, haemoglobin; Vit B12, vitamin B12; LFT, liver function test.

References

1. Bailey CJ (2000) Antidiabetic drugs. Brit. J. Cardiol. 7:350–360
2. DeFronzo RA (1999) Pharmacologic therapy for type 2 diabetes mellitus. Ann. Intern. Med. 131:281–303
3. Lebovitz HE (1999) Insulin secretagogues; old and new. Diabetes Revs. 7:139–153
4. Bailey CJ (2000) Potential new treatments for type 2 diabetes. Trends in Pharmacol. Sci. 21:259–265
5. Lebovitz HE (1998) α-Glucosidase inhibitors as agents in the treatment of diabetes. Diabetes Revs. 6:132–145
6. Bailey CJ, Day C (2001) Thiazolidinediones today. Brit. J. Diab. Vasc. Dis 1:7–13
7. Wiernsperger NF, Bailey CJ (1999) The antihyperglycaemic effect of metformin: therapeutic and cellular mechanisms. Drugs 58: suppl 1, 30–39
8. Ashcroft FM, Gribble FM (1999) ATP-sensitive K+ channels and insulin secretion: their role in health and disease. Diabetologia 42:903–919
9. Murphy GJ, Holder JC (2000) PPAR-γ agonists: therapeutic role in diabetes, inflammation and cancer. Trends in Pharmacol. Sci. 21:469–474

Oral Contraceptives

▶ Contraceptives

Orexins

O

Orexin A and orexin B (also known as hypocretins) are two hypothalamic neuropeptides derived from the same precursor by proteolytic processing. When injected into cerebral ventricles of rats, orexin A and orexin B stimulate food consumption. Inactivating mutations of orexins or the orexin receptor HCRTR2 cause narcolepsy in mice and dogs. Orexins act through high-affinity ▶ G-protein-coupled receptors.

▶ Appetite Control

Organic Cations

Organic cations are compounds that meet the two criteria of a single positive charge (no negative charge) and a significant degree of hydrophobicity (alkyl chains or aromatic rings, little capacity to form hydrogen bonds). Typical examples are tetraethylammonium (TEA), N^1-methylnicotinamide (NMN), and MPP^+.

▶ Organic Cation Transporters (OCT)

Organic Cation Transporters

DIRK GRÜNDEMANN, EDGAR SCHÖMIG
Department of Pharmacology,
University of Cologne, Cologne, Germany
dirk.gruendemann@uni-koeln.de,
edgar.schoemig@medizin.uni-koeln.de

Synonyms

Non-neuronal monoamine transporters

Definition

Cellular membranes are virtually impenetrable to charged organic compounds, so dedicated integral membrane proteins must be present to allow passage of a variety of endogenous organic compounds and drugs. Transport of ▶ organic cations across cellular membranes was first identified in the kidney. The proximal tubule efficiently clears model compounds like TEA and N^1-methylnicotinamide (see Fig. 1) from the blood by trans-epithelial secretion into urine. Secretion of organic cations is thought to serve in the elimination or detoxification of metabolites and xenobiotics (such as many drugs positively charged at physiological pH). The term "organic cation transporters" (OCT) originally refers to two distinct mechanisms identified and characterized by radiotracer experiments on membrane vesicles, isolated tubules, and tissue slices from various species such as dog, rat, rabbit, flounder, snake and human. At the basolateral (also called contraluminal or peritubular) membrane of proximal tubular cells, an electrogenic mechanism enhanced by the membrane potential (inside negative) facilitates entry of organic cations into the cytosol. At the brush border (also called luminal or apical) membrane, an organic cation/H^+ antiport mechanism allows electroneutral exit of organic cations in exchange for protons. Transport mechanisms with similar functional characteristics were also detected in other organs such as liver, intestine and choroid plexus, and in cell lines such as LLC-PK_1 (derived from pig kidney) and OK (opossum kidney). In addition, released monoamine neurotransmitters such as noradrenaline and 5-hydroxytryptamine are removed from the extracellular space into non-neuronal cells by a transport mechanism that

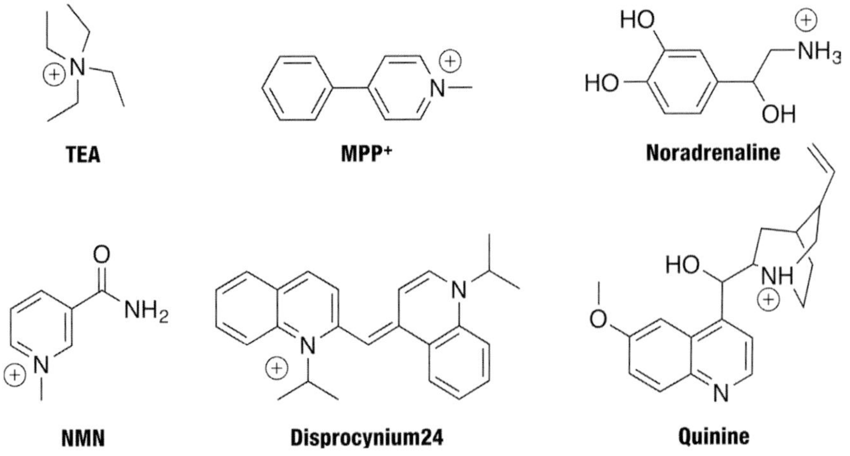

Fig. 1 Structures of some organic cations. TEA: tetraethylammonium; MPP^+: 1-methyl-4-phenylpyridinium; NMN: N^1-methylnicotinamide.

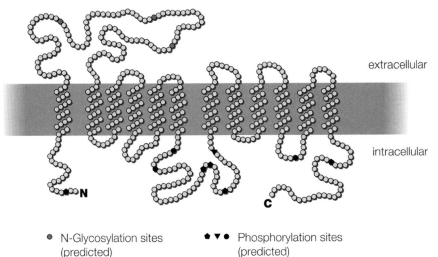

Fig. 2 Predicted membrane topology of EMT from human. Each symbol represents an amino acid. The model, based on hydropathy analysis, suggests a protein that contains, embedded within the membrane (gray bar), 12 transmembrane segments (probably α-helices as indicated).

extracellular

intracellular

• N-Glycosylation sites (predicted)

● ▼ • Phosphorylation sites (predicted)

pharmacologically resembles renal transport of organic cations.

In 1994, the first organic cation transporter, OCT1 from rat kidney, was cloned by functional expression in *Xenopus laevis* oocytes (1). Based on the amino acid sequence information of OCT1, two related transporters, OCT2 and EMT, were identified later by nucleic acid similarity cloning strategies.

▶ Neurotransmitter Transporters
▶ Vesicular Transporters

Basic Characteristics

Hydropathy analysis suggests that OCT1, OCT2 and EMT are integral membrane proteins. The predicted membrane topology of EMT from human, representative also of OCT1 and OCT2, is shown in Fig. 2. All carriers are around 555 amino acids long, which translates into 61 kD. Characteristic features are 12 predicted α-helical transmembrane segments, a large extracellular loop with multiple potential N-glycosylation sites between transmembrane segments 1 and 2, and multiple potential intracellular phosphorylation sites. There is some experimental evidence that phosphorylation may regulate transport activity of OCT1 and EMT. Both N- and C-terminus are exposed to the cytosol. Sequence analysis revealed corresponding amino acid motifs in the first and second half of the transporters, which suggests

that during evolution duplication of a primordial protein with only 6 transmembrane segments has occured.

EMT corresponds to the classical steroid-sensitive extraneuronal monoamine transport mechanism, first identified as "uptake$_2$" in rat heart, for noradrenaline and other monoamine transmitters such as histamine and 5-HT (Fig. 3) (2). It is clear, however, that OCT1 and OCT2 transport, e.g. noradrenaline and adrenaline, with an efficiency similar to EMT and may thus contribute to inactivation of released monoamine transmitters *in vivo*. Therefore, by reference to localization, these three transporters have been termed ▶ non-neuronal monoamine transporters. EMT from rat has also been called "OCT3". However, EMT from human does not accept typical organic cations such as TEA, guanidinium, creatinine and choline as substrates. Also, as indicated in Fig. 4, evolutionary distances (human amino acid sequences) of EMT to OCT1 (50% identity, 70% similarity) and OCT2 (50%, 73%) are considerably greater than between OCT1 and OCT2 (70%, 84%). Thus, the preferred and well established designation is extraneuronal monoamine transporter, EMT.

The non-neuronal monoamine transporters are part of the ▶ ASF family of transporters (gene symbol group *SLC22*, see Fig. 4), which in addition contains transporters for organic anions (OAT1–6), for zwitterions (OCTN1–3) and for unidentified substrates (RST1, UST1) (3). The ASF family itself is contained within the major facilita-

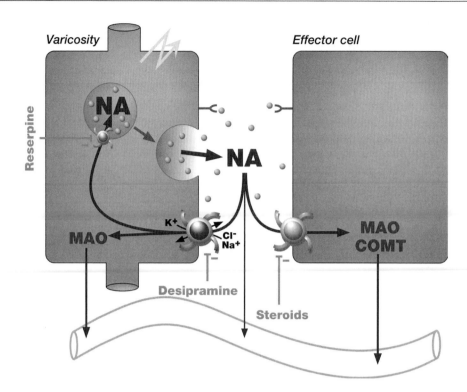

Fig. 3 Neuronal and extraneuronal transport mechanisms for noradrenaline (NA). The cartoon depicts noradrenaline-based signal transduction at a peripheral sympathetic synapse, e.g. in the heart. After release from its storage vesicles, noradrenaline stimulates pre- and postsynaptic adrenoceptors. This signal is terminated and thus controlled by two completely different transport mechanisms, originally called uptake$_1$ and uptake$_2$, which are located in neuronal (left) and non-neuronal (right) cells, respectively. Specific inhibitors are indicated. After carrier-mediated uptake, the transmitter is metabolized intracellularly (MAO, COMT) or transported into storage vesicles via the reserpin-sensitive vesicular monoamine transporter (VMAT).

tor superfamily (MFS). OCTN1, OCTN2 and OCTN3 have also been considered to represent organic cation transporters. However, the transport of, for example, TEA seems to be marginal with these carriers. Instead, the zwitterion carnitine is a relevant and specific substrate of OCTN2. Another transporter clearly involved in the phenomenon of organic cation transport is the multidrug resistance (MDR) efflux pump P-glycoprotein.

The genes of OCT1, OCT2, and EMT cluster closely together in a conserved region, on chromosome 6 in human (6q26–27) and on chromosome 17 in mouse. The precise order in the direction from telomer to centromer is IGF2R - OCT1 - OCT2 - EMT - APO(α)-similar gene - APO(α). This, together with the similarity of amino acid

sequences, suggests a common evolutionary origin, i.e. OCT1, OCT2 and EMT are descendants from a single gene. The intron exon structures of all three human genes have been elucidated. By contrast to OCT1 and OCT2, core promoter and exon 1 of EMT are part of a CpG island (i.e. a region with high content of guanine and cytosine bases and clustering of CpG dinucleotides).

▶ **Heterologous expression** in mammalian cell lines and oocytes from *Xenopus laevis* and subsequent functional characterization mostly with radiolabeled solutes has revealed that OCT1, OCT2 and EMT share some fundamental functional features: (i) ▶ MPP$^+$ is one of the best substrates for all, irrespective of species, in terms of transport efficiency. In general, a single positive charge is required on substrates, uncharged or doubly

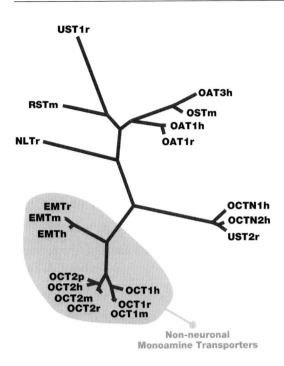

UST1r

OAT3h
RSTm
OSTm
OAT1h
NLTr
OAT1r

EMTr
OCTN1h
EMTm
OCTN2h
EMTh
UST2r

OCT2p
OCT2h
OCT2m   OCT1h
OCT2r   OCT1r
OCT1m

Non-neuronal
Monoamine Transporters

Fig. 4 Evolutionary tree of the ASF family of transport proteins. h, m, p, and r in conjunction with a protein name designate the species as being human, mouse, pig, or rat, respectively. The greater the sum of lengths of connective branches, the greater two transporters differ in amino acid sequences.

charged solutes are not transported. Since the non-neuronal monoamine transporters may be inhibited by a multitude of cationic compounds with a wide variety of structures, they have been called multispecific or polyspecific by some authors (4). It must be stressed, however, that it is not possible to judge from inhibition experiments whether a compound is actually transported. Thus, in comparison with other carriers e.g. for sugars or amino acids, it is probably more appropriate to attest a broad, but clear cut specificity with the focus on monoamine transmitters like adrenaline, noradrenaline, dopamine, tyramine, histamine, 5-HT, some derivatives like MPP^+ and cimetidine, and some smaller compounds such as TEA and guanidine. This broad spectrum resembles that of the vesicular monoamine transporters. (ii) Dependence of transport activity on membrane potential and pH is virtually identical, at least in heterologous expression systems with

intact cells. Decrease of extracellular pH and depolarization of membrane independently reduce velocity of uptake. Transport is independent of inorganic ion gradients of Na^+ and Cl^-. (iii) It has been shown by *trans*-stimulation that all three proteins are transporters, not just channels. Transport works in both directions (uptake and efflux). Thus, depending on substrate gradients across the cell membrane, OCT1, OCT2 and EMT may mediate electrogenic uniport of a substrate or electroneutral exchange of two substrates (antiport). (iv) Some compounds like quinine or mepiperphenidol inhibit all three carriers with similar potency.

However, the three non-neuronal monoamine transporters are not just redundant isoenzymes with marginal differences: (i) Localization differs widely; although knowledge is incomplete and sometimes inconsistent, marked differences are certain. OCT1 is expressed primarily in liver, and in rodents also strongly in kidney and intestine. OCT2 is strongly and almost exclusively expressed in the renal proximal tubule (S3 segment) and weakly in the brain. By contrast, EMT is expressed with substantial species differences in many but not all tissues. Expression levels vary widely between organs and during organ development (e.g. in placenta). Consistently high expression has been reported for placenta and heart. (ii) There are plain differences in substrate specificity (5). In contrast to OCT1 and OCT2, EMT does not transport TEA efficiently. Guanidinium and some derivatives like cimetidine or creatinine are particularly good substrates of OCT2. OCT1 alone does not accept histamine as a substrate, but accepts choline as a good substrate. (iii) Pharmacological characterization has revealed significant differences in sensitivity to inhibitors. OCT1 is relatively resistant to some steroids (such as 17β-estradiol and testosterone) and cyanine inhibitors, which are potent inhibitors of OCT2 and EMT. TEA inhibits OCT2 and OCT1 much better than EMT, but O-methylisoprenaline is more effective on EMT than on OCT1 and OCT2.

The physiological and pathophysiological significance of the non-neuronal monamine transporters remains to be fully resolved. Apart from the elimination of metabolites and xenobiotics, a role in monoamine transmitter inactivation seems likely.

O

Additional details for individual carriers are as follows:

- OCT1: gene symbol SLC22A1; cloned from human, rat, mouse and rabbit. Transported substrates include TEA, MPP+, dopamine, noradrenaline, adrenaline, tyramine, 5-HT and choline (radiotracer flux). There is indirect evidence (trans-stimulation or electric currents) that other short chain tetraalkylammonia compounds (with species differences) and procainamide are also transported. A fluorescent substrate is available. Quinine is not transported. Tissue distribution of OCT1 is narrow, with clear expression in liver, kidney, intestine and colon (OCT1 from rat); OCT1 from human and rabbit is absent from kidney and brain. There is unequivocal evidence that OCT1 from rat is located at the basolateral membrane in renal proximal tubule (S1 and S2 segments). By analogy, it is probably sorted to the sinusoidal membrane of hepatocytes. Cell lines expressing OCT1 are Fao (rat) and Caco-2 (human). A knock-out is available, as well as an antibody. Potent inhibitors include disprocynium24 (Ki = 100 nmol/l) and cyanine863.

- OCT2: gene symbol SLC22A2; cloned from rat, pig, mouse and human. Note that the sequence first published for rat contains an artifactual C-terminus. Most functional analyses have been performed with this erroneous clone. Radiolabeled substrates include TEA, MPP+, dopamine, noradrenaline, adrenaline, tyramine, 5-HT, histamine, cimetidine, propranolol and memantine; there is indirect evidence (intracellular pH-change or electric current) for metoprolol and amantadin. The zwitterion levofloxacin is not transported. Tissue distribution is very narrow; it is found almost exclusively in kidney, in the straight part of the proximal tubule (outer medulla, predominantly S3 segment, perhaps some late S2); much less mRNA is found in brain (demonstrated for rat, mouse and human) where the exact location is still under dispute. Some unconfirmed RT-PCR results suggest very weak expression in additional organs. Interestingly, OCT2 is expressed by a factor of about 1.5–3 (depending on the detection method) stronger in male versus female rat kidneys. No such differences have been found for OCT1 and EMT. The significance of this difference is unclear. Cell lines expressing OCT2 include LLC-PK1 (pig) and Caco-2 (human), and a knock-out has not been published. An antibody is available. Potent inhibitors include disprocynium24 (Ki = 10 nmol/l) and some steroids. There is still a debate over whether OCT2 corresponds to the apical (luminal) or basolateral organic cation transporter. The luminal transporter should be, according to membrane vesicle studies, an organic cation/H+ antiporter. Antibodies to an intracellular loop-epitope suggest a basolateral localisation, functional data indicate an apical localisation.

- EMT: gene symbol SLC22A3; cloned from human, rat and mouse. Radiolabeled substrates (in the order of decreasing transport efficiency for the human transporter): MPP+, histamine, tyramine, adrenaline, noradrenaline, cimetidine. Interestingly, sarcosinamide and a derived anti-cancer drug (SarCNU) are substrates of human EMT and may enter tumor cells via EMT. Localization is broad and probably includes (human RNA blot data) salivary gland, prostate, liver, placenta, adrenal, heart and probably brain and kidney. Expression in rodents seems to be somewhat different, with clear expression in placenta, intestine, heart and brain (expression in cerebellum and hippocampus is unconfirmed) and weak signals in kidney and lung but not in liver. Cell lines expressing EMT include Caki-1, HeLa, HKPT, Caco-2, ARPE-19 (human), and a knock-out has been published. An antibody is not available. Inhibitors include disprocynium24 (Ki = 15 nmol/l), O-methylisoprenaline and some steroids.

Drugs

Cimetidine is a competitive histamine receptor (H_2) antagonist that inhibits e.g. gastric acid secretion.

MPP+ is a potent neurotoxin that causes irreversible and selective destruction of dopaminergic neurons in primates; the resulting syndrome resembles Parkinson's disease.

Quinine is a natural alkaloid, first used as an antimalarial drug and still used in the treatment of severe malaria due to chloroquine-resistant or multidrug-resistant P. falciparum.

TEA is a selective ganglionic blocking agent.

References

1. Gründemann D, Gorboulev V, Gambaryan S, Veyhl M, Koepsell H (1994) Drug excretion mediated by a new prototype of polyspecific transporter. Nature 372:549–552
2. Gründemann D, Schechinger B, Rappold GA, Schömig E (1998) Molecular identification of the corticosterone-sensitive extraneuronal monoamine transporter. Nature Neurosci. 1:349–351
3. Sweet DH, Pritchard JB (1999) The molecular biology of renal organic anion and organic cation transporters. Cell Biochem. Biophys. 31:89–118
4. Koepsell H (1998) Organic cation transporters in intestine, kidney, liver, and brain. In: Hoffmann JF (ed) Annu. Rev. Physiol. Annual Reviews, Palo Alto, California, p243–266
5. Gründemann D, Liebich G, Kiefer N, Köster S, Schömig E (1999) Selective substrates for non-neuronal monoamine transporters. Mol. Pharmacol. 56:1–10

Organic Nitrates

Organic nitrates are polyol esters of nitric acid. This group of drugs includes glyceryl trinitrate (nitroglycerine), isosorbide mononitrate (ISMN), isosorbide dinitrate (ISDN) and amyl nitrite (AN). Organic nitrates release nitric oxide (NO), a process which involves an enzymatic step. NO release from organic nitrates activates the soluble form of guanylyl cyclase by interacting with a haem group in the enzyme. The formation of cyclic cGMP by guanylyl cyclase leads then to the relaxation of smooth muscle cells. Organic nitrates at clinical concentrations mainly lead to a relaxation of venous capacitance vessels. Organic nitrates are mainly used for the prophylaxis or acute treatment of anginal pain. The anti-anginal effect of organic nitrates decreases after repeated administration (tolerance). The main adverse effects are hypotension and headache.

▶ Guanylyl Cyclases

Organophosphates

Organophosphates are a group of pentavalent phosphorus compounds, which contain an organic group (e.g. parathion, malathion, tabun, sarin, soman). Organophosphates are irreversible acethylcholinesterase inhibitors. They are used as insecticides or "nerve gas".

▶ Acetylcholinesterase

ORL-1

The ORL-1 receptor was identified by its high homology to the other opioid receptor subtypes and termed "opioid receptor like", although none of the endogenous peptides or opiate drugs show a high affinitiy for this receptor. An endogenous peptide which binds to this "orphan" receptor with high affinity was identified and termed noceptin or orphanin FQ.

▶ Opioid System

Orphan Nuclear Receptor

An orphan nuclear receptor is a receptor protein belonging to the nuclear receptor superfamily, whose physiological ligand has not been identified.

▶ Nuclear Receptor Regulations of Drug-metabolizing P450 Enzymes

Orphan Receptors

Orphan receptors are receptors, for which a natural activating ligand has not yet been identified.

▶ P450-monooxygenase System

Osmotic Laxatives

▶ Laxatives

Osteoarthritis

Osteoarthritis is a disease of the load-bearing joints, characterised by gradual erosion of cartilage and deformation of bone. Pain is the main symptom, initially eased by rest, but later analgesics such as aspirin-like drugs are indicated.

▶ Non-steroidal Antiinflammatory Drugs

Osteoblast

An osteoblast is the cell forming new bone. Osteoblasts are derived from stromal bone marrow stem cells.

▶ Bone Metabolism

Osteoclast

An osteoclast is the cell which resorbs bone. Osteoclasts are derived from haematopoietic stem cells.

▶ Bone Metabolism

Osteopetrosis

Osteopetrosis is a rare disease in which bones are abnormally dense and fragile. Osteopetrosis is mostly due to defects in osteoclasts. In human patients with osteopetrosis, mutations have been found in a carbonic anhydrase isoform, in a subunit of the proton ATPase and in the chloride channel ClC-7.

▶ Cl⁻ Channels

Osteoporosis

Osteoporosis is a common condition, in which bone density is decreased as a consequence of an imbalance between bone formation (osteoblast) and bone loss (osteoclast). This leads to fragile bones, which are at an increased risk for fractures. The term "porosis" means spongy, which describes the large holes seen in these bones.

▶ Bone Metabolism
▶ Glucocorticoids
▶ Tyrosine Kinases

Ototoxicity

Ototoxicity describes a harmful effect on the inner ear, especially the sensory cells in the cochlea and the vestibular organ. Aminoglycosides are an example of drugs with ototoxic side effects.

▶ Ribosomal Protein Synthesis Inhibitors

Oxazolidinones

Oxazolidinones are a new class of synthetic antimicrobial agents, which have activity against many important pathogens, including methicillin-resistant *Staphylococcus aureus* and others. Oxazolidinones (e.g. linezolid or eperezolid) inhibit bacterial protein synthesis by inhibiting the formation of the 70S initiation complex by binding to the 50S ribosomal subunit close to the interface with the 30S subunit.

▶ Ribosomal Protein Synthesis Inhibitors

Oxidase, mixed function

▶ P450 Mono-oxygenase System

Oxytocin

▶ Vasopressin/Oxytocin

O

P

p53

p53 is a tumor suppressor protein which plays a key role in carcinogenesis. Inactivation of p53 is a common feature of the majority of human cancers. p53 is a transcriptional activator protein of 53 kD that regulates a variety of target genes. Under normal conditions, p53 is a short-lived protein that is rapidly degraded by the ubiquitin proteosome system (UPS). Conditions such as genetoxic stress result in a stabilization of p53 which leads to a suppression of growth.

▶ Ubiquitin/Proteasome System

PACAP

▶ Pituitary Adenylate Cyclase-activating Polypeptide

PAF

▶ Platelet-activating Factor

PAG

▶ Periaqueductal Grey

p24-family

The p24-family is a family of type I transmembrane proteins that function as coat receptors within the early secretory pathway.

▶ Intracellular Transport

P450 Mono-oxygenase System

ULRICH M. ZANGER, MICHEL EICHELBAUM
Dr. Margarete Fischer-Bosch Intitute of Clinical Pharmacology, Stuttgart, Germany
uli.zanger@ikp-stuttgart.de,
michel.eichelbaum@ikp-stuttgart.de

Synonyms

Mixed function oxidases

Definition

The cytochrome P450 mono-oxygenase system is a versatile enzyme system located in the membranes of the endoplasmic reticulum and mitochondria of eukaryotic cells that incorporates one atom of molecular oxygen into a substrate molecule and one atom into water (1). The general stochiometry of the reaction is as follows (S, substrate):

$$NADPH + H^+ + O_2 + S\text{–}H \rightarrow NADP^+ + H_2O + S\text{–}OH$$

A great variety of biotransformations including aromatic and aliphatic hydroxylations, dealkylations and oxidations of hetero-atoms, and epoxidations are based on this elementary reaction. Cytochromes P450 catalyze the phase I metabolism of most drugs and ► xenobiotics, often a prerequisite for a phase II conjugation reaction and subsequent elimination from the body, but they may also be required for ► prodrug activation. Other CYP enzymes participate in many critical physiological pathways leading to steroid hormones, bile acids, prostaglandines and many other endogenous compounds.

- ► Nuclear Receptor Regulation of Drug-metabolizing P450 Enzymes
- ► Pharmacogenetics
- ► Pharmacokinetics

Basic Characteristics

Cytochrome P450 Electron Transport Systems

The P450 mono-oxygenase system functions as an electron transport chain in which electrons are transferred from cellular pyridine nucleotides (NADPH/NADH) to the P450 hemoprotein. In vertebrates, there are two principal types of P450s and electron transfer chains. One is found in the mitochondrial inner membrane and the other in the endoplasmic reticulum (ER). The electron-donating protein of the ER system is called NADPH-cytochrome P450 oxidoreductase (CYPOR). It consists of two domains with two different prosthetic flavin groups FAD (flavin adenine dinucleotide) and FMN (flavin mononucleotide), which transfer two electrons acquired from NADPH directly, but only one at a time, to the P450 heme iron. CYPOR is bound to the ER membrane by its N-terminal tail, and the bulk of the protein is on the cytosolic side of the ER membrane. In humans, CYPOR is encoded by a single gene (*POR*) on chromosome 7q11.2, which encodes a protein of 677 amino acids. The crystal structure of CYPOR has been determined. In certain reactions catalyzed by microsomal P450s, the second electron can also be donated by cytochrome b_5, a smaller heme containing protein (MW ~15 kD), which accepts electrons from NADH via the flavoprotein NADH-cytochrome b_5-reductase.

In mitochondria, the electron acceptor protein is also a flavoprotein termed NADPH-adrenodoxin reductase (MW ~50 kD) because it was discovered in the adrenal cortex and because it donates its electrons not directly to the P450 but to the smaller redox protein adrenodoxin (MW ~12.5 kD) with two iron-sulfur clusters, which serve as electron shuttles between the flavoprotein and the mitochondrial P450.

Cytochrome P450 Structure

The name cytochrome P450 (P for pigment) derives from the unusual spectrum compared to other hemoproteins. Carbon monoxide strongly binds to the reduced (ferrous) heme iron inducing a strong absorption at 450 nm that was first discovered in 1958 and that can be used to quantitate cytochrome P450 via its reduced CO-difference spectrum (2). The structural difference between cytochrome P450 and other hemoproteins is the unusual 5th ligand to the heme iron, which is a histidine in other hemoproteins and a conserved cysteine thiolate in all P450s, located close to their C-termini. X-ray crystal structures now available for several bacterial P450s and for the mammalian (rabbit) CYP2C5 protein have confirmed the role of the conserved thiolate ligand (3). The many sequences available and the recent structural data indicate significant structural similarities between all P450s, which have about 500 amino acids and most likely evolved from a single common ancestor gene. Microsomal P450s are bound to the membrane by a single hydrophobic N-terminal transmembrane anchor and some hydrophobic parts of the heme moiety, which is colocalized with CYPOR at the cytoplasmic side of the ER. Mitochondrial P450s are synthesized as slightly larger precursors with an N-terminal signal sequence that is cleaved off during translocation of the protein to the inner mitochondrial membrane.

Cytochrome P450 Gene Superfamily

Whereas the electron transfer components of the P450 mono-oxygenases are usually encoded by single genes, cytochromes P450 are the products of a gene superfamily with currently more than 1200 known forms (isozymes) from all types of living organisms. A web site providing databases and many links to various aspects of P450 research can be found at http://drnelson.utmem.edu/CytochromeP450.html. Cytochrome P450 proteins are classified into families and subfamilies based on their sequence similarities. If more than

Tab. 1 Overview of the cytochrome P450 superfamily in humans.

Family	Subfamily, genes, pseudogenes (P)							Typical substrates/functions
CYP 1	A1	A2						PAHs, estrogens, aromatic amines
	B1							PAHs, estrogens, aromatic amines
	C1P							no function
CYP 2	A6	A7	A13	A18P				nicotine, coumarin, nitrosamines
	B6	B7P						cyclophosphamide, clopidogrel, bupropion
	C8	C9	C18	C19				taxol (2C8), NSAIDS, omeprazole (2C19)
	D6	D7P	D8P					antidepressants, opioids, beta-blockers
	E1							ethanol, halothane, aceton
	F1	F1P						naphtalene, styrene
	G1P	G2P						no function
	J2							arachidonic acid
	R1							unknown function
	S1							unknown function
	T2P	T3P						no function
	U1							unknown function
	W1							unknown function
CYP 3	A4	A5	A5P	A7	A43			cyclosporin, antidepressants, testosterone
CYP 4	A11	A20	A21P	A22				fatty acid omega-hydroxylation
	B1							fatty acids, clofibrate, steroids
	F2	F3	F8	F9P	F10P	F11	F12	arachidonic acid, leukotrienes, prostaglandines
	F22	F23P	F24P	F25P	F26P	F27P	F28P	
	V2	V5						unknown function
	X1							unknown function
CYP 5	A1							thromboxane A2 synthase
CYP 7	A1							steroid 7-alpha hydroxylase
	B1							brain-specific neurosteroid biosynthesis
CYP 8	A1							prostacyclin synthase
	B1							steroid 12-alpha hydroxylation
CYP 11	A1							cholesterol side chain cleavage
	B1	B2						cortisol and aldosteron biosynthesis
CYP 17								steroid 17-apha hydroxylase/17-20 lyase
CYP 19								steroid aromatase (estrogen biosynthesis)
CYP 20								unknown function
CYP 21	A1P	A2						steroid 21-hydroxylase
CYP 24								vitamin D degradation
CYP 26	A1							retinoic acid hydroxylation
	B1							retinoic acid hydroxylation
	C1							unknown function
CYP 27	A1							27-hydroxylation in bile acid biosynthesis
	B1							vitamin D3 1-alpha hydroxylase
	C1							unknown function
CYP 39								unknown function
CYP 46								cholesterol 24-hydroxylase
CYP 51		51P1	51P2	51P3				lanosterol 14-alpha demethylase

P

40% identity exists between two forms at the amino acid level, they belong to the same family (indicated by an Arabic numeral), whereas they belong to the same subfamily (indicated by a capital letter) if they share more than 55% of identical amino acids. Individual isozymes of the same subfamily are distinguished by an additional Arabic number. Based on the results of the human genome project, humans have about 60 individual functional cytochrome P450 genes that are organized in 18 families and 43 subfamilies and which are found dispersed over all autosomal chromosomes. Besides functional genes, there are also so-called ▶ pseudogenes, which harbour mutations that prevent the production of functional protein products. More than 20 *CYP* pseudogenes of different families have been identified in the human genome. Other mammals share the same 18 *CYP* families with humans, but the number of individual functional isozymes in each family or subfamily can be different. Based on their role in metabolism, the 18 *CYP* families can be broadly dichitomized into those catalyzing the metabolism of xenobiotics (families *CYP1*, *CYP2*, and *CYP3*), and those that are responsible for biotransformations of important endogenous substances (families *CYP4* to *CYP51*; Table 1). Whereas mutations in many *CYP* genes of the first category are frequent in the population and lead to polymorphic drug oxidation, mutations in CYPs catalyzing physiological reactions are rare inherited deficiencies that usually cause various diseases.

Drugs

Human Drug Metabolizing Cytochromes P450

Cytochrome P450s of families *CYP1* to *CYP3* are the principal enzymes catalyzing the oxidative metabolism of xenobiotics, especially for lipophilic drugs. Typical characteristics of these P450s are their extraordinarily broad and overlapping substrate specificities and their extremely variable expression and function both in terms of inter- and intraindividual variation. The *in vivo* activity of a specific P450 enzyme can principally be estimated by measuring metabolite concentrations of an ingested selective probe drug in urine, blood or breath of patients. Three basic mechanisms are responsible for variability in the activity of drug metabolizing enzymes: a) the existence of

genetic polymorphism; b) gene regulatory mechanisms that lead to enzyme induction or down-regulation; and c) direct inhibition of enzyme activity.

Polymorphisms in Drug Metabolizing P450s

▶ Genetic polymorphism is a difference in DNA sequence that has a frequency of at least 1% in a population. Many drug-metabolizing enzyme genes are highly polymorphic with consequences for expression and function of the gene product, such that they affect the disposition of drugs and xenobiotics. The best-studied example of a P450 genetic polymorphism is that of *CYP2D6* (4). It exists in two major phenotypes in the population, the extensive metabolizer (EM) phenotype and the ▶ poor metabolizer (PM) phenotype. The PM phenotype is inherited as an autosomal recessive trait and affects about 5 to 10% of Caucasians who are unable to metabolize a range of drugs that are substrates for CYP2D6. For drugs with narrow therapeutic window, these individuals may be at risk to develop adverse drug reactions when given normal drug doses. Further examples for polymorphisms in P450 genes are mentioned below. The Internet Home Page of the Human Cytochrome P450 (CYP) Allele Nomenclature Committee lists all known human cytochrome P450 alleles at http://www.imm.ki.se/CYPalleles/.

Gene Regulatory Mechanisms in Drug Metabolizing P450s

A variety of regulatory mechanisms act on different P450 genes in response to environmental stimuli to cause changes in gene expression. Members of the *CYP1* family and some other drug metabolizing enzymes including *UGT1A6* are collectively induced by polycyclic aromatic hydrocarbons (PAH) that serve as ligands to a specialized receptor called the Ah (aryl hydrocarbon) receptor, which translocates to the nucleus following binding of another protein component called arnt (arnt for Ah receptor nuclear translocator). In the nucleus these two proteins bind DNA and activate transcription. Another regulatory mechanism is responsible for the 40–50 fold induction of *CYP2B* enzymes of humans and rats following administration of phenobarbital and other barbiturates. The ▶ orphan nuclear receptor CAR (constitutively activated receptor) plays a central role in mediating the effect of phenobarbital. PXR, another orphan nuclear receptor, binds a different range of ligands including the antibiotic rifampin and leads to induction of a different set of enzymes, in particular CYP3A4. Both CAR and PXR bind to DNA in the form of heterodimers with the retinoic X-receptor, RXR, as binding partner (5). Other chemicals also induce P450s, e.g. ethanol induces the CYP2E enzymes. The general feature of these regulatory mechanisms is that substrates induce their own metabolism.

Direct Inhibition of P450

Direct inhibiton of P450 enzymatic activity is the most common reason for drug-drug interactions. P450 inhibitors can be either of the competitive or the mechanism-based type. Potent competitive inhibitors are often, but not always, substrates that have a high affinity for the enzyme. Mechanism-based or suicide enzyme inhibition occurs when a substrate is activated to a reactive intermediate that subsequently binds either to the P450 polypeptide or to the heme moiety thereby inactivating it irreversibly. Examples for both types of inhibitors are known for almost every drug-metabolizing P450. Substance interfering with P450 enzyme activity may also originate from food, e.g. grapefruit juice contains CYP3A4 inhibitors that have significant effects on *in vivo* drug concentrations lasting several days.

Direct Inhibition of P450

CYP1A1: Typical substrates are polycyclic aromatic hydrocarbons (PAHs) like benzo(a)pyrene or methylcholanthrene. The carcinogenicity of this substance depends on metabolic activation by CYP1A1. Some of the PAHs that induce CYP1 enzymes via the Ah receptor are found in cigarette smoke and charred food. CYP1A1 is expressed at very low levels in the liver of uninduced individuals but is found in extrahepatic tissues including placenta, lung and lymphozytes. CYP1A2 has broader substrate specificity than CYP1A2, including many aromatic and heterocyclic amines and is more abundantly expressed in human liver. Typical substrates are caffeine, phenacetine, clozapine, estrogens and others. Caffeine N3-demethylation can be used as a selective 1A2 marker activity, whereas 7-ethoxyresorufin O-deethylation or or phenacetin O-deethylation

reflect both CYP1A isozymes. Genetic polymorphisms have been found in all human *CYP1* genes and their associations with various forms of cancer were intensely studied. The *CYP1A1/2* genes are located on chromosome 15.

CYP1B1 (chromosome 5) has been linked to primary congenital glaucoma. CYP1B1 is not normally expressed in liver but is often found in various kinds of tumors. It metabolizes many aromatic amines and PAHs to potentially carcinogenic products.

The **CYP2** family is the largest CYP family in humans and it comprises about 15 functional genes and 10 pseudogenes.

CYP2A6 is the principal enzyme for nicotine metabolism. A selective probe drug for CYP2A6 is coumarin. Clinically important drug substrates are rare for this enzyme. Several genetic polymorphisms have been found in the *CYP2A6* gene that affects mainly expression levels. It has been suggested that smokers with genetically determined low CYP2A6 expression need to consume less nicotine to achieve the same satisfying blood levels of the drug.

CYP2B6 is the only functional isozyme of the 2B subfamily in humans, as *CYP2B7* appears to be pseudogene. Both genes are located within a large *CYP2* gene cluster on chromosome 19. CYP2B6 is inducible by barbiturates but its expression and function are also affected by frequent genetic polymorphisms. Clinically important substrates are the cytostatic cyclophosphamide, the antidepressant bupropion, the platelet aggregation inhibitor clopidogrel and the narcotic propofol. S-Mephenytoin N-demethylation and bupropion hydroxylation are selective marker activities that can be used both *in vitro* and *in vivo*.

The **CYP2C** subfamiliy comprises the four genes *CYP2C8, 2C9, 2C18* and *2C19*, which are localized on chromosome 10q1.24. The members of this subfamily show surprisingly large variation in substrate specificity and regulation. **CYP2C8** appears to have narrow substrate specificity with taxol 6-α hydroxylation being the most selective marker activity. **CYP2C9** is very abundantly expressed in human liver and has broad substrate specificity accepting many weakly acidic substances like the hypoglycemic agent tolbutamide, the anticoagulent warfarin, the anticonvulsant phenytoin and several NSAIDs (nonsteroidal anti-inflammatory drugs). **CYP2C19** substrates are (S)-mephenytoin, the 4-hydroxylation of which provides a very specific marker activity, the antiulcer drug omeprazole, the antimalarial proguanil, and diazepam. All *CYP2C* genes are genetically polymorphic. Clinically relevant are the two major variant alleles of CYP2C9, *2C9*2* and *2C9*3* that are associated with decreased enzyme activity, as well as the genetic polymorphism of *CYP2C19*, also known as the S-mephenytoin polymorphism, which affects about 3 to 5 % of Caucasians and up to 20% of Asian populations in the homozygous form. CYP2C18 is expressed as mRNA but not as protein in liver.

CYP2D6 was the first P450 for which a classical pharmacogenetic polymorphism became known. The enzyme and its gene, which is localized together with two pseudogenes on chromosome 22, have been very thoroughly studied. CYP2D6 is responsible for more than 70 different drug oxidations, mostly of substrates containing a basic nitrogen. They include antiarrhythmics (e.g. propafenone), antidepressants (e.g. amitriptyline, venlafaxine), antipsychotics (e.g. thioridazine), beta-Blockers (e.g. metoprolol), opioids (e.g. codeine) and more. Sparteine and debrisoquine, which are no longer in use, led to the discovery of the genetic *CYP2D6* polymorphism, also known as the sparteine/debrisoquine polymorphism. The molecular basis of this polymorphism is comprised in over 40 functionally distinct alleles that are associated with either complete lack of function (null-alleles) or with decreased or increased enzyme activity. The individual inherited allele combination determines whether an individual will have the ▶ **ultrarapid metabolizer** (UM), extensive (EM), intermediate (IM) or poor metabolizer (PM) phenotype. About 5 to 10% of Caucasians carry two null-alleles and are PMs, about 10 to 15% are IMs, and about 10% are UMs. In other ethnic populations, these percentages can be very different. Thus, in Asians the PM phenotype has a frequency of only 0.5 to 1%, whereas in certain Arabian and Eastern African populations, the frequency of the UM phenotype can be as high as 30%. The phenotype can be determined either by using one of several available specific probe drugs, e.g. dextrometorphan or metoprolol, or it can be predicted by genetic diagnosis.

CYP2E1 (chromosome 10) metabolizes small molecules including ethanol, halogenated hydrocarbons like halothane, as well as small aromatic and heterocyclic compounds, many of which also act as inducers. For example, it is known that CYP2E1 is induced in alcoholics. Only few drug substrates of CYP2E1 are known, but the enzyme activates many xenobiotic metabolites to toxic intermediates. Chlorzoxazone 6-hydroxylation has been proposed as a marker activity. Several polymorphisms were described in the *CYP2E1* gene, some of which were found to be more frequent in Asians and believed to be associated with increased cancer risk linked to smoking.

CYP2F1 appears to be expressed preferentially in lung where it bioactivates the selective pneumotoxins 3-methylindole and naphthalene. It is abundant in cardiovascular tissue and active in the metabolism of arachidonic acid to eicosanoids that possess potent anti-inflammatory, vasodilatory, and fibrinolytic properties.

Most of the other *CYP2* subfamilies and isozymes listed in Table 1 are poorly characterized, in part because most of them were discovered in the course of the human genome project.

The **CYP3A** subfamily is the most important drug metabolizing families in humans. **CYP3A4** plays the major role because it is the most abundantly expressed P450 not only of human liver but also of intestinal enterocytes. It has been estimated that CYP3A4 makes significant contributions to the metabolism of more than half of all clinically used drugs. They include large molecules like the immunosuppressant cyclosporin A, macrolid antibiotics like erythromycin, or anticancer drugs like taxol, and smaller molecules like benzodiazepines, HMGCoA reductase inhibitors, anaesthetics and many more. CYP3A4 expression levels are increased following exposure to a number of drugs that bind to the nuclear receptor PXR (pregnane X-receptor), which increases the rate of CYP3A4 gene transcription. Whereas genetic polymorphism does not appear to play a major role in determining CYP3A4 activity, expression of the two subfamily members, **CYP3A5** and **CYP3A7**, is confined to a smaller fraction of the population who carry particular alleles of these genes. CYP3A7 is more abundantly expressed in fetal liver than in adult liver. CYP3A43 is expressed at very low levels.

CYPs in Physiological Pathways

Most of these enzymes have steroids or fatty acids as their substrates. Many P450s in endogenous biotransformation pathways are characterized by narrow substrate and product specificity and by tight regulatory systems, especially those involved in steroid hormone biosythesis.

The **CYP4** family comprises a larger number of subfamilies and isozymes (Table 1). The major substrates for CYP4A forms are fatty acids that are hydroxylated at their omega position. The physiological significance of this is largely unknown. Non-fatty acid substrates may be metabolized by specific CYP4A forms. Expression of CYP4 enzymes is regulated by peroxisome proliferators like clofibrate (peroxisomes oxidize fatty acids), drugs that bind to another nuclear receptor termed PPAR (peroxisome proliferator activated receptor).

CYP5 synthesizes thromboxane A2, a fatty acid in the arachidonic acid cascade that causes platelet aggregation. Aspirin prevents platelet aggregation as it blocks the cyclooxygenases COX1 and COX2, which catalyze the initial step of the biotransformation of arachidonic acid to thromboxane and prostaglandins.

CYP7A catalyzes the first and rate-limiting step of bile acid synthesis. This is the principal way to eliminate cholesterol. **CYP7B** is primarily expressed in brain and catalyzes the synthesis of various neurosteroids.

CYP8A is the complementary enzyme to CYP5 in that it synthesizes prostacyclin in the arachidonic acid cascade. **CYP8B** catalyzes the steroid 12-α hydroxylation needed for bile acid biosynthesis.

CYP11A1 is known as the mitochondrial side chain cleavage enzyme that converts cholesterol to pregnenolone, the first step in steroid hormone biosynthesis. Steroid hormone levels are under tight endocrine control via the P450 enzymes involved in their biosynthesis, which are transcriptionally regulated by ACTH (adrenocorticotropic hormone) via intracellular cAMP. Genetic defects in CYP11A1 lead to a lack of glucocorticoids, feminization and hypertension. **CYP11B1** is the mitochondrial 11-β hydroxylase that synthesizes cortisol and corticosterone. Genetic defects in this gene lead to congenital adrenal hyperplasia. **CYP11B2**, aldosterone synthase, hydroxylates corticosterone at C-18. Genetic deficiency of CYP11B2 is the cause of congenital hypoaldosteronism.

CYP17 is a 17-α-hydroxylase and 17-20 lyase; two different reactions catalyzed by one enzyme and required for production of testosterone and estrogen. Defects in this enzyme affect development at puberty.

CYP19 is an aromatase that synthesizes estrogen, converting ring A of the steroid nucleus into an aromatic ring. Lack of this enzyme causes a lack of estrogen and failure of women to develop at puberty. Because estrogens are involved in breast cancer development, CYP19 is an important target to develop specific anti-breast cancer agents that inhibit the enzyme.

CYP20 is a newly identified P450 sequence and no function has yet been found.

CYP21 catalyzes steroid C21 hydroxylation required for cortisol biosynthesis. Genetic defects in this gene cause congential adrenal hyperplasia.

CYP24 is a 25-hydroxyvitamin D (3) 24-hydroxylase that degrades vitamin D metabolites.

CYP26 consists of three enzymes each representing a separate subfamily (Table 1), with probably all involved in retinoic acid hydroxylation. CYP26A1 is an all trans retinoic acid hydroxylase that degrades retinoic acid, an important signaling molecule for vertebrate development. It acts through retinoic acid receptors.

CYP27A1 catalyzes the side chain oxidation (27-hydroxylation) in bile acid biosynthesis. Because bile acid synthesis is the only elimination pathway for cholesterol, mutations in the CYP27A1 gene lead to abnormal deposition of cholesterol and cholestanol in various tissues. This sterol storage disorder is known as cerebrotendinous xanthomatosis. **CYP27B1** is the 1-α hydroxylase of vitamin D3 that converts the D3 precursor to the active vitamin form. The function of CYP27C1 is not yet known.

CYP46 hydroxylates cholesterol at the 24-position, a reaction that appears to play a role in cholesterol homeostasis in the brain.

CYP51 catalyzes lanosterol 14-α demethylation required in the biosynthesis of cholesterol. This enzyme is evolutionarily highly conserved in plants, fungi and animals, and bacteria and may be the ancestor of all eukaryotic P450s. Triazole antifungal drugs like ketoconazole act on CYP51. The enzyme appears to play critical functions.

P

References

1. Ortiz de Montellano (ed) Cytochrome P450. Structure, mechanism, and biochemistry. 2nd Edition 1995, Plenum Press, New York and London.
2. Omura T, Sato R (1964) The carbon monoxide-binding pigment of liver microsomes. I. Evidence for its hemoprotein nature. J Biol Chem 239:2370–2378
3. Williams PA, Cosme J, Sridhar V, Johnson EF, McRee DE (2002) Microsomal cytochrome P450 2C5: comparison to microbial P450s and unique features. J Inorg Biochem 81:183–190
4. Meyer UA, Zanger UM (1997) Molecular mechanisms of genetic polymorphisms of drug metabolism. Annu Rev Pharmacol Toxicol 37:269–296
5. Waxman DJ (1999) P450 Gene induction by structurally diverse xenochemicals: Central role of nuclear receptors CAR, PXR, and PPAR. Archives Biochem Biophys 369:11–23

p70S6 Kinase

p70S6 kinase is a serine/threonine protein kinase, which is involved in the regulation of translation by phosphorylating the 40S ribosomal protein S6. Insulin and several growth factors activate the kinase by phosphorylation in a phosphatidylinositol (PI) 3-kinase-dependent and rapamycin-sensitive manner. Phosphorylation of S6 protein leads to the translation of mRNA with a characteristic 5' polypyrimidine sequence motif.

▶ Insulin Receptor

Pain

The International Association for the Study of Pain (IASP) defines pain as "an unpleasant sensory and emotional experience associated with actual or potential tissue damage, or described in terms of such damage". This broad definition acknowledges that pain is more than a sensation subsequent to the activation of nociceptors. It includes cognitive, emotional and behavioral responses which are also influenced by psychological and social factors.

▶ Analgesics

Palmitoylation

Palmitoylation is the post-translational lipid modification of cysteine-residues in a variety of proteins.

▶ Lipid Modifications

Pancreatic β-cell

The predominant cell type in the pancreatic islets of Langerhans. The main secretory product of the β-cell is the peptide hormone insulin which has vital actions for the control of nutrient homeostasis and cellular differentiation.

▶ Diabetes Mellitus
▶ Oral Antidiabetic Drugs

Pancreatic Polypeptide

The hormone pancreatic polypeptide (PP) is a 36 amino acid peptide which is closely related to ▶ neuropeptide Y and ▶ peptide YY. PP is mainly found in pancreatic cells distinct from those storing insulin, glucagon or somatostatin. It acts on receptors which belong to the family of ▶ neuropeptide Y receptors, particularly on the Y_4 subtype.

Pantothenic Acid

▶ Vitamins, watersoluble

Parasympathetic Nervous System

The autonomic nervous system, which regulates functions that occur without conscious control, consists of two major divisions, the sympathetic and the parasympathetic nervous systems. In the periphery, it consists of nerves, ganglia, and plexuses that provide innervation to the heart, blood vessels, glands, other visceral organs and smooth muscle in various tissues. The parasympathetic nervous system is concerned primarily with conservation of energy and maintenance of organ function during periods of minimal activity. Acetylcholine is the neurotransmitter at all preganglionic autonomic fibers and at all postganglionic parasympathetic fibers.

▶ Muscarinic Receptors

Parasympatholytics

▶ Muscarinic Receptors

Parasympathomimetics

▶ Muscarinic Receptors

Parathyroid Hormone

As a major regulator of bone metabolism and calcium homeostasis, parathyroid hormone (PTH) is stimulated through a decrease in plasma ionised calcium and increases plasma calcium by activating osteoclasts. PTH also increases renal tubular calcium re-absorption as well as intestinal calcium absorption. Synthetic PTH (1-34) has been successfully used for the treatment of osteoporosis, where it leads to substantial increases in bone density and a 60–70% reduction in vertebral fractures.

▶ Bone Metabolism

Paraventricular Nucleus

The paraventricular nucleus in the hypothalamus is located adjacent to the third ventricle and has been identified as a satiety center. Neurons in the paraventricular nucleus produce neuropeptides which inhibit feeding when injected into the brain (thyrotropin-releasing hormone (TRH), corticotropin-releasing hormone (CRH), oxytocin).

▶ Appetite Control

Parkin

Parkin is a ubiquitin ligase encoded by a gene affected in autosomal recessive juvenile parkinsonism (AR-JP). This gene is located on chromosome 6 and encodes a protein of 465 amino acid residues with moderate similarity to ubiquitin at the amino terminus and a RING-finger motif at the carboxy terminus.

▶ Ubiquitin/Proteasome System

Parkinson's Disease

Parkinsons's disease (PD) is a progressive disease characterized by akinesia, muscle tremor and rigidity resulting from the degeneration of melanin-containing cells of the substantia nigra and the resulting reduction in brain dopamine levels. PD initially responds to L-DOPA therapy but the disease eventually enters a refractory phase possibly due to the continued loss of cells. Drugs that destroy dopaminergic neurons, block dopamine synthesis or antagonize D2-like receptors have PD-like effects.

► Dopamine System
► Ubiquitin/Proteasome System

PAS Domain

PAS domains are protein domains, encompassing about 250-300 amino acids, which in higher eukaryotes function as surfaces for both homotypic interactions with other PAS proteins and heterotypic interactions with cellular chaperones, such as the 90-kD heat shock protein (Hsp90). They are named according to the first letter of each of the three founding members of the family of PAS domain containing proteins, PER, ARNT and SIM. Most of the PAS proteins also contain basic-helix-loop-helix (bHLH) motifs immediately N-teminal to their PAS domain. The HLH domains participate in homotypic dimerization between two bHLH-PAS proteins, and they position the basic region to allow specific contacts with the major groove of target regulatory elements found in DNA. Important members of the PAS superfamily are the aryl hydrocarbon receptor (AHR), which together with ARNT forms the receptor for a class of co-planar polyhalogenated aromatic hydrocarbons like dioxins. Although structurally distinct from the group of nuclear receptors, the Ah receptor functions in similar fashion. In the absence of ligand, the receptor resides in the cytosol as an inactive complex with Hsp90. Binding of dioxins enables the receptor to translocate to the cell nucleus and to bind to specific DNA recognition motifs. Other members of the PAS superfamily include the products of the *period* and *clock* genes, which are involved in the regulation of circadian rhythms as well as hypoxia-inducible factor (HIF1), which mediates the effect of hypoxia on the regulation of the expression of a variety of genes, including those encoding erythropoietin or vascular endothelial growth factor.

Patch-clamp Method

The patch-clamp technique is based on the formation of a high resistance seal (10^9-$10^{10}\Omega$) between the tip of a glass micropipette and the cell membrane it touches (gigaohm-seal). This technique allows recordings of ionic currents through single ion channels in the intact cell membrane and in isolated membrane patches at a defined membrane potential (voltage-clamp). Variations of the technique include whole-cell voltage-clamp recording and recordings in inside-out or outside-out membrane configurations.

► ATP-dependent K^+ Channels

PCI

► Percutaneous Coronary Intervention

PDE

► Phosphodiesterase

PDGF

► Platelet-derived Growth Factor

PDK1

PDK1 (phosphoinositide-dependent kinase 1) contains a phosphatidylinositol 3,4-bisphosphate ($PtdIns$-3,4-P_2) and $PtdIns$-3,4,5-P_3-binding pleckstrin homology (PH) domain and contributes to activation of protein kinase B (PKB)/Akt through phosphorylation of a threonine residue.

▶ Phospholipid Kinases

PDZ Domain

PDZ domains were originally recognized as about 90 amino acid long, repeated sequences in the synaptic protein PSD-95/SAP-90, the Drosophila septate junction protein Discs-Larg and the epithelial tight junction protein ZO-1. PDZ domains interact specifically with peptide motifs (-E-T/S-D/E-V), which are found at the very C-terminus of a variety of proteins. They often function as scaffolding proteins, which hold together protein complexes at the inner side of the plasma membrane.

Pellagra

The clinically manifest form of niacin deficiency is called pellagra. Early symptoms are unspecific, including sleep disturbance, lack of appetite, weight reduction, diarrhoea and abdominal pain. Typical symptoms of more severe stages relate to skin (symmetrical pigmented and itching areas on sun-exposed skin), intestinal tract (glossitis, stomatitis, vomiting) and nervous system (pain and numbness of extremities, peripheral neuritis, psychological changes).

▶ Niacin

Pemphigus Blistering Disease

Pemphigus describes a group of rare autoimmune blistering diseases of the skin caused by autoantibodies to desmosomal components. These antibodies lead to a loss of adhesion between keratinocytes, called acantholysis. In pemphigus vulgaris, which is caused by autoantibodies to desmoglein 3, the blisters are located in the suprabasal layer, whereas in pemphigus foliaceus, which is caused by autoantibodies to desmoglein 1, the blisters occur within the upper layers of the epidermis. The major therapeutic strategy in pemphigus is chronic immunosuppressive therapy with glucocorticosteroids in combination with immunosuppressive adjuvants.

▶ Cadherins/Catenins
▶ Glucocorticoides
▶ Immunnosupressive Agents

Penicillin

▶ β-lactam Antibiotics

Penicillin-binding Protein

▶ β-lactam Antibiotics

Pentasaccharide

Heparin

▶ Anticoagulants

Peptide Mass Fingerprinting

Peptide mass fingerprinting (PMF) is a mass spectrometry based method for protein identification. The protein is cleaved by an enzyme with high specificity (trypsin, Lys-C, Asp-N, etc.) or chemical (CNBr). The peptide mixture generated is analyzed by matrix-assisted laser desorption/ionization (MALDI) or electrospray ionization (ESI) mass spectrometry. The determined set of masses (mass fingerprint) is characteristic for the protein present and is used to search peptide masses generated by theoretical fragmentation of protein sequences in databases.

▶ Proteomics

Peptide YY

The hormone peptide YY (PYY) is a 36 amino acid peptide which is closely related to ▶ neuropeptide Y and ▶ pancreatic polypeptide. PYY is predominantly synthesized and released by intestinal endocrine cells, and can also coexist with glucagon in pancreatic acini and enteroglucagon in endocrine cells of the lower bowel. It acts on the same receptors as ▶ neuropeptide Y. The endogenous long C-terminal PYY fragment PYY_{3-36} is a biologically active and subtype-selective metabolite.

Peptidoglycans

Peptidoglycans are covalently closed net-like polymers forming the rigid matrix of the bacterial cell wall. Glycan chains of alternating N-acetylglucosamine and N-acetylmuramic acid residues are substituted by L-alanyl-γ-D-glutamyl-L-diaminoacyl-D-alanine stem tetrapeptides, and cross-linked through direct interpeptide linkages or crossbridges. Bacteria that are actively multiplying (i.e. in the exponential phase of growth) manufacture a ($4{\rightarrow}3$) peptidoglycan in a penicillin-susceptible manner. Cross-linking involves the carbonyl of the D-alanine at position 4 of a stem peptide and the ω-amino group of the diaminoacid residue at position 3 of another stem peptide. Bacteria also manufacture a ($3{\rightarrow}3$) peptidoglycan in a penicillin-resistant manner, conferring intrinsic resistance to β-lactam antibiotics. Cross-linking involves the carbonyl of the diaminoacid residue at position 3 of a stem peptide and the ω-amino group of the diaminoacid residue also at position 3 of another stem peptide.

▶ β-lactam Antibiotics

Peptidyl Transferase Center

The peptidyl transferase center is the site of peptide bond formation on the ribosome and the target for a chemically diverse set of antibiotics. It is located in a cavity on the 50S subunit that leads into a peptide exit tunnel that passes through the body of the 50S subunit. The active site is in a deep cleft that is packed with nucleotides from the highly conserved internal loop in domain V of 23S ribosomal RNA (rRNA), termed the peptidyl transferase loop. In general, the single-stranded nucleotides in the loop are the closest to the active site, with the helices around the internal loop radiating away from the catalytic center. The peptidyl transferase loop has previously been implicated as a component of the catalytic site through the localization of chemical footprints and crosslinks from both antibiotics and transfer RNAs (tRNAs) to this region. In addition, for many of the peptidyl transferase antibiotics, mutations at single nucleotides in the peptidyl transferase loop produce antibiotic resistance.

▶ Ribosomal Protein Synthesis Inhibitors

Percutaneous Coronary Intervention

Percutaneous coronary intervention (PCI) is any of a number of techniques performed by use of a catheter inserted via a major limb artery that aims to relieve narrowing of coronary arteries. For example, percutaneous transluminal coronary angioplasty (PTCA) is the classic PCI that uses a catheter-directed balloon to dilate a stenotic coronary artery, more recent PCIs include stent implantation, rotational atherectomy and laser angioplasty.

▶ Anticoagulants

Periaqueductal Grey

The periaqueductal grey (PAG) is a major part of the descending inhibitory antinociceptive system. The periaqueductal grey area is localized in the midbrain, a small area of grey matter surrounding the central canal. Neurons of the PAG are excited by opioids leading to the stimulation of cells in the nucleus raphe magnus, which, *via* the dorsolateral funiculus, send projections to the dorsal horn which are mainly serotoninergic. These serotoninergic and opioidergic neurons lead to the inhibition of nociceptive transmission in the dorsal horn.

▶ Nociception

Pericytes

Pericytes are mural cells which stabilise capillaries and control functions of capillary endothelial cell properties.

▶ Angiogenesis and Vascular Morphogenesis

Peripheral Nerve

A peripheral nerve comprises different axons responsible for different modalities. It may contain efferent myelinated motor fibres, efferent unmyelinated autonomic fibres or afferent myelinated and unmyelinated sensory fibres. Depending on size, myelination and conduction velocity fibres are named A-, B- or C-fibres.

▶ Local Anaesthetics

Peripheral Neuropathy

Peripheral neuropathy is degeneration of peripheral nerves. Because motor and sensory axons run in the same nerves, usually both motor and sensory functions are affected in this disease. Neuropathies may be either acute (e.g. Charcot-Marie-Tooth disease) or chronic (e.g. Guillain-Barre syndrome) and are categorized as demyelinating or axonal.

Peroxisome Proliferator Activated Receptor

There are three types of peroxisome proliferator activated receptor (PPAR) molecules (PPARα, PPARβ/δ, PPARγ). They are nuclear receptor transcription factors belonging to the retinoid, steroid and thyroid receptor superfamily. They each exist as a heterodimer with the retinoid X receptor (RXR). PPARs are expressed to varying extents in most tissues, and were so-named because PPARα was originally shown to mediate peroxisome proliferation in rat liver. PPARα is expressed mostly in muscle, liver, heart and kidney and mediates lipid oxidation. Its ligands include eicosanoids, fatty acids and fibrate drugs. PPARγ is strongly expressed in adipocytes and mediates lipogenesis and adipocyte differentiation. Ligands for PPARγ

718 Peroxisome Proliferator Chemicals

include arachidonic acid and thiazolidinedione drugs. PPARβ is activated by some eicosanoids but its role is unclear.

▶ Nuclear Receptor Regulation of Drug-metabolizing P450 Enzymes

Peroxisome Proliferator Chemicals

Peroxisome proliferator chemicals (PPCs) are chemicals that activate the nuclear receptor PPARα (peroxisome proliferator-activated receptor-α) and induce the enlargement and proliferation of liver peroxisomes in susceptible rodent species, e.g., rats and mice. Persistent PPC exposure and PPARα activation is associated with hepatocarcinogenesis in these species.

▶ Nuclear Receptor Regulation of Drug-metabolizing P450 Enzymes

Pertussis Toxin

Pertussis toxin is naturally produced by the bacterium *Bordetella pertussis*. This substance is able to prevent the inhibition of adenylyl cyclase and other cellular effector molecules by mediating a covalent modification of certain G proteins (G_i/G_o).

▶ Somatostatin
▶ Transmembrane Signalling
▶ Heterotrimeric GTP-binding Proteins

PEST Sequences

PEST sequences are protein regions with a high content of the amino acid regions proline (P), glutamate (E), serine (S), and threonine (T). These sequences often serve as destruction signals recognized by the ubiquitin proteosome system (UPS). Phosphorylation of serine or threonine residues in these regions appears to be the trigger for recognition by certain SCF-RING ubiquitin (Ub) ligases.

▶ Ubiquitin/Proteasome System

PGI$_2$

Prostacyclin

▶ Prostanoids

P-glycoprotein

P-glycoprotein is a transporter/carrier protein, which actively pumps substances, including drugs, over cell membranes. It is also called "multi-drug resistance gene" (MDR1). P-glycoprotein/MDR1 belongs to the group of ABC transporters (ABCB1).

▶ Multidrug Transporter

PH Domain

▶ Pleckstrin Homology Domain

PHHI

Persistant Hyperinsulinemic Hypoglycemia of Infancy.

▶ Familial Persistant Hyperinsulinemic Hypoglycemia of Infancy

Phage

▶ Bacteriophage

Phagocyte/Phagocytosis

Phagocytes are a group of cells that may engulf and internalise antigens, pathogens or apoptotic cells and destroy them.

▶ Apoptosis
▶ Inflammation
▶ Immune Defense
▶ Hematopoietic Growth Factors
▶ Humanized Monoclonal Antibodies

Pharmacodynamics

Pharmacodynamics describe the effects elicited by a drug in the body.

Pharmacogenetics

JÜRGEN BROCKMÖLLER
Georg-August-Universität Göttingen,
Göttingen, Germany
jurgen.brockmoller@med.uni-goettingen.de

Definition

Pharmacogenetics is the study of genetically determined inter-individual variation within one species with respect to the response to drugs. Inherited genetic variations with frequencies above one percent are termed ▶ polymorphisms. In the human genome, there are more than 3 million polymorphisms. Some of these polymorphisms are the cause why some people do not respond to drugs or do respond extremely heavily or suffer from adverse events to drugs. Pharmacogenetics also includes the impact of genetic variability for an organisms response to any external chemical, physical or microbial influence (▶ ecogenetics), and some genetic polymorphisms affect internal processes of an organism. Therefore, pharmacogenetics may also provide explanations of individual differences in the ▶ susceptibility for a number of diseases. In contrast to inherited disease genes studied in human genetics, pharmacogenetic polymorphisms are not closely related to desease and typically the effect of genetic polymorphism become only apparent upon exposure to drugs or other conditions (▶ gene-environment interactions).

▶ Nuclear Receptor Regulation of Drug-metabolizing P450 Enzymes
▶ P450 Mono-oxygenase System

Basic Mechanisms

Pharmacogenetics is a rapidly evolving field of research (1,2,3,4,5). Fig. 1 illustrates the relationships of pharmacogenetics with other related disciplines. Historically, pharmacogenetic research started with the measurement of the ▶ phenotype, which is the apparent variability in structures or functions of one species (phenotyping). For instance, carriers of the deficiency of the drug metabolizing enzyme ▶ cytochrome P450 2D6 were identified as persons who did not excrete significant amounts of metabolites of drugs like debrisoquine or sparteine (i.e. they showed the deficient or ▶ poor metabolizer phenotype). The

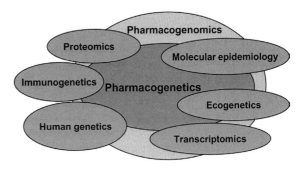

Fig. 1 Relationship between Pharmacogenetics and other disciplines illustrated using a Venn diagram.

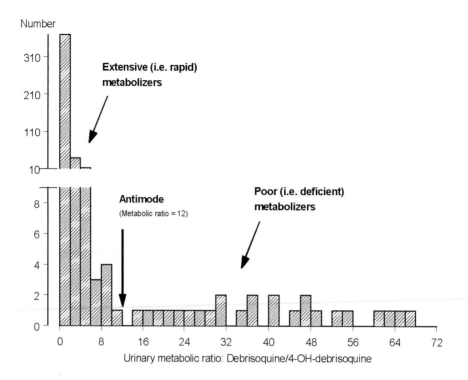

Fig. 2 Cytochrome P450 2D6 (*CYP2D6*) polymorphism as a prototype for a pharmacogenetic polymorphism. The activity was measured using the drug debrisoquine as a test drug and measuring the urinary excretion of the test drug and its 4'-hydroxylated metabolite. The bimodal frequency distribution of CYP2D6 in a human population (N=454) is shown with the rapid or so-called extensive metabolizers on the left side of the antimode and the deficient or so-called poor metabolizers on the right side. Poor metabolizers are unable to generate significant amounts of the 4'hydroxylated metabolite as indicated by the fact that their metabolic ratio is at least 12 corresponding to 12-times more parent drug than metabolite.

frequency distribution of this phenotype is illustrated in Fig. 2. For a monogenic determined polymorphism, the phenotype can typically be classified into two groups (▶ biomodal frequency distribution) or three groups (▶ trimodal frequency distribution). The values separating the two or three groups is termed ▶ antimode. For autosomal genes, a bimodal distribution would correspond to a dominant mode of inheritance. Trimodal distributions are more frequent in pharmacogenetics that mostly correspond to a ▶ codominant mode of inheritance. Nowadays, genetic polymorphisms are identified by molecular genetic analysis of genomic DNA (genotyping). The analysis of the correlation between a DNA variation and the phenotype (genotype-phenotype correlation) is an essential topic of current ▶ functional genomics research.

Essential to the definition of Pharmacogenetics is the term genetic polymorphism. It is extrapolated that there are at least 3 million genetic polymorphisms in the human genome. Historically, a genetic polymorphism was defined as a genetic variation with a population frequency of 1% and above, but the larger inter-ethnic variation of population frequencies makes a strict definition based on such frequencies impractical. The most common molecular type of polymorphism is the ▶ single nucleotide polymorphism (SNP). SNPs are classified according to their location in the coding region of exons as either synonymous SNPs (no change of the amino acid sequence) or non-synonymous SNPs (change of the amino acid sequence). Most SNPs are localized outside the protein coding sequences. Many of these non-coding SNPs may be absolutely silent, but some of these polymorphisms have significant effects on gene transcription or splicing. Other molecular types of genetic variation include insertions or deletions of one or several nucleotides or even entire genes. Some polymorphisms consist of duplications or higher number amplifications of entire functional genes (for instance, the gene duplication of *CYP2D6* results in a phenotype with very extensive expression of the enzyme and ultra-rapid biotransformation of *CYP2D6* substrates). Another distinct type of polymorphisms are the so called variable number of tandem repeat polymorphisms (VNTR) where a segments of repetitive DNA sequence exit with inter-individually variable number of repeats (also termed microsatellites).

Some authors use the term ▶ mutation as a synonym for genetic polymorphism. However, it is recommended to reserve the term mutation for genetic variations acquired within the life-span of an organism such as those mutations acquired in tumor-tissues during multi-step carcinogenesis.

Within a chromosome, genetic polymorphisms are inherited in a linked fashion and on average, the more closely two polymorphisms are located to each other the more tightly they are linked, but polymorphisms even located one base-pair apart may not be linked. The specific combination of genetic polymorphisms within one chromosome is termed ▶ haplotype. Compilations of genetic polymorphisms such as those for human cytochrome P450 enzymes (www.imm.ki.se/CYP-alleles) or those for ▶ N-acetyltransferases (http://www.louisville.edu/medschool/pharmacology/NAT.html) define the polymorphic alleles as much as possible as haplotypes of linked SNPs or other types of variants. Theoretically, medical studies on the function of polymorphisms should always be based on haplotypes, but complete experimental identification of haplotypes from the diploid cells is almost unfeasible with current technologies.

Genetic polymorphisms may affect the fate of a drug within the body of an organisms (▶ pharmacokinetics) and genetic polymorphisms may affect how the drug is acting on the molecular targets of the organism (▶ pharmacodynamics). Polymorphisms relevant for pharmacokinetic variability are in drug transporters relevant for active or facilitated transport through biological barriers and in the enzymes catalyzing drug biotransformation. The effect of polymorphisms in the enzymes of drug biotransformation has been the main focus of pharmacogenetic research in the past. Fig. 3 illustrates on the example of the ▶ cytochrome P450 2C19 polymorphism the genotype-phenotype correlation. In this example, the exposure of the human body to omeprazole differs about 15-fold depending on the cytochrome P450 polymorphism as expressed as the area under the blood plasma concentration time curve (▶ AUC) of the drug. In general, the rapid metabolizers may be prone to ineffective action of the drug and the deficient metabolizers (the so-called poor metabolizers) may be prone to adverse effects due to overdosage. The medical impact differs depending on the therapeutic index and other properties of each drug; in the given example of omeprazole, low efficacy in rapid metabolizers was identified as a problem.

There are only very few genes which do not carry any polymorphisms. And there exists even a significant number of polymorphic genes that are not expressed at all in part of the population due to genetic polymorphisms. Table 1 summarizes a few selected polymorphisms with their functional and medical impact.

Pharmacological Relevance

Individualization of Drug Treatment

If the genotype-phenotype correlation is sufficiently high, an individual's phenotype can be predicted by the genotype. Thus, genotyping can be used to predict in part an individual's response to specific drugs. A drug therapy optimized according to a number of genetic variants is likely to be more efficacious and will produce fewer or less severe adverse effects compared with current drug therapy. It is anticipated that in future non-responders to drugs who are explained by ultra-rapid drug biotransformation or by their less reactive receptors will receive higher drug doses or alternative drugs. Heavy responders to drug due to genetic receptor variation or due to poor drug biotransformation will receive lower doses or alternative drugs. In particular, subjects prone to idiosyncratic adverse drug reactions that are due to immunogenetic polymorphisms, impaired detoxification of reactive metabolites or other genetic variations will not be treated with the drugs which may be dangerous for this subgroup.

P

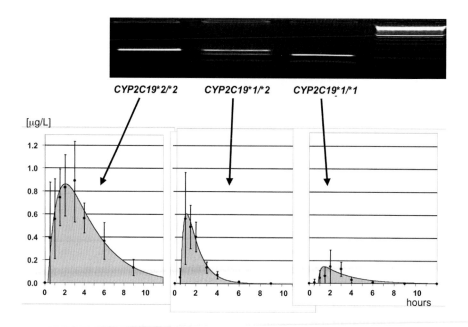

Fig. 3 Illustration of the genotype-phenotype correlation on the example of the cytochrome P450 2C19 polymorphism. The upper part illustrates a molecular analysis of this polymorphism using PCR and restriction fragment analysis resulting in a loss of the restriction site in carriers of the non-functional variant *2. The genotype *CYP2C19*2/*2* indicates poor metabolizers of substrates of the enzyme CYP2C19 and as shown below, the area under the concentration time curve of them is about 15-fold higher compared to homozygous extensive metabolizers (genotype *CYP2C19*1/*1*). The phenotype of the heterozygotes is in-between corresponding to an co-dominant mode of inheritance typical for polymorphisms in drug metabolizing enzymes.

In current daily medical practice, the concept of pharmacogenetic genotyping prior to drug treatment is not routinely used with a few exceptions. At some clinics, phenotyping or genotyping ▶ thiopurine S-methyltransferase (Table 1) is performed prior to therapy with azathioprine and the doses are adjusted accordingly. Currently routine application of pharmacogenetic testing in medicine is limited in part due to lack of knowledge about application and impact of pharmacogenetics among physicians and in part due to the limited availability of rapid genotyping methods. In some instances only moderate specificity or sensitivity depending on the relevant gene and the clinical problem may also be a problem. For instance, poor biotransformation of substrates of CYP2C19 or CYP2D6 can be predicted with a 100% specificity and positive predictive value, thus, low doses can be prescribed to poor metabolizers with sufficient certainty. But sensitivity and negative predictive value are less than 100% since other factors like drug-drug-interactions, rare unidentified polymorphisms or unidentified liver disease may also result in poor metabolism.

Pharmacogenetics as a Compound Selection Tool in Drug Development

In drug development the impact of frequent genetic polymorphisms particularly in genes involved in drug biotransformation is routinely studied by *in vitro* methods and by clinical trials in humans. Preference is given to those drugs not significantly affected by genetic polymorphisms, but existing effects of genetic polymorphisms is not necessarily a knock-out criterion if the drug has specific properties not available with other analogues of that class. In addition, pharmacogenetic testing during clinical drug trials may help to reduce variability and thus to more specifically identify the effects of a certain drug in smaller numbers of subjects.

Tab. 1 **Selected genetic polymorphisms and their medical impact.**

Enzyme	Functional effects of polymorphism and frequency	Examples for the medical impact
Glucose-6-phosphate dehydrogenase	Low or absent enzyme activity in about 10 % of African populations.	Hemolysis following intake of a number of drugs which have electrophilic reactive metabolites, but also, carriers of this enzyme deficiency have a partial protection from malaria.
Pseudocholine esterase	Low or absent activity in 0.05 % of Caucasian populations.	Prolonged action of succinylcholine and mivacurium.
Paraoxonase (PON1)	Low activity in carriers of the glutamine192 variant with a population frequency of about 50 % fort he homozygous glutamine genotype in Caucasians.	Carriers of low activity may show higher lipid peroxidation and higher toxificy from organophosphorothio-ate insecticides.
NADPH:quinone oxidoreductase 1	Pro187Ser variant occurring with about 5 % frequency is functionally almost completely deficient.	Impaired activity associated with benzene toxicity and cancer chemotherapy induced leukemia.
Cytochrome P450 2C9	Low activity in about 10 % (heterozygotes) and very low activity in about 0.8 % (homozygotes) of Caucasian populations.	Prolonged action of several CYP2C9 inactivated drugs like phenytoin, tolbutamide, ibuprofen, or S-warfarin.
Cytochrome P450 2C19	Deficient activity in about 3 % of Caucasian populations and in about 20 % of Asian populations.	Prolonged action of several CYP2C19 inactivated drugs like omeprazole or diazepam in the poor metabolizers.
Cytochrome P450 2D6	Extremely high activity in about 2 % of Caucasian populations and completely deficient activity in about 7 %.	Inefficiency in ultra-rapid metabo-lizers and extremely heavy effects in poor metabolizers for more than 50 drugs. A few drugs requiring bio-activation by CYP have low efficacy in poor metabolizers (example: codein is activated to morphine via CYP2D6).
N-acetyltransferase 2	Low activity in about 60 % of Caucasian populations.	High incidence of adverse events from the drug isoniazide in slow acetylators.
Glutathione S-transferase M1	Deficient activity in about 50 % of Caucasians.	Carriers of the deficiency may have a slightly increased risk for a number of smoking-related cancers.
Thiopurine S–methyl-transferase	Low activity in about 10 % of Caucasians and deficient activity in about 0.4 %.	High incidence of severe adverse events from azathioprine and 6-mercaptopurine in carriers of low activity.
β-adrenergic receptor 2	Amino acid variants appear to be associated with receptor function and agonist induced downregulation.	Some variants may predispose to some types of asthma and modulate action of β-2-adrenergic drugs.

P

Tab. 1   Selected genetic polymorphisms and their medical impact. (Continued)

Enzyme	Functional effects of polymorphism and frequency	Examples for the medical impact
Factor V Leiden	Factor V Leiden refers to a Arg506Gln replacement which occurs with about 5 % frequency in the heterozygous form in Caucasians. The variant is inactivated approximately ten times slower than normal factor V.	About 5-fold increased risk for thrombosis in heterozygous carriers of the glutamine variant. Extremely increased risk in homozygous carriers and in heterozygotes taking oral contraceptives. On the other hand, possibly protection from severe blood loss during accidents, surgery or child birth.
5-Lipoxygenase	A VNTR polymorphism in 100 bp upstream from the ATG start codon is associated with transcription efficiency.	Differences in response to 5-lipoxygenase inhibitors and leucotriene receptor antagonists.
β-adrenergic receptor 2	Amino acid variants moderately associated with receptor function and agonist induced downregulation.	Some variants may predispose to some types of asthma and modulate action of β-2-adrenergic drugs.
Cysteine-cysteine chemokine receptor 5 (CCR5)	A 32-bp deletion with a population frequency of about 0.1 in Caucasians results in truncated non-functional receptor.	Carriers of this variant are partially protected from HIV infection, particularly the homozygous carriers.
G protein β-3 subunit	Truncated protein with increased signal transduction in carriers of the 825T allele.	Associated with hypertension and with the response to thiazide diuretics.

Pharmacogenetics as a Discovery Tool for Mechanisms of Diseases and New Therapeutic Principles

The existence of naturally occurring variations in almost all genes in the human population provides a way to identify the genes involved in disease pathogenesis. This may be particularly helpful in those diseases or adverse drug effects where the mechanisms are unknown. By correlating genetic polymorphisms in possibly related genes (candidate gene approach) or in the entire genome (gene mapping approach) one may be able to identify genes and their polymorphisms that are causative for that disease. This may then allow to design new drugs or other therapeutic principles targeted at these genes.

References

1. Pharmacogenetics & Pharmacogenomics (2000) Recent Conceptual and Technical Advances. Pharmacology 61(3) (the entire issue)
2. W. W. Weber (1997) Pharmacogenetics. Oxford University Press, Oxford
3. W. Kalow (1992) Pharmacogenetics of Drug Metabolism. Pergamon Press, Oxford
4. Pharmacogenomics: The search for individualized therapies. edited by J. Licinio, M.L.Wong (2002) Wiley-VCH/John Wiley, Weinheim
5. The reader is also referred to a number of journals specifically devoted to this field of research: Pharmacogenetics published by Lippincott Williams and Wilkins; Pharmacogenomics published by Ashley Publications Ltd.; American Journal of PharmacoGenomics published by ADIS international; The Pharmacogenomics Journal published by Nature Publishing group.

Pharmacogenomics

Pharmacogenomics relates to the exploitation of genome data for the development of new drug treatments. Systematic (genomic) theoretical and experimental approaches are employed for the identification of new drug targets and the design and synthesis of new drugs (e.g., ▶ bioinfomatics, gene expression profiling, ▶ gene expression analysis). Compared with ▶ pharmacogenetics, which relates to inherited properties (polymorphisms) determining an individual's response to a certain drug, pharmacogenomics is a broader term, including both the genome-wide search for new drug targets and the correlation of polymorphisms with drug responses. Quite often, however, the two terms are used interchangeably.
(see also: Lindpaintner, K. (2002) The impact of pharmacogenetics and pharmacogenomics on drug discovery. Nature Reviews Drug Discovery 1, 463-469.)

Pharmacokinetics

PETER WELLING
University of Strathclyde, Glasgow, Scotland
peter@pwelling.freeserve.co.uk

Synonyms

Drug kinetics, ADME

Definition

Pharmacokinetics is the study of the rates of drug absorption, distribution, metabolism and excretion.

▶ Drug Interactions
▶ Nuclear Receptor Regulation of Drug-metabolizing P450 Enzymes
▶ P450 Mono-oxygenase System

Basic Mechanisms

Pharmacokinetics is one of the many disciplines that contribute to the discovery, development and use of drugs. Pharmacokinetics, and the closely related discipline of drug metabolism, have made a substantial contribution to the understanding and management of drug action. Prior to 1960, pharmacokinetics and metabolism made only a minor contribution to regulatory drug marketing submissions. Not only was there little appreciation of the importance of this type of information, but also little means to provide it. The situation has changed dramatically since then, and continues to evolve as greater emphasis is placed on concentration-effect relationships, both in drug research and in clinical practice.

Pharmacokinetics is a highly interactive discipline influencing a large spectrum of activities ranging from molecular structure determination during early drug discovery to designing optimal drug dosage regimens in clinical practice.

Four different approaches to to pharmacokinetics can be identified. These are ▶ compartment modeling, physiological modeling, model-independent pharmacokinetics and population or mixed-effect modeling (1).

In the compartment modeling approach, the body is assumed to consist of one or more compartments. These may be spatial or chemical in nature. If a drug is converted in the body to a metabolite then the metabolite may be considered to be a separate compartment to the parent drug. Alternatively, a compartment may be used to represent a body volume, or a group of similar tissues or fluids into which a drug distributes after absorption. Typical compartment models of this type are shown in Fig. 1.

In these models, the drug is assumed to distribute between compartments at rates controlled by first-order or saturable kinetics. For example, in the one compartment open model with bolus intravenous injection , plasma drug levels may be described in the form of Equation 1 in which Co is the concentration of drug in plasma at time zero, and t is time after drug dosing.

$$C = Co(EXP - k(el)t) \quad (1)$$

P

ONE-COMPARTMENT OPEN MODEL, BOLUS INTRAVENOUS INJECTION

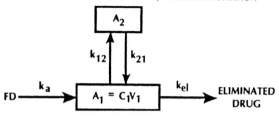

TWO-COMPARTMENT OPEN MODEL, ORAL ADMINISTRATION

Fig. 1 Top: One compartment open model after bolus intravenous injection. D is the dose, A is the amount of drug in the body, C is the concentration of drug in distribution volume V and k(el) is the first order rate constant for drug elimination. **Bottom: Two compartment open model after oral administration.** FD is the fraction of dose absorbed, k12 and k21 are first-order rate constants for transfer of drug between compartments, and ka is the first order rate constant for drug absorption. Subscripts denote first (central) or second (peripheral) compartments.

Appropriate equations may similarly be derived to describe drug disposition in other kinetic models.

In the physiological model approach, pharmacokinetic modeling is based on known anatomical and physiological values. Drug disposition is based on blood flow rates through organs and tissues, and experimentally determined drug blood-tissue concentration ratios at steady state. The basic unit model that describes the relationship between drug concentrations in blood and in a particular organ or tissue is shown in Fig. 2.

The main advantage of physiological modeling is that drug movement and drug concentrations in particular organs and tissues can be predicted, and changes in organ or tissue perfusion can be taken into account in pathological conditions when predicting drug levels. The physiological model approach has been used extensively for anticancer compounds and for agents where drug or metabolite concentrations in particular organs and tissues are important.

The main disadvantages of physiological modeling are that the mathematics can become complex and unwieldy, and that kinetic model parameter values, necessarily developed in experimental animals, may not apply in humans.

Model-independent pharmacokinetics represents a less complex approach based on simple mathematical description of blood or plasma profiles of drugs or metabolites without invoking a particular kinetic model. In many situations during drug discovery and development, and also in clinical practice, it is sufficient to characterise plasma drug or metabolite profiles in terms of maximum plasma levels, time of maximum levels, area under the drug or metabolite plasma curve, and elimination rate or half-life. Values for these parameters can generally be obtained by simple inspection of plasma profiles without fitting data to a particular kinetic model.

However, more complete kinetic modeling may be necessary for complete pharmacokinetic characterisation and to examine relationships between drug disposition and pharmacologic effects.

A fourth approach to pharmacokinetic data analysis uses a combination of pharmacokinetic and statistical methods. This is generally described as ▶ population pharmacokinetics or mixed-effect modeling. Whereas traditional pharmacokinetic analysis focuses on fairly complete data sets obtained from individual subjects, with averages of such data being used to find population tendencies, the population pharmacokinetics or mixed effect modeling method focuses on the central tendency of diverse and often sparse data obtained across a subject population (2).

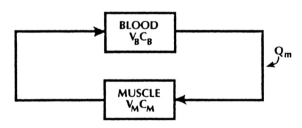

Fig. 2 Basic unit of the physiological model. Qm is blood flow through the organ, V is organ volume, and C is drug concentation. Subscript denotes the organ, in this case blood (B) or muscle (M).

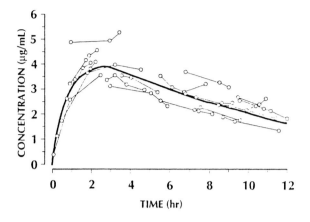

Fig. 3 Population pharmacokinetic analysis of simulated data from 25 individuals to yield a pharmacokinetic profile of central tendency (based on data in Reference 3).

An example of the latter approach to pharmacokinetic data analysis is shown in Fig. 3 that is based on a simulation in which 25 individuals each yielded 3–4 plasma drug concentration points at various times after oral drug administration. None of the individual data sets describes a complete plasma profile. However, using a population pharmacokinetics approach, a composite profile can be obtained that is highly characterised, both pharmacokinetically and statistically.

Population pharmacokinetics requires only a small number of data points from each individual and thus permits cost-effective sampling over a large population, thus generating a broad base of pharmacokinetic information. However, this carries with it the disadvantage of possible protocol deviations, lack of control over study conditions, and sample documentation problems.

Pharmacological Relevance

Pharmacokinetics and Pharmacodynamics
Current major emphasis in drug development programs is to establish and characterise relationships between drug pharmacokinetics and pharmacologic or therapeutic outcomes. Appreciation of the importance of pharmacokinetic-pharmacologic relationships has projected these disciplines into a central and critical position in drug discovery and development. This is particularly so in the case of clinical studies. During all phases of clinical drug development, blood level determinations and the relation of these values to pharmacologic or therapeutic end points are included in most study protocols. Much of the initiative for this has been the keen interest shown by regulatory bodies in drug level-effect relationships, and also the availability of appropriate mixed-effect modeling computer programs (4).

Toxicokinetics and Toxicodynamics
Blood drug levels were originally obtained during toxicity studies merely to ensure that drugs were administered and were to at least some extent systemically available. Drug safety assessments were based on dose-effect relationships. This situation has changed. Toxicokinetics is now a necessary component of toxicology studies, and the disposition of a drug or metabolite(s) must now be characterised in toxicity species at toxicological dose levels. Drug safety assessments are based on concentration-effect relationships. The very high doses generally used in toxicology studies, compared to those used in nonclinical pharmacology or clinical studies often give rise to marked differences in toxicokinetic and pharmacokinetic drug profiles.

The discipline of toxicodynamics is of more recent origin than ▶ pharmacodynamics, and few toxicokinetic-toxicodynamic relationships have been described. Nonetheless, this area is advancing rapidly and has presented a new perspective in the design and interpretation of toxicology studies.

Conclusions
Pharmacokinetics and toxicokinetics differ in terms of their goals and philosophical emphasis. Both are recognised as critical components in the drug development process. Pharmacokinetic studies require extensive collaboration with such disciplines as pharmacology, clinical pharmacology and clinical development. Toxicokinetics, on the other hand, requires collaboration principally with toxicology, as well as clinical pharmacology, and clinical development. These latter collaborations are frequently based on assessment of drug safety and therapeutic margins. These multidisciplinary interactions reflect the global impact of

P

the discipline of pharmacokinetics, together with the related disciplines of drug metabolism, transport and drug interactions, across the spectrum of pharmaceutical research and development, and in clinical medicine.

References

1. Welling PG (1997) Drug absorption, distribution, metabolism, and excretion, in Pharmacokinetics, Processes, Mathematics, and Applications. Am Chem Soc, Washington DC, p3–11
2. Olson SC (1992) The population approach, in European Cooperation in the Fields of Scientific Research. New Strategies in Drug Development and Clinical Evaluation. Office for Official Publications of the European Communities: Brussels, p143–152
3. Olson SC, Kugler AR (1990) Evaluation of sampling strategies (SS) for pharmacokinetic screening (PKS) in Phase III clinical trials. Pharm Res. 7:S262
4. Hochhaus G, Derendorf H (1995) Dose optimisation based on pharmacokinetic-pharmacodynamic modeling, in Pharmacokinetic/Pharmacodynamic Correlation. CRC Press, Boca Raton, p79–120

Pharmocodynamic Tolerance

Pharmocodynamic tolerance develops in response to continued application of drugs, by mechanisms that include reversible cellular adaptation processes, such as receptor desensitization, internalization and down-regulation as well as changes in the activity and levels of other components of the receptor's signal transduction pathways.

Pharmocokinetic Tolerance

Pharmocokinetic tolerance develops in response to continued application of drugs by pharmocokinetic mechanisms that include e.g. decreased absorption, increased rate of drug metabolism and excretion.

Phenothiazines

▶ Antipsychotic Drugs

Phenotype

The phenotype is the apparent form of a polymorphism measurable as function or structure by use of inspection, enzyme kinetic methods, or other methods.

▶ Pharmacogenetics

Phenylalkylamines

Phenylalkylamines are a family of compounds blocking dihydropyridine-sensitive high-voltage-activated (HVA) calcium channels.

▶ Ca^{2+} Channel Blockers
▶ Voltage-dependant Ca^{2+} Channels

Phorbol Esters

Phorbol esters are diterpene esters isolated from croton oil produced by the plant *Croton tiglium*. The prototypical phorbol ester, 12-O-tetradecanoyl-13-acetate (TPA) is a tumour promoter which activates various protein kinase C (PKC) isoforms.

▶ Phospholipases
▶ Protein Kinase C

Phosphatases

A phosphatase is an enzyme that hydrolyzes phosphomonoesterases, a reaction yielding free phosphate and alcohol. Substrates for phosphatases include both phospholipids and proteins. A wide variety of protein phosphatases exist and are generally classified according to their substrate specificities. For example, protein tyrosine phosphatases (e.g. SHP-2) dephosphorylate phosphotyrosine residues while dual specificity phosphatases dephosphorylate both phosphothreonine and phosphotyrosine residues (e.g. calcineurin). PTEN is a phosphatase that can dephosphorylate both lipids and proteins.

▶ MAP Kinase Cascades
▶ Growth Factors

Phosphatidic Acid

Phosphatidic acid is glycerol esterified at the sn-1 and sn-2 positions to two fatty acids and at the sn-3 position to phosphoric acid. It is a product of phospholipase D action that is also an intermediate in the biosynthesis of phosphatidylserine and phosphatidylinositol.

▶ Phospholipases

Phosphatidylinositol 3-kinase

Phosphatidylinositol 3 kinases (PI3-kinase) are a family of enzymes phosphorylating phosphatidylinositol (PtdIns), PtdIns(4)phosphate and PtdIns(4,5)phosphate in the 3-position. The PtdIns(3)phospholipids are second messengers in processes like cell growth, cytoskeletal rearrangement and vesicular transport. PI 3-kinases are heterodimers composed of a catalytic and a regulatory subunit. The enzymes are activated by insulin, many growth factors, and by a variety of cytokines. Their activity can be inhibited by wortmannin and LY294002.

▶ Phospholipid Kinases

Phosphatidylinositol 4,5-bisphosphate

Phosphatidylinositol 4,5-bisphosphate is a derivative of phosphatidylinositol in which the inositol ring is phosphorylated at positions 4 and 5.

▶ Phospholipases

Phosphatidylinositol Phophate

Phosphatidylinositol phosphates (PIPs) are phosphorylated derivatives of PI (phosphatidylinositol). PIPs that have been detected in cells include PI-3-P, PI-4-P(PIP), PI-5-P, PI-3,4-P_2, PI-4,5-P_2(PIP$_2$), PI-3,5-P_2, and PI-3,4,5-P_3(PIP$_3$). PIP and PIP$_2$ are the most abundant forms (~60%).

▶ ATP-dependent K^+ Channels
▶ Phospholipases

Phosphatodylinositol

Phosphatidylinositol is a phospholipid containing the inositol sugar head group.

▶ Phospholipases

P

Phosphodiesterases

JENNIFER L. GLICK, JOSEPH A. BEAVO
Depatartment of Pharmacology, University of
Washington, Seattle, WA, USA
jbelyea@u.washington.edu
beavo@u.washington.edu

Synonyms

Cyclic nucleotide phosphodiesterases, PDEs

Definition

Cyclic nucleotide phosphodiesterases are a class of
enzymes that catalyze the hydrolysis of 3′,5′-cyclic
guanosine monophosphate (cGMP) or 3′,5′-cyclic
adenosine monophosphate (cAMP) to 5′-guanos-
ine monophosphate (GMP) or 5′-adenosine monophosphate (AMP), respectively.

▶ Adenylyl Cyclases
▶ Guanylyl Cyclase
▶ Smooth Muscle Tone Regulation

Basic Characteristics

The cyclic nucleotide phosphodiesterases (PDEs)
are a superfamily of enzymes that hydrolyze cGMP
and cAMP to their respective 5′ monophosphates.
Cyclic nucleotide signaling is important in a large
number of processes including proliferation,
▶ chemotaxis, contraction, relaxation and inflammation. Therefore, together with the cyclases
(adenylyl and guanylyl cyclase), the PDE family is
crucial for survival and for maintaining quality of
life in eukaryotic organisms. Currently there are 11
known PDE gene families, all of which have
unique characteristics in terms of substrate specificity, expression patterns, kinetics and regulatory
properties (Table 1). The current nomenclature for
a PDE contains, in order, 2 letters to indicate species, a number indicating gene family, a letter to
represent an individual gene, and a letter to signify
splice variant. For example, MMPDE9A1 represents the mouse PDE9 gene family, gene A, splice
variant 1. In general, all PDEs share the same
structural organization. Each protein has an N-

terminal motif that is used to regulate the protein's
activity or localization, and a C-terminal catalyitic domain, followed by a short tail. The catalyic
domains of PDEs share approximately 35%
sequence identity, including the conserved signature sequence H-D-X_2-H-X_4-N.

Substrate Specificity

The substrate specificity of the PDEs range from
dual specificity enzymes (PDE1,2,10 and 11) to
those that hydrolyze either cGMP (PDE5,6 and 9)
or cAMP (PDE3,4,7 and 8) exclusively. In fact, the
relative substrate specificity can vary between
members of a gene family. For example, within the
PDE1 gene family PDE1A has a Km for cGMP that
is much lower than that for cAMP, while PDE1C
has roughly equal affinity for both nucleotides. In
addition, the activity of a PDE toward one cyclic
nucleotide can vary depending on the concen-
tratation of the other cyclic nucleotide. For
instance, PDE2 will hydrolyze cAMP and cGMP
with relatively similar Km values. However, the
presence of a small amount of cGMP (through
allosteric binding sites) stimulates the activity of
PDE2 towards cAMP. There are also PDEs for
which one cyclic nucleotide acts as a competitive
inhibitor for the other. Cyclic AMP is a competitive
inhibitor of PDE10 cGMP hydrolysis, and cGMP is
a potent inhibitor of PDE3's cAMP hydrolyzing
activity. Thus, with a wide variety of specificities
and affinities for the different nucleotides, the
PDEs are a group of enzymes that are well adapted
to fine tune the cyclic nucleotide pools within the
cell.

Regulatory Domains

All of the PDEs possess a significant amount of
sequence that is N-terminal to the catalytic
domain. In fact, the N-terminus can be larger than
the catalyitic domain itself. Within the N-terminus
there are domains used to regulate the activity of
the catalyic site (Fig. 1). The PDE1 family members have two Ca^{2+}/calmodulin-binding domains.
Binding of Ca^{2+}/calmodulin to these domains
stimulates the activity of the PDE1s several fold.
PDE2, PDE5, PDE6, PDE10 and PDE11 all have
allosteric, cGMP-binding GAF domains (named
after cyclic GMP-binding phosphodiesterase,
▶ adenylyl cyclase, FhlA) in their N-termini. Binding of cGMP to these domains have various effects

Tab. 1 **Characteristics of the individual PDE families.**

PDE Family	Genes	Splice Variants	Regulatory Domains / Role	Phosphorylation	Substrate(s)	Commonly used Inhibitors
PDE1	1A, 1B, 1C	9	CaM / activation	PKA	cGMP, cAMP	KS-505
PDE2	2A	3	GAF / activation	unknown	cAMP, cGMP	EHNA
PDE3	3A, 3B	1 each	transmembrane domains / membrane targeting	PKB	cAMP	Milrinone
PDE4	4A, 4B, 4C, 4D	>20	UCR1, UCR2 / unclear	ERK, PKA	cAMP	Rolipram
PDE5	5A	3	GAF / unclear	PKA, PKG	cGMP	Sildenafil, Dipyrimadole, Zaprinast
PDE6	6A, 6B, 6C	1 each	GAF / activation	PKC, PKA	cGMP	Dipyrimadole, Zaprinast
PDE7	7A, 7B	6	unknown	unknown	cAMP	none identified
PDE	8A, 8B	6	PAS / unknown	unknown	cAMP	none identified
PDE9	9A	4	unknown	unknown	cGMP	none identified
PDE10	10A	2	GAF / unknown	unknown	cAMP, cGMP	none identified
PDE11	11A	4	GAF / unknown	unknown	cAMP, cGMP	none identified

on PDEs. For PDE2, binding of cGMP to its GAF domain results in stimulation of its cAMP hydrolyzing activity. Binding of cGMP to PDE5 increases its susceptibility to phosphorylation, but it is not clear whether cGMP binding has a direct effect on activity. PDE10 and PDE11 have unusual GAF domains. The affinity of PDE10 for cGMP is low, with a reported Kd of greater than 10 μM. This high Kd value implies that the GAF domains in PDE10 might bind some other small molecule and therefore play a different role in regulation of PDE10 catalytic activity than the GAF domains of PDE2, 5 and 6. In the PDE11 family there are reported splice variants with one full length and one truncated GAF domain. It is unclear what role this truncated form might play, if any, in PDE11 function. The N-terminus of PDE8 has another small molecule binding domain, the PAS domain. PAS domains are found in a number of eukaryotic systems and are found within proteins that are involved in sensing their environment such as oxygen, energy or light levels. They also bind small molecules and can be involved in protein-protein interactions. PAS domains in other proteins com-

monly function either as protein interaction sites or small molecule binding domains. Occasionally they serve both functions. However, it is not known for PDE8 whether the PAS domain has either of these functions. It will be of great interest if a small molecule regulatory ligand that binds to the PAS domain can be identified.

PDEs are also regulated by targeting and phosphorylation. The PDE3 family members have six putative transmembrane domains in their N-terminal regions, the likely reason PDE3 activity is largely membrane associated. Some PDEs, such as PDE2A2 and PDE9A1, have putative N-myristoylation sites which presumably target these proteins to the membrane. While this has not been demonstrated for PDE9, a membrane associated form of PDE2 activity has been shown. PDE6, the PDE involved in retinal ▶ phototransduction, is prenylated and tightly associated with the disc membranes of the photoreceptor cells. Lipid modification, however, is not the only mechanism for localizing PDEs. Examples of proteins that associate with PDEs and likely target them to cellular compartments are emerging. Recently, RACK1, a

P

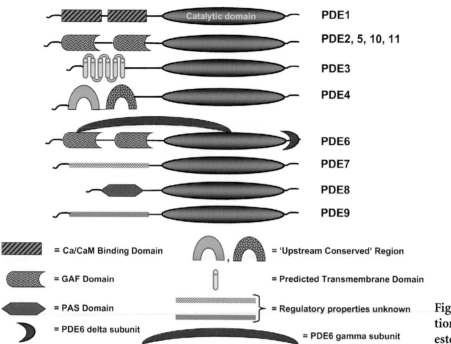

Fig. 1 Domain organization of the phosphodiesterase family.

▶ scaffolding protein that associates with PKC and Src, was also shown to bind PDE4D5. PDE4D also associates with a centrosomal protein, myomegalin, and a PKA anchoring protein, mAKAP. All of these associations with PDE4D are likely to be targeting this PDE to specific cAMP pools in the cell. Undoubtedly, more examples of this type of targeting will be discovered.

Compartmentalization of PDEs

Compartmentalization of cyclic nucleotide signaling within the cell is a notion that has been around for some 20 years, yet has been difficult to demonstrate for the PDEs. However, some examples of compartmentalization of PDEs in cells have been shown. The best studied example is in the photoreceptor, where PDE6 is concentrated on the membrane disks along with the other players in the phototransduction cascade. There, PDE6 is activated in response to light and hydrolyzes local cGMP, and resident cGMP-gated cation channels close, hyperpolarizing the cell. In kidney mesangial cells, the production of ▶ superoxide and mitogenesis are both stimulated through the elevation of cAMP. The production of superoxide is rolipram sensitive, indicating a role for PDE4 in this process. Mitogenesis is cilostamide sensitive,

implying a role for PDE3. Superoxide generation is not effected by cilostamide and mitogenesis is insensitive to rolipram. Thus, while both of these processes are cAMP-dependent, different cAMP pools and PDEs are involved in each. Another example of compartmentalization of PDE activities in the cell exists in the olfactory epithelium, where PDE1C2 and PDE4A are expressed. PDE1C2 is found in the cilia of the epithelium, where it colocalizes with adenylyl cyclase. PDE4A is found throughout the epithelial layer, but not in cilia. Therefore, as in the kidney mesangial cells, different PDEs must be working on different cyclic nucleotide pools.

Drugs

Currently, Viagra (Pfizer, Inc.) is the best example of a specific PDE inhibitor put to clinical use. Stimulation of the smooth muscle cells of the corpus callosum by nitric oxide results in the elevation of cGMP. This increase in cGMP levels results in relaxation of the vascular smooth muscle and engorgement of the penis. Viagra, through inhibition of PDE5 in the smooth muscle cells, potentiates this effect. And because it is highly selective for PDE5, Viagra has been used to treat male erectile disfunction with generally minor side effects.

Beyond Viagra, there are a number of other PDE inhibitors that are used clinically. In fact, the classic drugs papaverine and dipyridamole were used clinically before their effects on PDEs were known. Caffeine and theophylline (a compound found in tea) are also PDE inhibitors. However, all of these drugs most likely have multiple targets, making conclusions regarding the roles of PDEs in processes that are sensitive to these agents difficult to interpret. Certainly, some of their effects are due to their action on adenosine receptors.

The PDE3 inhibitor, cilostazol, has been used as an anti-thrombotic agent and is currently being used in patients being treated for intermittent claudication. Cilostazol is also used for the prevention of ▶ restenosis after treatments such as angioplasty. Another PDE3 selective inhibitor, milrinone, has been used in the treatment of congestive heart failure. Milrinone also has been shown to increase the conductance of the CFTR transporter *in vitro*. This observation, although preliminary, indicates that milrinone may have future applications in the treatment of cystic fibrosis.

PDE4 inhibitors may also serve as anti-inflammatory agents. Older PDE4 inhibitors tend to be limited by their emetic side effects, but newer drugs are now in clinical trials and may have milder side effects. These drugs (Ariflo; GlaxoSmithKline, and Roflumilast; Byk Gulden) are being tested for the treatment of asthma and chronic obstructive pulmonary disease with some success.

Dipyridamole is a PDE5/PDE6 selective inhibitor that is used widely in conjunction with aspirin to reduce clotting and prevent stroke. While the combination of dipyridamole and aspirin is commonly prescribed, the evidence for an added benefit of dipyridamole over aspirin alone is limited. The recent European Stroke Prevention Study 2 is the first clear demonstration of added benefit of this combination over aspirin, yet the patients reported high levels of neurological and gastrointestinal side effects.

And finally, IBMX is a methylxanthine derivative that has long been used *in vitro* as a general PDE inhibitor. IBMX is effective at inhibiting most PDEs, with an IC50 of 2–50 μM. However, the recently cloned PDEs, PDE8 and PDE9, are IBMX-resistant. It is therefore important to keep this in mind when using IBMX to investigate potential roles for PDEs.

References

1. Beavo JA (1995) Cyclic nucleotide phosphodiesterases: functional implications of multiple isoforms. Physiological Reviews 75:725–748
2. Gibson A (2001) Phosphodiesterase 5 inhibitors and nitrergic transmission – from zaprinast to sildenafil. European Journal of Pharmacology 411:1–10
3. Essayen DM (2001) Cyclic nucleotide phosphodiesterases. Journal of Allergy and Clinical Immunology 108:671–680
4. Soderling SH, Beavo JA (2000) Regulation of cAMP and cGMP signaling: new phosphodiesterases and new functions. Current Opinion in Cell Biology 12:174–179

Phospholipases

JOHN H. EXTON
Howard Hughes Medical Institute
and Department of Molecular Physiology
and Biophysics, Vanderbilt University
School of Medicine
john.exton@mcmail.vanderbilt.edu

Definition

Enzymes that hydrolyze ▶ phospholipids

▶ Phospholipid Kinases
▶ Transmembrane Signalling

Basic Characteristics

▶ Phospholipases are widely distributed in nature and carry out many important cellular functions. They are classified into four types: A_1, A_2, C and D. Phospholipase A_1 and A_2 act respectively on the ester bonds that link fatty acids to the sn-1 and sn-2 positions of the glycerol backbone of phospholipids (Fig. 1). Their action generates free fatty acids and lysophospholipids. Phospholipase C acts on the phosphodiester bond that links the headgroup of the phospholipid to the glycerol backbone. It yields phosphorylated headgroups and ▶ diacylglycerol (DAG). Phospholipase D acts on the other side of the phosphodiester bond to yield free headgroups and ▶ phosphatidic acid (PA). Phospholipases alter cell activities through their effects on membrane phospholipids. Their products also influence cellular functions by acting as intracellular and extracellular messengers. Thus the lipids (fatty acids, DAG, PA) released as a result of phospholipase activity can alter the activity of enzymes and other cellular proteins or they can be metabolized to other lipids, some of which are released and exert diverse effects (eicosanoids, lysophosphatidic acid). Mammalian phospholipase C acts on inositol phospholipids, principally ▶ phosphatidylinositol 4,5-bisphosphate (PIP$_2$) and the phosphorylated headgroup primarily released by phospholipase C action (inositol 1,4,5-trisphosphate, IP$_3$) plays a major role in Ca^{2+} mobilization in the cell, with subsequent important physiological consequences. As expected from their important physiological functions, many phospholipases are highly regulated by hormones, neurotransmitters, growth factors and cytokines.

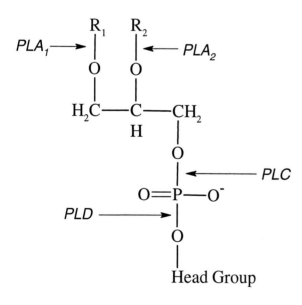

Fig. 1 Generic phospholipid with sites of action of phospholipases shown.

Phospholipase A1

Phospholipase A1 (PLA$_1$) is widely distributed. It has not been studied extensively and is not known to be regulated. Its major substrates are PA, phosphatidylcholine (PC) and phosphatidylethanolamine (PE) and it releases mainly saturated or monounsaturated fatty acids, which are predominantly present at position sn-1 of these phospholipids. Through the combined action of PLA$_1$ and lysophospholipase, arachidonic or other unsaturated fatty acids can be released from the sn-2 position also. A PA-preferring PLA$_1$ isozyme has been cloned. It has a molecular mass of 98 kD and is expressed in brain and testis. No other isozymes have been cloned. The function of PLA$_1$ relates to phospholipid remodeling i.e. the substitution of one fatty acid by another, which it accomplishes in combination with lysophospholipid acyltransferase.

Phospholipase A2

Phospholipase A2 (PLA$_2$) occurs in several forms as the products of different genes (Tables I and II). Some forms are of low molecular mass (~14 kD) and are secreted by cells, whereas others are of higher mass (26–114 kD) and are mainly located in the cytosol (1). The smaller forms are components of snake and bee venoms, but some are also present in mammalian tissues and are secreted into pancreatic juice and synovial fluid (1). They have a rigid crystal structure due to their high disulfide bond content (Table I). Catalysis involves a conserved His that, together with a conserved Asp, polarizes a bound H$_2$O to attack the substrate carbonyl group. They require millimolar Ca^{2+} for activity. The Ca^{2+} is bound to a conserved glycine-rich loop and interacts with the conserved Asp to stabilize the transition state. Secretory PLA$_2$s (sPLA$_2$s) act predominantly on PC and PE and have been classified into several groups (I, II, III, V and X) based on sequence differences (Table I). For conciseness, only the mammalian groups will be described. Group I sPLA$_2$ is present in pancreatic acinar cells as a proenzyme form. It is released into pancreatic juice and is converted by trypsin to the active form, which is involved in digestion. Group II sPLA$_2$ exists in several subgroups and is present in synovial fluid and many tissues. Group III sPLA$_2$ is present in several human tissues and has a preference for phosphati-

Tab. 1 Classification of low molecular mass phospholipase A₂ isozymes that use catalytic His.

Group	Sources	Molecular Mass [kDa]	Disulfides (No.)
I A, B	Snake venom, pancreas	13–15	7
II A–F	Snake venom, synovial fluid, pancreas, testis, spleen, brain, heart, uterus	13–17	6–8
III	Bee, lizard, scorpion, human	15–18	5
V	Heart, lung, macrophages	14	6
IX	Snail venom	14	6
X	Spleen, thymus, leukocytes	14	8
XI A, B	Rice	12–13	6

Adapted from Six and Dennis (1)

dylglycerol. Groups V and X are also widely distributed and are active on PC and PE. Serum levels of sPLA₂s are elevated in inflammatory conditions and trauma, and secretion of these isozymes into other body fluids occurs in specific diseases e.g. pancreatitis, inflammatory bowel disease and arthritis. The secretion and expression of sPLA₂s is increased by pro-inflammatory cytokines, e.g. tumor necrosis factor α and certain interleukins, resulting in the production of arachidonic acid that is subsequently converted to prostaglandins and other eicosanoids.

The cytosolic forms show no sequence homology to the secreted forms and have a different catalytic mechanism (1). They are widely distributed and occur as either Ca^{2+}-dependent and Ca^{2+}-independent forms (Table II). Ca^{2+}-dependent PLA₂ (Group IV or cPLA₂) occurs in three isoforms (α, β,γ). cPLA₂α is regulated by cytokines and growth factors and plays a major role in the regulated production of arachidonic acid. It shows marked specificity for phospholipids containing arachidonic acid in position sn-2 and also exhibits lysophospholipase activity. The arachidonic acid produced is subsequently metabolized to a variety of eicosanoids (e.g. prostaglandins, prostacyclin, thromboxanes, leukotrienes) that contributes to inflammation and a large variety of other physiological responses. These include changes in blood flow, platelet function, smooth muscle contractility, renal function, endocrine responses and gastrointestinal secretion. These effects may be positive or negative, depending on the specific eicosanoid and target tissue.

cPLA₂α (85 kD) has been much studied and contains a Ca^{2+}-lipid-dependent binding (CaLB) domain in its N-terminus (1). The structure of this domain is similar to that of the C-2 Ca^{2+}-binding domains found in ▶ protein kinase C, phospholipase Cδ and synaptotagmin. The catalytic mechanism is different from that of the low molecular mass PLA₂s and involves a Gly-Leu-Ser-Gly-Ser sequence which resembles that seen in many serine esterases and neutral lipases. The central Ser (Ser²²⁸) serves as the active site nucleophile and catalyzes hydrolysis in association with Asp⁵⁴⁹. Like other serine esterases in which the nucleophilic serine is on a 'nucleophilic elbow' (a turn between a β strand and α-helix), cPLA₂ has a central β-sheet with Ser²²⁸ located within this 'elbow'. However, other structural features of the catalytic site are quite different from those of other serine esterases. Surprisingly, the catalytic site is buried quite deeply in the catalytic domain core suggesting that the enzyme must become embedded in the lipid bilayer.

An increase in Ca^{2+} in the micromolar range induces translocation of cPLA₂ to the nuclear membrane. The translocation involves the CaLB domain that presents the catalytic domain to the phospholipid substrate, resulting in increased arachidonic acid release. The enzyme is also phosphorylated and activated by mitogen-activated protein kinases (MAPKs). The phosphorylation is

P

Tab. 2   Classification of higher molecular mass phospholipase A$_2$ isozymes that use catalytic Ser.

Group	Sources	Molecular Mass [kDa]	Ca^{2+} Requirement
IV A–C	Platelets, lymphocytes, kidney, pancreas, liver, heart, brain, skeletal muscle	61–114	<µM*
VI A, B	Macrophages, lymphocytes, heart, skeletal muscle	84–90	0
VII A, B	Plasma, kidney, liver	40–45	0
VIII A, B	Brain	26	0

Adapted from Six and Dennis (1).
*Group IVC does not require Ca^{2+}

catalyzed by both extracellular signal-regulated kinase (ERK) and p38 MAPK, and involves a specific residue (Ser^{505}). This Ser residue is located within the catalytic domain in close proximity to the C-2 Ca^{2+} binding domain. It has been proposed that phosphorylation of Ser^{505} improves the positioning of the catalytic site in relation to the lipid bilayer.

In addition to its rapid activation by agonists that elevate cytosolic Ca^{2+} and activate MAP kinase, cPLA$_2$ can be regulated at the transcriptional level by the proinflammatory cytokines interleukin 1 and tumor necrosis factor α, whose action is inhibited by glucocorticoids. Other factors (macrophage colony-stimulating factor, lipopolysaccharide, epidermal growth factor) also activate transcription of cPLA$_2$.

The Ca^{2+}-independent cytosolic PLA$_2$ (iPLA$_2$ or Group VI) isozymes are widely distributed and located predominantly in the cytosol (1), although there are some membrane-associated forms (Table II). Their molecular masses range between 84 and 90 kD due to multiple splice variants, and some forms contain ankyrin repeats. They contain the lipase consensus sequence and the active Ser found in cPLA$_2$s. They are involved in phospholipid fatty acid remodeling and may be involved in arachidonic acid release and prostaglandin formation, although this is limited compared with other PLA$_2$ isozymes.

Two other groups of PLA$_2$s (Groups VII and VIII) inactivate platelet-activating factor (PAF) (1). They are also called PAF-acetylhydrolases and are highly specific for PAF or PAF analogues with short-chain oxidized fatty acids in position sn-2.

PAF is a modified form of PC in which the sn-1 chain is linked by an ether linkage, and an acetyl group is present at sn-2. It has many potent effects including vasodilation, platelet activation, chemotactic action and smooth muscle contraction. These types of PLA$_2$ have the characteristic lipase catalytic sequence of cytosolic PLA$_2$s, but are of lower molecular mass (26–45 kD). They exist as either intracellular or secreted forms, and are found in many tissues.

Phospholipase C

In contrast to phospholipases of the A type, which have broad substrate specificity, phospholipase C (PLC) in mammalian cells acts only on inositol-containing phospholipids, in particular PIP$_2$, which is cleaved to form IP$_3$ and diacylglycerol (▶ PI Response). Mammalian PLC occurs as four different isozymes (β, γ, δ and ε) and there are several subtypes of these (β1–β4, γ1, γ2, δ1–δ4) (2). The β1, β3, γ1, δ1, δ4 and ε isozymes are widely distributed, whereas the β2 and γ2 forms are found predominantly in hematopoietic cells, and the β4 isozyme is confined to retina and brain. The β and γ isozymes are highly regulated by different agonists, whereas the δ isozymes are not subject to agonist control, but are stimulated by a rise in cytosolic Ca^{2+} (2). The β isozymes are activated by α- or βγ-subunits released from heterotrimeric proteins of the G$_q$ and G$_{i/o}$ families as the result of activation of certain receptors. The γ isozymes are activated by growth factor receptors that encode tyrosine kinase activity and by cytokines that induce tyrosine phosophorylation of their receptors. The PLCε isozyme contains a Ras guanine

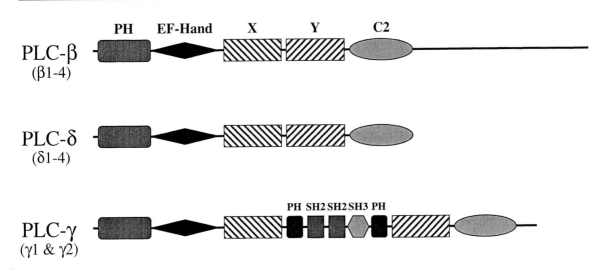

Fig. 2 Representation of the domains in the major isozymes of phospholipase C (adapted from Ref. 2).

nucleotide exchange factor domain (GRF CDC25) and two Ras binding domains. It is directly activated by active Ras, which also causes its membrane translocation.

All PLC isozymes have conserved catalytic domains designated X and Y, and a C2 domain similar to that in $cPLA_2$. (Fig. 2). In addition, the β-, γ- and δ-isozymes have pleckstrin homology (PH) domains and EF-hand domains located in the N-terminal region. The γ-isozymes differ in that they have Src homology domains (SH2 and SH3) and an additional PH domain split by the SH domains. The β- and γ-isozymes are of 140–155 kD mass, whereas the δ-isozymes are smaller (85 kD) and the σ-isozyme is larger (240 kD).

The three-dimensional structure of PLC-δ1 has been defined. The catalytic domain is in the form of an α/β or TIM barrel (discovered first in triosephosphate isomerase). The active site is in the cleft of the barrel and contains a coordinated Ca^{2+} that is required for catalysis. The proposed general mechanism is general base/general acid catalysis. Membrane binding of the enzyme depends on the PH domain, which is proposed to tether the enzyme through PIP_2 binding. The C2 domain is proposed to fix the catalytic domain so that it can penetrate the membrane, allowing PIP_2 hydrolysis to proceed.

The β isozymes are activated by G protein-coupled receptors through two different mechanisms (2). The first involves activated α-subunits of the G_q family of heterotrimeric G proteins (G_q, G_{11}, G_{14}, $G_{15/16}$). These subunits activate the β1, β3 and β4 PLC isozymes through direct interaction with a sequence in the C terminus. The domain on the $G_q\alpha$-subunit that interacts with the β isozymes is located on a surface α-helix that is adjacent to the Switch III region, which undergoes a marked conformational change during activation. The second mechanism of G protein activation of PLCβ isozymes involves βγ-subunits released from $G_{i/o}$ G proteins by their pertussis toxin-sensitive activation by certain receptors. The βγ-subunits activate the β_2 and β_3 PLC isozymes by interacting with a sequence between the conserved X and Y domains.

The physiological importance of PLC activation is to cleave PIP_2 into IP_3 and DAG. IP_3 induces the release of Ca^{2+} from Ca^{2+} stores in the endoplasmic reticulum, which results secondarily in increased Ca^{2+} influx into the cell. The resultant increase in cytosolic Ca^{2+} causes a variety of physiological responses including smooth muscle contraction in many organs, secretion of cellular constituents in many cells and glycogen breakdown and other metabolic responses in liver and other organs. The DAG that accumulates in the plasma membrane as a result of PLC activation causes membrane translocation and activation of most isozymes of protein kinase C (PKC). This kinase

P

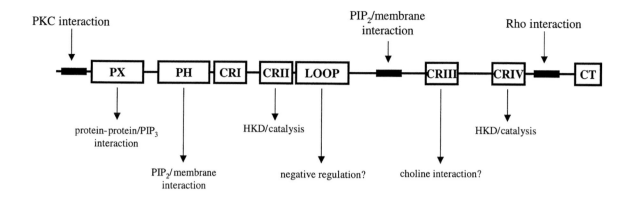

Fig. 3 Representation of the domain structure of phospholipase D1 (adapted from Frohman MA, Sung T-C, Morris AJ (1999) Biochim. Biophys. Acta 1439:175-186).

acts on many membrane proteins (e.g. receptors, ion channels, transporters) to modulate their activities and modify certain physiological responses.

Phospholipase D

Phospholipase D is widely distributed in bacteria, fungi, plants and animals, and is present in almost all mammalian cells (3). In mammals, it occurs as alternatively spliced products of two genes (PLD1 and PLD2) (Fig. 3). Most mammalian cells express different levels of both isoforms. Both PLD1 and PLD2 have four conserved sequences (I-IV), and sequences I and IV contain the $HXKX_4D$ (HKD) motif that is characteristic of the PLD super-family, which includes bacterial endonucleases, phospholipid synthases, viral envelope proteins and a murine toxin (Fig. 3) (3). Both HKD domains are required for catalytic activity and they dimerize to form the catalytic center. Catalysis occurs in a two-step reaction involving the two His residues of the dimer (3). The first step is a nucleophilic attack by one His on the substrate phosphorus to produce a phosphatidyl-enzyme intermediate. The second step involves the other His that protonates the oxygen of the leaving group. Both PLD isoforms require PIP_2 for activity, but are distributed in different cellular sites and are differentially regulated. PLD1 is activated *in vitro* by the α- and β-isozymes of PKC and by members of the Rho and ARF families of low Mr G proteins (3). Combinations of these proteins produce synergistic activation of the enzyme. In contrast, PLD2 is not regulated by these factors *in vitro*. The interaction site for PKCα is at the N-terminus of PLD1, while that for RhoA is at the C-terminus. The binding site for ARF is unknown.

PLD is highly regulated *in vivo* by hormones, neurotransmitters and other G protein-coupled agonists, and also by growth factors and cytokines. The regulation is not direct but involves signaling through PKC and Rho family proteins. The enzyme can be phosphorylated on Tyr and Ser/Thr residues *in vivo*, but the role of these phosphorylations in its regulation is unclear. The cellular roles of PLD include the regulation of Golgi function, exocytosis, endocytosis, the actin cytoskeleton, superoxide production and growth. It has been proposed that the role of ARF in vesicle trafficking in the Golgi involves not only coatomer formation, but also PLD activation, which stimulates vesicle budding through PA formation. PLD is implicated in catecholamine secretion, endocytosis of membrane receptors and glucose transport. The rearrangement of the actin cytoskeleton resulting in stress fiber formation also depends on PLD activity. The activation of NADPH oxidase that yields superoxide in neutrophils involves PA formation via PLD activity, and PLD has been implicated in ERK activation in some cells.

Drugs

Phospholipase A2

Glucocorticoids inhibit $cPLA_2$ at the level of transcription and this is part of their anti-inflammatory action. Antimalarial drugs (mepacrine, aminoglycosides and polyamines) inhibit PLA_2 activity, but they are too non-specific to be therapeutically useful. This is also true of covalent-modifying PLA_2 agents such as manoalide and p-bromophenacyl bromide, which are selective for $sPLA_2$ *in vitro*. Another agent 3-(3-acetamide-1-benzyl-2-ethylindol-5-oxy) propane sulfonic acid (LY311727) inhibits $sPLA_2$ selectively in cell studies, but there have been no reports of its use *in vivo*. Arachidonyl trifluoromethyl ketone and methylarachidonyl fluorophosphonate are potent $cPLA_2$ inhibitors. However, they are too toxic and insufficiently specific to be useful therapeutically. Bromoenol lactone, which is a potent inhibitor of $cPLA_2$, has actions on other lipid-metabolizing enzymes and therefore limits its use *in vivo*.

Phospholipase C

There are no specific inhibitors of PLC, but compounds that interact with PIP_2, e.g. neomycin can reduce its activity. However, such drugs interfere with other signaling processes involving this lipid. The aminosteroid 1-[6-[[17β-3-methoxyestra-1,3,5(10)-trien-17-yl]amino]hexyl]-1*H*-pyrrole-2,5-dione (U-73122) has been reported to inhibit PLC, but has other effects related to cell Ca^{2+} homeostasis.

Phospholipase D

There are no specific inhibitors of PLD. Xanthogenate tricyclodecan-9-yl (D609) and 1-O-octadeyl-2-O-methyl-sn-glycero-3-phosphocholine (ET-18-OCH_3) lack specificity since they act by competing with substrate (phosphatidylcholine). Primary alcohols such as ethanol, propanol and butanol inhibit the actions of PLD by reducing the formation of PA through the transphosphatidylation reaction that generates phosphatidylalcohols. Since PA is the primary signaling molecule produced by PLD action, the cellular actions of this lipid are curtailed.

References

1. Six DA, Dennis EA (2000) The expanding superfamily of phospholipase A2 enzymes: classification and characterization. Biochim. Biophys Acta 1488:1–19
2. Rhee SG, Bae YS (1997) Regulation of phosphoinositide-specific phospholipase Isozymes. J. Biol. Chem. 272:15045–15048
3. Exton JH (2002) Phospholipase D – structure, regulation and function. Rev. Physiol. Biochem. Pharmacol. 144:1–94

Phospholipid

A phospholipid is an amphiphilic lipid that is a derivative of glycerol-3-phosphate, with fatty acids esterified to the sn-1 and sn-2 positions of the glycerol and a head group (choline, ethanolamine, serine or inositol) esterified to the phosphate. Phospholipids are major constituents of membranes.

▶ Phospholipases
▶ Phospholipid Kinases

Phospholipid Kinases

BERND NÜRNBERG
Universitätsklinikum Düsseldorf,
Düsseldorf, Germany
Bernd.Nuernberg@uni-duesseldorf.de

Synonyms

Phosphoinositol kinases, Phosphatidylinositol kinases, Phosphatidylinositide kinases

Definition

Phospholipid kinases comprise a family of enzymes that phosphorylate phosphatidylinositol and phosphatidylinositides at positions 3', 4' or 5' but not at positions 2' and 6' of the inositol ring (Fig. 1). Phosphatidylinositides represent approxi-

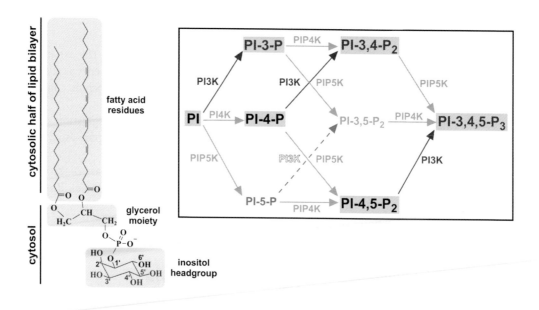

Fig. 1 Phosphoinositol (PtdIns [PI], left part) is found in the inner leaflet of the plasma membrane where it becomes a substrate for phospholipases and phosphoinositide kinases. Phosphorylation of PI by various phospholipid kinases results in the formation of distinct phosphoinositides (right part). *According to (1).*

mately 1% of all membrane lipids of the plasma membrane but are also found on endomembranes and in the nucleus. In unstimulated cells, more than 90% of all phosphoinositides correspond to unphosphorylated phosphoinositol (PtdIns), whereas the remaining 10% consist of roughly equal amounts of PtdIns-4-P and PtdIns-4,5-P_2 (1). These phosphoinositides were initially assumed to exclusively function as precursors for signaling molecules. For instance, PtdIns-4,5-P_2 serves as a substrate for phospholipases C and phosphoinositide-3-kinases. Interestingly, PtdIns-4,5-P_2 also interacts with intracellular proteins in a regulatory manner, thereby affecting their localization and activity. In resting cells, less than 0.25% of the phosphoinositides are 3'-phosphorylated. Stimulation of cells with ligands activating receptor tyrosine kinases or ▶ G-protein-coupled receptors results in the rapid and transient phosphorylation of PtdIns-4,5-P_2 to PtdIns-3,4,5-P_3. This 3'-phosphorylated phospholipid behaves as a typical second messenger. Hence, the responsible phosphoinositide-3-kinases are considered as important regulatory modules of the cell.

▶ **Phospholipases**

Basic Characteristics

Cellular phosphoinositide concentrations are under tight control by phospholipid kinases and phosphatases. Phospholipid kinases preferentially phosphorylate distinct positions of the inositol ring and hence are subdivided into phosphoinositide-3-kinases, phosphoinositide-4-kinases, and phosphoinositide-5-kinases. Moreover, phospholipid kinases exhibit some substrate specificity which allows further differentiation. Accordingly, enzymes responsible for generation of PtdIns-4-P are phosphatidylinositol-4-kinases (PI4K). They are grouped into two subfamilies, i.e. the type II and III PI4-kinases (2). In a canonical pathway, PtdIns-4,5-P_2 is generated from PtdIns-4-P by phosphatidylinositol-4-phosphate 5-kinase (PIP5K) enzymatic activity [see Fig. 1 and (3)]. The corresponding enzymes are also divided into two subfamilies, PIP5K class I and PIP5K class II, and operate by different mechanisms. Moreover, as shown in Fig. 1, additional pathways have been discovered which are regulated by poorly defined phospholipid kinase.

Of all phosphoinositides, PtdIns-3,4,5-P_3 and PtdIns-3,4-P_2 have been recognized as important

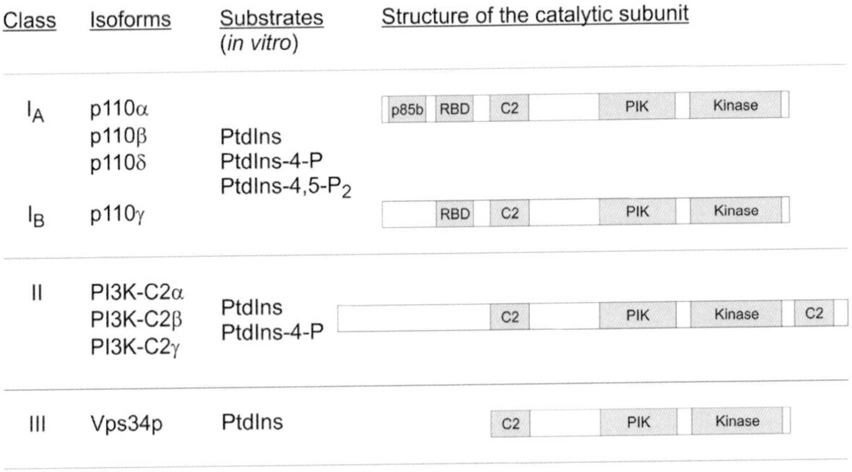

Class	Isoforms	Substrates (*in vitro*)	Structure of the catalytic subunit					
I$_A$	p110α p110β p110δ	PtdIns PtdIns-4-P PtdIns-4,5-P$_2$	p85b	RBD	C2		PIK	Kinase
I$_B$	p110γ			RBD	C2		PIK	Kinase
II	PI3K-C2α PI3K-C2β PI3K-C2γ	PtdIns PtdIns-4-P			C2		PIK	Kinase	C2
III	Vps34p	PtdIns			C2		PIK	Kinase

Fig. 2 Classification of the catalytic subunits of PI-3-kinases *(according to 1).* For details see text.

intracellular mediators of signalling processes. These molecules act as second messengers generated after stimulation of cells by extracellular stimuli. They are involved in cell survival pathways, the regulation of gene expression, cell metabolism and cytoskeletal rearrangements including cell movement (4). Correspondingly, the enzymes producing PtdIns-3,4,5-P$_3$ have been implicated in major human diseases such as diabetes, cancer and inflammatory processes. This has attracted high interest in establishing specific pharmacological interventions into PI3-dependent pathways. Based on their substrate specificity, phosphoinositide-3-kinases (PI3K) are subgrouped into three classes (Fig. 2).

Class I PI-3-kinases are capable of phosphorylating PtdIns, PtdIns-4-P and PtdIns-4,5-P$_2$ *in vitro*, whereas class II PI-3-kinases phosphorylate PtdIns and PtdIns-4-P but not PtdIns-4,5-P$_2$, and class III PI-3-kinases only utilize PtdIns as a substrate. Receptor-induced formation of PtdIns-3,4,5-P$_3$ from PtdIns-4,5-P$_2$ is therefore restricted to the enzymatic activity of class I kinases. In fact, it appears that class I members only use PtdIns-4,5-P$_2$ as a substrate *in vivo*. Accordingly, PtdIns-3-P concentrations remain unchanged following agonist stimulation and PtdIns-3,4-P$_2$ is most likely the result of PtdIns-3,4,5-P$_3$ degradation catalyzed by a PI-5-phosphatase (4).

Parallel to the difference in substrate specificity, important functional and structural differences are evident between the members of the three PI3K classes.

All class I members are heterodimers consisting of a p110 catalytic and a p85 or p101 type non-catalytic subunit (1,4). The class I$_A$ p110 isoforms α, β, and δ are relatively unstable and form a complex with p85 adapter subunits whereas the only class I$_B$ member p110γ is associated with a p101 non-catalytic subunit. The p85 subunit (Fig. 3) binds to tyrosine-phosphorylated RTKs. This interaction has two consequences and results in the activation of heterodimeric PI3K. First, the cytosolic enzyme translocates to the inner leaflet of the plasma membrane giving p110 access to its lipid substrate. Secondly, the interaction with the tyrosine-phosphorylated receptor induces a conformational change of p85 which results in disinhibition of the enzymatic activity of the p110 catalytic subunit. Since the p85 regulatory subunit inhibits the p110 subunit, it is feasible that constitutively membrane-associated class I$_A$ p110 mutants trigger downstream responses characteristic of growth factor action. Hence, the non-catalytic p85 subunits are important regulators of p110 activity (1,4). Seven isoforms exist which are the products of three distinct genes, α, β and γ (Fig. 3). Interestingly, specific interactions between p85 and p110 isoforms have not been reported so far. p85 proteins contain characteristic protein modules which allow multiple protein-protein interactions. With the exception of the shorter isoforms, they harbour an N-terminal SH3 domain, a proline-rich sequence (P1), and a ▶ BH domain (Bcr homology domain). These modules are followed by a second proline-rich domain and two SH

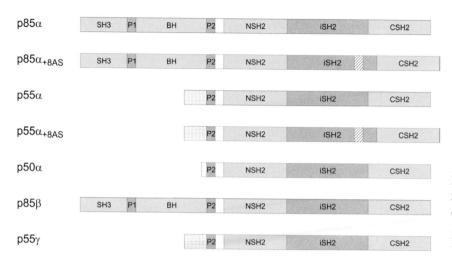

Fig. 3 Classification of the regulatory subunits of class I$_A$ PI-3-kinases *(according to 6).* For details see text.

domains which are distinguished by their relative position to the N- and C-termini. An inter-SH2-region (iSH2) between the two SH2 domains is responsible for the interaction with the catalytic p110 subunit. Interestingly, recently it became evident that cells contain excess p85 which may allow fine tuning of signalling processes.

Similar to class I$_A$ PI3Ks, unstimulated class I$_B$ PI3Kγ is predominantly localized in the cytosol, and GPCRs induce an increase of PI3Kγ in the membrane fraction (5). This membrane recruitment is accompanied by the activation of the enzyme, most likely through direct interaction with Gβγ dimers. In addition, Gβγ is able to stimulate membrane-targeted PI3Kγ which suggests that PI3Kγ can be activated synergistically by both membrane recruitment and interaction with Gβγ. There is some evidence that the catalytic p110γ subunit also occurs in the absence of the non-catalytic p101 subunit. Accordingly, Gβγ is able to stimulate both the monomeric and the heterodimeric PI3Kγ, although p101 functions as a Gβγ sensitizer for p110γ.

Class II PI3K are monomers and predominantly localized in the membrane fraction (1,6). They have a molecular weight of 170—210 kD and possess a characteristic C2-domain at their C-terminal end. Accordingly, the three mammalian class II PI3Ks are subdivided into PI3K-C2α, PI3K-C2β and PI3K-C2γ. There are recent indications that they are sensitive to stimulation by receptors specific for chemokines, insulin and growth factors.

Vps34p (*vacuolar protein-sorting protein*) represents the prototypical class III PI3K which was found in *S. cerevisae*. It apparently plays a major role in intracellular trafficking (1,6). The mammalian homolog Vps34p has been suggested to have similar functions. However, in contrast to class I enzymes, extracellular stimuli do not regulate the activity of Vps34p. It exists as a heterodimer together with a myristoylated serine/threonine kinase, Vps150p, which is responsible for its membrane association.

Despite marked differences between the various PI3-kinases, they all share characteristic structural features (1). They exhibit three conserved domains which are termed homology regions (HR). HR1 represents the C-terminal kinase domain harbouring the catalytic domain. This catalytic core shows considerable similarity to known serine/threonine kinases, in particular with respect to the ATP-binding region. In fact, PI3-kinases also exhibit protein kinase activity which results in autophosphorylation of the catalytic and/or p85 subunit. HR2 is shared by all lipid kinases and is also known as PIK domain as initially described for PI4-kinases. The PIK domain may serve as a backbone being surrounded by other domains. Furthermore, it is assumed to be involved in protein-protein interactions.

The HR3 domain is identical to a ▶ C2 domain. C2 domains mediate calcium-dependent and -independent binding of proteins to phospholipid membranes. In fact, recent data showed that p110γ

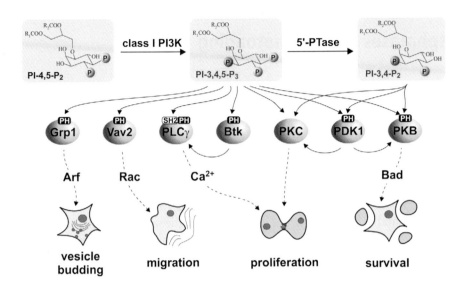

Fig. 4 Cellular functions of class I lipid products. (*according to 4*). For details see text.

interacts with phospholipid vesicles through its HR3 domain.

Most interestingly, all catalytic class I p110 subunits have a Ras binding domain (RBD) or HR4 domain in common (1). This domain, close to the N-terminus, shows some similarity with the RBD of the Ras effector ▸ Raf. Accordingly, several p110 members were shown to be activated by Ras, although there is some evidence that Ras may be under control of PI3K activity.

The 3'-phosphorylated phosphoinositides interact with specific domains of proteins thereby recruiting them to the membrane (4). For instance, PtdIns-3-P generated by class III PI3Ks interact with FYVE- and PX domains. The putative second messengers PtdIns-3,4,5-P_3 and PtdIns-3,4-P_2 bind to ▸ PH domains of different specificity (Fig. 4). PKB/Akt contains a PtdIns-3,4-P_2-specific PH domain whereas guanine nucleotide exchange factors such as GRP1 bind PtdIns-3,4,5-P_3 through a specific PH domain.

Drugs

PI3-kinases are involved in basic pathophysiological processes. They are involved in the development of a broad variety of dysfunctions including chronic proliferative and inflammatory diseases. Many pharmaceutical companies are currently screening for specific and potent inhibitors of these enzymes. Previously, some compounds have been identified which are for experimental work

(7). One example is the irreversible inhibitor Wortmannin, which shows a reasonable specificity for class I PI3Ks at nanomolar concentrations. Other inhibitors of the ATP-binding site are demethoxyviridiin and the reversible inhibitor LY294002, a morpholine derivative of the flavonol quercetin. Very recently, caffeine and theophyllin were also reported to selectively affect class I PI3K members.

References

1. Vanhaesebroeck B, Leevers SJ, Ahmadi K, Timms J, Katso R, Driscoll PC, Woscholski R, Parker PJ, Waterfield MD (2001) Annu. Rev. Biochem. 70:535–602.
2. Gehrmann T, Heilmeyer MG (1998) Phosphatidylinositol 4-kinases. Eur. J. Biochem. 253:357–370.
3. Anderson RA, Boronenkov IV, Doughman SD, Kunz J, Loijens JC (1999) Phosphatidylinositol phosphate kinases, a multifaceted family of signalling enzymes. J. Biol. Chem. 274:9907–9910.
4. Cantley LC (2002) The phosphoinositide 3-kinase pathway. Science 296:1655–1657.
5. Stephens LR, Jackson TR, Hawkins PT (1993) Agonist-stimulated synthesis of phosphoinositol(3,4,5)-trisphosphate: A new intracellular signalling system? Biochim. Biophys. Acta 1179:27–75.
6. Wymann MP, Pirola L (1998) Structure and function of phosphoinositide 3-kinases. Biochim. Biophys. Acta 1436:127–150.
7. Stein RC, Waterfield MD (2000) PI3-kinase inhibition: a target for drug development. Mol. Med. Today 6:347–357.

P

Phospholipid Phosphatases

Phospholipid phosphatases are enzymes such as SHIP (SH2-domain containing inositide-5-phosphatase) or PTEN (phosphatase and tensin homolog deleted on chromosome 10) which dephosphorylate phosphoinositides. Whereas SHIP removes phosphate from the 5' position, PTEN dephosphorylates the 3' position of the inositol. Therefore, PTEN has opposite effects to phosphatidylinositol (PI) 3-kinases and is considered to be a tumor suppressor.

▶ Phosphatases
▶ Phospholipid Kinases

Phosphorylation

Phosphorylation is the enzymatic process of introducing a phosphoric acid residue from ATP as a phosphoryl donor into a substrate protein. Predominant target residues are serine, threonine and tyrosine.

▶ Insulin Receptor
▶ JAK-STAT-pathway
▶ MAP Kinase Cascades
▶ Transmembrane Signalling
▶ Tyrosin Kinases

Phosphotyrosine-binding (PTB) Domain

The PTB domain is a phosphotyrosine binding domain (100-150 amino acids) with a different domain structure from that of SH2.

▶ Growth Factors

Photoaging

Photoaging and photodamage (dermatoheliosis) are terms used interchangeably to describe chronic changes in the appearance and function of the skin caused by repeated sun exposure rather than by the passage of time (the latter is called intrinsic or chronologic aging). Epidemiologic and laboratory evidence indicates that sun exposure and other sources of UV radiation (UVR) play the major role in causing the undesirable skin changes of fine and coarse wrinkles, roughness, laxity, mottled pigmentation, actinic lentigines, actinic keratoses, leathery texture/coarseness, scaling/xerosis, sallowness, and telangiectasia. Cigarette smoking is the only other environmental factor that has been related to the development of changes in the skin associated with aging.

Photoaging and photodamage are serious medical problems, not just cosmetic or aesthetic concerns, because prevention of photoaging and photodamage may prevent the progression of changes toward skin cancer.

The use of sunscreens that protect against UVB and UVA should be encouraged. There is no safe way to tan!

▶ Retinoids

Phototransduction

Phorotransduction is the detection of light and generation of a neuronal signal by the retina in the eye.

Phthalate Esters

Phthalate esters are di- and mono-esters of phthalic acid, an ortho-dicarboxylic acid derivative of benzene. These compounds are widely used as industrial plasticizers to coat polyvinylchloride surfaces of plastics used in food packaging and medical devices (i.v. drip bags, blood storage bags, etc.) and are common environmental contaminants. Several phthalate mono-esters are peroxisome proliferator chemicals and can activate the ▶ peroxisome proliferator-activated receptor PPAR.

▶ Nuclear Receptor Regulation of Drug-metabolizing P450 Enzymes

Physical Dependence

Physical dependence on a substance is characterized by the desire or compulsion to continue taking the substance, a tendency to increase the dose due to increasing tolerance, a dependence on the properties of the substance as manifested by somatic withdrawal symptoms and a negative influence on the individual and society.

▶ Drug Addiction/Dependence

PIAS

Protein inhibitors of activated signal transducer and activator of transcription (▶ STAT) are transcription factors mediating the interferon response. At least some PIAS proteins act as ▶ SUMO ligases.

▶ JAK-STAT Pathway

Picornaviruses

Picornaviruses are small, non-enveloped RNA viruses. Members of this family include rhino- and enteroviruses, which are responsible for a variety of human diseases (viral respiratory infection, viral meningitis, myocarditis, pericarditis, encephalitis, chronic meningoencephalitis, her-

pangina, otitis media, neonatal enteroviral disease and acute exacerbations of asthma).

▶ Antiviral Drugs

Picrotoxin

Picrotoxin is a mixture of pircotin (non-toxic) and picrotoxinin, which occurs in the seeds of the Asiatic climber *Anamirta cocculus* (levent berry, cockles). It is a non-competitive antagonist at the γ-aminobutyric acid$_A$ (GABA$_A$) receptor.

▶ GABA$_A$ Receptor

PI3-Kinase

▶ Phosphatidylinositol 3-kinase

PIP

▶ Phosphatidylinositol Phosphate

PI Response

Hormonal factors and other stimuli by activating phospholipase C-β or -γ isoforms stimulate the breakdown of phosphatidylinositol 4,5-bisphosphate to inositol 1,4,5-trisphosphate and diacylglycerol, a reaction called the PI response.

▶ Phospholipases
▶ Transmembrane Signalling

Pituitary Adenylyl Cyclase-activating Polypeptide

Pituitary Adenylyl Cyclase-activating Polypeptide (PACAP) is a 38-amino acid peptide (PACAP-38), which is widely expressed in the central nervous system. PACAP is most abundant in the hypothalamus. It is also found in the gastrointestinal tract, the adrenal gland and in testis. Its central nervous system functions are ill-defined. In the periphery, PACAP has been shown to stimulate catecholamine secretion from the adrenal medulla and to regulate secretion from the pancreas. Three G-protein coupled receptors have been shown to respond to PACAP, PAC_1 (PACAP type I) specifically binds PACAP, $VPAC_1$ and $VPAC_2$ also bind vasoactive intestinal peptide (VIP). Activation of PACAP receptors results in a G_s-mediated activation of adenylyl cyclase.

PKA

▶ Protein Kinase A

PKB/Akt

▶ Akt
▶ Insulin Receptor

PKC

▶ Protein Kinase C

PKD2

PKD2, also called polycystin 2, is a TRP-related protein defective in human autosomal polycystic kidney disease, the most common life-threatening genetic disease. PKD2 appears to be a cation channel in the plasma membrane, although there is evidence that it is an intracellular Ca^{2+} release channel. Mammalian homologues include "polycystin-like" (PCL).

▶ TRP Channels

Placenta Growth Factor

Placenta grwoth factor is a vascular endothelial growth factor (VEGF)-related molecule which binds to VEGF-R1.

▶ Angiogenesis and Vascular Morphogenesis

Plasmid

Plasmids are extrachromosomal, mainly circular genetic elements that reproduce autonomously within the bacterial cell. Their sizes vary from 1 to over 1000 kilobase pairs. Plasmids are not essential for growth but carry genes that may confer selective growth advantage in specific environments. Examples are genes controlling the production of toxins, virulence factors or enzymes allowing the catabolism of unusual substrates. R plasmids (resistance plasmids) confer resistance to antibiotics and various other inhibitors of growth e.g. heavy metals.

Plasmin

Plasmin is the serine protease that is responsible for degradation of fibrin during activation of the fibrinolytic system. Plasmin cleaves fibrin into soluble fibrin degradation products and is also capable of degrading other proteins in the coagulation cascade.

▶ Coagulation/Thrombosis

Platelet-activating Factor

Platelet-activasting factor (PAF) is a biologically active lipid, which is derived from its precursor, acyl-PAF, by phospholipase A_2 activity, resulting in lyso-PAF, which is then acetylated to give PAF, which in turn can be deacetylated to lyso-PAF. PAF is generated and released from inflammatory cells when they are stimulated and is believed to be an important mediator in both acute and persistent allergic and inflammatory processes. PAF acts on a specific G-protein coupled receptor, which mediates its actions like vasodilatation, increased vascular permeability, hyperalgesia and chemotaxis.

▶ Phospholipases

Platelet-derived Growth Factor

Platelet-derived growth factors (PDGFs) are a group of growth factors consisting of dimers, whose biological actions are mediated through two receptor tyrosine kinases PDGFR-α and PDGFR-β. PDGFs are produced by a wide variety of cells and function as mitogens for fibroblasts, smooth muscle cells or glia cells. They also play important roles in morphogenesis during development.

▶ Growth Factors

Platelets

Platelets are the formed elements of the blood which participate in hemostasis. Platelets are enucleated, discoid fragments which arise from mature megakaryocytes in the bone marrow. Under normal circumstances, platelets do not adhere to endothelial surfaces of blood vessels. However, platelets can adhere to damaged areas of blood vessels and become activated in such a way that they can also bind fibrinogen.

▶ Anti-platelet Drugs

Pleckstrin Homology Domain

Pleckstein homology (PH) domains are a large family of compact protein modules defined by sequences of approxmately 100 amino acides. Proteins containing the PH domain were found to be membrane-associated by virtue of their intrinsic ability to bind the phosphatidyl inositol 4,5 bisphosphate of the plasma membrane. PH domains are also capable of functioning as protein-protein interaction modules.

▶ Phospholipid Kinases

Plexins

Plexins are a group of transmembrane proteins, which mediate the effects of ▶ semaphorins.

PMF

▶ Peptide Mass Fingerprinting

Polyamines

Polyamines are low molecular weight aliphatic nonprotein nitrogenous bases. Putrescine (Put), cadaverine (Cad), spermidine (Spd) and spermine (Spm) are the most common natural polyamines. They are synthesized by decarboxylation of ornithine and methionine. At physiological pH, these polyamines can be considered as organic polycations, Put^{2+}, Cad^{2+}, Spd^{3+} and Spm^{3+}. Polyamines are essential for many growth-related processes such as DNA replication, RNA synthesis and translation, as well as for block of some ion channels. Putrescine and spermidine are ubiquitous in living organisms, while spermine is rare or even nonexistent in prokaryotes. In neurons they exert an activity-dependent block of the channel pore of Ca^{2+}-permeable AMPARs.

▶ Ionotropic Glutamate Receptors
▶ Inward Rectifier K^+ Channels
▶ Ionotropic Glutamate Receptors

Polyenes

▶ Antifungal Drugs

Polyethylene Glycol

Polyethylene glycol is a water-soluble polymer that can be covalently attached to certain molecules, e.g. filgrastim. Addition of polyethylene glycol does not change the identity, purity, or biological activities of filgrastim, but plasma clearance is decreased and the circulating half-life of filgrastim is increased.

▶ Hematopoietic Growth Factors

Polymorphism

▶ Genetic Polymorphism

POMC

▶ Prepro-opiomelanocortin

Poor Metabolizer

A poor metabolizer (PM) is a historically used pharmacogenetic term for a person with deficient metabolism with respect to substrates of a specified enzyme. Genetically, a PM is an autosomal recessively inherited drug metabolism phenotype resulting from homozygosity for null-alleles of drug metabolizing enzymes. For example, PMs for debrisoquine or sparteine, substrates of CYP2D6, are also PMs of certain antidepressants or beta-blockers which are substrates of the same enzyme.

▶ Pharmacogenetics

Population Pharmacokinetics

Population pharmacokinetics is the application of pharmacokinetic and statistical methods to sparse data to derive a pharmacokinetic profile of central tendency.

▶ Pharmacokinetics

Positron Emission Tomography

Positron emission tomography (PET) is an imaging technique that relies on the emission of positrons from radionucleotides tagged to an injectable compound of interest. Each positron emitted by the radioisotope collides with an electron to emit two photons at 180° from each other. The photons are detected and the data processed so that the source of the photons can be identified and an image generated showing the anatomical localization of the compound of interest.

▶ Antipsychotic Drugs

Post-translational Modification

Post-translational modification (PTM) is the enzymatic processing of a protein into the biologically active form following release from the ribosome. This includes removal and/or derivatization of specific amino acid residues, proteolytic cleavage, loss of signal sequences, and formation of disulfide cross-links. Other common post-translational modifications are phosphorylation, glycosylation, acetylation, hydroxylation, myristylation, isoprenylation, and many other reactions. All amino acid side chains except those of alanine, glycine, isoleucine, leucine and valine can be modified.

Potentiation

▶ Long-term Potentiation

PP

▶ Pancreatic Polypeptide

PPA

▶ Peroxisome Proliferator Activated Receptor
▶ Nuclear Receptor Regulation of Drug-metabolizing P450 Enzymes

PPCs

▶ Peroxisome Proliferator Chemicals

PR

Progesterone Receptor.

▶ Sex Steroid Receptors

Pregnane X Receptor

The pregnane X receptor (PXR) is a promiscuous nuclear receptor, that has evolved to protect the body from toxic chemicals. It is activated by a wide variety of xenobiotics including several drugs like rifampicin, hyperforin (the active ingredient of St. John's wort), clotrimazole and others. PXR heterodimerizes with the retinoid X receptor (RXR) and is also activated by various lipophilic compounds produced by the body such as bile acids and steroids. PXR heterodimerized with RXR stimulates the transcription of cytochrome P450 3A monooxygenases (CYP3A) and other genes involved in the detoxification and elimination of the potentially harmful substances. PXR appears to be the key regulator of CYP3A induction by xenobiotics.

▶ Nuclear Receptor Regulation of Drug-metabolizing P450 Enzymes

P

Preintegration Complex

The preintegration complex is a complex of retroviral DNA and proteins that translocates from the cytosol into the nucleus prior to integration.

▶ Gene Therapy

Prenylation

Prenylation is the post-translational addition of 15- or 20-carbon isoprenyl lipids to the C-terminus of proteins. Prenylation is an irreverable modification that anchors proteins to the membrane fraction of cells.

▶ Lipid Modifications

Prepro-opiomelanocortin

Prepro-opiomelanocortin (POMC) is a huge precursor protein, from which several peptides are generated by proteolytic cleavage (melanocyte-stimulating hormone, adenocorticotrophic hormone (ACTH), β-endorphin, methionine enkephalin).

▶ Anti Obesity Drugs
▶ Opioid System

Presynaptic Receptors

Presynaptic receptors are located in axon terminals and modulate the probability of transmitter release. Most are G protein-coupled.

▶ Synaptic Transmission

Primary Aldosteronism

Primary aldosteronism is a plasma aldosterone concentration above the normal range, usually due to abnormal secretion of aldosterone by benign or malignant adrenal tumors.

▶ Epithelial Na$^+$ Channel

Primary Hemostasis

Primary hemostasis is the first phase of hemostasis consisting of platelet plug formation at the site of injury. It occurs within seconds and stops blood loss from capillaries, arterioles and venules. Secondary hemostasis, in contrast, requires several minutes to be complete and involves the formation of fibrin through the coagulation cascade.

▶ Antiplatelet Drugs

Prodrug

A prodrug is a drug that is not by itself pharmacologically active but needs metabolic activation by an enzyme. Examples are the cytostatic cyclophosphamide, which is activated by hydroxylation catalyzed by CYP2B6, or the β-hydroxy-β-methylglutaryl-coenzyme A (HMGCoA) reductase inhibitor, lovastatin, which contains a lactone ring that must be cleaved by carboxylesterases to yield the active free carboxylic acid.

▶ P450 Mono-oxygenase System

Progesterone

Progesterone is a natural sex hormone, which is secreted mainly by the *corpus luteum* in the second part of the menstrual cycle. Small amounts are also secreted by the testis in the male and the adrenal cortex in both sexes, and large amounts are secreted by the placenta.

▶ Sex Steroid Receptors

Progesterone Receptor

▶ Sex Steroid Receptors

Progestins

Progestins are derived from the 21-carbon series and contain as a basic structure the pregnane nucleus. In the non-pregnant female they are mainly produced in the ovary.

▶ Contraceptives

Programmed Cell Death

▶ Apoptosis

Prolactin

Prolactin is peptide hormone secreted by the pituitary gland. It acts on prolactin receptors in breast tissue where it stimulates production of casein and lactalbumin. It also acts on the testes and ovaries to inhibit the effects of gonadotrophins. Since the secretion of prolactin is under tonic dopaminergic inhibition by the hypothalamus, dopamine D_2-receptor antagonists cause prolactin release through a process of disinhibition, leading to elevated prolactin levels resulting in gynaecomastia, galactorrhoea, anovulation, and impotence.

▶ JAK-STAT Pathway

Promoter

The promoter is the region of a gene that regulates initiation of transcription. It contains binding sites for transcription factors; their action allows RNA polymerase to access the start site of transcription.

Proopiomelanocortin

Proopiomelanocortin (POMC) is the precursor peptide of hormones and neuropeptides expressed in the pituitary and the hypothalamus (adrenocorticotropic hormone (ACTH), lipotropin, α-melanocyte-stimulating hormone (αMSH), γMSH, β-endorphin and others). The main clinical consequences of POMC deficiency are adrenal insufficiency (due to absence of ACTH), red hair pigmentation (due to absence of MSH) and severe early-onset obesity (due to the lack of αMSH).

▶ Appetite Control
▶ Opioid System

Prostacyclin

PGI_2

▶ Prostanoids

Prostaglandins

▶ Prostanoids

Prostanoids

RICHARD M. BREYER, MATTHEW D. BREYER
Vanderbilt University, Nashville; TN, USA
rich.breyer@mcmail.vanderbilt.edu

Synonyms

Prostaglandins; dinoprostone; ▶ eicosanoids

Definition

Prostanoids, or prostaglandins, are potent mediators of a wide range of physiological actions
including pain, inflammation, modulation of
smooth muscle tone as well as water and ion transport. Prostaglandins are oxygenated metabolites
of the essential fatty acid ▶ arachidonic acid. Four
of the principal prostaglandins are analogs of the
twenty carbon unnatural fatty acid prostanoic
acid, distinguished by its five carbon "prostane"
ring group comprised of carbons 5 through 8. The
fifth prostanoid, thromboxane, has an inserted
ether oxygen and thus has a six-member ring
structure and is an analog of the unnatural fatty
acid thrombanoic acid (1).

- ▶ Cyclooxygenases
- ▶ G-protein-coupled Receptors
- ▶ Nuclear Receptor Regulation of Drug-metabo-
  lizing P450 Enzymes

Basic Characteristics

Biosynthesis

PGs act locally in an autocrine or paracrine fashion in the tissues in which they are synthesized,
rather than as circulating hormones that act at a
distant site. For this reason, studies localizing the
enzymatic machinery that synthesize prostaglandins is informative with respect to the site of PG
actions. PG synthesis is initiated by
▶ cyclooxygenase (COX) mediated metabolism of
the unsaturated twenty carbon fatty acid arachidonic acid to PGG/H_2, generating five primary
bio-active prostanoids: PGE_2, $PGF_{2\alpha}$, PGD_2, PGI_2
(prostacyclin) and TXA_2 (thromboxane; Fig. 1).
Arachidonic acid is esterified in the lipid bilayer of
most cells, and is liberated by the action of specific
phopholipases e.g. PLA_2. Mobilization of arachidonic acid by phospholipases is regulated by a
number of hormones and signal transduction
pathways, and represents a critical control point of
prostanoid synthesis. Upon liberation, arachidonic
acid is rapidly metabolized by a number of enzymatic pathways including the cyclooxygenase
pathway. Cyclcooxygenase, also known as PGH
synthase, catalyzes two sequential reactions, a
*bis*oxygenase, or cyclooxygenase, reaction leading
to the formation of PGG_2 and a subsequent peroxidase activity at the C15 position leading to the conversion of PGG_2 to PGH_2 (2). Two isozymes of
cyclooxygenase have been identified, designated
COX-1 and COX-2, which catalyze the formation of
identical products but have different patterns of
expression and differential regulation. Differential blockade of the COX isozymes has proven to
be a clinically important pharmaceutical strategy,
as described below. PGH_2, the immediate product
of COX activity, is an unstable product that spontaneously degrades to other prostaglandin metabolites. However, *in vivo*, PGH_2 is acted upon by
specific PG synthases leading to differential shunt-
ing of PGH_2 to 1 of the 5 principal prostanoid
products. Following their formation, PGs cross the
cell membrane where local concentrations of PGs
may be modulated by specific transporters including the recently described specific PG transporter
(PGT). Although PGT's role is incompletely understood, it has been proposed to facilitate the reuptake of PGs to allow vectorial transport of PGs
synthesized in polarized cells.

Receptor Pharmacology

The local action of PGs depends in part on activation of a family of specific ▶ G-protein coupled
receptors (GPCRs), designated EP for E-prosta-
noid receptors, FP, DP, IP and TP receptors respectively, for the other prostanoids (3). The EP receptors are unique in that four receptors, designated
EP1 through EP4, have been described for PGE_2,
each encoded by a distinct gene. A second class of
prostaglandin D receptor designated **c**hemoat-
tractant **r**eceptor-homologous molecule expressed
on **T**h2 cells (CRTH2) has been identified which
has no sequence homology to the remaining PG
receptors. This receptor has been unofficially designated "DP2". Each of the other PGs has a single

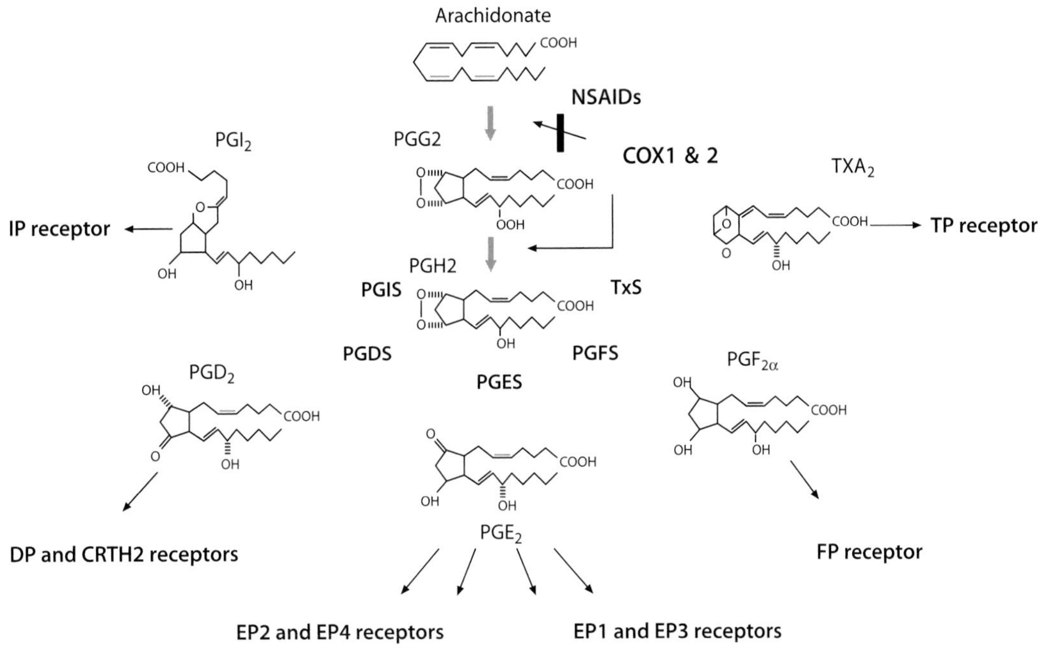

Fig. 1 Synthetic pathway of the prostaglandins. Arachidonate is metabolized by cyclooxygenases –1 and –2 (COX1 & COX2) to PGG_2 then PGH_2 in a two step reaction. PGH2 is relatively unstable and is then enzymatically converted to one of five known primary prostanoids: PGI_2, PGD_2, PGE_2, $PGF_{2\alpha}$, and TxA_2. Each prostanoid interacts with distinct members of a subfamily of the G-protein coupled receptors. PGI_2 activates the I-prostanoid (IP) receptor, PGD_2 activates the DP and CRTH2 receptors, $PGF_{2\alpha}$ the FP receptor and TxA_2 the TP receptor. PGE interacts with one of four distinct EP receptors each of which also couples to distinct signaling pathways.

receptor, and taken together there are nine PG GPCRs, each encoded by distinct genes (Table 1). Alternative mRNA splice variants have been cloned for the EP1, EP3, TP and FP receptors. In each case, these splice variants generate receptor sequence diversity in the intracellular C-terminal tail of the receptor protein (Fig. 2). Functionally, these splice variants appear to modulate the specificity of G-protein coupling, as well as regulation of receptor desensitization by encoding alternate phosphorylation sites. Pharmacologically, the PG receptors are distinguished by their ligand-binding selectivity as well as the signal transduction pathway they activate. In general, PG receptors may have significant affinity for PGs other than its principal ligand. Moreover, multiple PG receptors are frequently co-expressed in a single cell type or tissue. COX activation and resulting PG production may lead to complex effects in the target tissue by activation of multiple PG receptor subtypes. Thus, a given PG ligand may elicit multiple and at times apparently opposing functional effects on a given target tissue. For example, prostaglandin receptors were initially characterized by their actions on smooth muscle, where they may lead to either smooth muscle contraction or relaxation. The vasodilator effects of PGE_2 have long been recognized in both arterial and venous beds. Smooth muscle relaxation by PGE_2 is, however, not uniformly observed, and PGE_2 is a potent constrictor in other smooth muscle beds, including trachea, gastric fundus and ileum. Importantly, some structural analogs of PGE_2 are capable of reproducing the dilator effects of PGE_2 but are inactive on tissues where it is a constrictor. Conversely, analogs that reproduce the constrictor effects of PGE_2 may fail to affect tissues where PGE_2 is a dilator. The EP receptor mRNAs exhibit

P

differential expression in a number of tissues with distinct functional consequences of activating each receptor subtype. Functional antagonism among PGs can also be observed in platelet aggregation, where TXA_2 activation of the TP receptor causes platelet aggregation. Conversely, prostacyclin activates a platelet IP receptor that opposes this platelet aggregation. Thus, the balance of PGs synthesized as well as the complement of PG receptors expressed determines the COX effect on platelet function.

In addition to the GPCR-mediated effects, there is evidence that prostaglandin metabolites are capable of activating some nuclear transcription factors. This action is exemplified by the cyclopentenone prostaglandins of the J-series, e.g. 15-deoxy-Δ12,14-PGJ_2 (15d-PGJ_2), which are derived from PGD_2. 15d-PGJ_2 activates a nuclear hormone receptor designated ▶ perixisome proliferator activator receptor γ (PPARγ). There is also evidence that prostacyclin (PGI_2) also activates another member of this family designated PPARδ. It is unclear whether the PGs represent true endogenous ligands of these receptors, as their affinity is generally in the micromolar range. This is two to three orders of magnitude lower affinity than the nanomolar affinities observed for PGs at the GPCRs, yet nonetheless concentrations that could be achieved in the intracellular environment.

Prostanoid Catabolism

Prostaglandins are short-lived and endogenous PGs circulate only at extremely low levels. Once synthesized and released, PGs are rapidly inactivated by one pass through the pulmonary circulation. The principal inactivating step of PGs is the oxidation of the 15-OH group to the corresponding ketone by prostaglandin 15-OH dehydrogenase (4). Consequently many synthetic PG analogs have modifications at the 15 carbon to decrease inactivation of these compounds and increase their half-life *in vivo*.

Drugs

Two distinct classes of drugs are important in modulating PG signaling: There are those that inhibit PG synthesis, and those that act directly on the receptor as either agonists or antagonists.

Drugs that inhibit PG synthesis are a particularly widely utilized class of therapeutic agents designated as ▶ non-steroidal anti-inflammatory drugs (NSAIDs). These drugs act as either competitive inhibitors of COX (e.g. ibuprofen, indomethacin, diclofenac etc.), or as irreversible inactivators of COX enzymes (aspirin). Classical non-selective NSAIDs inhibit the cyclooxygenase activity of both COX-1 and COX-2, thereby suppressing PG synthesis. These drugs are utilized for their anti-pyretic, anti-inflammatory and analgesic properties, and as a class represent one of the most widely prescribed and economically important groups of drugs. Although generally safe and effective, because of their widespread use significant numbers of patients develop undesirable side effects from these drugs. The most common serious side effects are gastro-intestinal bleeding and renal failure. PGE_2 is a major PG in the gastro-intestinal (GI) tract, and NSAID-mediated suppression of PGE synthesis is thought to be responsible for NSAID-induced gastrointestinal injury. Co-administration of the PGE analog misoprostol with NSAIDs is cytoprotective. Nonetheless, misoprostol itself can have unwanted GI side effects such as cramping and diarrhea. An alternative approach for developing NSAIDs with decreased side effects has been the identification of isozyme selective inhibitors that selectively target the COX-2 enzyme, while leaving the COX-1 isozyme functional. COX-2 expression is inducible, and its expression level is elevated in response to many inflammatory stimuli. COX-2 selective inhibitors such as valdecoxib, rofecoxib and celecoxib (▶ COXIBs) have significantly reduced the unwanted side effects of NSAIDs such as gastro-intestinal bleeding, while retaining their anti-pyretic, analgesic and anti-inflammatory properties (5). Moreover these drugs can be administered at doses sufficient to allow essentially complete blockade of COX-2 without the acute side effects of dual COX-1 and COX-2 blockade. More recent studies have raised the theoretic possibility that selective inhibition of COX-2 may yet cause a unique profile of unwanted side effects. For example, studies suggest pro-thrombotic platelet derived TXA_2 is primarily synthesized by COX-1, whereas antithrombotic prostacyclin is at least in part, a COX-2 product. Thus selective COX-2 inhibition could potentially been suggested tip the

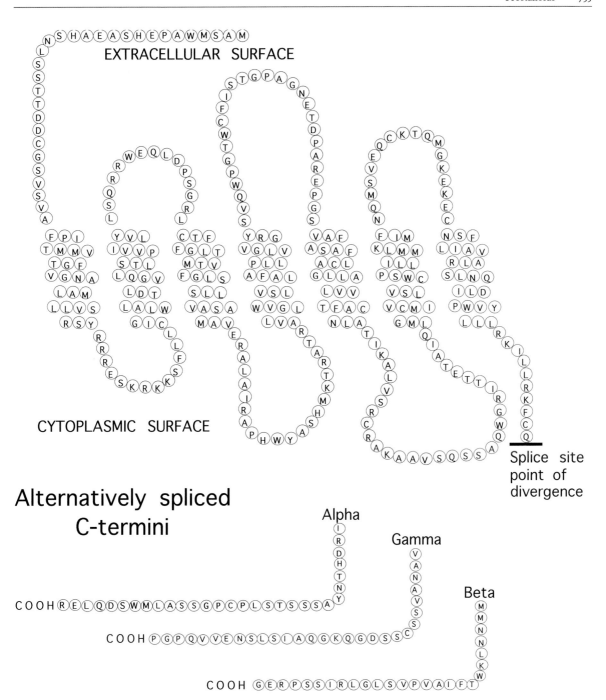

Fig. 2 Amino acid sequence of three mouse EP₃ receptor splice variants differing only in their intracellular carboxyl termini. The predicted amino acid sequences of each splice variant is represented by the one letter amino acid code. The carboxyl variable tails are designated alpha, beta and gamma.

Tab. 1 Prostanoid Receptor Pharmacology and Signaling

Prostanoid	Receptor		Agonist	Signaling
Thromboxane A$_2$	TP		I-BOP U46619 STA2	↑ IP3/DAG
PGI$_2$ (prostacyclin)	IP		Cicaprost AP-227 Iloprost	↑ cAMP
PGE	EP			
		EP1	17-phenyl-trinor PGE2 Iloprost Sulprostone	↑ IPE/DAG
		EP2	Butaprost AH13205 11-deoxy PGE1 19(R)-OH-PGE2 (?)	↑ cAMP
		EP3	M&B 38767 Sulprostone 11-deoxy-PGE1 Misoprostol	↑ cAMP
		EP4	Misoprostol	↑ cAMP
PGF$_{2\alpha}$	FP		Fluprostenol	↑ IP3/DAG
PGD	DP			
		DP ("DP1")	BW 245C	↑ cAMP
		CRTH2 ("DP2")	DK-PGD$_2$	↑ Ca^{2+}

TXA$_2$/PGI$_2$ balance towards the pro-aggregatory TXA$_2$ arm of PG modulation. This may causes a loss of the cardioprotective of aspirin, and may cause an increase in cardiac events. Other data in rodent models suggest that inhibition of microvascular derived COX2 activity could block angiogenesis, including that occurring in cancers. This has promoted studies designed to explore whether COX-2 inhibition may be beneficial in the treatment of cancer.

Because of the complexities resulting from use of these relatively broadly acting COX inhibitors, the use of selective PG receptor agonists and antagonists could provide therapeutic alternatives devoid of these side effects and therefore with therapeutic value. At this point there are no potent and selective PG receptor antagonists in routine clinical use (1). Development of selective agonists

for PG receptors has been limited. Use of PG receptor agonists is complicated because these ▶ autacoids normally act locally and systemic administration of PG agonists may have profound adverse side effects. Nonetheless several PG agonists are in clinical usage, and they are particularly effective when they can be delivered directly to the site of action.

For example PGF$_{2\alpha}$ agonists such as latanaprost have been developed as eye-drops to reduce intraocular pressure for the treatment of glaucoma. More recently the PGF$_{2\alpha}$ analog bimatoprost has also been approved for this indication. Topical instillation of these agonists is effective in lowering intraocular pressure and may be used as a first line therapy for the treatment of glaucoma.

PGE$_2$ was initially characterized by its actions on female reproductive tissue, and this has been an area of considerable pharmaceutical development activity. PGE$_2$ (dinoprostone) and PGE$_1$ (alprostadil) have been used as abortafacients in early pregnancy, and they facilitate labor at term by promoting ripening and dilatation of the cervix. PGE$_1$ may be used for the treatment of impotence by direct intracavernous injection. As noted above, PGE$_1$ analog misprostol has been utilized for the treatment of NSAID induced GI bleeding, and presumably acts by replacing the loss of the endogenous PGE$_2$.

Prostacyclin (epoprostanol) is one of the few drugs effective for the treatment of primary pulmonary hypertension (PPH), a rare but frequently fatal illness of young adults where increased blood pressure in the pulmonary circulation leads to right-heart failure. Continuous infusion of epoprostanol leads to a decrease in blood pressure, however it is unclear whether this is due to direct dilator activities of the IP receptor acting on smooth muscle or a more indirect mechanism.

It is worth noting that in many cases PG drugs have found greatest use where they may be applied locally and directly rather than systemically. Glaucoma is treated with latanprost eye drops, induction of labor with dinoprostone vaginal suppositories, GI ulcers are treated with oral misoprostol. In contrast, treatment of PPH with epoprostanol, and the use of PG analogs as abortafacients requires their systemic application.

References

1. Morrow JD, Roberts LJ, 2nd (2001) Lipid-Derived Autacoids. In: Hardman JG, Limbird LE, Gilman AG (eds) Goodman & Gilman's the pharmacological basis of therapeutics, 10th ed. McGraw-Hill, New York, pp 669–685
2. Marnett LJ (2000) Cyclooxygenase mechanisms. Curr Opin Chem Biol 4:545–552
3. Breyer RM, Bagdassarian CK, Myers SA, Breyer MD (2001) Prostanoid receptors: subtypes and signaling. Annu Rev Pharmacol Toxicol 41:661–690
4. Coggins KG, Latour A, Nguyen MS, Audoly L, Coffman TM, Koller BH (2002) Metabolism of PGE2 by prostaglandin dehydrogenase is essential for remodeling the ductus arteriosus. Nat Med 8:91–92
5. Turini ME, DuBois RN (2002) Cyclooxygenase-2: a therapeutic target. Annu Rev Med 53:35–57

Protamine Sulfate

Protamine sulfate is a mixture of basic polypeptides isolated from salmon sperm that is used to neutralize heparin *in vitro* or *in vivo*.

▶ Anticoagulants

Protease-activated Receptors

▶ Proteinase-activated Receptors

Proteases

▶ Proteinases
▶ Non-viral Proteases

Proteasome

The proteasome is a multi-subunit intracellular structure containing multiple threonine proteinases with different substrate specificities. The proteasome is responsible for degradation of ubiquitinated intracellular proteins and/or peptides.

▶ Ubiquitin/Proteasome System

Protein Folding

Proteins fold on a time scale from μseconds to seconds. Starting from a random coil conformation, proteins can find their stable fold quickly, although the number of possible conformations is astronomically high.

▶ Bioinformatics
▶ Molecular Modelling

Protein Kinase

▶ Table appendix: Protein Kinases

Protein Kinase A

Protein kinase A (PKA) is a cyclic AMP-dependent protein kinase, a member of a family of protein kinases that are activated by binding of cAMP to their two regulatory subunits, which results in the release of two active catalytic subunits. Targets of PKA include L-type calcium channels (the relevant subunit and site of phosphorylation is still uncertain), phospholamban (the regulator of the sarcoplasmic calcium ATPase, SERCA) and key enzymes of glucose and lipid metabolism.

▶ Voltage-dependent Ca^{2+} Channels

Protein Kinase C

The protein kinase C-family (PKC) consists of at least 12 isoforms of serine/threoine protein kinases, which possess distinct differences in structure, substrate requirement, expression and cellular localization. PKC isoforms have been grouped into three subfamilies. The subfamily of convential or classical PKCs (cPKCs) is activated by Ca^{2+}, diacylglycerol (DAG) or phorbol esters and includes the isoforms α, βI, βII and γ. The subfamily of so-called novel PKCs (nPKCs), comprises the isoforms δ, ε, η and θ. They are Ca^{2+}-independent but are also activated by DAG and phorbol esters. The third subfamily called "atypical" PKCs (aPKCs) consists of the isoforms ζ and θ/λ. Atypical PKC-isoforms are Ca^{2+} and DAG-independent.

▶ Phospholipases
▶ Tyrosin Kinases

14-3-3 Proteins

14-3-3 proteins are a family of conserved regulatory molecules, which are expressed in all eukaryotic cells and are able to bind a multitude of signaling proteins, including kinases and phosphatases as well as transmembrane receptors. They are involved in the coordination of cellular processes such as mitogenic signal transduction, apoptotic cell death and cell cycle control.

Protein Trafficking and Quality Control

RALF SCHÜLEIN, WALTER ROSENTHAL
Forschungsinstitut für Molekulare
Pharmakologie, and Institut für Pharmakologie,
Freie Universität Berlin, Berlin, Germany
schuelein@fmp-berlin.de,
rosenthal@fmp-berlin.de or
rosenthal@zedat.fu-berlin.de

Synonyms

Protein sorting, intracellular protein transport

▶ Intracellular Transport

Definition

Intracellular protein transport is the transport of proteins to their correct subcellular compartment or to the extracellular space (secretion). Endo- and exocytosis describe vesicle budding and fusion at the plasma membrane and are by most authors not included in the term protein transport.

▶ Intracellular Transport

Basic Mechanisms

General Transport Routes
Intracellular protein transport mechanisms ensure that proteins are delivered to their correct subcel-

lular compartment. An efficient intracellular protein transport is a prerequisite for the establishment of both cell architecture and function. In the past decade, transport processes have also drawn the attention of clinicians and pharmacologists since many diseases have been shown to be caused by transport deficient proteins.

The general transport routes of proteins are well established (Fig. 1). Initially, every protein is synthesized at cytoplasmic ribosomes. Its destination within the cell is then determined by transport signals. If the nascent chain does not contain transport signals, it becomes a cytosolic protein.

Transport signals can be of the import or the export type. Import signals are contained in proteins that are transported into the individual compartments of mitochondria (matrix, inner membrane, intramembrane compartment, outer membrane), peroxisomes (lumen, boundary membrane) and into the interior of the nucleus. They mediate transport to the target compartment when protein biosynthesis is complete (post-translational transport).

Export signals direct proteins to the secretory pathway that extends from the ▶ endoplasmic reticulum (ER) via the ▶ ER/Golgi intermediate compartment (ERGIC) and the different compartments of the ▶ Golgi apparatus to the plasma membrane. The occurence of export signals leads to the stop of the cytoplasmic protein translation (elongation arrest) by the binding of the ▶ signal recognition particle (SRP). The resulting nascent chain/ribosome/SRP complex is then targeted to the ▶ translocon at the ER membrane. Here translation restarts and the export signals mediate integration into (membrane proteins) or translocation across the ER membrane (secretory proteins). At the ER membrane, protein integration or translocation takes place simultaneously with protein sythesis (co-translational transport). Secretory proteins contain N-terminal signal peptides as export signals. The signal peptides are cleaved off by the ▶ signal peptidases of the ER after translocation of the nascent chain. Secretory proteins consequently become part of the ER lumen. In membrane proteins, two different types of export signals are found to mediate ER targeting/insertion (Fig. 2): a) proteins with an extracellular N terminus may contain cleavable signal peptides similar to that of secretory proteins (type I pro-

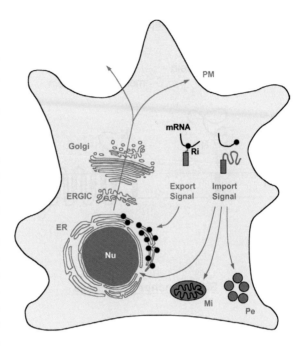

Fig. 1 Intracellular protein transport. General transport routes of proteins starting with the initial synthesis at cytoplasmic ribosomes (Ri). The export (secretory) pathway to the plasma membrane (PM) *via* the endoplasmic reticulum (ER), the ER/Golgi intermediate compartment (ERGIC) and the Golgi apparatus (Golgi) is indicated in red. The different import pathways are indicated in blue. Import pathways direct proteins into the individual compartments of mitochondria (Mi) (matrix, inner membrane, intermembrane compartment, outer membrane), peroxisomes (Pe) (lumen, boundary membrane) and into the interior of the nucleus (Nu). Note that transport is post-translational in the case of all import pathways but co-translational in the case of the export pathway.

teins); b) the vast majority, however, use the first transmembrane domain of the mature protein as a so-called signal anchor sequence (type III proteins). Membrane proteins with an intracellular N tail invariantly contain signal anchor sequences (type II proteins). In contrast to secretory proteins, membrane proteins become part of the ER membrane. Their extracellular domains are translocated into the ER lumen, their intracelluar domains remain in the cytoplasm.

Signal peptides

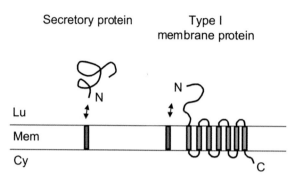

Signal anchor sequences

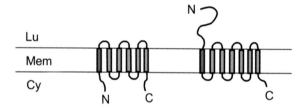

Fig. 2 Intracellular protein transport. Types of signal sequences in the export pathway for translocation across (secretory proteins) or integration into (membrane proteins) the ER membrane. The signal sequences are indicated in red. Lu, ER lumen; Mem, ER membrane; Cy, cytoplasm. Upper panel: secretory proteins contain signal peptides which are removed by signal peptidases in the ER lumen. A subset of the membrane proteins with an extracellular N terminus may also contain signal peptides (type I proteins). Lower panel: the second group of membrane proteins with an extracellular N terminus use signal anchor sequences for ER insertion (type III proteins). Membrane proteins with an intracellular N terminus contain invariantly signal anchor sequences (type II proteins).

In the secretory pathway, the ER is the compartment in which protein folding is established. Correct folding is mediated by proteins called ▶ molecular chaperones. The ER also contains a quality control system allowing only correctly folded proteins to leave the ER. Misfolded, or incompletely folded proteins are recognized, retained and finally subjected to proteolysis. Mutations in secretory and membrane proteins frequently lead to misfolded and transport deficient proteins and thereby to inherited diseases (see below).

The quality control system is mainly located in the ER. It consists of several components:
a) Molecular chaperones like BiP recognize misfolded proteins by exposed hydrophobic domains that are more likely present on the surface of misfolded molecules. Binding to these domains leads to a prolonged association with the chaperones and consequently to ER retention.
b) An yet unknown system in the ER recognizes misfolded proteins by dibasic ER retention signals (consensus sequence = RXR). These signals are not accessible in correctly folded forms but are exposed upon misfolding. The adaptor molecules for the RXR signals are not identified as yet.
c) Recent results indicate that the quality control of misfolded proteins is not restricted to the ER. If misfolded proteins escape from the ER, they are also recognized in the ERGIC. From there, misfolded proteins are transported back to the ER (retrograde transport). In the ERGIC, the misfolded proteins seem to be recognized by the molecular chaperone ▶ BiP.

Once the proteins have reached a correct and transport competent folding state, they are transported in vesicles from the ER via the ERGIC, the cis-Golgi region, the medial compartment of the Golgi apparatus, and the trans-Golgi network to the plasma membrane. Soluble proteins are transported in the vesicle lumen, membrane proteins in the vesicle membrane. Transport to the cell surface is the "default" pathway for secretory and membrane proteins. Proteins may also become part of one of the intracellular compartments along the secretory pathway, but only if they contain specific retention signals.

It is thought that soluble proteins enter the transport vesicles of the secretory pathway by bulk flow. In contrast, the recruitment of membrane proteins into the vesicles seems to require specific sorting signals. Whereas the sorting signals mediating the transport through the intracellular compartments seem to be identical in different cell types, those for the plasma membrane may be variable. In polarized epithelial cells, for example, the cell surface is not homogenous but consists of two different compartments, the apical and the basolateral membranes. Here, additional sorting information is required in the trans-Golgi network to deliver proteins correctly. The same holds true for neurons containing dentritical and axonal membranes or endothelial cells, containing luminal and abluminal membranes.

Diseases Caused by Transport-deficient Proteins

To date more than 90 diseases are known that are caused by the intracellular retention of mutant proteins or by the impairment of components of the secretory pathway (see 1 for an overview). The disease-causing mechanisms are variable and include:

a) Disorders caused by ER retention and degradation of mutant proteins (e.g. mutations of the cystic fibrosis transmembrane regulator protein (CFTR) causing cystic fibrosis)

b) Disorders caused by ER retention and accumulation of mutant proteins. The consequence are ER stress and cell damage (e.g. mutations in α_1-antitrypsin (PiZ) leading to α_1-antitrypsin deficiency and hereditary emphysema with liver injury).

c) Disorders caused by the impairment of the Golgi apparatus and further vesicular trafficking (e.g. mutations in the Rab escort protein Rep1 leading to choroideremia).

d) Disorders caused by mislocalization of lysosomal proteins (e.g. mutations in the N-acetylglucosamine 1-phosphotransferase leading to inclusion cell disease).

e) Disorders affecting the import pathways to mitochondria, peroxisomes and the nucleus (e.g. mutations in the peroxisomal Pex proteins leading to Zellweger syndrome).

Among the many diseases known to be caused by transport defective proteins, cystic fibrosis is one of the most frequent and best characterized. It is caused by mutations in the gene for the CFTR protein, a cAMP-regulated chloride channel belonging to the ABC transporter family. The CFTR protein is expressed in the apical membrane and in subapical endosomal compartments of secretory epithelial cells, where it regulates the chloride transport over the apical membrane. In about 70% of the patients, the ΔF508 mutation of the CFTR protein is found. The ΔF508 mutant is recognized by the quality control system, retained intracellularly and subjected to proteolysis. The quality control of the ΔF508 mutant is exerted by a) molecular chaperones like Hsp70, b) the exposure of RXR retention signals of the mutant protein, and c) the ERGIC which recognizes ΔF508 mutants that have escaped from the ER. The intracellularly retained ΔF508 mutant is functional, i.e. the quality control system seems to be overprotective in the case of this mutant.

Pharmacological Intervention

Most pharmacological strategies for the treatment of protein transport diseases aim to rescue mutant poteins retained by the quality control system of the ER. The idea is to develop substances favouring correct folding of the mutant proteins, thereby allowing them to pass the quality control system. Most studies were carried out with the ΔF508 mutant of the CFTR protein. Although the new pharmacological approaches for the causal treatment of protein transport diseases are promising, none of the substances made its way out of the experimental or the early clinical trial level as yet. Two groups of substances favouring correct protein folding are examined at the moment: the chemical and the pharmacological chaperones.

Chemical Chaperones

The observation that reduction of temperature sometimes favours correct protein folding led to the idea that this effect may also be achieved by the addition of chemical compounds acting as "chemical chaperones" which improve protein folding by unspecific interactions with target molecules. Indeed, it was shown for the ΔF508 CFTR mutant that the amount of correctly processed and functional protein could be increased if cells were treated with chemical chaperones such as glycerol, trimethylamine-N-oxide and 4-phenylbu-tyrate. These chemical chaperones were also able to correct misfolding of many other membrane and secretory proteins. The most important disadvantage of chemical chaperones is that they must be used in very high (toxic) concentrations (10–1000 mM) that precludes their application.

Pharmacological Chaperones

The disadvantages of the chemical chaperones led to the idea that correct protein folding may also be stabilized by compounds binding specifically to the patients target proteins. For example, addition of an agonist or an antagonist during the folding process of a mutant receptor protein may help to establish the correct conformation of the ligand binding pocket and consequently the correct structure of the full length protein. If such high affinity "pharmacological chaperones" interact with the extracellular domains of membrane proteins or with secretory proteins, they must, however, be hydrophobic enough to pass not only the the plasma but also the ER membrane.

In the case of the ΔF508 CFTR mutant, the A_1 adenosine receptor antagonist 8-cyclopentyl-1,2-dipropylxanthine (CPX) is such a compound that exhibits a more specific action. It binds to the first nucleotide binding domain of CFTR that is structurally related to an A_1 adenosine receptor binding site. In transfected cells, CPX leads to a restoration of the plasma membrane transport of the ΔF508 CFTR mutant, most likely by stabilizing correct folding. For this compound, phase II clinical trials with cystic fibrosis patients are underway. Likewise, the CFTR-activating benzo(c)quinolizinium drugs MPB-07 and MPB-91 restore the transport of the ΔF508 CFTR mutant This effect, too, appears to involve a specific binding site. The concept of pharmacological chaperones was recently extended to misfolded vasopressin V_2 receptors (rescue with the nonpeptidic antagonist SR121463A) and the α subunit of the rapidly activating delayed rectifier potassium channel (rescue with the antiarrhythmic drug E-4031).

Neither chemical nor pharmacological chaperones lead to wild-type expression levels of the mutant proteins at the cell surface. Alternative or additional strategies are needed to improve the intracellular transport of the mutant proteins. In the future drugs may be developed that influence those components of the quality control system that are involed in the retention of misfolded proteins. Among these are e.g. the yet unknown adaptor proteins for the exposed RXR signals.

References

1. Hong W, (1996) Protein trafficking along the exocytotic pathway (Molecular Biology Intelligence Unit). Springer-Verlag, Heidelberg, Germany
2. Brodsky JL (1998) Translocation of proteins across the endoplasmic reticulum membrane. Int. Rev. Cytol. 178:277–328
3. Ellgaard L, Helenius A (2001) ER quality control: towards an understanding at the molecular level. Curr. Opin. Cell Biol. 13:431–437
4. Aridor M, Hannan LA (2000) Traffic jam: a compendium of human diseases that affect intracellular transport processes. Traffic 1:836–851
5. Zeitlin P (2000) Future pharmacological treatment of cystic fibrosis. Respiration 67:351–357

Proteinase-activated Receptors

SCOTT MACFARLANE, ROBIN PLEVIN
Department of Physiology and Pharmacology, Strathclyde Institute for Biomedical Sciences, University of Strathclyde, Glasgow, UK
scott.macfarlane@strath.ac.uk;
r.plevin@strath.ac.uk

Synonyms

Protease-activated receptors

Definition

▶ Proteinase-activated receptors (PARs) are a subclass of G-protein coupled receptors activated by ▶ serine proteinase-mediated proteolysis of their N-terminal sequence leading to the formation of a new N-terminal sequence, or ▶ tethered ligand that intra-molecularly activates the receptor.

▶ Non-viral Proteases

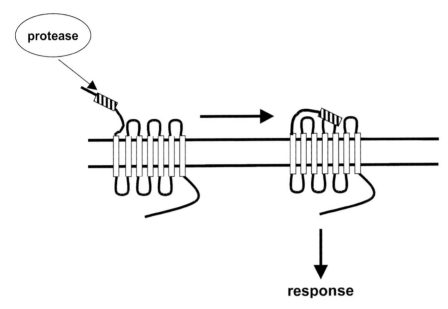

protease

response

Fig. 1 Schematic diagram of the 'tethered ligand' theory of activation characteristic of the PAR family.

Basic Characteristics

Proteinase-activated receptors (PARs) are defined by their mechanisms of activation: Unlike other G-protein coupled receptors (GPCRs) that are activated by a soluble ligand, ▶ serine proteinase enzymes activate PARs. The N-terminus of the receptor is cleaved at specific amino acid residues and the new terminus functions as an intra-molecular ligand to activate the receptor within the extracellular loops (ECL) (Fig. 1). This is known as the ▶ tethered ligand mode of activation. Correspondingly, synthetic PAR activating peptides (APs) can be generated that mimic the new N-terminus and activate PARs without the need for enzymatic cleavage of the receptor. The prototypic member of this class of receptor, PAR-1, is cleaved at Arg^{41} by thrombin to generate the N-terminal ligand sequence SFLLRN that then activates the receptor by binding principally to the N-terminal exodomain and the ECL-2 (1).

There are currently 4 members of the PAR family, PARs 1–4, although additional subtypes have been proposed. Each receptor is characterised by the preferred activating ▶ serine proteinase enzyme, the site of cleavage within the N-terminus and the peptide sequence that can activate the receptor exogenously (Fig. 2). ▶ Thrombin selectively activates PARs 1 and 3 through high affinity binding to a site within the receptor known as the

▶ hirudin-like binding domain. PAR-4 does not contain such a domain and is less selective for thrombin over ▶ trypsin and may also be activated by cathepsin G. PAR-2 is distinct from PARs 1, 3 and 4 in that it is selectively activated by trypsin and relatively insensitive to thrombin (Table 1). However, PAR-2 is also activated by other proteases such as α-tryptase (2), acrosin, the blood coagulation Factors VIIa and X, and other serine proteases such as neurosin and MT-SP-1 (1). Thus, relative to the other PARs, PAR-2 has a potentially complex mode of activation depending upon the tissue or cellular expression of the relevant activators.

Cellular Activation

Activation of PARs 1–4 results in increased $InsP_3$ formation and a rise in intracellular Ca^{2+} indicating coupling to the Gq/11 class of heterotrimeric G-proteins. PAR –1, and to a lesser extent PAR-2, has been shown to be coupled to multiple kinase signalling pathways including ERK, JNK and p38 MAP kinase and nuclear factor κ B (1). To date, no such events have been demonstrated for hPAR-3 or -4.

Functional Roles of the PARs

PAR-1. This receptor is recognised to play important roles in the regulation of cardiovascular func-

P

tethered ligand domain

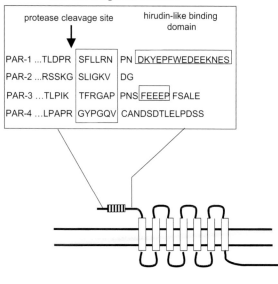

Fig. 2 Diagram showing the cleavage sites and tethered ligand sequences for the 4 known PAR family members.

tion particularly in response to vessel damage. Initially thrombin stimulates platelet aggregation and vascular smooth muscle contraction as part of an acute response. Thrombin also increases endothelial permeability, recruitment of white blood cells, in particular leucocytes, and release of inflammatory cytokines and induction of adhesion molecule expression. These events, combined with a marked increase in endothelial and smooth muscle proliferation, the synthesis of matrix proteins and other tissue factors, contribute to a co-ordinated wound healing response. Important non-vascular functions of PAR-1 include the regulation of neuronal cell survival, intestinal motility and bone remodeling (1).

PAR-2. In contrast to the other PARs, PAR-2 is strongly expressed in cells of epithelial origin including vascular endothelial cells, airway and kidney epithelia, intestinal smooth muscle and enterocytes and basal keratinocytes. PAR-2 is also expressed in neutrophils, leucocytes and mast cells. Stimulation of PAR-2 in vascular preparations and airways causes relaxation though NO or PGE_2 release whilst in the intestine, increases

intestinal motility and fluid release. In keratinocytes, PAR-2 activation results in a decrease in cell proliferation and an increase in cytokine release. PAR-2 is also associated with increased adhesion and rolling of leucocytes and mast cell degranulation. In neuronal cells, PAR-2 has been implicated in cell death (1).

PAR-3/PAR-4. Far fewer studies have shown functions for these novel thrombin-sensitive receptors. The function of hPAR-has proved difficult to elucidate due to the lack of a specific agonist for the receptor, although the distribution of the receptor has been well documented. In one study the mouse homologue of PAR-3 was unable to function as a receptor but was suggested to act as a tethering protein for thrombin to activate PAR-4 (3).

PAR-4 is also expressed in human platelets and functions to maintain the late phase of platelet coagulation. PAR-4 is also expressed in a number of smooth muscle preparations where it causes contraction (1).

Roles of PARs in Disease

PAR-1. Since thrombin plays a key role in wound healing, PAR-1 is strongly implicated in cardiovascular disease (Table 1). PAR-1 expression is up-regulated in coronary vessels following balloon injury, whilst in PAR-1-deficient mice reduced neointima formation is observed following injury. PAR-1 is also associated with vascular inflammation including crescentric glomerulonephritis, a renal inflammatory condition associated with fibrin deposition. Since thrombin is able to stimulate cellular proliferation, motility and increased expression of adhesion molecules, PAR-1 is implicated in some forms of cancers including pulmonary metastasis and breast cancers. Finally, PAR-1 is associated with some neurological disorders particularly those involving brain trauma (1).

PAR-2. The tissue and cellular distribution of PAR-2, its mechanisms of action and its cellular effects have strongly implicated PAR-2 in inflammation (Table 1). PAR-2 activators such as tryptase and trypsin are released by inflammatory challenge or during diseases such as psoriasis and pancreatitis. Indeed, in PAR-2-deficient mice, inflammatory

Tab. 1 Activators, tethered ligand sequences, known and proposed functions for human PAR family members. For more complete tables, see (1,5).

	PAR-1	PAR-2	PAR-3	PAR-4
Endogenous agonist	Thrombin	Trypsin, tryptase, acrosin	Thrombin	Thrombin, trypsin, cathepsin G
Specific peptide ligand	TFLLR	SLIGKV, SLIGRL	--	GYPGQV, AYPGKF
Known function	Platelet activation	--	--	Platelet activation
Proposed disease associations	Cancer, wound healing, vascular remodeling, inflammation, crescentric glomerulo-nephritis	Skin pigmentation, cancer, vascular remodeling, neuorogenic pain, inflammation	--	--

responses are delayed although not fully compromised. Recently, PAR-2 has been strongly implicated in mediating inflammatory pain, including thermal hyperalgesia and intestinal pain. In addition to psoriasis, PAR-2 is also associated with skin pigmentation and hair follicle development and implicated in diseases associated with disorders in these processes (1).

In some tissues, such as the lung, a role for PAR-2 in disease is not easily defined. In airway vessels PAR-2 promotes relaxation but may also promote airway smooth muscle and fibroblast proliferation and cytokine release. Thus the role of PAR-2 in disease states may be dependent on levels of receptor and expression of tissues specific proteases.

PAR-3/PAR-4. No definitive roles of PAR-3 or PAR-4 have been identified for these PARs to date.

Drugs

Serine Protease Inhibitors
Since thrombin plays an important role in initiating blood coagulation in addition to its receptor mediated actions, initial studies focused on the development of thrombin inhibitors. These included active site inhibitors and compounds based on the binding site of hirudin. Other antithrombin compounds, such as antithrombin II,

have been implicated as potential agents for inhibiting PAR-1 activation. However; such inhibition of thrombin in a global manner may not be desirable, the development and use of specific PAR-1 antagonists must remain the preferred option for the treatment of PAR-1 specific diseases.

▶ Serine proteinase inhibitors may be of use in PAR-2 related diseases. For example, work in both pigs and humans has indicated the potential usefulness of serine proteinase inhibitors, topically applied, in dealing with diseases of skin pigmentation (4). As is the case with thrombin inhibitors however; the widespread inhibition of proteinases within the body would prove highly undesirable, and is unlikely to be of overall use in the treatment of PAR-related disease.

PAR-1 Agonist/Antagonists
The distinct hexapeptides that activate PARs have been used as structural templates for the design and synthesis of receptor antagonists. For PAR-1, a series of substituted pentapeptides incorporating substitutions at positions 2, 3 and 4 of SFLLRN, e.g. A(pF)FRCha-HarY-NH$_2$. This template has also been used to synthesise antagonist peptides and peptoids including, N-trans (p-F)FpGu-Phe-Leu-Arg-NH$_2$ (BMS-197525), RWJ-56110 and SCH79797. RWJ-56110 has been shown to inhibit both thrombin and SFLLRN-stimulated responses including platelet aggregation and smooth muscle

P

Ca^{2+} mobilisation. However, an orally active antagonist with good bioavailability has not reached clinical trials. However, PAR-1 antagonists are likely to find uses as antithrombotic agents, inhibitors of vascular remodelling or possible anti-cancer agents (1).

It should be noted that several of these putative PAR-1 selective drugs require to be re-assessed following the discovery of PARs 2–4.

PAR-2. A similar approach has been used to identify PAR agonists and antagonists. No such agonist compounds have been identified with more than moderate potency. However pharmacological studies using one of these peptides, trans-cinnamoyl-LIGRLO-NH$_2$, have suggested the presence of PAR-2 subtypes. Recently a PAR-2 antagonist has been identified as part of a recent patent application displaying relatively low potency.

PAR-3/PAR-4. To date little progress has been made in the synthesis of highly selective PAR-3 or PAR-4 agonist/antagonists. However the observation that PAR-4 is activated in platelets by relatively high concentrations of thrombin, suggests that blockage of this receptor may be desirable in thrombosis.

References

1. Macfarlane SR, Seatter MJ, Kanke T, Hunter GD and Plevin R (2001) Proteinase-activated receptors. Pharmacological Reviews 53:254–282
2. Molino M, Barnathan ES, Numerof R, Clark J, Dreyer M, Cumashi A, Hoxie JA, Schechter N, Woolkalis M & Brass LF (1997a) Interactions of mast cell tryptase with thrombin receptors and PAR-2. Journal of Biological Chemistry 272:4043–4049
3. Nakanishi-Matsui M, Zheng YW, Sulciner DJ, Weiss EJ, Ludeman MJ & Coughlin SR (2000) PAR3 is a cofactor for PAR4 activation by thrombin. Nature 404:609–613
4. Hermanns JF, Petit L, Martalo O, Pierard-Franchimont C, Cauwenbergh C & Pierard GE (2000) Unraveling the patterns of subclinical pheomelanin-enriched facial hyperpigmentation: Effect of depigmenting agents. Dermatology 201:118–122
5. Vergnolle N, Wallace J L, Bunnet N W and Hollenberg M D (2001) Protease-activated receptors in inflammation, neuronal signalling and pain. TRENDS in Pharmacological Sciences 22:146–152

Proteinases

Proteinases are enzymes which catalyze the hydrolysis of peptide bonds in proteins. Many, but not all, proteinases require specific amino acid sequences around the preferred cleavage site.

▶ Non-viral Proteases

Proteome

The proteome is the protein complement expressed by a genome. While the genome is static, the proteome continually changes in response to external and internal events.

▶ Proteomics

Proteomics

EBERHARD KRAUSE
Forschungsinstitut für Molekulare Pharmakologie, Berlin, Germany
ekrause@fmp-berlin.de

Synonyms

Proteome analysis; proteome research

Definition

The proteome has been defined as the entire protein complement expressed by a genome. Thus the field of proteomics involves the extensive study of the dynamic protein products of the genome and includes the identification, characterization and quantitation of proteins and their interactions.

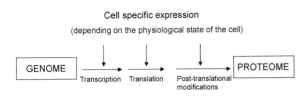

Cell specific expression
(depending on the physiological state of the cell)

GENOME → Transcription → Translation → Post-translational modifications → PROTEOME

Fig. 1 Genome versus proteome.

▶ Gene Expression Analysis
▶ Microarray Technology

Description

Genome and Proteome

The term proteome was introduced in 1995 (1) and has spread world wide within just a few years. Proteome is the linguistic equivalent of the term genome and describes the whole complement of proteins expressed by a cell at any given time. In contrast to the genome, the proteome is dynamic and very complex. The expression of a gene has no definitive relationship to the expression or abundance of its protein product. In addition, ▶ post-translational modifications (PTM), such as processing, phosphorylation and glycosylation as well as other modifications cannot be deduced from genomic data. PTMs are important for structure, localization, function and turnover of proteins, and have been shown to be involved in disease states. Proteomics involves extensive protein analysis and is intimately involved with protein chemistry. In the early work, proteomics was associated with the cataloging of a large number of proteins separated by two-dimensional gel electrophoresis. Now that the human genome and the genomes of several species have been determined, proteomics is expected to contribute to the understanding of gene function. The field of proteomics is currently in a rapid state of development (2). The main areas of research include: (i) identification of proteins; (ii) characterization of post-translational modifications; (iii) studies of protein interactions and complex formation; and (iv) differential display effects for the comparison of protein expression. Functional proteomics is defined as the use of the methods of proteomics to analyze the molecular networks in cells, for example the identification of specific proteins of these networks following functional stimulation.

The Tools of Proteomics

One of the most challenging steps in proteome research is the separation, visualization, and quantification of proteins. Current methodology suffers from the lack of an amplifying method analogous to the polymerase chain reaction. If a given cell at a given time expresses 5000 genes, approximately 15000 cellular proteins can be expected as a result of mRNA splicing and post-translational modifications. In addition, the broad dynamic range of protein expression (10^8 and higher) and the physico-chemical diversity of proteins makes the visualization of an entire proteome an unresolved problem. Unfortunately, there is no universal separation method, although ▶ two-dimensional gel electrophoresis, 2DE (3) is commonly used for the quantitative analysis of the state of expression of large numbers of proteins in a cell. Proteins are separated electrophoretically in the first dimension according to their isoelectric point (isoelectrofocusing, IEF) and in the second dimension according to their mobility in the porous polyacrylamide gel (SDS-PAGE). A standard 2DE of 150 μg of cell lysate allows the resolution of more than 2000 proteins on the basis of charge and mass. Sample pre-fractionation techniques prior to 2DE aim to reduce the complexity of protein mixtures found in cells or tissues and may enhance sensitivity for the more interesting low-abundance proteins by removing the housekeeping proteins that are present at higher concentrations. Sensitive silver staining methods that do not covalently modify proteins, or Coomassie Blue dye staining methods are available for the detection of gel-separated proteins. In particular, fluorescent staining methods that offer a broader dynamic range of detection than silver staining, and computer image analysis methods enable quantification of proteins at least over the range of a few orders of magnitude and allow comparative proteome mapping. The weakness of 2DE is that it does not work well with very large, very small, or hydrophobic proteins (especially membrane-bound and cytoskeletal proteins), and those exhibiting extreme isoelectric points. An alternative approach is to use affinity-based protein purification combined with one-dimensional SDS gel

P

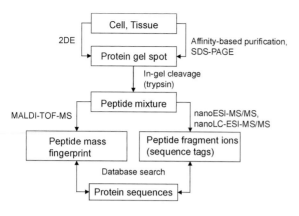

Fig. 2 A strategy for mass spectrometry-based identification and characterization of proteins.

electrophoresis, a technique that is able to visualize even extremely hydrophobic as well as acidic and basic proteins.

Non-gel separation techniques such as multidimensional capillary chromatography and the recently described isotope-coded affinity tag (ICAT) method circumvent the disadvantages of 2DE. The ICAT methods (4) are based on a class of cysteine-specific reagents that incorporate an isotopically coded linker and a biotin affinity tag. The method involves three steps: (i) site-specific covalent labeling of proteins with isotopically "light" or "heavy" deuterated ICAT reagents; (ii) proteolysis of the combined labeled protein samples; and (iii) isolation, identification and quantification of the tagged peptides by avidin affinity chromatography, reversed-phase chromatography, and ▶ tandem mass spectrometry followed by computational analysis. The isotope peak ratios of the labeled pairs of peptides give the relative amounts of the corresponding proteins. ICAT enables quantitative cataloging and comparison of protein expression by mass spectrometry and is therefore useful for differential display proteomics. However, at present 2DE gives the highest resolution of all separation methods and the broad applicability of non-gel approaches has yet to be proven. Further advances in proteomics can be expected from the miniaturization of separation techniques (nano methods) that lead to increased sample concentration, reduced loss of analyte and improved compatibility with mass spectrometry.

The study of proteomes also requires efficient methods for the identification and characterization of separated proteins. Recent advances in mass spectrometric instrumentation and techniques have revolutionized protein analysis; see (5) for review. The development of so-called "soft" ionization methods such as electrospray ionization (ESI) and matrix-assisted laser desorption/ionization (MALDI) have enabled the generation of gas-phase ions of peptides and proteins without significant fragmentation. Various mass analyzers such as the time-of-flight (TOF), quadrupole, ion trap and ion cyclotron resonance systems as well as various combinations thereof can be used. MALDI-TOF-MS provides very accurate and sensitive mass measurements of peptides as well as high molecular weight proteins. New instrumental designs such as delayed extraction ion sources and low-flow devices (nanoelectrospray, nanoESI) have improved the resolution and sensitivity of mass spectrometry. Triple quadrupole, ion trap, or in particular, hybrid mass analyzers such as quadrupole-TOF (Q-TOF) systems have been applied to tandem mass spectrometry in which peptide ions are selectively separated in the first step and then fragmented by collision-induced dissociation (CID) and analyzed in the second step in the mass spectrometer. These types of mass spectrometers typically use electrospray ionization. MALDI-MS including fragmentation of high-energy ions by post-source decay (PSD) techniques also may yield fragment ion spectra. Both CID and PSD spectra obtained by these methods mainly show sequence-specific N-terminal 'b' and C-terminal 'y' ions. Such fragmentation by mass spectrometry gives at least partial information about the peptide sequence and can be used to identify proteins from databases of expressed sequence tags. In contrast to Edman sequencing, which fails in the analysis of subpicomole quantities or of N-terminally blocked proteins, mass spectrometry provides accurate mass measurements at a very high level of sensitivity even of protein mixtures. Although it has been demonstrated that sample amounts at attomole (10^{-18} mol) levels can be analyzed by MS, for protein identification the sensitivity limit is in the low femtomole range and routine sensitivities are only in the low picomole range. Suitable sample volumes are in the range from 500 nL to 1 μL.

Although MS is now the method of choice for protein analysis, there is a need for instrumentation that allows greater sensitivity, reliability and speed. Thus sample preparation methods, the ionization process, mass analyzers and data processing are fields of rapid development. Besides sensitive methods for the analysis of proteins, bioinformatics is one of the key components of proteome research. This includes software to monitor and quantify the separation of complex samples, e.g. to analyze 2DE images. Web-based database search engines are available to compare experimentally measured peptide masses or sequence ions of protein digests with theoretical values of peptides derived from protein sequences. Websites for database searching with mass spectrometric data may be found at http://www.expasy.ch/tools, http://prospector.ucsf.edu/, and http://www.matrixscience.com.

Identification of Proteins, Post-translational Modifications and Protein-protein Interactions

Because knowledge of the molecular weights of proteins is insufficient for database identification, mass spectrometric identification of proteins requires enzymatic digestion of proteins into peptide mixtures. Trypsin is the most commonly used enzyme for digestion since it is inexpensive and the cleavage rules are well known (peptide bonds after lysine and arginine are cleaved selectively). Digestion can be performed directly in-gel, followed by elution of the peptide mixture. The enzyme normally generates peptides between 600 and 2000 D, a mass range suitable for sensitive and accurate mass spectrometry. Once digested, the peptide mixtures can either be directly analyzed by MALDI-MS or can be separated by capillary reversed-phase liquid chromatography coupled directly to a quadrupole-TOF MS. From the mass spectra a set of experimentally obtained peptide masses, the ▶ peptide mass fingerprint (PMF), can be extracted and used for database searches. Depending on protein molecular weight, the detection of even a small number of peptides (20 to 30% sequence coverage) provides sufficient data for reliable identification. Peptide mass mapping using MALDI-MS works satisfactorily if a complete genomic sequence database is available. The method can be automated and makes possible the identification of hundreds of 2DE separated proteins. In case peptide mass mapping is unsuccessful, tandem mass spectrometry (MS/MS) has to be used. The method utilizes the fragmentation of individual peptides of the protein digest by collision-induced dissociation in a collision cell of the mass spectrometer (see above). Protein identification using this approach is particularly useful for proteins from species with incompletely sequenced genomes. MS/MS spectra may yield an amino acid sequence or at least a partial sequence that is specific for a protein and can be used to search protein sequence databases or nucleotide databases (EST).

More than 200 different naturally occurring post-translational protein modifications (PTMs) have been described. Most of these modifications are accessible to analysis via mass spectrometry. Although mass spectrometry is the method of choice to determine the structure and site of modification, such an analysis is much more difficult than the determination of protein identity. Despite numerous reports of MS analysis of phosphorylation and glycosylation, the detection of such modifications in mass fingerprints still presents a serious challenge. Because the modification is frequently labile, mass spectrometry has to be performed under very mild conditions in terms of sample preparation and ionization. Furthermore, the identification of PTMs requires determination of the specific peptide that contains the modified amino acid. In principle, procedures used for protein identification are also applicable to the determination of PTMs. A mass difference compared to the expected mass after enzymatic degradation of the protein by specific endoproteinases (peptide mass mapping) can be used as a sign for the presence of modified peptides, even though this indication is not very specific. Selection and preconcentration of modified sequences by immunoprecipitation or binding to a chelating column are techniques that have been described for phosphopeptides. To determine the site of modification, i.e. the modified amino acid side chain, fragmentation by post-source decay MALDI-MS or collision-induced ▶ ESI-MS must be performed.

Because it is well accepted that cellular processes are controlled by multi-protein complexes and such complexes are actual molecular targets of drugs, a further key aim of proteomics is to study protein-protein interactions. The characterization of complexes in which several proteins are associated to perform their biological function can be achieved by purification of the entire protein complex using affinity based methods, such as glutathione S-transferase (GST)-fusion proteins. The tandem-affinity-purification-tag (TAP-tag) techniques use two high affinity binding sequences separated by a highly specific cleavage site for a protease to capture and purify a protein complex. After separation by gel electrophoresis the single proteins are identified either by their peptide mass fingerprints or via tandem mass spectrometry. As an example, several new factors of the human spliceosome were obtained by these techniques and analyzed further (2).

Pharmacological Relevance:

Extensive protein identifications has been performed in the framework of numerous proteome projects to study human pathogens (e.g. comparative proteome analysis of *Helicobacter pylori*), to identify disease-associated proteins (e.g. cancer or heart proteomics), and to analyze proteins involved in signal transduction cascades. Although the main goal of proteomics is the mapping of proteins of cells or tissues, there are further tasks beyond the identification of proteins. Post-translational modifications of proteins are important for biological processes, particularly in cellular signal transduction. The processing generates functional proteins, lipid modifications determine the location of proteins, and the attachment of phosphate can activate or inactivate reaction cascades. Because of its regulatory importance, protein phosphorylation, i.e. the formation of phosphate esters with the hydroxyl groups of serine, threonine, and tyrosine, has received the most attention. Kinases and phosphatases catalyze phosphorylation and dephosphorylation, respectively. Several receptor-mediated signal transduction pathways result in tyrosine phosphorylation of various proteins. A functional proteomics approach that focuses on the isolation, separation and identification of phosphorylated proteins following stimulation of wild-type and/or modified receptors provides insights into the quality and quantity of signaling proteins. Examples include EGF and PDGF receptor signaling, which involve activation or inactivation by endogenous or exoge-

nous factors and interactions between different signal pathways. Post-genomic proteomics also includes areas such as the determination of protein function, structural analysis, analysis of metabolic pathways, drug mode-of-action and toxicity studies. Proteomics directly contributes to the identification of diagnostic markers and drug targets.

References

1. Wilkins MR et al. (1996) From proteins to proteomes: large scale protein identification by two-dimensional electrophoresis and amino acid analysis. BioTechnology 14:61–65
2. Pandey A, Mann M (2000) Proteomics to study genes and genomes. Nature 405:837–846
3. Klose J (1975) Protein mapping by combined isoelectric focusing and electrophoresis of mouse tissues. A novel approach to testing for induced point mutations in mammals. Humangenetik 26:231–243
4. Gygi SP et al. (1999) Quantitative analysis of complex protein mixtures using isotope-coded affinity tags. Nature Biotechnol. 17:994–999
5. Aebersold R, Goodlett DR (2001) Mass spectrometry in proteomics. Chem. Rev. 101:269–295

Proteosomal Degradation

Proteosomal degration is the process by which improperly folded proteins or proteins with altered post-translational modifications are removed from a cell before they have a detrimental effect on cellular function. This is performed in small organelles known as proteosomes. Proteins are targeted for destruction in the proteosome by having a number of small ubiquitin molecules added.

▶ Glucocorticoids
▶ Ubiquitin/Proteasome System

Prothrombin Time

Prothrombin time (PT) is a coagulation assay which measures the time for plasma to clot upon activation by 'thromboplastin' (a mixture of tissue factor and phospholipids).

▶ Anticoagulants

Protocadherins

▶ Table appendix: Adhesion Molecules

Proton Pump Inhibitors and Acid Pump Antagonists

JAI MOO SHIN, BJÖRN WALLMARK[*], GEORGE SACHS
University of California at Los Angeles,
Los Angeles, USA, [*]Schering AG, Berlin, Germany
jaishin@ucla.edu, bjoern.wallmark@schering.de,
gsachs@ucla.edu

Synonyms

Gastric H, K-ATPase inhibitors

Definition

The ▶ gastric H, K-ATPase in the parietal cell secretes hydronium ions, H_3O^+, in exchange for K^+ into the secretory canaliculus generating a pH of <1.0 in lumen of the stomach.

Pump directed inhibitors of acid secretion can be classified into two groups: reversible (acid pump antagonists, APA's) and non-reversible covalent inhibitors (protn pump inhibitors, PPI's). The covalent binding inhibitors are substituted 2-(pyridinemethylsulfinyl) benzimidazoles and the reversible inhibitors are K^+-competitive. PPI's have dramatically influenced the management of acid-peptic disorders.

Mechanism of Action

The gastric H,K-ATPase consists of a α-subunit of about 1034 amino acids and a β-subunit having about 290 amino acids, and 6 or 7 N-linked glycosylation sites The H,K-ATPase α-subunit has ten transmembrane segments and β-subunit one transmembrane segment. The H,K-ATPase α-subunit has a strong association with the β-subunit at the luminal loop between the seventh segment (TM7) and the eighth transmembrane segment (TM8). The gastric H,K-ATPase transports H_3O^+ ions from the cytoplasmic region to lumen by conformational changes induced by phosphorylation and dephosphorylation. In the first step, the E_1 form of the H,K-ATPase binds hydronium ion and MgATP with the ion site facing the cytoplasm. The enzyme is then phosphorylated to form $E_1P \cdot H_3O^+$ and the conformation changes from $E_1P \cdot H_3O^+$ to the $E_2P \cdot H_3O^+$ form, where the ion site faces exoplasmically. H_3O^+ is released and K^+ binds on the extra-cytoplasmic surface of the enzyme, resulting in the $E_2P \cdot K^+$ conformation. This dephosphorylates, forming $E_2 \cdot K^+$ with the ion occluded and this conformation converts to E_1K^+ that releases K^+ to the cytoplasmic side with binding of MgATP. The H,K-ATPase has a very similar structural motif when compared with other P_2-type ATPases such as the Na,K- and ▶ Ca-ATPases.

Since a substituted benzimidazole was first reported to inhibit the H,K-ATPase, many PPI's have been synthesized and are in clinical use. These all have a similar core structure. Several APA's have been in clinical trial and these contain protonatable nitrogens but have a variety of core structures. One type is represented by the imidazo-pyridine derivatives, others are piperidinopyridines, substituted 4-phenylaminoquinolines, pyrrolo[3,2-c]quinolines, guanidino-thiazoles, 2,4-diaminopyrimidine derivatives, and scopadulcic acid (1). Some natural products such as cassigarol A and naphthoquinone also showed inhibitory activity.

Proton Pump Inhibitors

The first compound of this class with inhibitory activity on the enzyme and on acid secretion was the 2-(pyridylmethyl)sulfinylbenzimidazole, timoprazole, and the first pump inhibitor used clinically was 2-[[3,5-dimethyl-4-methoxypyridin-2-

P

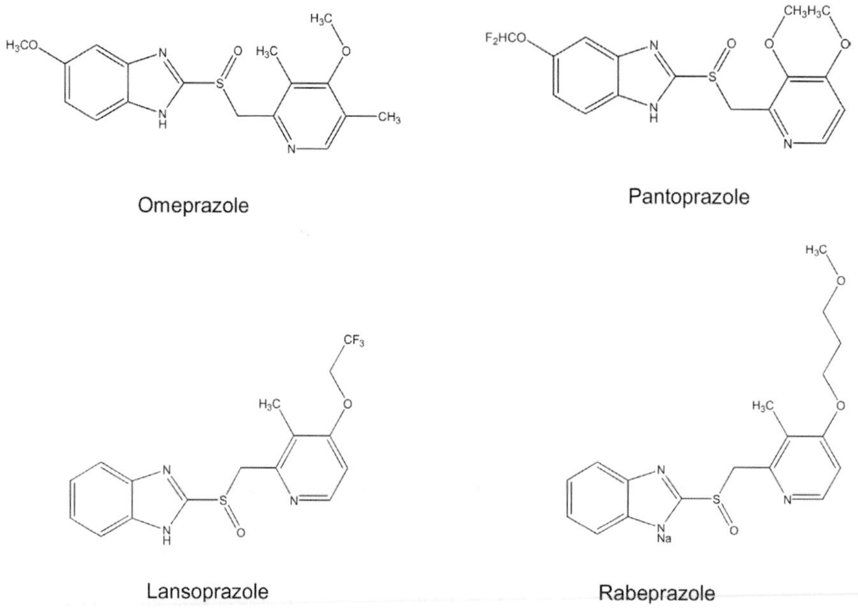

Omeprazole

Pantoprazole

Lansoprazole

Rabeprazole

Fig. 1 Proton Pump Inhibitors and Acid Pump Antagonists – Irreversible proton pump inhibitors used clinically.

yl]methylsulfinyl]-5-methoxy-1H-benzimidazole, omeprazole. Omeprazole is an acid-activated prodrug. Omeprazole can be accumulated in the acidic space of the parietal cell and there converts to a thiol-reactive cationic sulfenic acid and sulfenamide, which binds to -SH groups to form disulfides as shown in Fig. 2 (1).Substituted benzimidazole inhibitors show slightly different effects depending on the inhibitor structure. The omeprazole-bound enzyme is in the E_2 form. Another inhibitor, rabeprazole (E3810), 2-[[4-(3-methoxypropoxy)-3-methylpyridin-2-yl]methylsulfinyl]-1H-benzimidazole, stabilizes the E_1 form of the enzyme after binding. It is claimed that the K^+ dependent dephosphorylation of the phosphoenzyme is inhibited in the rabeprazole-bound enzyme but not in the omeprazole-bound enzyme, whereas phosphoenzyme formation in the absence of K^+ is inhibited in both the E3810- and omeprazole-bound enzyme.

Omeprazole binds to cysteines in the extracytoplasmic regions of M5/M6 (cys-813) and M7/M8 (cys-892). Pantoprazole binds only to both the cysteines in M5/M6, cysteine 813 and 822, and lansoprazole binds to cysteine 321 in M3/M4 and to cysteine 813 in M5/M6, and cysteine 892 M7/M8. These data suggest that of the 28 cysteines in the α-subunit only the cysteines present in the M5/M6

domain are important for inhibition of acid secretion by the PPI's (1,2).

Acid Pump Antagonists

SCH28080, a substituted imidazo[1,2α] pyridine, is the best defined among other reversible proton pump inhibitors. SCH 28080, 3-cyanomethyl-2-methyl-8-(phenylmethoxy) imidazo[1,2α]pyridine, inhibits the H,K-ATPase competitively with K^+ (1). SCH 28080 binds to free enzyme extracytoplasmically in the absence of substrate to form E_2(SCH 28080) complexes. SCH 28080 inhibits ATPase activity with high affinity in the absence of K^+. SCH 28080 has no effect on spontaneous dephosphorylation but inhibits K^+-stimulated dephosphorylation, presumably by forming a E_2-P•[I] complex. Hence SCH 28080 inhibits K^+-stimulated ATPase activity by competing with K^+ for binding E_2P. Steady state phosphorylation is also reduced by SCH 28080, showing that this compound also binds to the free enzyme.

MDPQ or other 2,4-diaminoquinazoline derivatives are also known to act like SCH28080.

Clinical Use

Proton pump inhibitors are used for the therapy of gastric ulcer, duodenal ulcer, ▶ gastroesophageal reflux disease, ▶ Zollinger-Ellison syndrome and

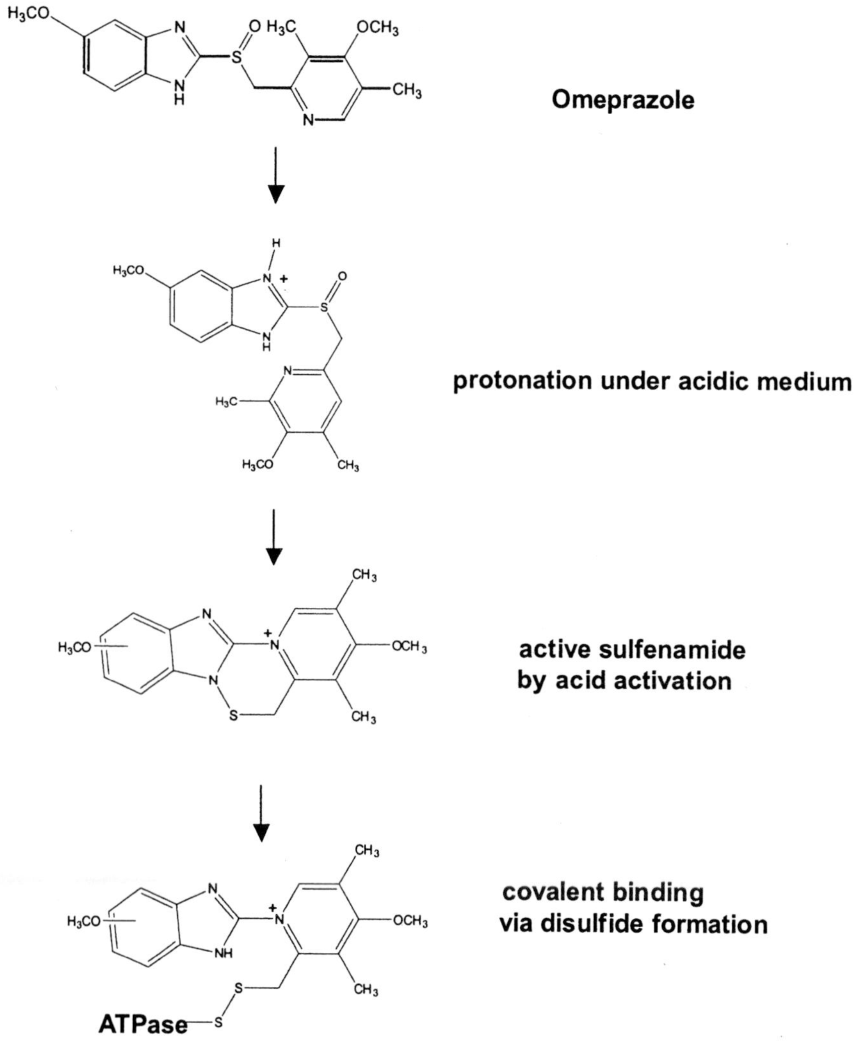

Omeprazole

protonation under acidic medium

active sulfenamide by acid activation

covalent binding via disulfide formation

Fig. 2 Proton Pump Inhibitors and Acid Pump Antagonists – Mechanism of irreversible proton pump inhibitor, Omeprazole. Omeprazole, one of substituted benzimidazole compounds, is accumulated in acidic lumen and converted to active sulfenamide, which binds extracytoplasmic cysteinesof the gastric H,K-ATPase.

for eradication of *Helicobacter pylori*. The primary effect of these proton pump inhibitors is gastric acid suppression. The degree of acid suppression correlates with healing rates for reflux oesophagitis and peptic ulcer. Omeprazole, lansoprazole, pantoprazole, and rabeprazole showed equivalent potency of gastric acid suppression (3).

Recently, S-omeprazole has become available for clinical use. Omeprazole is a racemate consisting of S- and R-enantiomers. The R-form of omeprazole is sensitive to CYPs 2C19 and 3A4 enzymes, while S-form is less sensitive to these ▶ CYP enzymes (4). S-omeprazole has longer plasma half-life compared to omeprazole, providing longer duration of acid suppression.

Proton pump inhibitors are successfully used in triple therapy (i.e. combined with two antibiotics) for eradication of ▶ *Helicobacter pylori*.

References

1. Shin JM, Bayle D, Bamberg K, Sachs G (1998) The gastric H,K-ATPase. In: Advances in Molecular and Cell Biology, JAI Press Inc., Connecticut 23A:101–142
2. Sachs G, Briving C, Shin JM, Hsersey S, Wallmark B (1995) The phamacology of the gastric acid pump, the H+,K+-ATPase. Ann. Rev. Pharmacol. Toxicol. 35:277–305
3. Stedman CAM, Barclay ML (2000) Review article: Comparison of the pharmacokinetics, acid sup-

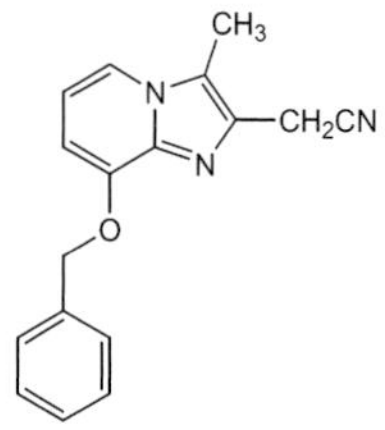

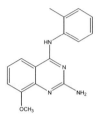

SCH28080

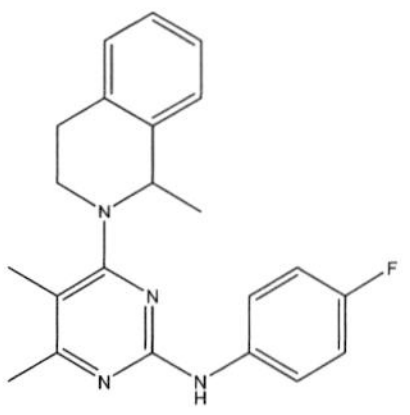

YH1885

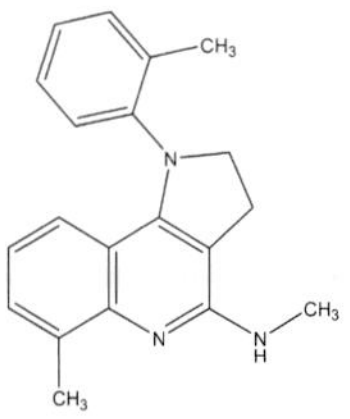

MDPQ (quinoline derivative: SK&F)

2,4-Diaminoquinazoline derivative (SK&F)

Fig. 3 Proton Pump Inhibitors and Acid Pump Antagonists – Some reversible proton pump inhibitors under investigation.

pression and efficacy of proton pump inhibitors. Aliment. Pharmacol. Ther. 14:963–978

4. Abelo A, Andersson TB, Antonsson M, Naudot AK, Skanberg I, Weidolf L (2000) Stereoselective metabolism of omeprazole by human cytochrome P450 enzymes. Drug Metab. Dispos. 28(8):966–972

Proto-oncogenes

A proto-oncogene is a normal cellular gene, usually concerned with the regulation of cell proliferation, that can be converted to a cancer promoting oncogene by mutation.

▶ Oncogenes

Pseudogene

A pseudogene is a defective gene which has accumulated mutations that interfere with the production of a functional protein. Pseudogene transcripts may however be expressed. The origin of pseudogenes are gene duplications. Because one of the copies can continue to provide the enzymatic activity, the other(s) often degenerates over time and loses its function. Alternatively, it may acquire a new catalytic function.

Pseudohypoaldosteronism Type I

Autosomal recessive pseudohypoaldosteronism type I is caused by loss of function mutations in any of the three subunits of the epithelial sodium channel. Disease manifestations are apparent shortly after birth and include failure to thrive, renal Na wasting and dehydration, hyperkalemia, metabolic acidosis, and elevated plasma renin and aldosterone. In addition, salt concentrations in sweat are elevated, and recurrent infections and wheezing indicate altered fluid transport in the lung. Autosomal dominant pseudohypoaldosteronism type I is the result of mutations in the mineralocorticoid receptor gene.

▶ Diuretics
▶ Epithelial Na$^+$ Channels (ENaC)

Psoralens

Psoralens are naturally occurring substances, which are used for photochemotherapy, e.g. for treatment of psoriasis or vitiligo. The local application of e.g. 8-methoxypsoralen on the skin and subsequent irradiation with UVA-light is called PUVA. Psoralens are absorbed rapidly after oral administration and photosensivity is maximal about 1–2 hours after ingestion.

Psychedelic Hallucinogen

The term "psychedelic" literally means "mind manifesting" and was applied to hallucinogens like LSD or mescaline to emphasize the intensification of awareness and sensory perception that is associated with these drugs.

▶ Psychotomimetic Drugs

Psychostimulants

ION ANGHELESCU, ISABELLA HEUSER,
Psychiatrische Klinik und Poliklinik,
Freie Universität Berlin, Berlin, Germany
ion.anghelescu@medizin.fu-berlin.de,
isabella.heuser@medizin.fu-berlin.de

Synonyms

Stimulants, stimulant drugs, psychomotor stimulant drugs.

Definition

Psychostimulants are drugs that substantially influence cognitive and affective functioning and behaviours. Effects are increased motivational desire, agitation, heightened vigilance, euphoria, hyperactivity and decreased sleepiness as well as appetite. Traditionally, mainly cocaine and amphetamines are considered psychostimulants. However, nicotine, coffeine and even certain antidepressants could be included in this class. Methylphenidate, amphetamine (like dextro-amphetamine) and also pemoline – the latter was newly retracted from the market due to hepatotoxicity – are or have been widely used for the treatment of ▶ attention deficit/hyperactivity disorder (ADHD). Another psychostimulant indicated in ▶ narcolepsy is modafinil.

▶ Psychotomimetic Drugs

Mechanism of Action

General Remarks

The final pathway of psychostimulants on the behavioural level is an increased mobilization of the normal fight/flight/fright reaction that is mediated by the biogene amines epinephrine, norepinephrine, serotonin and dopamine. The most widespread extra-clinically used psychostimulant is ecstasy (3,4-methylenedioxymethamphetamin; MDMA), which also exhibits perceptual distortions due to 5-HT_{2A}-receptor agonism like lysergic acid diethylamide (LSD).

The main target of action of methylphenidate, the most widespread clinically used psychostimulant, is the dopamine transporter (DAT); its inhibition increases intrasynaptic dopamine concentrations. The subcortical dopamine system (mesolimbic and nigrostriatal parts) mediates the unconditioned and conditioned responses toward reinforcement.

Within the striatum, dopamine terminals have direct synaptic contacts with the spines of striatal neurons. These synaptic contacts appear to provide the anatomical substrate for both compartmental (synaptic) and volume (extra-synaptic) transmission. The DAT is located intra- or perisynaptically, suggesting that dopamine has a limited ability to escape the striatal synapse. Moreover, dopamine D2 and, to a lesser extent, D1 receptors are located postsynaptically from dopamine terminals, suggesting compartmental transmission. However, there is a significant cohort of D1 and D2 receptors that are not directly opposed to dopamine terminals, suggesting some component of volume transmission within the striatum. Therefore, tonic and phasic changes in dopamine transmission are critical in producing behavioural effects associated

P

Tab. 1 Properties of cortical versus striatal dopamine system.

	Cortical	Striatal
Synthesis-regulating autoreceptors	0	++
Impuls-regulating autoreceptors	0	++
DAT expression	0/+	++
DAT localization	extrasynaptical	synaptical

with the striatum. In contrast, in cerebral cortex, volume transmission appears to be more critical in mediating the effects of dopamine. DAT density is reduced in the ▸ frontal cortex (FC) relative to the striatum, and it is localized extra-synaptically. Moreover, D1-immunoreactivity within FC is virtually never opposed to tyrosine hydroxylase-immunopositive terminals suggesting that the effects of dopamine on D1 receptors is by volume transmission. This hypothesis has direct relevance to the neurochemistry of ADHD because cognitive functions known to be affected in this disorder, namely working memory and inhibitory control, are sensitive to manipulations of D1 receptor-mediated dopamine transmission (1). Thus, the tonic component might be more critical for the behavioural functions of the FC.

Several classes of drugs modulate the firing rates or patterns of midbrain dopamine neurons by direct, monosynaptic, or indirect, polysynaptic, inputs to the cell bodies within the ventral mesencephalon (i.e. nicotine and opiates). In contrast, amphetamine, cocaine and methylphenidate act at the level of the dopamine terminal interfering with normal processes of transmitter packaging, release, reuptake and metabolism.

Methylphenidate, Amphetamine and Cocaine

Methylphenidate like cocaine largely acts by blocking reuptake of monoamines into the presynaptic terminal. Methylphenidate administration produces an increase in the steady-state (tonic) levels of monoamines within the synaptic cleft. Thus, DAT inhibitors, such as methylphenidate increase extracellular levels of monoamines. In contrast, they decrease the concentrations of the monoamine metabolites that depend upon monoamine oxidase (MAO), i.e. HVA, but not cat-

echoamine-o-methyltransferase (COMT), because reuptake by the transporter is required for the formation of these metabolites. By stimulating presynaptic autoreceptors, methylphenidate induced increase in dopamine transmission can also reduce monoamine synthesis, inhibit monoamine neuron firing and reduce subsequent phasic dopamine release.

The pharmacology of amphetamine is considerably more complex. It does not only block monoamine reuptake, but also directly inhibits the vesicular monoamine transporter, causing an increase in cytosolic but not vesicular dopamine concentration. This may lead to reverse transport of the amines via the membrane-bound transporters. Further mechanisms of amphetamine action are: direct MAO inhibition and indirect release of both dopamine and serotonin in the striatum.

Mild increases in tonic dopamine release – as a consequence of the administration of both methylphenidate and amphetamine – could have important impact on subsequent phasic release by feedback mechanisms (lowering the concentration).

As pointed out before there are some major differences between the striatal and cortical dopamine terminals (Table 1).

Therefore, dopamine transporter inhibitors exhibit less effect in the FC. There, dopamine seems to be reuptaken by the norepinephrine transporter, which dopamine actually has a higher affinity for than norepinephrine itself.

Amphetamine administration produces a marked increase in cortical dopamine, norepinephrine and serotonin release that is impulse-independent. Methylphenidate can produce significant increases in dopamine and norepinephrine release (Table 2).

Dopaminergic mechanisms within the ventral striatum (i.e., nucleus accumbens) subserve the ability of amphetamine and methylphenidate in low to moderate doses to increase locomotor activity. In contrast, very low dosages in animals seem to cause hypoactivity presumably by stimulation of autoreceptors, a finding that would be compatible with the clinical impression that methylphenidate might be useful in some patients with mania.

At low doses, both psychostimulants could theoretically stimulate tonic, extracellular levels of

Tab. 2 Influence of the psychostimulants amphetamine, cocaine and methylphenidate on the different biogene amines.

	Amphetamine	Cocaine	Methyl–phenidate
Dopamine	++	++	++
Norepi-nephrine	++	++	+
Serotonin	+	++	(+)

monoamines, and the small increase in steady state levels would produce feedback inhibition of further release by stimulating presynaptic autoreceptors. While this mechanism is clearly an important one for the normal regulation of monoamine neurotransmission, there is no direct evidence to support the notion that the doses used clinically to treat ADHD are low enough to have primarily presynaptic effects. However, alterations in phasic dopamine release could produce net reductions in dopamine release under putatively altered tonic dopaminergic conditions that might occur in ADHD and that might explain the beneficial effects of methylphenidate in ADHD.

Repeated intermittent exposure to psychomotor stimulants can produce sensitisation, where subsequent drug exposures produce increased behavioural and neurochemical responses. The ability of the drug and ultimately of related stimuli to elicit behaviour may be increased with repeated administration or intake of the drug. Dopaminergic sensitization within the amygdala has also been found after repeated exposure to amphetamine and this can enhance appetitive and aversive learning even after drug cessation.

Besides the dopaminergic system, the noradrenergic nucleus, locus coeruleus (LC) may be another structure involved in the mode of action of psychostimulants. Electrophysiological recordings from this area demonstrate a relationship between behavior and response of the LC to targets versus distractors in an attention task. Baseline firing shows a constant increase paralleling the conditions from drowsiness to hyperarousal. In contrast, phasic responses are maximal in an optimal alert attentive state and minimal in drowsiness as well as hyperarousal that may be associated with poor cognitive performance due to high distractability.

Finally, the cerebellum has recently become a focus of interest in the context of the pathophysiology of ADHD and as a possible target for psychostimulants since it is not only important for motor coordination but also for processing cognitive situations.

P

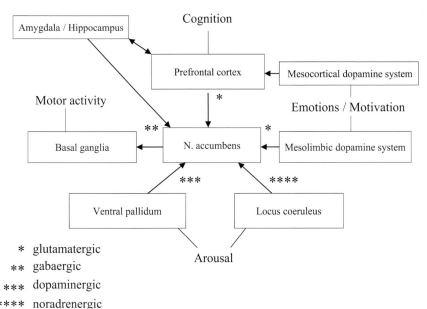

* glutamatergic
** gabaergic
*** dopaminergic
**** noradrenergic

Fig. 1 Nucleus accumbens as a major intersection of cognitive, motor and arousal processes.

Tab. 3 Acute effects of psychostimulants and the brain regions that are mainly involved in these effects.

Acute effects	Mainly involved brain region
Locomotion	Ventral striatum (i.e. nucleus accumbens)
Motor stereotypy	Dorsal striatum (i.e. caudate putamen)
Reinforcement	Ventral striatum
Conditioned reward	Ventral striatum / amygdala
Stimulus-reward learning	Amygdala

In summary, main structures involved in the action of psychostimulants can be divided into cortical (mainly prefrontal cortex) and subcortical (basal ganglia and related structures, LC and cerebellum) ones. Fig. 1 gives a schematic overview of the connections between these structures, omitting the cerebellum due to lack of precise information.

Modafinil

The mode of action of modafinil, a new arousal-promoting compound used in the treatment of sleepiness associated with narcolepsy, is not fully understood. It has been suggested that modafinil increases wakefulness by activating α_1 noradrenergic receptors or hypothalamic cells that contain the peptide ▸ hypocretin (3), or that it may act by modulating the GABAergic tone that might lead to an increased dopamine release in the nucleus accumbens. On the other hand, modafinil does not have any effect in DAT knockout mice.

Nicotine

Nicotine is the main psychoactive ingredient of tobacco and is responsible for the stimulant effects and abuse/addiction that may result form tobacco use. Cigarette smoking rapidly (in about 3 sec!) delivers pulses of nicotine into the bloodstream. Its initial effects are caused by its activation of ▸ nicotinic acetylcholine (nACh) receptors. nACh receptors are ligand-gated ion-channels and pre- and postsynaptically located. Reinforcement depends on an intact mesolimbic dopamine system (VTA). nACh receptors on VTA dopamine neurons are normally activated by cholinergic innervation from the laterodorsal tegmental nucleus or the pedunculopontine nucleus.

Clinical Use

The main indication for certain psychostimulants is ADHD in children and adults (4). Recent research shows that the clinical effect and benefit are dramatic even in adults. About 60% of adult patients receiving stimulant medication showed moderate-to-marked improvement, as compared with 10% of those receiving placebo. The core symptoms of hyperactivity, inattention, mood lability, temper, disorganization, stress sensitivity, and impulsivity have been shown to respond to treatment with stimulant medications.

The characteristic behavioural effects of acute and chronic psychomotor stimulant drugs are locomotor activation, stereotypy, and conditioned reward and stimulus-reward learning. The most important brain regions involved in these effects are summarized in Table 3.

Each of these processes depends upon increases in dopaminergic transmission within the striatum, and possibly, amygdala. Moreover, neurochemical actions within the FC may contribute to the ability to modulate some of these basic motivational processes. This data is based primarily on studies in rodents given systemic injections of moderate to high doses of stimulants, and it is not known whether lower doses applied orally would produce similar behavioural and neurochemical effects. Nevertheless, when given acutely or chronically to animals, psychomotor stimulants appear to alter the neurochemistry of the striatum in such a way as to augment the control of behaviour by conditioned or unconditioned stimuli associated with reinforcement processes. These effects may be consistent with the suggestion that amphetamine or methylphenidate may exert some of their beneficial clinical effects by augmenting conditioned reinforcement and stimulus-reward associations that could enhance aspects of task performance.

A simple decrease in striatal dopamine transmission produced by even low clinical doses of the drugs according to current data seems an untenable hypothesis. However, if the tonic control of

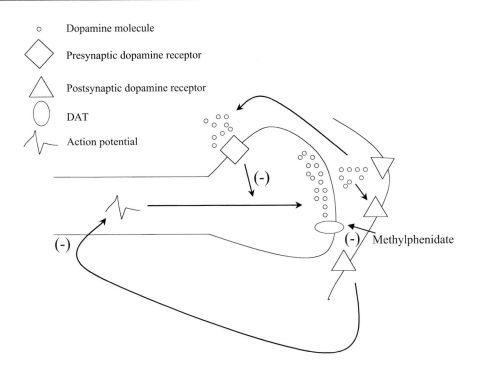

Fig. 2 Dopamine molecules have two different possible targets. Both ways are initially increased by DAT inhibition caused by methylphenidate: pre- and postsynaptic dopamine receptors. Stimulation of postsynaptic receptors results in inhibition of presynaptic action potential generation. On the other hand, presynaptic receptor stimulation leads to a transmission inhibition of action potentials. Therefore, both mechanisms are responsible for a decrease in vesicular depletion of dopamine into the synaptic cleft (adapted from 2).

phasic release by dopamine is abnormally low in ADHD, then a high phasic dopamine response may be associated with ADHD and treatment efficacy. Moreover, alterations in corticolimbic tonic/phasic balance may also provide an explanation of why chronically administered psychostimulants in ADHD produce a behavioural profile and response associated with subcortical dopamine neuronal hyperactivity and cortical hypoactivity, though issues of dose and route of administration should be considered in this context.

Another theory for the action of stimulant drugs in ADHD involves effects on nonstriatal monoamine systems. Frontal cortical dopamine, norepinephrine and serotonin are clearly important in cognitive functioning and impulse control. These neurotransmitters directly modulate reward-related behaviors associated with the striatal dopamine system. Moreover, the amygdala may be pharmacologically influenced leading to

enhanced associative learning and recall. Thus, the net behavioural effects of psychomotor stimulant drugs may promote changes in reward-motivated behaviors and impulsivity, as well as neuromodulation of inhibitory control (FC), working memory and incentive learning (amygdala).

Dysfunction of cortical-subcortical dopamine systems are associated with an impaired inhibitory control after chronic drug administration.

Since there is some evidence that the dopaminergic system might also play an important role in the pathophysiology of depression, methylphenidate has also been successfully used as an augmentation strategy in the treatment of depressive disorders. Modafinil might be useful in this indication, too, besides its effect in narcolepsy and ADHD (5).

Fig. 2 (adapted from 2) illustrates the acute and chronic actions of methylphenidate. By blocking DAT, methylphenidate causes an accumulation of dopamine in the synaptic cleft. Although this may initially increase the stimulation of postsynaptic DA receptors, in the long term the consequence is rather a down-regulation of dopamine release. First, there is feedback inhibition of dopamine neuron firing to decreased spike-dependent dopamine release. Second, much larger quantities of dopamine are enabled to escape from the cleft and accumulate in the extrasynaptic space. Presynaptic receptors are stimulated and thus firing rate is reduced. The amount of phasic dopamine that can be released is subsequently diminished.

Moreover, no significant differences could be found between the efficacy of methylphenidate and amphetamine. Methylphenidate is faster metabolized and seems to be associated with fewer side effects regarding appetite loss and insomnia. From a clinical point of view, dosage and route of administration are the most important features influencing the spectrum of effects and side effects.

An important clinical clue connected with the difference between tonic and phasic dopamine release is the so-called "rate dependence" of psychostimulant action. That means, it depends on the actual dopaminergic state (tonic and phasic) how an individual will react to psychostimulants. Fig. 3 illustrates this rule by some examples (adapted from 2). The arrows represent the response of each component to methylphenidate for each of the classes of subjects tested, with the horizontal dashed line representing the baseline tonic and phasic levels present in control individuals. Summarizing, methylphenidate tends to normalize dopamine transmission regardless what the baseline rate is.

Despite their clinical use, psychostimulants are strongly reinforcing, and their long-term use is linked to potential abuse and addiction, especially when they are rapidly administered. Nevertheless, long-term use is rather associated with emotional and motivational than with physical dependence. This is also true for cocaine and amphetamine. Methylphenidate might also be abused, although it is far less potent, possibly due to its specific mode of action (see above).

Nicotine differs from cocaine in that it is powerfully reinforcing in the absence of subjective euphoria. The high incidence of cancerinogenicity associated with long-term tobacco use is asso-

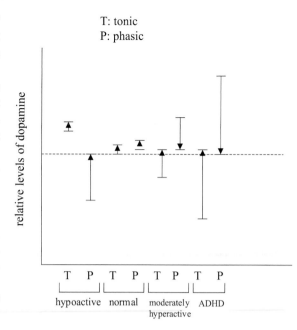

Fig. 3 **Effect of methylphenidate depending on baseline tonic (T) and phasic (P) dopamine levels.** In a "normal" state only minimal changes are noted (which points to a rather low abuse potential). From a "hypoactive" state, methylphenidate increases both T and P levels. However, this is much more true for the strongly lowered P tone. In contrast, in moderately hyperactive states and ADHD, T levels are increased and P levels are decreased, respectively, correlating with the baseline levels (adapted from 2).

ciated with compounds other than nicotine that are also contained in tobacco. Main short-term effects of nicotine are increased alertness, muscle relaxation, nausea and increased psychomotor activation. Typical withdrawal symptoms include dysphoria, increased appetite, hyperventilation and concentration difficulties.

References

1. Taylor JR, Jentsch JD (2001) Stimulant effects on striatal and cortical dopamine systems involved in reward-related behavior and impulsivity. In: Stimulant Drugs and ADHD, Solanto MV, Arnsten AFT, Castellanos FX, Oxford University Press, pp.104–133
2. Grace AA (2001) Psychostimulant actions on dopamine and limbic system function: relevance to

the pathophysiology and treatment of ADHD. In: Stimulant Drugs and ADHD, Solanto MV, Arnsten AFT, Castellanos FX, Oxford University Press, pp.134–157

3. Scammell TE, Estabrooke IV, McCarthy MT, Chemelli RM, Yanagisawa M, Miller MS, Saper CB (2000) Hypothalamic arousal regions are activated during modafinil-induced wakefulness. J Neuroscience 20:8620–8628

4. Wender PH, Wolf LE, Wasserstein J (2001) Adults with ADHD. An overview. Ann N Y Acad Sci. 931:1–16

5. Menza MA, Kaufmann KR, Castellanos A (2000) Modafinil augmentation of antidepressant treatment in depression. J Clin Psychiatry 61:378–381

Psychotomimetic Drugs

G.K. AGHAJANIAN
Yale School of Medicine, New Haven, USA
george.aghajanian@yale.edu

Synonyms

Hallucinogenic, psychotogenic

Definition

Psychto*mimetic* drugs can be defined as chemical agents that reliably and dose-dependently induce a psychosis, often including hallucinations and delusions in normal individuals. Implicit in this term is a *mimicking* of naturally occurring psychosis.

▶ Psychostimulants

Mechanism of Action

There are remarkable qualitative differences in the types of psychoses induced by different classes of psychotomimetic drugs. Some drugs cause such profound deficits in cognitive functioning that the resulting psychosis is associated with gross disorientation and confusion; a state sometimes called "dementia" or "organic psychosis". A psychotomimetic effect of this kind is seen, for example, after high doses of atropine or scopolamine, drugs which block muscarinic cholinergic receptors. Drugs of this type serve to mimic or model Alzheimer's disease and other severe brain disorders. There are other types of drugs that produce hallucinations and delusions without marked disorientation or confusion. Examples are ▶ psychedelic hallucinogens such as lysergic acid diethylamide (LSD) and mescaline and, in low doses, the ▶ dissociative anesthetics phencyclidine (PCP) and ketamine. This essay will focus upon the psychedelic hallucinogens and dissociative anesthetics, which are of special interest because they are believed to model some important features of ▶ schizophrenia (1, 2).

For many years it was believed that the brain mechanisms underlying the effects of psychedelic hallucinogens and dissociative anesthetics were separate and distinct. Indeed, there has been considerable debate about which represents the best drug model of schizophrenia. However, recent data shows that the two classes of psychotomimetic drugs share a common final pathway involving an increase in the release of the excitatory neurotransmitter ▶ glutamate.

Mechanism of Action of Psychedelic Hallucinogens

In the early 1950s, not long after the discovery of the powerful hallucinogenic properties of LSD, it was proposed that this drug interacted with a structurally related endogenous brain substance named ▶ serotonin. As seen in Fig. 1, LSD and serotonin (5-hydroxytryptamine; 5-HT) share an indolethylamine moiety, as do certain simpler indoleamine hallucinogens such as psilocin. On the other hand, the hallucinogen mescaline, despite having psychological or behavioral effects virtually identical to LSD, has a phenethylamine- rather than indoleamine-based structure. Nevertheless, mescaline does share certain other structural features with LSD (Fig. 1), consistent with the hypotheses that these two drugs have a common site of action. In the mid-1980s it was shown that the hallucinogenic potency of indoleamine and phenethylamine hallucinogens could be predicted by their affinity for a subtype of serotonin receptor, the 5-HT_{2A} receptor (3). The recognition of an association between hallucinogens and the 5-HT_{2A} receptor has formed the foundation for contemporary research in the field. Presently there is much

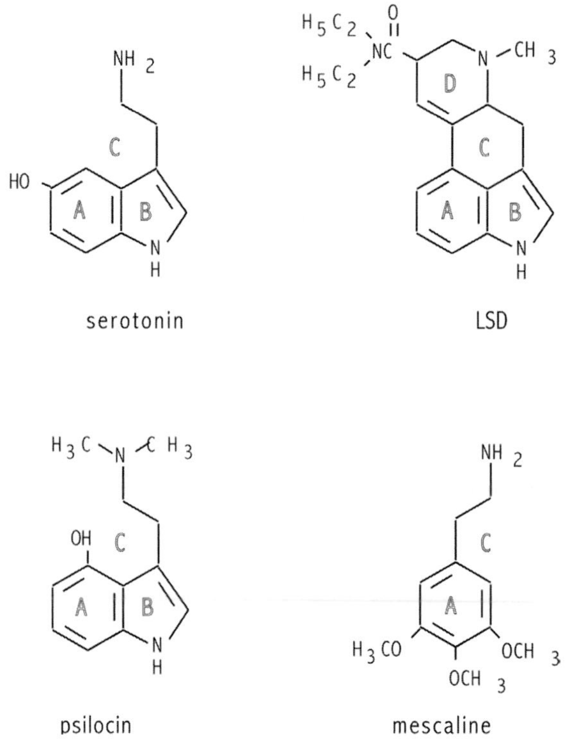

Fig. 1 Chemical structures of serotonin (5-hydroxytrptamine; 5-HT), the ergoline hallucinogen LSD (lysergic acid diethylamide), the simple indoleamine hallucinogen psilocin, and the phenethylamine hallucinogen mescaline. The letters A–D denote the four rings of LSD which are shared in varying aspects by the other hallucinogens as well as serotonin.

evidence from biochemical, electrophysiological, and animal as well as human behavioral studies that the effects of hallucinogens are mediated through a partial agonist action at 5-HT$_2$ receptors, particularly of the 5-HT$_{2A}$ subtype (4).

The effects of hallucinogens on an array of complex integrative processes such as cognition, perception and mood suggest the involvement of the cerebral cortex. In support of this idea, histochemical mapping by receptor autoradiography, mRNA *in situ* hybridization, and immunocytochemistry, shows a high expression of 5-HT$_{2A}$ receptors in the cerebral cortex, particularly within the apical dendrites of cortical ▶ pyramidal cells. At an electron microscopic level, an association has been observed between 5-HT$_{2A}$ immuno-

reactivity and the postsynaptic density of excitatory synapses in the neocortex.

The high density of 5-HT$_{2A}$ receptors in the cerebral cortex has stimulated study of the physiological role of this receptor in that region of brain (4). A striking effect of serotonin in the cerebral cortex is to increase the release of ▶ glutamate onto layer V ▶ pyramidal cells of neocortex, as measured by electrophysiological recording of "spontaneous" excitatory postsynaptic potentials (▶ EPSPs). *In vitro* studies in brain slices show that EPSPs are induced by serotonin through a focal action at the apical dendrites of pyramidal cells. This effect is blocked by low concentrations of highly selective 5-HT$_{2A}$ antagonists and is virtually absent in mice where there has been a genetic deletion of the 5-HT$_{2A}$ receptor. While a serotonin-induced increase in ▶ EPSPs occurs throughout the neocortex, this effect is most pronounced in frontal areas such as the medial prefrontal cortex where there is an increased density of 5-HT$_{2A}$ receptors as compared to more posterior regions. It has been postulated that the effect of serotonin is mediated indirectly by a ▶ retrograde messenger since 5-HT$_{2A}$ receptors have a predominantly postsynaptic localization. Recently, it has been found that LSD and other hallucinogenic drugs, while having relatively low efficacy in inducing spontaneous ▶ EPSPs, dramatically increase the probability of occurrence of a late component of EPSPs evoked by electrical stimulation of the subcortical white matter. In contrast, serotonin itself usually does not promote the late component of electrically-evoked EPSPs, probably due to opposing actions at 5-HT$_1$ or other non-5-HT$_{2A}$ receptors. It has been proposed that excessive induction of late EPSPs may underlie the disruptive effects of hallucinogens upon cortical function. The opposition by non-5-HT$_{2A}$ receptors of this effect may explain why treatments that elevate endogenous serotonin (e.g., monoamine oxidase inhibitors or selective serotonin uptake blockers) are not hallucinogenic and may in fact attenuate the subjective effects of hallucinogens in humans.

Mechanism of Action of Dissociative Anesthetics

The most commonly used (or abused) drugs in this category are the structurally-related drugs, PCP and ketamine (Fig. 2). At high doses these

phencyclidine   ketamine

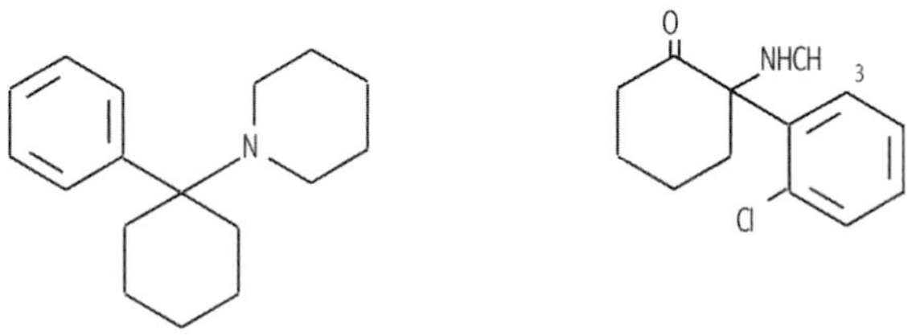

Fig. 2 Chemical structures of the dissociative anesthetics phencyclidine (PCP) and ketamine. Both are arylcycloalkylamine derivatives that are open channel blockers of the NMDA channel.

drugs produce a delerium-like state as seen in stage I anesthesia. Lower, subanesthetic doses are capable of producing a psychotomimetic state in normal subjects that stops short of frank delirium. Both PCP and ketamine are known to act as non-competitive antagonists of the ▶ NMDA receptor; a subtype of ionotropic ▶ glutamate receptor (5). The NMDA receptor belongs to the general class of ligand-gated non-selective cation channels and is distinguished within this group by its high permeability for calcium in addition to sodium and potassium ions. Because of it high calcium permeability, the NMDA receptor has been linked to various intracellular calcium signalling pathways. Another notable characteristic of NMDA receptor channels is blockade by magnesium ions under resting or hyperpolarized conditions, a block that is relieved under excitatory, depolarizing conditions. As suggested by the non-competitive nature of the blockade, these drugs do not act directly at the glutamate ligand-binding site, but rather interact with a separate site within the pore of the open channel, hence their designation as "open channel" blockers. While other actions also have been described, it is generally believed that the primary mechanism by which PCP and ketamine produce their adverse behavioral effects is through blockade of NMDA receptors. The net effect of these drugs has sometimes been thought of in terms of a general impairment of glutamatergic transmission. However, it should be noted that these drugs do not block non-NMDA glutamate receptors, including other ionotropic glutamate receptors (i.e., AMPA and kainate) and

all three major groups of metabotropic glutamate receptors. Recently, it has been shown that many of the effects of NMDA antagonists may be mediated through increased release of glutamate in prefrontal cortex and other regions, causing excessive activation of non-NMDA receptors. Suppression of excessive glutamate release ameliorates many of the resulting adverse behavioral effects. The mechanism by which NMDA antagonists increase glutamate release appears to be distinct from that of 5-HT_{2A} agonists since local application of phencyclidine to brain slices, in contrast to local serotonin application, does not result in an increase in EPSCs in layer V pyramidal cells of prefrontal cortex.

Conclusions

This essay has highlighted both differences and similarities in the mechanism of action of the psychedelic hallucinogens and ▶ dissociative anesthetics. The initial sites at which these two classes of psychotomimetics act are quite different: the psychedelic hallucinogens acting via 5-HT_{2A} receptors and dissociative anesthetics through blockade of NMDA receptors. However, recent evidence reveals intriguing common features downstream from the initial receptors. Most notably, both hallucinogens and dissociative anesthetics indirectly produce an enhancement of glutamate release in the cerebral cortex. However, it would not be expected that the effects of the two classes of drugs would be identical since in the case of the psychedelic hallucinogens, NMDA receptors are not be blocked. Blockade of NMDA receptors may account for the progressive disorientation or delirium seen clinically with near-anesthetic doses of the phencyclidine/ketamine class of drugs, effects that are not characteristic of the psychedelic hallucinogens. Nevertheless, evidence for an increase in glutamate transmission for both psychedelic hallucinogens and dissociative anesthetics points to a convergence upon a final common glutamatergic pathway to account for overlapping aspects of their psychotomimetic effects.

P

References

1. Abi-Saab WM, D'Souza DC, Moghaddam B, Krystal, JH (1998) The NMDA antagonist model for schizophrenia: promise and pitfalls. Pharmacopsychiatry (Supplement) 31:104–109
2. Gouzoulis-Mayfrank E, Hermle L, Thelen B, Sass H (1998) History, rationale and potential human experimental hallucinogenic drug research in psychiatry. Pharmacopsychiatry (Supplement) 31:63–68
3. Glennon RA (1990) Do classical hallucinogens act as 5-HT2 agonists or antagonists. Neuropsychopharmacology 3:509–517
4. Aghajanian GK, Marek GJ (1999) Serotonin and hallucinogens. Neuropsychopharmacology 21:16S–23S
5. Javitt DC, Zukin SR (1991) Recent advances in the phencyclidine model of schizophrenia. Am. J Psychiat. 148(10):1301–1308

PT

▶ Prothrombin Time

PTB Domain

▶ Phosphotyrosine-binding (PTB) Domain

PTEN

PTEN is a phosphatase, which is a product of a tumor suppressor gene. This phosphatase has a unusually broad specificity and can remove phosphate groups attached to serine, threonine and tyrosine residues. It is believed that its ability to dephosphorylate phosphatidylinositol (PI) 3,4,5-triphosphate, the product of PI-3 kinase, is responsible for its tumor suppressor effects.

▶ Phosphatases
▶ Phospholipid Kinases
▶ Phospholipid Phosphatases

PTM

▶ Post-translational Modification

P-type ATPase

▶ Table appendix: Membrane Transport Proteins

Pulmonary Hypertension

Primary pulmonary hypertension is a disease of unclear etiology that is characterized by abnormally high mean pulmonary arterial pressures, in the absence of a demonstrable cause. A wide variety of pulmonary and cardiac diseases can lead to secondary pulmonary hypertension.

Purinergic System

GEOFFREY BURNSTOCK
Autonomic Neuroscience Institute, Royal Free & University College Medical School, London, UK
g.burnstock@ucl.ac.uk

Definition

The purinergic system is a signalling system where the purine nucleotides, ▶ ATP and ADP, and the nucleoside, ▶ adenosine, act as extracellular messengers. This concept, which was first proposed over 30 years ago[1], met with considerable resistance for many years because ATP had been established as an intracellular energy source involved in various metabolic cycles, and it was thought that such a ubiquitous molecule was unlikely to be involved in selective extracellular signalling. However, ATP was one of the first molecules to appear in biological evolution so that it is not really surprising that it should have been utilized early for

Tab. 1 Characteristics of purine-mediated receptors (from 5).

Receptor		Main Distribution	Agonists	Antagonists	Transduction Mechanisms
P1 (adenosine)	A_1	Brain, spinal cord, testis, heart, autonomic nerve terminals	CCPA, CPA	DPCPX, CPX, XAC	G_i (1–3) $\downarrow$cAMP
	A_{2A}	Brain, heart, lungs, spleen	CGS 21680	KF17837, SCH58251	G_S $\uparrow$cAMP
	A_{2B}	Large intestine, bladder	NECA	Enprofylline	G_S $\uparrow$cAMP
	A_3	Lung, liver, brain, testis, heart	DB-MECA, DBX MR	MRS1222, L-268, 605	G_i (2,3) $G_{q/11}$ $\downarrow$cAMP $\uparrow$IP$_3$
P2X	$P2X_1$	Smooth muscle, platelets, cerebellum, dorsal horn spinal neurones	$\alpha\beta$meATP = ATP = 2meSATP (rapid desensitization)	TNP-ATP, IP$_5$I, NF023	Intrinsic cation channel (Ca^{2+} and Na^+)
	$P2X_2$	Smooth muscle, CNS, retina, chromaffin cells, autonomic and sensory ganglia	ATP $\geq$ ATPγS $\geq$ 2mSATP >> $\alpha\beta$meATP (pH + zinc sensitive)	Suramin, PPADS	Intrinsic ion channel (especially Ca^{2+})
	$P2X_3$	Sensory neurones, NTS, some sympathetic neurones	2mSATP $\geq$ ATP $\geq$ $\alpha\beta$meATP (rapid desensitization)	TNP-ATP, suramin, PPADS	Intrinsic cation channel
	$P2X_4$	CNS, Testis, colon	ATP >> $\alpha\beta$meATP		Intrinsic ion channel (especially Ca^{2+})
	$P2X_5$	Proliferating cells in skin, gut, bladder, thymus, spinal cord	ATP >> $\alpha\beta$meATP	Suramin, PPADS	Intrinsic ion channel
	$P2X_6$	CNS, motor neurones in spinal cord	(does not function as homomultimer)		Intrinsic ion channel
	$P2X_7$	Apoptotic cells in immune cells, pancreas, skin etc.	BzATP > ATP $\geq$ 2meSATP >> $\alpha\beta$meATP	KN62, KN04 Coomassie brilliant blue	Intrinsic cation channel and a large pore with prolonged activation
P2Y	$P2Y_1$	Epithelial and endothelial cells, platelets, immune cells, osteoclasts	2meSADP > 2meSATP = ADP > ATP	MRS2279, MRS2179	G_q/G_{11}; PLCβ activation
	$P2Y_2$	Immune cells, epithelial and endothelial cells, kidney tubules, osteoblasts	UTP = ATP	Suramin	G_q/G_{11} and possibly G_i; PLCβ activation
	$P2Y_4$	Endothelial cells	UTP $\geq$ ATP	RB2, PPADS	G_q/G_{11} and possibly G_i; PLCβ activation
	$P2Y_6$	Some epithelial cells, placenta, T-cells, thymus	UDP > UTP >> ATP	RB2, PPADS, suramin	G_q/G_{11}; PLCβ activation
	$P2Y_{11}$	Spleen, intestine, granulocytes	ARC67085MX>BzATP$\geq$ATPγS>ATP	Suramin, RB2	G_q/G_{11} and G_S; PLCβ activation
	$P2Y_{12}$	Platelets	ADP	ARC67085MX, ARC6993lMX	G_i (2); inhibition of adenylate cyclase

extracellular, as well as intracellular, purposes. The existence of potent extracellular enzymes that regulate the amount of ATP and adenosine available for signalling also provides support that ATP has extracellular actions.

Basic Characteristics

Purinoceptor Subtypes

Implicit in purinergic signalling is the presence of receptors for ATP[2]. A basis for distinguishing adenosine receptors (P1) from ATP/ADP receptors (P2) was proposed in 1978. This helped resolve some of the earlier ambiguous reports, which were complicated by the breakdown of ATP to adenosine by ectoenzymes so that some of the actions of ATP were directly on P2 receptors while others were due to indirect action via P1 receptors. Four subtypes of P1 receptors have been cloned, namely, A_1, A_{2A}, A_{2B} and A_3. P2 receptors belong to two families based on molecular structure and second messenger systems, namely P2X ionotropic ligand-gated ion channel receptors and P2Y metabo-

tropic G protein-coupled receptors. This framework allows for a logical expansion, as new receptors are identified. There are currently seven subtypes of P2X receptors and six subtypes of P2Y receptors identified and characterised in mammals (Table 1). P2X receptors are characterized by two transmembrane domains, short intracellular N- and C-termini and an extensive extracellular loop with conservation of 10 cysteines (Fig. 1a). Broadly, $P2X_1$ receptors are strongly represented in smooth muscle, $P2X_2$, $P2X_4$ and $P2X_6$ receptors in the central nervous system, $P2X_3$ receptors on sensory neurones, $P2X_5$ receptors associated with cell proliferation and differentiation and $P2X_7$ receptors with cell death. The ion pores appear to consist of three subunits forming homomultimers or heteromultimers, including $P2X_{1/5}$, $P2X_{2/3}$, $P2X_{2/6}$ and $P2X_{4/6}$. P2Y receptors, in common with other protein-coupled receptors, have seven transmembrane domains, an extracellular N, and intracellular C-terminus (Fig. 1b; ▶ G-protein-coupled Receptors). $P2Y_1$ receptors are ADP-selective in

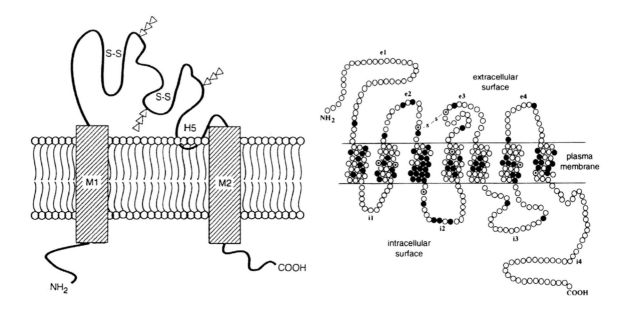

Fig. 1 a. Diagram depicting the transmembrane topology for P2X receptor protein showing both N- and C- terminals in the cytoplasm. Two putative membrane spanning segments (M1 and M2) traverse the lipid bilayer of the plasma membrane and are connected by a hydrophilic segment of 270 amino acids. This putative extracellular domain is shown containing two disulphide-bonded loops (S-S) and three N-linked glycosyl chains (triangles). **b. Schematic diagram of the sequence of the $P2Y_1$ receptor showing its differences from $P2Y_2$ and $P2Y_3$ receptors.** Filled circles represent amino acid residues that are conserved among the three receptors (from 1).

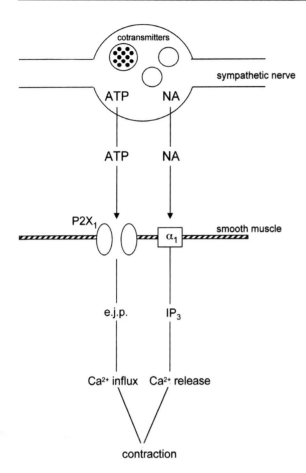

Fig. 2 Cotransmission in sympathetic nerves. ATP and noradrenaline (NA) from terminal varicosities of sympathetic nerves can be released together. With NA acting via the postjuctional α1-adrenoceptor to release cytosolic Ca^{2+} and ATP acting via $P2X_1$-gated ion channel to elicit Ca^{2+} influx, both contribute to the subsequent response (contraction). IP3, inositol triphosphate; e.j.p., excitatory junction potential (from 1).

Physiology

Short-term Neuronal Signalling. There was early evidence that ATP was a ► neurotransmitter in nonadrenergic, noncholinergic (NANC) nerves supplying the gut and bladder. There is now supporting evidence that ATP is a cotransmitter in many nerve types[1], probably reflecting the primitive nature of purinergic signalling. Thus, there is now evidence for ATP as a cotransmitter with:

► noradrenaline and neuropeptide Y in sympathetic nerves.
► ATP with acetylcholine and vasoactive intestinal peptide in some parasympathetic nerves.
► ATP with nitric oxide and vasoactive intestinal peptide in enteric NANC inhibitory nerves.
► ATP with calcitonin gene-related peptide and substance P in sensory-motor nerves.

There is also evidence for ATP as a cotransmitter with γ-aminobutyric acid in retinal nerves and/or ATP with glutamate, serotonin or dopamine in nerves in the brain.

In sympathetically innervated tissues, such as vas deferens or blood vessels, ATP produces fast responses mediated by P2X receptors followed by a slower component mediated by G protein-coupled α-adrenoceptors (Fig. 2); neuropeptide Y usually acts as a pre- or postjunctional modulator of the release and/or action of noradrenaline and ATP. Similarly, for parasympathetic nerves supplying the urinary bladder, ATP provokes a fast, short-lasting twitch response via P2X receptors, whereas the slower component is mediated by G protein-coupled muscarinic receptors. In the gut, ATP released from NANC inhibitory nerves produces the fastest response, nitric oxide gives a less rapid response, and vasoactive intestinal peptide produces slow tonic relaxations. In all cases of ► cotransmission, there are considerable differences in the proportion of the cotransmitters in nerves supplying different regions of the gut or vasculature, in different developmental or pathophysiological conditions and between species.

The first clear evidence for nerve-nerve purinergic ► synaptic transmission was in 1992, when it was shown that excitatory postsynaptic potentials in the celiac ganglion and in the medial habenula in the brain were reversibly antagonized by suramin, a P2 receptor antagonist. Since then,

mammals, and 2-methylthioADP and MRS 2179 are selective agonists and antagonists, respectively. At $P2Y_2$ and $P2Y_4$ receptors in the rat, ATP and UTP are equipotent, but the two receptors can be distinguished with antagonists. $P2Y_6$ is UDP-selective. $P2Y_{11}$ is unusual in that there are two transduction pathways, adenylate cyclase as well as inositol trisphosphate, which is the second messenger system used by the majority of the P2Y receptors. The $P2Y_{12}$ receptor is found on platelets.

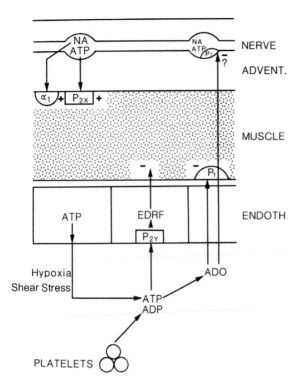

Fig. 3 A schematic representation of the interactions of ATP released from perivascular nerves and from the endothelium (ENDOTH). ATP is released from endothelial cells during hypoxia to act on endothelial P2Y receptors leading to production of EDRF (NO) and subsequent vasodilatation (-). In contrast, ATP released as a cotransmitter with noradrenaline (NA) from perivascular sympathetic nerves at the adventitia (ADVENT.)/muscle border produces vasoconstriction (+) via P2X receptors on the muscle cells. Adenosine (ADO) resulting from rapid breakdown of ATP by ecto-enzymes produces vasodilatation by direct action on the muscle via P1 receptors and acts on the perivascular nerve terminal varicosities to inhibit transmitter release (from 1).

there have been many articles describing either the distribution of various P2 receptor subtypes in the brain and spinal cord or electrophysiological studies of the effects of purines in brain slices, isolated nerves and glial cells. Synaptic transmission has also been found in the myenteric plexus and in various sensory, sympathetic and pelvic ganglia.

Short-term Non-neuronal Signalling. There are many examples of purinoceptor-mediated responses in non-neuronal cell types[3]. c Endothelial cells, which express P2Y₁, P2Y₂ and probably P2Y₄ receptors, when occupied, release nitric oxide leading to vasodilatation (Fig. 3). The more recent discovery of P2X receptors in endothelial cells suggests a role regulating gap and tight junctions involved in permeability and in cell adhesion. P2Y₁ receptors in pancreatic β-cells have been shown to be involved in insulin secretion, and P2Y₂ receptors are present on hepatocytes. P2Y₁₂, P2X₁ and P2Y₁ receptors are expressed in platelets and P2Y₁ and P2Y₂ receptors on non-myelinating and myelinating Schwann cells, respectively. Purinergic receptors are also involved in signalling to endocrine cells, leading to hormone secretion.

Long-term (trophic) Signalling. Purinergic signalling is also concerned with long-term events, such as cell proliferation, migration, differentiation and death associated with development and regeneration[1,3]. For example, αβ-meATP produces proliferation of glial cells, whereas adenosine inhibits proliferation. A P2Y₈ receptor was cloned from frog embryo that appears to be involved in the development of the neural plate. P2Y₁ receptors seem to have a role in cartilage development in limb buds and in development of the mesonephros. P2X₅ and P2X₆ receptors have been implicated in the development of chick skeletal muscle. In recent studies of purinoceptor expression in developing mouse myotubes, there was progressive expression of P2X₅, P2X₆ and P2X₂ receptors. The P2X₁ receptor is prominent in the contractile smooth muscle phenotype but is absent in the synthetic smooth muscle phenotype grown in culture, while P2Y receptor expression is substantially increased. There are several reports showing that P2X and P2Y receptors in ▶ osteoclasts and osteoblasts are involved in bone development and remodelling.

Pathophysiology and Therapeutic Potential

There is increasing interest in the therapeutic potential of purinergic compounds in relation to both P1 and P2 receptors[4]. A number of purine-related compounds have been patented.

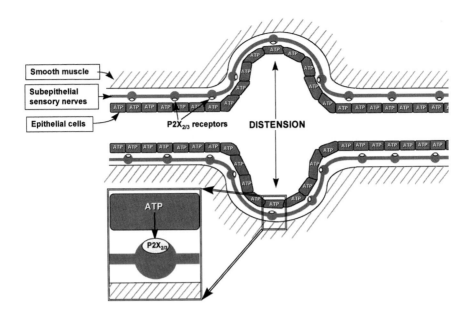

Fig. 4 Schematic representation of the hypothesis for purinergic mechanosensory transduction in tubes (e.g. ureter, vagina, salivary and bile duct and gut) and sacs (e.g. urinary and gall bladders, and lung). It is proposed that distension leads to release of ATP from the epithelium lining the tube or sac, which then acts on $P2X_{2/3}$ receptors on subepithelial sensory nerves to convey sensory (nociceptive) information to the CNS (from 5).

It is well established that the ▶ autonomic nervous system shows marked plasticity. The expression of cotransmitters and receptors shows dramatic changes during development and ageing, in nerves that remain after trauma or surgery and in disease conditions. There are now a number of examples where the purinergic component of cotransmission is increased in pathological conditions[4]. Purinergic nerve-mediated contractions of the human bladder are increased up to 40% in pathophysiological conditions such as interstitial cystitis, outflow obstruction and possibly also neurogenic bladder. ATP plays a significantly greater cotransmitter role in sympathetic nerves supplying hypertensive blood vessels. Upregulation of $P2X_1$ and $P2Y_2$ receptor mRNA in hearts of rats with congestive heart failure has been reported. Adenosine modulates long-term synaptic plasticity in the hippocampus; it attenuates long-term potentiation (LTP); P1 receptor antagonists facilitate LTP. It is suggested that adenosine-related compounds might prove helpful in the treatment of memory disorders and intellectual performance related to caffeine intake.

A new hypothesis for purinergic ▶ mechanosensory transduction in visceral organs involved in the initiation of pain has been proposed. It is suggested that distension of tubes (such as the ureter, salivary duct and gut) and sacs (such as urinary and gall bladder) leads to the release of ATP from the lining epithelial cells that diffuses to subepithelial sensory nerves with $P2X_3$ and/or $P2X_{2/3}$ nociceptive receptors, which mediate messages to pain centres in the central nervous system[5] (Fig. 4). Recording in $P2X_3$ knockout mice has shown that the micturition reflex is impaired and that responses of sensory fibres to $P2X_3$ agonists are gone, suggesting that $P2X_3$ receptors on sensory nerves in the bladder have a physiological as well as a nociceptive role.

P1 (adenosine) receptors were explored as therapeutic targets before P2 receptors. Adenosine was identified early and is in current use to treat ▶ supraventricular tachycardia. A_{2A} receptor antagonists are being investigated for the treatment of ▶ Parkinson's disease, and patents have been lodged for the application of P1 receptor subtype agonists and antagonists for myocardial

P

ischaemia and reperfusion injury, cerebral ischaemia, stroke, intermittent claudication and renal insufficiency.

Purinergic receptors have a strong presence in bone cells. P2X and P2Y receptors are present on osteoclasts, with P2Y receptors only present on osteoblasts. ATP, but not adenosine, stimulates the formation of osteoclasts and their resorptive actions *in vitro*, and can inhibit osteoblast-dependent bone formation. A recent study has shown that very low (nM) concentrations of ADP, acting through $P2Y_1$ receptors, turn on osteoclast activity. Modulation of P2 receptor function may have potential in the treatment of osteoporosis. The anticancer activity of adenine nucleotides was first described in 1983 and since then intraperitoneal injection of ATP into tumour-bearing mice has resulted in significant anticancer activity against several fast-growing aggressive carcinomas.

Purinergic signalling is important in the special senses. For example, $P2Y_2$ receptor activation increases salt, water and mucus secretion in the eye, and thus represents a potential treatment for dry eye disease. P2 receptor agonists have greater efficacy in reducing intraocular pressure than cholinergic and adrenergic agents, raising possibilities for novel treatment of glaucoma. It has been suggested that ATP may regulate fluid homeostasis, cochlear blood flow, hearing sensitivity and development, and thus may be useful in the treatment of Ménières disease, tinnitus and sensorineural deafness.

There have been very promising recent developments concerning purinergic drugs aimed at treating ▶ thrombosis. Clopidogrel and ticlopidine are antagonists to the $P2Y_{12}$ receptor and appear to reduce the risks of recurrent strokes and heart attacks, especially when combined with aspirin. Further therapeutic targets include: chronic renal failure, congestive heart failure, hypertension, stroke, angina, asthma, chronic obstructive pulmonary disease (COPD), epilepsy, sleep apnea, diabetes, inflammation, erectile function and wound healing.

References

1. Burnstock G (1997) The past, present and future of purine nucleotides as signalling molecules. Neuropharmacology 36:1127–1139
2. Ralevic V, Burnstock G (1998) Receptors for purines and pyrimidines. Pharmacol Rev. 50:413–492
3. Abbracchio MP, Williams M (eds) (2001) Purinergic and Pyrimidinergic Signalling, Handbook of Experimental Pharmacology, Vol. 151 (I/II) Springer, Berlin.
4. Abbracchio MP, Burnstock G (1998) Purinergic signalling: pathophysiological roles. Jpn J Pharmacol, 78:113–145
5. Burnstock, G. (2001) Purine-mediated signalling in pain and visceral perception. Trends Pharmacol. Sci. 22:182–188

Purinoceptor

A purinoceptor is a cell surface receptor for the purinergic nucleotides ATP and ADP and for the purine nucleotide, adenosine.

▶ Purinergic System

PXR

▶ Pregnane X Receptor
▶ Nuclear Receptor Regulation of Drug-metabolizing P450-Enzymes

Pyknosis

Pyknosis refers to a degenerative (thickening) process in a cell in which the nucleus shrinks in size and chromatin condenses to a solid mass that has no defined structure.

▶ Apoptosis

Pyramidal Cell

Pyramidal neurons are the principal long-projecting cells of the cerebral cortex and hippocampus. They are so named because of the characteristic large apical dendrite, giving them a pyramidal shape.

▶ Psychotomimetic Drugs

Pyrexia

▶ Fever

P

Q

QT Prolongation

The QT interval is measured in an electrocardiogram (ECG) between the onset of ventricular depolarisation (QRS) and the end of the repolarization process (T wave). The QT interval is rate-dependent and may be altered by numerous pathophysiologic and pharmacologic influences. The QT interval corrected for heart rate is termed QTc; its prolongation is known to be associated with various malignant tachy-arrhythmias and specifically ▶ torsades de pointes. Drugs which prolong the cardiac action potential, lead to a prolongation of the QTc interval on the electrocardiogram. This may for instance be the case for drugs, which delay cardiac repolarisation (e.g. class III antiarrhythmic drugs). In addition antibacterial agents, such as macrolides and quinolones, as well as drugs from other classes, have the potential to prolong the QTc interval. A slight prolongation does not represent a risk *per se*, but when these drugs are combined with other agents known to prolong the QT interval in at-risk patients possible untoward effects might occur.

▶ Antiarrhythmic Drugs
▶ Quinolones: Potent Inhibitors of Bacterial Topoisomerases

Quantitative PCR

Quantitative polymerase chain reaction, also called real-time RT-PCR or QPCR, is a method which employs insertion of a signal, such as fluorescence or enzyme activity, into PCR products generated by RT-PCR to determine the amount of messenger RNA (mRNA) in a tissue accurately.

▶ Gene Expression Analysis

Quinolinic Acid

▶ Kynurenine Pathway

Quinolones

RALF STAHLMANN
Institut für Klinische Pharmakologie und
Toxikologie, Freie Universität Berlin, Germany
ralf.stahlmann@medizin.fu-berlin.de

Definition

The term "quinolone antibacterials" describes a large group of drugs that are 4-quinolone derivatives with a carboxylic acid moiety in position 3 of the basic ring structure or 1,8-naphthyridone (8-aza-quinolone) derivatives. They are active against a broad spectrum of gram-negative and gram-positive pathogens. They exhibit their antibacterial action by inhibiting topoisomerase II (so-called ▶ gyrase) and topoisomerase IV, which are enzymes that control structure and function of bacterial DNA. ▶ Topoisomerases in eukaryotic, mammalian cells are not inhibited by quinolone antibacterial agents. Among the quinolones in clinical use today, four groups can be distinguished: those which inhibit gram-negative bacteria, but are not sufficiently active against pneumococci (groups I and II, e.g. ciprofloxacin), those which exhibit increased activity against a broad spectrum of bacteria, including pneumococci (group III, e.g. levofloxacin) and those which act against a broad spectrum with high anti-pneumococcal activity and are also active against some anaerobic bacteria (group IV, e.g. moxifloxacin and gatifloxacin). All of these compounds are fluorinated in position 6 of their basic heterocyclic structure and therefore are also termed "▶ fluoroquinolones". However, quinolones without 6-fluorination are under development (e.g. garenoxacin, PGE9262932) and thus the term "quinolones" seems to be more appropriate for the whole group of antibacterials. According to their differences in antibacterial activity and also their pharmacokinetic properties the indications differ for their clinical use. When used therapeutically, also their potential toxicities and possible adverse reactions have to be taken into account.

▶ β-lactam Antibiotics
▶ Microbial Resistance to Drugs
▶ Ribosomal Protein Synthesis Inhibitors

Mechanism of Action

The ▶ chromosomes of *Escherichia coli* and other bacteria are single, double-stranded DNA molecules with a total length of more than 1,000 µm. Relaxed DNA exists as a helical molecule, with one full turn of the helix occurring approximately every 10.4 base pairs. This molecule must undergo several folding and compaction steps to fit into an *E. coli* cell which is only 1 to 3 µm long. Despite this enormous compaction, bacterial DNA must be accessible for the bacterial enzymes that catalyze DNA replication and transcription into mRNA, the prerequisite for protein synthesis. These and other topological problems are solved by enzymes called

DNA topoisomerases. DNA gyrase (topoisomerase II) was the first quinolone target identified on the basis of genetic studies with *E. coli* mutants that were resistant against nalidixic acid (i.e. the first quinolone antimicrobial which is no longer in clinical use). DNA gyrase has a tetrameric A_2B_2 structure (Table 1); the two subunits of gyrase are encoded by the *gyrA* and *gyrB* genes. The enzyme is responsible for introducing negative ▶ supercoils into DNA - negatively supercoiled DNA contains slightly less than 1 helical turn per 10.4 base pairs. This is an ATP-dependent reaction that requires both strands of the DNA be cut to permit passage of a segment of DNA through the break; the cleavage is then resealed. Topoisomerase IV is a homologue of gyrase, which is encoded by the *parC* and *parE* genes. This enzyme catalyzes the unlinking of replicated daughter chromosomes, a process that is called decatenation. Both enzymes cause double strand breakage of DNA strands and are called "type II topoisomerases" in contrast to "type I topoisomerases" that catalyze single-stranded-DNA cleavage.

Quinolones inhibit bacterial DNA synthesis by their ability to bind to and to stabilize complexes of DNA and type II topoisomerases; there is strong evidence for a role of Mg^{2+} ions in this process. The enzymes break DNA and the quinolones prevent religation of the broken DNA strands. Inhibition of DNA synthesis by interaction with gyrase occurs rapidly, but inhibition due to interaction with topoisomerase IV occurs with some delay. This is thought to relate to differences in the localization of DNA gyrase and topoisomerase IV on the bacterial chromosome; gyrase works ahead of replication forks and topoisomerase IV is located behind replication forks. Differences exist with respect to the primary targets of quinolones in different bacteria. For *E. coli*, DNA gyrase is more sensitive to many quinolones than topoisomerase IV, but for the gram-positive pathogen *S. aureus* topoisomerase IV is the more sensitive of the two enzymes. The more sensitive enzyme usually represents the primary quinolone target for a given organism. Events in addition to interaction of the quinolone with its target enzyme DNA complex are necessary for the rapid bactericidal action of quinolones, but these events are poorly understood. Probably at least two different lethal modes of action exist, one that requires protein synthesis and one that does not.

Tab. 1 Quinolones – Classification of bacterial topoisomerases.

Topoisomerase	Type	Structure	Gene	Predominant function in cell
I	I	1 subunit		Relaxes negatively supercoiled DNA
II ("gyrase")	II	tetramer (2 GyrA; 2 GyrB subunits)	gyrA/gyrB	Introduces negative supercoils into DNA
III	I	1 subunit		Decatenation of replication intermediate
IV	II	tetramer (2 ParC; 2 ParE subunits)	parC/parE	Decatenation of linked daughter DNA molecules

Most of our knowledge about the targets of quinolone action is the result of extensive studies performed to understand (and possibly overcome) the phenomenon of bacterial ▶ resistance against quinolones, which represents an increasing problem with the use of these and other antimicrobial agents. In *E. coli* and other Gram-negative bacteria first step quinolone resistance mutations occur in *gyrA*, or less commonly, *gyrB*. In contrast, for many Gram-positive bacteria, as for *S. aureus*, first-step mutations occur in *parC*, less commonly *parE*. To avoid the development of double mutants, the quinolone should be active enough to destroy pathogens with reduced susceptiblity due to first step resistance. An optimal bactericidal effect requires the AUC/MIC ratio to be greater than 100, selection of resistant mutants is unlikely with a C_{max}/MIC ratio greater than 10.

Interestingly, rather slight modifications of the molecular structure of antibacterial quinolones can render them into substances that have the potential to inhibit mammalian topoisomerases. One of such compounds is CP-115,953 which is a more potent inhibitor for mammalian topoisomerases than etoposide, a drug that is used as a cytostatic agent in cancer patients. CP-115,953 and similar derivatives were not further developed for clinical use. Because any inhibition of mammalian topoisomerases is unwanted with drugs used for the treatment of bacterial infections, quinolones are tested at very early stages during their preclinical development as to whether they exhibit such a potential. However, these antineoplastic quinolones represent a potentially important source of new anticancer agents.

Clinical use

Besides the four most widely used fluoroquinolones (ciprofloxacin, levofloxacin, moxifloxacin and gatifloxacin) more than a dozen other derivatives of the same basic structure are available for clinical use. However, several shortcomings, such as relatively low antibacterial activity or poor pharmacokinetics, do not render them drugs of first choice. For example, enoxacin has a relatively low antibacterial activity and exhibits a pronounced potential for ▶ drug interactions by inhibition of CYP1A2 (theophylline metabolism). Another example is ofloxacin that represents a racemate consisting of equal parts of two substances (the R- and L-forms), but only one of these compounds – the L-form, also called levofloxacin – exhibits antibacterial activity. Thus, from a pharmacological point of view levofloxacin is the more rational choice than ofloxacin. The indications for the four most often used quinolones differ due to differences in their antimicrobial spectrum as well as their pharmacokinetics. Table 2 provides an overview of the indications of these drugs as licensed in Germany and many other countries. They are available for oral as well as for intravenous application (exception: the i.v. formulation of gatifloxacin is available in the USA, but not yet in Europe).

As with all drugs, the specific side effects of the quinolones must be considered when they are chosen for treatment of bacterial infections. Reactions of the gastrointestinal tract and the central nervous system are the most often observed adverse effects during therapy with quinolones. It should be underlined, however, that compared with many other antimicrobials, diarrhea is less

Q

Tab. 2 Quinolones

Indication	Ciprofloxacin	Levofloxacin	Moxifloxacin	Gatifloxacin
Uncomplicated UTI*	X	X		X
Complicated UTI	X	X		X
Gonorrhea	X	X		X
Community-acquired pneumonia		X	X	X
Acute exacerbation of chronic bronchitis		X	X	X
Sinusitis		X	X	X
Uncomplicated skin and skin structure infections	X	X	X	X
Pseudomonas infections	X			
Sepsis	X			

*UTI = urinary tract infection ("uncomplicated" = no obstruction)

frequently observed during quinolone treatment. Also, antibiotic-associated colitis has been observed only very rarely during quinolone therapy. Similarly, hypersensitivity reactions, as oberved during therapy with penicillins and other β-lactams, is more rarely caused by quinolones. Some other risks of quinolone therapy have been defined and must be considered if a drug from this class is chosen for treatment of bacterial infections.

Because quinolones can cause prolongation of the QTc-interval, they should not be used (i) in patients with inborn ▶ QT prolongation, (ii) in patients treated with other drugs that cause QT prolongation (e.g. antiarrhythmics), (iii) in patients with electrolyte disturbances, such as hypokaliemia or hypomagnesiemia or (iv) in patients with severe heart disease. Alterations of glucose homoestasis have been observed with quinolone use and strict glucose controls of diabetic patients are recommended, especially if they are treated with sulphonylurea agents. Damage of articular joint cartilage as well as the epiphyseal growth plate can be induced by quinolones in immature animals and these chondrotoxic effects have led to a restricted use of quinolones in pediatrics. Another manifestation of the connective tissue toxicity of quinolones is tendopathies.

▶ Tendinitis and tendon ruptures have occurred in rare cases as late as several months after treatment with quinolones.

A number of quinolones had to be taken off the market due to toxic effects on the liver, the heart or other organs, that became recognized only after marketing (e.g. temafloxacin, trovafloxacin, grepafloxacin). A risk for severe cardiotoxicity, hepatotoxicity or phototoxicity is not associated with the clinical use of those four quinolones (ciprofloxacin, levofloxacin, moxifloxacin, gatifloxacin) described as preferential quinolones in this chapter.

References

1. Gootz TD, Osheroff N (1993) Quinolones and eukaryotic topoisomerases. In: Quinolone Antimicrobial Agents. 2nd Edition. Hooper DC and Wolfson JS (eds). American Society for Microbiology, Washington, DC, pp139–160
2. Hooper DC (2001) Mechanism of action of antimicrobials: focus on fluoroquinolones. Clin Infect Dis 32 (Suppl 1) S9–S15
3. Hooper DC (2000) Quinolones. In: Mandell, Douglas, and Bennett's Principles and Practice of Infectious Diseases. Mandell GL, Bennett JE, Dolin R (eds). Churchill Livingstone, Philadelphia et al., pp404–423

4. Stahlmann R, Lode H (1999) Fluoroquinolones. In: Clinical Infectious Diseases: a Practical Approach. Root RK (ed). Oxford University, New York - Oxford, pp305–312

5. Stahlmann R, Lode H (2000) Safety Overview. Toxicity, adverse effects, and interactions. In: The Quinolones. 3rd Edition. Andriole V (ed). Academic Press, London, pp397–453

6. Wang JC (1996) DNA topoisomerases. Annu Rev Biochem 65:635–692

Q

R

Rab-GTPases

Rab proteins are a family of small GTPases related to ras. Rab proteins possess GTP-binding motifs, an effector loop that changes conformation concomitant with the GTP-GDP cycle and a C-terminal CXC or CC box that serves as attachment for the hydrophobic geranylgeranyl membrane anchors. Each intracellular membrane carries a specific set of Rab proteins. The GTP-GDP cycle of rab proteins is regulated by a complex network of protein-protein interactions. The GDP form of rabs is recognized by a soluble protein termed GDI (for GDP dissociation inhibitor). GDI dissociates GDP-rabs from the membrane and allows for rebinding, thus ensuring that rabs are not carried along the secretory pathway, which would result in a loss of membrane specificity.

Membrane-bound GTP rabs recruit effectors to the membrane. In neurons and neuroendocrine cells, the vesicle-associated Rab3 binds to rabphilin and to RIM. RIM is a component of the presynaptic cytomatrix and may thus serve as a docking receptor for synaptic vesicles at the active zone.

▶ Exocytosis
▶ Intracellular Transport
▶ Small GTPases

Radiocontrast Agents

ULRICH SPECK
Universitätsklinikum Charité,
Humboldt-Universität Berlin, Berlin, Germany
ulrich.speck@charite.de

Synonyms

X-ray contrast agents, contrast media, contrast materials

Definition

▶ Radiocontrast agents are compounds, compositions, or preparations aimed at modifying the X-ray absorption in a human or an animal undergoing an X-ray examination.

Although X-rays of suitable energy are able to penetrate the living organism without major scattering, thus providing a shadow image of their absorption by the body constituents, only the bones and gas-filled lungs are clearly visible. Soft tissues and liquid-filled cavities are too similar in X-ray absorption to be differentiated. X-ray contrast agents enhance the contrast between body cavities and soft tissues or between tissues of different quality, preferably between normal and diseased tissue.

Mechanism of Action

Basic physics
X-ray radiography relies on differences in the absorption of X-rays by the various body constituents. The absorption of X-rays depends in a com-

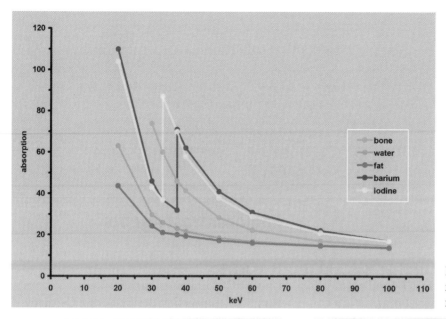

Fig. 1 Absorption of diagnostic X-rays by various materials and elements.

plex way on their energy (keV) and the atomic number of the absorbing materials (Fig. 1). X-rays used in diagnostic radiology range in energy from about 10–70 keV. They are produced by tube voltages of 20–140V. As a rule, elements with higher atomic numbers absorb X-rays more efficaciously than lighter elements. Furthermore, absorption depends on the amount of the material to be passed by the rays. Consequently, thick layers of dense material (e.g. large calcium-containing bones) absorb a greater proportion of X-rays than soft tissues consisting mainly of water (hydrogen and oxygen), protein, and fat (with carbon and nitrogen as the main additional elements). The X-ray absorption of different soft tissues is very similar. Only fat displays a somewhat lower absorption due to its low oxygen content and low density (g/ml).

Since, as a rule, contrast media cannot be administered in unlimited amounts or concentrations, they need to be very different in X-ray absorption from the usual body constituents in order to be effective. This can only be achieved by using heavy elements or introducing gas into body cavities normally filled with fluid. Iodine and barium are the preferred X-ray-absorbing elements in contrast agents. More recently, contrast media based on a lanthanide element (gadolinium) have

been introduced because of certain favorable features in their tolerance profile.

Radiographic techniques and sensitivity of detection
In projection radiography a certain part of the body is irradiated from one side (e.g. the chest) with a film or a screen behind the object to detect the radiation as it passes through the different structures within the body. Digital detectors allowing for quantification and various calculations based on the original data are gaining in importance. In the subtraction mode two images are obtained shortly after each other: the first one immediately before and the second one directly after contrast medium injection. The difference between the two images represents the distribution of the contrast medium without the interfering native contrast of the tissues and bones. In projection radiography the minimum amount of the radiation-absorbing element per square centimeter which may be detected is about 20 mg (this is very similar for iodine and barium and only slightly lower for elements such as gadolinium). The amount of 20 mg per square centimeter corresponds to a concentration of 20 mg per ml if a structure 1 cm thick in the direction of the rays is to be visualized or to 200 mg iodine/ml for a blood vessel with a diameter of 1 mm. Gas-filled structures may not be visible unless they are several

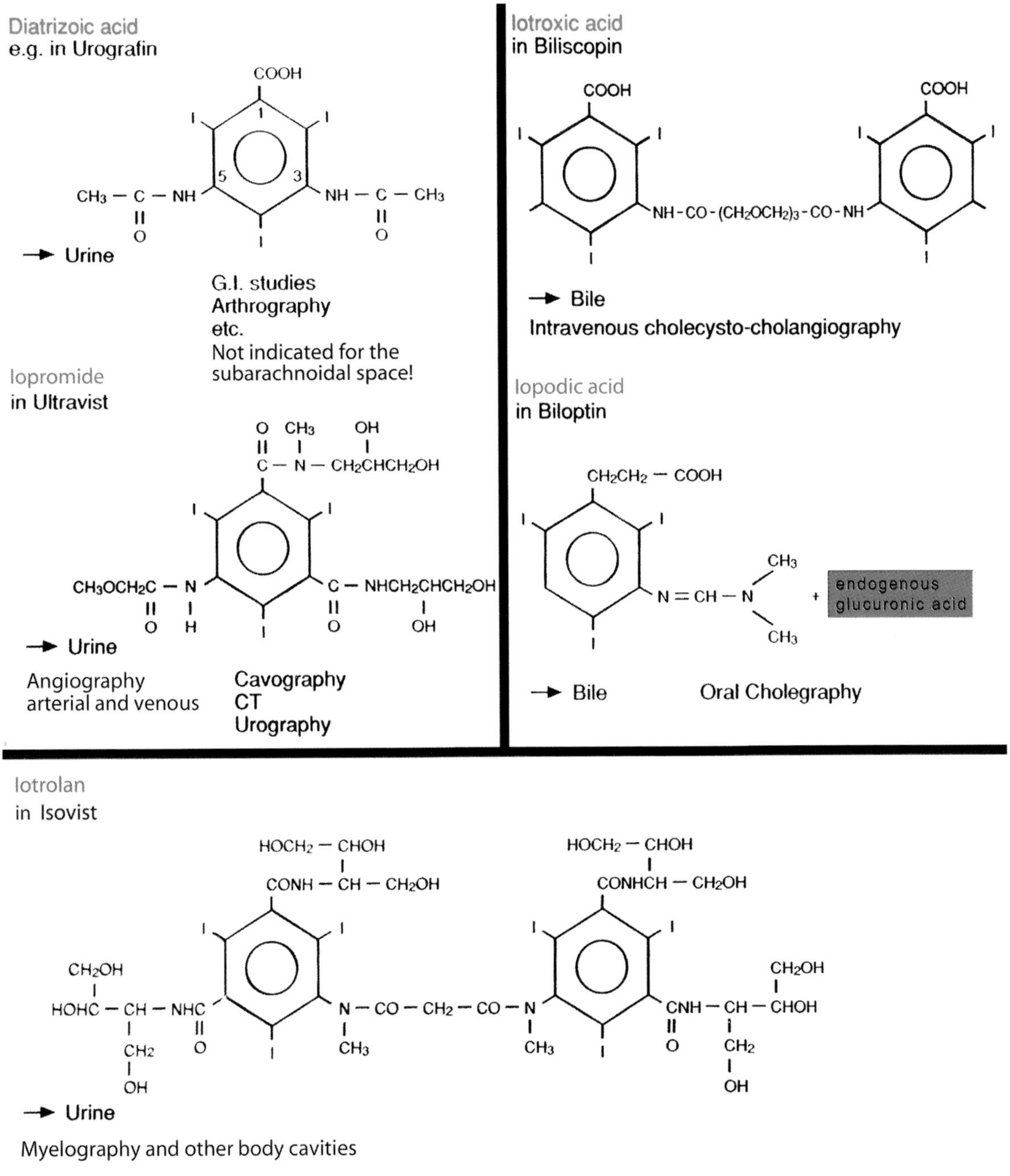
Diatrizoic acid
e.g. in Urografin
COOH
CH3 — C — NH
NH — C — CH3
→ Urine
G.I. studies
Arthrography
etc.
Not indicated for the
subarachnoidal space!
Iotroxic acid
in Biliscopin
COOH
COOH
NH-CO-(CH2OCH2)3-CO-NH
→ Bile
Intravenous cholecysto-cholangiography
Iopromide
in Ultravist
O CH3 OH
C — N — CH2CHCH2OH
CH3OCH2C — N
C — NHCH2CHCH2OH
→ Urine
Angiography
arterial and venous
Cavography
CT
Urography
Iopodic acid
in Biloptin
CH2CH2 — COOH
N = CH — N
CH3
CH3
endogenous
glucuronic acid
→ Bile
Oral Cholegraphy
Iotrolan
in Isovist
HOCH2 — CHOH
CONH — CH — CH2OH
HOCH2 — CHOH
CONHCH — CH2OH
CH2OH
HOHC — CH — NHC
N — CO — CH2 — CO — N
CNH — CH — CHOH
→ Urine
Myelography and other body cavities

Fig. 2 Chemical structure of common radiographic contrast media.

millimeters in size in the direction the X-rays are passing them.

In ▸ **computerized tomography** the radiation source as well as the detector circles around the subject collect quantitative data on the X-ray absorption of every line through the body from every direction. These data serve to calculate thin slices through the body.

The sensitivity of contrast detection is about 1 mg/ml or less for heavy elements such as iodine, barium, or gadolinium. Even small gas bubbles (less than 1 mm in diameter) are visible.

Doses of less than 1 g of the contrast-providing element may be necessary to visualize small body cavities following direct puncture and injection of the contrast agent. At the other end visualization of the whole gastrointestinal tract or of large blood vessels as well as tissue contrast enhancement in computerized tomography may require doses of more than 100 g of barium or iodine per patient.

Chemistry and pharmaceutical preparations

Iodinated contrast agents. The most frequently used X-ray contrast media are based on iodine as the heavy X-ray-absorbing element. Iodine has been selected because of its low toxicity and the capability of the organism to excrete free iodide but, most importantly, because it forms stable covalent bonds with organic molecules. The carriers of iodine have been optimized in terms of tolerance and pharmacokinetics. The currently used iodinated X-ray contrast media are almost exclusively derivatives of triiodobenzoic acid (Fig. 2). Originally, these were sodium or meglumine (an organic base somewhat similar to glucosamine) salts of the iodinated acids. Nowadays neutral (=non-ionic) molecules with a better safety profile are preferred for most conventional applications. The use of acidic molecules remains justified where the efficacy depends on a specific pharmacokinetic profile, requiring the accumulation of the molecules by an anion transport mechanism. An iodinated oil is the only contrast agent of some importance that is not a derivative of triiodobenzoic acid.

Water-soluble iodinated contrast agents are usually available as highly concentrated preparations containing up to 400 mg of organically bound iodine per ml, which is equivalent to about 800 mg of dry contrast material/ml. These solutions contain less than 0.7 ml of water/ml, resulting in a specific density of up to 1.4 g/ml or more. The osmolality and viscosity of these preparations are decisive criteria for practical application and tolerance. Viscosity should be as low as possible. The osmolality of modern products ranges between 300 and 1000 mosm/kg H_2O (blood and other body fluids: 300 mosm/kg H_2O).

Barium sulfate. Barium absorbs X-rays very well. The ion itself is rather toxic, and its excretion is extremely slow. Barium is used in the form of the largely insoluble sulfate.

Metal chelates. Heavy metal ions are effective absorbers of X-rays. However, their solubility at physiological pH, instability of covalent binding to organic molecules, inherent toxicity, and lack of excretion are significant drawbacks compared to iodide. Since the introduction of magnetic resonance imaging in medicine, stable chelates of paramagnetic ions have been developed which are surprisingly well tolerated at low doses. Their administration as radiocontrast agents is feasible if doses are limited in an appropriate way.

Gas. Because of its low density, gas of any composition is a weak absorber of X-rays compared to tissues and body fluids. Gas can serve as a contrast agent provided the contrast is sufficient for the diagnostic problem, the formation of different phases (layers) within the target location does not impair image quality, and the risk of embolism can be excluded. The preferred gas is carbon dioxide because of its almost immediate solubility in blood and, therefore, low risk of embolism.

Specificity
Whereas therapeutic agents may flood the whole organism and still exert specific effects on the heart, the pancreas, the central nervous system, or other targets, useful information provided by radiocontrast agents depends completely on their appropriate distribution within the field of view imaged during the X-ray examination. Several mechanisms have been found to be useful and suitable for routine clinical application:

▶ Direct filling of body cavities with contrast material through natural entrances or by percutaneous injection
▶ Injection of contrast agents into blood vessels and observation of their passage with the blood stream
▶ Renal or biliary excretion with opacification of the kidneys and the urinary and biliary tract
▶ Visualization of perfusion, capillary permeabili-

ty, and the proportion of the extracellular space of tissues.

The underlying pharmacokinetic principles are simple:

With the exception of the orally administered cholegraphic contrast media, all other compounds and preparations are practically not absorbed by the gastrointestinal tract, and they do not penetrate cell membranes (again with the exception of cholegraphic contrast media which enter the hepatocytes by a rate-limited active transport process). After intravascular injection, water-soluble iodinated contrast media (or metal chelates) just flow with the plasma, leave the capillaries where these are perforated, distribute within the extracellular space of the tissues, and diffuse back through the same pores through which they left the capillaries as the plasma level decreases due to excretion by glomerular filtration without undergoing biotransformation. If injected into body cavities, such as the subarachnoid space or synovial cavity or directly into solid tissue, they follow the bulk water flow to the general circulation, for example, through valve-like structures of spinal and arachnoid granulations or via the interstitial lymph. These contrast media are known as urographic or extracellular agents. Because they passively flow with the plasma or diffuse where pores allow them to pass membranes without interaction with active transport systems, specific-binding to receptors, transporters or enzymes, they are also called 'non-specific contrast media'.

They still provide very useful and often specific information, for example, on the shape of the lumen of a variety of organs, the perfusion of tissues (Fig. 3), the disruption of the blood-brain barrier at sites of inflammation in the central nervous system, the absence of the blood-brain barrier in tumours, or the increased interstitial space of diseased tissue. As markers of glomerular filtration they provide quantitative and spatially resolved information on renal function.

In contrast to ▶ urographic contrast agents, which serve many purposes, ▶ cholegraphic agents are solely applied in cases of known or suspected disease affecting the bile ducts or gall bladder. They have to meet three requirements regarding their molecular structure: A negative electrical charge (▶ ionic contrast media), a threshold

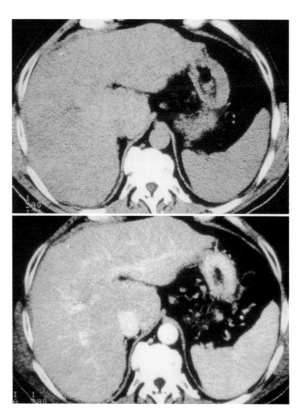

Fig. 3 Computed tomography of a patient before and after contrast agent administration.

molecular size and some lipophilicity. After oral ingestion (oral cholegraphic agents) or intravenous injection (i.v. cholegraphic agents), a large proportion of the iodinated molecules are reversibly bound to albumin, thus apparently increasing the molecular size beyond the limit of glomerular filtration. Uptake into hepatocytes and biliary excretion occur via the same anion transport mechanism which handles bilirubin glucuronide and many other acidic compounds. Therefore, elevated serum bilirubin reduces the efficacy of biliary contrast agents because of competitive inhibition of the transport system.

Clinical Use (Including Side Effects)

Indications, doses, concentrations, injection rates

Radiocontrast agents belong to several classes of products and are available for different clinical indications. Water-soluble iodinated non-ionic contrast agents are the most frequently used and

R

most versatile class of products. A few examples for indications are:

▶ Intravenous injection in computed tomography to visualize
  - blood vessels and cardiac cavities
  - perfusion of tissues/ischemia
  - tumours, inflammation, and other diseased tisues
  - the kidneys and the urinary tract.

▶ Doses range from about 1–2 ml/kg per injection; more than one injection per patient may be required. Doses should preferably be calculated in grams of iodine/kg body weight since it is possible in many cases to use higher volumes and injection rates rather than higher concentrations. Common concentrations are 300–370 mg of iodine/ml and injection rates of 1–5 ml/sec. Disruption of the blood-brain barrier, which may be caused by a tumour, can be detected with a similar effectiveness by infusion of less concentrated preparations.

▶ Angiography including selective opacification of arteries and veins for diagnostic or interventional radiologic or cardiologic procedures such as angioplasty and stent implantation, thrombolysis, embolization. In most cases injection is performed through catheters specially designed for the individual type of procedure. Depending on the size of the vessel and the type of imaging equipment (digital subtraction versus conventional), very different volumes (a few ml to about 80 ml), concentrations (150–400 mg iodine/ml), and injection rates (hand injection or automatic injector up to 20 ml/sec) are administered.

▶ Intravenous urography. Contrast agents are typically administered by fast intravenous injection of 50–10 ml of a preparation containing 300–37 mg iodine/ml.

▶ Contrast enhancement of open and closed body cavities for
  - gastrointestinal tract assessment
  - arthrography
  - myelography
  - endoscopic retrograde cholangiography.

Again, depending on the size of the cavity and the imaging modality (CT versus projection radiography), very different doses and concentrations may be used. In most cases slow administration is preferred.

Cholegraphic contrast media are far less important. Oral cholecystographic agents are administered 12 hours before the radiological examination to allow absorption, biliary excretion, and concentration in the gall bladder. Doses are low (about 2–4 g iodine). Intravenous agents require slow administration (infusion over 10 min or more) because of side effects and increased renal excretion in case of rapid injection. Doses are limited to about 5 g iodine. Due to rate-limited biliary excretion, higher doses do not improve contrast.

Carbon dioxide is used to visualize not only body cavities but also arteries below the diaphragm. It dissolves rapidly enough to avoid gas embolism. The absence of toxicity (no iodide, no hypersensitivity reactions, good renal tolerance) allows for its use in patients at high risk of reacting adversely to iodinated agents.

For the same reason, gadolinium chelates have been used in selected patients. However, there is as yet too little data to justify a general recommendation.

Barium sulfate may be used for gastrointestinal studies only. Patients at risk of gastrointestinal leaks must not receive barium sulfate because it may induce severe inflammatory reactions in the peritoneum and is not excreted. Doses are low in CT (up to about 10 g) but may reach several hundred grams for other applications.

Adverse events

Iodinated contrast agents contain or release traces of iodide sufficient to induce, in the worst case, a thyrotoxic crisis in patients prone to such a reaction.

Contrast media (even barium sulfate, most likely due to excipients or additives) may cause immediate or delayed hypersensitivity reactions. The incidence of minor reactions is in the range of several percent of the examinations. They include hot flushes, urticaria, nausea and vomiting, and slight cardiovascular reactions. More severe reactions such as bronchospasm with dyspnea and significant hypotension are rare (about 0.1%), the incidence of severe reactions requiring emergency resuscitation may be another order of magnitude lower. Fatal reactions occur but are too rare to give any relevant incidence even with the large number of contrast-enhanced procedures performed today. The main risk factors are previous reactions to contrast media, asthma and allergies in general but it is not possible to make a prediction for an individual patient. Prophylactic measures include administration of corticosteroids, the first dose at least 12 hours, a second dose two hours before contrast medium administration, and of H_1- and H_2-blockers.

High-dose intravascular contrast media may affect renal function; these effects are usually transient but may also become permanent. The risk is very low in patients with normal renal function and intravenous injection. It increases significantly with preexisting renal impairment, diabetes, dehydration, high dose of contrast agents, repeated examinations requiring contrast agents within a few days, and arterial injection. The only generally accepted prophylactic measure is hydration of the patients before and several hours after contrast agent injection.

In addition to the above-mentioned potential adverse events of contrast agents, there are procedure-related side effects, of which only a few are given:

Peripheral arteriography: local heat sensation and pain mainly due to the hypertonicity of certain contrast agents.

Cardioangiography: ECG disturbances such as bradycardia, negative but also positive inotropic effects.

Cerebral arteriography: neurologic deficits, in most cases transient.

Myelography: headache, neurologic deficits.

Gastrointestinal studies with barium sulfate: Barium sulfate may enter the lungs through aspiration or a leak in the peritoneal cavity causing severe, potentially fatal inflammatory reactions mixed with infections.

Overall, radiographic contrast media provide essential diagnostic information and cause few side effects. However, since severe reactions may reach a life-threatening grade, although very rarely, the administration of radiographic contrast media requires continuous attention.

References

1. Dawson P, Clauss W: Contrast media in practice. Questions and answers. 2nd Edition, Springer Berlin, Heidelberg, 1998.
2. Dawson P, Cosgrove DO, Grainger RG (eds.): Textbook of contrast media. Isis Medical Media, Oxford, 1999.
3. Speck U. (ed.): Contrast media. Overview, use and pharmaceutical aspects. 4th Edition, Springer Berlin, Heidelberg, 1999.

Radioiodine

The 131 isotope of iodine is used for treatment of thyroid disorders.[131]I-iodine is administered orally as a single dose. It is rapidly and completely absorbed and is accumulated in the thyroid gland *via* an active transport mechanism. Thereafter it is oxidized and organified by thyroid follicular cells. Its physiologic half life is 8 days. [131]I emits both beta and gamma radiation. The toxic effect on thyroid tissue is caused by the released beta particles, which have a path length of 1 to 2 mm. They destroy thyroid follicular cells. The additional fraction of gamma radiation is utilised for detection. When used for treatment of benign thyroid disorders (e.g. Graves' disease or thyroid autonomy), exposure of other organs is small. Infrequent side effects of radioiodine therapy are nausea, vomiting and anorexia. Although there is no established teratogenic risk, the use of radioiodine is contraindicated in pregnancy and breastfeeding women. It should be administered within 10 days of the onset of a menstrual period or after a negative pregnancy test and pregnancy should be avoided for 4 months after radioiodine treatment.

▶ Antithyroid Drugs

Radiomimetics

Radiomimetics are a class of agents that cause DNA damage of a similar quality to that resulting from exposure to ionising radiation.

▶ Cancer (molecular mechanisms of therapy)

R

Raf

Raf kinases such as Raf1 are serine/threonine-specific protein kinases which function in signal transduction pathways between the cell surface and the nucleus. It is a downstream target of the monomeric GTPase Ras.

▶ Phospholipid Kinases

Raphe Nuclei

Raphe nuclei are large clusters of cells in the pons and upper medulla, which lie close to the midline. These are the main serotonin-containing neurons in the central nervous system. The rostrally situated nuclei project to many parts of the cortex, hippocampus, basal ganglia, limbic system and hypothalamus. The caudally situated cells project to the cerebellum, medulla, and spinal cord.

Ras

▶ Small GTPases

Raynaud's Phenomenon

Raynaud's phenomenon is an exaggerated vascular response to cold temperature or emotional stress. Clinical symptoms are sharply demarcated color changes in the skin of the digits. The underlying disorder consists of abnormal vasoconstriction of digital arteries and cutaneous arterioles due to a local defect in normal vascular responses.

▶ Ca^{2+} Channel Blockers

Rb Gene

▶ Retinomablastoma (Rb) Gene

Reactive Oxygen Species

Reactive oxygen species are chemical species that possess an unpaired electron in the molecule such as the superoxide anion ($O_2 \cdot -$), hydroxyl radical ($\cdot OH$), and nitric oxide ($NO \cdot$), and peroxynitrite ($ONOO-$). They are very short-lived and can react with most molecules in their vicinity inducing inflammatory and growth-promoting actions.

▶ Apoptosis
▶ Renin-angiotensin-aldosteron System

Receptor Occupancy

Receptor occupancy refers to the ratio of receptors occupied by a ligand at equilibrium and the total number of receptors available, usually expressed as a percentage of the total number of receptors. Since it is often not possible to quantify the total number of receptors or the number of receptors occupied by a ligand, another parameter called binding potential is often used to measure receptor occupancy. Binding potential (BP) refers to the ratio of the maximum number of receptors and the equilibrium dissociation constant of the drug, so that % receptor occupancy equals to

$100 \times BP_{baseline} - BP_{post-treatment} / BP_{baseline}$.

Receptor Protein

▶ Table appendix: Receptor Proteins

Receptor Reserve

In terms of the relationship between ▶ receptor occupancy by an agonist and tissue response, if the maximal response to the agonist can be obtained with concentrations of agonist that do not occupy all of the receptors, then the system is said to have a receptor reserve. For example, if only 10% of the receptors need be occupied by a certain agonist to produce the system maximal response, then there is a 90% receptor reserve. Under these circumstances, 90% of the receptors could be irreversibly removed (i.e by an irreversible antagonist) and the agonist would still produce the maximal response. However, the dose-response curve to the agonist would be shifted to the right by the presence of the irreversible antagonist. It should be noted that receptor reserve is not a property of the system but rather that it varies with different agonist efficacies in different systems.

▶ Drug-receptor-interaction

Receptor Serine/Threonine Kinases

Receptor serine/threonine kinases function as hetero-oligomeric complexes, consisting of type I and type II serine/threonine kinase receptors. Ligand binding induces the oligomerization. Type II-receptors primarily bind the ligand and phosphorylate type I-receptors, which then specifically phosphorylate in turn receptor-regulated Smad-proteins (R-Smads). These then dimerize with Co-Smads in the cytosol. The R-Smad/Co-Smad complex then translocates to the nucleus where it binds to regulatory sequences in combination with specific transcription factors.

▶ Neurotrophic Factors
▶ SMADs
▶ Table appendix: Receptor Proteins

Receptor Subtype

Most hormones and neurotransmitters interact with more than one receptor subtype. The different receptor isoforms can differ in ligand binding and signal transduction pattern. This allows cell type- or tissue-specific targetting of drugs to receptor subtypes.

▶ Transmembrane Signalling

Receptor Tyrosine Kinase

Receptor tyrosine kinases (RTKs) are a family of membrane proteins which bind extracellular ligands like insulin and growth factors (e.g. platelet derived growth factor receptor, epidermal growth factor receptor). After binding of the ligand, the intracellular domain of the receptor catalyzes autophosphorylation and phosphorylation of specific substrates on tyrosine residues.

▶ Growth Factors
▶ Tyrosine Kinases
▶ Table appendix: Receptor Proteins

Receptors

Scientists in the nineteenth century realized that some chemicals produced effects at extremely low concentrations and that these effects could be modified by equally low concentrations of other chemicals with a strict adherence to chemical structural guidelines. Thus, they proposed that 'receptors' with strict recognition properties for these chemicals existed in biological systems. While receptors technically can be any biological entity such as enzymes, reuptake recognition sites and genetic material such as DNA, the term is usually associated with proteins on the cell surface that transmit information from chemicals to cells. The most therapeutically relevant receptor class are G Protein Coupled Receptors (GPCR's) presently comprising 45% of existing therapies.

► G Protein Coupled Receptors
► Transmembrane Signalling

Rectification

In many channels the relation between current and membrane potential is nonlinear. These channels show rectification i.e. the property of the channel to conduct ions more readily in one direction than in the other. Depending on the preferential current flow through channels, these are described as outward or inward rectifying.

► Inward Rectifying K^+ Channels
► Ionotropic Glutamate Receptors

Reelin

Reelin is an extracellular matrix protein, which is secreted by neuronal cells and binds to two lipoprotein receptors (VLDLR and ApoER2) that relay the reelin signal inside target neurons by docking with the tyrosine kinase adapter disabled-1 (Dab1). This allows neurons to complete migration and adopt their ultimate positions in laminar structures in the central nervous system. In addition, the integrins alpha 3/beta 1 and protocadherins of the CNR family may also modulate the reelin signal.

► Cadherins/Catenins

Reentrant Arrhythmia

Reentrant arrhythmia occurs when due to inhomogeneous repolarization or unidirectional block, heart tissue which is no longer refractory is close beside tissue which is still activated. This

may result in a circuit propagation of activation serving as a reverberator.

► Antiarrhythmic Drugs

Regulators of G-protein Signalling

Regulators of G-protein signalling (RGS) are a group of G-proteins which are able to act as GTP-activating proteins (GAPs) for heterotrimeric G-proteins. They are thus able to limit the signal generated by G-protein coupled receptors (GPCRs). RGS-proteins are a large family of structurally diverse proteins, which in addition to an RGS-domain carry variable sequence motifs, which are responsible for additional specific interactions.

► G-proteins
► Transmembrane Signalling

Regulatory Regions

Regulatory regions are transcriptional control sequences which consist of promoters, response elements, enhancers and possibly silencers located upstream of the start site of transcription. The overall effect on gene ttanscription is a sum of the contributions of these elements and the activities of proteins recruited to these sites. Promoters are located immediatedly upstream of the strat site and initiate transcription. They often contain tissue- or cell-specific elements if the gene is not ubiquitously expressed. Enhancers are positive regulatory elements which function independently of orientation and distance from the genes they regulate.

► Glucocorticoids

Reinstatement

The reinstatement model is the first choice for the measurement of craving and relapse behaviour. In this paradigm, animals are trained to self-administer a drug and are then subjected to extinction - that is, they are tested under conditions of non-reinforcement until operant responding appears to be extinguished. When the animals reach some criterion of unresponsiveness, various stimuli are presented. A stimulus is said to reinstate drug-seeking behaviour if it causes renewed responding, e.g. lever pressing, without any further response-contingent drug reward. At least three conditions can reinstate responding, drug priming i.e. the injection of a small dose of the drug, stress or conditioned stimuli.

▶ Drug Addiction/Dependence

Relative Potency

The affinity of a drug is the ability of that drug to bind to the receptor. The efficacy of an agonist is its ability to activate (or inactivate in the case of an ▶ inverse agonist) the receptor. The relative potency of an agonist (with respect to another agonist at the same receptor) is therefore determined by both its affinity and efficacy and only gives an indication of the relative concentrations at which they produce a particular response.

▶ G-Protein-coupled Receptors
▶ Histaminergic System
▶ Transmemebrane Signalling

Relaxin

Relaxin and its relative relaxin-like factor (RLF/INSL3) belong structurally to a group of peptide hormones, that includes insulin and insulin-like growth factor 1 (IGF1). Relaxin regulates the growth and remodeling of reproductive tissues during late pregnancy. It promotes expansion of the birth canal during parturition. In humans, the peak in circulating relaxin occurs during the first trimester. Relaxin is secreted by the ovary during pregnancy as well as by many other tissues. It may act as a vasoactive hormone, which has dilatory effects on blood vessels. The closely related relaxin-like factor is synthesized by Leydig cells in the fetal testis and appears to be responsible for the second phase of testicular descend by influencing the growth and differentiation of the cords, which connect the testes with the lower abdomen. The effects of relaxin and relaxin-like factors are mediated at least in part by G-protein coupled receptors (LGR7 and LGR8, which are coupled to G_s).

REM Sleep

REM is the abbreviation for rapid eye movement sleep. REM sleep is a sleep phase characterized by rapid eye movements, muscular atony and an activated electroencephalogram (EEG).

Renin

R

Renin is a proteolytic enzyme that is secreted into the circulation by cells of the juxtaglomerular apparatus, which lies in the afferent arteriole of the glomerula in the kidney. Renin release is stimulated by sympathetic activity, decreased renal perfusion pressure or a fall in the sodium concentration of the fluid in the distal tubules, which, in the form of the macula densa, are in close contact with the juxtaglomerular apparatus. Renin is cleared rapidly from plasma. It acts on angiotensinogen, from the N-terminus of which it splits off a decapeptide, angiotensin I. Angiotensin I, which has no major activity, can be converted by the angiotensin-converting enzyme (ACE) to an octapeptide, angiotensin II, which is a potent vasoconstrictor.

▸ Renin-angiotensin-aldosterone System

Renin-Angiotensin-Aldosterone System

MICHAEL BADER
Max Delbrück Center for Molecular Medicine (MDC), Berlin-Buch, Germany
mbader@mdc-berlin.de

Synonyms

RAAS, Renin-angiotensin system (RAS)

Definition

The renin-angiotensin-aldosterone system (RAAS) generates the peptide hormone angiotensin II and subsequently the mineralocorticoid aldosterone which both exert considerable impact on blood pressure (▸ Blood Pressure Control) and fluid homeostasis and have prime etiologic and therapeutic significance for cardiovascular diseases.

▸ ACE Inhibitors
▸ Blood Pressure Control

Basic Characteristics

General

Renin is a circulating enzyme formed in specialized smooth muscle cells in the kidney that cleaves its only, liver-born substrate, angiotensinogen, in the plasma to form the inactive decapeptide angiotensin I. Angiotensin I is then metabolized further into the octapeptide angiotensin II via the endothelium-bound angiotensin converting enzyme (ACE). Angiotensin II elicits an increase in blood volume and blood pressure by stimulating vasoconstriction, sodium retention, thirst, the sympathetic nervous system and aldosterone secretion from the adrenal gland. Aldosterone is a steroid hormone that binds to the mineralocorticoid receptor and amplifies the sodium-retaining effect. Physiologically this makes sense, since the RAAS is activated under conditions of acute volume loss by the induction of the rate-limiting enzyme renin. Major renin-inducing stimuli include a fall in renal perfusion pressure, a decrease in salt content in the distal tubule sensed and transmitted via the ▸ macula densa, an increase in the renal sympathetic tone, and a reduction in angiotensin II concentration employing a negative feedback mechanism. In addition to their haemodynamic actions, angiotensin II and aldosterone also induce growth- and fibrosis-related processes in several organs, such as vessels, heart and kidney.

To elicit these effects, angiotensin II binds to two main receptors, AT1 and AT2, which both belong to the ▸ G-protein-coupled receptor family. Most of the abovementioned effects of angiotensin II are however, mediated by the AT1 receptor, while the physiological function of the AT2 receptor is enigmatic. In most studied cases, the AT2 receptor counteracts the AT1 effects by exerting growth-inhibiting and vasodilatating actions partly by the stimulation of kinin generation.

Angiotensin II binding to the AT1 receptor stimulates via the G-protein, G_q, the activity of phospholipase C to generate the second messengers inositole phosphate (IP3) and diacylglycerol, and inhibits via G_i the activity of adenylyl cyclase to reduce the synthesis of cyclic AMP. Diacyglycerol activates protein kinase C and can be converted to arachidonic acid and ▸ eicosanoids. Furthermore, angiotensin II induces the generation of ▸ reactive oxygen species by the stimulation of membrane-bound NAD(P)H oxidase. One of the immediate consequences of these early signals is activation of tyrosine kinases that include PYK2, c-Src, JAK2, platelet-derived growth factor (PDGF) receptor and the epidermal growth factor (EGF) receptor, as well as of the serine/threonine kinases, ERK, Akt/protein kinase B and S6 kinase, and subsequent induction of ▸ immediate early genes and protein synthesis.

Besides the plasma renin-angiotensin system (RAS), intrinsic tissue RAS exist. Angiotensin II is generated not only in the circulation but also locally in organs from precursors and enzymes either locally synthesized or imported from the

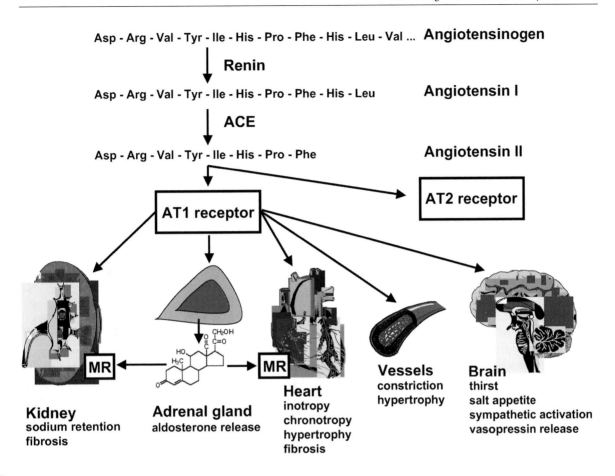

Fig. 1 The renin-angiotensin-aldosterone system. Angiotensin II is generated in a two-step enzymatic process from the liver-born protein angiotensinogen by the kidney-derived enzyme renin and the endothelium-bound angiotensin-converting enzyme (ACE). The octapeptide interacts with two receptors, AT1 and AT2. The AT1 receptor confers most of the known actions of angiotensin II such as the liberation of aldosterone from the adrenal gland. Aldosterone via the mineralocorticoid receptor (MR) and angiotensin II together induce sodium retention in the kidney and fibrotic processes in kidney and heart. Moreover, angiotensin II elicits constriction of vessels, has positive inotropic and chronotropic actions on the heart, promotes growth in vessels and heart, and induces thirst, salt appetite, vasopressin release, and the activation of the sympathetic nervous system in the brain. Some of these effects are also mediated by locally produced angiotensin II in the respective tissues.

plasma. These systems are autonomously regulated and have physiological functions inside the respective organs. Local RAS have been described for organs involved in cardiovascular control such as kidney, vessels, heart, adrenal gland and brain.

Adrenal Gland. In the ▸ zona glomerulosa of the adrenal gland, renin is locally synthesized and together with angiotensinogen and ACE generates angiotensin II, which acts as paracrine or intracrine hormone on adrenocortical cells. Circulating,

as well as this locally produced angiotensin II, stimulates aldosterone release by increasing the expression of aldosterone synthase, the rate-limiting enzyme of aldosterone synthesis.

Kidney. The kidney contains the major site of renin synthesis, the juxtaglomerular cells in the wall of the afferent arteriole. From these cells, renin is secreted not only into the circulation but also into the renal interstitium. Moreover, the enzyme is produced albeit in low amounts by proximal tubular cells. These cells also synthesize angiotensinogen and ACE. The RAS proteins interact in the renal interstitium and in the proximal tubular lumen to synthesize angiotensin II. In the proximal tubule, angiotensin II activates the sodium/hydrogen exchanger (NHE) that increases sodium reabsorption. Aldosterone elicits the same effect in the distal tubule by activating epithelial sodium channels (ENaC) and the sodium-potassium-ATPase. Thereby, it also induces water reabsorption and potassium secretion.

In the interstitium, angiotensin II induces proliferation of mesangial cells and fibroblasts and the synthesis of collagen and other matrix molecules by these cells via the AT1 receptor. Moreover, by the concomitant stimulation of chemoattractant ▶ cytokines, inflammation is induced. These processes are mediated by endothelin, ▶ transforming growth factorβ and reactive oxygen species and finally lead to interstitial fibrosis and glomerulosclerosis observed in hypertension and diabetes.

Heart and Vessels. In heart and vessels, angiotensin II is generated mostly by renin and angiotensinogen imported from the plasma and locally synthesized ACE. Additionally in the human heart, mast cells contain the enzyme chymase that also metabolizes angiotensin I to angiotensin II. The physiological relevance of this enzyme is controversial. Circulating as well as locally generated angiotensin II, induce vasoconstriction and exert direct inotropic and chronotropic actions on the heart. These effects are enhanced by a facilitation of noradrenaline release from sympathetic nerve endings.

Alike in the kidney, angiotensin II also in the heart induces inflammation and fibrosis by increasing endothelin, transforming growth factor β, reactive oxygen species and pro-inflammatory cytokines. Furthermore, angiotensin II induces hypertrophy of cardiomyocytes and smooth muscle cells in the heart and vessels, respectively, partially employing the same mediators. This is aggravated by increased circulating aldosterone levels that also elicit fibrotic processes in the heart by a yet unresolved mechanism.

Brain. Circulating angiotensin II can only reach the ▶ circumventricular organs of the brain, which express AT1 receptors and lack a blood-brain barrier normally limiting the access of peptides to brain receptor sites. However, areas beyond the blood-brain barrier have been shown to be responsive to angiotensin II and to express AT1 receptors. These sites are affected by locally synthesized peptide from renin, angiotensinogen and ACE present in the central nervous system. Possibly, also other enzymes may be involved in angiotensin II generation in the brain, e.g., cathepsins. Circulating and locally synthesized angiotensin II induces thirst, salt appetite, and ▶ vasopressin release, stimulates the sympathetic nervous system and moderates the ▶ baroreceptor reflex, and thereby increases blood volume and blood pressure.

Drugs

ACE inhibitors

Pharmacological intervention in RAS began in the late 1960s with the discovery that the venome of the brazilian snake *Bothrops jararaca* contains a substance that inhibits ACE. In first clinical trials this substance proved to be a potent antihypertensive agent but it had the disadvantage that it could only be taken by injection. By modelling the active site of ACE and designing drugs potentially binding to this site, the first orally available ACE inhibitor was discovered, captopril. In the meantime, at least a dozen -prils have been developed and marketed; captopril, enalapril, lisinopril, perindopril, cilazapril, benazepril, quinapril, fosinopril, ramipril, moexipril and trandolapril. ACE inhibitors are first choice antihypertensive drugs. Furthermore, a multitude of large scale clinical studies have proven a strong beneficial effect of these drugs on morbidity and mortality in congestive heart failure, e.g. after myocardial infarction, and chronic renal diseases, e.g. caused by diabetes or hypertension. In the heart, ACE inhibitors exert their beneficial actions by reducing preload and afterload and inhibiting myocardial fibrosis and remodelling processes. In the kidney, a reduction in glomerular pressure as well as antifibrotic and antiinflammatory actions contribute to the efficiency of the drugs.

ACE not only activates angiotensin but is also involved in the metabolism of other peptides, e.g., it is a major kinin-degrading enzyme. Therefore,

ACE inhibitors also increase kinin concentrations. Furthermore, it has recently been shown that these drugs potentiate kinin effects by modulating a direct interaction between the ACE protein and the kinin B2 receptor, which is independent from the enzymatic activity of ACE. Kinin potentiation may be involved in the beneficial action of ACE inhibition since ▶ kinins are known to exert cardio- and renoprotective actions. However, it is also the major reason for the adverse side effects of ACE inhibitors, namely cough and angio-oedema. Another observed side-effect, first-dose orthostatic hypotension, is probably due to both angiotensin inhibition and kinin potentiation.

Since angiotensin II is important for kidney development in mammals, ACE inhibitors and other drugs interfering with RAS should not be given during pregnancy.

AT1 antagonists

A second, newly developed group of drugs interfering with RAS are specific antagonists for the AT1 receptor. The first example of this class was losartan, which was followed by at least 5 other - sartans (telmisartan, candesartan, valsartan, eprosartan, irbesartan). These drugs exert a more complete angiotensin blockade, since alternative pathways of angiotensin generation not affected by ACE inhibitors and employing cathepsins or chymase become ineffective by AT1 antagonism. They are also more specific for RAS than ACE inhibitors since other peptide systems should not be affected. However, the compensatory increase in renin concentration after AT1 blockade leads to an accumulation of angiotensin II, which activates the AT2 receptor. It is yet unknown whether this AT2 stimulation often followed by kinin generation is involved in the action of AT1 antagonists.

In first clinical trials, AT1 antagonists have proven to be as effective in hypertension, congestive heart failure and renal failure as ACE inhibitors. However, large scale trials comparing both classes of drugs have to be awaited. If equipotency can be confirmed the favourable side-effect profile of AT1 antagonists would argue for a greater use of these drugs. At present, they are indicated in patients who do not tolerate ACE inhibitor treatment.

Renin Inhibitors

The most logical point to interfere pharmacologically with RAS would be the rate-limiting enzyme renin. Intervention at this step is expected to be more specific than ACE inhibition and AT1 antagonism since hardly any angiotensin peptide could be generated and no other peptide system would be directly affected. Therefore, fewer compensatory and unwanted effects would be expected, and thus renin inhibitors should be safe drugs. Nevertheless, the development of renin inhibitors has been stopped by most companies and only remikiren has been used for some clinical trials. Several reasons may be responsible for this: First, since the human renin protein is different from the rodent enzymes and only interacts with primate or human angiotensinogen, the testing of such drugs can not be performed in classical animal models. Second, the first renin inhibitors were difficult to synthesize and exhibited a low bioavailability. Third, it would be difficult to market a third class of drugs interfering with RAS, when the existing drugs are quite effective and safe.

Vasopeptidase Inhibitors

(▶ Vasopeptidase Inhibitors)A new class of drugs has been developed that inhibits ACE and neutral endopeptidase 24.11 (NEP). NEP degrades vasodilatory peptides such as kinins, ▶ natriuretic peptides, and adremomedullin, and, therefore, its inhibition should complement the vasodilatory action of ACE inhibition. Since ACE and NEP are very similar in structure it was possible to develop inhibitors with dual specificity for both enzymes such as omapatrilat, sampatrilat, and gemopatrilat. In first clinical trials, the -patrilats have proven to be even more effective than ACE inhibitors in blood pressure reduction and in improving congestive heart failure. Nevertheless, large trials are needed to confirm these encouraging results and have to assess safety issues, which may be more problematic because of the diversity of substrates metabolized by NEP.

Aldosterone Antagonists

ACE inhibitors do not completely block aldosterone synthesis. Since this steroid hormone is a potent inducer of fibrosis in the heart, specific antagonists, such as spironolactone and eplerenone, have recently been very successfully used in clinical trials in addition to ACE inhibitors to treat congestive heart failure. Formerly, these drugs have only been applied as potassium-saving diuretics in oedematous diseases, hypertension and hypokalaemia as well as in primary hyperaldosteronism. Possible side effects of aldosterone antagonists include hyperkalemia and, in case of spironolactone, which is less specific for the mineralocorticoid receptor than eplerenone, also antiandrogenic and progestational actions.

References

1. Pitt B, Zannad F, Remme WJ, Cody R, Castaigne A, Perez A, Palensky J, Wittes J (1999) The effect of spironolactone on morbidity and mortality in patients with severe heart failure. Randomized Aldactone Evaluation Study Investigators. N Engl J Med 341:709–717
2. Burnier M, Brunner HR (2000) Angiotensin II receptor antagonists. Lancet 355:637–645
3. Yusuf S, Sleight P, Pogue J, Bosch J, Davies R, Dagenais G (2000) Effects of an angiotensin-converting-enzyme inhibitor, ramipril, on cardiovascular events in high-risk patients. The Heart Outcomes Prevention Evaluation Study Investigators. N Engl J Med 342:145–153
4. Bader M, Peters J, Baltatu O, Müller DN, Luft FC, Ganten D (2001) Tissue renin-angiotensin systems: new insights from experimental animal models in hypertension research. J Mol Med 79:76–102
5. Weber MA (2001) Vasopeptidase inhibitors. Lancet 358:1525–1532

Repolarization

Repolarization is a return of membrane potential to its resting value. It refers mostly to repolarization of an action potential, although a more general meaning of returning a membrane potential back to a more negative value after (forced) depolarization is also common.

▶ Antiarrhythmic Drugs

Resiniferatoxin

Resiniferatoxin (RTX) is the toxin isolated from the spurge *Euphorbia resinifera* which is responsible for the powerful burning sensation and skin irritation induced by the milky sap of these plants. Like capsaicin, resiniferatoxin activates TRPV1 currents, but not the currents through other members of the TRPV subfamily.

▶ TRP Channels
▶ Vanilloid Receptor

Resistance

If the concentration of an antibacterial agent required to inhibit or kill a microorganism is greater than the concentration that can be safely achieved during therapy, the microorganism is considered to be resistant to the drug. Resistance most often is acquired by horizontal transfer of resistance determinants from a donor cell by transformation, transduction or conjugation and subsequently it may be rapidly and widely disseminated by clonal spread. The recent emergence of antibiotic resistance in bacterial pathogens (e.g. penicillin-resistant pneumococci) is a very serious development.

Respiratory Burst

The respiratotry burst is the ability of phagocytes to destroy pathogens by the release of a variety of toxic products including, hydrogen peroxide, superoxide anion and nitric oxide. Production of these toxic metabolites is induced by the binding of aggregatred antibodies to the Fc gamma receptors.

Response Elements

Response elements are short sequence motifs of promoter regions or enhancers which are recognized by regulatory transcription factors and mediate the transcriptional response of a cell to external stimuli. A gene can be under the control of one or more response elements.

Restenosis

Restenosis is the phenomenon of vascular re-occlusion post-angioplasty or stent.

Resting Potential

Resting potential is a stable membrane potential in non-excitable cells, or the most stable membrane potential between action potentials of excitable cells. In some excitable tissues, it is impossible to define a resting potential because of continuous changes in membrane potential.

Resting Tremor

Resting tremor is a tremor present at rest, which usually abates during voluntary movements. Its frequency in Parkinsonism is 4 to 8 Hz and it occurs most often in the distal extremities.

▶ Parkinson's Disease

Retinal

▶ Vitamin A

Retinitis Pigmentosa

Retinitis pigmentosa (RP) refers to a group of diseases which cause slow but progressive loss of vision. In each of them there is a gradual loss of photoreceptors (primarily of the rod photoreceptors).

▶ Cyclic Nucleotide-regulated Cation Channels

Retinoblastoma (Rb) Gene

The retinoblastoma protein was identified originally through studies of an inherited form of eye cancer in children, known as retinoblastoma. The loss of both copies of the Rb gene leads to excessive cell proliferation in the mature retina. This suggested that Rb is the product of a tumour suppressor gene. Later it was shown that the retinoblastoma protein is a key regulator of a gene regulatory protein called E2F which plays a key role in the regulation of the cell cycle. E2F function is controlled primarily by the Rb protein. Rb binds to E2F and blocks the transcription of S-phase genes. When cells are stimulated to divide by extracellular signals, active G_1-Cdk accumulates and phosphorylates Rb, reducing its affinity for E2F. The Rb protein then dissociates, allowing E2F to activate S-phase gene expression.

▶ Cell-cycle Control

Retinoic Acid

Retinoic acid (RA) describes a group of vitamin-A-acid (synonym Vitamin A1 acid) derivatives such as all-trans-retinoic acid (tretinoin), 9-cis-retinoic acid and13-cis retinoic acid (isotretinoin). Retinoic acids act through binding to retinoic acid and retinoid X response elements.

▶ Retinoic Acid Receptors

R

Retinoic Acid Receptors

Retinoic Acid receptors (RARs) are nuclear receptors. Nuclear receptors are a large family of structurally related ligand-inducible transcription factors, including steroid receptors (SRs), thyroid/retinoids receptors (TR, RARs and RXRs), vitamin D receptors (VDR), LXR, peroxisome proliferator activated receptors (PPARs), estrogen receptors (ERa and ERb), and orphan receptors for which no ligand has been yet identified. While having in common a modular structure, they are activated by distinct lipophilic small molecules such as glucocorticoids, progesterone, estrogens, retinoids, and fatty acid derivatives.

All nuclear receptors have a hydrophobic pocket into which its specific ligand binds, with helix 12 (H12) being the key response element of NR's. When an agonist is bound to a NR, H12 is oriented anti-parallel to H11, capping the ligand binding pocket. This leaves a hydrophobic groove exposed for the binding of coregulator proteins. When an antagonist is bound, H12 is displaced via an extended side chain. H12 moves outward, rotates, and packs into the hydrophobic groove between helices 3, 4, and 5. As a result, coactivators needed for transcription cannot bind.

Several loci encoding RAR isoforms have been identified in mammals, RAR-alpha, -beta and -gamma. They respond to at-RA, 9-cis-RA and 13-cis-RA. The RARs show spatially restricted distribution patterns during embryogenesis, which have led to speculation on a variety of roles for RA in developmental processes. As with other enhancer-binding proteins, nuclear receptors act as transcription factors by binding to specific DNA recognition sequences generally located upstream of responsive genes. Although RARs can activate gene expression through binding to thyroid hormone response elements, much more specific and potent RA response elements (RAREs) have been identified within the promoter of the RAR gene. These RAREs are essential for RA induction of the RAR-gene and, when linked to heterologous promoters, can confer transcriptional activation *via* all three RARs.

Retinoid-resistance

The major limitation to the application of retinoids is the retinoid resistance observed in cancer cells. This means that such cells do not respond either to physiological or therapeutic concentrations of retinoids. Silencing of RARβ has been suggested to contribute to the tumorigenicity and retinoid resistance of lung and breat cancer cells. RARβ silencing is caused by epigenetic changes, namely DNA methylation and repressive chromatin remodeling of the RARβ P2 promoter. Epigenetic changes can be reversed. Pili *et al.* developed a strategy to overcome the silencing at RARβ by specifically targeting the epigenetic defect at RARβ P2, using combinations of histone deacetylase inhibitors (HDACIs), a class of chromatin remodeling drugs and RARβ agonists.

Retinoids

Thomas C. Roos
Reha Klinik Neuharlingersiel, Interdisciplinary Center for Dermatology, Pneumology and Allergology, Neuharlingersiel, Germany
roos@rehaklinik-neuharlingersiel-klinik.de

Synonyms

Retinoids, vitamin A, carotinoids, retinylesters, ▶ retinol, ▶ retinal, ▶ retinoic acid, vitamin A acid

Definition

Vitamin A (retinol) and its naturally occurring and synthetic derivatives, collectively referred to as ▶ retinoids (chemical structure), exert a wide variety of profound effects in apoptosis, embryogenesis, reproduction, vision, and regulation of inflammation, growth, and differentiation of normal and neoplastic cells in vertebrates.

Retinoids are alcohols and accordingly soluble in ethanol, isopropanol, and polyethylenglycol. Major sources of natural retinoids are animal fats, fish liver oil (retinylesters) and yellow and green

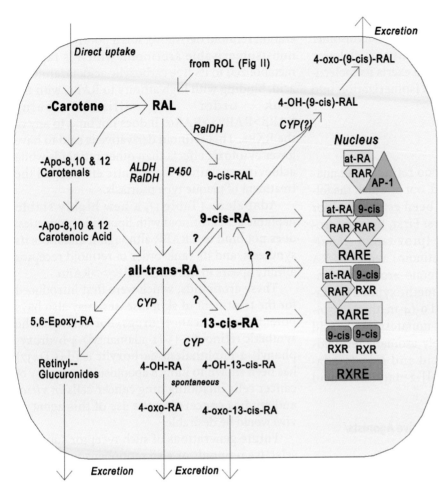

Fig. 1 Intracellular pathways and molecular action of retinoids.

vegetables (carotenoids). Ingested retinylesters (RE) are hydrolysed to retinol by enteral hydrolases in the intestine. ROL and carotenoids are absorbed by intestinal mucosa cells.

▶ Gluco-/Mineralocorticoid Receptors
▶ Sex Steroid Receptors

Mechanism of Action

Retinoids mediate their biological effects through binding to nuclear receptors known as ▶ retinoic acid receptors (RARs) and ▶ retinoid X receptors (RXRs), which belong to the superfamily of lig-and-inducible transciptional regulators that include steroid hormone receptors, thyroid hormone receptors, and vitamin D_3 receptors [reviewed in (1)]. RARs and RXRs act via polymorphic cis-acting responsive elements, the retin-oic acid responsive elements (RAREs) and retinoid X responsive elements (RXREs), present in the promoters of retinoid-responsive genes (Fig. 1).

The known beneficial effects of retinoids on malignancies are assumed to relate to retinoid receptor-mediated anti-promoting and anti-initiating effects. The latter appears to be influenced by interference of several xenobiotics with different steps of the retinoid metabolism in the target cell. Of the carotenoids, β-carotene is the most potent retinol precursor, yet being six-fold less effective than preformed retinol, resulting from incomplete resorption and conversion (one retinol equivalent is equal to 1 μg of retinol, 6 μg of β-carotene, or 12 μg of mixed carotenoids) [for retinoid metabolism review see (7)].

Although all-trans- and 9-cis-RA are only minor metabolites of ROL and β-carotene, they display 100 to 1000-fold higher biological activity.

Whereas *all-trans*-RA binds only to RARs, *9-cis*-RA binds both RARs and RXRs. The stereoisomer of *all-trans*-RA, *13-cis*-RA, exhibits a much lower affinity for RARs and RXRs and exerts its molecular effects mostly through its isomerization into *all-trans*-RA.

Clinical Use

Up to now, far more than 5000 retinoic acid analogues have been synthesized, out of which the following 3 generations have been established for therapy of various disorders: First, the non-aromatic retinoids β-carotene (provitamin A), *all-trans*-retinoic acid (RA) (tretinoin) and *13-cis*-RA (isotretinoin), second, the mono-aromatic retinoid-derivatives trimethyl-methoxyphenyl analogue of RA (etretinate) and 9-(4-methoxy-2,3,6-trimethylphenyl)-3-2,4,6,8-nonatetraenoic acid (acitretin), and third, the poly-aromatic retinoid-derivatives tazarotenic acid and 6-[3-(1-adamantyl)-4-methoxy-phenyl]-2-naphthoic acid (adapalene) (see Table 1).

Synthetic Retinoid Receptor Selective Agonists/Antagonists

The concept of drug development is based on the findings that retinoid receptors (RARs and RXRs) offer a new approach by targeting different genes depending on the activated retinoid receptor complexes. The multiplicity of these retinoid signaling pathways affords potential for therapeutic opportunity as well as retinoid therapy associated undesired side effects. It is possible that the indiscriminate activation of all pathways by non-specific retinoid ligands could lead to unacceptable side effects so that any enhanced efficacy would be obtained at the cost of enhanced toxicity.

The development of ligands selective for individual receptor subtypes relevant to a targeted disease could decrease these toxic effects thereby improving the therapeutic index. Two new arotinoids are already available for topical use in skin diseases. These are tazarotenic acid (tazarotene) and 6-[3-(1-adamantyl)-4-methoxyphenyl-2-naphtoic acid (adapalene) (Table 1), and other synthetic retinoid derivatives are in the pipeline. Also fenretinide, a synthetic amide of retinoic acid is available for systemic therapy in oncology.

Tazarotene (Table 1) is an acetylenic third generation retinoid derivative. It is a poorly absorbed, non-isomerisable arotinoid, which is rapidly metabolized to its free carboxylic acid, tazarotenic acid, binding with high affinity to RARs, with the rank order of affinity being RARβ>RARγ>>RARα. It does not bind to any of the RXRs. This retinoid derivative is said to have lower cytotoxic effects than other retinoids while achieving sustained therapeutic efficiacy in the treatment of plaque type psoriasis.

Adapalene (Table 1), a new highly stable naphtoic acid arotinoid with lipophilic properties, does not bind to CRABP, although it enhances its synthesis, and its rank-order of retinoid receptor affinity apears to be RARβ>RARγ>>RARα.

These arotinoids, which were first introduced for the treatment of skin diseases, may also have potential as anticancer drugs. For example, the synthetic retinoid 6-[3-(1-adamantyl)-4-hydroxy-phenyl]-2-naphthalene carboxylic acid (CD437) has been shown to induce apoptosis in a variety of cancer cells including lung cancer cells *in vitro*, and studies concerning the use of this agent *in vivo* would be desirable.

Future generations of such receptor subtype-selective retinoids or also retinobenzoic acids (3) may provide clinicians with more specific and less toxic drugs for dermatologic therapy.

Retinoids in Dermatology

Hyperkeratotic Disorders. The topical and oral use of retinoids for treatment of hyperkeratotic disorders such as psoriasis and Darier's disease has long been established. Systemic retinoid therapy is often combined with topical drugs such as corticosteroids, dithranol, tar, and also UVA/UVB phototherapies where synergistic effects have been reported.

Acne. Among retinoids, 13-cis-retinoic acid is known to have not only anti-inflammatory but also sebostatic effects. Therefore it is one of the most potent topical and also systemic agents for therapy of acne.

Photoaging and Wound Healing. Drug treatment of photoaged skin can be categorised as antioxidants, α-hydroxy acids and topical retinoids. Of these 3 approaches only topical retinoids, particularly retinaldehyde and *all-trans*-retinoic acid, have a well documented ability to restorethe repair function of photoaged skin at the clinical, histological and molecular level (4). According to these observations, retinoids were also shown to accelerate wound healing (4) and reduction of early striae distensae.

Skin and Oral Malignancies. Actinic keratoses were the first skin lesions to be treated topically with *all-trans*-retinoic acid. In various clinical trials, retinoids have been shown to be active in chemoprevention and treatment or prevention skin malignancies (7).

Currently, 13-cis-retinoic acid is the most studied chemopreventive agent that decreases the incidence of second primary tumors in patients with head-and-neck cancer, reverses premalignant lesions, and reduces appearance of non-melanoma skin cancer in patients with xeroderma pigmentosum. Unfortunately, this vitamin A derivative has a significant clinical toxicity, which limits its utility in a practice setting.

Molecular epidemiological studies to assess the risk associated with metabolic polymorphisms for cancers of head-and-neck and the lung have shown that the overall effect of common polymorphisms is moderate in terms of penetrance and relative risk. However, some gene combinations, such as mutated CYP1A1/GSTM1-null genotype, seem to predispose the lung and oral cavity of smokers to an even higher risk for cancer or DNA damage. These results require confirmation in larger studies that take into account the existence of ethnic variations even within the commonly defined groups.

Retinoids, isothiocyanates and tea polyphenols have been identified as possible chemopreventive agents for cancers of the lung and oral cavity. While a number of trials have been conducted with retinoids or β-carotene, the results were ambiguous and the causes are still being debated.

Newly acquired knowledge in the field of tumor biology and of the genetic changes underlying carcinogenesis through the use of new molecular technology represents the basis on which chemoprevention efforts should be based.

Retinoids in Oncology

Since retinoids play an important role in the molecular regulation of growth, differentiation and apoptosis of normal, premalignant and malignant cellls, especially epithelial cells, numerous studies have focussed on the effect of retinoids on a variety of malignancies. In animals, vitamin A deficiency has been shown to be associated with an increased incidence of cancer and an increased susceptibility of chemical carcinogens. On the molecular level, aberrant expression and function of nuclear retinoid receptors have been found in various types of premalignant lesions and cancers. Thus, aberrations in retinoid signalling appear to be early events in carcinogenesis, and retinoids at pharmacological doses have been shown to exhibit a variety of beneficial effects associated with cancer prevention and cancer therapy e.g. by suppression of transformation, inhibition of carcinogenesis in various organs in animal models.

Lung Cancer. Epidemiological and animal studies have demonstrated that retinoids are effective agents in preventing the development of tobacco-associated cancers. Unfortunately, clinical trials of retinoids on cigarette smokers have shown lack of efficacy in preventing lung cancer. A study investigated the effect of nicotine on the anti-cancer activity of all trans-retinoic acid (trans-RA) in human lung cancer cells and demonstrated that nicotine could abrogate the growth inhibitory effect of trans-RA by suppressing its ability to induce the expression of RA receptor β (RARβ), a tumor suppressor. The inhibitory effect of nicotine was accompanied with induction of orphan receptor TR3. Inhibition of TR3 expression by overexpression of TR3 anti-sense RNA in H460 lung cancer cells strongly prevented the suppressive effect of nicotine on *trans*-RA activity. These results suggest that nicotine suppresses the growth inhibitory effects of *all-trans*-RA by inhibiting RARβ expression through its induction of TR3 expression. Accordingly, RXR-selective retinoids may be more effective than classical retinoids for preventing and treating tobacco-associated cancers. Another study indicates the epidermal growth factor to be a target for the lung cancer preventive effect of retinoic acid.

R

Tab. 1 Indications and mode of administration of commercially available retinoids in dermatological therapy.

Generic Name	Chemical Structure	Mode of Administration	Principal Indication	Other Indications
Retinol (Vitamin A)		Oral	Vitamin Supplement	
Retinyl Palmitate		Topical 0.5–5% Emulsions	Cosmetic Agents	
β-Carotene (Provitamin A)		Topical	Hypopigmentations, Hyperpigmentations, Radical Protection	Nutritient Color
Tretinoin		Topical 0.025–0.1% Gels or Creams	Acne vulgaris, Parakeratosis, Hyperkeratosis	Photoaging, Actinic Keratosis
Isotretinoin		Topical 0.05% cream Oral 0.25–1.0 mg/kg/d	Cystic Acne, Recalcitrant Nodular Acne	Rosacea Gram-negative Folliculitis Pyoderma faciale Hidradenitis suppurativa Cancer Prevention
Etretinate		Oral 0.25–1.0 mg/kg/d	Generalized pustular Psoriasis, Exfoliative Psoriasis, Plaque Psoriasis	

Tab. 1 Indications and mode of administration of commercially available retinoids in dermatological therapy. (Continued)

Generic Name	Chemical Structure	Mode of Administration	Principal Indication	Other Indications
Acitretine		Oral 0.25–1.0 mg/kg/d	Psoriasis (erythrodermic, pustular, and severe recalcitrant)	Palmoplantar keratoderma Pustulosis palmoplantaris, Icthyosis, Darier's Disease, Pityriasis rubra pilaris, Lichen ruber planus
Tazarotene		Topical 0.05–0.1% gels	Psoriasis vulgaris	
Adapalene		Topical 0.1% gel	Acne vulgaris	

R

Encouraging findings concerning effective therapy strategies derive from combination studies in which retinoids, especially *all-trans*-retinoic acid, are added to either α-interferon or chemotherapy and radiotherapy. Here, more retinoid receptor-selective molecules may have a greater activity against lung cancer, with a more favourable toxicity profile, as recently suggested by preliminary data on Ro 41-5253 (2).

Breast Cancer. Studies with fenretinide in woman with stage I breast cancer did not show an overall effect of decreasing the risk of contralateral breast cancer. A protective effect could only be observed in premenopausal women, probably due to the modulation of the insulin-like growth factor 1 (IGF-1) by fenretinide in this population.

Liver Cancer. Hepatocellular carcinoma (HCC) develops in patients with chronic liver diseases associated with hepatitis B and hepatitis C virus infections with high incidences. Here, an acyclic retinoid has been shown to suppress the post-therapeutic recurrence after interferon-γ or glycerrhicin treatment in cirrhotic patients who underwent curative treatment of preceding tumors. The retinoid induced the disappearance of serum lectin-reactive α-fetoprotein (AFP-L3), a tumor marker indicating the presence of unrecognizable tumors in the remnant liver, suggesting a deletion of such minute (pre)malignant clones (clonal deletion). As a molecular mechanism of the clonal deletion, a novel mechanism of apoptosis induction by the retinoid via tissue transglutaminase has been implicated (5). In future, a combination of immunopreventive and chemopreventive therapies may give a clue to the further advances of cancer prevention, and thereby to the improvement of the prognosis of cirrhotic patients.

Leukaemia. Acute promyelocytic leukaemia (APL) is known as the most curable subtype of acute myeloid leukaemia in adults. Here, *all-trans*-retinoic acid induces differentiation of the leukemic cells into mature granulocytes. On the basis of clinical and *in vitro* studies, the following mechanisms have been proposed to explain the frequently occurring ATRA resistance: 1) induction of accelerated metabolism of ATRA, 2) increased expression of cellular retinoic acid-binding proteins (CRABPs), 3) constitutive degradation of PML-RARα, 4) point mutations in the ligand-binding domain of RARα of PML-RARα, 5) P-glycoprotein expression, 6) transcriptional repression by histone deacetylase activity, 7) isoforms of PML-RARα, 8) persistent telomerase activity, and 9) expression of type II transglutaminase. It is yet unclear which of these factors is mainly responsible for retinoid resistancies. Patients, who relapse after retinoic acid therapy, should be transferred to arsenic trioxide or stem cell transplantation therapy.

Neuroblastoma. Most recently, a phase-I-study defined a dose of 13-cis-retinoic acid that was tolerable in patients after myeloablative therapy, and a phase-III-trial showed that postconsolidation therapy with 13-cis-retinoic acid improved EFS for patients with high-risk neuroblastoma (6). Preclinical studies in neuroblastoma indicate that ATRA or 13-cis-RA can antagonize cytotoxic chemotherapy and radiation, such that use of 13-cis-RA in neuroblastoma is limited to maintenance after completion of cytotoxic chemotherapy and radiation. It is likely that recurrent disease seen during or after 13-cis-RA therapy in neuroblastoma is due to tumor cell resistance to retinoid-mediated differentiation induction. Studies in neuroblastoma cell lines resistant to 13-cis-RA and ATRA have shown that they can be sensitive, and in some cases collaterally hypersensitive, to the cytotoxic retinoid fenretinide. Here, fenretinide induces tumor cell cytotoxicity rather than differentiation, acts independently from RA receptors, and in initial phase-I-trials has been well tolerated. Clinical trials of fenretinide, alone and in combination with ceramide modulators, are in development.

Side Effects of Retinoids

Hypervitaminosis A is characterized by hepatomegaly, cerebral edema and bone structure alterations. β-Carotene causes yellow-orange coloring of the skin by binding to keratins. Topically applied retinoic acids can lead to irritation, rash and Xerosis. Also worsening of atopic dermatitis and increased light sensitivity has been reported.

Systemic treatment of 13-cis retinoic acid frequently leads to cheilitis and eye irritations (e.g.

unspecific cornea-inflammation). Also other symptoms such as headache, pruritus, alopecia, pains of joints and bone, and exostosis-formation have been reported. Notably, an increase of very low density lipoproteins and triglycerides accompanied by a decrease of the high density lipoproteins has been reported in 10 to 20% of treated patients. Transiently, liver function markers can increase during oral retinoid therapy. Etretinate causes the side effects of 13-cis retinoid acid at lower doses. In addition to this, generalized edema and centrilobulary toxic liver cell necrosis have been observed.

The most important clinical side effects of systemically applied retinoic acid therapy are teratogenity and embryotoxicity. Topical administration of retinoic acid does not appear to cause such effects. This is supported by the observation that nutritional retinoid administration can lead to higher plasma levels than topical treatment with retinoic acid. However in several countries, the topical administration during pregnancy is prohibited. In the USA, contraception during topical use of retinoic acid is recommended. This narrow therapeutic frame requires a pregnancy testing, measuring of liver enzymes, triglycerides, cholesterin and glucose before and frequent follow up examinations during retinoid therapy (every 3rd or 4th week).

Increased risk factors for suffering retinoid side effects are adipositas, alcohol abuse, diabetes, nicotine-abuse, familiar lipid-metabolism alterations and other concommittant therapies (see below).

Interactions with Other Agents

Dexamethasone, the macrolide antibiotic triacetyloleandromycin, and phenobarbital are all well established inducers of the CYP3A subfamily, and can increase microsomal 4-hydroxylation of RA in rat liver. To what extent this is also the case for humans is not completely clear.

Glucocorticoids (clobetasol) also induce the expression of CYP1A1 in human skin. This is mediated through glucocorticoid receptor responsive elements (GRE) that have been identified in the first intron of the rat and human *CYP1A1* genes. These findings suggest the possibility that skin changes caused by long-term treatment with topical or systemic glucocorticoids could be mediated

by a steroid-induced depletion of active retinoids. Therefore, we hypothesize that tandem treatment of patients with both glucocorticoids and low-dose RA may prevent some steroid side effects. In a mouse model this idea has already been confirmed. Interestingly, there retinoids showed a steroid-sparing effect.

Skin procarcinogens, such as 3-MC and the polycyclic aromatic hydrocarbon (PAH) benzo[a]pyrene, can increase RA catabolism in human skin and induce local tissue depletion of retinoids, respectively. This can be antagonized by high dietary intake of β-carotene or retinoid acid. This acceleration of retinoid cleavage is primarily due to the xenobiotic-mediated induction of CYP1A1, which is also involved in the inactivation of RA to *4-OH*-RA. Accordingly, retinoid-induced inhibition of basal as well as coal tar- and glucocorticoid-induced CYP1A1-expression in human skin as reported in (7) seems to reflect a competitive feedback-inhibition of CYP1A1 activity by RA. Interestingly, CYP1A1 is one major enzyme that converts the procarcinogens mentioned above into active carcinogenic metabolites in skin. The induction of this enzyme, leading to an acceleration of the turnover of RA to inactive metabolites and a local RA deficiency, might further explain the profound effect of these carcinogenic CYP1A1-inducers on cell proliferation and tumor formation. In support of this notion, 7,8-benzoflavone, an inhibitor of CYP1A1 activity, increases local vitamin A concentrations, and reduces tumor formation in mouse skin [review see (7)].

Imidazole antimycotics, ketoconazole, clotrimazole, and miconazole are potent inhibitors of various cytochrome P450-isoenzymes that also affect the metabolism of retinoids. They were first shown to inhibit the metabolism of RA in F9 embryonal carcinoma cells. When tested *in vitro* liarazole, a potent CYP-inhibitor, suppressed neoplastic transformation and upregulated gap junctional communication in murine and human fibroblasts, which appeared to be due to the presence of retinoids in the serum component of the cell culture medium. Furthermore, liarazole magnified the cancer chemopreventive activity of RA and β-carotene in these experiments by inhibiting RA-catabolism as demonstrated by absence of a decrease in RA-levels in the culture medium in the presence of liarazole over 48 h, whereas without

R

liarazole 99% of RA was catabolized. *In vivo*, treatment with liarazole and ketoconazole reduced the accelerated catabolism of retinoids and increased the mean plasma *all-trans*-RA-concentration in patients with acute promyelocytic leukemia and other cancers.

Vitamin D3 (VD3) and retinoids synergistically inhibit the growth and progression of squamous cell carcinomas and actinic keratoses in chronically sun exposed skin. One reason for this synergism may be the direct influence of VD3 on the isomerization and the metabolism of RA. Here, VD3 inhibits the isomerization of *13-cis*-RA to the more receptor active *all-trans* and *9-cis*-isomers. Moreover, the VD3 derivative secocholestratrien-1,3,24-triol (tacalcitol), used for the treatment of severe keratinizing disorders inhibits 4-hydroxylation of *all-trans*-RA.

Ethanol also inhibits ADH-catalyzed retinol oxidation *in vitro*, and ethanol treatment of mouse embryos has been demonstrated to reduce endogenous RA levels. The inhibition of cytosolic RolDH activity and stimulation of microsomal RolDH activity could explain ethanol-mediated vitamin A depletion, separate from ADH isoenzymes. Although the exact mechanism of inhibition of retinoid metabolism by ethanol is unclear, these observations are consistent with the finding that patients with alcoholic liver disease have depleted hepatic vitamin A reserves [review see (7)].

Different combinatory therapy regimens are known which additively or synergistically act in a variety of diseases:

Combinations of drugs displaying distinct effects on cell proliferation/ differentiation and immunomodulation (e.g.: retinoids and chemotherapy in advanced cutaneous T cell lymphoma).

Combinations of retinoids with ultraviolet A or B radiation (and other drugs). For example, RePUVA-therapy (retinoids and psoralen and UVA combination) is currently one of the most effective regimens for recalcitrant severe psoriasis.

Drugs with metabolic interactions that can enhance the half-life of active compounds. An example of this regimen is the interaction between azole- and vitamin D-derivatives that inhibit the metabolism of retinoids in skin cells leading to increased intracellular amounts of active RA-isomeres. Further study and the identification of novel interactions of this type of drug interaction is of great clinical interest since they may decrease the dose of retinoids required for efficacy thereby also reducing the risk of side effects of the retinoids.

Retinoid-resistance

(▶ Retinoid-resistance) Two possible explanations for accelerated clearance of retinoids in patients during long-term treatment with retinoids have been suggested: First, RA-mediated induction of CRABP-expression, which is known to lower the plasma and intracellular levels of active RA by binding RA, and second, the RA-mediated induction and/or constitutive overexpression of P-glycoprotein, which is encoded by the multidrug resistance gene-1, leading to decreased intracellular levels of RA by enhancing active transport of intracellular retinoids out of the target cells [review see (7)].

The knowledge concerning the molecular action of retinoids is steadily increasing but still the many steps of retinoid metabolism especially retinoid inactivation are not fully understood. The interaction of retinoids as the central agent with other drugs represents a new dimension of disease-therapy providing us with more specific and less toxic therapy approaches to influence cell proliferation and differentiation. Perhaps in no other area of pharmacology is the concept of using drug-drug interactions as a rationale for therapy more advanced than with retinoids in dermatology. It is likely that this strategy will prove useful in other areas as well.

References

1. Chambon P (1996) A decade of molecular biology of retinoic acid receptors. FASEB J 10:940-954
2. Elson ML (1998) The role of retinoids in wound healing. J Am Acad Dermatol Suppl 39:79-81.
3. Kagechika H (2002): Novel synthetic retinoids and separation of the pleiotrophc retinoidal activities. Curr Med Chem 9(5):591-608.
4. Kang S, Voorhees JJ (1998) Photoaging therapy with tretinoin: an evidence based analysis. J Am Acad Dermatol Suppl 39:55-61
5. Okuno M, Kojima S, Moriwaki H (2001) Chemoprevention of hepatocellular carcinoma: concepts,

progress and perspectives. J Gastroenterol Hepatol 16:1329-35.

6. Reynolds CP, Lemon RS (2001): Retinoid therapy for childhood cancer. Hematol Oncol Clin North Am 15(5):867-910.

7. Roos TC, Jugert FK, Merk HF, Bickers DR (1998) Retinoid Metabolism in the Skin. Pharmacol Rev. 1998 Jun;50(2):315-33.

Retinoids, chemical structure

Retinoids represent a class of compounds consisting of four isoprenoid units joined in a head-to-tail manner. All retinoids may be formally derived from a monocyclic parent compound containing five carbon-carbon double bonds and a functional group at the end of the acyclic portion. Notably, the so-called 'arotinoids' or 'retinoidal benzoic acid derivatives' as well as others, are not chemically retinoids. They contain, e.g., aromatic rings replacing either the basic-ionone-type ring structure or unsaturated bonds of the tetraene side chain of the retinoid skeleton.

▶ Retinoids

Retinoid X Receptor

The retinoid X receptor (RXR) is a nuclear receptor that binds and is activated by certain endogenous retinoids, such as 9-cis-retinoic acid. RXR is the obligatory heterodimerization partner for a large number of non-classic steroid nuclear receptors, such as thyroid hormone receptor, vitamin D3 receptor, peroxisome proliferator-activated receptor and pregnane X receptor.

Retinol

▶ Vitamin A

Retinyl Esters

▶ Vitamin A

Retrograde Messenger

A retrograde messenger is a chemical substance released by a postsynaptic neuron which can modify the release of neurotransmitter, either positively or negatively, from a nerve terminal input. It is designated "retrograde" because it is opposite to the usual forward direction of transmission from nerve terminal to postsynaptic cell.

▶ Synaptic Transmission

Retroviruses

▶ Gene Therapy
▶ Antiviral Drugs

Reuptake Transporter

Reuptake transporters are structures within the cell membranes of the presynaptic nerve terminal that serve to transport biogenic amines released from vesicles back into the nerve cell. These structures are targets for antidepressants, that block the transporter, thus increasing the bioavailability of neurotransmitters at postsynaptic receptors.

▶ Antidepressant Drugs
▶ Neurotransmitter Transporters

R

Reverse Transcription

Reverse transcription is the copying of an RNA molecule back into its DNA complement. The enzymes that perform this function are called reverse transcriptases. Reverse transcription is used naturally by retroviruses to insert themselves into an organism's genome. Artificially induced reverse transcription is a useful technique for translating unstable messenger RNA (mRNA) molecules into stable cDNA.

▶ Antiviral Drugs

Reward (pathways)

▶ Drug Addiction
▶ Dependence
▶ Psychostimulants

Reye's Syndrome

Reye syndrome is a rare disorder in children, characterized by a combination of severe liver disorder and encephalopathy (central nervous system (CNS) disturbances) that can follow an acute viral illness and which has a relatively high mortality. It has been found to be associated with the use of acetylsalicylic acid (aspirin). Although it is not completely clear to what extend aspirin is in fact implicated in the pathogenesis of the syndrome, aspirin is best avoided in children with viral infections.

▶ Non-steroidal Anti-inflammatory Drugs

RGS

▶ Regulators of G-protein signalling
▶ G-proteins

RGS Protein

▶ Regulators of G-protein signalling
▶ Table appendix: Receptor Proteins

Rhabdomyolysis

Rhabdomyolysis is disintegration and death of muscle cells (myocytes). It is an important, but rare, side-effect of treatment with statins.

▶ HMG-CoA-reductase Inhibitors

Rheumatoid Arthritis

Rheumatoid arthris is a chronic inflammatory condition of the synovial membranes lining the joints, probably of an autoimmune nature. It initially involves the peripheral joints in a symmetrical fashion. Monocytes and polymorphonucleocytes infiltrate the joints and release inflammatory mediators such as TNFalpha and interleukin-1. These in turn cause the generation of proteases, prostaglandins, leukotrienes and oxygen-derived free radicals which produce pain, swelling and tissue damage, resulting in cartilage erosion and synovial thickening.

▶ Immunosupressive Agents
▶ Non-steroidal Anti-inflammatory Drugs
▶ Glucocorticoids

Rho

Rho is a small monomeric GTPase that regulates a number of cellular functions (cell movement, cell adhesion, cytokinesis, cell growth).

▶ Small GTPases

Rho-kinase

Rho-kinase is the direct target for Rho. The enzyme is inhibited by Y-27632, a compound that lowers elevated blood pressure in animal models of hypertension.

▶ Small GTPases

Riboflavin

Riboflavin is vitamin B2.

▶ Vitamines, watersoluble

Ribosomal Protein Synthesis Inhibitors

Katherine S. Long
Department of Biological Chemistry, Institute of Molecular Biology, University of Copenhagen, Copenhagen, Denmark
long@mermaid.molbio.ku.dk

Synonyms

Translation inhibitors, ribosome-targeting antibiotics

Definition

Ribosomes and Protein Synthesis

Ribosomes are ancient ribonucleoprotein complexes that are the sites of protein synthesis in living cells. Their core structures and fundamental functional mechanisms have been conserved throughout the three domains of life: bacteria, archaea and eukaryotes. All ribosomes are organized into two subunits that are defined by their apparent sedimentation coefficient, measured in Svedberg units (S). There is a general increase in ribosome size with organism complexity from bacteria to archaea to eukaryotes. The smaller bacterial ribosome has a molecular mass of approximately 2.5 MD and is composed of a 30S small subunit, with 16S ribosomal RNA (rRNA; 1540 nucleotides) and 21 proteins, and a 50S large subunit, with 23S rRNA (2900 nucleotides), 5S rRNA (120 nucleotides) and over 30 proteins. Recent progress in the structural elucidation of the ribosome through X-ray crystallography has resulted in atomic resolution structures of ribosomal subunits and their complexes in association with antibiotics. These structures have begun to reveal molecular details of antibiotic binding to the ribosome and insights into the structural basis for antibiotic inhibition and resistance (1).

Protein synthesis is a complex multi-step process that can be divided into initiation, elongation and termination stages. In the initiation phase, the 30S subunit binds to messenger RNA (mRNA), along which triplet base codons specify the individual amino acids in a protein sequence that will be added via cognate transfer RNAs (tRNAs). tRNAs span the interface between the subunits, with the tRNA anticodon and aminoacylated ends interacting with the 30S and 50S subunits, respectively. The tRNA carrying the first amino acid (methionine) binds the mRNA on the 30S subunit through codon-anticodon base pairing, followed by positioning of the 3′-end in the peptidyl-donor site in a cavity on the 50S subunit. The second tRNA binds at the aminoacyl-acceptor site with its 3′-end positioned next to that in the donor site. Peptide bond formation occurs, catalyzed by the 50S subunit and resulting in transfer of the nascent peptide to the aminoacylated tRNA. The precise positioning of the 3′-ends of aminoacyl- and peptidyl-tRNA substrates is achieved in part through

R

base pairing interactions with the A-loop and P-loop of 23S rRNA, respectively. Although the mechanism of peptidyl transferase remains unclear, the atomic resolution structure of the archaeon *Haloarcula marismortui* 50S subunit complexed with a transition state analog reveals that there are no ribosomal proteins within 18 Å of the nascent peptide bond (2). Peptide bond formation is followed by translocation of the mRNA-tRNA complex, leaving a vacant A-site for the tRNA carrying the next encoded amino acid. Incoming tRNAs move through successive sites on the ribosome in a unidirectional manner, including aminoacyl-acceptor (A), peptidyl-donor (P) and exit (E) sites. This elongation cycle is repeated for each encoded amino acid. Termination occurs upon recognition of a termination codon, which triggers release of the nascent polypeptide along an exit channel through the 50S subunit, followed by subunit dissociation. The entire process is aided by protein factors at every stage, including aminoacyl-tRNA selection and translocation of the mRNA-tRNA complex.

The Ribosome as a Target for Antibiotics

The ribosome is an important target for a wide variety of antibiotics. Antibiotics inhibit protein synthesis at different functional steps and have served as valuable tools in determining the mechanisms of translation. Although a few universal antibiotics inhibit protein synthesis in most, if not all, living organisms, the majority of antibiotics exhibit selectivity for one or two domains of life. Consequently, many of the drugs have important medical applications in the treatment of serious bacterial infections. The wide clinical use of some antibiotics, however, has been curtailed in recent years due to problems of toxicity and antibiotic resistance. A detailed understanding of antibiotic inhibitory mechanisms has remained elusive despite the fact that many of the drugs have been known for decades. An important step forward has come with the recent breakthroughs in ribosome crystallography and the structural elucidation of ribosomal subunit-antibiotic complexes, obtained from crystals of ribosomal subunits through either soaking or co-crystallization with antibiotics. These complexes localize antibiotic binding sites and yield molecular insights into the

structural basis of antibiotic inhibition and resistance.

A number of general points can be made on antibiotic targeting of the ribosome: First, antibiotics bind to specific sites on the ribosome, with the majority targeting ribosomal RNA and not ribosomal proteins. This is consistent with crystallographic data showing that many functional centers on the ribosome are composed largely of rRNA. In addition, many antibiotics bind to regions of rRNA that are near mRNA template or tRNA substrate binding sites. Finally, antibiotics bind to regions of the ribosome that undergo conformational changes or rearrangements during translation. Most antibiotics that target the ribosome act at or near one of the following functional centers (Fig. 1). These are (1) the decoding center on 16S rRNA, (2) the GTPase-associated region, (3) the ribotoxin site and (4) the ▶ peptidyl transferase center, where the latter three involve 23S rRNA. This review will focus on antibiotics that target functional centers (1) and (4), on which there is high-resolution structural information available from ribosomal subunit-antibiotic complexes.

▶ β-lactam Antibiotics
▶ Microbial Resistance to Drugs
▶ Quinolones

Mechanism of Action

Antibiotics and the 30S Subunit

The two primary functions of the 30S subunit in protein synthesis are (1) decoding, the discrimination between cognate and non-cognate tRNAs by monitoring codon-anticodon base pairing in the ribosomal A site, and (2) translocation, where, together with the 50S subunit, tRNAs and the associated mRNA are moved by precisely one codon. The high degree of translational accuracy achieved by the ribosome is thought to involve both initial selection (via codon-anticodon base pairing) and proofreading steps, with the latter important for discrimination between cognate and near-cognate tRNAs. The structures of bacterial 30S-antibiotic complexes yield insights into how the following drugs interfere with 30S function: spectinomycin, streptomycin, paromomycin, tetracycline and pactamycin (3,4).

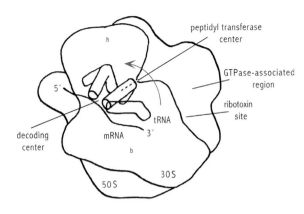

Fig. 1 Schematic drawing of the morphology of the ribosome. The ribosomal subunits are labeled, as are the approximate locations of their respective functional centers. The drawing is a transparent view from the solvent side of the small subunit. Transfer RNAs are shown in different binding states with the arrow indicating their direction of movement through the ribosome. The tRNA anticodon ends are oriented towards the viewer, whereas the 3'-ends of the tRNAs are oriented towards the peptidyl transferase region on the large subunit. The letters 'h' and 'b' denote the head and body regions on the 30S subunit, respectively.

Spectinomycin inhibits translocation of peptidyl-tRNA from the A- to the P-site. The antibiotic has a rigid structure composed of three fused rings that binds at one end of helix 34 in the minor groove, interacting mostly with nucleotides G1064 and C1192. Translocation requires movement of elements of the head of the 30S subunit, including helix 34. Through binding near a pivot point of the head, spectinomycin can interfere with movements of the head through steric hindrance and thereby block translocation.

Streptomycin is thought to make ribosomes error-prone by affecting proofreading and initial selection steps. The antibiotic interacts with four points of the phosphate backbone of 16S rRNA (at nucleotides 13, 526, 915 and 1490) through salt bridges and hydrogen bonds. It also contacts lysine 45 of protein S12. The binding site suggests that streptomycin affects the helix 27 accuracy switch by stabilizing the *ram* state of the ribosome. In the *ram* state there is a higher affinity for tRNA in the A-site, which increases binding of non-cog-

nate tRNAs. Stabilization of the *ram* state would make switching to the restrictive state more difficult and thereby affect proofreading. A number of streptomycin-resistance mutations in 16S rRNA and protein S12 result in a hyperaccurate phenotype. In general, these mutations disrupt interactions that contribute to stabilization of the *ram* state.

Paromomycin belongs to a subclass of aminoglycoside antibiotics that target an asymmetric internal loop element in helix 44 of 16S rRNA, where they decrease the fidelity of translation. These antibiotics contain a 2-deoxystreptamine ring and an aminoglycoside ring that is either 4,5-disubstituted (neomycin and paromomycin) or 4,6-disubstituted (gentamycin and kanamycin). Paromomycin binds in the major groove of helix 44, where rings i and ii direct the specific interaction with 16S rRNA (Fig. 2). Ring i stacks against G1491 and hydrogen bonds to A1408 and the backbone of A1493, to flip A1492 and A1493 out of the helix. The unstacked bases point into the A-site and are positioned to interact in the major groove of the codon-anticodon helix. The bases hydrogen bond to 2'-hydroxyl groups on both sides of the codon-anticodon helix and are thereby able to monitor the shape and width of the minor groove of three consecutive base pairs, allowing for discrimination between correct base pairing and mismatches. Structural data suggests that unstacking of A1492 and A1493 occurs during normal translation if favorable interactions can be made across the minor groove with both mRNA and cognate tRNA in the codon-anticodon helix. When paromomycin is bound, the bases are flipped out of the helix causing an increase in the affinity of cognate and near-cognate tRNAs, and also the error rate. NMR studies show that paromomycin and gentamycin interact with 16S rRNA in the same manner, indicating that other aminoglycosides induce errors in translation via the same mechanism.

Hygromycin B is an aminoglycoside composed of four rings (I-IV) that inhibits translocation by sequestering tRNA in the A-site. It binds above paromomycin in the major groove near the top of helix 44 (Fig. 2), contacting rRNA from both strands (nucleotides 1400–1410 and 1490–1500). Hygromycin B binds exclusively to RNA bases in a sequence-specific manner. The drug adopts an

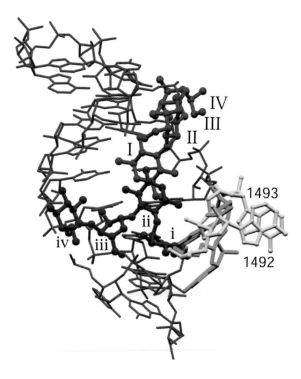

Fig. 2 The bound structures of paromomycin and hygromycin B in helix 44 of the 30S subunit. Two nucleotides in helix 44, A1492 and A1493, are labeled, as are rings i–iv of paromomycin and rings I-IV of hygromycin B (from (4) with copyright permission).

A magnesium ion is found in the binding site that mediates salt bridge interactions between the drug and the backbone of 16S rRNA. The binding site is not well conserved between bacteria and eukaryotes, providing a rationale for the specificity of the drug for bacteria. Tetracycline prevents binding of tRNA in the A-site through steric hindrance. The initial binding of tRNA in the ternary complex is not affected since its angle of approach is different from free tRNA in the A-site, avoiding a steric clash with the antibiotic.

Tetracycline has a secondary binding site in the H27 switch region that may also be functionally significant. The drug binds at the interface of the three domains of 16S rRNA, close to helix 44 and between helices 11 and 27. As with the primary binding site, contacts are made from the hydrophilic face of the drug to the backbone of 16S rRNA. In this binding site, tetracycline may function to stabilize the *ram* state.

The universal antibiotic pactamycin targets a highly conserved region of 16S rRNA, contacting the tips of helices 23b and 24a in the central domain. Pactamycin folds up to mimic a RNA dinucleotide in that its two distal aromatic rings

extended structure and makes base-specific hydrogen bonds spanning more than three bases along one strand of helix 44. Hygromycin B prevents movement from the A- to the P-site by interacting with regions of helix 44 that are known to be involved in translocation. Binding of the drug could also disrupt the switch between *ram* and restrictive states since this transition affects bases in the hygromycin B binding site.

▶ Tetracycline is known to block binding of aminoacyl-tRNA to the A-site, but not initial binding of the EF-Tu:aminoacyl-tRNA:GTP ternary complex. The primary binding site is located just above the binding site for aminoacyl tRNA, between the head and the body of the 30S subunit. The drug interacts with the sugar phosphate backbone of residues in helices 31 and 34 through hydrogen bonds with oxygen atoms and hydroxyl groups on the hydrophilic side of the drug (Fig. 3).

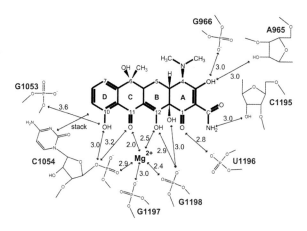

Fig. 3 The chemical structure of tetracycline and possible interations with 16S rRNA in the primary binding site. Arrows with numbers indicate distances (in Å) between functional groups. There are no interactions observed between the upper portion of the molecule and 16S rRNA, consistent with data that these positions can be modified without affecting inhibitory action (from (4) with copyright permission).

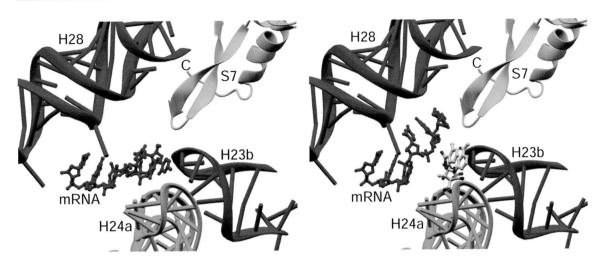

Fig. 4 The binding site of pactamycin on the 30S subunit. The positions of mRNA, the RNA elements H28, H23b, H24a, and the C-terminus of protein S7 are depicted in the E-site of the native 30S structure (left) and in the 30S-pactamycin complex (right). In the complex with pactamycin, the position of mRNA is altered (from (4) with copyright permission).

stack on each other and G693 (Fig. 4). The central ring of the drug interacts with nucleotides in helices 23b and 24a. The stacked aromatic rings lie in the position occupied by the last two bases of the E-site codon, displacing mRNA from its normal position and disrupting interactions with the E-site tRNA (Fig. 4). The position of the bound drug also suggests that it would disrupt the ▶ Shine-Dalgarno interaction, which is important for initiation in bacteria.

Antibiotics and the Peptidyl Transferase Center
The peptidyl transferase center is the site where peptide bond formation occurs, and is located in a cavity on the interface side of the 50S subunit that leads into the peptide exit channel. It is the binding site for the 3′-termini of both donor and acceptor tRNA substrates, and is targeted by a group of structurally diverse antibiotics that either inhibit peptide bond formation directly (including amicetin, chloramphenicol, puromycin and sparsomycin) or indirectly by interfering with movement of the nascent peptide (including erythromycin and the streptogramin B drugs). The structures of bacterial 50S-antibiotic complexes have localized binding sites of chloramphenicol, erythromycin and clindamycin that are consistent with biochem-

ical and genetic data (Fig. 5) and represent a forward step towards understanding their inhibitory mechanisms (5).

Chloramphenicol is a competitor of puromycin and thereby considered to be an inhibitor of the A-site. Several functional groups on the drug are within hydrogen-bonding distance of nucleotides in the peptidyl transferase cavity including G2061, C2452, U2504, G2505 and U2506 (Fig. 5). Two divalent magnesium ions are involved in chloramphenicol binding and mediate some interactions between the drug and the peptidyl transferase cavity. Chloramphenicol binds in the A-site and may interfere with the positioning of the aminoacyl moiety and formation of the transition state.

Erythromycin is a macrolide antibiotic composed of a 14-membered lactone ring, substituted with desosamine and cladinose sugars, which does not block peptide bond formation directly. The ▶ macrolides are believed to function primarily by blocking the nascent peptide from the exit tunnel. Reactive groups of the desosamine sugar and the lactone ring mediate all hydrogen bond interactions with the peptidyl transferase cavity. The second generation derivatives, clarithromycin and roxithromycin, bind to the ribosome in the same

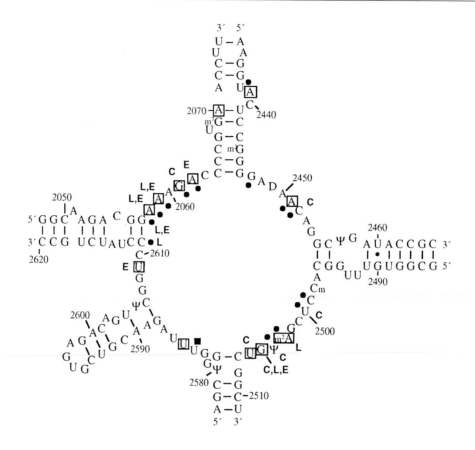

Fig. 5 Nucleotides at the binding sites of chloramphenicol, erythromycin and clindamycin at the peptidyl transferase center. The nucleotides that are within 4.4 Å of the antibiotics chloramphenicol, erythromycin and clindamycin in 50S-antibiotic complexes are indicated with the letters C, E, and L, respectively, on the secondary structure of the peptidyl transferase loop region of 23S rRNA (the sequence shown is that of *E. coli*). The sites of drug resistance in one or more peptidyl transferase antibiotics due to base changes (solid circles) and lack of modification (solid square) are indicated. Nucleotides that display altered chemical reactivity in the presence of one or more peptidyl transferase antibiotics are boxed.

fashion as erythromycin. The 2′-hydroxyl group of the desosamine sugar interacts with the N6 and N1 atoms of A2058, providing an explanation for why A2058 is essential for macrolide binding. Two common macrolide resistance mechanisms include 1) dimethylation of N6 of A2058, and 2) rRNA mutations at A2058. Dimethylation causes steric hindrance and prevents hydrogen bonds to the desosamine sugar. The importance of A2058 for macrolide binding explains the selectivity of macrolides for bacterial ribosomes. Position 2058 is one of a few nucleotides in the peptidyl transferase loop that is not conserved in all phyloge-

netic domains, with the mitochondrial and cytoplasmic 23S rRNAs of larger eukaryotes having a G at this position. Binding of erythromycin and an adjacent magnesium ion reduces the diameter of the peptide tunnel entrance by over 50%, suggesting that macrolides can sterically block progression of the nascent peptide into the tunnel.

Clindamycin, a lincosamide antibiotic, binds to the peptidyl transferase center so as to contact both A- and P-sites. The three hydroxyl groups and carbonyl group on the drug are positioned to interact with nucleotides A2058, A2059, A2503 and G2505 (Fig. 5). Two hydroxyl groups interact with the N6 group of A2058, explaining its importance in lincosamide binding and why modifications or mutations at this position lead to drug resistance. The binding site of clindamycin suggests that it can interfere with the positioning of the 3′-ends of tRNA in the A- and P-sites, while also blocking access to the peptide tunnel.

Summary

The ribosome is currently understood as a dynamic ribonucleoprotein assembly that is an active participant in protein biosynthesis. This view is strongly supported by images of the ribosome (7.5–20 Å resolution) in different functional states obtained from cryoelectron microscopy. Structures of ribosomal subunit-antibiotic complexes have made measurable contributions towards understanding both the universal mechanisms of translation and antibiotic inhibitory mechanisms. The structures illustrate the large diversity of binding sites and strategies to inhibit protein synthesis utilized by ribosome-targeting antibiotics.

In general, antibiotics interfere, either directly or indirectly, with movements of ribosomal components or the positioning of mRNA template or tRNA substrates that are critical for ribosome function. On the 30S subunit, several antibiotics inhibit the relative movement of ribosomal components, either those necessary for translocation (spectinomycin, hygromycin B) or the helix 27 accuracy switch (streptomycin). A family of aminoglycosides (including paromomycin and gentamicin) induces a conformational change in 16S rRNA that is normally induced by a cognate tRNA during the decoding process. Other antibiotics inhibit tRNA binding in the A-site (tetracycline) or displace mRNA (pactamycin), leading to disruption of the E-site tRNA interaction and the Shine-Dalgarno interaction in prokaryotes. In the peptidyl transferase cavity on the 50S subunit, antibiotics interfere with the proper positioning of tRNAs and their movement through the active site (chloramphenicol, clindamycin) or with movement of the nascent peptide into the peptide tunnel (erythromycin). The structures of the ribosome, ribosomal subunits, and their complexes have provided a wealth of molecular detail and have paved the way for rational drug design. This will be important in both modifying existing antibiotics to produce more potent inhibitors and identifying new target sites for drug action on the ribosome.

References

1. Ramakrishnan V, Moore PB (2001) Atomic structures at last: the ribosome in 2000. Curr Opin Struct Biol 11:144–154
2. Nissen P, Hansen J, Ban N, Moore PB, Steitz TA (2000) The structural basis of ribosome activity in peptide bond synthesis. Science 289:920–930
3. Carter AP, Clemons WM, Brodersen DE, Morgan-Warren RJ, Wimberly BT, Ramakrishnan V (2000) Functional insights from the structure of the 30S ribosomal subunit and its interactions with antibiotics. Nature 407:340–348
4. Brodersen DE, Clemons WM, Carter AP, Morgan-Warren RJ, Wimberly BT, Ramakrishnan V (2000) The structural basis for the action of the antibiotics tetracycline, pactamycin and hygromycin B on the 30S ribosomal subunit. Cell 103:1143–1154
5. Schlünzen F, Zarivach R, Harms J, Bashan A, Tocilj A, Albrecht R, Yonath A, Franceschi F (2001) Structural basis for the interaction of antibiotics with the peptidyl transferase centre in eubacteria. Nature 413:814–821

Ribozymes

Ribozymes are small RNA molecules with endoribonuclease activity. Under appropriate conditions, ribozymes exhibit sequence-specific cleavage of the target. The cleaved messenger RNA (mRNA) is destabilised and subject to intracellular degradation.

▶ Antisense Oligonucleotides

Rigidity

Rigidity is muscular stiffness throughout the range of passive movement in a limb segment.

R

Cogwheel rigidity, which is typical for parkinsonism, means that tremor is superimposed on muscle stiffness.

▶ Parkinson's Disease

RNA Editing

RNA-editing is a posttranscriptional mechanism mediated by RNA editases, which results in a site-selective deamination of adenosine to inosine. This alters codons and splicing in nuclear transcripts and thereby alters the structure and function of proteins.

▶ Ionotropic Glutamate Receptors

RNAi

▶ RNA Interference

RNA Interference

RNA interference (RNAi) describes the ability of double-stranded RNA (dsRNA) to induce sequence-specific gene silencing by degradation of messenger RNA (mRNA). RNAi has been discovered in the nematode *C. elegans*, but has been found to work also in a variety of other eukaryotic organisms including mammals. The current model for RNAi suggests that dsRNA is recognized and processed by a group of proteins (e.g. Dicer), which contain an RNA-binding domain and a dsRNA-specific endonuclease domain. These proteins bind to dsRNA and generate small (21-23 nucleotides) dsRNAs called short interfering RNAs (siRNAs). In the RNA-induced silencing complex (RISC), siRNAs bind specifically to mRNAs and direct the cleavage of the target RNA. The cleaved target RNA is then sequentially degraded. The physiological function of RNAi is not completely clear. It may play an important role in protecting the genome against instabilities caused by sequence repetitions and transposons and it may be an antiviral response/protection mechanism. It remains to be shown that RNAi has an integral function in the regulation of gene expression. RNAi has recently developed as a powerful tool to inactivate genes in a variety of organisms.

▶ Antisense Oligonucleotides and RNA Interference

RNA Polymerase II

RNA polymerase II is found in the nucleoplasm where it catalyzes the synthesis of an RNA chain with a sequence complementary to the template strand of DNA in a process known as transcription.

▶ Glucocorticoids

RNA Polymerase Inhibitors

The inhibitors of RNA polymerase, which generates RNA from DNA, inhibit a crucial step in gene expression. Inhibition of the eukaryotic form of RNA polymerase is used in cancer chemotherapy and is also an important experimental tool. For example, actinomycin D binds to the guanine residues in DNA and blocks the movement of the eukaryotic RNA polymerase. Specific inhibitors of bacterial RNA polymerase can be used as antibacterial agents. Most of these inhibitors like rifamycin bind to the prokaryotic enzyme.

RNA Polymerase III Promoter

RNA polymerase III promoters are promoters expressing transfer RNAs (tRNAs), U6 small nuclear (sn) RNAs, and adenovirus (Ad) virus associated (VA) RNAs which are transcribed by RNA polymerase III. They produce small, compact RNAs that possess stability in the intracellular environment.

▶ Antisense Oligonucleotides

RNAse

RNAse is an enzyme that catalyses the breakdown of RNA molecules into their component nucleotides. RNAses are extremely common in the modern world, resulting in very short lifespans for any RNA that is not in a protected environment.

▶ Antisense Oligonucleotides

RTK

▶ Receptor Tyrosine Kinase

RT-PCR

This acronym stands for Reverse Transcriptase Polymerase Chain Reaction, a method used to first copy a strand of RNA into cDNA, then amplify it through standard PCR methods.

▶ Gene Expression Analysis

RXR

▶ Retinoid X Receptor

Ryanodine Receptor

YASUO OGAWA, NAGOMI KUREBAYASHI, TAKASHI MURAYAMA
Department of Pharmacology, Juntendo University School of Medicine, Tokyo, Japan
ysogawa@med.juntendo.ac.jp,
nagomik@med.juntendo.ac.jp,
takashim@med.juntendo.ac.jp

Synonyms

Ca^{2+} release channel, Ca^{2+}-induced Ca^{2+} release (CICR) channel, foot or depolarization-induced Ca^{2+} release (DICR) channel

Definition

Ryanodine receptor is a Ca^{2+} release channel protein in the ▶ sarcoplasmic reticulum (SR) or the endoplasmic reticulum that binds [^{3}H]ryanodine, after which it is named, with high affinity in a Ca^{2+}-dependent way. A monomer of about 5000 amino acid residues (~560 kD) is divided into a large hydrophilic N-terminal domain on the cytoplasmic side and a small hydrophobic C-terminal domain (1/10–1/5) containing 4–8 transmembrane domains, with both N- and C-termini in the cytoplasm (Fig. 1). Its homotetramer (Fig. 2) is active as a Ca^{2+} release channel which can primarily be opened by Ca^{2+} that binds to the high-affinity activating Ca^{2+}-site (▶ CICR). In skeletal muscle, however, gating by the conformation change of the voltage sensor, i. e., the α1S subunit of ▶ dihydropyridine receptor (DHPR), is of physiological relevance (▶ DICR). CICR in skeletal muscle is involved rather in pathological conditions such as in malignant hyperthermia. CICR is physiologically important in cardiac and smooth muscle contraction.

▶ Voltage-dependent Ca^{2+} Channels

Basic Characteristics

There are three genetically distinct isoforms of the ryanodine receptor (RyR) in mammals: RyR1 pri-

R

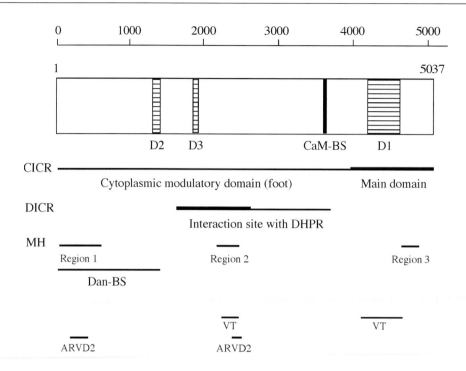

Fig. 1 Schematic illustration of characteristic structure and function of monomeric RyR. Common structural characteristics are depicted with RyR1 as the representative of the three isoforms. D1, D2, and D3 represent regions of high sequence diversity among RyR1-3 isoforms. D2 is characteristically missing in RyR3. CaM-BS, calmodulin binding sites. About 1000 residues in the C-terminal side compose the main channel-forming domain, which can essentially function as a Ca^{2+} channel, including putative ryanodine-, Ca^{2+}- and ATP-binding sites, and hydrophobic 4, 6 or 8 transmembrane segments. A large hydrophilic N-terminal region lies in the cytoplasm and serves as the regulatory (modulatory) domain. Both the N- and C-termini are detected in the cytoplasmic side. An amino acid mutation of RyR1 in malignant hyperthermia (MS) can be detected in regions 1–3. Dan-BS, dantrolene binding site. Recently, familial ventricular tachycardia in the absence of any evidence of structural myocardial disease (VT) and with accompanying right ventricular dysplasia (ARVD2) have been determined to be caused by a missense mutation in RyR2, whose functional changes are not yet examined. Notably, the mutated sites well correspond to those of MH in RyR1. Inositol trisphosphate (IP3) receptor, another Ca^{2+} release channel opened by IP3 that occurs mainly in cells other than striated muscles, shows similar characteristics in its primary structure: of the total ~2700 amino acid residues, a large hydrophilic N-terminal region that is further divided into IP3-binding domain (~600 N-terminal residues) and regulatory domain (~1600 residues), and a small hydrophobic C-terminal region containing 6 or 8 transmembrane segments which show a higher similarity to the counterparts of RyR. The unit conductance of RyR/Ca^{2+} release channel is ~600 pS with Na^+ or K^+ and ~100 pS wih Ca^{2+}, whereas that of IP3-R/Ca^{2+} release channel is about 5 times less than that of RyR.

marily in the skeletal muscles, RyR2 in the cardiac muscle and in the brain, albeit in a lesser amount, and RyR3 ubiquitously in various organs and tissues, but in such a miniscule amount that only the sensitive Western blot can detect occurrence of the isoform. This distribution of each isoform is also true in other vertebrates, except that their genetic loci have not yet been determined and two iso-

forms (RyR1 and RyR3 homologues, also referred to as α- and β-RyR, respectively) are detected in similar amounts in many vertebrate skeletal muscles. A huge integral membrane protein that shares the molecular characteristics described above was also detected in *C. elegans*, fruit fly and recently in sea urchin eggs. Descriptions, however, are limited to vertebrate RyRs.

cytoplasmic face   parallel to membrane

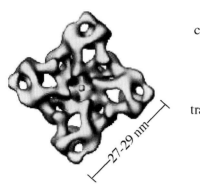

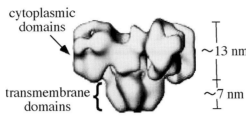

cytoplasmic domains

transmembrane domains

~13 nm

~7 nm

27-29 nm

Fig. 2 Ryanodine receptor (calcium release channel) viewed from the cytoplasmic face and parallel to the membrane. 3D reconstruction of tetrameric RyR/calcium release channel; courtesy of Dr. T. Wagenknecht (3).

Ryanodine, an alkaloid, is well known for its action of inducing a slowly appearing but robust and sustained ▶ contracture of vertebrate skeletal muscles. The underlying mechanism was found to be the binding of ryanodine to CICR channels at the open state, holding them at this state. Using these characteristics, the binding protein, i. e., RyR was isolated from skeletal (RyR1) and cardiac (RyR2) muscles. Electron microscopic observation of the isolated RyR1 (Fig. 2) proved that its cytoplasmic part is the foot, the electron dense material spanning between the ▶ T-tubule and the junctional face of ▶ SR (TC), which plays the most critical role in ▶ excitation-contraction coupling (▶ EC coupling) in skeletal muscle (see Fig. 3A). The myotube from DHPR-deficient mice (dysgenic mice), which die of asphyxia at birth, shows no muscle contraction or charge movements reflecting conformation change of the L-type Ca^{2+} channel molecules in the T-tubule by electrical stimulation. Nowadays, DHPR in the T-tubule of skeletal muscle serves as the voltage sensor, the conformation change of which is transmitted to RyR1 resulting in Ca^{2+} release, i. e., DICR.

Fig. 3B shows details of relative positions of feet and tetrads (four assembled DHPRs in a cluster). Two (in some cases three) rows of feet are aligned in the junctional face of the SR (TC), and tetrads are located in the T-tubule in precise register opposite alternate feet. In cardiac muscle and probably also in smooth muscle, however, neither this tight relationship between tetrads and feet nor tetrads themselves are observed, although feet are clustered around DHPRs which appear as large intramembranous particles. The myotube from

RyR1-deficient mice, which die of asphyxia at birth, shows loss of foot (dyspedic mice) that is recovered by expression of RyR1. Tetrads could be observed only when RyR1 was expressed in dyspedic myotubes, but not when RyR2 or RyR3 was expressed. This means that neither RyR2 nor RyR3 induces tetrad formation. DHPRs primarily act as channels for Ca^{2+} influx in cardiac and smooth muscles. In skeletal muscle, in contrast, they serve as voltage sensors rather than Ca^{2+} channels (see later). A RyR2-deficient embryo, incidentally, dies at an early stage of development, whereas RyR3-deficient mice do not show obvious abnormality.

The CICR activity of RyR is evaluated by Ca^{2+}-dependent [3H]ryanodine binding with a stoichiometry of 1 mol per mol of a tetramer with K_D of 2–3 nM or larger, depending on the experimental conditions, also by Ca^{2+}-activated channel activity on the lipid bilayer membrane, and by CICR from isolated SR vesicles in *in vitro* experiments, whereas by ▶ Ca^{2+} transients and ▶ Ca^{2+} sparks in *in situ* or *in vivo* experiments. Reliable determination of DICR is made in *in vivo* experiments.

The opening of RyR is activated by Ca^{2+} at a concentration lower than 0.1 mM (EC_{50} ~10 μM) and inhibited by Ca^{2+} at a concentration higher than this (IC_{50} ~3 mM). This biphasic Ca^{2+} dependence can be explained by Ca^{2+} binding to high affinity activating Ca^{2+} sites (A-sites) and to low affinity inactivating Ca^{2+} sites (I-sites) of RyR. RyR1 is more variable than RyR3 in Ca^{2+} sensitivity among animal species and muscle fiber types: EC_{50} is varied between 1 and 10 μM. RyR1 diversity is also found in the amino acid identity and in mobility on SDS-PAGE. Whereas RyR3 is more

R

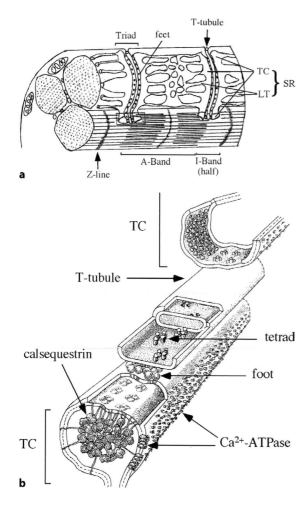

Fig. 3 Mammalian skeletal muscle (a) and the apparatus essential for EC coupling (b). The T-tubule invaginates at the A–I junction of mammalian skeletal muscle. TC, terminal cisternae of the SR; LT, longitudinal tubule of the SR. Panels A and B were partly modified from (6) and (7), respectively.

homogeneous in these properties, the content is varied among animal species, muscle fiber types and ages. Although there are many reports that the sensitivity to Ca^{2+} of RyR2 is higher in the A-sites and lower in the I-sites than RyR1, some investigators insist there is no significant difference between the two isoforms. It should be noted that channel activity of RyR (particularly RyR2 and RyR3) when incorporated into the lipid bilayer membrane may show a different Ca^{2+} dependence: It is much steeper, and there is higher sensitivity

to stimulating Ca^{2+} and weaker inhibition at higher Ca^{2+}. These differences are partly due to the greater vulnerability of RyR2 and RyR3 to oxidation in the lipid bilayer membrane.

The CICR activity including [^{3}H]ryanodine binding and channel activity on the lipid bilayer membrane is modulated by endogenous substances, particularly Mg^{2+} and ATP. Mg^{2+} serves as an antagonist to Ca^{2+} in the A-sites and as an agonist of Ca^{2+} in the I-sites. The A-site shows as much as 20–30 fold preference for Ca^{2+} over Mg^{2+}, but the I-site shows no preference between the two cations. Mg^{2+}, therefore, shifts the pCa-activity relationship to a higher Ca^{2+} concentration range with reduced peak activity. The inhibitory effect of Mg^{2+}, in other words, depends on the Ca^{2+} concentration where the effect is examined. Cytoplasmic Mg^{2+} concentration is estimated to be 1 mM in striated muscles and about 0.5 mM in smooth muscle or non-muscle cells. The EC_{50} for Ca^{2+} in CICR in the frog skeletal muscle myoplasm was estimated to be 30 µM, whereas in tension development of myofibrils it was around 2 µM.

AMPPCP, an unhydrolyzable analog of ATP, increases the peak activity alone without any change in the Ca^{2+} dependence of CICR. This effect is also observed with ATP, ADP and AMP, whose stimulating effects are irrespective of free, Ca^{2+}- or Mg^{2+}-complexed form. The CICR activity including [^{3}H]ryanodine binding and channel activity, A, can be expressed by the equation, $A = A_{max} * f_A * (1-f_I)$ where f_A and f_I stand for fractional ratios for A- and I-sites occupied by Ca^{2+} and/or Mg^{2+}, respectively, and A_{max} represents the maximum attainable activity under the experimental condition. The effect of an adenine nucleotide is to increase A_{max} alone without changing f_A or f_I. The maximum attainable activity (A_{max}), therefore, is not fixed but variable, depending on the experimental conditions. This finding means that occupation of the A-sites by Ca^{2+} is a necessary but not sufficient condition for CICR.

In skeletal muscle, Ca^{2+} influx is not necessary for contraction by electrical stimulation. As shown in Fig. 3B, half of RyR1s are coupled with DHPR, but the other half are uncoupled. Therefore it might be possible that the Ca^{2+} released from coupled RyR1 enhances CICR from uncoupled RyR1. The rate of CICR under conditions simulating the myoplasm, in the presence of 1 mM Mg^{2+} and 4–

8 mM ATP, was estimated to be $10-20$ min^{-1} at most in skinned frog skeletal muscle fibers, whereas DICR was estimated to be $1200-3000$ min^{-1}. Even if RyR were to become insensitive to Mg^{2+}, the rate of CICR would be no more than 100 min^{-1}. The rate of CICR in skeletal muscle is so low that its contribution to DICR that is of physiological relevance in electrical stimulation of muscle would be minor. CICR is, however, critically involved in the mechanism underlying ▶ malignant hyperthermia where missense mutation in a single amino acid residue of RyR1 is in many cases believed to be the cause (see Fig. 1).

In the SR membrane, RyR is complexed with FKBP12 (or 12.6) and calmodulin with a stoichiometry of each of 1 mol/mol of RyR monomer on the cytoplasmic side, and with calsequestrin and triadin in the luminal side, which can modulate CICR activity. These may be reflected in the finding that the affinities of A- and I-sites for Ca^{2+} and Mg^{2+} in [3H]ryanodine binding to purified RyR1 and 3 are lower than those of CICR channels in the native SR, keeping the selectivity of Ca^{2+} over Mg^{2+} unchanged. Notably, the native RyR1 in the SR is selectively suppressed in [3H]ryanodine binding, whereas purified RyR1 and RyR3 show indistinguishable binding. Scatchard plot analysis showed that the dissociation constant was greatly increased without change in the maximum number of binding sites. This means that all RyR1 channels are active, but their A_{max} is reduced; the mechanism underlying this remains to be elucidated. Therefore, CICR in frog skeletal muscle is largely performed by RyR3 or β-RyR.

In contrast, in cardiac and smooth muscles and non-muscle cells where the contraction or the biological responses depend largely on the Ca^{2+} inflow from the medium, CICR is critically important. Dimensions of these cells are small, and the response cannot be as fast as in DICR in skeletal muscles. Correspondingly, RyR2 and RyR3 accomplish CICR alone, whereas RyR1 performs not only CICR but also DICR. It should be mentioned that RyR2 appears to show much higher rate of CICR than RyR1, because CICR in cardiac ventricle muscles is too fast to determine its time course by the method adopted in skeletal muscle.

For DICR, RyR1 must closely interact with DHPR (see Fig. 3B); a conformation change in DHPR upon depolarization of T-tubule causes an opening of the gate of RyR1 (orthograde signaling) and the existence of RyR1 induces a tetrad formation of DHPR and enhances Ca^{2+} entry through the L-type channel (retrograde signaling). The critical site of DHPR for interactions is the cytoplasmic loop connecting domains (or repeats) II and III of α1S subunit (II-III loop) of DHPR. The counterpart in RyR1 is suggested to be a region between 1635 and 2636 amino acid residues. A region, $2569-3720$ of RyR1 also seems to be required for retrograde signaling (Fig. 1). The interaction sites are quite likely to be multiple and further investigations are required.

Drugs

Ryanodine and its derivatives (Ryanoids): A neutral alkaloid from the ground stem wood and root of *Ryania speciosa* Vahl. It specifically binds to the open state of the CICR channel/RyR, but not to the closed state, which enabled the isolation and identification of RyR.

This effect of sustained opening results in the increase of the cytoplasmic Ca^{2+} and robust, but characteristically slowly appearing contracture in skeletal muscles because the released Ca^{2+} remains within the myoplasm. In cardiac muscles, however, negative inotropism, i.e., decrease in cardiac contraction is the effect, because the released Ca^{2+} is rapidly extruded out of the sarcoplasm, largely by the Na^+-Ca^{2+}-exchange reaction. In the lipid bilayer membrane experiments, persistent subconductance state was observed. In a high concentration of 10 µM or more, the channel was reported to be closed again; but in the ▶ skinned fiber no closing was observed and the store remained depleted. The natural ryanodine is very slow in its binding and action, and faster derivatives are being synthesized as tools for investigation.

Caffeine

This drug increases CICR activity by two actions: increase in the affinity for Ca^{2+} alone in only the A-site and increase in the maximum attainable activity (A_{max}). The former effect reached the maximum at 10 mM, whereas the latter effect increased beyond this. The latter effect is more potent in frog than in mammalian skeletal muscles, whereas the former effect is similar. It also increases ► twitch response at a low concentration.

Caffeine-like drugs

Halothane and inhalation general anesthetics, phenols (thymol, 4-chloro-m-cresol, 4-chloro-3-ethyl-phenol and others), and quercetin stimulated CICR in a way similar to that of caffeine. The details, however, remain to be elucidated.

Imperatoxin A

Imperatoxin A is a basic peptide of 33 amino acid residues obtained from the venom of the African scorpion *Pandinus imperator*. It was first believed to be an activator specific to RyR1, but later it was realized that RyR2 and RyR3 were also stimulated.

-SH Modulators (oxidized form of glutathione, Ag2+, Hg-compounds, alkylating and NO producing chemicals)

Oxidation (or modifications) of some -SH thiols reversibly increased CICR activity, whereas more extensive modification inactivated the channel irreversibly. Stimulated channels show an increased sensitivity to activators such as Ca^{2+}, an adenine nucleotide and caffeine, whereas they show less inhibition by Mg^{2+} and a high concentration of Ca^{2+}.

FK506

FK506 removes FKBP12 or 12.6 from RyR1 or RyR2, resulting in activation of channel activity. At high concentration, FK506 shows a direct stimulatory effect on [^{3}H]ryanodine binding.

Procaine and Tetracaine

Procaine and Tetracaine decrease CICR activity. Their inhibition is independent of Ca^{2+}, and thus the reduction in the maximum attainable activity (A_{max}) is probably of primary importance.

Dantrolene

Dantrolene is an antidote for malignant hyperthermia without having impact on cardiac performance; therefore, there is no effect on RyR2.

[^{3}H]Ryanodine binding to RyR1 and RyR3 is decreased. It was reported that the drug was effective in suppression of twitch but was less effective on ► tetanus.

Ruthenium Red

Ruthenium Red inhibits CICR, [^{3}H]ryanodine binding and channel activity, but does not inhibit Ca^{2+}-pump activity. It also inhibits mitochondrial function.

Cyclic ADP Ribose (cADPR)

It was first shown that cADPR was increased in sea urchin eggs activated by fertilization, resulting in Ca^{2+} release through a RyR-like channel. In mammalian cells, the action of the reagent was reported to be dependent on the isoform; many investigators reported that RyR2 is sensitive to cADPR, but some investigators claimed that it is RyR3 that is sensitive to the reagent.

References

1. Franzini-Armstrong C, Protasi F (1997) Ryanodine receptor of striated muscles: a complex channel capable of multiple interactions. Physiol Rev 77:699–72

2. Zucchi R, Ronca-Testoni S (1997) The sarcoplasmic reticulum Ca2+ channel/ryanodine receptor: modulation by endogenous effectors, drugs and disease states. Pharmcol Rev 49:1–51

3. Wagenknecht T, Radermacher M (1997) Ryanodine receptor: structure and macromolecular interactions. Curr Opin Struct Biol 7:258–265

4. Ogawa Y, Kurebayashi N, Murayama T (1999) Ryanodine receptor isoforms in excitation-contraction coupling. Adv Biophys 36:27–64

5. MacLennan D H (2000) Ca2+ signaling and muscle disease. Eur J Biochem 267:5291–5297

6. Fawcett DW (1994) Bloom and Fawcett's A Textbook of Histology, 12th ed., Chapman & Hall, New York and London, p278

7. Block B, Imagawa T, Campbell KP, Franzini-Armstrong C (1988) J Cell Biol 107:258–2600 (The Rockefeller University Press)

S

S-adenosyl-L-methionine

S-adenosyl -L-methionine (AdoMet, SAM) is a cofactor and the most important donor of the methyl (CH_3-) group for methyltransferases, including COMT. When the methyl-group has been transferred, the remaining demethylated compound is called S-adenosyl-L-homocysteine.

► Catechol-O-Methyltransferase and its Inhibitors

Salicylate

► Non-steroidal Antiinflammatory Drugs

SAM

► S-adenosyl -L-methionine

Sarafotoxin

Sarafotoxin is a 21-amino acid peptide which has some structural similarity with endothelins and was isolated from the venom of the burrowing asp. Sarafotoxin is a selective agonist of the endothelin ET_B-receptor.

► Endothelins

Sarcolemma

The sarcolemma is the plasma membrane of muscle cells.

Sarcoplasmic Reticulum

The sarcoplasmic reticulum (SR) is equivalent to the smooth-surfaced endoplasmic reticulum (ER) which functions as an intracellular Ca^{2+} store. In skeletal muscle, it is notionally divided into two parts, the terminal cisternae (TC) and longitudinal tubules (LT) whose luminal space is assumed to be continuous. The Ca^{2+} release channel/ryanodine receptor (RyR) is located only in the junctional face of the TC, whereas the Ca^{2+} pump protein (SERCA protein) is closely packed over the entire area of the SR.

► Ryanodine Receptor

SARMs

► Selective Androgen Receptor Modulators

Saxitoxin

Saxitoxin (STX) is a toxin which is found in marine microorganisms. It is most likely synthesized by bacteria which live in symbiosis with dinoflagellates, a component of phytoplankton. Through the marine food chain, it can lead to poisoning of humans. The mechanism of toxicity of saxitoxin is very similar to that of tetrodotoxin. Saxitoxin binds from the outside of the membrane to various forms of voltage-sensitive Na^+ channels and blocks the channel in an activation state-independent manner.

▶ Voltage-dependent Na^+ Channels

Scaffolding Proteins

Scaffolding proteins are proteins, which are able to bind several other proteins in order to organize these interacting proteins into functional complexes. Scaffold proteins often guide the interactions between components in such complexes. This allows, for instance in signaling cascades, a precise relay of the signal with high speed and efficiency. Scaffolding proteins also avoid unwanted cross-talk between different functional protein complexes.

In *Drosophila* eyes, the light-activated TRP channel is organized into a supramolecular complex, the "transducisome", along with other transduction proteins, such as phospholipase C (PLC) and protein kinase C, through association with the scaffolding protein INAD, a multi PDZ domain-containing protein. The mammalian TRPC4 is associated with calmodulin, the inositol 1,4,5-triphosphate (IP_3)-receptor and, *via* the scaffolding protein ezrin-binding phospho protein 50 or NHERF, with PLC and the actin cytoskeleton.

▶ TRP Channels

Scatchard Plot

A Scatchard plot is a plot of *B*/x against B (where *B* is the amount of bound ligand and x is the ligand concentration), which is used to estimate the maximal binding, B_{max} as well as the binding affinity (*K*).

Schild Analysis

Schild analysis is a very powerful method to quantify the potency of a competitive antagonist and to test whether the blockade of response by a molecule is consistent with simple competitive antagonism. Devised by Arunlakshana and Schild (1959), it is based on the principle that the antagonist-induced dextral displacement of a dose-response curve is due to its potency (K_{eq} value, ▶ affinity) and its concentration in the receptor compartment. Since the antagonism can be observed and the concentration of antagonist is known, the K_{eq} (denoted K_B for antagonist) can be calculated. The relationship between antagonism and concentration must be log-linear with a unit slope to adhere to true competitive kinetics.

▶ Drug-receptor Interaction

Schizophrenia

Schizophrenia is a psychiatric disorder characterized by a number of psychotic manifestations including delusions, hallucinations, disorganized thinking and behaviour, amotivation, paucity of thought and speech, flat affect and anhedonia. The aetiology of schizophrenia is thought to involve a combination of genetic and environmental factors. While florid symptoms most commonly present in adolescence or early adulthood, they are usually preceded by premorbid changes in personality and social functioning. Diagnosis is made after exclusion of other causes of psychotic symptoms (e.g. head injury, cerebrovascular accident, substance intoxication) and based on the presence of at least two clinical manifestations present for at least six months in the presence of social dysfunction (DSM-IV criteria). Classical antipsychotic drugs (dopamine D2-like receptor blockers) are effective in reducing the positive symptoms of schizophrenia (delusions, hallucinations) but are less useful in treating the negative symptoms of the disorder (loss of affect, withdrawal).

▶ Antipsychotic Drugs

Secondary Aldosteronism

In secondary aldosteronism, the plasma aldosterone concentration is above the normal range, due to various pathophysiological states (cardiac congestive failure, cirrhosis).

▶ Epithelial Na$^+$ Channel

Second Messenger

A second messenger is an intracellular metabolite or ion whose concentration is altered when a receptor is activated by an agonist (or "first messenger").

Secretory Pathway

Transport of proteins and lipids occurs between the organelles of the secretory pathway, i.e. endoplasmic reticulum (ER), Golgi, endosomes, lysosomes and the plasma membrane.

▶ Intracellular Transport

Sedatives

Sedatives decrease activity, moderate excitement and calm the recipient. In contrast to hypnotic drugs, they do not produce drowsiness and do not facilitate the onset and maintenance of sleep. The most important group of sedatives are the benzodiazepines given at low or moderate doses.

▶ Benzodiazepins

Seizure

A seizure is an abnormal behavioural (often motoric) activity caused by abnormal electrical activity of the brain. Seizures can be the symptom of a chronic neurological malfunction, i.e. ▶ epilepsy, or can appear as single events, e.g. during fever in infants.

▶ Antiepileptic Drugs

Selectins

The three selectins are related both structurally and functionally. They are transmembrane proteins, with an N-terminal C-type actin domain, followed by an EGF repeat and a variable number of complement control protein (CCP) domains. Selectins bind carbohydrates, which are present in various glycoproteins.

▶ Inflammation
▶ Table appendix: Adhesion Molecules

S

Selective Androgen Receptor Modulators

Selective Androgen Receptor Modulators (SARMs) are androgen receptor (AR) ligands that display tissue-specific androgenic/antiandrogenic activities.

▶ Selective Sex-steroid Receptor Modulators

Selective Estrogen Receptor Modulators

Selective estrogen receptor modulators (SERMs) are synthetic compounds with partially agonistic and partially antagonistic estrogenic properties. In bone, selective estrogen receptor modulators (SERM) inhibit bone resorption *via* the mechanisms known for estrogens. Major SERMs are tamoxifen, a triphenylethylene compound, and raloxifene. In postmenopausal women, the latter has been shown to prevent bone loss and to reduce fracture risk by 40%.

▶ Selective Sex-steroid Receptor Modulators

Selective Noradrenaline Reuptake Inhibitors

Selective noradrenaline reuptake inhibitors (SNRIs) are a group of drugs, which act as antidepressants by the selective inhibition of the reuptake of noradrenaline from the synaptic cleft *via* the selective blockade of the noradrenaline-specific neurontransmitter transporter (e.g. reboxetine).

▶ Antidepressants
▶ Neurotransmitter Transporters

Selective Progesterone Receptors Modulators

Selective progesterone receptor modulators (SPRMs, mesoprogestins) are progesterone receptor (PR) ligands that exhibit agonistic and antagonistic activities. Examples are J876 and J1042.

▶ Selective Sex-steroid Receptor Modulators

Selective Serotonine Reuptake Inhibitors

Selective serotonine reuptake inhibitor (SSRI) is an abbreviation for the class of antidepressants known as the Selective Serotonin Reuptake Inhibitors. Examples of SSRIs include fluoxetine (Prozac), paroxetine (Paxil), citalopram (Celexa) and sertraline (Zoloft). These drugs selectively inhibit the serotonin transporter thus prolonging the synaptic lifespan of the neurotransmitter serotonin.

▶ Antidepressants
▶ Neurotransmitter Transporters

Selective Sex-steroid Receptor Modulators

JULIE M. HALL, KENNETH S. KORACH
National Institute of Environmental Health Sciences, Research Triangle Park, NC USA
hall8@niehs.nih.gov, korach@niehs.nih.gov

Synonyms

Mixed agonists/antagonists; tissue-specific agonists/antagonists

Definition

Selective sex-steroid receptor modulators are compounds that mimic the effects of sex steroids in some tissues, while at the same time can oppose endogenous hormone action in other tissues.

▶ Gluco-/Mineralocorticoid Receptors
▶ Sex Steroid Receptors

Background

The sex steroids comprise a class of hormones including ▶ estrogens, ▶ progestins and ▶ androgens that play important roles in the development and maintenance of the male and female reproductive systems. In addition, sex steroids have functions in tissues other than those related to reproduction. For example, estrogen is involved in the development and maintenance of skeletal integrity and is an important regulator of triglyceride and cholesterol homeostasis. Not all of the biological functions of the sex steroids are beneficial, however, as chronic simulation by estrogens, progestins and androgens has been implicated in the genesis and progression of cancers in a number of tissues. The necessity for compounds that retain the beneficial effects of sex steroids in some tissues but oppose the action of endogenous hormone in others has resulted in the generation of a novel class of pharmaceuticals termed selective steroid receptor modulators (SSRMs). This chapter will focus primarily on known ▶ selective estrogen receptor modulators (SERMs), which represent a class of pharmaceuticals used clinically for cancer and osteoporosis, and for sustaining beneficial effects of estrogen in postmenopausal women (1,4,5). The general mechanisms of SERMs are similar to that of ▶ selective progesteron receptor modulators (SPRMs) and ▶ selective androgen receptor modulators (SARMs), which are currently in development for the treatment of progesterone- and androgen-associated pathologies, respectively.

Mechanism of Action

Targeting Estrogen Action in a Tissue-Specific Manner: The SERM Concept

The ovarian hormone estrogen is a key regulator of the processes involved in the growth, differenti-ation and function of a wide variety of tissues of diverse functions. The importance of estrogen in sustaining overall health is evidenced by the adverse effects of hormone deficiency in postmenopausal women who experience increased hot flashes, depression, cardiovascular disease, and losses in bone mineral density that often lead to osteoporosis. These observations have led to the development of ▶ estrogen replacement therapies (ERT), where premenopausal estrogen levels are restored and the symptoms of menopause are alleviated. The best studied responses are in bone, where ERT can decrease the incidence of hip fractures by 50%, and in the central nervous system, where up to 90% inhibition of hot flashes is observed. ERT has also been shown to be associated with improvement in cognitive function in postmenopausal women and may delay the onset of Alzheimer's disease (1,4).

Although the positive effects of ERT have been well established, it has been shown that the cell proliferative actions of estrogen can increase the incidence of breast cancer in some patients. In addition, duration of exposure to physiological levels of unopposed estrogens is an established risk factor for breast, uterine and ovarian cancer. In an effort to attain pharmaceutical agents that oppose the carcinogenic actions of estrogens, ▶ antiestrogens have been developed, and are being used clinically for the treatment of ▶ estrogen receptor (ER)-positive breast cancers. The necessity for compounds that retain the beneficial effects of estrogen in some tissues has resulted in the generation of a novel class of antiestrogens (SERMs) that display tissue-specific ▶ agonist and ▶ antagonist activities (1,4,5).

Molecular Mechanisms of SERM Action as a Means of Understanding their Tissue-Selective Activities

The molecular pharmacology of estrogens and antiestrogens is complex. It is clear, however, that all of these compounds mediate their biological activities through two intracellular receptors, the ERs (ERα and ERβ) that function as ligand-inducible transcription factors in target cell nuclei (4). Hormone binding to the receptors transduces the endocrine signal into genomic responses, resulting in the up-regulation or down-regulation of specific genes at the messenger RNA (mRNA) level. The mRNAs are then translated into pro-

S

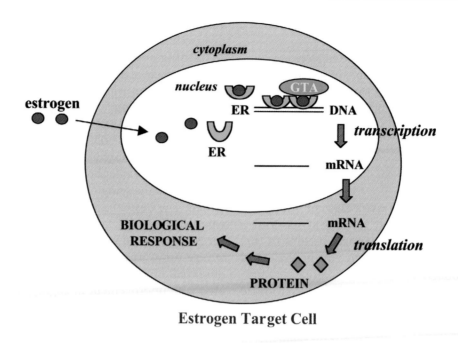

Estrogen Target Cell

Fig. 1 The Biological Effects of Estrogens are Mediated through Nuclear Estrogen Receptors. Hormone diffuses into target cells where it binds to nuclear estrogen receptors (ER). This event induces a conformational change in ERs that enables the receptor to bind to the regulatory region of estrogen-responsive genes. The DNA-bound ER interacts with components of the general transcriptional apparatus (GTA) to induce gene transcription. The resultant mRNAs are transported into the cell cytoplasm where they are translated into proteins. These proteins function with the cell to mediate biological responses.

teins that function within the cells of hormone-responsive tissues to regulate proliferation, differentiation and homeostasis (Fig. 1).

Ligand binding is the event that initiates ER signaling. According to classical receptor theory, agonists (such as endogenous estrogens) act as molecular switches, converting ER from an inactive to an active form. Antiestrogens, synthetic compounds developed to oppose the action of natural hormone, were thought to competitively inhibit agonist binding and in doing so were able to lock the receptor in a latent state. Thus, it was considered that when corrected for affinity that all agonists were functionally indistinguishable, and likewise, antagonists were all the same. However, the existence of SERMs indicated that this model is oversimplified, as it does not account for the biology of known antiestrogens. Some of the first evidence that antiestrogens do more than freeze ER in a latent state and thus play a more active role in ER action came from clinical studies of patients

that were administered tamoxifen (see below, SERMs) as adjuvant therapy for estrogen-dependent breast tumors. Strikingly, while tamoxifen blocked the actions of estrogen in breast cancer cells, it was shown to function as an agonist in bone and the uterus, mimicking the actions of estrogen. The observation that tamoxifen displays tissue-specific agonist/antagonist activities was inconsistent with the classical definition of antagonist action, and furthermore, suggested that this compound may alter ER in such a way that the ligand-bound receptor would be recognized differently in distinct cell types (4).

The concept that different ligands play an active role in ER function is apparent at the biochemical level. In addition to competitive inhibition of estrogen binding, antiestrogens induce unique conformations/structures of both ERα and ERβ. This provides a structural basis for the unique biological activities displayed by the different compounds (4).

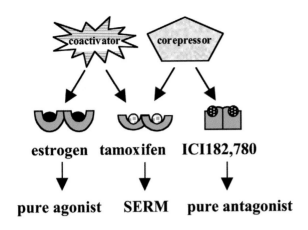

Fig. 2 Cofactor Binding is Regulated by the Structure of the Ligand-ER Complex. Different ligands induce distinct conformations of ER (estrogen receptor), leading to differential cofactor recruitment. Pure agonists like estrogen, drive the receptor into a structure compatible with coactivator binding, whereas pure antagonists (ICI182,780) induce a conformation recognized by corepressors. SERMs such as tamoxifen, which display both agonist and antagonist activities on ER, permit the receptor to interact with either coactivators or corepressors.

The understanding of diversity in ligand-mediated ER activity was advanced by the discovery of transcriptional cofactors. These proteins, termed ▶ co-activators and ▶ co-repressors, bind the ligand-bound ER and enhance or decrease ER-mediated transcription of target genes, respectively. The ability of different ER agonists and antagonists to induce different conformations of the receptors influences the binding of coactivators and corepressors to the receptors (Fig. 2). Different ligands induce unique structural changes in ER that result in differential recruitment of coactivators and corepressors, leading to diversity in biological response. This provides a mechanism by which different ligands acting through the same receptor can mediate unique biological effects (4). For example, estrogen induces coactivator recruitment to ER, whereas when bound to the pure antiestrogen ICI 182,780, the conformation of ER is compatible with corepressor (but not coactivator) binding. Correspondingly, estrogen is a full agonist of ER, while ICI functions as a pure antagonist

on the receptor. In contrast, when bound to the SERM tamoxifen, which displays both agonist and antagonist activities, ER is capable of interacting with either coactivators or corepressors. It is likely that diversity in the availability of coactivators or corepressors in different target cells may be the mechanism underlying the tissue-specific agonist/antagonist activities of tamoxifen and other SERMs. Thus, it will be important to identify the cofactor proteins present in different ER target cells in order to allow mechanistic screening for new tissue-targeted SERMs.

Clinical Use

Mechanistic Classes of Antiestrogens and SERMs

ER antagonists comprise two broad categories: pure antiestrogens and SERMs. A summary of the different biological functions associated with some of the known antiestrogens is displayed in Table 1.

Pure Antiestrogens

Pure antiestrogens, represented by ICI 182,780, oppose estrogen and ER activity in all tissues (4). In theory, these properties make Type I antiestrogens useful in cancer therapy since they block the carcinogenic effects of estrogen in the breast and reproductive system. However, since ICI 182,780 lacks the beneficial agonist effects of estrogen in bone and in the cardiovascular and central nervous systems, the clinical use of this compound is limited. Another pure antiestrogen, EM-800, has

Tab. 1 Biological Activities of ER Ligands in Selected Target Tissues.

	bone	breast	cardio-vasculature	uterus
estrogen	+++	+++	+++	+++
ICI182,780	-	-	-	-
tamoxifen	+	-	+	+
raloxifene	+	-	+	-
lasoxifene	++	-	++	-

+ denotes agonist activity
- denotes antagonist activity

benefits in breast cancer patients who have become resistant to tamoxifen (see below). Since EM-800 also prevents bone loss and lowers serum lipids, it is currently being used in late-stage clinical trials in breast cancer patients (2).

SERMs

First Generation. The triphenylethylene tamoxifen (Nolvadex) is the best characterized SERM, used clinically since 1971. The notable antagonist effects of tamoxifen in the breast make it a first line therapy for the treatment of pre- and postmenopausal women with estrogen-responsive advanced (stage IV) breast cancer. In addition to the use in the prevention and treatment of cancer, tamoxifen has very beneficial effects in the maintenance of bone mineral density and decreases serum triglyceride (LDL) levels in postmenopausal women. Unfortunately, the estrogenic activity of tamoxifen provides for undesirable uterotrophic effects, leading to an increased risk for endometrial cancer in women undergoing prolonged tamoxifen therapy. Similar to that seen in women on ERT, tamoxifen also induces ovarian cysts due to its agonist activity in the ovary. An additional concern has been the observed development of "tamoxifen resistance" in a significant proportion of women after 5 years of antiestrogen therapy. This term refers to the phenomenon by which certain breast cancers alter their biology and recognize the compound as an agonist for growth. Other tamoxifen-derived compounds such as toremifene, droloxifene and idoxifene are currently being evaluated in clinical studies for their potential long-term beneficial effects in antagonizing ER-positive breast tumor growth (1,3,5).

Second Generation. Second generation SERMs were developed with the objective of obtaining ER-targeted pharmaceuticals that lacked the uterotrophic and carcinogenic effects of tamoxifen. The best characterized second generation SERM is raloxifene (EVISTA). This compound functions as an estrogen in bone and the cardiovascular system, but acts as a pure antagonist in the breast and uterus. Type II antiestrogens are currently in clinical use; raloxifene was shown to prevent bone loss in preclinical trials of postmenopausal osteoporosis. Consequently, raloxifene received FDA approval for the prevention and treatment of osteoporosis in 1999 and is now widely used in the clinic (1,4). The utility of raloxifene in the prevention and treatment of breast cancer is currently under investigation. Also demonstrating promise is a compound termed lasofoxifene, which clinically appears to possess the favorable qualities of raloxifene, but is even more effective in enhancing bone mineral density and decreasing serum LDL and cholesterol levels (5).

Quest for the "Perfect" SERM

Recently, leaders in the pharmaceutical industry have developed a list of desired properties for a third generation of SERMs (Table 2). In general, future SERMs must oppose endogenous hormone action in the breast and reproductive system while displaying full estrogenic effects in the cardiovasculature, bone and central nervous systems. An additional criterion is that third generation SERMs will be effective in males in prevention of age-related bone loss and in decreasing serum lipid and cholesterol levels (5).

Selective Progesterone Receptor Modulators (SPRMs)

Progestins (progesterone and related compounds) are ovarian hormones that mediate their biological effects through an intracellular ▶ progesterone receptor (PR), a hormone-inducible transcription factor. Progesterone is involved in the development of the female reproductive system, pregnancy and fertility, and in regulation of gonadotropin hormone secretion. Progestins are used clinically in oral contraceptives, to induce abor-

Tab. 2   Criteria for 3rd Generation SERMs.

1. Antagonize estrogen action in the breast and ovary.

2. Display no uterotrophic activity.

3. Bone protective to the full extent of estrogen.

4. Possess better cardiovascular and central nervous system profiles than current SERMs.

5. Contain potential benefits for men in protection against age-related bone loss and increases in cholesterol levels, without displaying estrogen-like proliferative effects in the prostate.

tion and missed menses, and in treatment of endometriosis and fibroids (3). Since progestins function as antiestrogens in the uterus, yet display proliferative effects in the breast, pharmaceutical companies are currently engaged in efforts to develop compounds that display tissue-targeted progestin/antiprogestin activities. This should provide for an additional class of anticancer agents that retain the beneficial effects of progesterone in selected tissues.

Selective Androgen Receptor Modulators (SARMs)

Androgens (testosterone and related compounds) comprise a class of male steroid hormones secreted by the testes. Androgens are essential for spermatogenesis, formation of reproductive organs and development of secondary sexual characteristics. In addition, androgens are involved in bone and muscle growth, regulation of hypothalamic-pituitary hormone secretion, reproductive behaviour, and neural regeneration (6). Unfortunately, prolonged exposure to unopposed androgens is an established risk factor for prostate cancer, a serious health concern among middle-aged and elderly men. The proliferative effects of androgens in the prostate are mediated through the ▶ androgen receptor (AR), which like ER and PR, functions as a hormone-inducible transcription factor in target cells (6). In an effort to attain pharmaceutical agents that oppose the carcinogenic actions of androgens in the prostate, AR antagonists (antiandrogens) are currently in development. To retain the beneficial effects of androgens in some organs, it will be important to develop tissue-targeted antiandrogens termed SARMs. It is the hope that such compounds can be used clinically for both the prevention and treatment of prostate cancer.

Summary

The sex steroids comprise a family of hormones that share a similar mode of action through binding nuclear receptors and regulating the expression of genes involved in cell proliferation, differentiation and function. Sex steroids have a wide range of biological roles in reproduction and in other organ systems. While many hormone functions are critical for homeostasis, chronic stimulation of sex steroid-mediated pathways has also been implicated in cancer and other pathologies.

The necessity for compounds that retain the beneficial effects of sex steroids in some tissues but oppose the action of endogenous hormone in others has resulted in the generation of SSRMs, which display tissue-specific agonist and antagonist activities. Further investigation into the mechanisms by which different cells recognize ligand-bound receptor complexes in a unique manner will provide for mechanistic screening for new pharmaceuticals that display more specific and effective tissue-targeted activities.

References

1. Avioli LV (1999) SERM drugs for the prevention of osteoporosis. TEM 10:176–179
2. Labrie F, Labrie C, Belanger A, Simard J, Giguere V, Tremblay A, Tremblay T (2001) EM-652 (SCH57068), a pure SERM having complete antiestrogenic activity in the mammary gland and endometrium. J. Steroid Biochem Mol Biol 79:213–225
3. McDonnell DP (1995) Unraveling the human progesterone receptor signaling pathway: Insights into antiprogestin action. TEM 6:133–138
4. McDonnell DP (1999) The molecular pharmacology of SERMs. TEM 10:301–311
5. Negro-Vilar A (2001) Third-generation SERMS: partial agonists with full benefits. The Endocrine Society's 83rd Annual Meeting, Denver, CO, p 36
6. 6. Roy AK, Tyagi RK, Song CS, Lavrovsky Y, Ahn SC, Oh TS, Chatterjee B (2001) Androgen receptor: structural domains and functional dynamics after ligand-receptor interaction. Ann N Y Acad Sci 949:44–57

Semaphorins

Semaphorins are a large family of secreted and transmembrane signaling proteins, that were first described as regulating axonal guidance in the developing nervous system. Recent studies suggest that semaphorin receptors (plexins) also act in such diverse processes as lymphocyte activation, control of vascular endothelial cell motility, and lung morphogenesis.

Senescence

Senescence is defined as cellular ageing resulting in an irreversible cell-cycle arrest. Primary cells divide about 50 times and then arrest due to senescence. Senescence is associated with shortening of telomeres.

▶ Telomerase

Sensitization (drug abuse)

Sensitization has been implicated in the development of compulsive drug use and involves a dramatic augmentation of behavioral and neurochemical responses associated predominantly with mesolimbic dopamine transmission that often develops with intermittent exposure to drugs of abuse. Whether sensitization of mesolimbic dopamine neurons is linked to enhanced rewarding efficacy remains unclear. Indeed, current conceptualizations of the significance of sensitization in compulsive drug-seeking behavior hold that, rather than enhancing "reward", repeated drug use leads to a progressive and persistent hypersensitivity of neural systems that mediate "incentive salience", resulting in excessive craving.

▶ Drug Addiction/Dependence

Septicemia

Septicemia is a generally serious illness caused by the presence of bacteria and/or bacterial toxins in the blood ('blood poisoning').

Sequence Profile

A sequence profile represents certain features in a set of aligned sequences. In particular, it gives position-dependent weights for all 20 amino acids and for insertion and deletion events at any sequence position.

▶ Bioinformatics

Sequential Preparations

Sequential preparations contain only estrogens in the first and a fixed estrogen/progestin combination in the second phase of the application period.

▶ Contraceptives

SERCA

Sarcoplasmic calcium ATPase; this enzyme utilizes the energy gained from hydrolysis of ATP to pump calcium from the cytosol into the stores of the ▶ sarcoplasmic reticulum. Its activity is negatively regulated by the closely associated protein phospholamban, and this inhibition is relieved upon phosphorylation of phospholamban by ▶ protein kinase A (PKA).

▶ β-adrenergic System

Serine-hydroxymethyltransferase

The amino acid glycine, a neurotransmitter at inhibitory synapses throughout the central nervous system (CNS), is preferentially synthesized by the tetrahydrofolate and pyridoxal phosphate-dependent enzyme serine-hydroxymethyltransferase. In the CNS, glycine synthesis involves the mitochondrial isozyme. While serine-hydroxymethyltransferase may also contribute to glycine catabolism, the preferred degradation is via the glycine cleavage system, resulting in the formation of to CO_2 and ammonia.

▶ Glycine Receptors

Serine Proteinases

Serine proteinases are proteinases that utilize the terminal hydroxyl group of the side chain of serine to effect peptide bond hydrolysis.

▶ Non-viral Proteases

Serine/Threonine Kinase

▶ Table appendix: Protein Kinases

SERM

▶ Selective Estrogen Receptor Modulators
▶ Sex Steroid Receptors

Serotonin

Serotonin or 5-hydroxytryptamine is an important biogenic amine, which is synthesized *via* 5-hydroxytryptophan from the amino acid tryptophan. The highest concentration of serotonin occurs in the wall of the intestine. About 90% of the total amount is present in enterochromaffin cells, which are derived from the neural crest, similarly to those of the adrenal medulla. Enterochromaffin cells are interspersed with mucosal cells

mainly in the stomach and small intestine. In the blood, serotonin is present at high concentrations in platelets, which take up serotonin from the plasma by an active transport process. Serotonin is released on platelet activation. In the central nervous system, serotonin serves as a transmitter. The main serotonin-containing neurons are those clustered in form of the Raphe-nuclei. Serotonin exerts its biological effects through the activation of specific receptors. Most of them are G-protein coupled receptors (GPCRs) and belong to the 5-HT_1-, 5-HT_2-, 5-HT_4-, 5-HT_5-, 5-HT_6-, 5-HT_7-receptor subfamilies. The 5-HT_3-receptor is a ligand-operated ion channel.

▶ Serotoninergic System

Serotonin (vomiting)

Serotonin, also known as 5-hydroxytryptamine (5-HT), is both a neurotransmitter and an autacoid depending on its location. In the central nervous system, serotonin functions as a neurotransmitter liberated from serotonergic neurons. When stored in enterochromaffin cells in the gastrointestinal tract, serotonin acts as an autacoid. It can be liberated from enterochromaffin cells by a number of stimuli and then acts on serotonin 5-HT_3 receptors located on vagal afferent nerves to cause depolarization, thereby activating the neurons. Centrally, 5-HT_3 receptors are located in the area postrema, nucleus tractus solitarius, dorsal motor nucleus of the vagus and the spinal trigeminal nerve complex and may contribute to emesis in some circumstances. The serotonin 5-HT_3 receptor is a ligand-gated cation channel. Long and short splice variants of the receptor exist in a number of species, including humans. There are also 5-HT_{3A} and 5-HT_{3B} subunits of the receptor and co-expression of these two subunits has been detected in central neurons and in small populations of cells in the small and large intestine. These findings raise the possibility that the various 5-HT_3 receptors involved in vomiting may not be a uniform population. Serotonin 5-HT_{1A} receptors in the brainstem may also be involved in vomiting mecha-

S

nisms. Activation of this receptor subtype inhibits vomiting.

▶ Serotoninergic System
▶ Emesis

Serotoninergic System

Daniel Hoyer
Novartis Pharma AG, Basel, Switzerland
daniel1.hoyer@pharma.novartis.com

Synonyms

Serotonin = 5-Hydroxytryptamine = 5-HT (= enteramine)

Definition

The serotoninergic system is one of the oldest neurotransmitter/hormone systems in evolution, which may explain why ▶ 5-HT interacts with such a diversity of receptors of the G protein coupled family and the ligand gated family, similarly to acetylcholine, GABA or glutamate. 5-HT was discovered in the gut in the 1930s and called enteramine, then rediscovered in the 1940s in the blood and called serotonin, as it had vasoconstrictor features. 5-HT is synthesised from L-tryptophan, the tryptophan hydroxylase forming 5-hydroxytrytophan (5-HTP), which by the L-amino acid decarboxylase leads to 5-HT; serotonin can be conjugated with glucuronide or sulfate or in nerves metabolised via monoamine oxydase to 5-hydroxyindolacetaldehyde and finally to 5-hydroxyindolacetic acid (via aldehydedehydrogenase). It can also lead to 5-hydroxytryptophol by an aldehydereductase in some peripheral nerves. Thus, 5-HT acts both as a neurotransmitter with all the features, such as intracellular storage, activity dependent release, the existence of both pre- and post-synaptic receptors, an active uptake system, via the serotonin transporter and metabolising/inactivating enzymes and a hormone, released into the blood or gut to work more distantly.

▶ Antidepressant Drugs

▶ Antipsychotic Drugs
▶ Emesis

Basic Characteristics

Physiology

The main source of 5-HT is in the gut, more precisely enterochromaffin cells, where it is synthesised from tryptophan. It can be released into the gut lumen e.g. as a reaction to pressure and act on receptors located on the smooth muscle, or into the portal blood circulation, by a variety of nervous or alimentary stimuli. 5-HT is also found in enteric neurons. In the blood, the vast majority of 5-HT is not free but found in the platelets, which are endowed with a very active uptake system (they probably do not synthesise 5-HT) and 5-HT is stored in storage granules. Large amounts of 5-HT are released during platelet aggregation, and it can act locally on endothelial cells and vascular smooth muscle. 5-HT is also found in mast cells. In the central and peripheral nervous system, 5-HT acts as a neurotransmitter on a large variety of receptors, which may be located pre- or post-synaptically. 5-HT is also found in the pineal gland, where it is believed to serve essentially as a precursor for the synthesis of melatonin by 5-HT-N-acetyltransferase and hydroxyindole-O-methyltransferase, under the control of the clock in the suprachiasmatic nucleus which during the circadian rhythm modulates enzyme activity levels up to 50 fold.

Multiple 5-HT Receptor Subtypes

There are at least 14 different 5-HT receptors, and the system is probably much more complex (see Tables 1-3 and Fig.1). With the exception of 5-HT_3 receptors, (ligand-gated ion channels), 5-HT receptors belong to the ▶ G-protein-coupled receptor (GPCR) superfamily and, with at least fourteen distinct members, represents one of the most complex families of neurotransmitter receptors. Multiple splice variants (5-HT_4, 5-HT_7) or RNA edited isoforms (5-HT_{2C}) have been described; there is also evidence that homo- and hetero-dimerisation ($5\text{-HT}_{1B/1D}$) can occur. Furthermore, peptide or lipid modulators of 5-HT receptors have been described such as 5-HT moduline (Leu-Ser-Ala-Leu (LSAL), a putative product

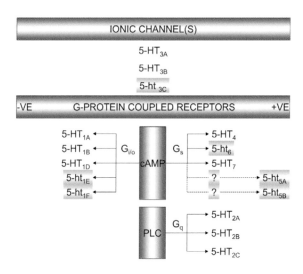

Fig. 1 Graphical representation of the current classification of 5-hydroxytryptamine (5-HT) receptors.
Receptor subtypes represented by shaded boxes and lower case designate receptors that have not been demonstrated to definitively function in native systems. Abbreviations: 3'-5' cyclic adenosine monophosphate (cAMP); phospholipase C (PLC); negative (-ve); positive (+ve).

of a chromogranin), which has selectivity for the 5-HT$_{1B}$ and 5-HT$_{1D}$ receptors, or oleamide, which acts on several receptors (e.g. 5-HT$_{2A/2C}$ and 5-HT$_7$). Before the era of cloning three classes of 5-HT receptors were proposed (1). However, as molecular biology started to play a prominent role in the discovery of additional receptors, the Serotonin Club Receptor Nomenclature Committee proposed a classification system based on operational, structural and transductional information (5). The current classification (3) is progressively adapted to incorporate new information, obtained with both recombinant and native receptors, and favours an alignment of nomenclature with the human genome to avoid species differences (2,4). Currently, seven families of 5-HT receptors have been recognised, 5-HT$_1$ to 5-HT$_7$.

The 5-HT$_1$ receptor class comprises five receptors (5-HT$_{1A}$, 5-HT$_{1B}$, 5-HT$_{1D}$, 5-ht$_{1E}$ and 5-ht$_{1F}$) which, in humans, share 40–63% overall sequence identity and couple somewhat preferentially to G$_{i/o}$ to inhibit cAMP formation (see Tables 1-3). The 5-ht$_{1E}$ and 5-ht$_{1F}$ receptors are given a lower case

appellation to denote that endogenous receptors with a physiological role have not yet been found. In contrast, 5-HT$_{1A}$, 5-HT$_{1B}$ and 5-HT$_{1D}$ receptors have been demonstrated functionally in a variety of tissues. The 5-HT$_{1C}$ designation is vacant, as the receptor was renamed 5-HT$_{2C}$ due to structural, operational and transductional similarities with the 5-HT$_2$ receptor family.

5-HT$_{2A}$, 5-HT$_{2B}$ and 5-HT$_{2C}$ receptors exhibit 46–50% overall sequence identity and couple preferentially to G$_{q/11}$ to increase inositol phosphates and cytosolic [Ca^{++}] (see Tables 1-3).

5-HT$_3$ receptors belong to the ligand-gated ion channel receptor superfamily, similar to the nicotinic acetylcholine or GABA$_A$ receptors and share electrophysiological and structural patterns. The receptors are found on central and peripheral neurons where they trigger rapid depolarisation due to the opening of non-selective cation channels (Na$^+$, Ca^{++} influx, K$^+$ efflux). The response desensitises and resensitises rapidly. The native 5-HT$_3$ receptor, as revealed by electron microscopy in neuroblastoma-glioma cells, is a pentamer, and there may exist 3 different subunits.

5-HT$_4$, 5-ht$_6$ and 5-HT$_7$ receptors all couple preferentially to G$_s$ and promote cAMP formation, yet they are classified as distinct receptor classes because of their limited (<35%) overall sequence identities. This subdivision is arbitrary and may be subject to future modification.

Two subtypes of the 5-ht$_5$ receptor (5-ht$_{5A}$ and 5-ht$_{5B}$), sharing 70% overall sequence identity, have been found in rodents. The human 5-ht$_{5B}$ receptor gene does not encode a functional protein due to the presence of stop codons in its coding sequence. Human recombinant 5-ht$_{5A}$ receptors inhibit forskolin-stimulated cAMP production, although the receptor may also couple positively to cAMP. Currently, a function for this receptor is still being investigated.

Several endogenous 5-HT receptors have been defined pharmacologically, although a corresponding gene product encoding the receptor has yet to be identified. As long as their structure is unknown, these receptors are regarded as orphans in the current nomenclature. One of these however, the so-called '5-HT$_1$-like' receptor mediating direct vasorelaxation corresponds to the 5-HT$_7$ receptor. On the other hand, the situation with the remaining ► orphan receptors (see 3) has not

Tab. 1 5-HT$_1$ receptors.

Nomenclature	5-HT$_{1A}$	5-HT$_{1B}$	5-HT$_{1D}$	5-ht$_{1E}$	5-ht$_{1F}$
Selective Agonist	8-OH-DPAT	L 694247	PNU 109291	None	LY 334370, LY344864
Rank order	Di-nPr-5-CT>5-CT >8-OH-DPAT>5-HT >buspirone>sumatriptan	Human: 5-CT>5-HT >sumatriptan >RU-24969>CP-93,129 >8-OH-DPAT Rodent : RU-24969 >5-CT = CP-93,129 >sumatriptan>8-OH-DPAT		5-HT>RU-24969>5-CT>sumatriptan	
Antagonists (pK_B)	(±)WAY 100635 (8.7)	GR 55562 (7.4) SB 224289 (8.5) SB 236057 (8.9)	BRL 15572 (7.9)	-	-
Radioligands	[^{3}H]WAY100635 [^{3}H]8-OH-DPAT	[^{125}I]GTI [^{125}I]CYP (rodent) [^{3}H]Sumatriptan [^{3}H]GR 125743	[^{125}I]GTI [^{3}H]Sumatriptan [^{3}H]GR 125743	[^{3}H]5-HT	[^{125}I]LSD [^{3}H]LY 334370
Effector	G_i/G_o Preferentially inhibits cAMP formation Increases inwardly rectifying K$^+$ current, PLC activation with increased IPs and elevated [Ca^{++}]$_i$ observed in recombinant systems.	G_i/G_o Preferentially inhibits cAMP formation; PLC activation with increased IPs and elevated [Ca^{++}]$_I$ observed in recombinant systems.	G_i/G_o Preferentially inhibits cAMP formation; PLC activation with increased IPs and elevated [Ca^{++}]$_i$ observed in recombinant systems.	G_i/G_o Preferentially inhibits cAMP formation (in recombinant system).	$G_{i/o}$ Preferentially inhibits cAMP formation (in recombinant system).
Localisation	CNS: Hippocampus (CA1, CA3, DG), septum, amygdala, raphé nuclei Peripheral: Cholinergic heteroreceptor - myenteric plexus	CNS: Striatum, hippocampus (CA1), substantia nigra, globus pallidus, superior colliculi, spinal cord, raphé nuclei Peripheral: Vascular smooth muscle, autonomic terminals	CNS: like 5-HT1B but at lower densities. Peripheral: autonomic and trigeminal nerve terminals	CNS: Caudate putamen, parietal cortex, fronto-parietal motor cortex, olfactory tubercle, amygdala Peripheral: None identified	CNS: Cortex, Thalamus, olfactory bulb (rat), claustrum (g-pig), hippocampus (CA3), spinal cord. Peripheral: Uterus, mesentery

Tab. 2 5-HT$_{2,3,4}$ receptors.

Nomenclature	5-HT2A	5-HT2B	5-HT2CΦ	5-HT3	5-HT4
Selective Agonist Rank order	DOI 5-HT = α-me-5-HT > 5-CT = 2-me-5-HT > sumatriptan > BW723C86	BW 723C86 5-HT = α-me-5-HT > BW723C86>5-CT = 2-me-5-HT >>sumatriptan	Ro 600175 5-HT = α-me-5-HT >DOI>RU-24969 = quipazine>5-CT >sumatriptan	SR 57227, mCPB m-CPB>5-HT >2-me-5-HT>>5-MeOT	BIMU 8, SC53116 ML10302, RS 67506 SC53116>BIMU 8 >5-MeOT>α-me-5-HT >cisapride>(S)-zacopride >5-CT
Selective antago- nists (pK$_B$)	Ketanserin (8.5-9.5) MDL 100907 (9.4)	SB 200646 (7.5)†† SB 204741 (7.8)	Mesulergine (9.1) SB 242084 (9.0) RS 102221 (8.4)	Granisetron (10) Ondansetron (8-10) Tropisetron (10-11)	GR 113808 (9-9.5) SB 204070 (10.8) RS 100235 (11.2)
Radioligands	[^{125}I]DOI [^{3}H]Ketanserin [^{3}H]MDL 100907	[^{3}H]5-HT	[^{125}I]LSD [^{3}H]Mesulergine	[^{3}H](S)-zacopride [^{3}H]tropisetron [^{3}H]granisetron [^{3}H]GR 65630 [^{3}H]LY 278584	[^{125}I]SB 207710 [^{3}H]GR 113808 [^{3}H]RS 57639
Effector	G$_{q/11}$ Preferentially increases Pi hydrolysis and elevates [Ca^{++}]$_i$	G$_{q/11}$ Preferentially increases Pi hydrolysis and elevates [Ca^{++}]$_i$ (in recombinant systems)	G$_{q/11}$ Preferentially increases Pi hydrolysis and elevates [Ca^{++}]$_I$	Intrinsic ligand-gated ion channel Promotes increased [Na+][Ca^{++}]i	G$_s$ Preferentially increases cAMP formation.
Localisation	CNS: Cortex, hippocam-pus, striatum, olfactory bulb, spinal cord Peripheral: GI, vascular and bronchial smooth muscle, vascular endothelium, platelets	CNS: not present in adult. Peripheral: Smooth muscle of ileum, stomach fundus (rat), uterus, vasculature, endothelium	CNS: Choroid plexus, medulla, pons, striatum, hippocampus (CA1, CA3), hypothala-mus, spinal cord Peripheral: None identified	CNS: Striatum, hippoc-ampus (CA1), substantia nigra, globus pallidus. Peripheral: Post-ganglionic sympathetic neurones, sensory neurones	CNS: Striatum, brainstem, thalamus, hippocampus, olfactory bulb, substantia nigra Peripheral: Cariac muscle, post-ganglionic parasympa-thetic neurones (myenteric plexus), oesophageal and vascular smooth muscle

S

Tab. 3 5-HT$_{5,6,7}$ receptors.

Nomenclature	5-ht5A	5-ht5B	5-ht6	5-HT7
Selective Agonist *Rank order*	-	-	-	- *5-CT>5-HT>8-OH-DPAT >sumatriptan*
Selective antagonists (*pK$_B$*)	-	-	Ro 630563 (7.9) SB 271046 (7.8) SB 357134 (8.5)	SB 258719 (7.9) SB 269970 (9.0)
Radioligands	[^{125}I]LSD [^{3}H]5-CT	[^{125}I]LSD [^{3}H]5-CT	[^{125}I]SB 258585 [^{125}I]LSD [^{3}H]5-HT	[^{125}I]LSD [^{3}H]SB 269970 [^{3}H]5-CT [^{3}H]5-HT
G protein effector	Gs Gi? increases (decreases) cAMP formation	not identified	G$_s$ Preferentially increases cAMP formation	G$_s$ Preferentially increases cAMP formation
Localisation	*CNS:* Hippocampus (CA1, CA3, DG), cortex, cerebellum (granular layer), olfactory bulb, habenula, spinal cord *Peripherl*: None identified		*CNS:* Caudate putamen, olfactory tubercle, nucleus accumbens, cortex, hippocampus (CA1, CA3, DG) *Peripheral:* Superior cervical ganglion	*CNS:* Hippocampus (CA1, CA2), hypothalamus, thalamus, superior colliculus, raphé nuclei *Peripheral:* GI and vascular smooth muscle, sympathetic ganglia

evolved further and thus the status quo ante remains. In particular, no progress has been made with the so-called 5-HT$_{1P}$ receptor, which is present in the gut and whose pharmacology is reminiscent of the 5-HT$_4$ receptors, with the restriction that some of the ligands described, like the 5-HT dipeptides do not affect 5-HT$_4$ receptors.

Pathophysiology/Clinical Applications

5-HT has been implicated in the aetiology of numerous disease states, including depression, anxiety, social phobia, schizophrenia, obsessive compulsive disorders, panic-disorders, migraine, hypertension, pulmonary hypertension, eating disorders, vomiting and ▶ irritable bowel syndrome (IBS) by interacting at different receptors.

5-HT is also a substrate for the 5-HT transporter, itself an important player in the treatment of depression and social phobia. It is the target for ▶ SSRIs (selective serotonin reuptake inhibitors) such as fluoxetine, paroxetine, fluvoxamine and citalopram or the more recent dual reuptake inhibitors (for 5-HT and noradrenaline) such as venlafaxine.

5-HT$_{1A}$ receptor agonists, such as buspirone or gepirone, are being used/developed for the treatment of anxiety and depression. Furthermore, the 5HT$_{1A}$ receptor and β-adrenoceptor antagonist, pindolol, was reported to enhance the therapeutic efficacy and shorten the onset of action of SSRIs upon co-administration in severely depressed patients. However, both positive and negative findings have been reported, as is common in depression trials. Flesinoxan, a 5-HT$_{1A}$ receptor agonist, was initially developed as an anti-hypertensive agent, however its effects in patients were disappointing and this approach has now been abandoned.

Interest in 5-HT$_{1B}$ receptor agonists has been triggered by the anti-migraine properties of sumatriptan, a non-selective 5-HT$_{1D/1B}$ receptor agonist; various agonists have been developed for this indication (dihydroergotamine (DHE), zolmitriptan, naratriptan, rizatriptan, elitriptan, almotriptan, donitriptan and others. The putative 5HT$_{1B}$ receptor agonist, anpirtoline, has analgesic and antidepressant-like properties in rodents and interestingly, 5-HT$_{1B}$ receptor knockout mice were reported to be highly aggressive and show an increased preference for alcohol. However, the development of 5-HT$_{1B}$ agonist 'serenics' such as eltoprazine was not successful; the expected anti-aggressive effects were not observed in patients.

The anti-migraine 5-HT$_{1B/1D}$ agonist sumatriptan labels 5-ht$_{1F}$ sites with high affinity. The binding site distribution obtained was very similar to that for 5-ht$_{1F}$ mRNA. Naratriptan also has affinity for 5-ht$_{1F}$ receptors and it has been hypothesised that they might be a target for anti-migraine drugs. 5-ht$_{1F}$ receptor mRNA has been detected in the trigeminal ganglia, stimulation of which leads to plasma extravasation in the dura, a component of neurogenic inflammation thought to be a possible cause of migraine. LY 334370, a selective 5-ht$_{1F}$ receptor agonist, inhibits trigeminal stimulation-induced early activated gene expression in nociceptive neurons in the rat brainstem. 5-ht$_{1F}$ selective ligands i.e. LY 344864 and BRL 54443, are currently in development (migraine), however they also have affinity for 5-ht$_{1E}$ receptors.

Ketanserin and MDL 100907 are selective antagonists. Ketanserin was developed for the treatment of hypertension, but 5-HT$_{2A}$ receptor antagonism as a valid anti-hypertensive principle is now questioned since ketanserin is a potent $α_1$ adrenoceptor antagonist. LSD and other hallucinogens most probably produce hallucinations via 5-HT$_{2A}$ receptors. Although their selectivity vis-a-vis 5-HT$_{2B}$ and 5-HT$_{2C}$ receptors is rather limited this represents currently the best possible explanation. 5-HT$_{2A}$ receptor antagonists such as risperidone, ritanserin, seroquel, olanzapine or MDL 100907 have been indicated/developed for the treatment of schizophrenia. However, development of MDL 100907 for acute schizophrenia was stopped. The combination of dopamine D$_2$ and 5-HT$_{2A}$ receptor antagonism may still explain the anti-psychotic activity of drugs such as clozapine, olanzapine, seroquel and others.

BW 723C86 has agonist selectivity at the rat 5-HT$_{2B}$ receptor, although less marked at human receptors. 5-HT$_{2B}$ receptor antagonists such as SB 200646 may be indicated for the treatment of migraine prophylaxis, given the vasodilatatory role of this receptor and that a number of 'older' antimigraine drugs share 5-HT$_{2B}$ receptor antagonism. Activation of the 5-HT$_{2B}$ receptor is most probably responsible for the valvulopathies reported for appetite suppressant preparations containing dex-fenfluramine.

The anxiogenic component of mCPP may be mediated by 5-HT_{2C} receptor activation, and selective 5-HT_{2C} receptor antagonists such as SB 242084 display anxiolytic properties in various animal models. However, additional studies utilising selective agonists are required (e.g. Ro 600175). mCPP or Ro 600175 cause additional behavioural responses attributed to central 5-HT_{2C} receptor activation, e.g. hypoactivity, hypophagia, increased penile grooming/erections and oral dyskinesia. 5-HT_{2C} receptor activation produces a tonic, inhibitory influence upon frontocortical dopaminergic and adrenergic, but not serotonergic transmission and, in part, play a role in neuroendocrine function. 5-HT_{2C} receptor knockout mice have spontaneous convulsions, cognitive impairment, increased food intake and obesity, but similar effects are not reproduced by selective antagonists, suggesting that these changes may result in part from neuroadaptation. Nevertheless, the 5-HT_{2C} receptor is an attractive target for the discovery of novel treatment for feeding disorders.

The 5-HT_3 receptor antagonists ondansetron, granisetron and tropisetron are used clinically in chemotherapy- and radiotherapy-induced nausea and vomiting. Since 5-HT_3 receptor activation in the brain leads to dopamine release, and 5-HT_3 receptor antagonists produce central effects comparable to those of anti-psychotics and anxiolytics, schizophrenia and anxiety were considered as potential indications. 5-HT_3 receptor antagonists have been reported to induce cognition enhancing effects. However, there are not enough clinical data to substantiate such activities. Similarly, that 5-HT_3 antagonists should prove useful in the treatment of migraine did not materialise in clinical studies. More recently, alosetron was developed for the treatment of women suffering from ▶ IBS with diarrhoea, but had to be withdrawn due to safety reasons.

Selective 5-HT_4 receptor ligands may have therapeutic utility in a number of disorders, including cardiac arrhythmia, neuro-degenerative diseases and urinary incontinence. Cisapride, a gastroprokinetic agent, acts as an agonist at the 5-HT_4 receptor. Tegaserod (HTF-919, Zelmac/Zelnorm), a new generation 5-HT_4 receptor partial agonist, is used to treat constipation predominant IBS, and its therapeutic activity in functional motility disorders of the upper G.I. tract is currently under clinical investigation.

Antipsychotics (clozapine, olanzapine, fluperlapine and seroquel) and antidepressants (clomipramine, amitryptyline, doxepin and nortryptyline) are 5-ht_6 receptor antagonists. This attribute tempted speculation of an involvement of the 5-ht_6 receptor in psychiatric disorders, although these drugs are by no means selective.

Indeed, atypical antipsychotics e.g. clozapine, risperidone and antidepressants have also high affinity for the 5-HT_7 receptor. 5-HT_7 receptor down-regulation occurs after chronic anti-depressant treatment, and acute, but not chronic, stress regulates 5-HT_7 receptor mRNA expression. The presence of 5-HT_7 sites in the limbic system and thalamocortical regions, suggest a role in the affective disorders, which however will need clinical confirmation.

References

1. Bradley, P. B., Engel, G., Feniuk, W., Fozard, J. R., Humphrey, P. P. A., Middlemiss, D. N., Mylecharane, E. J., Richardson, B. P. & Saxena, P. R. (1986). Proposals for the classification and nomenclature of functional receptors for 5-hydroxytryptamine. Neuropharmacol. 25:563–576
2. Hartig, P., Hoyer, D., Humphrey, P. P. A. & Martin, G. R. (1996). Alignment of receptor nomenclature with the human genome. Effects on classification of 5-HT1D/5-HT1B receptor subtypes. Trends Pharmacol. Sci. 17:103–105
3. Hoyer, D., Clarke, D. E., Fozard, J. R., Hartig, P. R., Martin, G. R., Mylecharane, E. J., Saxena, P. R. & Humphrey, P. P. A. (1994). International Union of Pharmacology classification of receptors for 5-hydroxytryptamine (Serotonin). Pharmacol. Rev. 46:157–204
4. Hoyer D., Hannon J., & Martin G.R. (2002) Molecular, pharmacological and functional diversity of 5-HT receptors. Pharmacol. Biochem. Behav. 71:533–554
5. Humphrey, P. P. A., Hartig, P. R. & Hoyer, D. (1993). A new nomenclature for 5-HT receptors. Trends Pharmacol. Sci. 14:233–236

Serum Sickness

Serurm sickness is an inflammatory condition caused by the deposition of immune complexes in blood vessel walls and tissues.

▶ Allergy
▶ Humanized Monoclonal Antibodies

Seven Transmembrane Span Proteins

▶ G-Protein Coupled Receptors

Sex Steroid Receptors

JUDITH M. MÜLLER, ROLAND SCHÜLE
Universitäts-Frauenklinik und Zentrum für
Klinische Forschung, Klinikum der Universität
Freiburg, Freiburg, Germany
jmueller@frk.ukl.uni-freiburg.de,
schuele@frk.ukl.uni-freiburg.de

Definition

Sex steroid receptors are members of the steroid hormone receptor family that ligand-dependently regulate functions of the sexual organs. Sex steroid receptors are the androgen receptor (AR), the estrogen receptor α and β (ERα, ERβ), and the progesterone receptor (PR).

▶ Contraceptives
▶ Gluco-/Mineralocorticoid Receptors
▶ Selective Sex-steroid Receptor Modulators

Basic Characteristics

The subgroup of steroid hormone receptors (SHRs) belong to the superfamily of ▶ nuclear receptors (NRs), which transactivate target genes ligand-dependently. Unliganded SHRs are associated with large multiprotein complexes of ▶ chaperones in the cytoplasm, in contrast to other NRs. SHRs comprise the glucocorticoid receptor and the mineralocorticoid receptor and the sex ▶ steroid receptors.

SHRs are built in a modular structure with similar structure elements. They contain a DNA-binding domain (DBD), a hinge region with a nuclear location signal (NLS), a ligand-binding domain (LBD) and several transcriptional activation functions (Fig. 1). Their ligands are fat-soluble steroid hormones derived from cholesterol that bind to the LBD of their specific intracellular SHR after diffusing into the cell. After binding of the steroid hormone (Kd between 0.1 to 4 nM) the conformation of the SHR changes, exposing the NLS and the complex of steroid hormone and SHR gains access to the nucleus (Fig. 2). Utilising the two zinc fingers of their DBD, SHRs bind as homodimers to unique DNA sequences called hormone response elements (HREs). The HRE is comprised of two half-sites organised as palindrome with a 3 nucleotide spacer. SHRs regulate the expression of target genes after association with large multisubunit complexes that contain ▶ transcriptional co-activators such as histone acetylases and several other proteins that facilitate transcription. Several signalling pathways furthermore influence the activity of SHRs, by modifying either SHRs directly or partner proteins. SHRs can also act without binding to DNA via interaction with other transcription factors, thereby altering their own or their partner's properties.

The physiological and pathophysiological roles of the sex steroid receptors are diverse and will be summarised separately for AR, ERα, ERβs, and PR in the following paragraphs. Estrogen related receptors (ERRs) share structural and functional similarities with ERs. They are orphan receptors indicating that there is no known ▶ ligand and therefore there are not grouped as SHR.

The Androgen Receptor (AR)

Androgens act via the AR and play an important role in the development and differentiation of the male sexual organ. Furthermore, they are involved in several diseases, the most important being partial and complete androgen insensitivity syndrome (formerly known as the testicular feminiza-

S

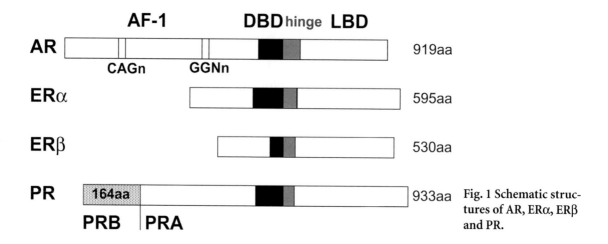

Fig. 1 Schematic structures of AR, ERα, ERβ and PR.

tion syndrome), bulbar and spinal muscle atrophy (Kennedy's disease), and the neoplastic transformation of the prostate. The two natural occurring androgens are testosterone (T) and the more potent 5α-dihydrotestosterone (DHT). T is mainly produced by the Leydig cells of the testis and can also be produced in most peripheral tissues from the adrenal-produced inactive steroid precursors dehydroepiandrosterone, its sulfate, and androstenedione. T is converted into DHT by the 5α-reductase enzyme expressed in the urogenital tract. Besides positive regulation of target genes by the androgen-loaded AR, there is growing evidence of additional regulation pathways and indirect regulation mechanism of the AR. The expression of specific transcriptional coactivators of the AR in different tissues may fine-tune the transcriptional AR-activity. Ligand-independent activation of the AR by protein kinase pathways can circumvent the need for androgens. In addition, protein-protein interactions of the AR with other transcription factors regulate the transcriptional activity of these partner proteins.

The 8 exons of the AR gene encode a protein of around 917aa depending on two polymorphic regions of polyglutamines and polyglycines in the N-terminal activation domain. Two isoforms are detected in tissues; the predominant (80%) 110kD (B isoform) and 87kD (A isoform). It is not clear whether the 2 isoforms also serve different functions.

The structure of the AR comprises an N-terminal transactivation domain of around 500aa, a DBD of 66–68aa, and a LBD of 250aa. The hinge region contains the lysine-rich NLS. The AR posesses two activation functions (AFs): AF-1 in the N-terminal region and the AF-2 core domain in the LBD.

The AF-1 contains two polymorphic regions of polyglutamine (CAG) and polyglycine (GGN) repeats. Normally the number of the 5' CAG repeats is 11–31 (average 21) whereas up to 50 repeats are found in individuals affected with bulbar and spinal muscle atrophy. Since the number of glutamines inversely correlates with the transcriptional activity of the AR these amplified repeats lead to a reduced activity of the AR. The increased size of a polymorphic tandem CAG repeat is associated with the X-linked spinal and bulbar muscular atrophy and may also be associated with oligospermic infertility and with low serum androgens in a subset of anovulatory female patients. On the other hand, a shorter CAG length correlates with a higher risk, more severe and earlier onset of prostate cancer probably resulting from a higher activity of the AR. Experimental evidence also correlates increased or prolonged induction of AR activation with a higher incidence or acceleration of prostate cancer.

In the beginning, prostate cancer cells are largely dependent on androgens for growth and survival. Observations, that castration is beneficial in prostate cancer made androgen ablation and antiandrogen therapy a standard treatment for patients with metastatic prostate cancer following surgery of the tumor tissue. Antiandrogen therapy includes inhibition of androgen synthesis by aminoglutethimide or ketoconazole, inhibition of

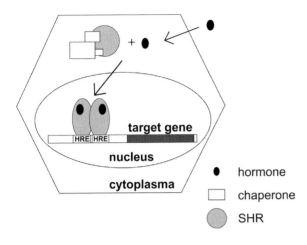

hormone

chaperone

SHR

Fig. 2 The classical activation pathway of SHR. SHRs (grey circle) are associated with chaperones (rectangles). After binding of steroid hormones (black circle) SHRs activate target genes in the nucleus. Additional regulation mechanisms e.g. phosphorylation are described in the text.

▶ 5α-reductase by finasteride in combination with AR ▶ antagonists such as flutamide, or cyproterone acetate.

Unfortunately, remaining prostate cancer cells eventually adapt to grow in the low-androgen enviroment, rendering the tumor growth independent of androgens. Androgen-independent prostate cancer may result from one or more of the following mechanism: increased gene copy number, altered interaction of the AR with coregulatory proteins e.g. resulting from AR mutations, bypassing of the AR pathway, or ligand-independent activation of AR e.g. by protein kinase pathways.

The Estrogen Receptor (ER)

Estrogens mainly affect the growth and maturation of the female reproductive system and the maintenance of its reproductive capacity. In addition, estrogens act on several other tissues e.g. on lipid and bone metabolism. Uterus, placenta and testis are the principal sites of 17β-estradiol (E2) production. ▶ Agonists and antagonists of ERs are used for treatment of breast cancer, menopausal symptoms, osteoporosis and cardiovascular diseases.

The main isoforms of the human ERs are ERα and ERβ, which display distinct expression patterns. Additional ER isoforms, generated by alternative mRNA splicing, have been identified in several tissues. A cell-specific localization for each of the ER subtypes is found in the majority of the reproductive organs studied. The role of the different ER isoforms in modulating the estrogen response or in tumorigenesis is not completely understood. ERs bind most ligands with similiar affinities and display equal transcriptional activation. However, in some assays ER isoforms respond differently to ligands. The naturally occuring phytoestrogen genistein or antiestrogens, such as tamoxifen or raloxifen are examples of these selective ERs modulators (▶ SERMs). The characterisation of SERMs that specifically regulate defined functions promises to increase efficacy and reduce side effects in estrogen-regulated processes.

ERα (also called ESR1 and ESRA)

ERα is involved in the differentiation and maintenance of reproductive, neural, skeletal and cardiovascular tissues. Two separate AFs mediate transcriptional activation, the ligand-dependent AF-2 in the LBD, and the ligand-independent AF-1 in the N-terminus. After binding of estrogen to the LBD, ERα activates target genes such as the progesterone receptor gene by association to estrogen response elements (EREs). Besides this classical activation, non-estrogen dependent activation of ERα has been described. Signalling pathways and extracellular signals such as EGF, IGF-I or insulin, stimulate phosphorylation of the receptor. Phosphorylation of ERα affects all steps of transcriptional activation, such as ligand binding, dimerization, DNA binding and interaction with cofactors. Heregulin is an example of an extracellular signal modulating ER activity. After binding to its receptor HER-2 ER is rapidly phosphorylated on tyrosine residues, followed by transcription of the PR gene. Since heregulin promotes hormone-independent growth of breast cancer cells, activation of ER by heregulin or HER-2 may be involved in the development of E2-independent cancer cells growth.

ERα can also regulate gene expression by interacting with different transcription factors. For example, interaction of ERα with the c-Rel subunit

S

Tab. 1 Basic characteristics of sex steroid receptors.

SHR	Gene map locus	cDNA size	Natural agonist	Binding halfsite	Main expression
AR	Xq11-q12	ca. 919 aa (see text)	5α-dihydro-testosterone (DHT), testoterone (T)	AGAACA	Prostate, male urogenital system, muscle
ERα	6q25.1	595 aa	17β-estradiol (E2)	AGGTCA	Ovary, uterus, mammary gland, vagina, testis (Leydig cells), bone
ERβ	14q	530 aa, 583 aa, further isoforms	17β-estradiol (E2)	AGGTCA	Ovary, testis (Sertoli and Leydig cells, efferent ducts), prostate, bone, thymus, spleen, brain
PR	11q22	2 isoforms: PR-A 769 aa, PR-B 933 aa	Progesterone	AGAACA	Uterus, ovary, central nervous system

of NF-κB prevents binding to NF-κB response element resulting in reduced interleukin-6 transcription. Here, ERα acts E2-dependently but without directly binding to DNA. However, the complex formation of ER with the transcription factor Sp1 is hormone independent and enhances Sp1 binding to DNA. ERα as well as ERβ thereby enhance transcription of the retinoic acid receptor α1 gene. Other partner proteins are fos/jun family members, which regulate gene expression via AP-1 sites. In this situation E2 can either act as agonist in the presence of ERα or as antagonist in the presence of ERβ. Another possibility to modulate ER signalling is the aryl hydrocarbon receptor (AhR). Ligands for AhR mediate antiestrogenic effects by several pathways.

The measurement of ER has become a standard assay in the clinical management of breast cancer. The presence of ERα identifies those breast cancer patients with a lower risk of relapse and better clinical outcome. Receptor status also provides a guideline for those tumors that may be responsive to hormonal intervention. But only about half of ER-positive patients respond to hormonal therapies. Of those who respond initially, most will eventually develop an estrogen unresponsive disease following a period of treatment even though ERα is often still present. Mutant receptors and constitutively active receptors as well as hormone independent activation of the ERα are discussed.

The involvement of ERβ isoforms is under investigation.

Analysis of ERα-deficient mice showed that both sexes are infertile and display a variety of phenotypic changes associated with the gonads, mammary glands, reproductive tracts, and skeletal tissues. In addition, a hyperplasia and hypertrophy of adipocytes was found in these mice.

In females, ovariectomy or menopause leads to rapid loss of trabecula bone and the osteoporosis indicating that E2 maintains bone mass. E2 enhances bone formation by osteoblasts and supresses bone resorption by osteoclasts by regulating several important growth factors. In mice, ERα seems to induce growth but not maintenance of trabecular bone whereas ERβ terminates growth during late puberty. However, while in humans the role of ERα and ERβ in bone is not completely clear, ESRA polymorphism is related to bone density and height during late puberty and at attainment of peak bone density in young men.

ERβ (also called ESR2 and ESRB)

In 1995 the discovery of ERβ explained many actions of estrogens in ERα free tissues. ERβ shows high homology to ERα in the DNA- and lig-and-binding domains, but encodes a distinct transcriptional AF-1 domain. At least 5 isoforms, designated ERβ-1 through ERβ-5, are decribed that differ in their C-terminal sequences and tissue expression patterns, or have extended N-termini.

This new complexity of isoforms is further enhanced by the fact that ERβ isoforms cannot only heterodimerize with each other but also with ERα. The functional consequences for the action of estrogens depending on the expression pattern are only beginning to be evaluated.

ERβ is highly expressed in ovary, male organs, and parts of the central nervous system (CNS), but also in other organs such as spleen and thymus.

The phytoestrogen genistein binds better to ERβ than to ERα and the partial ERα agonists tamoxifen, raloxifen and ICI-164, 384 are antagonists for ERβ.

It has been postulated that co-factor recruitment is different for the ERs, however knowledge about this interesting field of selective ER regulation is only beginning to accumulate.

Since only ERβ is expressed widely in the male urogenital tract of several animals it is now under evaluation whether the pronounced effects of E2 in men are caused by direct action of E2 on ERβ in these reproductive organs. The view that E2 acts only indirectly by reducing androgen levels via the central nervous system clearly has to be corrected.

Analysis of ESRB -/- mice showed fewer and smaller litters than wildtype mice as well as abnormal vascular function and hypertension. The reduction in fertility was attributed to reduced ovarian efficiency. Mutant females had normal breast development and lactated normally. Older mutant males displayed signs of prostate and bladder hyperplasia. The results indicated that ESRB is essential for normal ovulation efficiency but is not essential for lactation, female or male sexual differentiation or fertility.

The Progesterone Receptor (PR)

The PR is involved in diverse functions in female reproduction, such as implantation of the embryo, and in the maintainance of pregnancy. Progesterone is mainly produced in the corpus luteum in the second half of the menstrual cycle and in early pregnancy, later in the placenta. The PR is expressed in the uterus, ovary and the CNS. In men there is no known function. Estrogens induce expression of the PR gene. PR agonists such as medroxyprogesterone or the sythetic R5020 are called progestins or gestagens.

The human PR exists as 2 functionally distinct isoforms PRA and PRB transcribed from 2 promoters from a single gene. PRA lacks the N-terminal 164aa and is a 769aa protein. PRB functions as a transcriptional activator in most cell and promoter contexts. In contrast, PRA is transcriptionally inactive and functions as a strong ligand-dependent transdominant repressor of steroid hormone receptor transcriptional activity. Different co-factor interactions were demonstrated for PRA and PRB, probably due to an inhibitory domain within the first 140aa of PRA, which is masked in PRB. Both PR isoforms however, repress estradiol-induced ER activity when liganded.

PRs also interact with other signalling pathways, which can e.g. be regulated by phosphorylation. Independent of transcriptional activation of PR, progestins can activate cytoplasmic signalling molecules including SRC and downstream MAP kinase in mammalian cells via interaction by a specific polyproline motif in the N-terminal domain of PR.

Mice models reveal that both PR forms are physiologically important. Mice lacking the PR gene fail to ovulate, are infertile and have impaired thymic function. Selective PRA deficient female mice are infertile due to reduced oocyte and uterine deficiency in implantation. However, these mice had normal mammary epithelium proliferation and differentiation and showed normal thymic involution. In mice, PR regulates expression of proteases that degrade the follicular wall thereby facilitaing ovulation.

In breast cancer patients, total PR status is measured for hormonal treatment. The presence of PR is associated with increased survival rates and hormonal responsiveness of mammary tumors. PR agonists are widely used in contraception, ▶ hormone replacement therapy (HRT), breast cancer and endometrial hyperplasia. ▶ Antiprogestins such as RU486 are used for blocking ovulation and preventing implatation, and in addition they are in clinical testing for the induction of labor and to control various neoplastic transformations.

▶ Selective progesterone receptor modulators (SPRM) (mesoprogestins) are PR ligands with agonistic and antagonistic activities. Some SPRM show weak antiglucocorticoid or mixed andro-

S

genic/antiandrognic activites. SPRM are currently tested and may be useful e.g. for the treatment of endometriosis.

Drugs

In clinical use are pure and partial agonists and antagonists (see individual SHR) as contraceptives, treatment for hormonal ablation in breast and prostate cancer and hormonal replacement therapy (HRT) in osteoporosis.

References

1. Beato M, Herrlich P, Schütz G (1995) Sex steroid receptors: many actors in search of a plot. Cell 83:851–857
2. Nilsson S et al. (2001) Mechanism of estrogen action. Physiological Reviews 81:1535–1565
3. OMIM *313700 ANDROGEN RECEPTOR; AR
4. OMIM *133430 ESTROGEN RECEPTOR 1; ESR1
5. OMIM *601663 ESTROGEN RECEPTOR 2; ESR2
6. OMIM *264080 PROGESTERONE RESISTANCE; PGR

Sex Steroids/Hormones

▶ Sex Steroid Receptors
▶ Contraceptives

SGLT

▶ Na$^+$-dependent Glucose Cotransporter

SH2 Domain

▶ Src-homology 2 Domain

SH3 Domain

▶ Src-homology 3 Domain

Shaker-channels

Shaker-channels, eag (*ether-à-go-go*)-channels, slo (*slow-poke*)-channels were cloned from behavioral *Drosophila melanogaster* mutants. The channels were named according to the *Drosophila* mutant phenotype, *Shaker, ether-à-go-go, slow-poke*. Subsequently, eag-cDNA was used to clone related voltage-gated potassium channel subunits erg (eag-related) and elk (eag-like). The human erg ortholog (HERG) mediates cardiac I$_{KS}$.

▶ Voltage-gated K$^+$ Channels

Shine-Dalgarno Interaction

The Shine-Salgano interaction is a base pairing interaction that occurs during translation initiation in prokaryotes between the Shine-Dalgarno sequence on messenger RNA (mRNA) and the anti-Shine-Dalgarno sequence on 16S ribosomal RNA (rRNA). The Shine-Dalgarno sequence is a purine-rich sequence located four to seven bases upstream of the initiation codon in prokaryotic mRNAs. It has variable length and complementarity to the anti-Shine-Dalgarno sequence found in the 3'-end region of all bacterial 16S rRNAs (and in archaeal and chloroplast 16S rRNAs).

▶ Ribosomal Protein-synthesis Inhibitors

SIADH

SIADH, the syndrome of inappropriate antidiuretic hormone, is defined by water retention, dilutional hyponatremia and decreased volume of highly concentrated urine. There are several causes for SIADH, neoplasms, ectopically secreted arginine vasopressin (AVP), eutopic release of AVP by various diseases or drugs, exogenous administration of AVP, dDAVP, lysipressin or large doses of OT (iatrogenic SIADH).

▶ Vasopressin/Oxytocin

Sialic Acid

Sialic acid is a carbohydrate that can be attached to certain molecules, e.g. epoetin alfa.

▶ Hematopoietic Growth Factors

Sialin

Sialin was first identified as the product of the gene defective in sialidosis, a lysosomal storage disorder. The transporter mediates the movement of sialic acid out of lysosomes by coupling to the proton electrochemical gradient across the lysosomal membrane. Unlike the vesicular ▶ neurotransmitter transporters which are antiporters, sialin is a symporter with ▶ sialic acid and protons both moving out of the lysosome.

σ-Opioid Receptors

σ-Opiod receptors are postulated receptors, which mediate the "dysphoric" effects (anxiety, hallucinations, bad dreams etc.), which are produced by some opioids. They are not true opioid receptors,

as many other drugs also interact with them. Of the opioids, only benzomorphans, such as pentazozine, interact with sigma-receptors. The molecular identity of sigma-receptors is not known.

Signal Peptidases

Signal peptidases are specific proteases located on the luminal side of the endoplasmic reticulum. They cleave the amino-terminal peptides from the precursor forms of membrane and secretory proteins.

▶ Protein Trafficking

Signal Recognition Particle

The signal recognition particle (SRP) is a cytosolic ribonucleoprotein complex which binds to signal sequences of nascent membrane and secretory proteins emerging from ribosomes. The SRP consists of a 7S RNA and at least six polypeptide subunits (relative molecular masses 9, 14, 19, 54, 68, and 72 kD). It induces an elongation arrest until the nascent chain/ribosome/SRP complex reaches the translocon at the endoplasmic reticulum (ER) membrane.

▶ Protein Trafficking

S

Signal Transducer and Activator of Transcription

▶ STAT
▶ JAK-STAT Pathway

Simple Diffusion

Simple diffusion is permeation of a drug through biological membranes according to the electro-chemical gradient. This type of drug transport can be explained by the pH-partition theory.

▶ Drug Interaction

Simulated Annealing

Simulated annealing is a type of molecular dynamics experiment in which the temperature of the system is cycled over time with the goal of widely sampling conformational space. There are two basic ideas. The first is to create a computational analogue of experimental annealing techniques and the second is to use controlled mechanisms for obtaining different initial structures by using temperature to surmount torsional barriers. Heating to a higher temperature (e.g.1000K) allows the system to rearrange from the present state, cooling to a lower temperature brings the system into a stable state. The cycle is repeated several times (e.g. 100), so that multiple conformations may be obtained. Favourable and stable geometries occur in clusters of similar conformations. During the cooling phases it is possible to introduce constraints between atoms coming from experiments. This procedure is applied to calculate structures based on atom distances like nuclear Overhauser effect (NOE) distances and other geometrical data produced by nuclear magnetic resonance (NMR) spectroscopy.

▶ Molecular Modelling
▶ NMR-based Ligand Screening

Single Channel

The number of nAChR at the neuromuscular junction per square micrometer is ~ 10,000. The flow of ions through a single channel and transitions between open and closed states of a channel can be monitored with a time resolution of microseconds by the patch-clamp technique introduced by Erwin Neher and Bert Sakmann in 1976.

▶ Non-selective Cation Channels
▶ Tolerance and Desensitization

Single Nucleotide Polymorphisms

Single nucleotide polymorphisms (SNPs) are single base pair positions in genomic DNA at which normal individuals in a given population show different sequence alternatives (alleles), with the least frequent allele having an abundance of 1 % or greater. SNPs occur once every 100 to 300 bases and are hence the most common genetic variations.

▶ Microarray Technology
▶ Pharmacogegentics

Sinus Rhythm

The sinus rhythm is the heart rhythm in which the sinus node generates an electrical impulse which travels through specialized cells (that form a conduction system) and leads to a ventricular contraction.

▶ Antiarrhythmic Drugs

siRNAs

Small interfering RNAs (siRNA) are the mediators of gene-specific silencing by RNA interference. SiRNA stands for small interfering RNA duplexes They are typically 21-23 bp in length. SiRNA were either chemically synthesised for experimental purposes or produced by Dicer-mediated cleavage of long double-stranded RNA.

▶ Antisense Oligonucleotides

Skinned Fiber

A skinned fiber is a muscle fiber, the sarcolemma of which has been mechanically removed or which is made freely permeable to small molecules, such as Ca^{2+}, Mg^{2+}, EGTA, ATP, soluble enzymes and others by a chemical agent (saponin, β-escin or *Staphylococcus* α-toxin). The organization of the sarcoplasmic reticulum (SR) and myofibrils is kept as they are in the living muscle.

▶ Ryanodine Receptor

SMADs

Smads are a group of proteins, which serve as substrates for type I receptor serine/threonine receptor kinases. The ubiquitously expressed Smad proteins fall into three subfamilies, receptor-activated Smads (R-Smads), e.g. Smad 1, Smad 2, Smad 3, Smad 5, Smad 8, which become phosphorylated by the type I receptors, common mediator Smads (Co-Smads), e.g. Smad 4, which oligomerise with activated R-Smads and inhibitory Smads (I-Smads), e.g. Smad 6 and Smad 7, which are induced by TGF-β family members. These last exert a negative feedback effect by competing with R-Smads for receptor interaction and by marking the receptors for degradation. Activation of type I serine/threonine receptor kinases results in the phosphorylation of R-Smads. The consequence of R-Smad phosphorylation is the formation of oligomeric complexes with the Co-Smad, Smad 4. Substrate specificity is determined by the structural properties of the R-Smads; e.g. TGF-β and activin receptors phosphorylate Smad 2 and Smad 3, while bone morphogenetic protein receptors phosphorylate Smad 1, Smad 5 and Smad 8. The R-Smad/Co-

Smad complex translocates to the nucleus, where it binds to regulatory sequences of the DNA together with specific transcription factors.

▶ Receptor Serine/Threonine Kinases
▶ Neurotrophic Factors

Small GTPases

GUDULA SCHMIDT, KLAUS AKTORIES
Institut für Experimentelle und Klinische Pharmakologie und Toxikologie, Albert-Ludwigs-Universität Freiburg, Freiburg, Germany
gudula.schmidt@pharmakol.uni-freiburg.de, klaus.aktories@pharmakol.uni-freiburg.de

Synonyms

Low molecular mass GTPases, small G-proteins

Definition

Small GTPases are monomeric 20 to 40 kD GTP-binding proteins that interconvert between an active (GTP bound) and an inactive (GDP bound) state. As molecular switches they are involved in the regulation of complex cellular processes.

▶ Bacterial Toxins
▶ Exocytosis
▶ Intracellular Transport

Basic Characteristics

Regulation

Activation of small GTPases occurs by GDP/GTP exchange catalysed by ▶ guanine nucleotide exchange factors (GEFs). They stimulate the dissociation of GDP in response to an upstream signal and results in the binding of GTP. In the GTP-bound form the GTPases are active, and bind to and activate a number of effector molecules. The small G proteins are able to hydrolyse the bound nucleotide to GDP. This inactivation step is accelerated by ▶ GTPase activating proteins (GAPs). In the GDP bound form Rho is inactive and binds to

S

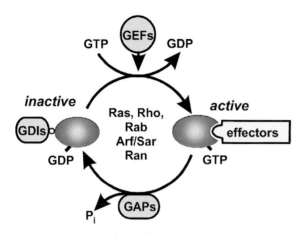

Fig. 1 The GTPase cycle: GTPases are inactive in the GDP-bound form. In a complex with guanine nucleotide dissociation inhibitors (GDIs) the inactive form is stabilized. Guanine nucleotide exchange factors (GEFs) cause the release of GDP and binding of GTP and thereby the activation of the proteins. The active state of the GTPases is turned off by GTP hydrolysis catalysed by GTPase activating proteins (GAPs).

▶ guanine nucleotide dissociation inhibitors (GDIs) that stabilize the inactive form. In mammalian cells, each family of GTPase regulating proteins comprise numerous members, which are more or less specific for individual GTPases, cell types, GTPase functions and signal pathways.

General Structural Properties

All small GTPases are folded in a similar way. They possess 4 consensus amino acid sequences in common, which are involved in nucleotide binding and hydrolysis: GXXXXGK, DXXG, NKXD and EXSAX. Two highly flexible regions (Switch I-and Switch II regions) determine the nucleotide-dependent activity state of the GTPases and the protein-protein-interactions with effectors and regulatory proteins.

Post-translational Modification

All small GTPases (except Ran) are posttranslationally modified. Most important is the isoprenylation of the C-terminus. The type of modification is determined by the COOH-terminal amino acid sequence. GTPases with a C-terminal CAAX-box (A=aliphatic amino acid, X=any amino acid)

are farnesylated at the cysteine residue followed by the proteolytic degradation of the last three amino acids and subsequent methylation of the carboxy-terminus. In the case of a CAAL or CAC, the cysteines are modified by geranylgeranylation. In some cases an additional cysteine is palmitoylated or N-terminal myristoylation occurs. All these posttranslational modifications allow the interaction of GTPases with the phospholipid bilayer. Lipid modification of the GTPases is required for their membrane localization. For example, for Ras it has been shown that farnesylation is needed for the contact with the GEF at the membrane and thus for activation of Ras.

Families

The superfamily of small GTPases consists of more than 100 members from yeast to human with more than 80 members expressed in mammalian cells. Based on structural and functional similarities the GTPases are subdivided into 5 major classes.

Ras GTPases

The mammalian family of Ras GTPases consists of more than 15 members, which share high homology to each other and include Ha-Ras, Ki-Ras, N-Ras, R-Ras, Rap, Ral, Rheb, Rin and Rit proteins. Ras proteins have achieved attention with the discovery that they contain point mutations in 15% of all human tumours (more than 90% in pancreatic tumours), leading to the exchange of conserved amino acids e.g., at positions 12 and 61. Amino acid exchanges at these positions block the GTP hydrolase activity of the GTPases, resulting in constitutive activation. Ras GTPases are involved in signal transduction of proliferation and/or differentiation. They couple receptor tyrosine kinases with a protein kinase cascade termed Raf/ERK kinase pathway (also known as MAP kinase cascade). Activation of this pathway leads to phosphorylation and activation of transcription factors like Elk-1, and stimulate gene expression. Activated Ras has been shown to transform culture cells and to produce tumours in nude mice. Besides the Raf kinase, the RalGDS, which is an activator of the Ral subfamily proteins, and the PI3 kinase, which is involved in inositol signalling, are important effectors of Ras. Ral GTPases (~50% identical with Ras) control cell proliferation, Ras-mediated cell transformation, vesicle traffic, phospholipase D and cytoskeleton organization. Ral is suggested to link the Ras pathway to the Rho family of GTPases and activates a GAP for Cdc42. Rap GTPases have been identified in a screen for cDNAs that are able to revert the transforming phenotype of Ki-Ras (Kirsten Ras) and, therefore, were also termed K-rev proteins.

Rho GTPases
Members (>15) of the Rho family of GTPases, including RhoA, B, and C, Cdc42 and Rac1 and 2, share more than 50% sequence identity. The GTPases are important regulators of the actin cytoskeleton. RhoA regulates the formation of actin stress fibers whereas Cdc42 is known to induce filopodia. Rac is involved in the formation of lamellipodia and membrane ruffles. Rho-GTPases are involved in migration, phagocytosis, endo- and exocytosis, cell-cell and cell-matrix contact. Rac regulates NADPH oxidase. Furthermore, Rho GTPases are involved in transcriptional activation, cell transformation and apoptosis.

Many Rho GTPase effectors have been identified, including protein- and lipid kinases, phospholipase D, and numerous adaptor proteins. One of the best characterized effector of RhoA is Rho kinase, which phosphorylates and inactivates myosin phosphatase; thereby RhoA causes activation of actomyosin. Rho proteins are preferred targets of bacterial protein toxins (▶ Bacterial Toxins).

Rab GTPases
The largest family of small GTPases with more than 40 members identified are the Rab GTPases. Rab proteins are important regulators of specific steps of vesicle trafficking, including budding, targeting, docking and fusion with acceptor membranes. Each Rab protein has a organelle-specific subcellular localization and seems to be functionally specialized. Rab1A and Rab1B are two of the most extensively studied members of the Rab family. Both proteins are found in membranes of the ER, Golgi apparatus and intermediate vesicles between these compartments. They appear to function in the anterograde trafficking of proteins from the ER to the Golgi compartment. Rab4 and Rab5 are present on early endosomes and are involved in the endocytic process, whereas Rab6 is localized at the Goli apparatus regulating processes of the secretory pathway. One of the best studied member of the Rab protein family is Rab3a. This GTPase is a key regulator of Ca^{2+}-induced exocytosis, particularly in nerve terminals. Several effectors of Rab proteins like Rabphilin, Rabaptin and Rim have been identified and characterized as essential for vesicle trafficking. Recently, the Rab effector Rabkinesin6 has been identified that links Rab proteins to the microtubule cytoskeleton. Rabkinesin6 may be the motor driving vesicles along microtubules from the Golgi apparatus to the periphery.

Arf/Sar1 GTPases
The name Arf (ADP ribosylation factor) stems from its discovery as a cytosolic factor with the ability to enhance the ADP-ribosylation of the α-subunit of the G protein G_S by ▶ cholera toxin. Arf is known to stimulate the activity of phospholipase D. Studies with dominant active or dominant negative mutants of Arf proteins in mammalian cells suggest the involvement of these GTPases in the trafficking of coated vesicles, and it is now known that Arf1 regulates the formation of COPI-coated vesicles for retrograde transport between Golgi apparatus and endoplasmic reticulum. Sar1, which is 37% identical to Arf1, is needed for the assembly of COPII proteins for vesicle transport in the opposite direction. Taken together, Arf and Sar proteins play crucial roles in the recruitment of COP components to vesicles thereby regulating vesicle budding. In contrast to the other small GTPases Arf/Sar1 proteins are not regulated by GDI-proteins, whereas different GEF- and GAP proteins have been identified.

Ran GTPases
In mammalian cells there is only one Ran gene, which was discovered as a Ras-like gene (Ran: Ras-related nuclear protein). In contrast, in yeast more than one related Ran genes have been identified. The predominant nuclear localization of the GTPase was the first hint that Ran is involved in nucleo-cytoplasmic transport processes. Interestingly, the only Ran GEF present in mammalian cells, RCC1 (regulator of chromatine condensation), is localized exclusively in the nucleus, whereas the single Ran GAP (Ran GAP1) is in the cytoplasm. This specialized localization of the reg-

ulators is the prerequisite for the asymmetric distribution of the GDP- and GTP-bound form of Ran and for its role as a nucleo-cytoplasmic transporter. In contrast to other GTPases, the activity of Ran is dependent on the gradient of the GTP-bound GTPase from cytoplasm to nucleoplasm that allows the transport of cargo proteins. Ran is involved in nuclear import as well as in export of proteins through the ▶ nuclear pore complex. Both processes require the formation of protein complexes, including Ran, the cargo protein and Ran binding proteins like ▶ importins or ▶ exportins.

In addition to its transporter function, Ran has been shown to participate in microtubule organization during the M phase of the cell cycle.

Cascades and Cross-talk

Small GTPases are not isolated molecular switches regulating cellular processes. Signalling cascades within one subfamily as well as cross-talk between members of different subfamilies are known. For example, Cdc42/ Rac/ Rho are sequentially activated after extracellular stimuli in quiescent Swiss 3T3 cells. Moreover, reciprocal modulation between Rho GTPases have been described. Ras and Rho proteins act in a cooperative manner in Ras-induced transforming. A further example of cross-talk between GTPase families is the cooperative function of Rho and Rab proteins during cell migration, with Rho proteins controlling the actin cytoskeleton and Rab proteins regulating vesicular traffic for the recruitment of membrane material and the recycling of proteins like integrins. Arfaptin connects signalling via Arf and Rac.

Drugs

Small GTPases, among other activities, regulate cell growth, neurite outgrowth and signalling of immune cells involved in inflammation. Pharmacological modulation of the activity of small GTPases is thus a useful aim in cancer and anti-inflammatory therapies. Farnesyltransferase inhibitors can be used to block the posttranslational modification of the GTPases, which for example is essential for the transforming activity of Ras or Rho GTPases. Such agents are at present in clinical trials.

References

1. Matozaki, T., H. Nakanishi, and Y. Takai (2000) Small G-protein networks; their crosstalk and signal cascades. Cell. Signalling 12:515–524
2. Takai, Y., Sasaki, T., and T. Matozaki (2001) Small GTP-binding proteins. Physiological Reviews 81:153–208

Smooth Muscle Tone Regulation

FRANZ HOFMANN
Technische Universität München, Germany
Pharma@ipt.med.tu-muenchen.de

Synonyms

Regulation of smooth muscle contractility

Definition

The following organs contain smooth muscles layers as a major functional part: arterial and venous vessels; lung and bronchia; oesophagus, stomach, small and large intestine; urinary tract and bladder; uterus. Hormones, locally released transmitters, and shear stress or pressure regulate the tonus of these organs. Each organ has a slightly different regulation of its contractility, but the basis for this regulation, i.e. the intracellular signalling pathways, are very similar or identical. This article will focus on major findings that may be similar for all smooth muscles.

▶ Blood Pressure Control
▶ Guanylyl Cyclase
▶ NO Synthases

Basic Mechanisms

Key mechanism of smooth muscle tone regulation is the phosphorylation of Ser-19 of the regulatory myosin light chain II (rMLC) (1). Phosphorylation and dephosphorylation is catalysed by ▶ myosin light chain kinase (MLCK) and the type 1 ▶ myosin phosphatase (MLCP), respectively. Calcium-dependent and calcium-independent signal

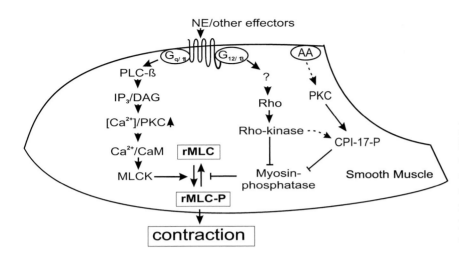

Fig. 1 Mechanisms leading to agonist stimulated calcium-dependent and calcium-independent contraction of smooth muscle. NE, norepinephrine. See text for the other abbreviations.

pathways regulate the activity of both enzymes and thereby the phosphorylation status of rMLC. An increase in the cytosolic calcium concentration leads to phosphorylation of the rMLC and contraction within 4 s. The correlation between percent phosphorylated rMLC and developed force is quite variable. Maximal force can be attained at 0.2–0.3 mol phosphate per mol rMLC. Phosphorylation can decline during maintenance of tension suggesting that even dephosphorylated cross-bridges can contribute to force maintenance.

Calcium-dependent Regulation

Calcium-dependent regulation involves the calcium-calmodulin complex that activates smooth muscle MLCK, a monomer of approximately 135 kD. Dephosphorylation is initiated by MLCP. MLCP is a complex of three proteins: a 110–130 kD myosin phosphatase targeting and regulatory subunit (MYPT1), a 37 kD catalytic subunit (PP-1C) and a 20 kD subunit of unknown function. In most cases, calcium-independent regulation of smooth muscle tone is achieved by inhibition of MLCP activity at constant calcium level inducing an increase in phospho-rMLC and contraction (Fig. 1).

Calcium-dependent Contraction

Different agonists such as norepinephrine, acetylcholine or angiotensin II activate smooth muscle contraction by binding to a heptahelical receptor, i.e. α-adrenergic, muscarinergic or AT-1 receptors, followed by an increase in cytosolic calcium (Fig. 1 and 2). The activation of the trimeric G Pro-

teins G_q or G_{11} increases the activity of phospholipase Cβ (PLC) generating inositol trisphosphate (IP_3) and diacylglycerol (DAG) and other fatty acid derived compounds. Classical findings suggested that IP_3 stimulates calcium release from intracellular stores that binds to calmodulin and activates MLCK. This simple scheme is not in line with the fact that a block of the ▶ L-type calcium channel inhibits contraction. The importance of the L-type calcium channel is further supported by genetic deletion of the corresponding $Ca_V1.2$ gene. Mice lacking the smooth muscle $Ca_V1.2$ channel have severe difficulties to contract intestinal and other smooth muscle. It is therefore likely that activation of a heptahelical receptor leads to depolarisation of the membrane and activation of the L-type calcium channels (Fig. 2). Possible candidates are ▶ TRP channels (most likely TRPC6) activated either by DAG or by interaction with empty IP_3-stores. The inflowing cations may depolarise the membrane to potentials that activate T- and thereafter L-type calcium channels or directly L-type channels. A second channel depolarising the membrane is the calcium-activated chloride channel present in many smooth muscle cells. Calcium released from IP_3-stores or flowing in through TRP channels could activate this chloride channel and depolarise the membrane. The L-type calcium channel provides calcium to trigger calcium release from ryanodine receptor controlled calcium stores and for refilling various intracellular calcium stores (2). The mechanism behind pressure or shear stress induced contraction is not known, but may again involve TRP channels.

S

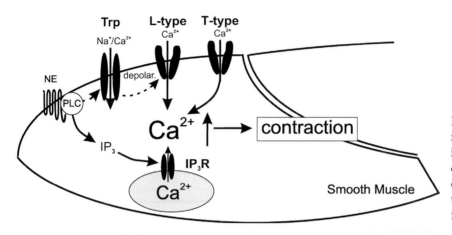

Fig. 2 Membrane mechanisms leading to an increases in cytosolic calcium concentration. depolar., depolarisation of the membrane; See text for abbreviations.

Calcium-independent Contraction

Agonist-activated receptors can induce contraction at a constant intracellular calcium concentration (3) if the receptor activates the G proteins G_{12} or G_{13} (Fig. 1). Activation of these G proteins recruits the monomeric GTPase ► Rho to the membrane, where Rho exchanges GDP against GTP and activates ► Rho-kinase. By a still unsolved cascade eventually involving ZIP kinase, the MYPT1 subunit of MLCP is phosphorylated at Thr-697 (rat MYPT1), which inhibits MLCP activity. Since the activity of MLCK is not affected by this cascade, rMLC is phosphorylated to a higher level. Phosphorylation and inhibition of MLCP activity is only observed if a central exon of MYPT1 is present. These results could explain the old finding that certain agonists induce calcium sensitation of the contractile machinery in most but not all smooth muscles. MLCP activity is also affected by a smooth muscle specific inhibitor protein of PP-1C, named ► CPI-17. Protein kinase C (PKC) phosphorylates CPI-17, which becomes a high affinity inhibitor of the catalytic subunit of MLCP. The nature of the PKC subtype is not clear. It is possible that it is one of the atypical PKC enzymes that is activated directly by arachidonic acid (AA). Rho-kinases that phosphorylate CPI-17 in vitro apparently does not affect directly in vivo the phosphorylation status of CPI-17. Arachidonic acid inhibits dephosphorylation of MLCs, i.e. by a second mechanism by dissociating the MLCP holoenzyme.

Relaxation of Smooth Muscle

The major relaxing transmitters are those that elevate the cAMP or cGMP concentration (Fig. 3). Adenosine stimulates the activity of cAMP kinase. The next step is not clear, but evidence has been accumulated that cAMP kinase decreases the calcium sensitivity of the contractile machinery. *In vitro*, cAMP kinase phosphorylates MLCK and decreases the affinity of MLCK for calcium-calmodulin. However, this regulation does not occur in intact smooth muscle. Possible other substrate candidates for cAMP kinase are the heat stable protein HSP 20, Rho A and MLCP that are also phosphorylated by ► cGMP kinase I (Fig. 3).

A major relaxing factor is ► NO, a signal molecule synthetized by three different ► NO synthases (NOS). NO synthesised in the endothelial layer of the vessels diffuses into the smooth muscle layer, where NO activates soluble guanylate cyclase (GC) and generates high concentrations of cGMP. In non-vascular systems such as the intestinal smooth muscle, NO is released from non-adrenergic, noncholinergic neurons. An alternative pathway for the production of cGMP is the stimulation of particulate GC by the ► natriuretic peptides ANF and BNF. ANF and BNF are released from cardiac atrial and ventricular muscle, respectively, and lower blood pressure. The effects of the natriuretic peptides are mediated through cGMP and cGMP kinase I, whereas NO has effects which are not mediated by cGMP kinase I.

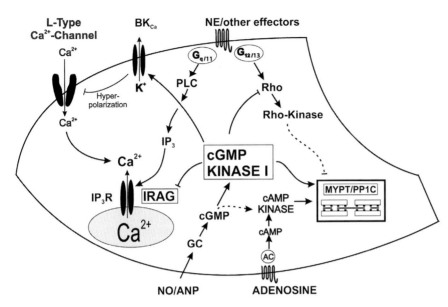

Fig. 3 Major mechanisms leading to relaxation of smooth muscle. See text for abbreviations.

Smooth muscle contains the two cGMP kinase isozymes Iα and Iβ and a number of identified substrates (4). The NO/cGMP/cGMP kinase pathway interferes with the calcium-dependent and the calcium-independent contraction. A number of researchers have shown that cGMP-dependent phosphorylation of the BK_{Ca} channel increases its open probability resulting in hyperpolarization of the membrane potential and closure of voltage-dependent calcium channels (▶ BK channel). The activity of the BK_{Ca} channel is upregulated by the intracellular calcium concentration establishing a negative feedback loop. It is well established that cGMP kinase decreases the release of calcium from intracellular stores. Recently, it was found that cGMP kinase Iβ is associated with the IP_3 receptor type 1 and the 130 kD protein ▶ IRAG. Phosphorylation of IRAG inhibits the release of calcium from IP_3-sensitive stores in COS cells. However, reconstitution of cGMP kinase I deficient cells suggested that, in murine aortic smooth muscle cells, cGMP kinase Iα and not Iβ lowers norepinephrine-stimulated increases in the cytosolic calcium concentrations. This result is in line with the recent notion, that calcium-dependent contraction of smooth muscle requires membrane depolarisation and calcium influx through menbrane localized ion channels (see above). It is possible that the IP_3-sensitive calcium pool associated with IRAG and cGKIβ controls other smooth muscle functions such as phenotype changes and smooth muscle growth.

Recently, it was demonstrated that cGMP kinase I inhibits smooth muscle contraction due to a calcium-insensitive pathway. A possible mechanism could be phosphorylation of Rho by cGMP kinase I. The phosphorylation site is identical to a cAMP kinase site identified in Rho from non-smooth muscle cells. It was reported that phosphorylation of Rho by cGMP kinase I prevents membrane association of Rho, which is required to stimulate the GDP/GTP exchange. Alternatively, phosphorylation of telokin may interfere with the calcium sensitisation of contraction. cGMP kinase Iα interacts specifically with a leucine zipper present at the C-terminus of MYPT1. Depending on the tissue, this leucine zipper is present or not. However, so far no change in MLCP activity has been found when MYPT1 is phosphorylated by cGMP kinase Iα.

Pharmacological Intervention

A large number of drugs interfere with smooth muscle contraction. These compounds lower blood pressure and are referred to as antihypertensive. In this section, only those coumpounds will be mentioned that have a direct effect on smooth muscle tone. Phenylephrine is an agonist on most smooth muscles and activates α_1 adrenoceptors. Carbachol is an agonist on some smooth muscles and activates contraction through muscarinic receptors. Blockers of the α_1-adrenoceptors such as prazosin and urapidil are competitive inhibitors of the α_1-receptor in vascular and bladder smooth muscle. Phenoxybenzamine is an irreversible blocker of α_1 receptors and phentolamine blocks α_1 and α_2 receptors. ▶ Calcium channel blockers such as the dihydropyridines, phenylalkylamines and benzothiazepines lower smooth muscle tone by blocking the L-type calcium channel.

▶ Nitrates (glycerol trinitrate, isosorbit dinitrate, pentaerythritol tetranitrate, molsidomine, sodium nitroprusside), which generate NO, increase cGMP concentrations and lower smooth muscle tone by activation of cGMP kinase I. Nitrates relax *in vivo* mainly the capacitative part of the circulation system, i.e. the veneous part. Sidenafil, a specific inhibitor of phosphodiesterase V, a cGMP hydrolysing enzyme, increases cGMP in the corpus cavernosum and lowers, together with nitrates, the blood pressure by the combined effect on cGMP level. An additional potentially important drug family are compounds that stimulate the soluble guanylyl cyclase independent of NO (5) and lower elevated blood pressure. The inhibitor of Rho-kinase,Y-27632, lowers elevated blood pressure in hypertensive animals, without affecting significantly the blood pressure of non-hypertensive animals (6).

References

1. Pfitzer G (2001) Invited review: regulation of myosin phosphorylation in smooth muscle. J Appl Physiol 91:497–503
2. Jaggar JH, Porter VA, Lederer WJ, Nelson MT (2000) Calcium sparks in smooth muscle. Am J Physiol Cell Physiol 278:C235–C256
3. Somlyo AP, Somlyo AV (2000) Signal transduction by G-proteins, rho-kinase and protein phosphatase to smooth muscle and non-muscle myosin II. J Physiol 522:177–185
4. Hofmann F, Ammendola A, Schlossmann J (2000) Rising behind NO: cGMP-dependent protein kinases. J Cell Sci 113:1671–1676
5. Stasch JP, Becker EM, Alonso-Alija C, Apeler H, Dembowsky K, Feurer A, Gerzer R, Minuth T, Perzborn E, Pleiss U, Schroder H, Schroeder W, Stahl E, Steinke W, Straub A, Schramm M (2001) NO-independent regulatory site on soluble guanylate cyclase. Nature 410:212–215
6. Uehata M, Ishizaki T, Satoh H, Ono T, Kawahara T, Morishita T, Tamakawa H, Yamagami K, Inui J, Maekawa M, Narumiya S (1997) Calcium sensitization of smooth muscle mediated by a Rho-associated protein kinase in hypertension. Nature 389:990–994

SNAPs

SNAPs is an acronym for soluble NSF attachment proteins. They were originally discovered as cofactors for NSF that mediate the membrane binding of NSF in *in-vitro* transport assays. Several isoforms of SNAPs exist in mammalian cells. SNAPs are also highly conserved proteins. Crystallographic studies indicated that the proteins form a very stiff and twisted sheet that is formed by a series of antiparallel and tightly packed helices connected by short loops.

▶ Exocytosis

SNARE Proteins

SNAREs is an acronym for solubleNSF acceptor protein receptors. They are a superfamily of small and mostly membrane-bound proteins that are distinguished by the presence of a conserved stretch of 60 amino acids referred to as a SNARE motif. With few exceptions, a single transmembrane domain is located adjacent to the SNARE motif at the C-terminal end. Many SNAREs possess in addition an independently folded N-terminal domain whose structures are more diverse.

SNARE motifs spontaneously assemble into SNARE complexes. These consist of a bundle of four intertwined α-helices that are connected by a total of 16 layers of mostly hydrophobic amino acid side chains. In the middle of the bundle, there is a highly conserved and polar "o-layer" consisting of three glutamine and one arginine residue. These residues are among the most conserved in the SNARE superfamily and led to a classification of SNAREs into Q- and R-SNAREs, respectively. Different fusion steps require different sets of SNAREs but some SNAREs can participate in different complexes, and some fusion steps involve several SNARE complexes that appear to operate in parallel and independently.

In vitro, SNARE-complex formation is irreversible. Disassembly requires the concerted action of the chaperone-like ATPase NSF and SNAPs.

▶ Exocytosis

SNPs

▶ Single Nucleotide Polymorphisms

SNRIs

▶ Selective Noradrenaline Reuptake Inhibitors

SOCS

Suppressors of cytokine signaling are a family of cytokine-inducible proteins that inhibit JAK kinases.

▶ JAK-STAT Pathway

SOD

▶ Superoxide Dismutase

Solid Phase Synthesis

Solid phase synthesis is a polymer-supported or solid-supported synthesis, i.e. stepwise construction of product molecules attached to an insoluble organic or inorganic polymer.

▶ Combinatorial Chemistry

Soluble Guanylyl Cyclase

The enzyme guanylyl cyclase produces the second messenger guanosine monophosphate (3',5'-cyclic GMP, cGMP) from guanosine triphosphate (GTP). The soluble isoform is the primary target of the signaling molecule NO.

▶ Guanylyl Cyclase

Solute Carrier

▶ Table appendix: Membrane Transport Proteins

Somatomedins

Somatomedins are polypeptide mediators produced in response to growth hormone in the liver, e.g. insulin-like growth factors (IGFs). In particular, IGF-1 is the main mediator of growth hormone action.

S

Somatostatin

GISELA OLIAS, WOLFGANG MEYERHOF
German Institute of Human Nutrition,
Department of Molecular Genetics,
Potsdam-Rehbrücke, Germany
Olias@mail.dife.de, meyerhof@mail.dife.de

Synonyms

Somatostatin, SOM, SST14, SST28, somatotropin
release inhibitory factor (SRIF), growth hormone
release-inhibiting factor

Definition

Somatostatin is a regulatory cyclic peptide that
was originally described as a hypothalamic growth
hormone release-inhibiting factor. It is produced
throughout the central nervous system as well as
in secretory cells of the periphery and mediates its
regulatory functions on cellular processes such as
neurotransmission, smooth muscle contraction,
secretion and cell proliferation via a family of
seven ▶ transmembrane domain ▶ G-protein-coupled receptors termed sst_1-sst_5.

▶ G-protein-coupled Receptors

Basic Characteristics

Biosynthesis
The human somatostatin gene is located on chromosome 3q28 and contains a single intron of 876
base pairs (bp) in its coding sequence. Its 5′
upstream region includes several regulatory
domains such as a cAMP ▶ response element
(CRE). The intracellular mediator camp is one of
the activators of somatostatin gene transcription,
but also many other factors such as Ca^{2+}, glucocorticoids and growth hormones are able to influence somatostatin gene expression (1).

As with other neuropeptides, somatostatin is
synthesized as a prepro-hormone on ribosomes of
the rough ▶ endoplasmic reticulum (RER). The
translation product of the 351 bp long mRNA coding sequence is prepro-somatostatin, a peptide of
116 amino acids. After translocation of the precursor molecule into the ER lumen and cleavage of
the signal peptide the prohormone is further
transported by transfer vesicles through the Golgi
stacks into the *trans* compartment of the ▶ Golgi
apparatus. Differential posttranslational processing of prosomatostatin on the way from the ER to
the *trans*Golgi network results in two biologically
active isoforms, the tetradecapeptide somatosta-
tin-14 and the amino-terminally extended octa-
cosapeptide somatostatin-28, respectively. Cleavage of the C-terminal region of prosomatostatin at
a dibasic Arg-Lys site produces somatostatin-14
and cleavage at a monobasic Gln-Arg site results in
somatostatin-28. Candidates for somatostatin-14
converting enzymes are prohormone convertases
PC1 and PC2, whereas ▶ furin is a candidate soma-
tostatin-28 convertase. The amounts of the isoforms produced are tissue specific. Whereas the
hypothalamus synthesizes both, somatostatin-14
and somatostatin-28 in a ratio of 4:1, the intestinal
mucosal cells produce mainly somatostatin-28.

In the *trans* Golgi compartment the peptide is
sorted via secretory vesicles into a regulated pathway. In contrast to vesicles of the constitutive
pathway, vesicles of the regulated pathway are
stored in the cytoplasm until their stimulated
release. Membrane depolarisation as well as a wide
range of substances such as intracellular mediators, neuropeptides, neurotransmitters, classical
hormones, cytokines, growth factors, ions and
nutrients induce somatostatin secretion. General
inhibitors of somatostatin release are opiates,
GABA, leptin and TGF-β.

Tissue Distribution
High amounts of somatostatin are found in the
central nervous system (CNS), the peripheral
nervous system, the gut and the endocrine pancreas whereas the kidneys, adrenals, thyroid, sub-
mandibular glands, prostate and placenta produce
rather low amounts. In particular, the hypothalamus, all limbic structures, the deeper layers of the
cerebral cortex, the striatum, the periaqueductal
central gray, and all levels of the major sensory
pathway are brain areas that are especially rich in
somatostatin. 80% of the somatostatin immunoreactivity in the hypothalamus is found in cells of
the anterior periventricular nucleus (1). In the gut
δ cells of the mucosa and neurons, which are
intrinsic to the submucous and myenteric plex-

Tab. 1   Somatostatin effects in different tissues (adapted from references 1, 3, 4).

Site	Effects
Hypothalamus	Inhibition of norepinephrine, GHRH, TRH, and CRH release. Inhibition of endogenous SST release.
Other Brain Regions	Effects on cognitive, locomotor, sensory and autonomic functions, analgesic effects. Inhibition of dopamine release from the midbrain. Stimulation of dopamine release in basal ganglia.
Pituitary	Inhibition of basal and stimulated release of GH. Inhibition of TSH release. **No** effects on LH, FSH release. **No** effect on ACTH release in normal subjects, but suppresses elevated levels in Addison's disease and in ACTH producing tumours. **No** effect on prolactin release in normal subjects, but diminishes increased prolactin levels in acromegaly.
Gastrointestinal Tract	Inhibition of most gut hormones, gastric acid, pepsin, bile and colonic fluid secretion. Suppression of motor activity in general, inhibition of gallbladder contraction, gastric emptying. Stimulation of migrating motor complex activity.
Thyroid	Inhibition of TSH-stimulated T4 and T3 release. Inhibition of calcitonin secretion from thyroid parafollicular cells.
Adrenal	Inhibition of angiotensin II stimulated aldosterone release. Inhibition of acetylcholine stimulated medullary catecholamine release.
Kidney	Inhibition of hypovolemia stimulated renin secretion. Inhibition of ADH-mediated water absorption.
Immune Cells	Diminishing IFN-γ secretion from lymphocytes.
Lymphocytes, Inflammatory Cells, Intestinal Mucosal Cells, Cartilage Cells, Bone Precursor Cells	Inhibition of proliferation.
Other Tissues/Cells	Inhibition of growth factor (IGF1, EGF, PDGF) and cytokine (IL6, IFN-γ) secretion.

uses, produce somatostatin. Furthermore, somatostatin has been found in δ cells of the pancreas and within the thyroid where somatostatin has been detected in a subpopulation of C cells that additionally contain calcitonin. Somatostatin has also been localized in the inner part of the retina and in cells and organs of the immune system, for example, within macrophages, lymphocytes and the thymus.

Somatostatin Receptors

Somatostatin acts on various organs, tissues and cells as a neurotransmitter, paracrine/autocrine and endocrine regulator on cell secretion, smooth muscle contractility, nutrient absorption, cell growth and neurotransmission (1, 2, 3). Some of its mainly inhibitory effects are listed in Table 1. Somatostatin mediates its function via a family of heptahelical G-protein-coupled receptors termed sst_1, sst_2, sst_3, sst_4 and sst_5, which were cloned almost 10 years ago. Despite a high degree of sequence homology the receptors derive from separate genes localized on different chromosomes (Table 2). The genes of sst_1, sst_3, sst_4 and sst_5 do not contain any introns in their protein coding regions. In contrast to this, the sst_2 gene contains a cryptic splice site at the 3′ end of its coding region giving rise to two splice variants, sst_{2A} and sst_{2B}.

Studies investigating the distribution of *sst* mRNAs have shown that *sst* gene expression varies during ontogeny. Moreover, all five genes are tissue specifically expressed. However, expression pattern overlap and different mRNA levels have been demonstrated in brain, pituitary, pancreas, adrenals, kidneys, liver, lung, placenta, stomach, gut, thyroid and immune cells. In addition to the *sst*gene expression in organs, many tumour cell lines, such as AtT20 and GH3 pituitary cells, and numerous human tumours, benign or malignant, have been shown to be a rich source of sst subtypes. *sst2*mRNA is highly expressed in many tumours, while *sst5* mRNA is abundant in breast tumours and *sst1* appears to be preferentially expressed in primary prostate cancers (1, 2, 3). Laboratories investigating neuroendocrine tumours, such as gastrinomas and insulinomas, reported general expression of *sst1*, *sst2*, but also varying levels of *sst3*, *sst4*, and *sst5* mRNAs have been observed. Interestingly, in gastrinomas and carcinoids only low amounts of *sst3* mRNA have been detected so far. However, it should be noted that these results may not automatically mirror functional receptor levels, since to date nearly all investigations of sst subtypes in tumours are based on mRNA studies.

Besides developmental and tissue specific regulation of *sst* gene expression, regulation by extracellular signals such as estrogen and thyroid hormone has been observed. The underlying mechanisms still remain to be elucidated, although ▶ promoter studies of various laboratories have begun to work out the molecular basis for a better understanding. All sst subtype promoters investigated to date contain consensus sequences for several common transcription factors. For example, the sst_2 gene contains estrogen response elements whereas progesterone/glucocorticoid and thyroid response elements were found in the *sst1* and *sst5* genes (1, 3).

The human sst receptor protein isoforms range in size from 364 amino acids to 418 amino acids (Table 2). The sst subtypes show highest sequence identity in their putative transmembrane domains and can be divided on the basis of amino acid homologies and by their ability to bind somatostatin analogues (Table 3) into two subclasses, termed $SRIF_1$ and $SRIF_2$. The $SRIF_1$ group comprises sst_2, sst_3 and sst_5 ($SRIF_{1A}$, $SRIF_{1B}$ and $srif_{1C}$) and the $SRIF_2$ group includes sst_1 and sst_4 ($SRIF_{2A}$ and $srif_{2B}$). Receptors of the $SRIF_1$ group bind seglitide and octreotide with high (sst_2 and sst_5) to moderate (sst_3) affinity while members of the $SRIF_2$ group are insensitive to these compounds.

All six receptors seem to couple to ▶ pertussis toxin-sensitive ▶ G proteins of the G_i/G_0 type (4). Depending on the sst subtype, cell type and species, different G-proteins couple the individual receptor isoforms to various second-messenger systems, which include ▶ adenylyl cyclase, K^+ and Ca^{2+} channels, Na^+/H^+ exchanger, phospolipase C, phospolipase A2, mitogen activated protein kinase, serine-threonine phosphatase and phosphotyrosine phosphatase (Table 2). The fact that sst subtypes share transduction mechanisms, bind their endogenous ligands with nanomolar affinities, and that more than one receptor isoform can be expressed in a single cell, might indicate a functional interaction between the different receptor isoforms. In this respect it should be noted that heterodimerization of sst subtypes has been reported.

Physiological functions for sst subtypes have not yet been unequivocally determined. It appears, however, that sst_2 mediates inhibition of glucagon release from pancreatic α-cells, whereas sst_1 and sst_5 seem to be responsible for the inhibition of insulin secretion from pancreatic β-cells. Furthermore, it is thought that sst_2 contributes to the regulation of gastric acid release and that sst_1, sst_2 and sst_5 inhibit hormone-stimulated and/or basal level secretion of GH secretion from the pituitary (1,4).

Somatostatin Related Peptides
Natural binding partners of all sst subtypes cloned to date are somatostatin-14 and somatostatin-28, which are bound with nanomolar affinity; sst_{1-4} bind somatostatin-14 with comparable affinities, while sst_5 may have a slight preference for somatostatin-28. Cortistatin, a recently discovered closely related peptide of somatostatin, also binds sst subtypes with high affinity *in vitro*. In contrast to

Tab. 2 Properties of sst subtypes (adapted from references 1, 3, 4).

Receptor Type	sst$_1$/SRIF$_{2A}$	sst$_2$/SRIF$_{1A}$	sst$_3$/srif$_{1C}$	sst$_4$/srif$_{2B}$	sst$_5$/SRIF$_{1B}$
Chromosomal Localization	14q13	17q24	22p13.1	20p11.2	16p13.3
Length of Human Receptor	391 aa	369 aa (sst$_{2A}$) 356 aa (sst$_{2B}$)	418 aa	388 aa	364 aa
Reported Transduction Mechanism	Inhibition of adenylyl cyclase. Stimulation of tyrosine phosphatase activity. Stimulation of MAP kinase activity. Inhibition of Ca^{2+} channel activation. Stimulation of Na$^+$/H$^+$ exchanger. Stimulation of AMPA/kainate glutamate channels.	Inhibition of forskolin-stimulated adenylyl cyclase. Activation of phosphoinositide metabolism. Stimulation of tyrosine phosphatase activity. Inhibition of Ca^{2+} channel activation. Activation of K$^+$ channel. Inhibition of AMPA/kainate glutamate channels. Inhibition of MAP kinase activity.	Inhibition of adenylyl cyclase. Stimulation of phosphoinositide metabolism. Stimulation of tyrosine phosphatase. Activation of K$^+$ channel. Inhibition/stimulation of MAP kinase activity.	Inhibition of adenylyl cyclase. Stimulation of MAP kinase. Activation of tyrosine phosphatase. Stimulation of K$^+$ channels and phospholipase A$_2$.	Inhibition of adenylyl cyclase. Activation/ inhibition o phosphoinositide metal lism. Inhibition of Ca^{2+} influ Activation of K$^+$ chann Inhibition of MAP kina Stimulation of tyrosine phosphatase.

S

Tab. 3   Selected somatostatin analogues (adapted from references 1, 2, 4, 5).

sst Subtype Ligands and Analogues	Binding Properties
Endogenous Ligands	
Somatostatin-14	Binding to all sst subtypes with high affinity.
Somatostatin-28	Binding to all sst subtypes with high affinity, but slightly higher preference for sst_5.
Human cortistatin-17	Binding to sst_{2-5} with high affinity, slightly lower preference for sst_1.
Rat cortistatin-29	Binding to sst_3 with high affinity, slightly lower preference for sst_1 and sst_4 and sst_2, and lower preference for sst_5 (i. e. ~ 100-fold lower than that of somatostatin-14).
Synthetic Peptide Analogues	
Octreotide (SMS201-995)	Binding to sst_2 with high affinity, slightly lower affinity to sst_5 and sst_3.
Vapreotide (RC-160)	Binding to sst_5 and sst_2 with high affinity, moderate affinity for sst_3 and sst_4.
Lanreotide (BIM23014)	Binding to sst_2 and sst_5 with high affinity, moderate affinity for sst_3 (and sst_4).
Seglitide (MK678)	Binding to sst_2 and sst_5 with high affinity, moderate affinity for sst_3.
BIM23268	Binding to sst_5 with high affinity, slightly lower preference for sst_2, sst_4 and sst_1, moderate affinity for sst_3.
NC8-12	Binding to sst_3 and sst_2 with very high affinity.
BIM23197	Binding to sst_2 and sst_5 with high affinity, moderate affinity for sst_3.
CH275	Binding to sst_1 and sst_4 with high affinity.
Nonpeptide Agonists	
L-797,591	Binding to sst_1 and sst_2 with high affinity.
L-779,976	Binding to sst_2 with very high affinity.
L-796,778	Binding to sst_3 with moderate affinity.
L-803,087	Binding to sst_4 with high affinity.
L-817,818	Binding to sst_5 with high affinity, with slightly lower affinity to sst_1, moderate affinities for sst_2, sst_3 and sst_4.
Radioligands	
[123]I-Tyr[3]-octreotide	Binding to sst_2 and sst_5 with high affinity, lower affinity to sst_3.
^{111}In-DTPA-DPhe[1]-octreotide*	Binding to sst_2 and sst_5 with high affinity, lower affinity to sst_3.
[111]In/^{90}Y-DOTA-lanreotide**	Binding to sst_2, sst_3, sst_4 and sst_5 with high affinity, lower affinity to sst_1.
^{111}In-DOTA-DPhe[1]-Tyr[3]-octreotide	Binding to sst_2 and sst_5 with high affinity, lower affinity to sst_3.
[99m]Te-depreotide	Binding to sst_2, sst_3 and sst_5 with high affinity.

* DTPA, diethylenetriaminepentaacetic acid
**DOTA, 1,4,7,10-tetraazacyclododecane-N,N',N",N"-tetraacetic acid

Tab. 3   Selected somatostatin analogues (adapted from references 1, 2, 4, 5). (Continued)

sst Subtype Ligands and Analogues	Binding Properties
^{111}In-DTPA-Tyr^3-octreotate	Binding to sst$_2$ and sst$_5$ with high affinity.
Antagonists	
BIM23056	sst$_5$ selective.
sst$_3$-ODN-8	sst$_3$ selective.
Cyanamid 154806	sst$_2$ selective.

*   DTPA, diethylenetriaminepentaacetic acid
**DOTA, 1,4,7,10-tetraazacyclododecane-N,N',N",N"-tetraacetic acid

somatostatin, the presence of cortistatin is restricted to the cerebral cortex and the hippocampus. It shows functional characteristics that have not been demonstrated for somatostatin, such as sleep modulating properties. So far a cognate cortistatin receptor has not been identified.

Drugs

The diverse effects of somatostatin, such as inhibition of cell proliferation and hormone release, led to the suggestion that it could be used for the treatment of various diseases. However, its short plasma half-life (less than 3 minutes) and its relative low receptor subtype selectivity make it less useful for therapeutic purposes. Therefore, several synthetic analogues (Table 3) with a higher stability to enzymatic degradation and a higher selectivity for specific sst subtypes have been synthesized. The synthetic peptide analogues have a decisive amino acid motif in common, since pharmacological studies have shown that the amino acid residues 7 to 10 (Phe^7-Trp^8-Lys^9-Thr^{10}) of somatostatin are the responsible segment for receptor binding. In particular Trp^8 and Lys^9 are essential, while the remaining two amino acids may be replaced. Phe^7 can be exchanged with tyrosine and Thr^{10} can be substituted by serine or valine. To date, only a few potential antagonists, such as cyanamid 154806, sst$_3$-ODN-8 and BIM-23056 are available, which preferentially bind to human sst$_2$, sst$_3$, and sst$_5$, respectively (4,5).

To date three analogues, octreotide, lanreotide and vapreotide are clinically used. All three substances display high affinity for sst$_2$ and sst$_5$.

Already in the 1980s octreotide was used in the therapy of acromegaly and other neuroendocrine tumours. Acromegaly is a chronic disease of growth hormone (GH) hypersecretion and in most cases is caused by a pituitary adenoma. Somatostatin analogues have been shown to improve the clinical symptoms of acromegaly, for example gigantism in children, disfigurements of the hands, feet and the face in adults, headache and perspiration. Moreover, tumour shrinkage has been observed in about 50% of the patients, even though the tumour size reduction is reversible. The decreased tumour volume is presumably caused by a shrinkage of individual tumour cells. Recently, sustained release formulations of octreotide and lanreotide have been developed. These new drugs are administered by intramuscular injections only every 7–28 days making life of patients easier, who need a long-term therapy. Octreotide treatment achieves good results in patients with insulinomas, gastrinomas, glucagonomas, ▸ VIPomas and metastatic carcinoids expressing *sst2* and *sst5*. Symptoms such as peptic ulceration, diarrhea, dehydration and necrolytic skin lesions rapidly improve giving the life of patients a higher quality. Despite the successful reduction of symptoms only in about 20% of the patients, tumour shrinkage was observed and, in contrast to acromegalic patients, most patients suffering from carcinoids became insensitive to octreotide therapy within weeks to months. The desensitisation might be explained by a downregulation of sst subtypes or more likely by an outgrowth of sst subtype-negative cell clones.

S

Other tumours, such as ACTH-secreting pituitary adenomas, prolactinomas, pancreatic and prostate cancer, which express no or other *sst* subtypes than *sst2* and *sst5* are rather unresponsive to octreotide therapy. Therefore, the development of new sst-subtype-selective analogues is required. Transfer of genes encoding *sst2* or *sst5* into such tumour types might also be a strategy, since clinically used somatostatin analogues exert the majority of their antineoplastic effects via these receptor subtypes. Furthermore, stable transfection of human pancreatic cancer cell lines with human sst_2 cDNA resulted in a significant reduction of tumour cell growth, indicating that the loss of *sst2* expression in pancreatic cancer could be responsible for the growth advantage of this kind of tumour.

Clinical studies of somatostatin analogues in combination with other substances, such as tamoxifen, which is used for the treatment of estrogen-positive metastatic breast cancer were rather disappointing. No benefit of the additional administration of octreotide was observed and, moreover, the combination of both compounds caused higher side effects in patients. Despite this, the combination of octreotide with interferon-α improved the sensitivity of neuroendocrine gastroenteropancreatic tumours, which responded only marginally to the individual application of the drugs. Although a significant reduction of tumour size was not detectable, in 18% of the patients a complete, and in more than half of them a partial, normalization of hormone levels was observed (2).

Somatostatin Receptor Scintigraphy and Receptor-targeted Radiotherapy

Radiolabeld somatostatin analogues, such as ^{111}In-DTPA-DPhe[1]-octreotide or ^{111}In-DOTA-lanreotide are employed for somatostatin receptor scintigraphy (SRS), an imaging technique that is nowadays used in many hospitals to visualize sst subtype positive tumours *in vivo*. The high sensitivity of this method can be explained by an accumulation of radioligands within the tumours, which is presumably caused by the internalisation of the agonist-receptor complex (2). Many human tumours seem to contain high mRNA levels for specific sst subtypes. For example, sst_2 is the predominant isoform expressed by neuroendocrine tumours,

whereas intestinal adenocarcinomas mostly contain sst_3 and sst_4. Therefore, in particular ^{111}In-DOTA-lanreotide is a very suitable tool for the detection of a wide range of tumours, since it binds not only sst_2 and sst_5 with high affinity but also sst_3 and sst_4 and to a lesser extent sst_1.

Furthermore, some of these radioligands have been used in first trials of receptor-targeted radiotherapy. Although ^{111}In is not the most favourable substance for radiotherapy, large amounts of[111]In-DTPA-DPhe[1]-octreotide were used for the treatment of patients suffering from neuroendocrine tumours. In a patient with an inoperable metastasised glucagonoma, treatment with[111]In-DTPA-DPhe[1]-octreotide led to a small but significant reduction of tumour size and transiently lowered plasma glucagon levels (2). Two further analogues,[90]Y-DOTA-lanreotide and[90]Y-DOTA-D Phe[1]-Tyr[3]-octreotide, have also been tested for tumour therapy. In a phase II study investigating more than 60 tumour patients treated with ^{90}Y-DOTA-lanreotide about 35% of the patients showed a stabilization of tumour growth and in 15% of the cases a tumour regression was observed. However, clinical long-term trials are still needed to evaluate the therapeutic effectiveness of somatostatin analogues in cancer treatment.

References

1. Patel YC (1999) Somatostatin and its receptor family. Frontiers in Neuroendocrinology 20:157–198
2. Hofland LJ and Lamberts SWJ (1997) Somatostatin analogs and receptors. Diagnostic and therapeutic applications. Cancer Treatment and Research 89:365–382
3. Baumeister, H and Meyerhof, W (2000) Gene regulation of somatostatin receptors. Journal of Physiology (Paris) 94:167–177
4. Hoyer D, Epelbaum J, Feniuk W, Humphrey PPA, Meyerhof W, Patel Y, Reisine T, Reubi JC, Schonbrunn A, Vezzani A (2000) Somatostatin receptors. In: The IUPHAR Compendium of Receptor Characterization and Classification. International Union of Pharmacology Committee on Receptor Nomenclature and Drug Classification, IUPHAR Media London.
5. Reubi JC, Schaer J-C, Wenger S, Hoeger C, Erchegyi J, Waser B, and Rivier J (2000) SST3-selective potent

peptidic somatostatin receptor antagonists. Proceedings of the National Academy of Sciences of the U S A 97:13973–13978

Spermine/Spermidine

Spermine and spermidine are the most common natural polyamines with the structures $NH_2(CH_2)_3NH(CH_2)_4 NH(CH_2)_3NH_2$ and $NH_2(CH_2)_3NH(CH_2)_4NH_2$, respectively.

▶ Polyamines
▶ Inward Rectifier K$^+$ Channels

Sphingosine Kinase

Sphingosine kinase catalyses the phosphorylation of sphingosine to ▶ sphingosine-1-phosphate (S1P). Sphingosine kinase activity and/or formation of S1P are stimulated by several G protein-coupled receptors, growth factor receptors and antigen receptors and by depolarization. The product, S1P, may act intracellularly or may be secreted. Recent data suggest that sphingosine kinase can also occur extracellularly. Until now, two distinct sphingosine kinases (SPK1, SPK2) have been identified on the molecular level, and more are likely to exist. The catalytic domain of these enzymes has a homology to that of the diacylglycerol kinases. Overexpression of SPK1 promotes cell growth and protects from apoptosis.

▶ Lysophospholipids

Sphingosine-1-phosphate

Sphingosine-1-phosphate (S1P) is a versatile bioactive lipid which can act as first and second messenger. Extracellular S1P is a ▶ lysophospholipid mediator and activates specific G protein-coupled receptors. On the other hand, stimulation of many

cells with diverse agonists causes a rapid and transient increase in intracellular S1P formation, and inhibition of this S1P formation by ▶ sphingosine kinase inhibitors abrogates e.g. agonist-induced Ca^{2+} mobilization. Different approaches, e.g. intracellular microinjection of S1P or overexpression of sphingosine kinase, support the hypothesis that intracellular S1P mediates mobilization of Ca^{2+} from intracellular stores as well as proliferation and survival. The sphingosine kinase/S1P signal transduction pathway has been compared to the phospholipase C/inositol-1,4,5-trisphosphate Ca^{2+} mobilization pathway but intracellular target sites of S1P have not been identified so far.

▶ Lysophospholipids

Splice Variant

A splice variant can arise when a gene contains at least 2 ▶ introns leading to the possibility that the DNA between them (an ▶ exon) may not be included in the final messenger RNA (mRNA) and protein product. Thus, the final protein product may exist in 2 forms, one containing the amino acid sequence encoded by the exon that is located between the introns in the original DNA, and the other in which the amino acid sequence encoded by that exon has been 'spliced out'. These two products are referred to as splice variants.

▶ Histaminergic System

S

Split-and-recombine Synthesis

Split-and-recombine synthesis is the simultaneous preparation of many products with one reaction vessel per coupled building block. Consequently, complex defined mixtures of product compounds are obtained.

▶ Combinatorial Chemistry

Sporotrichosis

Sporotrichosis is the fungal disease caused by *Sporotrix schenckii* and involves the lymphatic and subcutaneous tissues. The lesions spread *via* the lymphatics from the original wound and form nodules or pustules that quickly ulcerate. Dissemination is rare.

▶ Antifungal Drugs

SPRM

▶ Selective Progesterone Receptor Modulators

SR

▶ Sarcoplasmatic Reticulum

Src Gene

The c-src gene encodes the non-receptor tyrosine kinase pp60$^{c\text{-}src}$ that is involved in signal transduction. The pp60$^{c\text{-}src}$ protein consists of a tyrosine kinase domain, a src homology 2 (SH2) domain that can bind to receptor tyrosine kinases, and a ▶ src homology 3 (SH3) domain that binds to proline rich sequences. The viral homolog of c-src, v-src, from the Rous sarcoma virus is a potent oncogene.

▶ Tyrosin Kinases

Src-homology 2 Domain

The Src-homology 2 (SH2) domain is a protein domain of roughly 100 amino acids found in many signalling molecules. It binds to phosphorylated tyrosines, in particular peptide sequences on activated receptor tyrosine kinases or docking proteins. By recognizing specific phosphorylated tyrosines, these small domains serve as modules that enable the proteins that contain them to bind to activated receptor tyrosine kinases or other intracellular signalling proteins that have been transiently phosphorylated on tyrosines.

Src-homology 3 Domain

The Src homology 3 domain is a 60 amino acid long domain that binds to proline-rich sequences, thereby enabling protein-protein interactions.

▶ Growth Factors

SRP

▶ Signal Recognition Particle

SSRIs

▶ Selective Serotonin Reuptake Inhibitors

S-stereoisomer

Carbon atoms with four different substituents are called chiral. Drugs which contain a chiral carbon can exist in two stereoisomeric forms named S or

R, depending on the sequence of the substituents at the chiral carbon.

▶ Local Anaesthetics

STAT

STATs (**s**ignal **t**ransducers and **a**ctivators of **t**ranscription) constitute a highly conserved family of proteins with the dual function of transducing signals from the cell surface into the nucleus as well as activating transcription of target genes. They convert extracellular stimuli into a wide range of appropriate cellular processes, such as immune response, antiviral protection, and proliferation.

▶ JAK-STAT Pathway

State-dependent Block

State-dependent block describes the binding of a drug to a certain state of an ionic channel. Thus, the fast Na^+ channel switches between a resting, open and inactivated states, the latter being the state to which antiarrhythmic drugs like lidocaine bind.

▶ Antiarrhythmic Drugs

Statins

▶ HMG CoA Reductase Inhibitors

Steroid Hormones

▶ Steroids

Steroid Receptors

Steroid receptors belong to the nuclear receptor superfamily and bind steroid hormones. They are cytoplasmic when inactive and associated with chaperones.

▶ Sex Steroid Receptors
▶ Gluco-/Mineralcorticoid Receptors

Steroids

Steroids are a group of natural substances which share a common basic structure consisting of four condensed rings (sterane). Cholesterol is the precursor for the group of steroid hormones which are mainly formed in the adrenal medulla and in the gonads, including androgens, progesterone and estrogens as well as the mineralocorticoids. Steroid Hormons are lipophilic substances which bind to intracellular receptors. Other important steroids include the bile acids and the D-vitamins. Many related substances are found in plants, often present as glycosides. An important example of plant steroids are the cardiac glycosides.

▶ Contraceptives
▶ Gluco-/Mineralcorticoid Receptor
▶ Sex Steroid Receptor

Store-operated Ca^{2+} Entry

Ca^{2+} entry across the cell membrane is activated by a reduction in the stored Ca^{2+} within the cell. The Ca^{2+}-release-activated current (I_{CRAC}) represents a Ca^{2+} current carried through the prototype of a store-operated plasma membrane channel.

▶ TRP Channels

Stress Proteins

DAVID S. LATCHMAN
Institute of Child Health,
University College London, London, UK
d.latchman@ich.ucl.ac.uk

Synonyms

Heat shock proteins (HSPs)

Definition

Stress proteins are a diverse group of proteins that are synthesised at increased levels by cells exposed to a variety of stressful stimuli and which have a protective effect against the stress.

▶ Protein Trafficking and Quality Control

Basic Characteristics

When, in 1962, Ritossa reported the appearance of a new puffing pattern in the salivary gland polytene chromosomes of *Drosophila busckii* following exposure to elevated temperature, he can hardly have foreseen that this phenomenon would ultimately be of interest to those concerned with processes as diverse as protein folding and human ▶ autoimmune diseases. Yet, this finding represented the first step in the study of a group of proteins whose synthesis is induced by exposure of cells to elevated temperature or other stresses and which are therefore known as the stress or heat shock proteins. Studies over the past thirty five years have revealed the importance of these proteins in fundamental cellular processes such as protein folding as well as elucidating their role in a variety of different human diseases.

Following the initial report of Ritossa, subsequent studies revealed that similar elevated synthesis of a few proteins following exposure to heat or other stresses occurs in all organisms studied ranging from prokaryotic bacteria such as *E.coli* to mammals. Initially, the major stress or heat-inducible proteins were identified simply by exposing cells to such stresses in the presence of radiolabelled amino acids and identifying newly labelled proteins by autoradiography of polyacrylamide gels. Subsequently, following the cloning of the genes encoding stress proteins identified in this manner, other genes encoding related stress proteins were identified on the basis of their homology. It then became clear that many stress proteins are encoded by multi-gene families encoding proteins with similar but distinct features. In addition, other proteins that were identified in other situations were also subsequently shown to be induced by specific stresses when they were analyzed in detail.

In this manner, a number of different stress-inducible proteins have been defined. The major stress proteins which are normally referred to as hsp N where N is the molecular weight in kilo-Daltons are listed in Table 1 together with brief details concerning their features (for detailed review see reference 1).

Functions of Stress Proteins

Although the stress proteins were initially defined on the basis of their enhanced synthesis in response to exposure to heat or other stresses, many of these proteins are also expressed in normal unstressed cells. Thus, for example, hsp90 constitutes approximately 1% of the total protein in unstressed cells and is induced 2–5 fold following exposure to elevated temperature. Indeed, even where a specific stress protein is absent in unstressed cells, a homologous protein exists in normal unstressed cells. This is seen in the case of the hsp70 family where the major stress inducible protein (known either as hsp70 or hsp72) is absent in unstressed cells, which contain large amounts of another member of the family (known as hsc70 or hsp73) which is only mildly induced by exposure to stress.

This indicates therefore the function of the hsps is likely to be one which is required in normal cells but is of even greater importance in stressed cells. Moreover, this function is likely to be of great importance in all cells ranging from bacteria to man since it has been highly conserved in evolution. Thus, not only does exposure to stress induce the synthesis of specific proteins in all organisms, but these proteins themselves have been highly conserved in evolution as indicated in Table 1 which shows that prokaryotic homologues of most eukaryotic hsps can be identified in bacteria.

Tab. 1 Major eukaryotic stress proteins.

Family	Members	Prokaryotic homologues	Functional role	Comments
Hsp100	Hsp104, Hsp100	ClpA, Clpβ	Protein turnover	Have ATPase activity
Hsp90	Hsp90, Grp94	C62.5	Maintenance of proteins such as steroid receptors in an inactive form until appropriate	Drosophila and yeast proteins known as hsp83
Hsp70	Grp78 (= Bip), Hsp70, Hsc70, Hsx70	dnaK	Protein folding and unfolding, assembly of multi-protein complexes	Hsx70 only in primates
Hsp60	Hsp60	groEL (*E.coli*) Mycobacterial 65 kD antigen	Protein folding and unfolding, organelle translocation	Major antigen of many bacteria and parasites which infect man
Hsp56	Hsp56 (aka FKB52)	None	Protein folding, associated with hsp90 and hsp70 in steroid receptor complex	Have peptidyl prolyl isomerase activity, target of immuno-suppressive drugs
Hsp47	Hsp47	None	Protein folding of collagen and possibly other proteins	Has homology to protease inhibitors
Hsp32	Hsp32		Cleaves heme to yield carbon monoxide and the protective anti-oxidant molecule biliverdin	Also known as heme oxygenase-1
Hsp27	Hsp27, Hsp26 etc.	Mycobacterial 18 kDa antigen	Protein folding, actin binding proteins	Very variable in size (12–40 kD) and number in different organisms
Ubiquitin	Ubiquitin	None	Protein degradation	Also found conjugated to histone H2A in the nucleus

Numerous studies have indicated that the primary role of the majority of hsps lies in producing proper folding of other proteins so that they can fulfil their appropriate functions. This is required in all normal cells but will be of greater importance in stressed cells where exposure to elevated temperature or other noxious stimuli will result in the production of aberrant proteins that are improperly folded. Some of the roles of the hsps in proper protein folding include preventing the inappropriate associations of other proteins with each other, the correct intracellular transport of other proteins and the maintenance of specific proteins in an inactive form until the correct signal for their activation is received. These functions are evidently of importance in the normal cell, whilst in the stressed cell, abnormal interactions that are highly undesirable increase and must be dealt with by the increased concentrations of hsps produced by the stress.

Evidently, in some situations the damaged proteins produced by the stress will be too abnormal to be refolded properly. For this reason, some stress-inducible proteins such as the small hsp ubiquitin are involved in protein degradation and therefore assist in the destruction of damaged proteins in the stressed cell whilst also playing a role in normal protein turnover in unstressed cells.

S

Hsp Expression and Regulation

The dual role of stress proteins in both normal and stressed cells requires the existence of complex regulatory processes which ensure that the correct expression pattern is produced. Indeed, such processes must be operative at the very earliest stages of embryonic development since the genes encoding stress proteins such as hsp70 and hsp90 have been shown to be amongst the first genes transcribed from the embryonic genome.

A number of studies have shown that a specific ▶ transcription factor known as heat shock factor 1 (HSF1) is responsible for the induction of the stress protein genes following exposure to heat or other stresses. Thus, this factor exists in an inactive monomeric form in unstressed cells. Following exposure to heat or other stresses, it forms a trimeric form that is able to bind to appropriate DNA sequences in the promoters of the stress protein genes known as heat shock elements (HSE). Subsequently, HSF1 becomes phosphorylated and then activates transcription of these genes (for review see 2).

Much less is known about the regulation of these genes in response to non stressful stimuli or in normal cells. It has been shown that a second form of HSF known as HSF2, which also binds to the HSE, mediates the induction of the hsp70 gene that occurs when an erythroleukaemia cell line is induced to differentiate following exposure to hemin. However, it is now becoming clear that transcription factors which bind to sites within the stress protein gene promoters that are distinct from HSE sequences, also play a role in the regulation of these genes in normal cells and in response to specific non-stressful stimuli. Thus, for example, it has been shown that the enhanced synthesis of hsp70 and hsp90 following exposure of cells to ▶ cytokines such as interleukin-6 (IL-6) is mediated by transcription factors such as ▶ NF-IL6 and STAT-3, which bind to sites in their gene promoters adjacent to HSE sequences (for review see 3). Hence, the expression of the stress proteins in normal and stressed cells is parallelled by their regulation by transcription factors that are activated by non-stressful and stressful stimuli, respectively.

Stress Proteins and Protection

The important role of the stress proteins in processes such as protein folding and their expression in normal embryonic development suggests that they are likely to be essential for the survival of cells and organisms. Thus, although the inactivation of an individual stress protein gene may not be lethal in all cases since another member of the family might substitute for its functions, the complete elimination of the function of a specific family of stress proteins is likely to be lethal in the vast majority of cases.

As always, in discussing stress proteins it is necessary to consider not only their function in normal cells but their function in stressed cells. A very wide variety of studies have left no doubt that induction of the stress proteins by a specific stress does have a protective effect and enhances the ability of the organism to deal with that stress. Such a conclusion was initially reached on the basis of experiments showing that a mild stress sufficient to induce the hsps was able to protect cells against a subsequent more severe stress. Subsequently, such studies were supplemented by the overexpression of individual hsps in cultured cells which showed that this made the cells more resistant to a subsequent stress. Conversely, the elimination of a particular stress protein by micro-injection of an antibody to it or the use of an anti-sense approach resulted in a reduced tolerance to stress. These experiments were brought to their logical conclusion by the finding that transgenic animals overexpressing hsp70 showed enhanced resistance to cardiac ischaemia (for review see 4,5).

Stress Proteins and Human Disease

As described above, the stress proteins play a critical role in the functioning of normal cells and particularly in their stress resistance. These effects are obviously of great benefit to the organism. In addition, however, stress proteins have also been implicated in specific human diseases. Somewhat surprisingly, unlike the situation with most other essential proteins, such alterations in stress proteins in human diseases do not generally involve the reduction in their expression or the abolition of their function.

Rather, the enhanced expression of stress proteins has been reported in a number of different human diseases. Evidently, many such reports will simply arise from the fact that particular cells in a specific disease are exposed to stress due to the effects of the disease and therefore respond by inducing the synthesis of the stress proteins. In other cases, however, the specific synthesis of an individual stress protein has been reported with no effects on other stress proteins suggesting that the effect is a specific one which may be related to the nature of the disease. Thus, for example, hsp90 has been reported to be specifically overexpressed in a subset of patients with the autoimmune disease systemic lupus erythematosus (SLE) where the expression of other stress proteins is unaffected.

Probably the greatest significance of such general or specific overexpression of stress proteins in particular diseases is that they can provoke an autoimmune response leading to the production of antibodies or T cells that recognise these proteins and can produce a damaging immune response. Such immune responses to individual stress proteins, particular hsp60, have been reported in diseases as diverse as rheumatoid arthritis, multiple sclerosis and type 1 diabetes. Similar autoimmune responses to endogenous mammalian stress proteins can be provoked by exposure of animals to bacterial pathogens such as the Mycobacteria whose major antigen is homologous to hsp60.

Although such autoimmune responses appear to play a critical role, for example, in animal models of rheumatoid arthritis involving Mycobacterial infection, it is at present unclear whether they play a similar role in the pathogenesis of human rheumatoid arthritis and other autoimmune diseases such as type 1 diabetes or multiple sclerosis. This possibility needs to be borne in mind, however, in developing therapeutic procedures involving the enhanced expression of these protective proteins (see below).

Drugs

The protective effect of overexpressing stress proteins in cells or transgenic animals (described above) is of obvious therapeutic importance. Thus, if drugs could be developed that could induce enhanced stress protein expression without producing stress, they could potentially be used, for example, to minimise the damage that occurs in human diseases such as cerebral ischaemia or cardiac ischaemia. Evidently, the finding that naturally occurring non-stressful stimuli such as cytokines can induce enhanced stress protein synthesis (see above) offers hope that this can be achieved. Indeed, several drugs able to induce enhanced stress protein synthesis have been synthesised and such compounds or their derivatives may ultimately be of clinical use (for review see 4,5). Similarly, experiments in which a protective effect has been achieved by delivering stress protein genes using viral or non-viral vectors (4,5) indicates that delivery of exogenous stress protein genes by a ▶ gene therapy approach may be an alternative to the up-regulation of endogenous stress protein genes using a pharmacological approach. Of course, in considering these therapies one should bear in mind the potential role of stress protein overexpression in autoimmune diseases. Thus, not only will therapy of such diseases potentially require decreased rather than increased stress protein expression but care will be required to ensure that therapeutic overexpression of stress proteins in, for example, cerebral or cardiac ischaemia does not induce a damaging autoimmune response. Despite this caveat, however, it is likely that the phenomenon of stress proteins discovered nearly forty years ago in the fruit fly will one day be used for therapeutic benefit in human disease.

References

1. Latchman, D. S. (ed.) (1998) Stress Proteins. pp. 422 Springer Verlag.
2. Morimoto, R. I. (1998) Regulation of the heat shock transcriptional response: cross talk between a family of heat shock factors, molecular chaperones, and negative regulators. Genes and Development 12:3788–3796
3. Stephanou, A. S. and Latchman, D. S. (1999) Transcriptional regulation of the heat shock protein genes by STAT family transcription factors. Gene Expression 7:311–319
4. Latchman, D. S. (1998) Heat shock proteins: protective effect and potential therapeutic use. International Journal of Molecular Medicine 2: 375–381
5. Latchman, D. S. (2001) Heat shock proteins and cardiac protection. Cardiovascular Research 51:637–646

S

Structural Genomics

The genome projects produce an enormous amount of sequence data that needs to be annotated in terms of molecular structure and biological function.

Structural genomics aims to use high-throughput structure determination and computational analysis to provide structures and/or three-dimensional models of every tractable protein. The intention is to determine as many protein structures as possible and to exploit the solved structures for the assignment of biological function to hypothetical proteins.

▶ Bioinformatics
▶ Molecular Modelling

Strychnine

The convulsant alkaloid strychnine from the Indian tree *Strychnos nux vomica* is highly toxic. Strychnine poisoning causes hyperreflexia, increased muscle tone, convulsions, and finally death. Strychnine binds to the inhibitory glycine receptor with high affinity ($K_D \approx 10$ nM), efficiently displacing the neurotransmitter glycine. Glycine-displaceable binding of [^{3}H]strychnine is a highly specific probe for the glycine receptor.

▶ Glycine Receptors

STX

▶ Saxitoxin

Substance K

Neurokinin A.

▶ Tachykinins
▶ Neuroleptics

Substance P

Substance P is a member of a group of polypeptides known as neurokinins or tachykinins. It is thought to be the primary neurotransmitter for the transfer of sensory information from the periphery to the spinal cord and brain. Substance P as well as neurokinin NK_1 receptors have been detected in vagal afferent neurons in the area postrema, nucleus tractus solitarius and dorsal motor nucleus of the vagus. Substance P has been shown to increase the firing rate of neurons in the area postrema and nucleus tractus solitarius and to produce retching when applied directly to these areas in animal studies.

▶ Nociception
▶ Tachykinins

Substantia Gelatinosa

The substantia gelatinosa is part of the dorsal horn of the spinal cord, also called "lamina II". The substantia gelatinosa is made up almost exclusively of interneurons (both excitatory and inhibitory), some of which respond only to nociceptive inputs, while others respond also to non-noxious stimuli.

▶ Nociception

Substantia Nigra

▶ Nigrostriatal Tract/Pathway
▶ Anti-parkinson Drugs

Sulfonamides

Suphonamides are a group of anti-microbial agents which interfere with the synthesis of folate. Sulphonamides are structural analogues of p-aminobenzoic acid, which is essential for the synthesis of folic acid in bacteria. Folate is required for the synthesis of the precursors of DNA and RNA, both in bacteria and mammals. Mammals obtain their folic acid from their diet, whereas bacteria need to synthesize it. Sulphonamides compete with p-aminobenzoic acid for the enzyme dihydropteroate synthase. Sulphonamides inhibit the growth of bacteria (bacteriostatic), but are not bactericidal. Important sulfonamides in clinical use are sulphadiazine, sulphamethoxazole and sulphasalazine. Sulphonamides are often combined with trimethoprim (a combination called co-trimoxazole). Trimethoprim has some structural resemblance to folate and functions as a competitive inhibitor of dihydrofolate reductase, which synthesizes tetrahydrofolate from folate.

Sulfonylurea Receptor

The sulfonylurea receptor (SUR) is a regulatory subunit of the ATP-dependent potassium channel. It forms heterodimers with the channel subunit Kir 6.2, the channel is presumably composed of 4 SUR/Kir 6.2 heterodimers. Two isotypes, SUR1 and SUR2, and two splicing variants, SUR2A and SUR2B, have been identified and characterized. SUR contains multiple transmembrane domains and two nucleotide-binding folds. ATP and β-cytotropic agents bind to SUR1 and block the channel, ADP produces the opposite effect. Loss of SUR or of the whole channel results in spontaneous depolarization and loss of the effect of ADP.

▶ ATP-dependent K^+ Channels
▶ Oral Anti-diabetic Drugs

Sulfonylureas

Sulfonylureas are oral hypoglycemic drugs widely used in treatment of type2 diabetes. The first generation of sulfonylureas includes tolbutamide, acetohexamide, and chlorpropamide. The second includes glibenclamide, gliclazide, and glimepiride, which are considerably more potent than the earlier agents.

▶ ATP-dependent Potassium Channels
▶ Oral Anti-diabetic Drugs

Sulfotransferase

Sulfotransferases are a group of cytosolic enzymes, which catalyze the transfer of the sulfonate group from 3'-phosphoadenosine-5'-phosphosulfate (PRPS) to an acceptor substrate to form either a sulfate or sulfonate conjugate. Sulfotransferases metabolize a variety of small lipophilic endobiotics (e.g. estrogen, corticoid, thyroxin) as well as a variety of xenobiotics. Genes of cytosolic sulfotransferases (SULT) have been identified and several genetic polymorphisms have been observed in human sulfotransferases, such as ST1A2, ST1A3 and ST2A3.

Sulphonylureas

▶ Sulfonyureas

SUMO

SUMO is an abbreviation for 'small ubiquitin-related modifier'. Other names are GMP1, sentrin, SMT3, PIC1 or Ubl1. SUMO is a small protein of 98 residues that is covalently conjugated to other proteins. Vertebrate cells have at least three different

SUMO proteins, SUMO-1, SUMO-2 and SUMO-3, the two latter being very similar and conjugated especially under stress conditions.

▶ Ubiquitin-related Modifiers

Superantigen

A superantigen is a bacterial or viral protein which links T-cell receptors and MHC molecules through simultaneous interaction with the constant domains of all MHC class II molecules and of T-cell receptor β–chains. Hence, superantigens are polyclonal T-cell activators, most likely involved in the development of autoimmune diseases.

▶ Interferons

Supercoils

Bacterial as well as eukaryotic chromosomes contain too much DNA to fit easily into a cell. Therefore, the DNA must be condensed (compacted) to fit into the cell or nucleus. This is accomplished by supercoiling the DNA into a highly condensed form. When relaxed circular DNA is twisted in the direction that the helix turns, the DNA becomes positively supercoiled, if it is twisted in the opposite direction, it is called negatively supercoiled. Bacterial DNA is normally found in a negatively supercoiled state. Supercoiling reactions are catalyzed by topoisomerases.

▶ Quinolones, potent inhibitors of bacterial topoisomerases

Superfamily

The term superfamily is used to include in the classical sequence-based families, proteins with no statistically significant sequence similarities but with similar three-dimensional structures.

Superoxide

Superoxide is a free radical form of oxygen (O_2^-) that is damaging to cells. Superoxide is scavenged by the enzyme superoxide dismutase used by neutrophils to destroy microbes in the body.

Superoxide Dismutase

Superoxide dismutase (SOD) enzymes are metalloproteins that detoxify superoxide anions (O_2^-) by converting them to H_2O_2, which is subsequently reduced to water. SOD enzymes include the manganese (Mn) enzyme in mitochondria (SOD2) and the Cu/Zn enzyme that is present in the cytosol (SOD1) or on extracellular surfaces (SOD3). As superoxide anions play an important role in a variety of pathophysiological conditions, such as tissue injury and inflammation, the capacity of SOD enzymes may be important for the cause of the disease. SOD mimetics are under investigation for their potential use as anti-inflammatory agents.

Supraventricular Tachycardia

Supraventricular tachycardia is a heart condition characterised by fast arrhythmias involving the atrioventricular (AV) node.

▶ Antiarrhythmic Drugs

SUR

▶ Sulfonylurea Receptor

Susceptibility

Susceptibility in the context of pharmacogenetics is a marginally to moderately increased risk for a disease.

▶ Pharmacogenetics

Swiss-Prot

Swiss-Prot ia a curated databank of information on protein sequence, structure and function. It can be found under: http://www.ebi.ac.uk/swissprot/

▶ Bioinformatics
▶ Molecular Modelling

SxxK Acyl Transferases

The acyl transferases of the SxxK superfamily have a specific bar code in the form of three motifs SxxK, SxN or analogue and KTG or analogue (with x denoting a variable amino acid residue). The motifs occur at equivalent places and roughly with the same spacing along the polypeptide chains, and close to each other at the immediate boundary of the catalytic centre. A constellation of bacterial genes code for SxxK acyl transferases of varying amino acid sequences, functionalities and modular designs. They occur as free-standing polypeptides and as protein fusions. Those involved in bacterial wall (4→3) peptidoglycan assembly and metabolism bind penicillin in the form of stable and inactive penicilloyl derivatives in which the penicilloyl moiety is linked as an ester to the serine residue of the SxxK motif.

▶ β-lactam Antibiotics

SxxK β-lactamases

SxxK β-lactamases are uncoupled SxxK acyl transferases that work as β-lactam antibiotic hydrolases. They represent a mechanism of defense of great efficiency. On good β-lactam substrates, their catalytic centres can turn over 1000 times per second.

▶ β-lactam Antibiotics

SxxK Free-standing Penicillin-binding Protein

SxxK free-standing penicillin-binding proteins (PBPs) are uncoupled SxxK acyl transferases that work mainly as bacterial wall peptidoglycan-hydrolases and function as auxiliary cell-cycle proteins. They are not essential.

▶ β-lactam Antibiotics

SxxK PBP Fusions

Class A penicillin-binding protein (PBP) fusions combine in a single polypeptide chain a class A SxxK acyl transferase linked to a glycosyl transferase module having its own five-motif bar code, itself linked to a membrane anchor. They catalyse the conversion of disaccharide-peptide units, borne by a C_{55} undecaprenyl carrier, into polymeric (4→3) peptidoglycan. Class B PBP fusions are composed of a class B SxxK acyl transferase, a linker module having its own three-motif bar code and a membrane anchor. They are members of the morphogenetic apparatus. They are implicated in the remodelling of (4→3) peptidoglycan throughout the bacterial cell cycle. PBP fusions of classes

S

A and B are, globally, the lethal targets of β-lactam antibiotics.

▶ β-lactam Antibiotics

Sympathetic System

The sympathetic system is the part of the autonomic nervous system that utilizes noradrenaline (norepinephrine) and adrenaline (epinephrine) as its transmitters.

▶ β-lactam Antibiotics

Sympatholytic Drugs

Sympatholytic drugs are a group of drugs, which decrease the activity of the sympathetic nervous system, mainly by blocking the action of adrenaline and noradrenaline at adrenoceptors.

▶ α-adrenergic system
▶ β-adrenergic system

Sympathomimetic Drugs

Direct sympathomimetic drugs act as agonists on adrenergic receptors. In contrast, indirectly acting sympathomimetic drugs act by increasing the concentration of noradrenaline. Indirectly acting sympathomimetics like tyramine, amphetamine or ephedrine are take up into sympathetic nerve terminals and are transported into the vesicles by the vesicular monoamine transporter in exchange for noradrenaline, which escapes into the cytosol. Most of the noradrenaline in the cytosol escapes via the transporter in the presynaptic membrane in exchange for the indirectly acting sympathomimetic monoamine. By this mechanism as well as by partly inhibiting the reuptake of noradrenaline and partly by inhibiting the degradation of noradrenaline by monoamine oxidase (MAO), they increase the concentration of noradrenaline in the synaptic cleft.

▶ α-adrenergic system
▶ β-adrenergic system

Synapse

A synapse is a contact site between two neurones, where information is communicated from the axon of one neurone (the presynaptic) to the cell body, the dendrites or the axon of the second neurone (the postsynaptic). In most synapses, the information is communicated chemically; the presynaptic neurone releases a neurotransmitter substance, which then acts on receptors of the postsynaptic neurone. Most chemical synapses are characterized morphologically by an increase in diameter of the presynaptic axon to form a varicosity or bouton, by transmitter-storing vesicles inside the bouton and by a synaptic cleft crossed by cell adhesion molecules. In a relatively few synapses, the information is transmitted electrically. In a wider sense, sites of transmission between neuronal axons and peripheral effector cells, such as smooth muscle cells, are also synapses.

▶ Synaptic Transmission

Synaptic Transmission

Klaus Starke
Institut für Experimentelle
und Klinische Pharmakologie und Toxikologie,
Universität Freiburg, Freiburg, Germany
Klaus.starke@pharmakol.uni-freiburg.de

Definition

Synaptic transmission is the transfer of biological information across ▶ synapses. Drugs that influence synaptic transmission play an eminent role in therapy, for two reasons. Firstly, the nervous system controls all tissues. Second, with few exceptions synaptic transmission is chemical, operating by means of transmitter substances, and synapses therefore provide a large number of drug targets, such as the enzymes that synthesize the transmitter. However, the importance of synaptic pharmacology extends beyond therapy: many poisons act at synapses, as do the every-day drugs caffeine, ethanol and nicotine.

There are numerous transmitter substances. They include the amino acids glutamate, GABA and glycine; acetylcholine; the monoamines dopamine, noradrenaline and serotonin; the ▶ neuropeptides; ATP; and NO. Many neurones use not a single transmitter but two or even more, a phenomenon called ▶ cotransmission. Chemical synaptic transmission hence is diversified. The basic steps, however, are similar across all neurones, irrespective of their transmitter, with the exception of NO: transmitter production and vesicular storage; transmitter release; postsynaptic receptor activation; and transmitter inactivation. Fig. 1 shows an overview. ▶ Nitrergic transmission, i.e. transmission by NO, differs from transmission by other transmitters and is not covered in this essay.

▶ α-Adrenergic System
▶ Catechol-O-Methyltransferase and its Inhibitors
▶ Exocytosis

Basic Mechanisms

Transmitter Production and Vesicular Storage

All non-peptide transmitters are produced in the axon terminals, which possess the necessary machinery. Cholinergic terminals contain choline acetyltransferase, which acetylates choline to acetylcholine. Dopaminergic terminals contain tyrosine hydroxylase, which converts tyrosine into levodopa, and aromatic L-amino acid decarboxylase, which decarboxylates levodopa to dopamine. Noradrenergic terminals contain in addition dopamine β-hydroxylase, which oxidizes dopamine to noradrenaline. Following synthesis, the transmitters (except NO) are taken up into ▶ synaptic vesicles by means of a transport system consisting of two components: an ATP-driven H^+ pump that generates a proton gradient (ΔpH; vesicle lumen acidic) and a potential gradient ($\Delta\psi$;

vesicle lumen positive); and the Vesicular Neurotransmitter Transporter (VNT) (▶ Neurotransmitter Transporters, ▶ Vesicular Transporters), which exchanges intravesicular H^+ with axoplasmic transmitter (Fig. 1 inset). There are several VNT families. One is the Vesicular Monoamine Transporter (VMAT)/Vesicular Acetylcholine Transporter (VAChT) family. VMAT is responsible for the vesicular transport of dopamine, noradrenaline and serotonin (1).

In contrast to the small transmitter molecules, the neuropeptides are synthesized in the rough endoplasmic reticulum of the neuronal perikarya. They are enclosed in vesicles in the Golgi apparatus. The vesicles travel down to the terminals by axonal transport.

Transmitter Release

All transmitters (except NO) are released by the following cascade: arrival of the nerve action potential at the terminal → opening of voltage-sensitive Ca^{2+} channels → exocytosis → recycling of the vesicle membrane. The nerve action potential is mainly carried by Na^+ entry through voltage-dependent Na^+ channels. Axon terminal voltage-sensitive Ca^{2+} channels are mainly of the N- and P/Q-types.

The action potential-induced increase in axoplasmic Ca^{2+} is the physiological trigger for exocytosis. Exocytosis consists of the fusion of the vesicle membrane with the plasmalemma, the opening of a pore in the fused membranes, and outward diffusion of the neurotransmitter or neurotransmitters. Three proteins, the so called ▶ SNARE proteins, are essential in exocytosis (Fig. 1 inset). One, synaptobrevin, is a protein of the vesicle membrane; the other two, syntaxin and SNAP-25 (synaptosome-associated protein of 25 kD), are proteins of the plasmalemma (Fig. 1 inset). Upon an increase in cytoplasmic Ca^{2+} from about 0.1 to about 100 µM, the vesicular synaptobrevin grabs hold of the plasmalemmal SNAREs, and the three proteins intertwine into a complex that then tightens like a zipper. This "zippering" of the SNAREs pulls the vesicle and plasma membranes together so that the lipid bilayers merge. An additional vesicular protein, synaptotagmin, may be the Ca^{2+} sensor that detects the increase in cytoplasmic Ca^{2+}. Ca^{2+} channels and SNAREs lie closely together. Syntaxin and SNAP-25 in fact

Presynaptic terminal   **Postsynaptic cell**

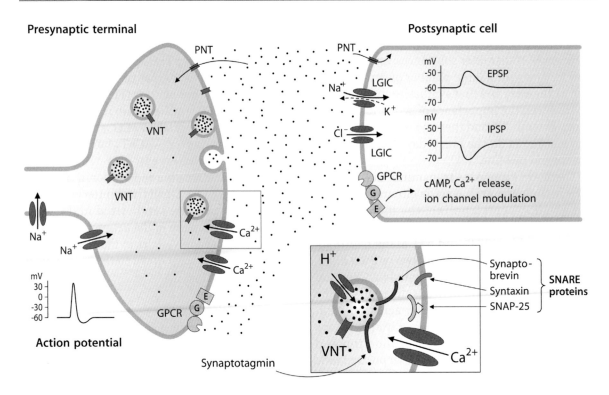

Fig. 1 Synaptic transmission. The presynaptic terminal contains voltage-dependent Na^+ and Ca^{2+} channels, vesicles with a Vesicular Neurotransmitter Transporter VNT, a Plasmalemmal Neurotransmitter Transporter PNT, and a presynaptic G protein-coupled receptor GPCR with its G protein and its effector E; the inset also shows the vesicular H^+ pump. The postsynaptic cell contains two ligand-gated ion channels LGIC, one for Na^+ and K^+ and one for Cl^-, a postsynaptic GPRC, and a PNT. In this synapse, released transmitter is inactivated by uptake into cells.

interact physically with the α1 subunit of N- and P/ Q-type Ca^{2+} channels. The close neighbourhood permits the quickness of exocytosis; the time from the arrival of the action potential to pore formation is only 100 μs or less.

After exocytosis, the vesicle membrane with its lipids and proteins is recycled, either by immediate re-filling with transmitter or by passing through a vesicle resting pool deeper inside the axon terminal.

Action potential-elicited neurotransmitter exocytosis is variable. First, action potentials trigger release from a given axon terminal only unreliably, with one or two release events per ten action potentials, resulting in a low overall release probability. Secondly, the probability of release is modulated by ▶ presynaptic receptors in the axon termi-

nal membrane (Fig. 1). Through these receptors, transmitter substances from neighbouring neurones and hormones can increase or reduce the release probability (2). Axon terminals thus integrate (1) the release command of the action potential and (2) various modulatory chemical messages from the neighbourhood to release an appropriate amount of transmitter.

Postsynaptic Receptor Activation

Of the several classes of receptors for endogenous chemical signals (4), two are used as postsynaptic receptors in synaptic transmission: ligand-gated ion channels (LGICs) and ▶ G protein-coupled receptors (GPCRs; Fig. 1). Due to the large number of transmitters and the existence of several receptor types for almost all, postsynaptic receptor acti-

Tab. 1 Selected neurotransmitter receptors.

Transmitter	Receptor[1]	Effector mechanisms[2]	Agonists	Antagonists
Glutamate	AMPA (LGIC)	↑ Na^+ and K^+ conductance	α-amino-3-hydroxy-5-methyl-4-isoxazolepropionic acid (AMPA)	
GABA	$GABA_A$ (LGIC)	↑ Cl^- conductance	muscimol	bicuculline
	$GABA_B$ (GPCR)	$G_{i/o}$	baclofen	
Glycine	glycine receptor (LGIC)	↑ Cl^- conductance		strychnine
Acetylcholine	nicotinic (LGIC)	↑ Na^+, K^+ and Ca^{2+} conductance	nicotine, suxamethonium	tubocurarine, α-conotoxins, α-bungarotoxin
	muscarinic M_{1-5} (GPCR)	M_1, M_3, M_5: $G_{q/11}$; M_2, M_4: $G_{i/o}$	muscarine, carbachol	atropine, scopolamine
Dopamine	D_{1-5} (GPCR)	D_1, D_5: G_s; D_2, D_3, D_4: $G_{i/o}$	D_2: bromocriptine	D_2: chlorpromazine D_4: clozapine
Noradrenaline	$α_{1A,B,D}$ (GPCR)	$G_{q/11}$	phenylephrine	prazosin
	$α_{2A-C}$ (GPCR)	$G_{i/o}$	clonidine	yohimbine
	$β_{1-3}$ (GPCR)	G_s	isoprenaline	propranolol
Serotonin	$5\text{-}HT_{1A-F}$ (GPCR)	$G_{i/o}$	$5\text{-}HT_{1B,D}$: sumatriptan	
	$5\text{-}HT_3$ (LGIC)	↑ Na^+ and K^+ conductance		ondansetron
Opioid peptides	μ, δ, κ (GPCR)	$G_{i/o}$	μ: morphine	naloxone

[1] LGIC, ligand-gated ion channel; GPCR, G protein-coupled receptor
[2] Activation of $G_{i/o}$ leads to ↓ cyclic AMP (inhibition of adenylyl cyclase) and ↓ Ca^{2+} conductance (N- and P/Q-type Ca^{2+} channels). Activation of $G_{q/11}$ leads to ↑ inositol trisphosphate and ↑ diacyl glycerol (stimulation of phospholipase C). Activation of G_s leads to ↑ cyclic AMP (stimulation of adenylyl cyclase).

vation is the most diversified step of synaptic transmission. Table 1 shows selected neurotransmitter receptors.

LGICs are hetero- or homo-oligomeric proteins consisting or 3, 4 or 5 peptide chains, of which each spans the membrane several times. The 3 to 5 subunits surround a pore, which in the absence of transmitter is closed. The nicotinic receptor for acetylcholine, the $GABA_A$-receptor, the glycine receptor and the $5\text{-}HT_3$-receptor for serotonin are pentamers. The ionotropic glutamate receptors are tetramers. The P2X-receptors for ATP are trimers. When transmitter is bound to a ligand-gated ion channel receptor, the open probability of the pore is increased. Ions may then enter or leave the cell, but a selectivity filter in the channel lets only certain ions pass.

The AMPA receptors for glutamate, the nicotinic acetylcholine receptor and the 5-HT$_3$-receptor for serotonin are cation channels (Table 1). When they open, the major consequence is a sudden entry of Na$^+$, depolarization and an excitatory postsynaptic potential (EPSP; Fig. 1).

The GABA$_A$-receptor and the glycine receptor are Cl$^-$ channels (Table 1). When they open at a resting membrane potential of about −60 mV, the consequence is an entry of Cl$^-$, hyperpolarization and an inhibitory postsynaptic potential (IPSP; Fig. 1).

All these postsynaptic events last only for a few milliseconds; synaptic transmission through LGICs is fast. When the postsynaptic cell membrane is sufficiently depolarized, voltage-dependent Na$^+$ channels open and an action potential is generated.

GPCRs are proteins that span the postsynaptic cell membrane seven times (heptahelical receptors). Small ligands are usually bound within a pocket formed by the seven transmembrane helices. The large neuropeptides bind to the extracellular domains. When the receptors are activated, they interact with the appropriate G proteins that are bound to the inner surface of the cell membrane. The G proteins then pass the information on to various effectors (Fig. 1).

The GABA$_B$-receptors, the muscarinic M$_2$- and M$_4$-receptors for acetylcholine, the dopamine D$_2$-, D$_3$- and D$_4$-receptors, the α_2-adrenoceptors for noradrenaline, the 5-HT$_{1A-F}$-receptors for serotonin, and the opioid μ-, δ- and κ-receptors couple to G proteins of the G$_{i/o}$ family and thereby lower (1) the cyctoplasmic level of the second messenger cyclic AMP and (2) the open probability of N- and P/Q-type Ca^{2+} channels (Table 1). The muscarinic M$_1$-, M$_3$- and M$_5$-receptors for acetylcholine and the α_1-adrenoceptors for noradrenaline couple to G proteins of the G$_{q/11}$ family and thereby increase the cytoplasmic levels of the second messengers inositol trisphosphate and diacyl glycerol (Table 1). The dopamine D$_1$- and D$_5$-receptors and the β-adrenoceptors for noradrenaline, finally, couple to G$_s$ and thereby increase the cytoplasmic level of cyclic AMP.

These cascades of reactions need time in the range of seconds: synaptic transmission through GPCRs is slow. All further postsynaptic changes depend on the type of postsynaptic cell. For example, activation of β_2-adrenoceptors causes: in the heart an increase of the rate and force of contraction; in skeletal muscle glycogenolysis and tremor; in smooth muscle relaxation; in bronchial glands secretion; and in sympathetic nerve terminals an increase in transmitter release.

Transmitter Inactivation

Once released, transmitters are inactivated by diffusion into the neighbouring extracellular space, combined with one of two specific pathways: either extracellular degradation by enzymes that face the extracellular space, or uptake into cells.

Extracellular degradation removes acetylcholine, the neuropeptides and ATP. Acetylcholine is rapidly hydrolyzed to choline and acetate by acetylcholinesterase. The enzyme is localized in both the presynaptic and the postsynatic cell membrane and splits about 10,000 molecules of acetylcholine per second.

Glutamate, GABA, glycine, dopamine, noradrenaline and serotonin are taken up into adjacent cells. The uptake is mediated by Plasmalemmal Neurotransmitter Transporters (PNTs; Fig. 1). The main driving force for all PNTs is the Na$^+$ concentration gradient across the axolemma. There are several PNT families. One is the Na$^+$/Cl$^-$-Dependent Neurotransmitter Transporter (SCDNT) family, which comprises transporters for GABA, glycine, dopamine, noradrenaline and serotonin. The GABA transporters are located partly in the GABAergic, and the glycine transporters are located partly in the glycinergic terminals themselves. The dopamine, noradrenaline and serotonin transporters are located almost exclusively in the dopaminergic, noradrenergic and serotoninergic terminals, respectively. In all these cases, cellular uptake means re-uptake into the presynaptic neurone. Re-uptake by the PNTs may be followed by vesicular re-uptake by the VNTs; an economical way of inactivation, reminiscent of the recycling of the storage vesicle membrane (1).

Pharmacological Interventions

Transmitter Production and Vesicular Storage
Drugs affecting transmitter production and storage include the following, all acting on monoamine neurones. Levodopa is administered as the precursor of dopamine to compensate for the loss of dopaminergic neurones in ▶ Parkinson's disease. Benserazide is an inhibitor of aromatic L-amino acid decarboxylase that does not pass the blood-brain barrier. It is given together with levodopa in Parkinson's disease to prevent the decarboxylation of levodopa in peripheral tissues. Reserpine specifically blocks VMAT, thus depletes monoamines from the axon terminals, and is occasionally used to treat hypertension.

Transmitter Release
So central is exocytosis from neurones for animal life, that evolution has made it the target of a large number of natural poisons, used by the producing organisms for defence or attack. The puffer fish produces tetrodotoxin and some dinoflagellates produce saxitoxin, both of which occlude voltage-gated Na^+ channels by binding to the external side of the channel pore. The cone snail *Conus geographus* produces the ▶ conotoxin ω-conotoxin GVIA, a small cysteine-rich peptide, which blocks N-type Ca^{2+} channels. P/Q-type Ca^{2+} channels are insensitive to ω-conotoxin GVIA but selectivley blocked by the funnel-web spider venom ω-agatoxin IVA, also a small cysteine-rich peptide. Tetrodotoxin and ω-conotoxin GVIA are the two most widely used toxins in neuroscience.

The most ingenious exocytosis toxins, however, come from the anaerobic bacteria *Clostridium botulinum* and *Clostridium tetani*. The former produces the seven botulinum neurotoxins (BoNTs) A to G; the latter produces tetanus neurotoxin (TeNT). All eight toxins consist of a heavy (H) chain and a light (L) chain that are associated by an interchain S-S bond. The L-chains enter the cytosol of axon terminals. Importantly, BoNT L-chains mainly enter peripheral cholinergic terminals, whereas the TeNT L-chain mainly enters cerebral and spinal cord GABAergic and glycinergic terminals. The L-chains are the active domains of the toxins. They are zinc-endopeptidases and specifically split the three core proteins of exocytosis, i.e. the SNAREs (Fig. 1 inset). Each of the eight toxins splits a single SNARE at a single site. Destruction of synaptobrevin, syntaxin or SNAP-25 in cholinergic terminals by the BoNTs leads to cessation of acetylcholine release followed by flaccid paralysis, the main symptom of ▶ botulism. Destruction of synaptobrevin in GABAergic and glycinergic terminals by TeNT leads to cessation of GABA and glycine release followed by spastic paralysis, the main symptom of ▶ tetanus. BoNT and TeNT are the most potent toxic substances known, able to kill vertebrates at a dose of 0.1 to 1 ng/kg body weight (3).

Postsynaptic Receptor Activation
The most diversified step of synaptic transmission is also the target of the greatest variety of drugs. Some are included in Table 1. Many are natural poisons such as muscimol, bicuculline, strychnine, nicotine, tubocurarine, muscarine, atropine, scopolamine, yohimbine and morphine, all of which stem from plants; the α-conotoxins; and α-bungarotoxin from the bungar snake. Tubocurarine, the α-conotoxins and α-bungarotoxin cause flaccid paralysis by blocking the postsynaptic nicotinic receptor of the skeletal muscle endplate- the same symptom that BoNTs produce by preventing the release of acetylcholine.

The therapeutic impact of drugs acting at transmitter receptors is enormous. All volatile and intravenous anaesthetics and also ethanol act primarily on cerebral LGICs, above all GABA$_A$-receptors. All neuromuscular blocking agents are agonists or antagonists at the skeletal muscle nicotinic receptor. There would be no surgery worth mentioning without these drug actions on neurotransmitter receptors. Morphine and related opioid agonists are the most effective analgesics. The β-adrenoceptor antagonists such as propranolol have become the most successful group of cardiovascular drugs. The benzodiazepine anxiolytics, which promote the effect of GABA on GABA$_A$-receptors, and the dopamine receptor-blocking ▶ neuroleptics such as chlorpromazine and clozapine are two major drug classes used in psychiatry.

Transmitter Inactivation
The cholinesterase inhibitors are the classical drugs that interfere with transmitter inactivation. The prototype was physostigmine, a plant poison and later a therapeutic agent in ▶ myasthenia

gravis. The highly toxic nerve gases such as sarin also are cholinesterase inhibitors. The GABA transporter is blocked by tiagabine, an antiepileptic that owes its effect to the ensuing increase of the concentration of GABA in the synaptic cleft. Cocaine is abused because it blocks the dopamine transporter and, hence, enhances dopaminergic transmission in the mesolimbic dopaminergic "reward system". Blockers of the noradrenaline transporter and blockers of the serotonin transporter are the main ▶ antidepressant drugs, i.e. the main members of the third major drug class in psychiatry.

References

1. Masson J, Sagné C, Hamon M, El Mestikawy S (1999) Neurotransmitter transporters in the central nervous system. Pharmacol Rev 51:439–464
2. Starke K (2001) Presynaptic autoreceptors in the third decade: focus on α2-adrenoceptors. J Neurochem 78:685–693
3. Schiavo G, Matteoli M, Montecucco C (2000) Neurotoxins affecting neuroexocytosis. Physiol Rev 80:717–766
4. Hofmann F (2001) Wirkungen von Pharmaka auf den Organismus: Allgemeine Pharmakodynamik. In: Forth W, Henschler D, Rummel W, Förstermann U, Starke K (eds) Allgemeine und spezielle Pharmakologie und Toxikologie. Urban & Fischer, München, p 4–25

Synaptic Vesicles

Synaptic vesicles are the organelles in axon terminals that store neurotransmitters and release them by exocytosis. There are two types, the large dense-core vesicles, diameter about 90 nm, that contain neuropeptides, and the small synaptic vesicles, diameter about 50 nm, that contain non-peptide transmitters. About 10 vesicles per synapse are 'docked' to the plasma membrane and ready for release, the 'readily releasable pool'. Many more vesicles per synapse are stored farther away from the plasma membrane, the 'resting pool'. When needed, the latter vesicles may be recruited into the readily releasable pool. Neuronal depo-

larization and activation of voltage-sensitive Ca^{2+} channels increases intracellular Ca^{2+} levels that promotes exocytosis and fusion of the vesicles with the presynaptic membrane allowing the vesicular neurotransmitter to be released into the synaptic cleft.

▶ Exocytosis
▶ Synaptic Transmission

Synaptotagmin

Synaptotagmin is an integral type I transmembrane glycoprotein that possesses two C2 calcium-binding domains. C2-domains are present in several other proteins such as the calcium-dependent isoforms of protein kinase C and phospholipase D where they are known to regulate Ca-dependent binding to phospholipid membranes. More than 10 different synaptotagmins are known, that are widely expressed in many tissues. Best characterized is synaptotagmin I, a resident of synaptic vesicles and neurosecretory granules. Synaptotagmin I probably functions as an exocytotic Ca-receptor that links the calcium signal to membrane fusion by means of Ca-dependent binding to membranes and (possibly) to SNAREs.

▶ Exocytosis

Syndecans

Syndecans are transmembrane proteins, which are modified by the addition of heparan sulphate glycosaminoglycan (GAG) chains and other sugars. Syndecans bind a wide variety of different ligands via their heparan sulphate chains. Binding specificities may vary depending on cell-type specific modifications of the heparan sulphate chains.

▶ Table appendix: Adhesion Molecules

Synergistic Interaction

Synergistic action is interaction in which the combined effect is greater than the sum of the effects of each drug administered separately.

▶ Drug Interactions

Systolic and Diastolic Blood Pressure and Pulse Pressure

Systolic pressure, or maximum blood pressure, occurs during left ventricular systole. Diastolic pressure, or minimum blood pressure, occurs during ventricular diastole. The difference between systolic and diastolic pressure is the pulse pressure. While diastolic blood pressure has been historically been used as the most relevant clinical blood pressure phenotype, it has now been clearly established that systolic blood pressure is the more important clinical predictor for cardiovascular morbidity and mortality. More recently, additional attention is focussed on the importance of pulse pressure, i.e. the blood pressure amplitude, as a predictive factor for cardiovascular disease.

▶ Blood Pressure Control

S

T

T3

▶ Triiodothyronine

T4

▶ Thyroxine

t1/2 or t1/2β

▶ Half-life /Elimination Half-life
▶ Pharmacokinetics

Tachykinins

Tachykinins are a group of related endogenous peptides, substance P, neurokinin A and neurokinin B, which are widely distributed in the central and peripheral nervous systems. Substance P and neurokinin A are formed by cleavage of a larger protein precursor, pre-pro-tachykinin. Nociceptive sensory neurons express substance P and neurokinin A and release these mediators in the periphery as well as in the dorsal horn of the spinal cord. Inflammation increases substance P expression. Activation of nociceptors results in the release of substance P in the periphery, which con-tributes to neurogenic inflammation. Substance P release in the dorsal horn contributes to the development of chronic pain. The effects of tachykinins are mediated by a group of G-protein coupled receptors called NK_1, NK_2 and NK_3, which serve as receptors for substance P, neurokinin A and neurokinin B, respectively.

▶ Analgesics
▶ Nociception

Tachyphylaxis

Tachyphylaxis is a loss of drug efficiency which develops in minutes or hours. Transmitter depletion and receptor desensitization are the basic mechanisms of this phenomenon.

▶ Tolerance and Resensitization

Tamoxifen

▶ Selective Sex Steroid Receptor Modulators

Tandem Mass Spectrometry

Tandem mass spectrometry (MS/MS) is a method to obtain sequence and structural information by measurement of the mass-to-charge ratios of ionized peptide molecules before and after dissociation reactions within a mass spectrometer which consists essentially of two mass spectrometers in tandem. In the first step, a mass filter (quadrupole) allows only selected ions (parent or precursor ions) to reach the collision cell. In the collision cell, the peptide is further fragmented by energy impact with a collision gas (argon). The generated daughter or product ions can be analyzed by a second mass filter (quadrupole, time-of-flight). MS/MS measurements can be performed with triple quadrupole mass spectrometry (MS), ion trap MS or more recently with quadrupole-time-of-flight MS. MS/MS spectra of peptides mainly show sequence-specific N-terminal 'b' and C-terminal 'y' ions and can be used to identify proteins from databases.

▶ Proteomics

Tardive Dyskinesia

Tardive dyskinesia (TD) refers to a neurological syndrome caused by the long-term use of antipsychotic medications. It is characterized by repetitive involuntary movements of the face, limbs, or trunk. The incidence of tardive dyskinesia is greater with conventional antipsychotic drugs than atypical antipsychotic drugs, and clozapine may even have an ameliorative effect on established TD. There is no known treatment for TD, though dose reduction, discontinuation of the offending drug or substituting with an atypical antipsychotic drug may be beneficial.

▶ Antipsychotic Drugs

Target

A target is a protein or protein assembly whose function is believed to be important for promoting health or treating disease.

▶ High-throughput Screening

Targeted Mutant

A targeted mutant is a mutation introduced into an endogenous gene by homologous recombination, typically in embryonic stem cells.

TATA Box

A TATA box is a consensus sequence in the promoter region of many eucaryotic genes that binds a general transcription factor and hence specifies the position where transcription is initiated by the RNA polymerase.

Taxanes

Taxanes are a group of antineoplastic agents including paclitaxel and docelatel which are derivatives of yew tree bark. Taxanes possess the ability to promote microtubule formation in the absence of GTP. They bind specifically to the β-tubulin subunit of microtubules and antagonize the disassembly of this cytoskeletal protein, resulting in an arrest of cells in mitosis.

▶ Antineoplastic Agents
▶ Cytoskeleton

T-cells

▶ T-lymphocytes

Telomerase

Telomerase is an enzyme which in growing tissue maintains and stabilizes the telomeres, which are specialized structures on the ends of each chromosome. The shortening and possibly disappearance of telomeres is believed to be the basis for cessation of cell division in many cells, which eventually leads to senescence. One reason why continuously proliferating cancer cells are immortal is thought to be that their telomeres do not shorten with each round of cell division due to the action of telomerase. Most differentiated cells do not express telomerase, while most cancer cells do express the enzyme. Inhibitors of telomerase are currently being explored as potential anti-neoplastic agents.

► Antineoplastic Agents
► Senescene

Temporal Lobe

The temporal lobe is the inferior middle portion of the cerebral cortex of both hemispheres. The temporal lobes are involved in the analysis of visual and acoustic information and in memory formation. The ► hippocampus is part of the inner, medial side of the temporal lobes.

► Antiepileptic Drugs

Tendinitis

Tendinitis is an inflammatory painful tendon disorder which can be caused by quinolones. Typical cases are characterized by acute onset, palpation and sharp pain mostly of one or both Achilles tendons, but other tendons may also be affected. Magnetic resonance imaging (MRI) is used to support the diagnosis. Estimates for the incidence of quinolone-induced tendinitis range from approximately 1:100 to 1:10,000. The etiology remains unknown, concomitant use of corticosteroids, end stage renal disease and age older than 60 years are recognized as risk factors. The latency period ranges from 2 to 60 days after start of treatment, but tendon ruptures may occur as late as 6 months after cessation of therapy.

► Quinolones, potent inhibitors of bacterial topoisomerases

Teratogen

Teratogens are agents which produce gross structural malformations of the foetus, such as absence of limbs or misdevelopment of organs. Teratogens act primarily during organogenesis, which occurs between day 17 and day 60 in the human pregnancy. Well known teratogens are thalidomide, coumarins, anticonvulsants like phenytoin or valproate, cytotoxic drugs and retinoids.

Testosterone

► Sex steroid receptors

Tetanus

Tetanus is a disease caused by the release of neurotoxins from the anaerobic, spore-forming rod *Clostridium tetani*. The clostridial protein, tetanus toxin, possesses a protease activity which selectively degrades the presynaptic vesicle protein synaptobrevin, resulting in a block of glycine and γ-aminobutyric acid (GABA) release from presynaptic terminals. Consistent with the loss of neurogenic motor inhibition, symptoms of tetanus include muscular rigidity and hyperreflexia. The clinical course is characterized by increased muscle tone and spasms, which first affect the masseter muscle and the muscles of the throat, neck and shoulders. Death occurs by respiratory failure or heart failure.

► Bacterial Toxines
► Exocytosis
► Glycine Receptors
► Ryanodine Receptor

Tethered Ligand

A tethered ligand is the new N-terminal formed following serine proteinase-mediated cleavage of the original N-terminal of a PAR family member, which is responsible for activation of the receptor.

▶ Proteinase-activated Receptors

Tetracycline

Tetracycline is an antibiotic with a flat structure of four fused rings with hydrophilic groups on one side and hydrophobic groups on the other side. It exhibits a broad spectrum of activity against Gram-positive and Gram-negative bacteria. It has been used widely in human and veterinary medicine until the recent spread of antibiotic resistance. Resistance to tetracycline, unlike many other antibiotics, is not caused by mutation of ribosomal RNA (rRNA) or ribosomal proteins or modification of a rRNA target site. It is rather caused by enzymes that result in 1) efflux of the drug across the cell membrane, 2) modification of the drug or 3) mimicry of elongation factors and release of the bound drug from the ribosome.

▶ Ribosomal Protein Synthesis Inhibitors

Tetrahydrocannabinol

THC ist the most abundant and most active cannabinoid found in the hemp plant *Cannabis sativa*. It constitutes about 1-10 % of *Cannabis sativa* preparations like marijuana or hashish.

▶ Endocannabinoid System

(6R)-5,6,7,8-tetrahydro-L-biopterin

Biopterin (2-amino-4-hydroxy-6-(1',2'-dihydroxy-propyl)-pteridine) is a pteridine derivative. The reduced form (6R)-5,6,7,8-tetrahydro-L-biopterin functions as a coenzyme in hydroxylation reactions of amino acids.

Tetrodotoxin

Tetrodotoxin (TTX) is a toxin derived from bacteria which is concentrated in the gonads and liver of certain pufferfishes (fugu). Similar to saxitoxin, tetrodotoxin is a very potent blocker of most voltage-sensitive Na^+ channels.

▶ Voltage-dependent Na^+ Channels

TF

▶ Tissue Factor

Tg

▶ Thyroglobulin

TGFβ

▶ Transforming Growth Factor β

TH

▶ Tyrosine hydroxylase

THC

▶ Tetrahydrocannabinol

Therapeutic Drug Monitoring

Therapeutic drug monitoring (TDM) is advised for the individualization of dosage of drugs with a narrow therapeutic index and broad inter-individual pharmacokinetic variability. This is routinely done by determination of blood levels.

▶ Pharmocogenetics
▶ Pharmacokinetics

Thiamin

Vitamin B1

▶ Vitamins, watersoluble

Thiazide Diuretics

Thiazide diuretics, a group of drugs with moderate diuretic activity, includes hydrochlorothiazide, chlorthalidone and xipamide. They decrease active reabsorption of sodium and accompanying chloride by binding to the chloride site of the electroneutral Na^+/Cl^- co-transport system in the distal convoluted tubule and inhibiting its action.

▶ Diuretics

▶ Epithelial Na^+ Channel

Thiazolidinediones

▶ Oral Antidiabetic Drugs

Thienopyridines

Thienppyridines are a Group of antiplatelet agents including ticlopidine and clopidogrel, which after oral administration are converted to active metabolites. The active metabolites in turn are able to block the P_2Y_{12}-receptors, which physiologically mediate part of the action of ADP on platelets.

▶ Antiplatelet Drugs

Thiopurine S-methyltransferase

Thiopurine S-methyltransferase is an enzyme which inactivates the anti-cancer drug 6-mercaptopurine by S-methylation.

▶ Pharmacogenetics

Thioxanthene

Thioxanthenes are a group of antipsychotic drugs (e.g. chlorprothixene).

▶ Antipsychotic Drugs

Threading

Threading techniques try to match a target sequence on a library of known three-dimensional structures by 'threading' the target sequence over the known coordinates. In this manner, threading tries to predict the three-dimensional structure starting from a given protein sequence. It is sometimes successful when comparisons based on sequences or sequence profiles alone fail due to too low a sequence similarity.

▶ Bioinformatics

Thrifty Gene Hypothesis

The thrifty gene hypothesis postulates that specific sets of genes, which optimized energy utilization and storage, prepared our ancestors for 'feast and famine' by efficiently protecting energy reserves when supplies were low and by rapidly replenishing them when supplies increased again. With unlimited food resources, the thrifty gene haplotype is responsible for a metabolic syndrome of obesity, insulin resistance, hypertension, and dyslipidemia. This dependence of the phenotype on 'lifestyle' was first observed in Polynesian and American Indian populations.

▶ Antiobesity Drugs

Thrombin

Thrombin (factor IIa) is an enzyme of 295 amino acids derived from prothrombin (vitamin K-dependent zymogen) that converts soluble fibrinogen into insoluble fibrin; other procoagulant activities of thrombin include activation of factor XIII to factor XIIIa (which irreversibly crosslinks fibrin polymers) and activation of the nonenzymatic coagulation factors V and VIII to Va and VIIIa, respectively (greatly amplifying thrombin generation). Thrombin also activates platelets. In addition, thrombin binds to thrombomodulin on endothelium, which causes thrombin to lose its procoagulant activities, and instead to convert protein C to activated protein C (APC), which down-regulates thrombin generation by proteolyzing factors Va and VIIIa.

▶ Anticoagulants
▶ Coagulation/Thrombosis
▶ Proteinase-activated Receptors

Thrombocytopenia

Thrombocytopenia is a decrease in the number of circulating blood platelets (below 150×10^9/L). Although severe thrombocytopenia can lead to spontaneous bleeding, a few disorders (e.g., heparin-induced thrombocytopenia) are paradoxically associated with an increased risk of thrombosis.

▶ Anticoagulants
▶ Hematopoietic Growth Factors
▶ Antiplatelet Drugs

Thrombolysis

Thrombolysis is fibrinolysis.

▶ Fibrinolytics

Thrombopoietin

▶ Hematopoietic Growth Factors

Thrombosis

Thrombosis is the development of a "thrombus", consisting of platelets, fibrin, red and white blood cells in the arterial or venous circulation. Platelet-rich "white thrombi" are found in the arterial system and can be prevented by antiplatelet drugs.

► Anticoagulants
► Antiplatelet Drugs
► Coagulation/Thrombosis
► Fibrinolytics

Thromboxane

► Prostanoids
► Cyclooxygenase

Thrombus

A thrombus is a mass of cells and protein composed principally of platelets and fibrin, but also containing red and white blood cells. A thrombus which forms in the circulatory system can become occlusive in that the thrombus can physically block flowing blood.

► Thrombosis

Thymoleptics

► Antidepressant Drugs

Thyroglobuline

Thyroglobulin (Tg) provides the matrix for thyroid hormone biosynthesis. It is a dimeric glycoprotein with a molecular weight of 660,000. Most of the thyroglobulin is present in the thyroid follicular lumen. Thyroglobulin contains 0.1–2.0% iodine and, as a glycoprotein, it contains 8–10% total carbohydrate, with galactose, mannose, fucose, N-acetyl glucosamine and sialic acid residues. The carbohydrate in the protein is distributed as three distinct units, A, B and C. Tg is synthesized on polysomes on the endoplasmic reticulum near the basal portion of the cell. After phosphorylation and gylcosylation it is vectorially transported to the apical membrane of the cell and deposited into the follicular lumen.

► Antithyroid Drugs

Thyroid Autonomy

Thyroid autonomy appears as a solitary toxic nodule or toxic multinodular goitre. In toxic thyroid, the nodule's synthesis and secretion of thyroid hormones is autonomous from the thyroid-stimulating hormone (TSH), which is produced in the pituitary gland. Accordingly TSH is suppressed and the extranodular thyroid tissue is functionally down-regulated. Thyroid autonomy occurs frequently in iodine-deficient countries whereas it is much less common in iodine-sufficient areas. Constitutively activating mutations in the ► TSH receptor and in the Gs α protein are the major molecular etiology of toxic thyroid nodules.

► Antithyroid Drugs

T

Thyroid Peroxidase

Thyroid peroxidase (TPO) is a membrane-bound, glycosylated, hemoprotein enzyme. It catalyzes iodination of tyrosyl residues and the coupling of iodotyrosyl residues in thyroglobulin to form thyroxine and triiodothyronine. All mammalian peroxidases belong to the same gene family. The human TPO gene consists of 17 exons and 16 introns and covers at least 150 kb pairs. The heme iron in native peroxidases including TPO and LPO, is in the ferric form (Fe III). In model systems, TPO has no catalytic activity in the absence of H_2O_2 and there is little doubt that H_2O_2 production plays an essential role in thyroid hormone formation *in vivo*. The H_2O_2 generating system is Ca^{2+} dependent and involves a nicotinamide ADPH (NADPH) oxidase.

▶ Antithyroid Drugs

Thyrotoxicosis

▶ Hyperthyroidism

Thyroxine

Thyroxine (3',5',3,5-L-teraiodothyronine, T4) is a thyroid hormone, which is transformed in peripheral tissues by the enzyme 5'-monodeiodinase to triiodothyronine. T_4 is three to eight times less active than triiodothyronine. T_4 circulates in plasma bound to plasma proteins (T_4-binding globulin, T_4-binding prealbumin and albumin). It is effective in its free non-protein-bound form, which accounts for less than 1%. Its half-life is about 190 hours.

▶ Antithyroid Drugs

Tissue Factor

Tissue factor (TF) is an integral membrane glycoprotein which is tightly associated with phospholipid (molecular weight 44 kD). It is located on most vascular cells and by functioning as a receptor for factor VII initiates the extrinsic pathway of the blood coagulation cascade. The formation of a 1 to1 complex with factor VII in the presence of Ca^{2+}-ions facilitates the conversion of factor VII to factor VIIa by minor proteolysis.

▶ Coagulation

Tissue Plasminogen Activator

Tissue plasminogen activator is a naturally occurring serine protease that can be secreted by endothelial cells in response to injury to the artery walls. This enzyme promotes the conversion of plasminogen into plasmin, a serine protease which ultimately effects clot dissolution by degradation of fibrin.

▶ Fibrinolytics

T-lymphocytes

T-lymphocytes are hematopoietic cells belonging to the adaptive immune system. The prefix 'T' indicates that immature precursors migrate to the thymus and are released as mature T-cells. During the maturation process in the thymus, a selection process eliminates both inactive and self-reactive cells. Each T-cell displays a specific receptor for antigen. From a functional point of view, T-cells are classified into cytokine-producing CD4+ or helper T-cells that provide growth and activation factors to neighbouring cells, and CD8+ or cytotoxic T-cells, that specifically attack and kill target cells expressing the specific antigen. The composition of cytokines released by CD4+ cells allows a classification into Th1 and Th2 populations. The term 'Memory cells' describes a population of sensitized T- or B-cells that persist in the host and can rapidly be reactivated upon exposure with the specific antigen.

▶ Immune Defense
▶ Immunosuppressive Agents

TNF

Tumor Necrosis Factor

▶ Tumor Necrosis Factor α
▶ TNF Receptor Superfamily

TNFα

▶ Tumor Necrosis Factor α
▶ TNF Receptor Superfamily
▶ Inflammation
▶ Cytokines

TNF Receptor Associated Factors

Tumor necrosis factor receptor associated factors are a group of at least 6 proteins (TRAF1-6), which are major signal transducers for the TNF receptor superfamily and the the interlukin-1 receptor / toll-like receptor (IL-1R/TLR) superfamily. TRAF proteins are characterized by the presence of the TRAF domain at the the C-terminus, which mediates self-association and upstream interaction with receptors and other signaling proteins. They function as adaptor proteins, which elaborate receptor signal transduction by serving as both a convergent and divergent platform.

▶ Tumor Necrosis Factor α
▶ TNF Receptor Superfamily
▶ Cytokines

▶ Inflammation
▶ Table appendix: Receptor Proteins

TNF Receptor Superfamily

The TNF receptor superfamily is a group of receptors, which share some structural similarities. Best-studied examples are the receptors for tumor necrosis factor α (TNFα) and the Fas receptor. Binding of the inherently trimeric ligands induces receptor trimerisation and results in the recruitment of several signaling proteins to the cytoplasmic domains of the receptors. TNF receptors recruit the "TNFR1-associated death domain protein" (TRADD), which serves as a platform to recruit several other mediators including "receptor-interacting protein 1" (RIP1), "Fas-associated death domain protein" (FADD) and "TNF-receptor associated factor 2 "(TRAF2). TRAF2 plays a central role in the induction of downstream events like activation of IκB-kinase (IKK) and MAP-kinases. Activation of Fas receptor does not result in the recruitment of TRAF2, but recruits FADD and subsequently leads to activation of caspase 8.

▶ Apoptosis
▶ Tumor Necrosis Factor α
▶ TNF Receptor Associated Factors
▶ Cytokines
▶ Inflammation
▶ Table appendix: Receptor Proteins

Tocolytics

Tocolytics are drugs such as the selective β_2-adrenoceptor agonists, e.g. salbutamol or terbutaline, which inhibit both the spontaneous and oxytocin-induced contractions of the pregnant uterus by relaxing the muscles of the uterus (myometrium). Tocolytics are used in selected patients to prevent premature labor.

▶ β-adrenergic System
▶ Smooth Muscle Tone Regulation

Tolerance

The term tolerance is used to describe a gradual decrease in responsiveness to a drug, typically developing over days or weeks. A fast loss of responsivess developing e.g. over a few minutes is called desensitisation or tachyphylaxis. It is important to note that tolerance does not only develop with drugs of abuse but also after repeated administration of a wide variety with drugs that are not self-administered by animals or used compulsively by man. Examples of the phenomenon of tolerance to opioids is described. Opioid tolerance is not associated with changes in affinity and/or density of opioid receptors. Opioid receptor desensitization is also not associated with receptor internalisation but underlies uncoupling of the G-protein.

▶ Drug Addiction/Dependence
▶ Tolerance and Desensitization

Tolerance and Desensitization

TORSTEN SCHÖNEBERG
Institut für Pharmakologie,
Universitätsklinikum Benjamin Franklin,
Freie Universität Berlin, Berlin, Germany
schoberg@zedat.fu-berlin.de

Definition

▶ Tolerance is the reduction in response to a drug after repeated administration. Clinically, a higher dose is required to obtain the original response. The time course and extent of tolerance developments varies between different drugs. At least two types of tolerance, ▶ pharmacokinetic and ▶ pharmacodynamic tolerance, can be distinguished. Tolerance development is a reversible process. The phenomenon of ▶ cross tolerance may develop to the effect of pharmacologically-related drugs, particularly to those acting at the same receptor.

▶ Desensitization describes the rapid signal attenuation in response to stimulation of cells by receptor agonists. Changes in the coupling efficiency of receptors to signal transduction pathways and receptor internalization can account for ▶ desensitization and the development of pharmacodynamic tolerance.

▶ Drug Addiction/Dependence
▶ Drug-Receptor Interaction
▶ G-protein-coupled Receptors

Basic Mechanisms

I. Removal of the Agonist

The action of an agonist can be terminated by its removal from the extracellular fluid. This includes simple dissociation and diffusion as well as the re-uptake and metabolic inactivation of the agonist. Latter mechanisms are fast and powerful and underlay a fine-tuned regulation that can adapt its capacity to maintain a physiological homeostasis. Many clinically used agonists are inactivated by similar mechanisms as the physiological ligands. Therefore, continued agonist treatment can induce an increased drug degradation. Such mechanisms may contribute to the development of a pharmacokinetic tolerance. For example, barbiturates induce their own metabolic inactivation in the liver, a process that leads to a reversible pharmacokinetic tolerance. Chemical modifications of an agonist that prevent re-uptake and metabolic degradation can help to circumvent this form of tolerance.

II. Receptor Desensitization

Receptor desensitization summarizes pharmacodynamic processes that lead to an inactivation of receptor signalling within seconds to minutes. The rapid attenuation of extracellular signals mediated by G-protein-coupled receptors (GPCRs) and their signalling pathways belong to the best-studied systems. The uncoupling of the receptor from its G protein involves receptor phosphorylation by different classes of protein kinases. Two types of receptor desensitization can be distinguished. ▶ Homologous desensitization is mediated by agonist-induced activation of the same receptor, whereas ▶ heterologous desensitization is caused by activation of a different receptor. The so-called

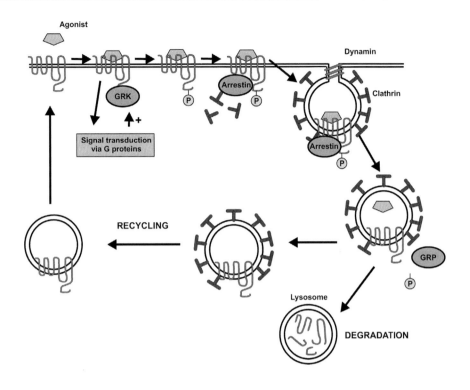

Fig. 1 Agonist-induced internalization of GPCRs. The model depicts the agonist-induced regulation of GPCR phosphorylation, internalization, recycling and degradation. Agonist activation of many GPCRs results in receptor phosphorylation by GPCR-specific kinases (GRK). The phosphorylated GPCR recruits β-arrestin, which initiates receptor targeting to clathrin-coated pits. Endosomal acidification permits dissociation of the ligand. The GPCR is dephosphorylated by a G-protein-coupled receptor specific phosphatase (GRP). Internalized receptors can recycle to the cell surface or are degraded in lysosomes.

► G-protein-coupled receptors kinases (► GRKs) are responsible for homologous agonist-induced receptor phosphorylation. So far, seven GRKs have been cloned. GRK2, GRK3 and GRK6 are the most widely distributed GRKs, but expression and knockout studies also implicate more distinct roles of individual GRKs. The phosphorylation sites, which are mainly serine residues, are located within the third intracellular loop and the intracellular C-terminus of GPCRs. Following receptor activation by an agonist, GRKs translocate from the cytosol to the plasma membrane. The efficacy of receptor phosphorylation by GRKs is greatly enhanced by binding to an activated receptor, depending on a specific phosphorylation consensus site as well as on the three-dimensional structure of the intracellular receptor surface. Once the receptor is phosphorylated, the functional cofactors of GRKs, the ► arrestins bind to the GPCR

and thereby quench the signal transduction by disrupting the interaction of the receptor and the G protein. At least three arrestins – the visual arrestin, β-arrestin-1 and β-arrestin-2 – can be distinguished. β-Arrestins are essential in the ► internalization of many GPCR. They act as adaptor proteins that link the receptors to the clathrin-coated pit endocytosis pathway (see III).

Second messenger-dependent kinases such as protein kinase A (PKA) and protein kinase C (PKC) are mainly involved in heterologous agonist-independent receptor desensitization. The heterologous desensitization includes receptors that use similar signal transduction pathways and simply depends on the overall kinase activity regulated by many different stimuli. Phosphorylation-induced conformational changes of the receptor reduce the affinity to the G protein, thereby leading to receptor/G-protein uncoupling.

T

Many GPCRs contain one or more conserved cysteine residues within their C-terminal tails which are modified by covalent attachment of palmitoyl or isoprenyl residues. The palmitoyl moiety is anchored in the lipid bilayer forming a fourth intracellular loop. There is evidence that palmitoylation of a GPCR is a dynamic process and may affect receptor desensitization.

Desensitization is also a general property of other receptor families such as receptor tyrosine kinases and ligand-gated ion channels. For example, receptor tyrosine kinases undergo agonist-induced dimerization and autophosphorylation that initiates receptor internalization (see III). Phosphorylation of serine and tyrosine residues may also modulate the desensitisation of ion channels such as the nicotinic acetylcholine receptor at the neuromuscular junction. Nevertheless, the molecular mechanism that mediates channel opening by agonist binding, and then allows the channel to close (desensitize) even though agonist remains bound is not understood in detail.

It should be noted that fast inactivation of receptor signalling not only involves the desensitisation of the receptor but also the components of the downstream signalling cascade. The deactivation of active $G\alpha$ subunits is controlled by the intramolecular hydrolysis of bound GTP, allowing it to reform the inactive heterotrimer. Termination of G-protein-mediated signalling *in vivo* is 10–100 fold faster than the *in vitro* rate of GTP hydrolysis by $G\alpha$ subunits, suggesting the existence of GTPase-activating proteins (GAPs). Indeed, so-called "regulators of G-protein signalling" (RGS), have been identified as potent GAPs for $G\alpha$ subunits which are required to achieve timely deactivation.

III. Receptor Internalization

Agonist-induced receptor ▸ internalization (also called receptor endocytosis or sequestration) has been observed for many membranous receptors including GPCRs. Following GRK-mediated receptor phosphorylation, arrestins bind to the receptor and recruit other proteins such as AP-2, dynamin and clathrin. Then, clathrin-coated pits are formed and the receptors internalize. Subsequently, endosomal acidification permits dissoziation of the ligand and dephosphorylation of the receptor by cytosolic phosphatases (Fig). Internal-

ized receptors can recycle to the cell surface or can degraded in lysosomes, a process known as receptor down-regulation (see IV). The predominant pathway for internalization requires a concerted action of dynamin, arrestin and clathrin, but it should be noted that there are additional pathways of GPCR endocytosis which are independent from the latter two proteins. Internalization of the M_2 muscarinic acetylcholine receptor also requires dynamin, but proceeds in an apparent β-arrestin- and clathrin-independent manner.

In some cases, receptor inactivation, e.g. of the V_2 vasopressin receptor, is mediated by agonist-induced enzymatic cleavage of the GPCR. This non-endocytic proteolysis is promoted by a plasma membrane-associated metalloprotease. Proteinase-activated receptors (PARs) such as the thrombin receptor also follow a distinctly different pathway. PARs require the enzymatic cleavage of their N terminus, and the newly generated N terminus activates the receptor. Once activated, PARs are internalized into endosomes and sorted to lysosomes for degradation. Recovery of functional receptors at the plasma membrane requires synthesis of new receptors or mobilization of intact receptors from intracellular pools.

Receptor tyrosine kinases such as the epidermal-growth factor (EGF) receptor also undergoes agonist-induced endocytosis, which is assumed to follow a two-step process. First, the agonist induces receptor dimerization and conformational changes that allow for cross-phosphorylation of tyrosine residues. In a second step, the phosphorylated receptor tyrosine kinase recruits adaptor proteins such as Cbl protein and endophilin, which promote receptor internalization by forming clathrin-coated pits. Receptor activation also induces ubiquitination, a sorting signal for receptor degradation in lysosomes. Interestingly, GPCRs can cross-desensitize receptor tyrosine kinases through clathrin-mediated endocytosis.

Ligand-gated ion channels such as GABA type A receptor can also undergo clustering and internalization that is evoked when receptors are occupied by agonists. Internalized receptors can be rapidly recycled to the cell surface, a process that is regulated by protein kinase C. On the other hand, a portion of the intracellular GABA type A receptors derived from ligand-dependent endocytosis is targeted to degradation pathways.

IV. Receptor Down-Regulation

The decrease in the total cellular receptor number is a process known as receptor down-regulation. It is caused by chronic agonist exposure and occurs in hours or days. This process is mainly agonist-mediated but there is also evidence for agonist-independent pathways of cell surface receptor depletion. Recovery from receptor down-regulation is reversible but slow. One mechanism of receptor down-regulation involves lysosomal targeting and the accelerated degradation of internalized receptors (Fig.). The factors that determine the fate of an internalized receptor (recycling pathway vs degradation) are currently unknown. Conjugation of proteins with ubiquitin, an abundant intracellular protein, is a signal for the rapid degradation of many cytosolic and membranous proteins. It has been demonstrated that receptor tyrosine kinases and GPCRs undergo agonist-induced ubiquitination.

The regulation of receptor synthesis is a second component of receptor down-regulation. It involves processes that reduce gene transcription, mRNA stability and receptor half-life time. It should be noted that mechanisms in addition to the regulation of the receptor number may account for tolerance development. Second messenger levels and enzyme activities that participate in the signalling of a given receptor are found to be up- or down-regulated to compensate for chronic over stimulation of a distinct signal transduction cascade.

Pharmacological Relevance

Desensitization, internalization and down-regulation of receptors are mechanisms that eventually lead to a loss of agonist efficacy. These processes together with agonist removal have been implicated in ► tachyphylaxis and in the development of tolerance and drug ► dependence. *Vice versa*, chronic administration of antagonists dramatically increase the number of receptors and may account for super sensitivity seen e.g. after rapid termination of a long-term treatment with β-adrenergic receptor antagonists. Understanding the molecular mechanisms of long-term receptor expression regulation may help to influence or even prevent therapeutically undesired effects.

Many mechanistic questions are still puzzling, but recent studies with genetically engineered mice have provided some new insights in the processes of desensitization and tolerance development. The desensitization of the μ-opioid receptor and development antinociceptive tolerance was abolished in mice lacking β-arrestin-2. As a result of gene deletion, these mice showed a remarkable potentiation and prolongation of the analgesic effect of morphine. Interestingly, the deletion of β-arrestin-2 does not prevent the chronic morphine-induced up-regulation of adenylyl cyclase activity, a cellular marker of dependence, and the mutant mice still became physically dependent on the drug. In concert with this finding, several studies indicate that highly addictive opiate drugs such as morphine are deficient in their ability to induce the desensitization and endocytosis of receptors. Therefore, the development of physical dependence and addiction appears to be independent from desensitization and endocytosis of opiate receptors.

Agonist-dependent and -independent changes in receptor density can contribute to pathological situations. There is a down-regulation of cardiac β-adrenergic receptors in dilated cardiomyopathy, probably as a consequence of increased sympathetic tone. A rapid up-regulation of β-adrenergic receptors is characteristic of myocardial ischemia and hyperthyreosis. Blockade of β-adrenergic receptors inhibits the basal receptor activity and action of endogenous catecholamine and may explain part of the beneficial effects of β-blockers in both diseases.

Taken together, the regulation of time course and extent of receptor desensitization and tolerance development involves complex cellular processes. Detailed understanding of the molecular mechanisms of receptor inactivation may improve the chronic drug treatment of patients and may offer new targets of therapeutic interventions.

References

1. Grady EF, Bohm SK, Bunnett NW (1997) Turning off the signal: mechanisms that attenuate signaling by G protein-coupled receptors. Am J Physiol 273:G586–601

2. Pierce KL, Lefkowitz RJ (2001) Classical and new roles of β-arrestins in the regulation of G-protein-coupled receptors. Nat Rev Neurosci 2:727–733
3. Bohn LM, Gainetdinov RR, Lin FT, Lefkowitz RJ, Caron MG (2000) μ-opioid receptor desensitization by β-arrestin-2 determines morphine tolerance but not dependence. Nature 408:720–723
4. Tsao PI, von Zastrow M (2001) Diversity and specificity in the regulated endocytic membrane trafficking of G-protein-coupled receptors. Pharmacol Ther 89:139–147
5. Danner S, Lohse MJ (1999) Regulation of β-adrenergic receptor responsiveness modulation of receptor gene expression. Rev Physiol Biochem Pharmacol 136:183–223

Toll-like Receptors

Toll-like receptors are proteins present on cells of the immune system that recognize DNA of prokaryotic origin containing unmethylated CpG motifs. These receptors are part of a familiy of related receptors that mediate innate immunity against a variety of microbes. Activation of toll-like receptors leads to secretion of immunostimulatory cytokines, leading to an enhanced immune response biased to a cytotoxic T-cell response.

▶ Cytokines
▶ Immune Defense
▶ Genetic Vaccination
▶ Table appendix: Receptor Proteins

Tonic-clonic Convulsions

Tonic-clonic convulsions are abnormal motor behaviour during a ▶ seizure characterised by slow movements with high muscle tension (tonic phase) and subsequent repetitive oscillating movements of limbs (clonic phase).

▶ Antiepileptic Drugs

Topoisomerase

Topoisomerase enzymes control and modify the topologic states of DNA. The mechanisms of these enzymes involve DNA cleavage and strand passage through the break, followed by religation of the cleaved DNA. Two main forms of topoisomerase exist. The type I topoisomerase of mammals is a 100 kD monomeric protein whose actvity is ATP-independent. This enzyme binds to double-stranded DNA and cleaves one of the DNA strands of the duplex, simultaneously forming an enzyme-DNA covalent bond between a tyrosine residue and the 3'-phosphate of the cleaved DNA. The type II topoisomerases are dimeric enzymes, which are ATP-dependant. Two isoforms of topoisomerase II exist, topoisomerase α and β, with apparent molecular weights of 170 and 180 kD. Topoisomerase II cleaves the two complementary strands of DNA four base pairs apart and the resulting 5'-phosphoryl groups become covalently linked to a pair of tyrosine groups, one in each half of the dimeric topoisomerase II enzyme. Several groups of drugs are known that selectively inhibit topoisomerases in bacteria (quinolones) or mammalian cells (etoposide, tenoposide). Quinolones are used to treat bacterial infections; inhibitors of mammalian topoisomerases are cytostatic drugs used for the treatment of cancer.

▶ Quinolones

Torsade de Pointes

Torsade de pointes is a life-threating polymorphic ventricular tachycardia which occurs in inherited long QT syndrome and as a side effect of the action potential prolonging drugs.

▶ Antiarrhythmic Drugs

TPO

▶ Thyroid peroxidase

Trace Amines

Trace amines are a group of substances including tyramine, tryptamine and β-phenylethylamine, which are derived from the metabolism of amino acids and are present in many tissues of the body including the brain. They may function as neuromodulators although they are usually present at relatively low levels. It has recently been shown that trace amines act on G-protein-coupled receptors called TA1 or TA2. Trace amine receptors are also activated by amphetamines, including 3,4-methylenedioxymethamphetamine (MDMA, "ecstasy").

▶ Psychostimulants

TRAF

▶ TNF Receptor Associated Factors
▶ TNF Receptor Superfamily
▶ Table appendix: Receptor Proteins

Trafficking

Trafficking is controlled movement of a protein from one subcellular location to another.

Tranquilizers

Tranquilizers (also called antianxiety drugs) are used to treat a variety of psychiatric disorders which go along with anxiety (anxiety disorders).

Serotonin-reuptake inhibitors and the benzodiazepines are the most commonly employed drugs for the treatment of common clinical anxiety disorders.

▶ Benzodiazepines

Transcription

Transcription is the synthesis of RNA by RNA polymerases using DNA as a template. Transcription factors facilitate this process through the recruitment of the RNA polymerase complex to gene promoters.

Transcriptional Co-activators

Transcriptional co-activators form a bridge between transcription factors, such as NF-κB and AP-1 and general transcription factors (GTFs), and RNA polymerase II. They do not bind DNA themselves but enable the transduction of the regulatory signal (e.g. NF-κB) to the basal transcriptional complex, enabling initiation of gene transcription. There are two types of coactivators, ubiquitous or general coactivators and more specialised coactivators that are tissue-specifically expressed and/or specifically bind to certain transcription factors. Co-activators contain histone acetyltransferase activity.

Coactivators enhancing the transcriptional activity of steroid hormone receptors activators include SRC-1 (steroid-receptor co-activator 1) or TIF2 (transcriptional intermediary factor 2), which are recruited by the DNA/steroid hormone receptor complex. Their main role is to attract other transcriptional coactivators with histone acetyltransferase activity in order to decondense chromatin and allow for the binding of components of the general transcription apparatus.

▶ Glucocorticoids
▶ Sex Steroid Receptors
▶ Contraceptives

T

Transcription Factor

Transcritpion factor is a term loosely applied to any protein required to initiate or regulate transcription in eucaryotes through binding to defined DNA regions. It includes both gene-regulatory proteins and the general transcription factor.

- ▶ Nuclear Receptor
- ▶ JAK-STAT Pathway
- ▶ MAP Kinase Cascade
- ▶ Interferons

Transduction

Transduction is the introduction and expression of genes in a cell.

Transfection

Transfection is the introduction of DNA or RNA into eukaryotic cells *in vitro* and *in vivo*.

Transforming Growth Factor β

Transforming growth factor β (TGFβ) consists of two 110-140 amino βacid peptides and belongs to a large family of cytokines. The spectrum of functions of TGF ranges from control of cell proliferation and differentiation, production of extracellular matrix components, chemotaxis and immunosuppression to regulation of cell death.

- ▶ Neurotrophic Factors

Transforming Oncogenes

The growth of tumours can be regarded as the result of an accumulation of genetic changes in a wide variety of genes, the incorrect activation of oncogenes and the loss of function of tumour suppressor genes. Oncogenes are defined on the basis of their gain of function. The number of oncogenes isolated since about the end of the 1970s has grown to over 250.

- ▶ Antisense Oligonucleotides

Transgene

A transgene is an additional extra gene which is introduced into the germline of an animal.

- ▶ Transgenic Animal Models

Transgenic Animal Models

UWE RUDOLPH
Institute of Pharmacology and Toxicology, University of Zurich, Zurich, Switzerland
rudolph@pharma.unizh.ch

Definition

Transgenic animals are genetically engineered animals which allow the functional assessment of specific genes or proteins in health and disease.

Description

It is a major goal in biomedical research to identify control elements that regulate complex physiological functions such as regulation of blood pressure or behaviour. These molecular control elements are of interest since they represent potential therapeutic targets for various disease states. Three different strategies have been employed to assess gene functions in terms of providing the determinants for a particular phenotype: a) Analysis of naturally occuring mutations in humans and animals, b) random chemical mutagenesis with subsequent screening for phenotypes and c) the generation of transgenic and targeted mutant animals, which are the subject of this contribution. In these approaches, an additional gene ("▶ transgene") is transferred to an animal or an inherent gene is mutated in order to assess the respective phenotypes. For the purpose of clarity, a clear distinction between "transgenic" (i.e. non-targeted) and "targeted mutant" animals is made here, although many scientists use the term "trangenic" in a broader sense to encompass all genetically engineered animals.

Generation of Transgenic Animals
Transgenic animals express a foreign gene, the "transgene", which is typically introduced into the mouse germline by microinjection of DNA into fertilized eggs. This technique is applicable to mice, rats and other species. The DNA will be integrated at random, frequently as concatamers. The tissue distribution and the level of expression vary between mouse lines depending on integration sites and copy number, even when the same DNA was used for injection. Transgenic mice may constitutively and tissue-specifically overexpress the transgene, or may carry gain-of-function mutations in the transgene. Alternatively, they may also contain dominant negative mutations, ribozyme or antisense constructs. Thus, both gain-of-function and loss-of-function approaches can be pursued with transgenes.

Generation of Targeted Mutant Animals
For the ▶ targeted mutant approach, targeting vectors are constructed that contain DNA sequences derived from the gene to be targeted. They are specifically integrated at the desired genomic location by homologous recombination in murine embryonic stem cells. These cells are then injected into ▶ blastocysts, which in turn are reimplanted into pseudopregnant foster mothers. The embryonic stem cells contribute to the developing embryo, which may carry the mutation in its germ line. This technique is currrently available only for mice. The target gene may be disrupted by introduction of a neomycin resistance cassette or by deletion of one or more, or even all, exons (classical or global ▶ knockouts). Since regulatory elements in the neomycin resistance cassette may affect the expression of neighbouring genes, it is advisable to eliminate this cassette e.g. by cre/loxP-mediated recombination. Knockout mutations may also be studied in the heterozygous state to assess potential gene dosage effects (1). The phenotypic consequences of the knockout mutation are expected to provide information on the normal function of the respective gene in wild type animals. Targeted mutagenesis is not limited to gene knockouts. Virtually any desired subtle mutation, e.g. a point mutation, or replacement of a gene with another gene, can be introduced into the mouse germline in this way ("knock-in"). The potential advantage of introducing a point mutation using a "knock-in" approach compared to a transgenic approach is that with a gene-targeted point mutation the gene harboring the mutation is expressed under the control of the endogenous promoter. In contrast, in transgenic aproaches the expression level and epression pattern may be different, making it more difficult to interpret a potential phenotype. In general, targeted point mutations permit more precise modelling of many human disease mutations.

Tissue-specific and Inducible Transgenes
The expression of transgenes in time and space is dependent on the promoter used in the transgene construct and the site of DNA integration. Many transgenes are expressed constitutively, which may perturb development and even cause lethality. To avoid these problems, transgenes may be expressed in an inducible fashion. Mice carrying an inducible transgene grow up normally. The acute effect of transgene expression can then be reversibly induced in adult animals. The same animal may be studied before and after the expression of the transgene and thus serve as its own control, e.g. in behavioural studies. Several systems have been developed to achieve inducible expression, of which the tet system appears to be the most widely used (Fig. 1). The reverse tetracycline-controlled transactivator (rtTA) consists of a rtTA fusion protein composed of the mutant version of the Tn10 tetracycline-resistance operon of *E. coli* and a C-terminal portion of protein 16 of herpes simplex virus, which functions as a strong

T

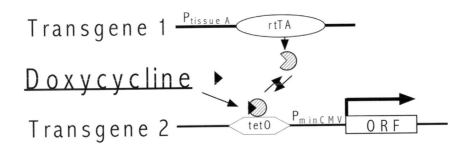

Fig. 1 Tissue-specific inducible transgene expression using the rtTA system. To achieve an inducible tissue-specific expression of a transgene, a mouse carrying two transgenes may be generated: Transgene 1 codes for rtTA, driven by a promoter expressed in tissue A ($P_{tissue\ A}$). Transgene 2 contains the open reading frame (ORF) of the gene that is to be expressed inducibly, preceded by a CMV minimal promoter (P_{minCMV}) and a tet operator (tetO). Only when doxycycline is present rtTA binds to tetO and the open reading frame (ORF) of interest is be expressed in tissue A.

transcriptional activator. The rtTA is placed under the contol of a tissue-specific promoter. Only in the presence of doxycycline, rtTA binds to the tetO that is placed on a separate construct and activates transcription from a minimal CMV promoter, which itself is inactive. This minimal promoter drives the expression of the desired gene. In summary, when doxycycline is added to the drinking water, the transgene is expressed in a tissue-specific fashion. Conversely, it is also possible to shut down the expression of a transgene using the tetracycline-controlled transactivator (tTA) system (2). A refined system by which two genes can be simultaneously regulated in opposite directions is provided by a recent extension of this strategy (3). More recently, a *lac* repressor transgene was developed that resembles a typical mammalian gene both in codon usage and structure and expresses functional levels of repressor in the mouse. This repressor was used to regulate the expression of a mammalian reporter gene containing *lac* operator sequences. The *lac* repressor can repress the activity of a reporter gene, which subsequently can be derepressed by the lactose analog IPTG (4).

Tissue-specific and Inducible Knockouts

Classical global knockouts may have a developmental or lethal phenotype and thus preclude the analysis of the phenotypic consequences of the lack of a gene in specific tissues in adult animals. With the development of the ▶ cre/loxP and ▶ flp/FRT systems it has become possible to excise defined DNA fragments from the genome of specified cells. Cre and Flp are bacterial and yeast recombinases, respectively, which recognize loxP and FRT sequences, respectively. The most common application is where the DNA fragment to be deleted is flanked by two parallel loxP or FRT sites. Expression of cre or flp, respectively, then leads to the excision or loss of the flanked fragment. This expression can be achieved in cell culture or in mice. In order to get rid of the neomycin resistance marker, this marker may be flanked by two FRT sites. Flp expression in embryronic stem cell culture or in mice expressing an appropoate flp transgene will eliminate the neo marker. In a typical example, essential exons of a gene are flanked by loxP sites ("floxed") (Fig. 2). These loxP sites most likely do not have a functional activity on their own, so that the "floxed" mice can be considered functional wild type mice (which however may have to be confirmed in each case). Crossing the "floxed" mouse with a transgenic mouse carrying a *cre* transgene that is expressed in tissue A will result in some mice carrying both the targeted "floxed" allele and the *cre* transgene. Only in tissue A will the *cre* transgene be expressed and the

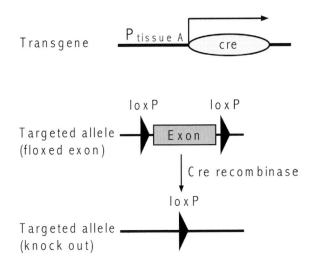

Fig. 2 Tissue-specific knockout using the cre/loxP system. To achieve a tissue-specific knockout, mice carrying a cre transgene ("Transgene") and a targeted allele characterized by a "floxed" exon in the gene of interest are generated. In this example, the cre transgene is expressed under the control of a promoter that is expressed in tissue A ($P_{tissue\ A}$). The Cre protein is synthesized in tissue A, recognizes the two parallel loxP sites and excises the exon that is flanked by the two loxP sites. If the floxed and later deleted exon is essential for gene function, the mouse will display a tissue-specific gene knockout.

exons flanked by loxP will be removed. In all other tissues, the loxP-fllanked DNA fragment will be retained.

One major problem with this strategy is that the cre expression has to be strong enough and highly tissue- or even cell type-specific. Many *cre* transgenes currently in use have been constructed as standard transgenes using promoter elements of limited size via pronucleus injection, with the expression level and pattern being dependent on the integration site. Frequently, these transgenes lack the specificity of cre expression that would be expected from the respective promoter that was used; in other words, the expression pattern of the *cre* transgene frequently does not match the expression pattern of the endogenous gene from which the promoter was isolated. It may be preferable to "knock-in" the *cre*-cDNA into the gene whose expression pattern one wants to replicate; potential disadvantages of this approach are that

the cre expression via the endogenous promoter may be too weak for complete excision of flanked sequences and that this approach is experimentally the most time-consuming one. An alternative approach to achieve cre expression from endogenous promoters utilizes bacterial artificial chromosomes (▶ BACs). BACs contain e.g. 150 kb–200 kb genomic DNA fragments. BAC libraries spotted on nylon membranes are commercially available. Clones hybridizing to a probe of interest can then be purchased individually. Positive clones are mapped to determine the approximate position of the gene of intererst in the BAC. A BAC can then be selected that contains the gene of interest roughly in the center and contains >50 kb of upstream sequence. Via homologous recombination in *E. coli* the *cre* cDNA can be introduced into the ATG start codon of the respective gene of interest. The BAC is then injected into a fertilized mouse egg and frequently integrated as a single copy. The integrity of the BAC ends can be confirmed e.g. by polymerase chain reaction. Though the integration occurs at a random position in the genome, it is hoped that the BAC contains all regulatory elements of the gene of interest (5). In contrast to the "knock-in" approach, the BAC transgene typically does not change the function of endogenous genes. Other genes present in the BAC may be overexpressed. The BAC approach has the advantage that it is usually much less time-consuming than the "knock-in" approach.

Transgenic and Knockout Mice in Functional Genomics Approaches

The linking of genomic sequence information to biological function is of major relevance for the identifcation of novel drug targets. Instead of analyzing the function of one gene at a time, entire sets of genes can be analyzed by multiplexing genes using "*in vivo* libraries". In this approach, overlapping yeast artificial chromosomes ("▶ YACs") covering a specific chromosomal region, which has been implicated in a specific biological function, are introduced into the mouse germline. The resulting mouse lines will be analyzed with respect to the phenotype in question, which has to be sensitive to gene dosage. The presence or absence of the phenotype in various mouse lines permits functional mapping of the gene of interest. In another approach, cDNAs of unknown function can be overexpressed in mice. However, a gene inactivation approach may frequently reveal more about the normal function of genes than the overexpression of cDNAs.

ES Cell Libraries

Both in the private and the public sector projects are ongoing in which random mutations are generated in murine embryonic stem cells on a large scale (ES cell libraries). Tagged and presumably inactivated genes are easily identified by sequencing. These stem cells can be used to generate the respective knockout mice.

Pharmacological Relevance

Transgenic and gene targeted animals have a significant impact in providing fundamental insights into biological systems and their pharmacological regulation. They provide valuable information relevant for target discovery and validation, e.g. by clarifying the functional roles of potential drug targets or by generating animal models for human diseases that allow testing potential therapeutic strategies. Genetically modified animals may also be useful for the development of novel assays for toxicolagal testing. Tissue-specific and inducible gene expression greatly increases the selectivity with which these analyses can be performed.

References

1. Crestani F, Lorez M, Baer K, Essrich C, Benke D, Laurent JP, Belzung C, Fritschy J-M, Lüscher B, Mohler H (1999) Decreased GABAA-receptor clustering results in enhanced anxiety and a bias for threat cues. Nat Neurosci 2:833–839
2. Kistner A, Gossen M, Zimmermann F, Jerecic J, Ullmer C, Lübbert H, Bujard H (1996) Doxycycline-mediated quantitative and tissue-specific control of gene expression in transgenic mice. Proc Natl Acad Sci USA 93:10933–10938
3. Baron U, Schappinger D, Helbl V, Gossen M, Hillen W, Bujard H (1999) Generation of conditional mutants in higher eukaryotes by switching between the expression of two genes. Proc Natl Acad Sci USA 96:1013–1018
4. Cronin CA, Gluba W, Scrable H (2001) The lac operator-repressor system is functional in the mouse. Genes Dev 15:1506–1517
5. Heintz N (2001) Bac to the future: The use of BAC transgenic mice for neuroscience research. Nat Rev Neurosci 2:861–870

Transient Receptor Potential

The founding member of the TRP channel family, TRP, was identified as the product of a gene locus, which was referred to a *transient receptor potential* (*trp*), because *trp* mutant flies display a defect in light induced Ca^{2+} influx .

▶ TRP Channels

Transition State

A transition state is an unstable, high-energy configuration assumed by reactants in a chemical reaction on the way to making products. Enzymes can lower the activation energy required for a reaction by binding and stabilizing the transition state of the substrate.

Translocon

A translocon is a multi-functional protein complex in the endoplasmic reticulum (ER) membrane. It translocates secretory proteins across and integrates membrane proteins into the ER membrane. The protein conducting channel protein Sec61p is the most important component of the translocon.

▶ Protein Trafficking and Quality Control

Transmembrane Domain

A transmembrane domain is a region of an integral membrane protein that is usually thought to form alpha helices and spans the lipid bilayer. A protein can have several transmembrane domains.

▶ G-Protein-coupled Receptors
▶ Somatostatin

Transmembrane Signalling

GÜNTER SCHULTZ
Institut für Pharmakologie,
Freie Universität Berlin, Berlin, Germany
gschultz@zedat.fu-berlin.de

Synonym

Membrane signal transduction

Definition

Cellular functions are controlled by extracellular signals such as hormones, neurotransmitters, odorants, light and other chemical or physical stimuli. Only a few of these signal molecules, e.g. the highly lipid-soluble steroid and thyroid hormones, permeate the plasma membrane to interact with their intracellular receptors. Most regulatory factors are water-soluble, interact with membrane receptors and induce a signal transduction process that leads to the formation of intracellular signals and to the stimulation of signalling cascades that result in the cellular reaction to the stimulus.

▶ Adenylyl Cyclases
▶ G-protein-coupled Receptors
▶ Guanylyl Cyclase
▶ Phospholipases
▶ Tolerance and Desensitization

Basic Mechanisms

Transmembrane signalling processes involve the recognition and reversible binding of an extracellular signal by an integral membrane receptor protein and the generation of intracellular signals by one or more ▶ effector protein. Receptor and effector can be domains on one and the same transmembrane protein or can be located on separate protein entities. On the basis of different molecular interactions of the signal-receiving receptor to the signal-generating effector protein (or effector domain), receptors can be divided into several groups (Figure).

Receptor Classification

Receptors Permanently Linked to an Effector. Receptors permanently linked to an effector consist of proteins with an extracellular ligand-binding receptor domain and a signal-generating effector domain. Most of these receptors are constituted by two to five structurally related or identical subunits. Effectors can be enzymes or ion channels whose activities are stimulated by agonist binding without significant delay.

1) Enzyme-linked receptors possess an extracellular domain with receptor function and another intracellular one possessing catalytic activity. Receptors can be linked to tyrosine kinases (like the receptors for growth factors, acting through the Ras-Raf-MEK-ERK pathway, and the insulin receptor), to phosphotyrosine phosphatases (e.g. CD45), to serine/threonine kinases (like the transforming growth factor receptor β, activin and inhibin receptors, acting via Smads) or to guanylyl cyclases (e.g. the receptors for natriuretic factors and guanylin). Some of these enzyme-linked receptors form homodimers, e.g. the receptor-tyrosine-kinases and the guanylyl cyclases.

2) Ligand-gated ion channels consist of several similar subunits that together form an extracellular ligand-binding domain and a pore acting as the regulated effector. The nicotinic acetylcholine receptors and the 5-HT$_3$ serotonin receptors (both consisting of five structurally related subunits with four transmembrane domains each), ionotropic glutamate receptors (consisting of four structurally related subunits

T

with three transmembrane domains each) and the P2X purinergic receptors (consisting of three subunits with two transmembrane domains each) are members of this family; they are connected to a cation channel. On the other hand, $GABA_A$ receptors and glycine receptors (consisting of five structurally related subunits with four transmembrane domains each, similar to the nicotinic acetylcholine and the $5\text{-}HT_3$ serotonin receptors) are members that are connected to anion channels.

Receptors Associated with an Effector System. Receptors associated with an effector system consist of two or more protein components. Two groups can be differentiated.

1) G-protein-coupled receptors (GPCRs, seven-transmembrane, 7TM or heptahelical receptors) that interact with regulatory heterotrimeric G proteins and regulate a variety of signal-generating enzymes and ion channels. These receptors represent the largest protein family. For about 200 of them the ligands are known, another 200 are orphan receptors with unknown ligands, and about 900 are olfactory receptors (but two thirds of the human olfactory receptor genes are pseudogenes). Activated GPCRs interact with membrane-attached G proteins, consisting of one α-, β- and γ-subunit each. The β- and γ-subunits form a functional complex ($G\beta\gamma$) that is released from the GTP-bound α-subunit within the receptor-mediated activation process. $G\alpha_{GTP}$ and free $G\beta\gamma$ regulate the activity of effector proteins such as enzymes (e.g. adenylyl cyclases, phospholipases $C\beta$, phosphatidylinositol 3-kinases and, in the retina, the cGMP phosphodiesterase type 6) and ion channels (e.g. voltage-gated calcium channels and inwardly rectifying potassium channels). G proteins are subdivided into four G-protein subfamilies according to structural similarities of their α-subunits. The G_s subfamily (including G_s and G_{olf} proteins) is involved in adenylyl cyclase stimulation, whereas the activated $G\alpha$- and $G\beta\gamma$-subunits of the $G_{i/o}$ subfamily (including three G_i isoforms, G_o, G_z, transducin and gustducin) mediate adenylyl cyclase inhibition (G_i), cGMP phosphodiesterase type 6 stimulation (transducin), calcium channel inhibition ($G\beta\gamma$ from G_o) and potassium

channel stimulation ($G_{\beta\gamma}$ from G_i). Beside $G\beta\gamma$, the various members of the G_q subfamily (largely G_q and G_{11}, but in some cellular systems also G_{14} and $G_{15/16}$) by their activated α-subunits cause activation of phospholipase $C\beta$ isoforms, thereby inducing a ▸ PI response. The α-subunits of the G_{12} subfamily, consisting of G_{12} and G_{13}, can stimulate guanine nucleotide exchange factors (GEFs) of Rho, thereby leading to activation of Rho and Rho-kinase (ROCK). This results in myosin phosphatase phosphorylation and inactivation with increased myosin light chain phosphorylation, cytoskeletal changes and contraction, e.g. of vascular smooth muscle. Most GPCRs interact with and activate more than one G protein subfamily, e.g. with G_s plus $G_{q/11}$ (histamine H_2, parathyroid hormone and calcitonin receptors), G_s plus G_i (luteinising hormone receptor, β2-adrenoceptor) or Gq/11 plus G12/13 (thromboxane A_2, angiotensin AT_1, endothelin ETA receptors). Some receptors show even broader G-protein coupling, e.g. to Gi, $G_{q/11}$ plus $G_{12/13}$ (protease-activated receptors, lysophosphatidate and sphingosine-1-phosphate receptors) or even to all four G-protein subfamilies (thyrotropin receptor). This multiple coupling results in multiple signalling via different pathways and in a concerted reaction of the cell to the stimulus.

2) Cytokine receptors (including those of various interleukins, prolactin, growth hormone and erythropoietin) are homo- or heterodimers that after ligand binding activate receptor-associated tyrosine kinases (JAKs) which phosphorylate transcription factors (STATs).

Cell Adhesion Molecules. ▸ Cell adhesion molecules (such as integrines, cadherins and selectins) do not only act as transmembrane proteins involved in cell-cell or cell-matrix interactions but are also involved in signal transduction processes. Integrins even mediate inside-out signalling.

Low Density Lipoprotein (LDL) Receptors and Transferrin Receptors. Low density lipoprotein (LDL) receptors and transferrin receptors are transmembrane proteins that are involved in the transmembrane transport of the ligands they bind rather than in signal transduction processes.

Receptors permanently linked to effectors

ligand-gated ion channels

enzyme-linked receptors

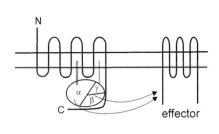

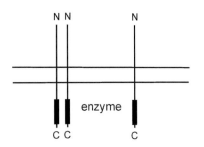

Receptors associated with effectors

Cell adhesion proteins

G-protein-coupled receptors

cytokin receptors

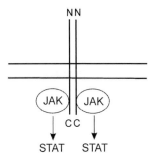

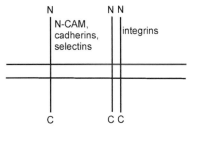

Fig. 1 Membrane topology of different groups of membrane receptors. Shown are single subunits of ligand-gated ion channels, which are actually composed of three, four or five structurally related subunits. For other receptors, the occurrence of homo- or heterodimers is indicated. α, β and γ stand for G-protein α-, β- and γ-subunits, respectively.

Whereas transmembrane topologies of most receptors have been well established, the three-dimensional structures of almost all receptors are unknown. The first resolved 3D structure of a GPCRs was that of rhodopsin. It is assumed that most transmembrane parts of receptors have α-helical structures; β-sheet transmembrane structures have only been reported for some transmembrane segments of ligand-operated ion channels.

Quantitative and Temporal Aspects

The number of receptor molecules is generally restricted to a few thousands per cell, and ligands are in most cases bound with nano- to micromolar affinities. The effectors coupled to a receptor, independently of being an enzyme or ion channel, act catalytically, causing the generation of many more intracellular signal molecules than those involved in transmembrane signal transduction. Therefore, the relative number of such effector proteins can be much smaller than that of receptors. On the other hand, G proteins occur at much higher abundances than receptors and effectors ($G_{i/o}$ proteins are generally found > G_s /$G_{q/11}$ > $G_{12/13}$).

The ligand-induced signal transduction process mediated by a ligand-operated ion channel, e.g. by the nicotinic receptor in muscle, results in an almost immediate (msec) cellular response as the number of components is very small and almost no enzymatic step is involved. In comparison, the onset of cellular reactions to ligands interacting with GPCRs and inducing the formation of intracellular signals that stimulate protein phosphorylation is slower (sec). Cellular responses induced by growth factors or cytokines acting via phosphorylation cascades on transcription factors take much longer.

Transmembrane signalling by one type of receptor, e.g. GPCR/G-protein signalling, affects signalling pathways used primarily by other receptor types, e.g. the Ras-Raf-MEK-ERK pathway controlled by receptor-tyrosine kinases. This means that the signalling typically induced by a given receptor cannot be seen as an event separate from other regulations but has to be considered as part of a signalling network within the cell.

Pharmacological Intervention

The naturally occurring as well as many synthetic ligands of membrane receptors, i.e. hormones, neurotransmitters, growth factors and cytokines, act as ▶ agonists, i.e. upon binding they induce the generation of intracellular signals leading to a cellular response. Partial agonists are compounds with less than the full intrinsic activity of an agonist but more intrinsic activity than that of an antagonist (they act as partial antagonists when applied in the presence of a full agonist). For receptors coupling to more than one G protein, the development of pathway-selective agonists may become possible. Antagonists that act as blockers of the effects of agonist have been developed as drugs.

The pharmaceutical industry has developed drugs that act as ▶ inverse agonists, i.e. these compounds through the same receptor cause opposite cellular reactions. Agonists are supposed to shift the equilibrium between the inactive and active (effector-coupled) forms towards the latter one, inverse agonists do the opposite; they can be used to silence a constitutively active receptor. Histamine H_2, H_3 and H_4 receptors are examples of receptors with high constitutive activity, and H_2 blockers such as cimetidine and ranitidine actually are powerful inverse agonists. Similarly, naloxone acts as an inverse agonist at δ-opiate receptors.

Most hormones and neurotransmitters act via more than one ▶ receptor subtype. Subtypes that are products of different genes can show differences in agonist and antagonist binding, a property that can be used for cell- or tissue-specific action. In addition, receptor subtypes often act on different effectors. The pharmaceutical industry has developed numerous compounds discriminating between receptor subtypes, thus providing higher selectivity for certain receptors than the naturally occurring agonists. Among receptor subtypes, the occurrence of ▶ ionotropic receptors (linked to ligand-gated ion channels) in parallel to the existence of ▶ metabotropic receptors (i.e. G-protein-coupled receptors) for the same neurotransmitters is most striking, i.e. nicotinic versus muscarinic acetylcholine receptors, 5-HT$_3$ versus the other serotonin receptors, GABA$_A$ versus GABA$_B$ receptors and P2X versus P2Y purinergic receptors.

▶ Organic Cation Transporters
▶ Vesicular Transporters

References

1. U. Gether (2000) Uncovering molecular mechanisms involved in activation of G protein-coupled receptors. Endocrin. Rev. 21:90–113
2. E. J. M. Helmreich (2001) The biochemistry of cell signalling. Oxford University Press, Oxford, New York.
3. T. Kenakin (2001) Inverse, protean, and ligand-selective agonism: matters of receptor conformation. FASEB J. 15:598–611
4. Palczewski K, Kumasaka T, Hori T, Behnke CA, Motoshima H, Fox BA, Le Trong I, Teller DC, Okada T, Stenkamp RE, Yamamoto M, Miyano M. (2000) Crystal structure of rhodopsin: A G protein-coupled receptor. Science 289:739–745
5. T. Schöneberg, A. Schulz, T. Gudermann (2002) The structural basis of G-protein-coupled receptor function and dysfunction in human diseases. Rev. Physiol. Biochem. Pharmacol. 144:143–227

Transport ATPase

▶ Table appendix: Membrane Transport Proteins

Transporter

▶ Table appendix: Membrane Transport Proteins

Transposon

Transposons are mobile DNA elements (sizes around 2.5 to 23 kb pairs) that move from one place to another in the chromosome or on to extrachromosomal genetic elements within the same cell. They are flanked by inverted repeats at their ends and encode among other proteins a transposase that is needed for the transposition process. Resistance genes in the transposon are often parts of integrons. These are structures that carry an integrase responsible for the insertion of the resistance gene cassettes into the integron.

▶ Microbial Resistance to Drugs

Trichomonas Vaginalis

Trichomonas vaginalis is a ubiquitous sexually transmitted anaerobic flagellate causing vaginitis in women and prostate gland infection in men.

▶ Antiprotozoal Drugs

Tricyclic Antidepressants

Tricyclic antodepressants are an important group of antidepressants. They block the uptake of monoamines by nerve terminals by competing for the binding site of the reuptake carrier protein.

▶ Antidepressant Drugs

Triglycerides

Triglycerides are composed of three fatty acids attached to a skeleton of glycerol. Most of the fat eaten by humans is triglyceride. Triglycerides are also produced by the liver and circulate in very-low-density-lipoproteins (VLDL).

▶ HMG-CoA-reductase Inhibitors

Triiodothyronine

Triiodothyronine (3',5,3-L-triiodothyronine, T_3) is a thyroid hormone. It is produced by outer ring deiodination of thyroxine (T_4) in peripheral tissues. The biologic activity of T_3 is three to eight times higher than that of T_4. T_3 is 99.7 % protein-bound and is effective in its free non-protein-bound form. The half-life of triiodothyronine is about 19 hours. The daily turnover of T_3 is 75 %. Triiodothyronine acts *via* nuclear receptor binding with subsequent induction of protein synthesis. Effects of thyroid hormones are apparent in almost all organ systems. They include effects on the basal metabolic rate and the metabolisms of proteins, lipids and carbohydrates.

▶ Antithyroid Drugs

Trimodal Distribution

A trimodal distribution is a frequency distribution of a certain phenotype with three peaks separated by two antinodes.

▶ Pharmacogenetics

T

Trophoblast

The trophoblast is the external layer of the embryonic blastocyst - a stage during early embryo development - containing a group of large secretory cells that establish contact with the uterine mucosa.

▶ Interferons

Tropism

A viral tropism is the specifity of a virus for particular host tissues and cells.

▶ Gene Therapy

TRP Channels

VEIT FLOCKERZI
Universität des Saarlandes, Homburg, Germany
veit.flockerzi@uniklinik-saarland.de

Definition

A superfamily of cation channels conserved in mammals, flies, worms and yeast. The various TRP-proteins bear sequence and predicted structural similarities to the founding member of this superfamily, ▶ transient receptor potential (TRP), a light activated cation channel in the *Drosophila* photoreceptor.

▶ Table appendix: Membrane Transport Proteins
▶ Non-selective Cation Channels
▶ Voltage-dependent Ca^{2+} Channels

Basic Characteristics

So far, more than twenty TRP genes have been identified in mammals (1,2). Almost all TRPs are supposed to form ion channels that are widely

Tab. 1 The Superfamily of Mammalian TRP Channels

TRPC subfamily	TRPV subfamily	TRPM subfamily
TRPC1	TRPV1	TRPM1
TRPC2	TRPV2	TRPM2
TRPC3	TRPV3	TRPM3
TRPC4	TRPV4	TRPM4
TRPC5	TRPV5	TRPM5
TRPC6	TRPV6	TRPM6
TRPC7		TRPM7
		TRPM8

expressed in the nervous system, and which may be the primary site of Ca^{2+} entry in non-excitable cells. A TRP protein contains six segments, predicted to cross the cell membrane, and a putative pore loop within the extracellular linker separating the fifth and sixth transmembrane segments (Fig. 1, top left), but lacks the voltage-sensing element (S4) present in voltage-gated channels. Almost all TRPs are activated by as yet unclear mechanisms (see below) involving phopholipase C (PLC) and phosphatidylinositol pathways. Four or five TRP proteins form homooligomeric and heterooligomeric channels (Fig. 1, top right) and evidence is steadily emerging that these channels are integrated into signal transduction complexes by ▶ scaffolding proteins. Based on their structural similarities the TRP proteins fall into three subfamilies of channels, TRPC, TRPV and TRPM (Table 1). Two additional subfamilies, TRPP and TRPML, which are more distantly related to TRP, include ▶ PKD2 and ▶ mucolipin.

Ion Channel Properties

Essential molecular determinants of ion permeation through TRP channels should reside within a protein domain, which participates in the formation of the ion permeable pathway of the channel. This domain is therefore called the pore loop. So far this region has only been characterized for TRP channels formed by members of the TRPV group. Here, ▶ TRPV1, TRPV2, TRPV3 and ▶ TRPV4 channels do only poorly discriminate

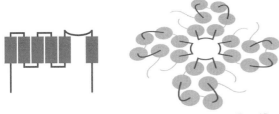

	P_{Ca}/P_{Na}
TRPV 1 YNSLYSTCLELFKFTIG *M* GDLEFT	<10
TRPV 2 YRGILEASLELFKFTIG *M* GELAFQ	<10
TRPV 3 YGSFSDAVLELFKLTIG *L* GDLNIQ	<10
TRPV 4 SETFSAFLLDLFKLTIG *M* GDLEML	<10
TRPV 5 YPTALFSTFELF-LTII **D** GPANYS	>100
TRPV 6 YPMALFSTFELF-LTII **D** GPANYD	>100

Fig. 1 TRP Protein Topology and Pore Loops of the Members of the TRPV Subfamily. Top, left: TRP proteins comprise six predicted transmembrane segments linked by extracellular and cytosolic protein domains. The pore loop resides within the extracellular linker separating the fifth and sixth transmembrane segments. **Top, right: View perpendicular to the surface of the plasma membrane.** Four TRP proteins assemble to form an ion channel. The four pore loops line the ion permeant pathway. Circles represent transmembrane segments. **Bottom: Amino acid sequence alignment of the pore loops of the members of the TRPV subfamily.** The D shown in bold represents the negatively charged aspartic acid residue responsible for the high Ca^{2+} selectivity of channels formed by TRPV5 and, presumably, TRPV6. P_{Ca} and P_{Na}, relative permeability to Ca^{2+} (P_{Ca}) and to Na^+ (P_{Na}).

between monovalent and divalent cations, especially Na^+ and Ca^{2+}, and accordingly, are called "non-selective" cation channels. In contrast, ▶ TRPV5 and ▶ TRPV6 form highly selective Ca^{2+}-channels. Thus the relative permeability to Ca^{2+} (P_{Ca}) is more than 100-fold higher than to Na^+ (P_{Na}) in these two channels. A single negatively charged aspartic acid residue (D, shown in bold in Fig. 1 bottom) in the pore loop of TRPV5, which is conserved in TRPV6, but not in the other members of the TRPV subfamily, has been shown to be responsible for the high Ca^{2+} selectivity of channels formed by TRPV5 (3).

For all other members of the TRP family it still has to be shown whether the presumptive pore loop or other protein domains actually line the ion conducting pathway of the channel. Based on the results showing that expression of most TRPC channels yields currents carried by Na^+ and Ca^{2+}, and that expression of ▶ TRPM4 and ▶ TRPM7 channels yields currents carried by Na^+ but not by Ca^{2+} (TRPM4) or even currents carried by Mg^{2+} or Ca^{2+} (TRPM7), it seems likely that the pore structures of these channel proteins vary considerably.

Modes of Activation

TRP channels vary significantly in their modes of activation (4). Given that *Drosophila* TRP requires PLC for activity *in vivo*, mammalian TRPs were predicted to be PLC-dependent ion channels. Activation of PLC could be coupled to TRP channel activation via relief of phosphatidylinositol-4,5-bisphosphate (PIP_2)-mediated channel repression and/or production of inositol-1,4,5-trisphosphate (IP_3) and diacylglycerol (DAG). According to one mechanism, referred to as ▶ store-operated Ca^{2+} entry, transient IP_3 induced release of Ca^{2+} from intracellular stores induces sustained Ca^{2+} influx by activation of a plasma membrane Ca^{2+} entry channel. Leading contenders for channels activated by the latter mechanism are TRPC1, TRPC3, TRPC4 and TRPC5, although none of the published reports have unequivocal evidence for such a mechanism. In addition, members of the TRPC subfamily could be activated by diacylglycerol (TRPC3, TRPC6), by direct interaction with the IP_3 receptor (TRPC3), and – like TRPV1 and TRPM7 – by relief of (PIP_2)-mediated repression of the channel, to mention a few.

Members of the TRPV subfamily are activated by a broad range of stimuli including heat (TRPV1, TRPV2, TRPV3 and TRPV4), ligands such as ▶ capsaicin (TRPV1) and ▶ endocannabinoids (TRPV1, TRPV4, see below), osmolarity and cell volume (TRPV4), hydrolysis of PIP_2 and protons (TRPV1). Sofar, TRPV5 and TRPV6 channels are unique in that they represent the only highly Ca^{2+} selective channels within the TRP superfamily (see above) and are activated by low intracellular Ca^{2+}.

Three TRPM proteins, ▶ TRPM2, TRPM6 and TRPM7, are distinguished from other TRPs and other known ion channels, in that they consist of enzyme domains linked to the C termini of the ion channel domains resulting in "Chanzymes".

TRPM6 and TRPM7 encode TRP proteins linked to functional atypical protein kinases; however, at least TRPM7 channel activity does not require the kinase domain for activation (5). Currents through channels formed by TRPM6, TRPM5, TRPM1 and TRPM3 have not been identified electrophysiologically so far. Currents through TRPM2 channels are activated by ADP-ribose and changes in the redox status within the cell. TRPM4 is a Ca^{2+}-activated channel (EC_{50}~0.3 to 0.4 μM), non-permeant for Ca^{2+}, whereas ▶ TRPM8 can be activated by a drop in temperature below 26°C or by agents, such as menthol and icilin, that evoke a cool sensation.

Pharmacology

A clear limitation of studies on TRP channels is the lack of specific channel blockers. Organic compounds (e.g. ruthenium red, econazole, miconazole, SK&F96365) and anorganic blockers (e.g. La^{3+}, Gd^{3+}) have generally found to be of insufficient potency and specificity. The few exceptions include compounds such as capsaicin (EC_{50}~0.7 μM) and ▶ resiniferatoxin (EC_{50}~0.04 μM) as activators and capsazepine (IC_{50}~0.3 μM) as blockers of the TRPV1 currents, the endogenous cannabinoid receptor agonist anandamide ($EC_{50} \geq 4.9$ μM) and related endocannabinoids as activators of TRPV1 and TRPV4 currents and 4α-PDD, a phorbol derivative, as activator of TRPV4 currents (EC_{50}~0.2 μM).

Biological Relevance and Emerging Roles for Mammalian TRP Channels

Most of the TRP channels have only been characterized in recombinant systems but not as functional channels in a physiological context; still others have not even been characterized as functional channels. Firm data on their biological relevance will emerge basically by the combination of three routes: 1. By the development and identification of toxins and agents that can be used to specifically block currents through a given TRP channel in primary cells and tissues (see above "Pharmacology"). 2. By linking diseases to mutations in TRP genes; e.g. familial hypomagnesemia with secondary hypocalcemia is caused by mutations in TRPM6, implicating a role for TRPM6 in renal Mg^{2+} uptake. Other examples are mucolipidosis type IV, a neurodegenerative disease caused by disruption of the mucolipin gene, a TRP of the TRPML subfamily, and common causes of polycystic kidney disease are mutations within PKD2, a TRP of the TRPP subfamily. 3. By transgenic mice with targeted disruption of single TRP genes or a combination of TRP genes; so far three TRP-deficient mice have been described that underline the biological roles of TRPC2, TRPC4 and TRPV1 in social and sexual behaviour (TRPC2), vasorelaxation and microvascular endothelial permeability (TRPC4) as well as nociception and thermal hyperalgesia (TRPV1). There are suggestions that a number of TRP-related proteins may also have roles in growth control, and changes in the expression of these channels may contribute to certain forms of cancer. A decrease in expression of TRPM1 appears to be a prognostic marker for metastasis in patients with localized malignant melanoma. Alterations of TRPM5 may be associated with Beckwith-Wiedemann syndrome, a predisposition to a variety of neoplasms, whereas expression of TRPM8 and TRPV6 appears to be upregulated in prostate cancers; these two TRPs may represent prognostic markers for prostate cancer and targets for new drugs to treat this disease.

References

1. Montell C, Birnbaumer L, Flockerzi V. (2002) The TRP channels, a remarkable functional family. Cell 108:595–598
2. Montell C, Birnbaumer L, Flockerzi V, Bindels RJ, Bruford EA, Caterina MJ, Clapham DE, Harteneck C, Heller S, Julius D, Mori Y, Penner R, Prawitt D, Scharenberg AM, Schultz, Shimizu N, Zhu MX (2002): A unified nomenclature for the superfamily of TRP cation channels. Molecular Cell 9:229–231
3. Vennekens R, Voets T, Bindels RJ, Droogmans G, Nilius B (2002) Current understanding of mammalian TRP homologues. Cell Calcium 31:253–264
4. Minke B, Cook B (2002) TRP channel proteins and signal transduction. Physiol Rev 82:429–472
5. Clapham DE (2002) Sorting out MIC, TRP, and CRAC ion channels. J Gen Physiol 120:217–220

TRPM2

TRPM2, also known as TRPC7 or LTRPC2, is responsible for a non-selective cation current activated by ADP-ribose, H_2O_2 and other agents that produce reactive oxygen and nitrogen species and possibly by nicotinamide ADP (NAD). Like TRPM7 and TRPM6, TRPM2 is an ion channel and an enzyme, an ADP-ribose-pyrophosphatase, raising the possibility that the enzyme is involved in channel deactivation.

▶ TRP Channels

TRPM4

TRPM4 also known as the Ca^{2+}-activated non-selective cation (CAN-) channel, mediates cell membrane depolarisation in many excitable and non-excitable cells.

▶ TRP Channels

TRPM7

TRPM7, also known as mTRP-PLIK, ChaK1 or LTRPC7, is a Mg^{2+}-permeable, non-selective cation channel, expressed in kidney, placenta, heart and seemingly, every cell examined, including blood cells and cell lines commonly used for expression studies. The monovalent current is inhibited by Mg^{2+} (IC_{50} ð 0.6 mM) - hence Mag-Num (magnesium- and nucleotide-regulated metal current) or MIC (Mg^{2+} inhibited current) - whereas activation involves reduction of local phosphatidylinositol 4,5-bisphosphate (PIP_2) concentrations. TRPM7 has been identified as a protein interacting with phospholipase Cβ1 (PLCβ1) and has, like TRPM6, the unique feature of being an ion channel and a protein kinase, although TRPM7 channel activity appears not to require the kinase domain for activation.

▶ TRP Channels

TRPM8

TRPM8 is also known as trp-p8 or the cold receptor.

▶ TRP Channels

TRPV1

TRPV1, also known as the capsaicin- or vanilloid-receptor, is a non-selective cation channel expressed e.g. in neurons of the dorsal root and trigeminal ganglions, which integrates multiple pain-producing stimuli including heat, protons, capsaicin and resiniferatoxin. In addition, TRPV1 currents can be activated by anandamide, protein kinase C (PKC) and by hydrolysis of phosphatidylinositol 4,5-bisphosphate (PIP_2).

▶ TRP Channels

TRPV4

TRPV4, also known as TRP12, OTRPC4 or VROAC, is a non-selective cation channel, predominantly expressed in endothelium, kidney, heart and brain. It is activated by a decrease in extracellular osmolarity, by cell swelling, arachidonic acid, anandamide, and by 4α-PDD, a phorbol derivative.

▶ TRP Channels

T

TRPV5 and TRPV6

TRPV5 and TRPV6, also known as the epithelial Ca^{2+} channel or ECaC (TRPV5) and Ca^{2+} transporter 1 or Ca^{2+} transporter-like (TRPV6), are the only two Ca^{2+}-selective TRP channels identified so far. They may function in vitamin D-dependent transcellular transport of Ca^{2+} in kidney, intestine and placenta. TRPV6 is also expressed in pancreatic acinar cells, and in prostate cancer, but not in healthy prostate or in benign prostate hyperplasia.

▶ TRP Channels

Trypsin

Trypsin is a major proteolytic digestive enzyme and the identified endogenous ligand for proteinase-activated receptor 2.

▶ Proteinase-activated Receptors

Trypsin-like proteinases

Trypsin-like proteinases are serine proteinases that recognized peptide residues with positively charged side chains (arginyl or lysyl residues) and that effect hydrolysis of the polypeptide chain on the carboxy-terminal side of these residues. All clotting and compliment cascade proteinases are trypsin-like.

▶ Non-viral Proteases

TSH Receptor

Thyrotropin (TSH) regulates the production and secretion of thyroid hormones as well as thyroid epithelial cell growth *via* the TSH receptor. The TSH receptor belongs to the family of G protein-coupled receptors. It is composed of 764 amino acids. The receptor contains a long hydrophilic region orientated toward the exterior of the cell (ectodomain), 7 hydrophobic transmembrane domains and a short cytoplasmic region.

▶ Antithyroid Drugs

T-tubule

A T-tubule is a transverse invagination of the sarcolemma, which occurs at characteristic sites in animal species and organs, i.e. at the Z-membrane in cardiac ventricle muscle and non-mammalian vertebrate skeletal muscle and at the A-I junction in mammalian skeletal muscle. It is absent in all avian cardiac cells, all cardiac conduction cells, many mammalian atrial cells and most smooth muscle cells. It serves as an inward conduit for the action potential. The surface area in the skeletal muscle can reach 6–8 times that of a cylinder with the same radius. In the T-tubule, Na-channel, Ca-channel and other important channels and transporters can be detected.

▶ Ryanodine Receptor

TTX

▶ Tetrodotoxin

Tubulin

Tubulin is a major component of the cellular cytoskeleton. Tubulin polymers (microtubules) are important for cell division (mitotic spindle) and the chemotaxis and phagocytosis of neutrophils. Prevention of tubulin polymerisation by colchicine accounts for the therapeutic effects of this drug in acute gouty arthritis and its anti-mitotic effects.

▶ α and β tubulin
▶ Cytoskeleton

Tumor Necrosis Factor

TNF

▶ Tumor Necrosis Factor α
▶ TNF Receptor Associated Factors
▶ TNF Receptor Superfamily

Tumor Necrosis Factor α

Tumor necrosis factor α (TNF α) is a potent proinflammatory cytokine that plays an important role in immunity and inflammation and in the control of cell proliferation, differentiation and apoptosis. Binding of TNF α to its two receptors, TNFR1 and TNFR2 results in signaling to at least three distinct effector pathways and to activation of caspases and two transcription factors, AP-1 and NF κB.

▶ TNF Receptor Superfamily
▶ TNF Receptor Associated Factors
▶ Cytokines
▶ Inflammation
▶ Table appendix: Receptor Proteins

Tumor Suppressor Gene

Tumor suppressors genes are defined by their loss of function mutations in tumors. According to the two-hit model by Knudsen, a mutation in only one allele of a tumor suppressor ("first hit") has no phenotype unless followed by a further mutation of the second allele ("second hit"). Frequently, mutation of one allele consists of a specific alteration in the coding sequence of a tumor suppressor resulting in a nonfunctional protein, whereas mutation of the other allele involves larger chromosomal alterations, such as deletions, gene conversion or others. Sometimes, mutations of tumor suppressors occur in an inherited, familial form resulting in a predisposition for patients to develop multifocal tumors when young. Prominent tumor suppressors are APC and p53.

▶ Cadherin/Catenin

TUNEL

TUNEL is the name given to the *in-situ* DNA end-labelling technique which serves as a marker of apoptotic cells. This method is based on the specific binding of terminal de-oxy nucleotidyl transferases to the 3-hydroxy ends of DNA. The technique is normally used for examination under the light microscope but can also be adapted for examination under the electron microscope.

▶ Apoptosis

Twitch

Twitch is muscle contraction caused by a single action potential, whereas tetanus is caused by a series of repetitive action potentials.

▶ Ryanodine Receptor

T

Two-dimensional Gel Electrophoresis

Two-dimensional electrophoresis (2DE) is a two-dimensional technique for protein separation, which combines isoelectric focusing and sodium dodecyl sulphate (SDS) electrophoresis. The high resolving power results from separation according to charge (isoelectric point) in the first dimension and size (mobility in a porous gel) in the second dimension. Depending on the gel size, from several hundred to more than 5,000 proteins can be separated.

▶ Proteomics

Two Metal Sites

Two metal sites were identified in the structure solved of the chimeric $VC_1 \cdot IIC_2$ adenylyl cyclase in complex with β-L-2',3'-dd-5'-ATP (A). One is associated with the pyrophosphate moiety of the inhibitor (metal B) and the other coordinates the attack of the 3'-OH group at the α-phosphate, thereby catalyzing the cyclizing reaction, when 5'ATP is bound (modeled in (B)). The amino acids participating in the binding of substrate are indicated. (C) represents an enlargement of (A) and depicts the loci for Zn^{2+} and Mn^{2+} used in the crystal (Figure).

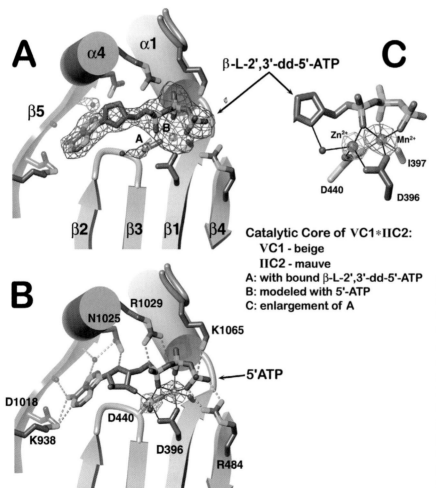

Catalytic Core of VC1∗IIC2:
VC1 - beige
IIC2 - mauve
A: with bound β-L-2',3'-dd-5'-ATP
B: modeled with 5'-ATP
C: enlargement of A

Fig. 1 **Two Metal Sites** – Structure of the catalytic active site of the $VC_1 \cdot IIC_2$ chimeric adenylyl cyclase. A) with β-L-2',3'-dd-5'-ATP showing loci for two metal sites (A and B); B) with ATP modeled and the amino acids identified with which it interacts; and C) an enlargement with the Zn^{2+} (metal A) and Mn^{2+} (metal B) used in forming the crystal.

Type I Allergic Reaction

Type I allergic reactions are inappropriate immune responses to an allergen with preferential synthesis of immunoglobulin E (IgE), a special antibody class, which binds to mast cells and basophilic granulocytes via Fcε receptors. Binding of the allergen to the cell-bound IgE initiates the rapid release of allergic mediators, most prominently histamine, and the *de novo* synthesis of arachidonic aicd metabolites and cytokines, which are responsible for the clinical symptoms.

▶ Allergy

Type II Allergic Reaction

A Type II allergic reaction occurs when antibodies specific for foreign substances recognize the body's own cells after they have firmly bound these foreign substances and initiate the cell's destruction by immune mechanisms.

▶ Allergy

Type III Allergic Reaction

A Type III allergic reaction occurs when antibodies of the immunoglobulin G class (IgG) form immune complexes which are slowly eliminated and thus may elicit an inflammatory reaction by binding to the Fcγ receptors of leukocytes resulting in their activation.

▶ Allergy

Type IV Allergic Reaction

Type IV allergic reactions are cell-mediated hypersensitivity reactions which are characterized by the expansion of T lymphocytes specific for foreign substances exposed on cell surfaces. In type IVa allergic reactions, this results in the cell-mediated destruction of the cells, whereas in type IVb allergic reactions an inflammatory reaction results after release of cytokines (delayed-type hypersensitivity reaction, DTH).

▶ Allergy

Tyrosine Hydroxylase

Tyrosine hydroxylase (TH) is an enzyme that catalyzes the hydroxylation of tyrosine to 3,4-dihydroxyphenylalanine in the brain and adrenal glands. TH is the rate-limiting enzyme in the biosynthesis of dopamine. This nonheme iron-dependent monoxygenase requires the presence of the cofactor tetrahydrobiopterin to maintain the metal in its ferrous state.

▶ Dopamine System

Tyrosine Kinases

ANDREE BLAUKAT
Oncology Research Darmstadt, Merck KGaA,
Darmstadt, Germany
Andree.Blaukat@merck.de

Synonyms

Protein tyrosine kinases, non-receptor tyrosine kinases, cytoplasmic tyrosine kinases, tyrosylprotein kinase, hydroxyaryl-protein kinase

T

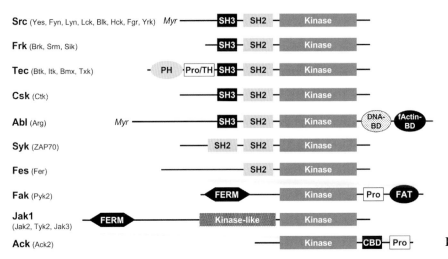

Src (Yes, Fyn, Lyn, Lck, Blk, Hck, Fgr, Yrk) Myr ——— SH3 — SH2 — Kinase —

Frk (Brk, Srm, Sik) SH3 — SH2 — Kinase —

Tec (Btk, Itk, Bmx, Txk) - PH - Pro/TH - SH3 - SH2 — Kinase —

Csk (Ctk) SH3 — SH2 — Kinase —

Abl (Arg) Myr ——— SH3 — SH2 — Kinase — DNA-BD fActin-BD

Syk (ZAP70) SH2 — SH2 — Kinase —

Fes (Fer) SH2 — Kinase —

Fak (Pyk2) FERM — Kinase — Pro - FAT

Jak1 (Jak2, Tyk2, Jak3) FERM — Kinase-like — Kinase —

Ack (Ack2) — Kinase — CBD - Pro -

Fig. 1 Tyrosine Kinases

Definition

Protein tyrosine kinases (PTKs) are enzymes (EC 2.7.1.112) that catalyze the transfer of the γ-phosphate group of ATP to tyrosine residues of protein substrates. The activity of PTKs is controlled in a complex manner by posttranslational modifications and by inter- and intramolecular complex formations.

▶ Table appendix: Protein Kinases
▶ Growth Factors
▶ Hematopoietic Growth Factors
▶ JAK-STAT Pathway
▶ Neurotrophic Factors

Basic Characteristics

PTKs have been implicated in the regulation of a variety of biological responses such as cell proliferation, migration, differentiation and survival. They have been demonstrated to play significant roles in the development of many disease states, including immunodeficiency, ▶ atherosclerosis, psoriasis, ▶ osteoporosis, diabetes and cancer. In recent clinical trials impressive anti-tumor effects of PTK inhibitors have been observed. In future, PTK inhibitors may therefore become important drugs for the treatment of specific cancers.

PTKs can be subdivided into two large families, receptor tyrosine kinases (RTKs) and non-receptor tyrosine kinases. The human genome encodes for a total of 90 tyrosine kinases of which 32 are

non-receptor PTKs that can be placed in 10 subfamilies (Fig. 1). All non-receptor PTKs share a common kinase domain and usually contain several additional domains that mediate interactions with protein binding partners, membrane lipids or DNA (Table 1). These interactions may affect cellular localization and the activation status of the kinase or attract substrate proteins for phosphorylation reactions.

c-Src

c-Src was the first cellular homologue of a viral oncoprotein (v-Src from the Rous sarcoma virus) to be discovered. It is involved in mitogenic signaling from many types of transmembrane receptors and has been implicated in a variety of cancers. c-Src and the Src-like kinases Fyn and Yes are expressed in most tissues and are at least partially redundant in their function. Hck, Fgr and Blk are primarily found in hematopoietic cells, whereas Lyn and Lck are also expressed in neuronal cells.

The inactive, closed conformation of Src is maintained by intramolecular interactions of the SH2 and SH3 domains (Fig. 2). The N-terminal SH3 domain binds to a proline-rich sequence in the linker region between the SH2 and the kinase domain. In addition, the SH2 domain binds to a phosphorylated tyrosine residue (Y527 in chicken, Y530 in human) in the C-terminal part of the protein. The kinase executing this phosphorylation is called Csk (C-terminal c-Src kinase) and is member of a distinct PTK family (Fig. 1). Both intracellular interactions together repress Src kinase activ-

Tab. 1   Tyrosine Kinases

Domain		Function
CBD	Cdc42-binding domain	Binding to the small G protein Cdc42
DNA-BD	DNA-binding domain	Binding to DNA
fActin-BD	fActin-binding domain	Binding to fActin
FAT	Focal adhesion targeting domain	Binding to focal adhesions complexes
FERM	4.1/ezrin/radixin/moesin domain	Binding to cytoplasmic regions of transmembrane proteins
Myr	Myristoylation site	Tethering to membranes
PH	Pleckstrin homology domain	Binding to membrane phospholipids, such as phosphoinositides
Pro	Prolin-rich sequences	Binding to SH 3 domains
PTB	Phospho-tyrosine binding domain	Binding to phosphorylated tyrosine residues
SH1	Src homology 1 domain, Kinase domain	Kinase activity
SH2	Src homology 2 domain	Binding to phosphorylated tyrosine residues
SH3	Src homology 3 domain	Binding to prolin-rich sequences
TH	Tec homology domain	SH3-binding prolin-rich sequences and Zn^{2+}-binding motif

ity by blocking access to the active site. Src can be activated by dephosphorylation of $pY527$ and by intermolecular interactions with SH2 and SH3 binding partners. A variety of cytosolic and receptor-type protein tyrosine phosphatases (PTPs), such as PTPα, PTP1B and SHP-1/2 has been shown to dephosphorylate $pY527$ and subsequently activate c-Src. Among the SH2 ligands that can activate Src are autophosphorylated RTKs (e.g. epidermal growth factor (EGF) and platelet derived growth factor (PDGF) receptors) and non-receptor PTKs (e.g. Fak and Pyk2) as well as tyrosine phosphorylated adaptor proteins (e.g. Shc). For full activation of Src a trans-autophosphorylation of a conserved tyrosine residue in the activation loop (Y416) has to occur. This model is supported by the elevated Src activity in transformed cells with increased PTP activity; a Src mutant with truncated C-terminus lacking Y530 that has been found in human colorectal cancers and is constitutively activated, and v-Src, which in addition to several point mutations lacks a large part of the C-terminal domain, has transforming potential.

Among the substrates of Src are other non-receptor PTKs (e.g. Fak, Syk and Tec kinases), RTKs (e.g. EGF and PDGF receptors), phospholipase Cγ, PI3-kinase, phosphatases (e.g. SHP-2 and PP2A) and adaptor (e.g. Shc and Cbl) as well as focal adhesion proteins (e.g. paxillin, $p130^{Cas}$ and tensin). Src-mediated phosphorylation either modulates enzymatic activity of target proteins or creates docking sites for SH2 or PTB domain containing proteins promoting the assembly of multimeric protein complexes that function in cellular signaling.

Given its involvement in many receptor-mediated signaling pathways, Src was thought to be an important regulator of cell proliferation, migration and adhesion. However, the most striking phenotype of c-Src deficient mice is an osteopetrosis suggesting a role for c-Src in bone remodeling and a compensation of c-Src-deficiency by other Src family members in other organs. Indeed, combined deletion of c-Src, Yes and Fyn in mice results in a lethal phenotype.

T

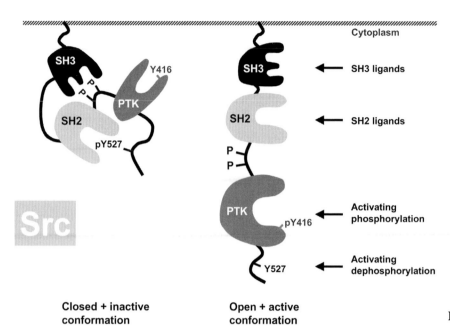

Closed + inactive conformation

Open + active conformation

Fig. 2 Tyrosine Kinases

c-Abl

c-Abl was first identified as the cellular homologue of the transforming gene product of the Abelson murine leukemia virus (v-Abl) and found to encode a non-receptor PTK. Mammalian c-Abl is expressed ubiquitously and in most cells is primarily localized in the nucleus where it has a role in DNA damage-induced apoptosis.

c-Abl is activated by ionizing radiation in a manner dependent on phosphorylation by ATM (ataxia telangiectasia-mutated), a nuclear protein serine/threonine kinase. c-Abl kinase activity in Go and G1 phase of the cell cycle is repressed by binding of Rb (retinoblastoma protein) to the activation loop, which is released during S-phase when Rb becomes hyperphosphorylated by cyclin-dependent kinases. Furthermore, c-Abl is negatively controlled by intramolecular SH3 domain interactions and by SH3-binding proteins, such as Pag/MSP23 (human proliferation-associated gene/macrophage 23-kD stress protein).

Nuclear substrates of c-Abl include DNA-PK (DNA-dependent protein kinase, an enzyme critical for DNA repair), Rad51 (a homologue of bacterial RecA involved in recombination/repair by catalyzing strand exchange between homologous DNAs), the tyrosine phosphatase SHPTP1 and the p85 subunit of PI3-kinase, negatively regulating their respective activity. In contrast, c-Abl activates JNK (c-Jun N-terminal kinase) and p38 mitogen-activated protein kinases (MAPKs). c-Abl also functions in the cytoplasm, where it is involved in PDGF-induced motility responses and cell adhesion.

In chronic myelogenous leukemia (CML) as well as in a subset of acute lymphoblastic leukemia (ALL) Bcr-Abl, a fusion protein of c-Abl and the breakpoint cluster region (bcr), is expressed in the cytosol of leukemic cells. This fusion protein forms homo-oligomeric complexes that display elevated kinase activity and is the causative molecular abnormality in CML and certain ALL. The transforming effect of Bcr-Abl is mediated by numerous downstream signaling pathways, including ▸ protein kinase C (PKC), Ras-Raf-ERK MAPK, JAK-STAT (see below) and PI3-kinase pathways.

Fak

Fak (focal adhesion kinase) is expressed in most tissues and is evolutionary conserved across species. Fak is activated by integrin clustering and by stimulation of several G protein-coupled receptors and RTKs. Fak is associated with focal adhesions and regulates cell spreading and migration. The kinase is essential for embryonic development since the homozygote Fak knockout is embryonic lethal. Pyk2 (proline-rich tyrosine kinase 2), the second member of the Fak kinase family has a more restricted expression pattern (primarily neuronal and hematopoietic cells) and does not localize to focal adhesions.

An early step in Fak activation is a high stoichiometry autophosphorylation of a tyrosine residue (Y397) proximal to the kinase domain. Phosphorylated Y397 is a high affinity ligand for the SH2 domain of Src, thereby recruiting Src kinases and stimulating their catalytic activity. In a second step, several other tyrosine residues in Fak become phosphorylated, either by Fak itself or by recruited Src. As a consequence, Fak kinase activity is further increased or docking sites for SH2 domain-containing proteins are created, e.g. for Grb2-Sos complexes that link Fak to the Ras-Raf-▶ MAPK cascade. N-terminal sequences containing the FERM domain anchor Fak to integrins or RTKs and the C-terminal FAT domain mediates binding to cellular focal adhesions. Among the substrates of Fak are the adaptor proteins paxillin and p130^{Cas} and the focal adhesion-associated protein tensin that bind to C-terminal sequences of Fak and, after their phosphorylation, promote the assembly of signaling complexes at discrete sites within cells.

Fak kinases could be modulators of some aspects of human cancers and may also contribute to the development of vascular diseases involving hyperproliferation and migration of vascular smooth muscle cells.

Jak

Jak1 and 2 were identified, among others, by PCR using degenerate oligonucleotides spanning the conserved kinase domain of Src and therefore initially named Jak, for "Just another kinase". When full length clones were isolated it was recognized that they differ markedly from other PTKs by the presence of an additional (pseudo)-kinase domain of unknown function. To denote this unique feature they were renamed as "Janus kinases" in reference to the ancient two-faced Roman god. Jak1, 2 and Tyk2 are ubiquitously expressed, whereas Jak3 is predominantly found in hematopoietic cells. Jak family PTKs mediate signaling primarily downstream of cytokine receptors. In response to ligand stimulation, cytokine receptors oligomerize and recruited or constitutively bound Jak kinases become activated and phosphorylate receptors.

Some of the receptors' phosphotyrosine residues subsequently bind to SH2 domains of STATs (signal transducers and activators of transcription), which are then phosphorylated by Jaks on a C-terminal tyrosine residue. This leads to STAT oligomerization through a reciprocal interaction between SH2 domains and phosphotyrosines. Dimeric STATs translocate to the nucleus where they initiate transcription of target genes. Alternatively, STATs can be activated by Src kinases that are recruited to Jak-phosphorylated cytokine receptors via their SH2 domain. Jak kinase signaling is negatively regulated by PTPs and by SOCS (suppressors of cytokine signaling) proteins that inhibit Jaks by binding to the activation loop and by targeting the kinases for protein degradation.

STAT 3 and 5 are overexpressed or overactivated in several human malignancies, such as breast, head and neck cancer. An aberrant activation of Jak kinases by fusion with the TEL transcription factor and subsequent constitutive dimerization has been observed in T-cell acute lymphocytic leukemia.

▶ JAK-STAT Pathway

Tec

Tec family kinases participate in signal transduction in response to virtually all types of extracellular stimuli that are transmitted by growth factor receptors, cytokine receptors, G protein-coupled receptors, antigen-receptors and integrins. Tec kinases are involved in the regulation of growth, differentiation, apoptosis and cell motility. They are primarily found in hematopoietic lineages but some family members (Btk, Etk/Bmx) have a somewhat broader expression pattern. The defining feature of Tec family kinases is the presence of a PH domain at their N-terminus. The PH domain has a broad binding capacity ranging from lipid products of PI3-kinase, heterotrimeric G protein subunits ($\beta\gamma$ as well as $G\alpha_q$ and $G\alpha_{12}$), PKC isoforms (βI and δ) to STATs and Fak kinases. These interactions may either be involved in Tec activation (phospholipids and G proteins) or recruit potential substrates of Tec kinases (PKC and STATs).

The current understanding on activation of Tec kinases fits into a two-step model. In the first step an intramolecular interaction between the SH3

T

domain and a proline-rich region in the TH domain is disrupted by binding of the PH domain to phosphoinositides, G protein subunits or the FERM domain of Fak. These interactions lead to conformational changes of Tec and translocation to the cytoplasmic membrane where, in a second step, Src kinases phosphorylate a conserved tyrosine residue in the catalytic domain thereby increasing Tec kinase activity. Autophosphorylation of a tyrosine residue in the SH3 domain further prevents the inhibitory intramolecular interaction resulting in a robust Tec kinase activation.

Among the substrates and downstream effectors of Tec kinases are phospholipase Cγ2 and PKCβI resulting in a sustained calcium influx and eventual activation of MAPKs. The interaction with the GDP/GTP exchange factor Vav can potentially activate Rac/Cdc42/Rho pathways, which can modulate actin cytoskeleton dynamics and also lead to JNK and p38 MAPK activation eventually inducing apoptosis. Paradoxically, Tec kinases may also trigger anti-apoptotic signals by stimulating PI3-kinase ▶ Akt and promote proliferation by activating STATs.

Naturally occurring mutations of Btk were identified in human immunodeficiency diseases and X-linked agammaglobulinemia, where a lack of mature circulating B cells and immunoglobulins are observed, supporting a central role for Btk in B cell maturation. In contrast, the knockout of Itk results in a lack of mature T cells and defects in T-cell receptor signaling. Furthermore, Btk and Etk/Bmx are able to complement a weakly oncogenic Src in transformation of hepatocytes and fibroblasts suggesting their participation in anchorage-independent growth and development of cancer.

Syk

Syk and ZAP-70 are early intermediates in the transduction of signals from immune receptors, including the B- and T-cell receptors for antigen, activatory natural killer-cell receptors, the mast cell and basophil receptor for IgE and the widely distributed receptors for the Fc portion of IgG. Immune receptors control checkpoints in lymphocyte development and serve to integrate the responses of innate and acquired immunity.

The current model proposes that upon engagement of immune receptors Src-family kinases are recruited that phosphorylate tyrosine residues in specific regions of the receptors, the immunoreceptor tyrosine-based activation motifs (ITAMs). These phosphotyrosines serve as docking sites for the SH2 domains of Syk and ZAP-70 that subsequently autophosphorylate and generate binding sites for SH2 domain containing proteins, like phospholipase Cγ, Vav and the adaptor protein Cbl. Furthermore, Syk and ZAP-70 phosphorylate a number of cytosolic and transmembrane linker proteins, such as SLP-76 (SH2-containing leukocyte protein of 76 kD), LAT (transmembrane linker for activation of T cells), TRIMM (T cell receptor-interacting molecule) and SIT (SHP2-interacting transmembrane adaptor protein) that function as scaffolds to localize and assemble signaling complexes. In addition to being a major player in immune receptor signaling, Syk has a role in the "inside-out" integrin activation signal that is necessary for fibrinogen binding and subsequent aggregation of platelets during hemostasis.

Drugs

PTKs have been shown to play significant roles in the development of many disease states, including immunodeficiency, atherosclerosis, psoriasis, osteoporosis, diabetes and cancer. Therefore, in the last years numerous PTK inhibitors have been developed that a currently undergoing clinical trials. The majority of them are directed against RTKs, however, most impressive clinical results have been obtained with the compound STI571 (signal transduction inhibitor 571, Gleevec™) that in addition to its action against PDGF and c-Kit receptors, potently inhibits the activity of the nonreceptor PTK c-Abl. STI571 is a phenylamino-pyrimidine that, as for almost all kinase inhibitors, competes for binding of ATP to the catalytic domain. In CML as well as in a subset of ALL Bcr-Abl fusion proteins with elevated kinase activity are the causative molecular abnormality. In clinical trials with CML patients, impressive response rates of up to 98% without severe adverse effects have been observed with once-daily oral doses of 400 mg of STI571. However, as with almost all chemotherapeutics, resistance to STI571 as a single agent was observed in patients that were irresponsive or relapsed after initial successful treatment. Major mechanisms for this resistance are Bcr-Abl amplifications and mutations in the kinase domain that reduce affinity for STI571. It became therefore obvious that a combination of kinase inhibitor with other drugs is necessary to achieve maximal therapeutic benefits for CML patients. STI571 was approved for the treatment of CML in about twenty countries by June 2001. Based on its ability to inhibit other PTKs such as c-Kit and PDGF receptors the spectrum of diseases that may respond to STI571 is growing. Preliminary remarkable activity and clinical responses in patients with gastrointestinal stromal tumors expressing gain-of-function mutants of c-Kit have been reported. Furthermore, STI571 could be used to treat other types of malignancies, such as small cell lung cancers overexpressing c-Kit, CML that express a constitutively active PDGF receptor fusion protein and glioblastomas associated with an autocrine growth loop involving PDGF and its receptor.

Currently, no other inhibitor of non-receptor PTKs has entered clinical trials. However, there are several candidates that have shown activity on cultured tumor cells and in animal experiments. For instance, PP1 is a pyrazolo-pyrimidine that blocks Src kinases and inhibits the anchorage-independent growth of Ras-transformed cells and the rapid growth of Ras-induced sarcomas in mice. More recently, peptidomimetic SH2 domain inhibitors for Src have been designed that decrease bone resorption and may be promising drugs to treat osteoporosis and other bone diseases, such as Paget's disease and osteolytic bone metastasis.

Other drugs against non-receptor PTKs with therapeutical potential are Jak2 inhibitors, such as AG490, a benzenmalononitrile that was shown to suppress the growth of leukemic cells and ovarian as well as breast cancer cell lines, to reduce myocardial infarct size and cardiomyocyte apoptosis in ischemia/reperfusion injury and to prevent experimental allergic encephalomyelitis.

Future basic research and clinical studies will show whether other inhibitors of non-receptor PTKs may be as successful drugs as STI571 for the treatment of fatal diseases such as cancer.

References

1. Blume-Jensen P, Hunter T (2001) Oncogenic kinase signalling. Nature 411:355–365
2. Hubbard SR, Till JH (2000) Protein tyrosine kinase structure and function. Annu. Rev. Biochem. 69:373–398
3. Thomas SM, Brugge JS (1997) Cellular functions regulated by Src family kinases. Annu. Rev. Cell Dev. Biol. 13:513–609
4. Mauro MJ, O'Dwyer M, Heinrich MC, Druker BJ (2002) STI571: A paradigm of new agents for cancer therapeutics. J. Clin. Oncol. 20:325–334
5. Morin M (2000) From oncogene to drug: development of small molecule tyrosine kinase inhibitors as anti-tumor and anti-angiogenic agents. Oncogene 19:6574–6583

Tyrosine Phosphatase

Tyrosine phosphatases are a group of enzymes catalyzing the dephosphorylation of tyrosine residues in protein substrates.

▶ JAK-STAT Pathway
▶ Tyrosin Kinases

Tyrphostins

Tyrphostins are a group of substances, which block a variety of tyrosine kinases. Some of them have a relative selectivity for defined tyrosine kinase subtypes.

▶ Tyrosin Kinases

Ubiquinone

▶ Coenzyme Q_{10}

Ubiquitin

Ubiquitin is a small protein of 76 residues that is conjugated posttranslationally to other proteins. It is ubiquitously present in all eukaryotes, hence its name, and is one of the most highly conserved proteins, with only 3 residue changes between yeast and humans. A poly-ubiquitin chain serves as a tag that marks proteins for degradation by the proteasome.

▶ Ubiquitin/proteasome System

Ubiquitin/Proteasome System

R. JÜRGEN DOHMEN
Institute for Genetics, University of Cologne, Germany
j.dohmen@uni-koeln.de

Definition

The ▶ ubiquitin/proteasome system (UPS) selectively targets proteins for degradation in a variety of processes in cell biology and development.

▶ Ubiquitin-related Modifiers

Basic Characteristics

Ubiquitin(Ub)-mediated proteolysis is the main pathway for ATP-dependent non-lysosomal degradation of short-lived proteins in eukaryotic cells. Naturally short-lived proteins as well as misfolded, damaged or otherwise abnormal proteins are marked for degradation by the attachment of poly-Ub chains. Poly-ubiquitylated proteins are recognized and degraded by the 26S proteasome. The UPS operates in the cell nucleus as well as the cytoplasm, and is in addition responsible for ER-associated degradation ('ERAD'). ERAD requires retrograde transport of proteolysis substrates from the ER to the cytoplasm through the ER translocon.

The Ubiquitin System

The Ub system is composed of a set of enzymes that mediate or reverse the conjugation of Ub to protein substrates (Fig. 1). Ub precursors are synthesized as the products of several genes, all of which encode fusions of Ub either to ribosomal subunits or to itself (1,2). In the latter case, a stress-inducible polyubiquitin gene encodes multiple Ub moieties in head to tail fusion. From these precursors, mature Ub is liberated by Ub-specific processing proteases. Covalent attachment of Ub to its substrates (ubiquitylation) requires the activity of at least three enzymes: First, the C-terminus of Ub needs to be activated by the Ub-activating enzyme (E1) in an ATP-dependent reaction. The transfer of Ub to substrates is catalyzed by complexes of Ub-conjugating/carrier enzymes (Ubc, E2) and substrate recognizing Ub ligases (recognin, E3). A cell contains a number of different Ubc enzymes (11 in yeast) and a multitude of

Ubiquitin system

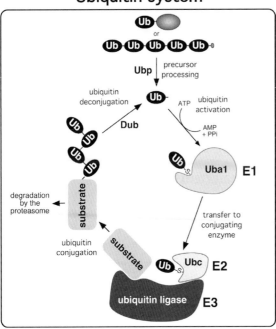

Fig. 1 Ubiquitin (Ub) is synthesized in precursor form in which it is either fused to ribosomal subunits or to itself. Mature Ub is generated from these precursors by specific Ub processing proteases termed Ubps. For conjugation, the C-terminus of mature Ub needs first to be activated by the Ub-activating enzyme Uba1 (E1). Activation is ATP-dependent, proceeds via a Ub-adenylate intermediate, and results in Ub being linked via a thioester to a cysteine residue in Uba1. Activated Ub is then transferred in a transesterification reaction to a cysteine residue of a Ub-conjugating enzyme (Ubc, E2). In conjunction with substrate recognizing ligases (E3 enzymes) Ubcs conjugates Ub to a variety of substrate proteins. A major function of ubiquitylation is to target proteins for degradation by the proteasome.

Ub ligases that are specific for certain substrates and processes (1,2).

Whereas the Ubc proteins are closely related in sequence and structure, there is only limited similarity between the Ub ligases. Two classes are distinguished (2): One class is characterized by a so-called HECT domain of about 80 residues including an active site cysteine that forms a thioester with Ub. A common feature of the second class of E3 proteins is a so-called RING finger domain.

This domain has been implicated in mediating functional interactions with E2 proteins. E3 proteins of the latter class facilitate the direct transfer of Ub from E2 enzymes to substrates without an E3-Ub thioester intermediate. Some important RING-type Ub ligases, such as the cell cycle-controlling complexes APC and SCF-RING, are multisubunit assemblies that can associate with alternative substrate-selecting subunits. Other RING-type Ub ligases, such as ▶ Parkin (see UPS and diseases) or N-recognin (see below), are single polypeptides. Different Ub ligases recognize a variety of distinct destruction signals ('degrons') of their substrates. One such signal can be a 'destabilizing' amino acid residue at the N-terminus ('▶ N-end rule') of a protein which mediates its ubiquitylation by N-recognin/E3-α (1). Other ligases, such as certain SCF-RING complexes, recognize phosphorylated '▶ PEST sequences'. Proteins ubiquitylated by APC typically contain a short sequence element of 9 residues ('destruction box') close to their N-termini (3).

E2/E3 complexes catalyze the conjugation of Ub to other proteins by formation of amide (isopeptide) bonds between the C-terminal glycine residue of Ub and the ε-amino group of internal lysine residues (1). A substrate-linked poly-ubiquitin chain, in which Ub moieties are themselves linked to each other via isopeptide bonds involving certain lysine residues (Lys48 or Lys29), serves as a tag that targets a protein for degradation by the 26S proteasome. In contrast, mono-ubiquitylation appears to serve other functions, e.g. as a modification of histones or as a translocation signal in the endocytic pathway. Poly-Ub chains linked via Lys63 have been implicated in non-proteolytic functions of the Ub system such as a cell cycle-regulated modification of the ribosome and DNA damage repair. The formation of some types of poly-Ub chains is enhanced by a processivity factor termed E4.

De-ubiquitylation enzymes (Dub or isopeptidases), which are in part overlapping in function with Ub-specific processing proteases, deconjugate Ub from its substrates and thereby recycle Ub. Cells contain a large number of different Dubs whose specific functions are only poorly understood.

The Proteasome

The 26S proteasome of eukaryotic cells is the main protease system responsible for the degradation of short-lived and abnormal proteins in the cytosol and nucleus as well as of the endoplasmic reticulum. In most cases studied, the proteasome degrades its substrate down to small peptides (Fig. 2). In some case, however, the proteasome has been shown to serve the function of a processing protease. An important example is the p50 subunit of NF-κB, a transcription factor mediating inflammatory responses, whose generation from a p105 precursor protein is mediated by the UPS. The proteasome, as the ubiquitin system, is essential for viability in eukaryotes. Among the substrates of the proteasome are many regulatory proteins including important regulators of the cell cycle, cell proliferation or ▶ apoptosis. It is for that reason that inhibitors that block the active sites of the proteasome have received attention as potential drugs to treat cancer or stroke (5).

The 26S proteasome is a complex protease with a molecular weight around 2000 kD (4). It is composed of a 19S activator complex that is specifically required for the degradation of ubiquitylated proteins and of a 20S complex (termed 20S proteasome) that is the catalytic core of the 26S structure. 20S proteasomes of similar structure have been found in eukaryotes as well as in the archaeons and eubacteria. The eukaryotic complex is composed of 14 different but related subunits, 7 of the 'α-type' and 7 of the 'β-type'. The active sites are located on the inner surface of a central chamber that is formed by the two rings of β subunits. In eukaryotic proteasomes, only 3 of the 7 different β subunits are active. A common feature of active site subunits are N-terminal threonine (Thr) residues that act as nucleophiles attacking peptide bonds of the substrates. This property characterized the proteasome as a novel type of Thr protease and placed it into a family of 'Ntn hydrolases' that are characterized by an N-terminal nucleophile. The 3 active site β subunits are synthesized as inactive precursors containing a propeptide that is thought to be cleaved off autocatalytically to yield the mature form with a N-terminal Thr. These 3 subunits provide the active site nucleophiles for the three different types of activities characteristic of eukaryotic proteasomes, namely 'chymotrypsin-like' (cleavage after hydrophobic

residues), 'trypsin-like' (cleavage after basic residues) and post-acidic activity (cleavage after acidic residues). In the human proteasome, the active subunits, upon immune stress, can be replaced by interferon-γ-induced subunits. Incorporaton of these subunits alters the cleavage specificity of the proteasome (see 'Function of UPS in Antigen Presentation'). The cleavage pattern of the proteasome is moreover modulated by an alternative interferon-γ-induced activator complex termed PA28 (4).

Structural analysis of the proteasome revealed that it has only a small opening formed in the center of the ring of α subunits. It is therefore only able to degrade peptides or structurally unstable proteins that can penetrate these pores. The degradation of more complex substrates requires the presence of the 19S activator complexes that are attached at both sides of the eukaryotic 20S proteasome (Fig. 2). This assembly step requires the presence but not the hydrolysis of ATP. Besides binding sites for multi-Ub chains and isopeptidase activity that releases them, the base of the 19S regulator contains a ring of six subunits with ATPase activity that are thought to unfold substrate proteins and to push them into the 20S cylinder.

The 20S proteasome is assembled via a half-proteasome intermediate containing a specific maturation factor and all 14 subunits, some of which are in the precursor form (Fig. 2). When two such half-proteasomes join to form the 20S complex, conformational changes that depend on the presence of the maturation factor trigger the autocatalytic processing of active site β subunits. The enclosed maturation factor is subsequently degraded by the activated proteasome (4).

Role of UPS in the Regulation of Cell Division

Three fundamental steps of the cell division cycle are regulated by UPS (3). The G1/S transition, i.e. the initiation of DNA replication, is triggered by the timed degradation of a cyclin-dependent kinase (Cdk) inhibitor. Phosphorylation of the inhibitor mediates its recognition by the F-box subunit of an SCF-RING complex, a multi-subunit Ub ligase. In mitosis, two key steps are controlled by ubiquitin-mediated degradation. The metaphase to anaphase transition is initiated by the degradation of an anaphase inhibitor called

Biogenesis of the proteasome

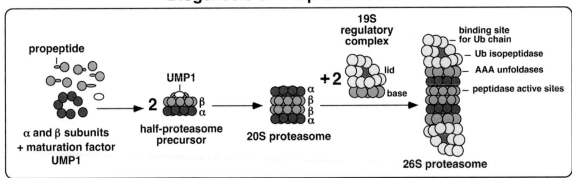

Functions of the proteasome

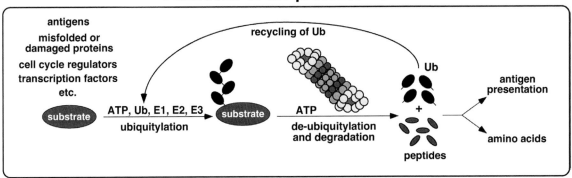

Fig. 2 *Upper part:* **Biogenesis of the proteasome:** seven α-type and seven β-type subunits assemble, possibly via an α-ring intermediate, into a half-proteasome precursor complex. This complex also includes a dedicated chaperone, termed Ump1 because of its function to 'underpin the maturation of the proteasome'. Two such half-proteasome precursor complexes join to form the 20S proteasome. In this process, with the help of Ump1, the three active β-subunits mature autocatalytically by release of their propeptides. The enclosed maturation factor is subsequently degraded within the proteasome. In order to be able to degrade poly-ubiquitylated proteins, the 20S catalytic core complex has to assemble with two 19S activator complexes to form the 26S proteasome. The base of each activator complex contains six AAA-type ATPase subunits, which are thought to mediate the unfolding of substrate proteins and their threading into the catalytic core. The lid of the activator complexes contains poly-Ub binding sites and de-ubiquitylation (Dub or isopeptidase) activity. *Lower part:* **Functions of the proteasome:** the main function of the proteasome is the degradation of ubiquitylated substrates ranging from antigens and abnormal proteins to important regulators. Such proteins are degraded to small peptides that can either be presented on MHC class I molecules or be degraded further by other peptidases. Ub is recycled by proteasome-associated and cytosolic isopeptidase activity.

'securin'. It inhibits a specific endoprotease termed 'separin' until the time comes to separate the sister chromatides. Timed degradation of securin activates separin which then cleaves 'cohesins' that keep the sister chromatides together. Ubiquitylation of securin is mediated by the APC complex in association with the substrate-selecting component CDC20. At the end of mitosis, the APC complex is also responsible for the degradation of mitotic cyclins and factors controlling spindle disassembly. To mediate this function, APC associates with another substrate-selecting component (CDH1/HCT1).

In response to DNA damage or to other perturbations of the cell such as viral infections, cell-cycle progression is inhibited by the activation of the tumor suppressor ▶ p53, a transcriptional activator. If damage to a cell's DNA exceeds a critical level, p53 also participates in the induction of programmed cell death (apoptosis). In normal cells, p53 is an unstable protein that is stabilized in response to DNA damage. Its turnover by the UPS is mediated by the Mdm2 ubiquitin ligase. Certain high risk forms of the human papillomavirus (HPV16) that cause cervical carcinomas encode a protein termed E6 that recruits the cellular ubiquitin ligase 'E6-associated protein' (E6-AP) to p53 thereby mediating its rapid degradation even under conditions where targeting by Mdm2 is inhibited (2). This function of the E6 protein is part of the viral strategy to allow induction of malignant proliferation of the infected host cell by preventing p53-induced apoptosis.

Function of UPS in Antigen Presentation

The UPS has an important role in the adaptive immune response (4). It generates antigenic peptides from proteins of intracellular pathogens such as bacteria or viruses. These peptides, some of which require additional processing by other peptidases, are translocated via the 'transporter associated with antigen processing' (TAP) into the ER where there are loaded onto major histocompatibility (MHC) class I molecules. Once loaded they are transported to the cell surface where the antigenic peptides are presented to cytotoxic T cells. According to a recent concept by Yewdell (6), a fast generation of breakdown products even of otherwise long-lived proteins is ascertained by the fact that a significant fraction of newly synthesized proteins are degraded even before or shortly after their completion. The underlying inaccuracy of protein synthesis and folding thus results in a constant generation of defective ribosomal products (DRiPs), which are degraded by the UPS and therefore are a source of antigenic peptides.

To increase the generation of certain antigenic peptides, a specialized proteasome subtype, termed 'immunoproteasome', is generated. It is distinguished from its house-keeping counterpart by an incorporation of interferon-γ-induced variants of the active site subunits. These 'immuno-subunits' confer an altered cleavage specificity to the proteasome that favors the generation of antigenic peptides with C-terminal hydrophobic or basic residues that are recognized by TAP and MHC class I molecules. In addition, the 20S proteasome can associate with an alternative interferon-γ-induced 11S activator complex termed PA28. The resulting complex, however, is not capable of degrading ubiquitylated proteins but may function in the processing of products generated by the 26S proteasome (4).

UPS and Disease

A variety of neurodegenerative diseases including Alzheimer's disease, Parkinson's disease, Amyotrophic Lateral Sclerosis (ALS), as well as diseases caused by expansion of polyglutamine tracts such as Huntington's disease and Spinocerebellar Ataxias are characterized by the formation of intracellular inclusions of abnormal proteins. Proteins found in these aggregates are often ubiquitylated and associated with chaperones and the proteasome. The accumulation of abnormal forms of the proteins underlying these processes is thought to eventually cause the induction of apoptosis in affected neurons.

One hereditary form of juvenile Parkinsonism has been tracked to mutations in a gene encoding Parkin, a RING-type Ub ligase. Recent work has shown that α-synuclein, a protein that accumulates in so-called 'Lewy Bodies' in the brains of most patients with Parkinson's disease (not the ones with Parkin mutations), is a substrate of this ligase. These observations suggest that impairment of the UPS contributes to this disease.

Angelman's syndrome, a neurological disorder characterized by mental retardation, has been linked to mutations affecting the human E6-AP gene encoding another Ub ligase (see above).

As an example of a link between the UPS and cancer, the targeted destruction of p53 mediated by the viral E6 protein as an aspect of the transforming effect of certain human papillomaviruses has been described above. Other examples are the breast and ovarian cancer susceptibility gene 1 (BRCA1) that appears to be a RING-type Ub ligase, and the tre-2 oncogene that encodes an inactive form of a de-ubiquitylation enzyme (2).

U

Muscle atrophy is associated with various pathological or physiological states such as denervation, injury, joint immobilization, sepsis, HIV infection, cancer or aging. Muscle wasting in such cases has been shown to be due to an up-regulation of the UPS. Recently, a RING-type Ub ligase and an F-box component of an SCF-RING-type Ub ligase were identified that are up-regulated in a rat model of muscle atrophy. Inactivation of the respective genes in mice resulted in resistance to atrophy.

Drugs

Aside of the lactone-based metabolite lactacystin or related compounds, a variety of synthetic peptide-based inhibitors of the proteasome, such as peptide aldehydes (e.g. MG132), peptide vinyl sulfonates, peptide boronates, as well as epoxyketone- or glyoxal-based peptide derivatives, have been described (5). All of these compounds inhibit the peptidase activity of the proteasome. Proteasome inhibitors are currently in clinical trials as anti-cancer drugs and as treatment for strokes because of their ability to reduce reperfusion injury. They are also considered as inhibitors of muscle wasting that occurs e.g. in patients with cancer, AIDS, or muscular dystrophies, and as immunosuppressive agents in the treatment of autoimmune disease and in transplantation medicine. In the future, more specific drugs that inhibit individual Ub ligases may provide important additional therapeutics for the treatment of variety of diseases.

References

1. Hershko A, Ciechanover A, Varshavsky A (2000) The Ubiquitin System. Nature Med.6:1073–1081
2. Weissman AM (2001) Themes and variations on ubiquitylation. Nature Rev. Mol. Cell Biol 2:169–178.
3. Zachariae W, Nasmyth K (1999) Whose end is destruction: cell division and the anaphase-promoting complex. Genes Dev. 13:2039–2058
4. Voges D, Zwickl P, Baumeister W (1999) The 26S proteasome: a molecular machine designed for controlled proteolysis. Annu. Rev. Biochem. 68:1015–1068
5. Lee DH, Goldberg AL (1998) Proteasome inhibitors: valuable new tools for cell biologists. Trends Biochem. Sci. 8:397–403
6. Yewdell JW (2001) Not such a dismal science: the economics of protein synthesis, folding, degradation and antigen processing. Trends Cell Biol. 11:294-297.

Ubiquitin-dependent Protein Degradation

Ubiquitin tags proteins for protein degradation. The ubiquitination requires three different enzymatic activities, a ubiquitin-activating enzyme (E1), a ubiquitin-conjugating enzyme (E2 or Ubc) and a ubiquitin ligase (E3). The action of all three enzymes leads to the establishment of a poly-ubiquitin chain on target proteins which are then recognized and proteolyzed by the 26S proteasome.

▶ Ubiqitin/Proteasome System

Ubiquitin-related Modifiers

R. JÜRGEN DOHMEN
Institute for Genetics, University of Cologne, Germany
j.dohmen@uni-koeln.de

Definition

▶ Ubiquitin-related modifiers are proteins such as ▶ SUMO, NEDD8/RUB and URCP/ISG15, which are structurally related to ubiquitin and posttranslationally attached to other proteins. These modifiers are linked to their substrates via amide (isopeptide) bonds formed between their C-terminal glycine residue and the ε-amino group of internal lysine residues (1).

▶ Ubiquitin/Proteasome System

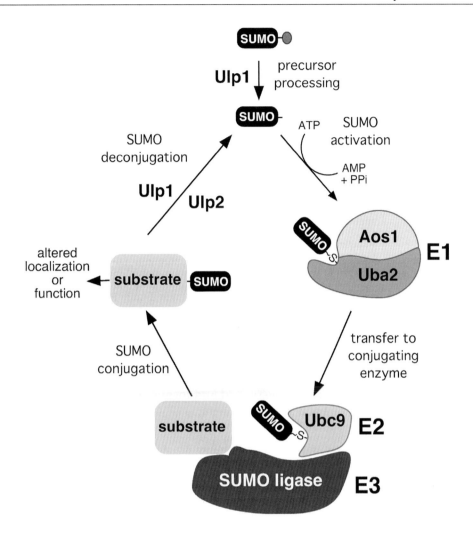

Fig. 1 Like ubiquitin, SUMO is synthesized as a precursor with a short C-terminal extension, which is cleaved off by a specific processing protease termed Ulp1. For conjugation, the C-terminus of mature SUMO needs first to be activated by the SUMO-activating enzyme (E1), a heterodimeric protein composed of Uba2 and Aos1. Both subunits have similarity to distinct regions of the ubiquitin-activating enzyme. Activation is ATP-dependent, proceeds via a SUMO-adenylate intermediate, and results in SUMO being linked by a thioester to a cysteine residue in Uba2. Activated SUMO is then transferred, in a transesterification reaction, to a cysteine residue of Ubc9, a conjugating enzyme (E2) specific for SUMO. In conjunction with substrate recognizing ligases (E3 enzymes), Ubc9 conjugates SUMO to a variety of substrate proteins. SUMO ligases constitute a protein family including several PIAS proteins that are involved in interferon-induced or β-catenin-dependent signaling.

U

Basic Characteristics

The first modifier described, aside of ubiquitin, was the interferon-induced UCRP, discovered by its cross-reaction with anti-ubiquitin antibodies. UCRP becomes conjugated to cytosolic endome-

trial proteins in response to interferon and pregnancy. NEDD8, also called RUB1, is the modifier whose sequence is most closely related to ubiquitin (50% identity). The only characterized substrates are proteins of the cullin/Cdc53 family. Cullins are components of ubiquitin ligases (E3s)

Tab. 1 Ubiquitin-related Modifiers

SUMO targets	Function/description	Effect of SUMO modification
RanGAP1	Nuclear transport	Interaction with nuclear pore
p53	Transcription factor/tumor suppressor	Regulation of activity
c-jun	Transcription factor/proto-oncogene	Regulation of activity
IκBα	Inhibitor of NF-κB/inflammatory response	Protection against ubiquitylation
PML	Affected by translocation causing APL	Localization to nuclear domains
HCMV IE2	Human Cytomegalovirus protein regulating infections.	Localization to nuclear domains
Septins	Polarized cell growth and cytokinesis	Unknown
Werner's syndrome protein	Mutations cause premature aging	Unknown
Androgen receptor	Hormone receptor	Unknown

known as SCF complexes that, among other functions, regulate the cell cycle transition from G1 to S phase.

SUMO is the modifier that, since its discovery in 1996, has received most attention because of its intriguing and essential functions (see below).

SUMO Modification System

Although the sequence identity between SUMO and ubiquitin is relatively low (~18% identity) the three-dimensional structures are very similar (2). The enzymes required for SUMO conjugation (sumoylation) were first characterized in yeast (Fig.1). Some of these enzymes, such as the SUMO-activating enzyme (E1) and SUMO-conjugating enzyme (E2), have similar primary structures as their counterparts in the ubiquitin system, and are conserved from yeast to humans (1,3). The genes for several enzymes of the SUMO modification system, such as E1, E2, and Ulp1 as well as the gene encoding SUMO itself, are essential for viability in baker's yeast (3). The phenotypes of mutants with conditional defects in these genes have uncovered the essential role of SUMO modification for a transition of the cell cycle from the G2 phase into mitosis. The relevant targets underlying this process are still unknown. Several enzymes of the SUMO system, including E1, E2, some E3s and deconjugating enzymes (Ulp2), as well as most SUMO-conjugates, are found enriched within the cell nucleus, whereas the

processing protease Ulp1 is associated with the nuclear pore. This distribution is consistent with functions of sumoylation in cytosol/nucleus transit and formation of subnuclear structures (see below).

An intriguing example of deregulation of the SUMO system by a human pathogen has been described recently (4). *Yersinia pestis* secretes a SUMO-deconjugating enzyme homologous to Ulp enzymes that inhibits the host immune response by preventing activation of MAP kinase and NF-κB pathways.

Functions and Targets of SUMO

SUMO was first discovered as a modifier of RanGAP1, a GTPase-activating protein for the cytosol/nucleus shuttling factor Ran (5). Sumoylation of RanGAP1 leads to its interaction with the cytoplasmic fibrils of the nuclear pore complex (Table 1).

In mammals, aside of modified RanGAP1, a large fraction of SUMO conjugates are associated with subnuclear structures known as ND10, in which several SUMO targets including PML and Sp100 accumulate (Table 1). ND10 are cell cycle-regulated, matrix-associated multiprotein aggregates that are detectable as punctate foci in interphase nuclei. The integrity of these structures appears to be important for normal cell growth and development since their disruption leads to human diseases such as acute promyelocytic leukaemia (APL) and spinocerebellar ataxia type I (SCA1). A variety of viral proteins, some of which themselves are SUMO targets, interfere with the formation of ND10 structures.

Another SUMO target is IκBα, which inhibits NF-κB, the transcriptional activator of the inflammatory response, by keeping it in the cytosol. Upon stimulation, IκBα is degraded by the ubiquitin/proteasome system allowing NF-κB to enter the nucleus. Sumoylation antagonizes IκBα ubiquitylation. Sumoylation of the tumor suppressor p53 appears to increase its capacity for transcriptional activation.

Septins are a family of GTPases involved in determining cell shape and future sites of cell division. In yeast, septins have been shown to be sumoylated in a cell cycle-regulated manner, which might influence their assembly or disassembly.

Further examples of a growing number of SUMO targets include a variety of other proteins implicated in human diseases, some of which are listed in Table 1. The effect of their modification by sumoylation, however, is still unclear.

What appears to emerge from the analysis of SUMO targets is that their modification alters their activities or subcellular localization.

Drugs

At present, there are no drugs known to specifically inhibit components of the SUMO system.

References

1. Jentsch S, Pyrowolakis G (2000) Ubiquitin and its kin: how close are family ties. Trends Cell Biol. 10:335–342
2. Melchior F (2000) SUMO – Nonclassical ubiquitin. Annu. Rev. Cell Dev. Biol. 16:591–626
3. Johnson ES, Schwienhorst I, Dohmen RJ, Blobel G (1997) The ubiquitin-like protein Smt3p is activated for conjugation to other proteins by an Aos1p/Uba2p heterodimer. EMBO J. 16:5509–5519
4. Orth K, Xu Z, Budgett MB, Bao ZQ, Palmer LE, Bliska JB, Mangel WF, Staskawicz B, Dixon JE (2000) Disruption of signaling by Yersina effector YopJ, a ubiquitin-like protein protease. Science 290:1594–1597
5. Mahajan R, Delphin C, Guan T, Gerace L, Melchior F (1997) A small ubiquitin-related polypeptide involved in targeting RanGAP1 to nuclear pore complex protein RanBP2. Cell 88:97–107

UDP-glucuronyl Transferase

UDP-glucuronyl transferases (UGTs) are a group of enzymes which catalyze the transfer of UDP-glucuronyl moieties from UDP-glucuronic acid into a variety of small lipophilic agents, which can be xenobiotics (drugs, environmental toxicants, carcinogens), as well as endogenous substances (steroids, bile acids, bilirubin, hormones, dietary constituents). Genes encoding UGTs have been cloned, and there are at least 15 UGTs in the mammalian system. Genetic polymorphisms have been observed in a variety of UGTs, which are responsible for differences in drug metabolism as well as for diseases like Crigler-Najjar's and Gilbert's syndrome.

Ultrarapid Metabolizer

An ultrarapid metabolizer (UM) is a drug metabolism phenotype that describes the ability to metabolize a drug at much faster rates than expected. The term was originally created for individuals who carry an allele of CYP2D6 with two or more functional gene copies, which results in increased enzyme protein being expressed in the liver. This condition can lead to lack of response and therapeutic failure, e.g. during treatment with antidepressants that are CYP2D6 substrates. Reliable prediction of the UM phenotype is not possible based on the genotype alone but requires phenotype determination using a probe drug.

▶ P450 Mono-oxygenase System

U

Unwanted Effects

Adverse Reaction

Urate

▶ Uric Acid

Urea Transporter

UT1, the urea transporter, is an integral membrane protein which is highly selective for urea and is expressed at the apical plasma membrane of principal cells of the collecting duct. The apical plasma membrane is the rate-limiting membrane for overall transcellular urea transport. The UT1 is activated by vasopressin through the V_2 receptor, urea is then transported through the cell into the interstitium. In this way urea contributes to the corticocapillary osmolality gradient, which provides the driving force for water reabsorption in the inner medulla of the kidney.

▶ Vasopressin/Oxytocin

Uric Acid

Uric acid is the endproduct of purine metabolism in man. Uric acid has a lower solubility than its progenitor metabolites, hypoxanthine and xanthine. Impaired uric acid elimination and/or increased uric acid production result in hyperuricemia and increase the risk of gouty arthritis. At physiological pH, 99% of the uric acid molecules are actually in the form of the urate salt. A decrease in pH increases the fraction of uric acid molecules relative to urate molecules. Uric acid possesses lower solubility than urate.

Uricostatic Drug

Uricostatic drugs inhibit the production of uric acid through the inhibition of xanthine oxidase. Allopurinol is the only therapeutically used uricostatic drug.

▶ Anti-gout Drugs

Uricosuric Drug

Uricosuric drugs increase the renal excretion of uric acid by inhibiting its renal reabsorption. Therapeutically used uricosuric drugs are benzbromarone, probenecid and sulfinpyrazone.

▶ Anti-gout Drugs

Urodilatin

Urodilatin is a peptide similar to atrial natriuretic peptide, which is produced in the distal tubule of the kidney and promotes sodium excretion and diuresis by acting on receptors localized on the luminal site of the collecting duct of the nephron.

▶ Guanylyl Cyclases

Urographic Contrast Agents

Urographic contrast agents are contrast agents which possess the characteristics of very little enteral absorption, almost no protein binding or uptake into cells, an extracellular (interstitial) distribution and glomerular filtration. These pharmacokinetics are due to very little interaction with the organism, resulting in very low toxicity, preferably nonionic (neutral) molecules.

▶ Radiocontrast Agents

Urotensin

Urotensin is a cyclic peptide of 11 amino acids, cleaved from a larger prepro-urotensin II precursor peptide of about 130 amino acids. The cyclic region of the peptide, which confers biological activity, has been highly conserved in evolution from fish to mammals. In humans, prepro-urotensin II is expressed mainly in the brain and spinal cord; it is also detected in other tissues, such as kidney, spleen, small intestine, thymus, prostate, pituitary and adrenal gland. In contrast, the receptor for urotensin II is found predominatly in the heart and arterial vessels. Urotensin II is the most potent mammalian vasoconstrictor yet identified, being of the order of 10-fold more potent than endothelin-1. The receptor of urotensin II has recently been identified (GPR14) and belongs to the group of ▶ G-protein-coupled receptors.

Urticaria

Urticaria is a usually transient skin reaction marked by edema and the formation of ▶ wheals, smooth, raised areas.

▶ Histaminergic System
▶ Allergy

UT1

▶ Urea Transporter

U

V

Vaccination

▶ Genetic Vaccination/Nucleic Acid Vaccination

VAChT

Vesicular Acetylcholine Transporters

▶ Vesicular Transporters

Vacuolar-type Proton Translocating ATPase

Vacuolar-type proton translocating ATPase is a heteromeric protein complex which appears to translocate two protons across the vesicle membrane for each ATP molecule that is hydrolyzed, generating chemical (ΔpH) and electrical ($\Delta\Psi$) gradients. Although the ATPases present on different classes of intracellular vesicle have similar functional properties, there are some differences in subunit composition.

▶ Vesicular Transporters

Vanilloid Receptor

The vanilloid receptor is named for its ability to respond to molecules that contain a vanillyl moiety, such as capsaicin, the "hot" component of chili peppers or resiniferatoxin. The vanilliolid receptor mediates the pain evoked by capsaicin. It has been shown to be an ion channel, which belongs to the group of "transient-receptor-potential" (TRP) cation channels. Together with at least four other TRP-channels, it forms the subgroup of TRPV channels. TRPV1 (the vanilloid receptor; VR1) is mainly expressed in the sensory nerves and is activated physiologically by heat (> 43°C), anandermide, phosphatidylinositol 4,5-bisphophate (PIP$_2$) and H$^+$ ions.

▶ TRP Channels

Varizella Zoster Virus

Varizella zoster virus (VZV) is a highly contagious herpesvirus causing chickenpox upon primary infection. After recovery, the virus stays dormant in nerve roots. Weakening of the immune system, e.g. in people over the age of 60 or under immunosuppressive therapy, can lead to reactivation of VZV. This recurrence causes shingles (herpes zoster), a painful rash that develops in a well-defined band corresponding to the area ennervated by the affected nerve cells.

▶ Antiviral Drugs

Vascular Endothelial Growth Factor

Vascular endothelial growth factors are a group of at least 4 growth factors VEGF-A, -B, -C and -D. They exert their biological functions as homodimers, and act almost exclusively on endothelial cells. VEGFs are expressed by almost all cell types and their expression is controlled by a number of different mechanisms including growth factors, cytokines, oncogenes or hypoxia. VEGF expression is controlled by these factors in a time- and tissue-specific fashion during embryonic development and physiological angiogenesis. VEGFs play important roles in embryonic vasculogenesis as well as in embryonic/adult angiogenesis by their effect on endothelial cells. The effects of VEGFs are mediated by the VEGF receptor family, consisting of the 3 members VEGF-R1, -2 and -3, which are receptor-tyrosine-kinases which become activated upon ligand binding. Since VEGF and its receptors have been involved in pathological processes like tumor angiogenesis, rheumatoid arthritis and diabetic retinopathy, monoclonal antibodies or small molecular weight compounds which block the action of VEGFs have been developed as new potential drugs.

▶ Angiogenesis and Vascular Morphogenesis

Vasoactive Intestinal Peptide

Vasoactive Intestinal Peptide(VIP) is a 28-amino acid peptide, which has a variety of actions as a neuroendocrine hormone and a putative neurotransmitter. It stimulates prolactin secretion from the pituitary and catecholamine release from the adrenal medulla. It acts also on cells of the immune system, stimulates electrolyte secretion and relaxes smooth muscles. VIP is produced from a precursor polypeptide (prepro-VIP). Two G-protein coupled receptors have been described which mediate the actions of VIP, $VPAC_1$ (VIP_1, PACAP type II) and $VPAC_2$ (VIP_2, PACAP-3). Both receptors also respond to pituitary adenylate cyclase-activating polypeptide (PACAP) and are coupled via G_S in a stimulatory fashion to adenylyl cyclases. In the autonomic nervous system, VIP is part of the NANC transmitter system. It is typically coexpressed with acetylcholine in postganglionic parasympathetic neurons, and functions as a cotransmitter which is involved in the induction of vasodilatation or bronchodilatation.

▶ Synaptic Transmission
▶ Cotransmission

Vasoconstrictor

Vasoconstrictors are drugs which increase the tone of smooth muscle cells in the vasculature. They include sympathomimetic amines and certain eicosanoids and peptides (angiotensin, vasopressin, urotensin or endothelin).

▶ Smooth Muscle Tone Regulation

Vasodilator

Vasodilators are a group of drugs, which relax the smooth muscle cells of the blood vessels and lead to an increased local tissue blood flow, a reduced arterial pressure and a reduced central venous pressure. Vasodilators reduce the cardiac pre-load as well as after-load and thereby reduce cardiac work. They are used in a variety of conditions including hypertension, cardiac failure and treatment/prevention of angina pectoris. Major groups are Ca^{2+}-channel blockers (e.g. dihydropyridines), NO-donors (e.g. organic nitrates), K^+-channel openers (minoxidil), phosphodiesterase inhibitors (e.g. sildenafil), Rho-kinase inhibitors (e.g. Y27632) or substances with unknown mechanism of action (e.g. hydralazine). Inhibitors of the renin-angiotensin-system (e.g. ACE inhibitors, angiotensin II receptor antagonists or renin inhibitors) also act as vasaldilators.

▶ Smooth Muscle Tone Regulation

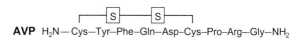

AVP H₂N—Cys—Tyr—Phe—Gln—Asp—Cys—Pro—Arg—Gly—NH₂

Vasopeptidase Inhibitors

Vasopeptidase inhibitors are a group of drugs (e.g. omapatrilat, sampatrilat) which have a dual mechanism of action in that they inhibit two metalloprotease enzymes, neutral endopeptidase (NEP) and angiotensin converting enzyme (ACE). This results in increased availability of natriuretic peptides that exhibit vasodilatory effects (NEP-inhibition) and in reduced formation of angiotensin II (ACE-inhibition). Since these peptidases are intimately concerned with regulating the structural and functional properties of the heart and circulation, they were named "vasopeptidases". Vasopeptidase inhibitors have been developed for the treatment of hypertension or congestive heart failure.

▶ Renin-angiotensin-aldosteron System

Vasopressin/Oxytocin

RICARDO HERMOSILLA
Forschungsinstitut für Molekulare
Pharmakologie, Berlin, Germany
hermosilla@fmp-berlin.de

Synonyms

Vasopressin: 8-arginine-vasopressin (AVP), antidiuretic hormone (ADH), lysipressin
Oxytocin (OT): 8-leucine-vasotocin

Definition

AVP plays a central role in water homeostasis of terrestrial mammals leading to water conservation by the kidney. OT is primarily involved in the event of milk ejection, parturition and in sexual and maternal behavior. Both hormones are peptides secreted by the neurohypophysis and both

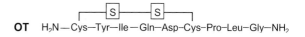

OT H₂N—Cys—Tyr—Ile—Gln—Asp—Cys—Pro—Leu—Gly—NH₂

Fig. 1 Amino acid sequence of AVP and OT. The disulfide bridge between Cys 1 and Cys 6 is shown.

act also as neurotransmitters in the central nervous system (CNS). The mayor hormonal targets for AVP are the renal tubules and vascular myocytes. The hormonal targets for OT are the myoepithelial cells that surround the alveolar channels in the mammary gland and the uterus. AVP plays a central role in pathological processes like ▶ diabetes insipidus (DI) and the syndrome of inappropriate antidiuretic hormone secretion (▶ SIADH).

▶ Diuretics

Basic Characteristics

AVP and OT are cyclic nonapeptides with a disulphur bridge between the cysteine residues 1 and 6, resulting in a six-amino acid ring and a COOH-terminal α-amidated three-residue tail. OT differs only in two amino acids from AVP: Ile in position 3, which is essential for OT receptor (OTR) stimulation and Leu in position 8. AVP has a Phe in position 3 and an Arg in position 8. Arg 8 is essential for acting upon vasopressin receptors (Fig. 1). Lysipressin, found in pigs and some marsupials, has a Lys in position 8 (1).

AVP and OT are synthesized initially as prepro-hormones consisting of a signal peptide, the hormone, the binding protein neurophysin and the glycosylated peptide copeptin (only for vasopressin). This single protein is processed into the final products in neurons located with their cell bodies in the supraoptic (SON) and paraventricular nuclei (PVN) of the hypothalamus. The axons of these cells project to form the neurohypophysis, or posterior pituitary gland, where AVP and OT are secreted after appropriate stimuli. Two

V

populations of neurons exist in the PVN, magnocellular neurons (with large cell bodies) terminating in the neurohypophysis, and parvocellular neurons (with smaller cell bodies) terminating elsewhere in the central nervous system, e.g. median eminence, brain stem, spinal cord, limbic and olfactory areas. Parvocellular neurons terminating in the median eminence are the major source of hypophysiotropic corticotrophin releasing factor (CRF), which is released together with AVP (and possibly also OT) into the hypophysial portal circulation. High concentrations of CRF and AVP are transported by this route to the anterior pituitary gland where they regulate the secretion of adrenocorticotropic hormone (ACTH). The SON contains exclusively magnocellular neurons. Magnocellular and parvocellular neurons produce either AVP or OT (2).

Several other areas of the CNS have also been described to possess non-magnocellular OT-secreting neurons, like the hypothalamic nucleus, thalamic nuclei, hippocampus, amygdala, olfactory bulbs and others, suggesting a role for OT as neurotransmitter in these areas. In addition, several other organs, like the heart, ovary, amnion, chorion, decidua, testis, epididymis and prostate, have been reported to synthesize OT, suggesting a paracrine role for this hormone in these tissues. Ectopic AVP production by lung cancer cells or other neoplasms has been described in humans, leading to SIADH.

The stimuli for AVP secretion are plasma hyperosmolality (sodium), hypovolemia and hypotension. In addition, potent stimuli are nausea and vomiting, less potent are situations leading to acute hypoglycemia. Several drugs induce AVP secretion, either directly, indirectly or by unknown mechanisms, like vincristine, cyclophosphamide, tricyclic antidepressants, apomorphine, nicotine, high doses of morphine and lithium. Lithium however also inhibits the renal effects of AVP. The secretion of AVP is suppressed by ▸ atrial natriuretic peptide, ethanol, opioids (particularly dynorphin), low doses of morphine, phenitoin, dopaminergic antagonists (fluphenazine, haloperidol, promethazine) and carbamazepine which also has a renal antidiuretic action.

The stimuli for OT secretion are the stimulation of the nipples, resulting in the milk ejection reflex, and the distension of cervix and vagina during labor. OT release is also stimulated by plasma hyperosmolality (sodium) and hypervolemia, suggesting a regulatory role in natriuresis and blood volume for this hormone. Secretion also occurs during sexual arousal and ejaculation. OT secretion is suppressed by alcohol and opioids.

AVP and OT elicit their physiological and pharmacological roles through cell surface receptors. The receptors for AVP and OT form a subfamily within the large protein family of G protein-coupled receptors (GPCR). Three different subtypes of AVP receptors are known ($V_{1a}R$, $V_{1b}R$, V_2R). So far, there is only one type of OTR known.

AVP receptors

The $V_{1a}R$ and $V_{1b}R$ selectively couple to G proteins of the $G_{q/11}$ family, which mediate the activation of distinct isoforms of phospholipase Cβ (PLCβ) (Fig. 2). Both receptors have been reported to activate PLD and PLA$_2$. The interaction between the activated GPCR and G protein leads ultimately to the dissociation of the G protein into the active $G\alpha_{(q/11)}$ subunit and the G$\beta\gamma$ heterodimer. The activated $G\alpha_{(q/11)}$ subunit stimulates PLCβ, which catalyses the hydrolysis of phosphatidylinositol 4,5-biphosphate into the second messengers inositol 1,4,5-triphosphate (IP$_3$) and 1,2-diacylglycerol (DAG). IP$_3$ diffuses through the cytosol and binds to the IP$_3$ receptor (IP$_3$R), an intracellular ion channel that mediates the release of calcium from the endoplasmic reticulum (ER). DAG activates protein-kinase C (PKC) which then stimulates the expression of the proto-oncogenes c-fos and c-jun and thereby cell growth. The V_2R activates a G_s protein leading to the activation of adenylyl cyclase (AC) and consequently to a cytosolic cyclic adenosine-monophosphate (cAMP) increase (Fig. 2).

The extrarenal actions of AVP, vasoconstriction, platelet aggregation, and hepatic glycogenolysis are mediated by the $V_{1a}R$ by increasing cytosolic calcium concentrations. This receptor is expressed in the liver (hepatocytes surrounding central veins), vascular and gastrointestinal smooth muscle, bladder, myometrium, platelets, the renal medulla and throughout the brain. It is believed that $V_{1a}R$ function is essential for an efficient response to hypovolemic stress conditions, e.g.: hemorrhagic shock, where AVP is secreted

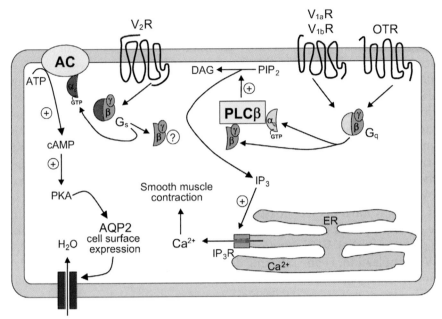

Fig. 2 Schematic representation of the two major signal transduction pathways of AVP and OT receptors. Current pharmacological intervention of both systems is based on selective agonists (AVP or OT analogues) or antagonists, which block the effects of AVP or OT at receptor sites.

copiously. The $V_{1a}R$ in the brain is proposed to mediate the effects of AVP on memory, learning, antipyresis, brain development, selective aggression, partner preferences in rodents, cerebrospinal fluid production and analgesia.

$V_{1b}R$ is mainly expressed in the anterior pituitary, adrenal medulla and kidney. In rats, several other tissues have been found to express this receptor, such as the brain, uterus, thymus, heart, breast, lung and adrenal medulla. The activation of $V_{1b}R$ together with CRF receptors in the anterior pituitary lobe leads to ACTH secretion into the systemic circulation.

V_2R is expressed in epithelial cells of renal collecting ducts; in rodents it is also expressed in cells of the thick ascending limb of Henle's loop (TAL). The antidiuretic function of AVP is mediated by V_2Rs that are located in the basolateral membrane of collecting duct principal cells. V_2R induced G_s-mediated activation of AC, the subsequent increase in cytosolic cAMP, and the stimulation of PKA, lead to the final step of the antidiuretic action of AVP: the exocytic fusion of intracellular vesicles bearing the selective water channel aquaporin-2 (AQP2) (▶ Aquaporins) with the apical membrane of principal collecting duct cells (short-term regulation). The water permeability of the cells increases dramatically (10–20 fold), allowing not only the entry of water via the apical membrane but also the exit across the basolateral membrane through constitutively expressed water channels (AQP3 and AQP4). Due to the osmotic gradient of the inner medulla, water accumulates in the interstitium and is removed by local circulation. AVP withdrawal is associated with endocytic retrieval of AQP2 back into intracellular vesicles. Activation of V_2Rs also stimulates the synthesis of mRNA encoding AQP2 (long-term regulation) in principal cells; it also regulates the apical expression of the urea transporter 1 (UT1) (▶ Urea Transporter). In addition, it regulates the long-term expression and the activation of the Na^+-K^+-$2Cl^-$ symporter in the TAL. These effects contribute to an increase in medullary osmolality and thereby to an enhanced renal water conservation. There is strong evidence for extrarenal V_2R expression; several organs have been implicated, like lungs, heart, skeletal muscle, inner ear and endothelial cells. The administration of a selective V_2R agonist (desmopressin) to patients suffering from X-linked congenital nephrogenic diabetes insipidus (V_2R gene defect) does not result in an expected increase of factor VIII, von Willebrand factor, and tissue plasminogen activator in the blood. The therapeutic utilisation of desmopressin for coagulation disorders like haemophilia A and von Willebrand's disease relies on the existence of extrarenal V_2R.

Congenital Nephrogenic Diabetes Insipidus (X-linked, autosomal)

Congenital nephrogenic diabetes insipidus (NDI) is a rare disease, characterized by an inability to concentrate urine despite normal or elevated AVP plasma concentrations. The syndrome is characterized by polyuria and polydipsia. If not treated, episodes of dehydration can result in mental retardation in newborn. Other symptoms include vomiting, anorexia, failure to thrive and constipation. The more common form is the X-linked NDI, caused by mutations in the V_2R gene. More than 150 different mutations of the V_2R have been found in NDI patients. The excessive water loss through the kidney is due to an improper V_2R function. Mutations of the V_2R can lead to: 1) an altered affinity for AVP (K_D decreased) or 2) an altered coupling to the G_s protein (▶ EC_{50} increased), 3) an altered mRNA synthesis or stability, and 4) the most common form, an altered transport to the cell surface (intracellular retained receptor). The autosomal NDI form, caused by mutations in the AQP2 gene, is extremely rare (3). In contrast to patients suffering from the X-linked NDI form, patients with the autosomal form show the typical coagulation response to desmopressin.

OT Receptor

The multiple hormonal and neurotransmitter functions of OT are mediated by the specific OTR which activates PLCβ and increases cytosolic calcium (see Fig. 2). These effects are mediated by the activation of the G protein $G_{q/11}$. The increase in cytosolic calcium concentrations is the main trigger for smooth muscle contraction. The OTR also binds AVP with relatively high affinity.

There is only one OTR known so far. Nevertheless, ▶ posttranslational modifications and interactions with downstream signal transduction components may modify OTR signaling. The OTR is differentially expressed in various tissues, mainly in myoepithelial cells of the galactiferus channels and the myometrium. The endometrium, ovary, decidua, amnion, testis, epididymis, prostate, thymus, and hypothalamus also express OTR, reaffirming the concept of a paracrine role of this peptide. Osteoblasts, a breast cancer cell line (MCF7) and vascular endothelium cells are also described to express OTRs. Expression of the OTR

has also been described in the brain (neurons and astrocytes), with patterns differing in sex, age and species, which may be related to different patterns of sexual and maternal behavior.

There are several hints indicating a strong interaction between the OTR and sexual hormones. During pregnancy, high plasma progesterone levels promote uterine relaxation and inhibit the function of the OTR system by both genomic and nongenomic mechanisms. The myometrial OTRs are more abundantly expressed after estrogen secretion, in the last days of pregnancy. It is possible that progesterone and estrogens act in opposing manner on the function, expression, and/or regulation of OTRs. However, despite the striking dependence of the OT system on gonadal hormones, the human OTR gene does not contain a classical steroid responsive element and nongenomic mechanisms are not well characterized. Although OT plasma concentrations remain relatively constant until labor itself, uterine sensitivity to OT is markedly increased around onset of labor. This is associated with both an upregulation of OTR mRNA levels and a strong increase in the density of myometrial OTRs, reaching a peak during early labor (200 times higher than in the nonpregnant state). Thus, at onset of labor, OT can stimulate uterine contractions at plasma concentrations that are ineffective in the nonpregnant state. After parturition, the concentrations of uterine OTRs rapidly decline. This downregulation of OTRs may be necessary to avoid unwanted contractile responses during lactation when OT plasma levels are raised (1).

Although the OT system may be regarded as a key regulator of parturition, in OT-deficient mice, parturition remains unaffected. Moreover, OTR knockout mice deliver in a normal fashion, but the offspring die during the very first days of life due to starvation as the milk ejection reflex is absent in these animals. These experiments show that the OT system is not essential for labor or reproductive behavior (at least in mice) but for the milk ejection reflex, which is fundamental for litter survival.

OTRs are also expressed in male reproductive tissues, like testis, epididymis and in the prostate. OT increases the resting tone of prostatic tissue from guinea pig, rat, dog and human. The activation of these receptors by OT could lead to the contraction of the prostate and the resulting expulsion of prostatic secretions during ejaculation.

Drugs

AVP receptors

Agonists. AVP is mainly used in the replacement therapy in ▶ central diabetes insipidus (CDI), but has only a short effect of 4–6 h. It is also used in the therapy of gastrointestinal hemorrhage (e.g. bleeding from esophageal varices), as a vasopressor during cardiac arrest and in the treatment of adult shock-refractory ventricular fibrillation. The major disadvantages of AVP in CDI therapy are its non-selective effects ($V_{1a}R$ stimulation), short duration and contraction of the uterus and gastrointestinal tract. Otherwise, former effects of AVP are useful to treat postoperative ileus and abdominal distension and to eliminate gas before abdominal radiographs.

The synthetic AVP analogue 1-deamino,8-D-arginine vasopressin (dDAVP) or desmopressin, is a selective V_2R agonist. Its antidiuretic effect is longer than AVP and it does not cause vasoconstriction and is better tolerated than AVP. Desmopressin is used in the treatment of CDI, by intranasal spray application. It is also used in the therapy of nocturnal enuresis. Another important clinical application of desmopressin is the treatment of hemophilia A (factor VIII) and von Willebrand's disease. Lysipressin is also available for intranasal application. The major complication of AVP, lysipressin and desmopressin is water intoxication with hyponatremia (iatrogenic SIADH).

OPC-51803 is a novel nonpeptide and a highly selective V_2R agonist that may be proven useful in treating CDI, urinary incontinence, enuresis and poliakiuria. It has a much higher bioavailability after oral ingestion than desmopressin.

Antagonists. There are several nonpeptide, orally active V_2 selective receptor antagonists under development (OPC-31260, SR-121463A, VPA-985), also known as ▶ aquaretic agents. Their main applications could be the treatment of water disorders caused by congestive heart failure, liver cirrhosis, nephrotic syndrome and SIADH. Dual V_{1a}/V_2R antagonists (YM-087) could also become useful for diseases such as congestive heart failure, in which increased peripheral resistance and dilutional hyponatremia are both present (4).

OTR

Agonists. OT is mainly used intravenously for labor induction without major side effects. It is also used in postpartum bleeding and to facilitate milk ejection in mastitic cows. Carbetocin, a long-acting OT analogue with modifications in the terminal cystein residue and in the disulphur bridge, is used to control bleeding after delivery, mainly in veterinary medicine.

Antagonists. Atosiban is an antagonist peptide of OTR and $V_{1a}R$. It is successfully used intravenously as an OTR antagonist in preterm labor. This peptide antagonist was shown to inhibit uterine contractions in women with threatened and established preterm labor, with an improved side effect profile when compared to ritodrine (β_2-simpathomimetic). Another potential use of atosiban is in benign prostate hyperplasia, as it is known, that OTRs play an important role in prostate contraction. Other nonpeptide OTR antagonists are under development (5).

References

1. Gimpl G, Fahrenholz F (2001) The oxytocin receptor system: structure, function, and regulation. Physiol Rev 81:629–683
2. Burbach JP, Luckman SM, Murphy D, Gainer H (2001) Gene regulation in the magnocellular hypothalamo-neurohypophysial system. Physiol Rev 81:1197–1267
3. Oksche A, Rosenthal W (1998) The molecular basis of nephrogenic diabetes insipidus. J Mol Med 76:326–337
4. Thibonnier M, Coles P, Thibonnier A, Shoham M (2001) The basic and clinical pharmacology of nonpeptide vasopressin receptor antagonists. Annu Rev Pharmacol Toxicol 41:175–202
5. Thorton S, Vatish M, Slater D (2001) Oxytocin antagonists: clinical and scientific considerations. Exp Physiol 86:297–302

V

Vasorelaxant

▶ Vasodilator

Vav

Vav proteins are guanine nucleotide exchange factors (GEF) for monomeric GTPases. The Vav proteins belong to the DBL family of Rho GEFs and have an important role in regulating early events in receptor signalling.

▶ Phospholipid Kinases
▶ Small GTPases

Vegetarian

There are different degrees of vegetarianism. Ovo-lacto vegetarians avoid meat and fish, but consume eggs and milk. Lacto-vegetarians only consume milk, but no eggs. Vegans or strict vegetarians eat no animal-derived products whatsoever, some even excluding honey from their diets.

VEGF

▶ Vascular Endothelial Growth Factor

Venus Flytrap (VFT) Module

The VFT module is a protein module first characterized in bacteria, where it is involved in the transport through the periplasm of small molecules like amino acids, ions, peptides and sugars. Since then, a similar protein module has been

shown to regulate the activity of operons (like the amidase operon that controls the expression of the amidase enzyme) and to be in the ▶ guanylyl cyclase and ▶ metabotropic glutamate receptors, for which it constitutes the ligand binding domain. This module is composed of two lobes interconnected by two or three linkers. In most cases, the two lobes are separated by a wide cleft in which the ligand binds. Binding of the ligand stabilizes a closed form of the protein, so that the ligand is trapped like an insect trapped between the two lobed of the leaves of the carnivorous plant "Venus Flytrap".

▶ G-protein Coupled Receptors

Very Low Density Lipoprotein

Very low density lipoprotein (VLDL) is a type of lipoprotein that mainly carries triglycerides (neutral fat) in the blood circulation.

▶ HMG-CoA-reductase Inhibitors

Vesicle

Vesicles are transport containers that are formed upon recruitment of coat proteins from a donor membrane and that fuse with an acceptor membrane.

▶ Intracellular Transport
▶ Exocytosis

Vesicular Acetylcholine Transporter

VAChT

▶ Vesicular Transporters

Vesicular Transporters

RICHARD REIMER AND ROBERT EDWARDS
Departments of Neurology and Physiology,
University of California at San Francisco,
San Francisco, USA
rjreimer@stanford.edu, edwards@itsa.ucsf.edu

Synonyms

Synaptic vesicle neurotransmitter transporters,
▶ VMAT1, VMAT2, ▶ VGAT/VIAAT, ▶ VGLUT1,
VGLUT2, ▶ VAChT

Definition

The exocytotic release of neurotransmitters from
synaptic vesicles underlies most information
processing by the brain. Since classical neurotransmitters including monamines, acetylcholine,
GABA and glutamate are synthesized in the cytoplasm, a mechanism is required for their accumulation in synaptic vesicles. Vesicular transporters
are multitransmembrane domain proteins that
mediate this process by coupling the movement of
neurotransmitters to the proton electrochemical
gradient across the vesicle membrane.

▶ Neurotransmitter Transporters
▶ Organic Cation Transporters

Basic Characteristics

Synaptic vesicles isolated from brain exhibit four
distinct vesicular neurotransmitter transport
activities: one for monoamines, a second for acetylcholine, a third for the inhibitory neurotransmitters GABA and glycine and a fourth for glutamate. Unlike Na^+-dependent plasma membrane
transporters, the vesicular activities couple to a
proton electrochemical gradient ($\Delta\mu_{H+}$) across the
vesicle membrane generated by the vacuolar H^+-
ATPase (▶ vacuolar type proton translocating
ATPase). Although all of the vesicular transport
systems rely on $\Delta\mu_{H+}$, the relative dependence on
the chemical and electrical components varies.
The vesicular monoamine and acetylcholine

transport systems depend primarily on the chemical component of this gradient (ΔpH), whereas
transport of GABA relies on both ΔpH and the
electrical component of the gradient ($\Delta\psi$), and
glutamate transport almost exclusively on $\Delta\psi$.
These bioenergetic differences appear to reflect
differences in protein structure.

Vesicular Monoamine Transport

The vesicular monoamine transporters were identified in a screen for genes that confer resistance to
the parkinsonian neurotoxin MPP^+. The resistance apparently results from sequestration of the
toxin inside vesicles, away from its primary site of
action in mitochondria. In addition to recognizing MPP^+, the transporters mediate the uptake of
dopamine, serotonin, epinephrine and norepinephrine by neurons and endocrine cells. Structurally, the vesicular monoamine transporters
(VMATs) show no relationship to plasma membrane monoamine transporters.

VMAT1 is expressed in the adrenal medulla, by
small intensely fluorescent cells in sympathetic
ganglia, and by other non-neural cells that release
monoamines. In contrast, VMAT2 is expressed by
neuronal populations in the nervous system. The
substrate specificity for the two isoforms is similar, but VMAT2 has a somewhat higher apparent
affinity for all monoamines than VMAT1. In addition, only VMAT2 appears able to transport histamine, consistent with its expression by mast cells.

Transport by the VMATs involves the exchange
of two lumenal protons for one cytoplasmic,
apparently protonated molecule of transmitter,
predicting accumulation of transmitter inside vesicles 10^4–10^5 the concentrations in cytoplasm.
Using reserpine binding (see below), a number of
residues appear to be required for substrate recognition; reserpine still binds to these mutants, but
cannot be displaced by substrates. In addition,
$\Delta\mu_{H+}$ accelerates reserpine binding to wildtype
VMAT2, suggesting that H^+ efflux reorients the
substrate recognition site to the cytoplasmic face
of the membrane. The substrate recognition
mutants do not affect this stimulation by $\Delta\mu_{H+}$.
However, substition of an aspartate in predicted
transmembrane domain (TMD) 10 of the VMATs
by a neutral residue abolishes reserpine binding
even in the presence of $\Delta\mu_{H+}$, and replacement by
glutamate shifts the pH sensitivity of transport,

V

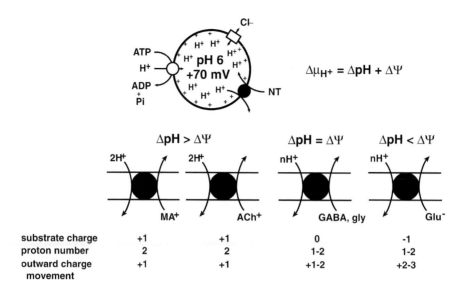

$$\Delta\mu_{H^+} = \Delta pH + \Delta\Psi$$

	$\Delta pH > \Delta\Psi$	$\Delta pH > \Delta\Psi$	$\Delta pH = \Delta\Psi$	$\Delta pH < \Delta\Psi$
	$2H^+$ / MA^+	$2H^+$ / ACh^+	nH^+ / $GABA, gly$	nH^+ / Glu^-
substrate charge	+1	+1	0	-1
proton number	2	2	1-2	1-2
outward charge movement	+1	+1	+1-2	+2-3

Fig. 1 Stoichiometry and bioenergetic dependence of the vesicular neurotransmitter transporters. The proton electrochemical gradient ($\Delta\mu_{H^+}$) that drives neurotransmitter transport into secretory vesicles is generated by the vacuolar-type proton translocating ATPase and consists of a 1–2 unit pH gradient (ΔpH) and a transmembrane potential ($\Delta\Psi$) ~+70 mV (inside positive). The different families of transport proteins exhibit different dependences on these two components of the gradient, with VMATs and VAChT most dependent on ΔpH, VGLUTs on $\Delta\Psi$, and VGAT dependent on both. These differences in dependence on $\Delta\mu_{H^+}$ reflect differences in the stoichiometry of transport.

suggesting that this residue contributes to H^+ translocation. In terms of structure, a lysine in TMD2 also appears to form a charge pair with an aspartate in TMD11.

Vesicular Acetylcholine Transport

Closely related to the VMATs, the vesamicol-sensitive vesicular acetylcholine transporter (VAChT) was identified in a screen for mutants resistant to inhibition of acetylcholinesterase in *C. elegans*. Like VMATs, VAChT recognizes a cationic substrate and depends primarily on ΔpH. In contrast to VMATs, with substrate affinities in the low or sub-micromolar, the mammalian VAChT exhibits an apparent affinity around 1 mM. The higher affinity of VMATs may reflect the need to lower cytoplasmic levels of potentially toxic monoamine transmitters. However, VAChT has been postulated to have a similar stoichiometry for 2 H^+, but to exhibit as well a H^+ leak not present with the VMATs.

Vesicular GABA Transport

Genetic and behavioral studies in the nematode *C. elegans* led to identification of the vesicular GABA transporter (VGAT.) As predicted from studies with purified synaptic vesicles, VGAT mediates uptake of GABA with an apparent affinity in the low millimolar range and can be driven by ΔpH or $\Delta\psi$. VGAT also recognizes glycine as a substrate, suggesting that these two inhibitory neurotransmitters can be stored in and released from the same vesicle.

VGAT shows no sequence similarity to VMATs or VAChT. Rather, it belongs to a large family of transporters that includes H^+-coupled amino acid permeases in *Arabidopsis thaliana* and several mammalian proteins. One of the related mammalian transport proteins corresponds to classical amino acid transport System N, and others correspond to classical System A, which is responsible for much of the active amino acid uptake by mammalian cells. These glutamine transporters appear to mediate aspects of the glutamine-glutamate cycle involved in nitrogen metabolism by the liver and in the regeneration of glutamate from glutamine required for excitatory neurotransmission. The System N transporter SN1 mediates glutamine efflux readily under physiological conditions and is expressed by astrocytes. In contrast, System A transporters SA1 and 2 primarily mediate glutamine uptake, and the expression of SA2 by neurons positions it to facilitate the uptake of glutamine released from astrocytes by SN1. The principal difference between System N and A transporters appears to be the translocation of H^+; SN1 mediates the exchange of H^+ for Na^+ and an amino acid whereas SA1 and 2 mediate only Na^+ cotransport.

Vesicular Glutamate Transport

Glutamate is the principal excitatory neurotransmitter in the mammalian central nervous system, yet the vesicular glutamate transporter eluded identification until recently. Initially isolated in a screen for genes upregulated by subtoxic doses of the excitotoxin N-methyl-D-aspartate, the brain-specific Na^+-dependent phosphate transporter (BNPI) resembled a class of ▶ inorganic phosphate transporters and conferred Na^+-dependent phosphate transport in *Xenopus* oocytes. Although suggested to participate in the regeneration of ATP at nerve terminals, BNPI expression is restricted to excitatory neurons, suggesting a more specific role in glutamate release. Indeed, the enzyme glutaminase that produces glutamate for release as an excitatory transmitter requires inorganic phosphate for activity. Further, studies in *C. elegans* indicated a specific role for the BNPI orthologue EAT-4 in glutamate release. Recent work has suggested that other type I phosphate transporters related to BNPI mediate the transport of organic anions with higher affinity than phosphate. Together with the determination that BNPI localizes to synaptic vesicles, this suggested an alternative role for the protein in vesicular glutamate transport.

Heterologous expression of BNPI in a variety of cell systems indeed confers vesicular glutamate uptake with all of the properties demonstrated using synaptic vesicles from brain. In particular, glutamate uptake by BNPI depends primarily on $\Delta\psi$ rather than ΔpH, does not recognize aspar-

tate, has an apparent affinity in the low millimolar, and shows a biphasic dependence on chloride with an optimum at 2–10 mM. BNPI has thus been renamed VGLUT1. In addition, vesicular glutamate transport by VGLUT1 leads to vesicle acidification, as previously demonstrated using native synaptic vesicle preparations. Presumably, a reduction in electrical potential caused by influx of the anionic glutamate secondarily activates the H^+-ATPase. However, VGLUT1 and other related proteins also appear to exhibit a substantial chloride conductance that is blocked by substrate.

Although the expression of VGLUT1 is limited to a subset of glutamatergic neurons in the brain, a highly homologous protein, also initially characterized as a phosphate transporter and named differentiation-associated Na^+-dependent phosphate transporter (DNP1), has a complementary pattern of expression. DNP1 also localizes to synaptic vesicles, mediates the vesicular uptake of glutamate and has been renamed VGLUT2. Although VGLUT2 exhibits transport activity very similar to VGLUT1, VGLUT2 appears to be expressed by a subset of glutamate neurons with a higher probability of release, and differences in subcellular location suggest differences in trafficking. In particular, the presence of two polyproline domains in the C-terminal cytoplasmic tail of VGLUT1 may mediate interactions with proteins containing SH3 domains that have been shown to be involved in synaptic vesicle recycling.

Vesicular Storage of Zinc, ATP and Neuropeptides

Synaptic vesicles mediate the release of small molecules other than classical neurotransmitters and neuropeptides. Of these, zinc and ATP are the best characterized. NMDA and GABA receptors contain binding sites for zinc, and zinc exerts a direct effect on excitatory and inhibitory neurotransmission. ATP activates both ionotropic and G protein-coupled receptors. As with the classical neurotransmitters, the exocytotic release of these compounds requires transport into synaptic vesicles.

Indirect evidence supports a role for ZnT3 in zinc uptake by synaptic vesicles. ZnT3 belongs to a family of zinc transporters and localizes to synaptic vesicles. Further, mice deficient in ZnT3 show a loss of zinc staining from hippocampal neurons. However, it has not been demonstrated that ZnT3 mediates zinc uptake in heterologous expression

V

systems. On the other hand, ZnT3 targeting to synaptic vesicles has been shown to depend on the adaptor protein AP3. In *mocha* mice deficient in AP3, synaptic vesicles accumulate normally, but no longer contain ZnT3 or zinc.

Chromaffin granules, platelet dense core vesicles and synaptic vesicles accumulate ATP. ATP uptake has been demonstrated using chromaffin granules and synaptic vesicles and the process appears to depend on $\Delta\mu_{H+}$. It has generally been assumed that ATP is costored only with monoamines and acetylcholine, as an anion to balance to cationic charge of those transmitters. However, the extent of ATP storage and release by different neuronal populations remains unknown, and the proteins responsible for ATP uptake by secretory vesicles have not been identified.

Unlike classical neurotransmitters, neuropeptides enter the lumen of the secretory pathway in the endoplasmic reticulum, through cotranslational translocation. They then sort to large dense core vesicles (LDCVs) in the trans-Golgi network (TGN) and undergo processing to form the biologically active species. LDCV exocytosis exhibits a different dependence from synaptic vesicles on stimulation and calcium concentration. After release, neuropeptides undergo degradation; they are generally not repackaged, although certain lumenal contents of dense core vesicles can remain tethered to the plasma membrane.

Regulation of Vesicular Transporters

Regulation of transmitter release may involve changes in the probability of release, or in the amount of transmitter per synaptic vesicle. A variety of mechanisms are known to regulate the probability of vesicle release. Similarly, changes in the amount of transmitter per vesicle, or quantal size, occur in several systems, including the neuromuscular junction. The mechanisms by which quantal size changes, however, remain less well characterized. Nonetheless, modulation of vesicular transport can clearly influence quantal size. VMAT2 knockout mice die shortly after birth, but heterozygous animals also exhibit substantial reductions in monoamine release, and alterations in behavior relative to wildtype litter mates. Conversely, over-expression of either VMAT2 or VAChT can increase quantal size.

Regulation of transporter expression may occur at the transcriptional level. Both VGLUTs were identified as genes upregulated by specific stimuli; VGLUT1 in response to an excitotoxin and VGLUT2 to the growth factor activin. The organization of the VAChT gene within an exon of the biosynthetic enzyme choline acetyl transferase further indicates a remarkable level of transcriptional coordination. In addition to transcriptional regulation of the VGLUTs, VMATs appear to be regulated by G proteins. Activation of the G protein $G\alpha_{O2}$ down-regulates their activity independent of $\Delta\mu_{H+}$, but the mechanism remains unclear.

The major mechanisms for regulation of vesicular neurotransmitter transport appear to involve changes in membrane trafficking. VMATs undergo phosphorylation by casein kinase and this posttranslational modification influences their retrieval from maturing LDCVs. In addition, phosphorylation of VAChT upstream from a dileucine-like motif influences sorting into LDCVs at the level of the TGN. Since sorting to LDCVs versus synaptic vesicles will determine the site and mode of transmitter release, the regulation of transporter trafficking has great potential to influence signalling. In particular, it is well known that midbrain neurons release dopamine from their cell bodies and dendrites as well as from their terminals, and the trafficking of VMAT2 presumably contributes to these two very different modes of release.

Drugs

VMATs are irreversibly inhibited by the potent antihypertensive drug reserpine. The depressive effects of reserpine helped to formulate the original monoamine hypothesis of affective disorders. Reserpine also appears to interact with the transporters near the site of substrate recognition. Tetrabenazine, which is used in treatment of movement disorders, inhibits VMAT2 much more potently than VMAT1, consistent with the less hypotensive action of this agent.

VMATs are not inhibited by drugs such as cocaine, tricyclic antidepressants and selective serotonin reuptake inhibitors that affect plasma membrane monoamine transport. Amphetamines have relatively selective effects on monoaminergic cells due to selective uptake by plasma membrane monoamine transporters, but their effect appears to be mediated by their ability as weak bases to reduce ΔpH, the driving force for vesicular monoamine transport that leads to efflux of the vesicular contents into the cytoplasm.

The vesicular acetylcholine transport can be inhibited by vesamicol and several related compounds. Vesamicol competitively inhibits transport by binding to a cytoplasmic domain on VAChT with a K_d of approximately 5 nM. Vesamicol binding can be used to estimate transporter number, but neither vesamicol nor its analogues are currently used clinically.

Vesicular GABA transport can be competitively inhibited by amino acids including glycine and β-alanine. Transport can also be competitively inhibited by γ-vinyl GABA, a derivative of GABA. γ-Vinyl GABA has been used in the clinical treatment of epilepsy and is known to inhibit GABA transaminase, an enzyme that metabolizes GABA. The mode of action for γ-vinyl GABA as an antiepileptic drug is thought to be through its effects on GABA transaminase, but inhibition of vesicular GABA transport could have an effect by increasing the non-vesicular release of GABA.

Several compounds that inhibit vesicular glutamate transport have been identified: These include the dyes Evans Blue and Rose Bengal. In addition, the stilbene derivative 4,4′-diisothiocyanatostilbene-2,2′-disulfonic acid (DIDS), a compound commonly used as a specific inhibitor of anion channels, inhibits vesicular glutamate transport. Most known inhibitors have limited use as they are membrane impermeant.

In addition to direct inhibition of the vesicular transport protein, storage of neurotransmitters can be reduced by dissipation of the proton electrochemical gradient. Bafilomycin (a specific inhibitor of the vacuolar H^+-ATPase), as well as the proton ionophores carbonyl cyanide m-chlorophenylhydrazone (CCCP) and carbonylcyanide p-(trifluoromethoxy) phenylhydrazone (FCCP) are used experimentally to reduce the vesicular storage of neurotransmitters. Weak bases including amphetamines and ammonium chloride are used to selectively reduce ΔpH.

References

1. Liu Y, Edwards RH (1997) The role of vesicular transport proteins in synaptic transmission and neural degeneration. Annu Rev Neurosci. 20:125–156
2. Parsons SM (2000) Transport mechanisms in acetylcholine and monoamine storage. FASEB J. 14(15):2423–2434
3. Reimer RJ, Fon EA, Edwards RH (1998) Vesicular neurotransmitter transport and the presynaptic regulation of quantal size. Curr Opin Neurobiol. 8(3):405–412
4. Reimer RJ, Fremeau RT Jr, Bellocchio EE, Edwards RH (2001) The essence of excitation. Curr Opin Cell Biol. 13(4):417–421
5. Schuldiner S, Shirvan A, Linial M (1995) Vesicular neurotransmitter transporters: from bacteria to humans. Physiol Rev. 75(2):369–392

VGAT/VIAAT

Vesicular GABA transporter; vesicular inhibitory amino acid transporte.

▶ Vesicular Transporters

VGLUT

VGLUT is short for vesicular glutamate transporter.

▶ Vesicular Transporters

V

Vinca Alkaloids

Vinca alkaloids are derived from the Madagascar periwinkle plant, *Catharanthus roseus*. The main alkaloids are vincristine, vinblastine and vindesine. Vinca alkaloids are cell-cycle-specific agents and block cells in mitosis. This cellular activity is due to their ability to bind specifically to tubulin and to block the ability of the protein to polymerize into microtubules. This prevents spindle formation in mitosing cells and causes arrest at metaphase. Vinca alkaloids also inhibit other cellular activities that involve microtubules, such as leukocyte phagocytosis and chemotaxis as well as axonal transport in neurons. Side effects of the vinca alkaloids such as their neurotoxicity may be due to disruption of these functions.

▶ Antineoplastic Agents

VIP

▶ Vasoactive Intestinal Peptide

Viral Proteases

CHRISTIAN STEINKÜHLER
IRBM - Merck Research Laboratories,
Pomezia, Italy
Christian_Steinkuhler@Merck.Com

Synonyms

Viral proteinases

Definition

Viral proteases are enzymes (endopeptidases EC 3.4.2) encoded by the genetic material (DNA or RNA) of viral pathogens. The role of these enzymes is to catalyze the cleavage of specific peptide bonds in viral polyprotein precursors or in cellular proteins. In most cases these proteolytic events are essential for the completion of the viral infectious cycle. Viral proteases may use different catalytic mechanisms involving either serine, cysteine or aspartic acid residues to attack the scissile peptide bond. This bond is often located within conserved sequence motifs extending for up to 10 residues. Selective recognition of these sequence patterns by a complementary substrate

binding site of the enzyme ensures a high degree of specific recognition and cleavage.

▶ Antiviral Drugs
▶ Non-viral Proteases

Basic Characteristics

The majority of approved antiviral pharmaceuticals belong to the category of nucleoside analogs that target viral polymerases. Adverse side effects, moderate clinical efficacy and especially the rapid emergence of drug-resistant mutant strains limits the efficacy of these inhibitors in monotherapy of chronic viral infections. Proteolytic maturation of large precursor proteins, catalyzed by virally encoded proteases, is a widespread strategy especially in viruses using RNA as genetic material. Since 1995, protease inhibitors have been successfully added to the therapeutic regimens of ▶ HIV infected individuals, and protease inhibitors are presently being developed to control other chronic viral infections such as ▶ hepatitis C (HCV). The infectious cycles of a retrovirus (such as the human immunodeficiency virus HIV), and of a (+)-strand-RNA virus (such as the hepatitis C virus, HCV) are schematically shown below. Both viruses use RNA as genetic material but in contrast to (+)-strand RNA viruses, retroviral genomes are back-transcribed into a double stranded DNA molecule by a reverse transcriptase contained inside the viral particle and delivered to the cell during infection (▶ reverse transcription).

The HIV genome is organized into three major coding elements called *gag, pol* and *env* (1). Upon integration of the provirus into the host cell genome, multiple copies of viral RNA are produced by hijacking the cellular transcription machinery. This RNA may have one of three different fates: A fraction of viral RNAs is reserved as genomes for new viral particles. Another fraction is spliced to yield subgenomic mRNA species that will be translated on membrane-bound polysomes to give rise to the *env* protein gp160, which is subsequently cleaved by cellular proteases into the envelope glycoproteins gp120 and gp41. Finally, a third fraction is used as mRNA for *gag* and *pol*. These gene products are produced as a nested set of precursor polyproteins such that the relative amount of *gag-pol* peptides (p160) is only 5% as

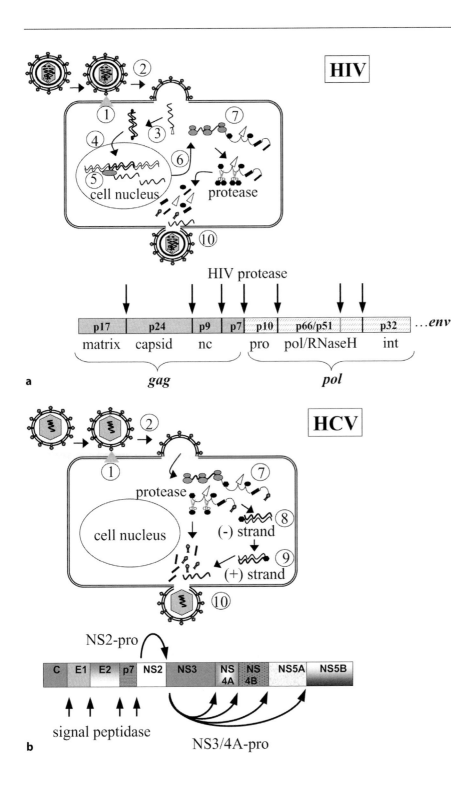

cell nucleus

protease

HIV protease

p17	p24	p9	p7	p10	p66/p51	p32	...*env*

matrix   capsid   nc   pro   pol/RNaseH   int

a $\underbrace{\qquad\qquad}_{\textit{gag}}$ $\underbrace{\qquad\qquad}_{\textit{pol}}$

HCV

protease

cell nucleus

(-) strand

(+) strand

NS2-pro

C	E1	E2	p7	NS2	NS3	NS 4A	NS 4B	NS5A	NS5B

signal peptidase

b   NS3/4A-pro

Fig. 1 Role of virally-encoded proteases in the replication cycle of a retrovirus (HIV, part a) and of a (+)-strand RNA virus (HCV, part b). The numbers correspond to the following steps in the infectious cycle: (1) binding to cell surface receptor; (2) fusion; (3) reverse transcription; (4) integration; (5) transcription by host cell RNA polymerase; (6) RNA export and splicing; (7) translation; (8) (-)-strand synthesis; (9) (+)-strand synthesis; (10) assembly and budding of new viral particle. The proteolytic cleavage sites in the HIV gag-pol precursor and in the HCV polyprotein are schematically shown.

abundant as *gag* peptides (p55). This relationship is maintained by partial bypassing of a translational stop signal at the end of *gag*. The *pol* gene encodes the viral enzymes protease, reverse transcriptase and ▶ integrase. Following a not well-

understood autocatalytic event, the protease is released and performs nine different cleavages in the *gag* and *gag-pol* precursor proteins. Mutations in the protease lead to the generation of defective, noninfectious particles, demonstrating the essential role of this enzyme in the viral infectious cycle. The HIV protease belongs to the family of aspartic acid proteases (E.C.3.4.23) and is closely related to cellular enzymes such as renin, cathepsin D or pepsin. The structure of the HIV protease has been extensively studied by X-ray crystallography both, in its free form and complexed to inhibitors. It is a homodimer consisting of two identical polypeptide chains of 99 residues each. Each monomer contributes one catalytic aspartic acid residue in the active site, which is located at the dimer interface. Well-defined subsites and two flexible flap regions protruding over the active site contribute to specific recognition of substrates and inhibitors.

Reverse transcriptase and protease inhibitors interfere at different stages within the viral replication cycle. The former class of compounds (nucleoside analogs or non-nucleoside inhibitors) blocks infection at an early step prior to integration of the retro-transcribed viral genome into the genome of the host cell. Consistent with this mode of action, reverse transcriptase inhibitors are ineffective in arresting the spread of viruses from cells that are already infected. This is in contrast to protease inhibitors that act at a late stage of the infectious cycle. Many present therapeutic regimens simultaneously target both HIV enzymes by combining protease inhibitors with nucleoside analogs such as AZT, ddC, ddI, d4T or 3TC or nonnucleoside reverse-transcriptase inhibitors (nevirapine, efavirenz, delavirdine).

The infectious cycle of a (+)-strand RNA virus such as the hepatitis C virus differs by the fate of the viral RNA genome in the infected cell. Upon entry into the cell, the HCV genome is used as a messenger RNA to drive the synthesis of a large polyprotein precursor of about 3000 residues (2). The structural proteins are excised from the precursor by host cell signal peptidase. The nonstructural region of the precursor, harboring the viral replication machinery, is cut into its mature components in a maturation reaction in which two viral proteases (NS2-pro and NS3/4A-pro) cooperate. Site-directed mutagenesis of an otherwise infectious cDNA has shown that both HCV-encoded proteases are necessary for viral infectivity, but most of the attention has so far been focused on one of them; a member of the serine protease family (EC 3.4.21) located in the N-termi-

nal region of the viral NS3 protein. The proteolytic activity of NS3 is turned on only upon binding to the cofactor NS4A, generating the active NS3/4A heterodimeric protease, and is used to perform a total of four different cleavages. The mature viral RNA-dependent RNA polymerase, the protein NS5B, also arises from one of these processing events. This enzyme subsequently replicates the viral genome in a two-step process involving a (–)-strand intermediate.

In contrast to retroviruses, proteolysis is an early event in the replication cycle of (+)-strand RNA viruses and both protease and polymerase inhibitors can be expected to halt the propagation of infectious viral particles from already infected cells.

The three-dimensional structure of the NS3 protease, either alone or in complex with its NS4A cofactor, was solved by both X-ray crystallography and by NMR spectroscopy. The enzyme adopts a chymotrypsin-like fold with two β-barrel domains contributing the residues that make up the catalytic triad; a histidine an aspartic acid and a serine residue. Comparison of structures obtained in the presence or in the absence of the cofactor lead to the conclusion that NS4A serves to stabilize the fold of the N-terminal beta-barrel of the protease thereby promoting the correct positioning of the catalytic machinery. In striking contrast to the HIV protease, there are no pronounced pockets or cavities in the proximity of the active site of NS3 that could serve to anchor inhibitors or substrates. Nevertheless, this protease is highly specific in binding to and processing of peptides with a consensus sequence spanning over ten residues. Specificity is conferred to this molecular recognition event by a series of weak interactions which are dispersed along a very extended interaction surface that involve hydrogen bonds, hydrophobic interactions and a crucial electrostatic complementarity between enzyme and active site ligand.

Drugs

HIV Protease inhibitors

So far, 5 different protease inhibitors have been approved by the FDA for the treatment of HIV infection (3, 4). Clinical trials in which protease inhibitors were evaluated in monotherapy demonstrated the potency of this class of inhibitors (decrease in HIV RNA levels, increase in CD4 cell counts). Treatment regimens were subsequently broadened to include reverse transcriptase inhibitors in combination with protease inhibitors. The result of these clinical trials has led to a list of guidelines with recommendations for the optimal treatment options. Prolonged control of the infection with combination therapy (highly active antiretroviral therapy, "HAART") could be shown.

Saquinavir (SQV, Invirase). Saquinavir was the first HIV protease inhibitor to obtain FDA approval in 1995 for the treatment of HIV infection in combination with nucleoside analogs. Phase I clinical trials revealed low oral bioavailability due to limited gastro-intestinal absorption and extensive first-pass metabolism by human intestinal cytochrome P_{450} 3A4 (CYP3A4) that may be limited by concomitant administration of CYP3A4 inhibitors (indinavir, ritonavir, ketoconazole, troleandomycin). Pharmacokinetics could also be improved by administration with a high-fat diet or in a novel soft gelatin capsule formulation (Fortovase). Saquinavir is generally well tolerated with mainly gastrointestinal side effects, including diarrhea, nausea and abdominal discomfort.

Ritonavir (RTV, Norvir). Clinical evaluation of Ritonavir demonstrated good absorption from the gastrointestinal tract and high plasma drug levels. When given in combination with reverse transcriptase inhibitors, Ritonavir showed significant reduction of disease progression in clinical efficacy trials enrolling patients with advanced HIV disease, as compared to therapy with reverse transcriptase inhibitors alone. Ritonavir has a high affinity for several cytochrome P_{450} isoenzymes and is a potent inhibitor of CYP3A4. This limits the concurrent use of ritonavir with agents that are metabolized by CYP3A such as various analgetics, antiarrhythmic agents, antibiotics, anticoagulants, anticonvulsants, antiemetics and antifungal agents. While such interactions may be clinically detrimental, simultaneous administration of low doses of Ritonavir was shown to boost plasma levels of other HIV protease inhibitors allowing for lower dosages or increasing dosing intervals. The most common adverse effects of Ritonavir are nausea, diarrhea, vomiting, muscular weakness, taste disturbance, anorexia, abnormal functioning of tissue and abdominal pain.

Indinavir (IDV, Crixivan). Indinavir is a modified hydroxyethylamine peptidomimetic developed by rational drug design. In clinical trials, Indinavir was shown to significantly lower HIV RNA levels in plasma and to increase CD4 cell counts in both monotherapy and in combination drug regimens. Indinavir is generally well tolerated and in phase II clinical studies less than 6% of subjects taking Crixivan alone discontinued therapy due to drug-related adverse experiences. Nephrolithiasis was reported in 12.4% of adults and 29% of children, during clinical trials involving patients on Crixivan. As with other protease inhibitors, changes in body fat, increased bleeding in some patients with hemophilia, and increased blood sugar levels or diabetes have been reported. Additionally, severe muscle pain and weakness have occurred in patients also taking cholesterol-lowering medicines called "statins".

Nelfinavir (NFV, Viracept). Nelfinavir is a nonpeptidic, rationally designed HIV protease inhibitor. Nelfinavir has demonstrated efficacy in both monotherapy and in combination with the reverse transcriptase inhibitors stavudine (d4T) or zivudine +3TC. The major side effect is mild to moderate diarrhea.

Amprenavir (APV, Agenerase). Amprenavir (APV, Agenerase) is the most recently approved HIV protease inhibitor. It is smaller and stereochemically less complex than the other drugs in this class. Adsorption of this compound was found to be impaired by high fat meals. Common side effects of Amprenavir are nausea, vomiting, diarrhea, rash and a tingling sensation around the mouth.

As with reverse transcriptase inhibitors, resistance to protease inhibitors may also occur. Mutations in the HIV protease gene were shown to confer resistance to each of the aforementioned molecules. In addition, passaging of virus in the presence of HIV protease inhibitors also gave rise to strains less susceptible to the original inhibitor or cross-reactive to other compounds in the same class.

V

New Drug Targets

Hepatitis C Virus Serine Protease (5). Hepatitis C is a predominantly chronic infection affecting 1–3% of the world population. The infectious cycle of the hepatitis C virus has been outlined above. Inhibitors against the key viral protease, the NS3/4A serine protease are currently in clinical trials. This enzyme proved to be a particularly difficult target due to the peculiar architecture of its substrate recognition site (see above). An unusual feature of the NS3 protease is the property to undergo potent inhibition by its cleavage products. This property was exploited to generate a family of highly active peptide inhibitors that may serve as a basis for the development of peptidomimetics with improved pharmacokinetic properties. Also, mechanism-based inhibitors are being exploited.

Rhinovirus Protease (3). Rhinoviruses, which represent the single major cause of common cold, belong to the family of picornaviruses that harbors many medically relevant pathogens. Inhibitors of the 3C protease, a cysteine protease, have shown good antiviral potential. Several classes of compounds were designed based on the known substrate specificity of the enzyme. Mechanism-based, irreversible Michael-acceptors were shown to be both potent inhibitors of the purified enzyme and to have antiviral activity in infected cells.

References

1. Luciw P (1996) Human immunodeficiency viruses and their replication. In: Fields, B N, Knipe, D N, Howley, P M (eds) Virology, Lippincott-Raven publishers Philadelphia, New York p1881–1952
2. Lohmann V, Koch J O, Bartenschlager R (1996) Processing pathways of the hepatitis C virus proteins. J. Hepatol. 24(Suppl 2):11–19
3. Patick A K, Potts K E (1998) Protease inhibitors as antiviral agents. Clin. Microbiol. Rev. 4:614–627
4. Tavel J A, (2000) Ongoing trials in HIV protease inhibitors. Exp. Opin. Invest. Drugs 9:917–928
5. Steinkühler C, Koch U, Narjes F, Matassa V G (2001) Hepatitis C virus serine protease inhibitors: current progress and future challenges. Curr. Med. Chem. 8:919–932

Viremia

Viremia is the presence of viruses in the blood.

▶ Antiviral Drugs

Vitamin A

Vitamin A describes a group of substances (retinol, retinyl esters, and retinal) with defined biological activities. Certain metabolites of vitamin A, such as *all-trans* and *cis*-isomeric retinoic acids, can perform most of the biological functions of vitamin A; they are incapable of being metabolically reversibly converted into retinol, retinal, etc. The unit of measurement is the Vitamin A International Unit (IU) which measures growth in rat pups (1 mg retinol = 3333 IU Vitamin A).

Vitamin B1

Thiamin

▶ Vitamins, watersoluble

Vitamin B2

Riboflavin

▶ Vitamins, watersoluble

Vitamin B6

▶ Vitamins, watersoluble

Vitamin B12

▶ Vitamins, watersoluble

Vitamin C

▶ Vitamins, watersoluble

Vitamin D

Calcitriol is the active hormone form of vitamin D that promotes the absorption of calcium and phosphate in the intestines, decreases calcium excretion by the kidneys, and acts along with parathyroid hormone to maintain bone homeostasis. Other names frequently used for calcitriol are 1α,25-dihydroxychole-calciferol, 1,25-dihydroxyvitamin D_3, 1,25-DHCC, $1,25(OH)_2D_3$ and 1,25-diOHC. Chemically, calcitriol is 9,10-seco(5Z,7E)-5,7,10(19)-cholestatriene-3β-ol. It is is active in the regulation of the absorption of calcium from the gastrointestinal tract and its utilization in the body.

The usual recommended amount for vitamin D is 400 International Units (IU) per day.

▶ Bone Metabolism

Vitamin E

J. FRANK, H.K. BIESALSKI
University of Hohenheim, Stuttgart, Germany
frank140@uni-hohenheim.de,
biesal@uni-hohenheim.de

Synonyms

The term vitamin E describes a family of eight antioxidants, four tocopherols (α, β, γ, δ) and four tocotrienols (also α, β, γ, δ). α-tocopherol is present in nature in only one form, RRR α-tocopherol. The chemical synthesis of α-tocopherol results in eight different forms (SRR, SSR, SRS, SSS, RSR, RRS, RSS, RRR), only one of which is RRR α-tocopherol. These forms differ in that they can be "right" (R) or "left" (S) at three different places in the α-tocopherol molecule. RRR α-tocopherol is the only form of vitamin E that is actively maintained in the human body and is therefore, the form of vitamin E found in the largest quantities in the blood and tissue. A protein synthesized in the liver (α-TTP: α-tocopherol transfer protein) preferentially selects the natural form of vitamin E (RRR-α-tocopherol) for distribution to the tissues. However, the mechanisms for the regulation of vitamin E in tissues are not known.

Definition

In 1922 Evans and Bishop named the animal nutritional factor essential of reproduction "vitamin E". In the 1960s, vitamin E was associated with antioxidant function. 25 years later, vitamin E has been found to possess functions that are independent of its antioxidant and free radical scavenging ability. α-tocopherol specific molecular mechanisms were discovered which are still under investigation.

▶ Vitamin K
▶ Vitamins, watersoluble

Mechanism of Action

The main function of α-tocopherol in humans appears to be that of a non-specific chain-breaking antioxidant that prevents the propagation of lipid peroxidation (Fig. 1). Reactive oxygen species (ROS) are formed primarily in the body during normal metabolism and also upon exposure to environmental factors such as pollutants or cigarette smoke. Fats (first of all several fold polyunsaturated fatty acids; PUFAS), which are an integral part of all cell membranes, are vulnerable to destruction through oxidation by ROS. The fat-soluble vitamin, α-tocopherol, is uniquely suited to intercepting free radicals and preventing a chain reaction of lipid destruction (Fig. 1). Aside from maintaining the integrity of cell membranes

V

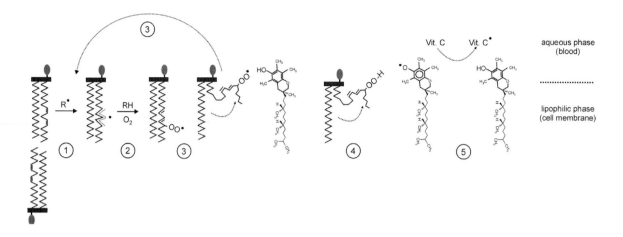

Fig. 1 The role of vitamin E in the mechanism of lipid peroxidation.
1. Initiation: a radical (R•) must be present.
2. Hydrogen abstraction from a weakened C H bond on carbon atoms adjacent to double bounds in a PUFA, forming a carbon centered radical.
3. Propagation: rearrangement to a conjugated diene followed by reaction with molecular oxygen (O_2) produces a highly reactive peroxyl radical which simultaneously propagates the reaction by hydrogen abstraction from another PUFA (chain reaction).
4. Termination: hydrogen abstraction from α-tocopherol form a lipid hydroperoxide and a tocopheroxyl radical. The chain reaction is broken since α-tocopheroxyl radical will not react with an adjacent PUFA.
5. The α-tocopheroxyl radical can be recycled by vitamin C.

throughout the body, α-tocopherol also protects the fats in low density lipoproteins (LDL) from oxidation. Oxidized LDL have been implicated in the development of cardiovascular diseases. When a molecule of α-tocopherol neutralizes a free radical, it is altered in such a way that its antioxidant capacity is lost. However, other antioxidants, such as vitamin C, are capable of regenerating the antioxidant capacity of α-tocopherol. If the rate of oxidation is greater than the rate of regeneration, α-tocopherol concentrations in the body will decrease. Low levels of α-tocopherol have been associated with increased incidence of cardiovascular diseases (heart disease and stroke), cancer, cataracts and immune function. Several other functions of α-tocopherol have been identified which are probably not related to its antioxidant capacity.

Potential, Non-antioxidant, α-Tocopherol Specific Effects

A specific role for vitamin E in a required metabolic function has not been found. In addition to its direct antioxidant effects, α-tocopherol has been reported to have specific molecular functions (2-4): The proposed molecular mechanisms of α-tocopherol are associated with transcriptional and post-transcriptional events. Activation of diacylglycerol kinase and protein phosphatase 2A (PP_2A) and the inhibition of protein kinase C (PKC), cyclooxygenase-I, 5-lipoxygenase and cytokine release by α-tocopherol are all examples of post transcriptional regulation. Protein kinase C inhibition by α-tocopherol was reported to be involved in cell proliferation and differentiation in smooth muscle cells, human platelets, and monocytes. The inhibitory effect of α-tocopherol on PKC can be correlated to a dephosphorylation of PKCα. Dephosphorylation of PKC occurs via the

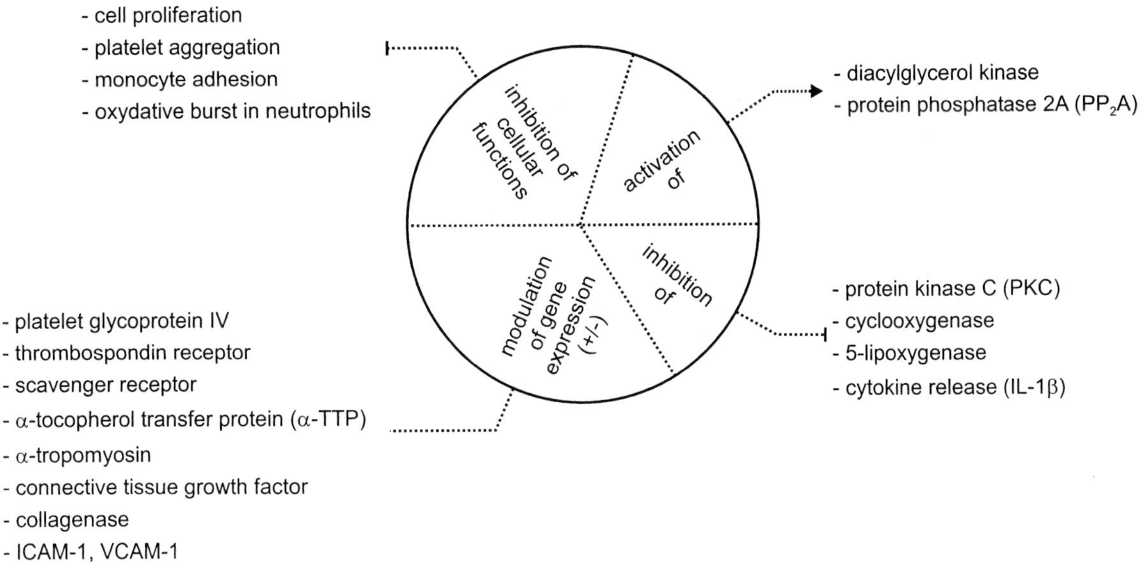

- cell proliferation
- platelet aggregation
- monocyte adhesion
- oxydative burst in neutrophils

- diacylglycerol kinase
- protein phosphatase 2A (PP$_2$A)

- protein kinase C (PKC)
- cyclooxygenase
- 5-lipoxygenase
- cytokine release (IL-1β)

- platelet glycoprotein IV
- thrombospondin receptor
- scavenger receptor
- α-tocopherol transfer protein (α-TTP)
- α-tropomyosin
- connective tissue growth factor
- collagenase
- ICAM-1, VCAM-1

(circle labels: inhibition of cellular functions / activation of / inhibition of / modulation of gene expression (+/-))

Fig. 2 Non-antioxidant properties of α-tocopherol.

protein PP$_2$A, which has been found to be activated *in vitro* by treatment of α-tocopherol.

Liver collagen α1, the α-tocopherol transfer protein gene (α-TTP), the α-tropomyosin gene and the collagenase (metallo-proteinase 1) gene have been found to be modulated at the transcriptional level by α-tocopherol. However, the mechanisms of transcriptional regulation of certain genes by α-tocopherol remain unclear. α-tocopherol also inhibits cell proliferation, platelet aggregation, monocyte adhesion and the oxidative burst in neutrophils. Vitamin E enrichment of endothelial cells down regulates the expression of intercellular cell adhesion molecule (ICAM-1) and vascular cell adhesion molecule-I (VCAM-I), thereby decreasing the adhesion of blood cells to the endothelium.

The observed immunomodulatory function of α-tocopherol may also be attributed to the fact that the release of the proinflammatory cytokine interleukin-1β can be inhibited by α-tocopherol via inhibition of the 5-lipoxygenase pathway. In addition, the inhibition of PKC activity from monocytes by α-tocopherol is followed by inhibition of phosphorylation and translocation of the cytosolic factor p47 (phox) and impaired assembly of the NADPH-oxidase and of superoxide produc-

tion. An overview of the non-antioxidant effects of α-tocopherol is summarized in Fig. 2.

Clinical Use (disease treatment)

Role in Cardiovascular Diseases
Low levels of vitamin E have been associated with increased incidence of coronary artery disease. Observational studies have therefore suggested that supplemental α-tocopherol might have value in the treatment of cardiovascular disease. Four large-scale, randomized, double-blind clinical intervention studies have tested the ability of vitamin E to prevent myocardial infarction. One was strongly positive (9), the other three were neutral (1,7,10). Therefore, the role of α-tocopherol supplementation in the treatment of cardiovascular disease is unclear and the results of further large intervention trials must be bided to clarify the role of vitamin E in the pathogenesis of cardiovascular diseases.

Role in Diabetes Mellitus
It has been proposed that the development of the complications of diabetes mellitus may be linked to oxidative stress and therefore might be attenuated by antioxidants such as vitamin E. Further-

V

more, it is discussed that glucose-induced vascular dysfunction in diabetes can be reduced by vitamin E treatment due to the inactivation of PKC. Cardiovascular complications are among the leading causes of death in diabetics. To our knowledge, to date no clinical intervention trials have tested directly whether vitamin E can ameliorate the complication of diabetes.

Role in Alzheimer's Disease

Alzheimer's disease is a degenerative disease of the brain in which oxidative stress appears to play a role. Vitamin E is thought to prevent brain cell damage by destroying toxic free radicals. In a 2-year, double blind, placebo-controlled, randomized, multicenter trial, supplementation of 341 patients who had moderate neurological impairment with 2000 IU synthetic α-tocopherol daily resulted in a significant slowing of the progression of Alzheimer's disease (8). Although these results are promising, it is too early to draw any conclusions about the usefulness of vitamin E in Alzheimer's disease or other neurological diseases. Therefore, further studies are required to determine the role of vitamin E supplementation in central nervous system disorders.

Note: A review in the September 2001 issue of Arteriosclerosis, Thrombosis, and Vascular Biology (6) concluded that there is little convincing evidence that vitamin E increases antioxidant defenses in the body. This would also question a benefit of vitamin E in the prevention and management of the diseases mentioned above.

Friedrich Ataxia

Ataxia with vitamin E deficiency is a very rare genetic disease. The Friedrich ataxia is the most frequent form of this disease. These patients lack a key protein in the liver (α-TTP) that is responsible for putting the vitamin E in the blood lipoproteins for transport to the tissues. For this reason, these patients develop serious deficiency that cause major neurological and muscle damage. In a study with 24 patients, supplementation with high levels of vitamin E (800 IU) increased the blood concentration and stabilized the neurological signs especially in early stages of the disease (5).

Side Effects

Due to bleeding risk, individuals on anticoagulant therapy or individuals who are vitamin K deficient should not take vitamin E supplementation without close medical supervision. Despite that, vitamin E is a well-tolerated, relatively non-toxic nutrient. A tolerable upper intake level of 1000 mg daily of α-tocopherol of any form (equivalent to 1500 IU of RRR-α-tocopherol or 1100 IU of all-rac-α-tocopherol) would be, according to the Food and Nutrition Board of the Institute of Medicine, the highest dose unlikely to result in hemorrhage in most adults.

References

1. Dietary Supplementation with N-3 Polyunsaturated Fatty Acids and Vitamin E after Myocardial Infarction: Results of the GISSI-Prevenzione Trial. (1999) Gruppo Italiano Per Lo Studio Della Sopravvivenza Nell'Infarto Miocardico. Lancet 354: pp 447–455.
2. Azzi A, Breyer I, Feher M, Pastori M, Ricciarelli R, Spycher S, Staffieri M, Stocker A, Zimmer S and Zingg J M (2000) Specific Cellular Responses to α-Tocopherol. J Nutr 130:1649–1652
3. Azzi A, Breyer I, Feher M, Ricciarelli R, Stocker A, Zimmer S and Zingg J (2001) Nonantioxidant Functions of α-Tocopherol in Smooth Muscle Cells. J Nutr 131:378S–381S
4. Azzi A and Stocker A (2000) Vitamin E: Non-Antioxidant Roles. Prog Lipid Res 39:231–255
5. Gabsi S, Gouider-Khouja N, Belal S, Fki M, Kefi M, Turki I, Ben Hamida M, Kayden H, Mebazaa R and Hentati F (2001) Effect of Vitamin E Supplementation in Patients with Ataxia with Vitamin E Deficiency. Eur J Neurol 8:477–481
6. Heinecke JW (2001) Is the Emperor Wearing Clothes? Clinical Trials of Vitamin E and the LDL Oxidation Hypothesis. Arterioscler Thromb Vasc Biol 21:1261–1264
7. Lonn E, Yusuf S, Dzavik V, Doris C, Yi Q, Smith S, Moore-Cox A, Bosch J, Riley W and Teo K (2001) Effects of Ramipril and Vitamin E on Atherosclerosis: the Study to Evaluate Carotid Ultrasound Changes in Patients Treated with Ramipril and Vitamin E (SECURE). Circulation 103:919–925
8. Sano M, Ernesto C, Thomas R G, Klauber M R, Schafer K, Grundman M, Woodbury P, Growdon J, Cotman C W, Pfeiffer E, Schneider L S and Thal L J (1997) A Controlled Trial of Selegiline, α-Tocophe-

rol, or Both as Treatment for Alzheimer's Disease. The Alzheimer's Disease Cooperative Study. N Engl J Med 336:1216–1222

9. Stephens NG, Parsons A, Schofield P M, Kelly F, Cheeseman K and Mitchinson M J (1996) Randomised Controlled Trial of Vitamin E in Patients With Coronary Disease: Cambridge Heart Antioxidant Study (CHAOS). Lancet 347:781–786

10. Yusuf S, Sleight P, Pogue J, Bosch J, Davies R and Dagenais G (2000) Effects of an Angiotensin-Converting-Enzyme Inhibitor, Ramipril, on Cardiovascular Events in High-Risk Patients. The Heart Outcomes Prevention Evaluation Study Investigators. N Engl J Med 342:145–153

Vitamin K

D. NOHR, H.K. BIESALSKI
University of Hohenheim, Institute of Biological Chemistry and Nutrition (-140-),
Stuttgart, Germany
nohr@uni-hohenheim.de,
biesal@uni-hohenheim.de

Synonyms

Vitamin K is a major term for two groups of substances named "phylloquinones" (vitamin K1; produced by plants) and menaquinones-n (MK-n; vitamin K2). Menaquinones are synthesized by bacteria, using repeated 5-carbon units in the molecules side chain (n stands for the number of 5-carbon units). Interestingly, MK-4 is synthesized only in small amounts by bacteria but can be produced by animals (including humans) from phylloquinones and is found in a number of organs. For an overview see (2, 4).

Definition

Vitamin K belongs to the group of fat-soluble vitamins. The term "K" refers to its main actions in blood-clotting, coagulation, in German named "koagulation". In the coagulation cascade (▶ Antiplatelet Drugs) seven coagulation factors depend on Vitamin K, which acts as coenzyme for a vitamin K-dependent carboxylase that catalyzes

the carboxylation of glutamic acid. This specific carboxylation occurs only in a small number of proteins but is essential for their ability to bind calcium (7). Vitamin K is light-sensitive but almost resistant to heat.

Vitamin K carboxylase is a transmembraneous protein in the lipid bilayer of the endoplasmatic reticulum (ER). It is highly glycosylated and its C-terminal is on the luminal side of the membrane. Besides its function as carboxylase it takes part as an epoxidase in the vitamin K cycle (Fig. 1). For the binding of the γ-carboxylase the vitamin K-dependent proteins have highly conserved special recognition sites. Most vitamin K-dependent proteins are carboxylated in the liver and in osteoblasts, but also other tissues might be involved, e.g. muscles (cf. 4).

▶ Vitamin E
▶ Vitamins, watersoluble

Mechanism of Action

General aspects

Although vitamin K is a fat soluble vitamin, only little stores are found in the body, which have to be refilled permanently via dietary input. The role of vitamin K derived from bacteria in the colon is controversially discussed, as the concentration of biliary acids for the resorption the fatsoluble vitamin K is very low in the colon. In addition, only diseases of the small intestine lead to a deficit in vitamin K concentration that cannot be restored by K2 production of colonic bacteria. However, watersoluble vitamin Ks can be resorbed by the colonic mucosa. Maybe because of the little stores for vitamin K, the process of vitamin K-dependent carboxylation of proteins is part of a cycle with several steps during which vitamin K normally is regenerated (see Fig. 1) and thus can be used several times.

Coagulation

Binding calcium ions (Ca^{2+}) is a prerequisite for the activation of seven clotting factors in the coagulation cascade that are dependent on vitamin K. The term cascade indicates, that the factors involved depend from each other to become activated and to fulfil their special part to stop bleeding. Prothrombin (factor II), factors VII, IX, and X

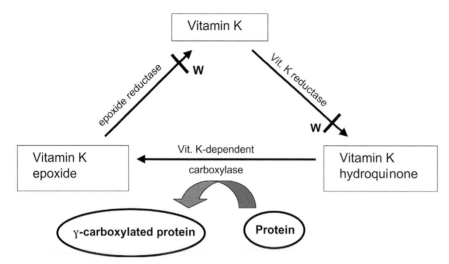

Fig. 1 The vitamin K cycle. w indicates where warfarin, a vitamin K antagonist, inhibits the cycle.

play central roles in the coagulation cascade, protein Z seems to enhance the thrombin action via promoting its association with phospholipids in cell membranes. The proteins C and S act as anticoagulant proteins such providing a vitamin K-dependent control and balance of the whole cascade. With both, coagulant and anticoagulant factors present in the cascade in the liver, uncontrolled bleeding and/or clotting can be well prevented. On the other hand, liver damage or diseases can disturb this well controlled cascade e.g. via reduced clotting factors in the circulating blood resulting in uncontrolled bleeding (hemorrhage) (5).

▶ Coagulation/Thrombosis

Bone mineralization

In bone, three proteins have been described which are vitamin K-dependent, osteocalcin (bone Gla protein), matrix Gla protein (MGP), and protein S. Osteocalcin is synthetized by osteoclasts, regulated by the active form of vitamin D, calcitriol. Its capacity to bind calcium needs a vitamin K-dependent γ-carboxylation of three glutamic acid residues. The calcium binding capacity of osteocalcin indicates a possible role in bone mineralization, but its exact function is still unclear. Protein S, a coagulant, is also vitamin-K dependent in its synthesis by osteoclasts, and its role in bone metabolism is unclear. However, children with reduced protein S levels express enhanced blood

clotting and a reduced bone density. MGP has been found in several supportive tissues (bone, cartilage) and in soft tissues including blood vessels. At least animal studies gave hints that MGP prevents soft tissues as well as cartilage from calcification while on the other hand it facilitates bone development and growth. Even the phenotype of mice lacking MGP supports this description, but the molecular mechanisms are still unknown. Rat studies with warfarin (vitamin K antagonist, see Fig. 1) led to prominent deformations of the skeleton of fetuses as well as newborns including excessive mineralisation of growth plates and nasal cartilage, and stunted growth. Comparable effects were seen in humans after a therapy with vitamin K antagonists during pregnancy. The so called warfarin-embryopathy includes hypercalcification of the growth plates (Chondroplasia punctata), a nasal hypoplasia and disturbances in the growth of facial and hollow bones.

Cell growth

Growth arrest-specific gene 6 (Gas6) is a γ-carboxylated protein found throughout the nervous system, in the heart, lung, stomach, kidneys, and cartilage. It is regarded as a ligand for several families of receptor tyrosine kinases (RTKs) which, when overexpressed, have effects on malignant cell survival (6). The exact mechanisms of Gas6 function have not yet been clarified but it is discussed as a cellular growth regulation factor with cell signaling activities as well as a supporter of hematopoetic cells in the bone marrow. In addition, a role in the developing and the aging nervous system is under dicussion (3,9). An enhanced proportion of neurite-bearing PCD12 cells and acetylcholinesterase activity were described when cells were treated with nerve growth factor (NGF) and vitamin K (1 or 2), in comparison to NGF treatment only which could be blocked by protein kinase A or MAP kinase inhibitors (10).

Clinical Use (incl. side effects)

Vitamin K deficiency

There are clearcut differences in deficiencies concerning infants, especially newborns, and adults. Deficiencies of vitamin K are seen seldom in healthy adults because the supply through daily food is (more than) enough, vitamin K is repeatedly recycled and therefore only a small loss appears, and – although not really accepted – the K2 production by intestinal bacteria (see above). On the other hand, those people with severe liver diseases or taking vitamin K antagonist anticoagulants have a risk of vitamin K deficiency. Symptoms are impaired blood clotting as revealed by routine tests measuring clotting time, unusual bleeding after smaller wounding, nose bleeding, heavy menstrual bleeding or a great susceptability to hematoma.

The picture is different concerning infants during the first days of life, especially for those being breast fed (8). Coagulation-related (vitamin K-dependent) plasma proteins develop slowly during pregnancy resulting in markedly reduced levels after birth. In addition, human milk is a low-vitamin K nutrient, the newborns intestine almost totally lacks menaquinone-synthetising bacteria, and the vitamin K cycle might not yet be established. These deficiencies can lead in healthy newborns to uncontrolled, in worst cases lethal intracranial bleedings. Due to that risk, in most countries newborns are supplied with phylloquinones, normally by injections, or by bottle feeding. Although there have been some hints in retrospective studies in the early 1990s on a correlation of vitamin K supplementation of newborns with the development of leucaemia, other retrospective studies found no correlations (cf. 2). Therefore, a routine vitamin K prophylaxis of newborns is still recommended because the risk of early postnatal bleedings is much greater than the (unproven) risk of cancer.

Osteoporosis

This illness is mainly characterized by an age-related bone loss. The detection of osteocalcin in bone was the starting point for a series of studies on the role of vitamin K-dependent proteins in bone development and maintenance and on possible supplementation therapies. Epidemiologic studies found differences in the risk of hip fractures depending on the dietary vitamin K intake (35% risk at 250 µg/day of those with 50 µg/day), although no association between dietary intake and bone density could be found. Osteocalcin has been found to be a reliable marker of bone formation and vitamin K is necessary for the carboxylation of this protein. Therefore, the degree of carboxylation of osteocalcin is a reliable marker for the respective vitamin status (1). Blood levels of undercarboxylated osteocalcin were found to be higher in postmenopausal women and markedly higher in women over 70. Studies with elderly women resulted in a positive correlation of the blood level of undercarboxylated osteocalcin and the risk of bone fractures. Interestingly, also a correlation of undercarboxylated osteocalcin with the vitamin D nutritional status were described.

Application of vitamin K-antagonistic anticoagulants like warfarin gave no clearcut results concerning bone density or a changed risk for bone fractures.

Supplementation with high doses of vitamin K1 (1 mg/day for 14 days) or MK-4 (45 mg/day) resulted in decreased levels of undercarboxylated osteocalcin and increase of bone formation markers and in a significant reduction in bone loss, respectively. Using such high doses, any kind of effects besides vitamin K can not yet be ruled out and have to be further elucidated by long term studies.

Atherosclerosis

In contrast to the formation and calcification of bones, vitamin K seems to lower the risk of aortic calcification. The mechanisms for these "antagonistic" effects is not known but a participation of osteocalcin as well as of matrix Gla protein (MGP) are discussed.

Tab. 1 Vitamin K content of selected nutrients in alphabetical order*.

Nutrient	Vitamin K content [μg/100g]
Bovine meat	210
Broccoli	130
Brussels sprouts	570
Butter	60
Cauliflower	300
Chicken	300
Chicken egg	45
Mayonnaise	81
Milk (3.5% fat)	3.7
Oil (sunflower)	500
Porcine meat	18
Rice, white	1
Sauerkraut	1540
Soyabeans (semen)	190
Spinach	810
Tea, black leaves	262
Tea, green leaves	1428
Tomatoes	8
Wheat (germs)	350
Wheat (grains)	17

*The adequate intake level (AI) for the US given by the FNB of the Institute of Medicine is 120 μg/day and 90 μg/day for men and women elder than19 years, respectively. In Germany, 60–80 μg/day for adults, 4 μg/day for sucklings < 4 months, and 50 μg/day for children < 15 years are proposed by the german nutrition society (DGE).

Safety and Toxicity

As the above mentioned studies with high supplementation dosages exemplarily show, there is no known toxicity for phylloquinone (vitamin K1). This is NOT true for menadione (vitamin K3) that can interfere with glutathione, a natural antioxidant, resulting in oxidative stress and cell membrane damage. Injections of menadione in infants led to jaundice and hemolytic anemia and therefore should not be used for the treatment of vitamin K deficiency.

People using warfarin should try to consume the recommended daily intake very regularly to avoid interferences with their anticoagulant dosage adjusted by the physician. Interestingly, high doses of vitamins A and E seem to antagonize vitamin K, vitamin A interfering with vitamin K absorption and vitamin E (tocopherol quinone) inhibiting vitamin K-dependent carboxylase enzymes.

Food sources

Phylloquinone (vitamin K1) is the form of vitamin K synthesized by mainly green leafy vegetables and such also appears in plant oils (soybean, cottonseed, canola, olive). Both are good sources for a daily supply, although the need of such a supply is still under discussion. Table 1 shows some good sources and their content of vitamin K1.

References

1. Booth, SL, Suutie JW (1998) Dietary intake and adequacy of vitamin K. J Nutrition 128:785–788
2. Booth, SL (2001) Vitamin K. Homepage of the Linus Pauling Institute at Oregon State University.
3. Ferland G (1998) The vitamin K-dependent proteins: an update. Nutrition Reviews 56:223–230
4. Jakob F (2002) Vitamin K. In: Biesalski HK et al. (eds) Vitamine, Spurenelemente und Mineralstoffe. Thieme Verlag, Stuttgart, pp33–40
5. Olson RE (1999) Vitamin K. In: Shils M et al. (eds) Nutrition in health and disease. 9th edition, Williams and Wilkins, Baltimore, pp 363–380
6. Saxena SP, Israels ED, Israels LG (2001) Novel vitamin K-dependent pathways regulating cell survival. Apoptosis 6(1–2):57–68
7. Shearer MJ (1997) The roles of vitamin D and vitamin K in bone health and osteoporosis prevention. Proc Nutrition Soc 56:915–937
8. Suzuki S, Iwata G, Sutor AH (2001) Vitamin K deficiency during the perinatal and infantile period. Semin Thromb Hemost 27(2):93–98
9. Tsaioun K (1999) Vitamin K-dependent proteins in the developing and aging nervous system. Nutrition Reviews 57:231–240
10. Tsang CK, Kamei Y (2002) Novel effect of vitamin K(1) (phylloquionone) and vitamin K(2) (menaquinone) on promoting nerve growth factor-mediated

neurite outgrowth from PC12D cells. Neurosci Lett. 323:9–12.

Vitamins, watersoluble

E. BACK, H. K. BIESALSKI
University of Hohenheim, Institute of Biological Chemistry and Nutrition, Stuttgart, Germany
evelback@uni-hohenheim.de
biesal@uni-hohenheim.de

Vitamin B1 (Thiamin)

Synonyms

Fig. 1 shows the chemical structure of vitamin B1 or thiamin (3-(4-amino-2-methyl-pyrimidin-5-ylmethyl)-5-(2-hydroxyethyl)-4-methylthiazolium) and its coenzyme form thiaminpyrophosphate (TPP).

Definition

Free thiamin is a base that is stable under acidic conditions up to pH 7, moderately light-sensitive and susceptible to oxidative degradation as well as inactivation by irradiation. For use in pharmaceutical and other preparations the vitamin is handled in the form of solid water-soluble thiazolium salts (thiamin chloride hydrochloride, thiamin mononitrate). There are also synthetic lipophilic derivatives of the vitamin, termed allithiamins. They can pass biological membranes more easily and in a nearly dose-linear fashion. Due to their improved bioavailability they can be used to build up high thiamin stores in certain target organs (drug targeting). In the human body, thiamin concentration is highest in the heart, followed by kidney, liver and brain. Yeast, pulses, wholemeal cereals, nuts and pork are good dietary sources for thiamin (1).

Some kinds of fish and crustacea contain thiaminases. These enzymes cleave thiamin and thus inactivate the vitamin. Some plant phenols, e.g. chlorogenic acid, may possess antithiaminic properties, too, though their mechanism of action is so far not well understood (1).

▶ Vitamin E
▶ Vitamin K

Mechanisms of Action

Several enzymes of the intermediary metabolism require thiaminpyrophosphate (TPP, Fig. 1) as coenzyme, e.g. enzymes of the pyruvate dehydrogenase complex, α-ketoglutarate dehydrogenase complex or pentose phosphate pathway.

TPP-dependent enzymes are involved in oxidative decarboxylation of α-keto acids, making them available for energy metabolism. Transketolase is involved in the formation of NADPH and pentose in the pentose phosphate pathway. This reaction is important for several other synthetic pathways. It is furthermore assumed that the above mentioned enzymes are involved in the function of neurotransmitters and nerve conduction, though the exact mechanisms remain unclear (2).

Clinical Use (incl. side effects)

Thiamin has a very low toxicity (oral LD_{50} of thiaminchloride hydrochloride in mice: 3–15 g/kg body weight). The vitamin is used therapeutically to cure polyneuropathy, ▶ beri-beri (clinically

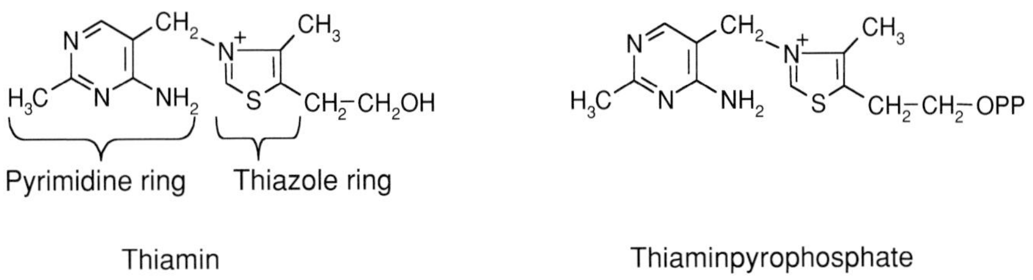

Pyrimidine ring   Thiazole ring

Thiamin

Thiaminpyrophosphate

Fig. 1 Structure of thiamin and its coenzyme form thiaminpyrophosphate (TPP).

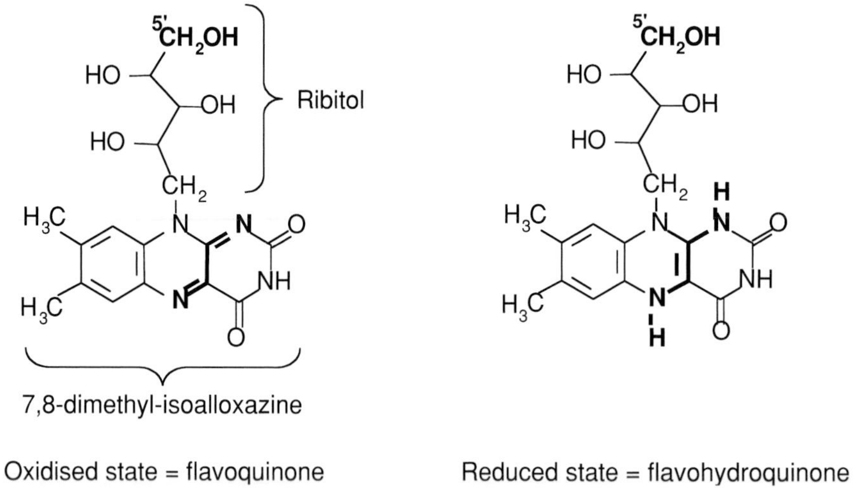

Oxidised state = flavoquinone   Reduced state = flavohydroquinone

Fig. 2 Structure of oxidised and reduced riboflavin.

manifest thiamin deficiency) and Wernicke-Korsakoff Syndrome. In mild polyneuropathy 10–20 mg/d water-soluble or 5–10 mg/d lipid-soluble thiamin are given orally. In more severe cases 20–50 mg/d water-soluble or 10–20 mg/d lipid-soluble thiamin are administered orally. Patients suffering from beri-beri or from early stages of Wernicke-Korsakoff Syndrome receive 50–100 mg of thiamin two times a day for several days subcutaneously or intravenously until symptoms are alleviated. Afterwards, the vitamin is administered orally for several weeks (3).

Vitamin B2 (Riboflavin)

Synonyms

Vitamin B2 or riboflavin is chemically defined as 7,8-dimethyl-10-(1′-D-ribityl)isoalloxazine. Fig. 2 shows the oxidised and reduced form of the vitamin. The ending "flavin" (from the the latin word flavus = yellow) refers to its yellowish colour.

Definition

Riboflavin is heat stable in the absence of light, but extremely photosensitive. It has a high degree of natural fluorescence when excited by UV light. This property can be used for detection and determination. Two coenzymes (Fig. 3), flavin mononucleotide (FMN) and flavin adenine dinucleotide (FAD), are derived from riboflavin.

Milk, milk products and foods of animal origin contain high amounts of (free) riboflavin with good bioavailability. In foods of plant origin, most riboflavin is protein-bound and therefore less bioavailable. Cereal germs and bran are plant sources rich in riboflavin (4).

Mechanisms of Action

The formation of FMN and FAD is ATP-dependent and takes place predominantly in liver, kidney and heart. It is controlled by thyroid hormones (5).

So far, about 60 flavoenzymes have been identified, the majority containing FAD. Examples for flavoenzymes are the mitochondrial enzymes of the respiratory chain, succinate dehydrogenase, L-gulonolactone oxidase, monoamino oxidase, xanthinoxidase, thioreduxin reductase and glutathione reductase. Flavin coenzymes are involved in both one- and two-electron transfer reactions and catalyse hydroxylations, oxidative decarboxylations, dioxygenations as well as reductions of oxygen to hydrogen peroxide. Through their function as coenzymes, FMN and FAD are involved in the metabolism of glucose, fatty acids, amino acids, purines, drugs and steroids, folic acid, pyridoxin, vitamin K, niacin and vitamin D.

The FAD-dependent enzyme glutathione reductase plays a role in the antioxidant system. Glutathione reductase restores reduced glutathione (GSH), the most important antioxidant in

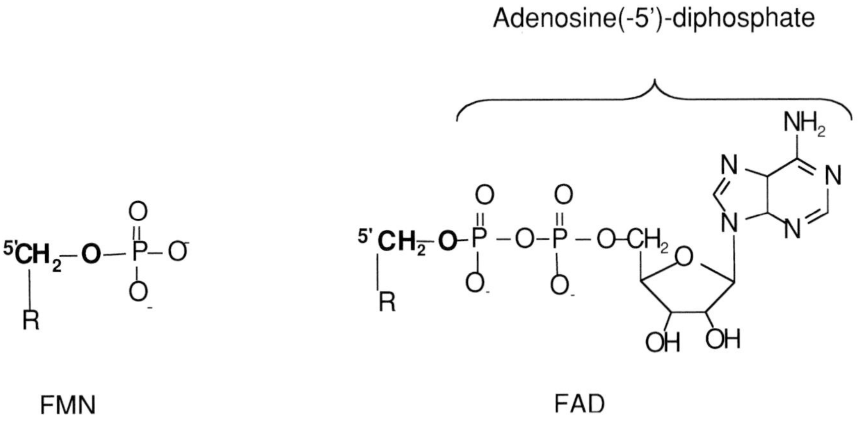

Adenosine(-5')-diphosphate

FMN

FAD

Fig. 3 Structure of flavin
mononucleotide (FMN)
and flavin adenine dinu-
cleotide (FAD).

erythrocytes, from oxidised glutathione (GSSG)
(4,5).

Clinical Use (incl. side effects)

Up to date, no case of riboflavin intoxication has
been described in the literature and riboflavin
intake is considered safe even at higher doses.

The vitamin is administered therapeutically to
reverse riboflavin deficiency symptoms or to prevent deficiency in high risk groups. Among the
high risk groups to develop riboflavin deficiency
count persons who regularly take certain drugs
(e.g. antidepressants, oral contraceptives), mal-
nourished patients, patients after trauma, patients
suffering from malabsorption and chronic alcoholics. The doses given are >10 mg/d. Two other
groups who benefit from riboflavin supplementation are newborns with hyperbilirubinemia who
are treated with phototherapy. The supply of
0.5 mg riboflavin/kg body weight and day can here
accelerate the photodegradation of bilirubin. Furthermore, persons with congenital methemoglobinemia might profit from the intake of high doses
of riboflavin (20–40 mg/d) (6).

Vitamin B6

Synonyms

Vitamin B6 (Fig. 4) is the collective name for all 3-
hydroxy-2-methylpyridine-derivatives with vitamin B6 function, including pyridoxin (= PN, alco-

hol), pyridoxal (= PL, aldehyde), pyridoxamine (=
PM, amine) and their 5'-phosphorylised forms.

Definition

In general, pyridoxamine and pyridoxin are more
stable than pyridoxal. All vitamers are relatively
heat stable in acid media, but heat labile in alkaline media. All forms of vitamin B6 are destroyed
by UV light in both neutral and alkaline solution.
The majority of vitamin B6 in the human body is
stored in the form of pyridoxal phosphate in the
muscle, bound to glycogen phosphorylase.

Plants contain to some extend less bioavailable
forms of vitamin B6, e.g. glycosylates, or biologically inactive metabolites, e.g. ε-pyridoxin-lysin-
complexes. In addition, the release of vitamin B6
from foods rich in fibre is probably delayed. The
bioavailability of vitamin B6 from animal-derived
foods is therefore overall higher than from plant-
derived foods. Good dietary sources of vitamin B6
include chicken, fish, pork, beans and pulses (7).

Mechanisms of Action

Pyridoxal phosphate mainly serves as coenzyme
in the amino acid metabolism and is covalently
bound to its enzyme via a Schiff base. In the enzymatic reaction, the amino group of the substrate
and the aldehyde group of PLP form a Schiff base,
too. The subsequent reactions can take place at the
α-, β-, or γ-carbon of the respective substrate.
Common types of reactions are decarboxylations
(formation of biogenic amines), transaminations
(transfer of the amino nitrogen of one amino acid

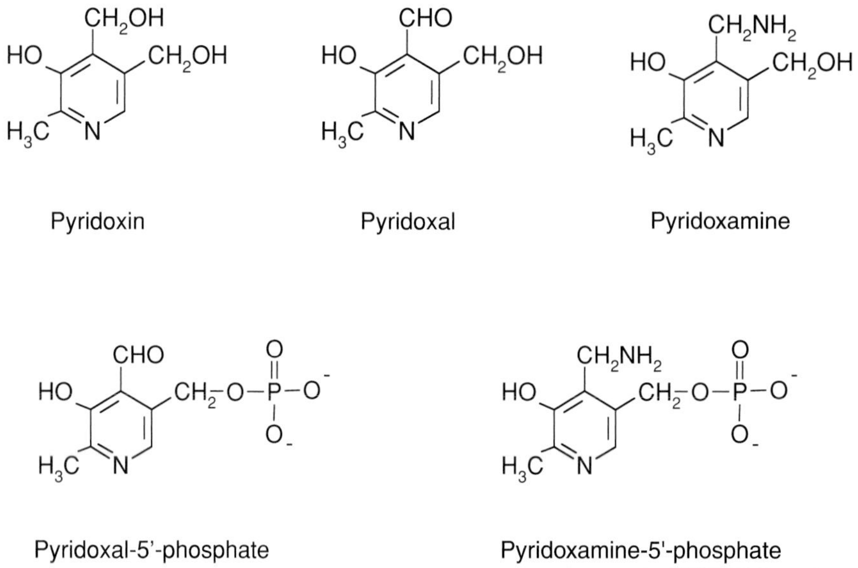

Pyridoxin

Pyridoxal

Pyridoxamine

Pyridoxal-5'-phosphate

Pyridoxamine-5'-phosphate

Fig. 4 Structure of pyridoxin, pyridoxal, pyridoxamine and the coenzymes pyridoxal-5'-phosphate and pyridoxamine-5'-phosphate.

to the keto analog of another amino acid), and eliminations.

Pyridoxamine phosphate serves as a coenzyme of transaminases, e.g. lysyl oxidase (collagen biosynthesis), serine hydroxymethyl transferase (C1-metabolism), δ-aminolevulinate synthase (porphyrin biosynthesis), glycogen phosphorylase (mobilisation of glycogen), aspartate aminotransferase (transamination), alanine aminotransferase (transamination), kynureninase (biosynthesis of niacin), glutamate decarboxylase (biosynthesis of GABA), tyrosine decarboxylase (biosynthesis of tyramine), serine dehydratase (β-elimination), cystathionine β-synthase (metabolism of methionine), and cystathionine γ-lyase (γ-elimination).

Vitamin B6-coenzyme is involved in a variety of reactions, e.g. in the immune system, gluconeogenesis, erythrocyte function, niacin formation, nervous system, lipid metabolism, and in hormone modulation/gene expression (8).

Clinical Use (incl. side effects)

Compared to other B-vitamins, pyridoxin has a high chronic toxicity. This is mainly attributable to the fact that, in contrast to the other water-soluble vitamins, intestinal absorption of vitamin B6 takes partially place via a nonsaturable, passive process. When more than 150 mg pyridoxin/d are adminis-

tered for several months, a reversible peripheral neuropathy with gait disturbances, dysreflexia and insensibility frequently develops (9).

The administration of vitamin B6-megadoses has yet proven beneficial in cystathioninuria (400 mg/d), homocystinuria (250–1250 mg/d), primary oxalosis type I, "spine-syndrome" (150 mg/d) and isoniazid intoxication (1 g PN per g isoniazid per os). Other fields of application, like carpal tunnel syndrome, rheumatic diseases, premenstrual syndrome and chinese restaurant syndrome, lack scientific evidence (9).

Vitamin B12

Synonyms

Vitamin B12 (Fig. 5) is defined as a group of cobalt-containing corroids known as cobalamins. The common features of the vitamers are a corrin ring (four reduced pyrrole rings) with cobalt as the central atom, a nucleotide-like compound and a variable ligand. Vitamin B12 is exceptional in as far as it is the only vitamin containing a metal-ion. The vitamers present in biological systems are hydroxo-, aquo-, methyl- and 5'-deoxyadenosylcobalamin.

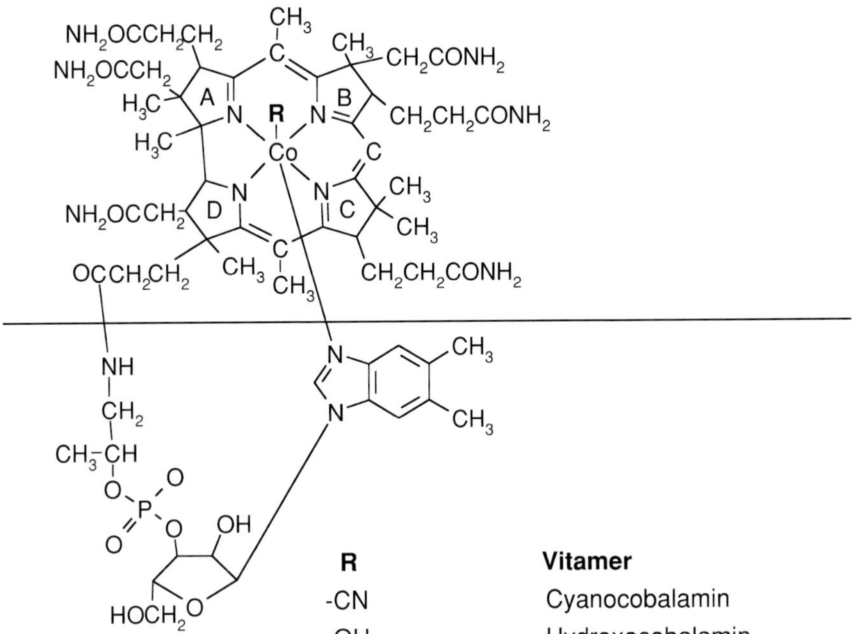

R	Vitamer
-CN	Cyanocobalamin
-OH	Hydroxocobalamin
-5'-Deoxyadenosyl	5'-Deoxyadenosylcobalamin
-CH₃	Methylcobalamin
-H₂O	Aquacobalamin
-NO₂	Nitritocobalamin

Fig. 5 Structure of the different vitamin B12 vitamers.

Definition

Only microorganisms are able to synthesise vitamin B12. Microbiological vitamin B12 synthesis in humans, however, takes place in the lower intestine where the body cannot sufficiently absorb the vitamin. Therefore, humans have to supply the vitamin via the diet. The vitamers differ in their photosensitivity, but they are all sooner or later inactivated when exposed to visible light. Good dietary sources of vitamin B12 comprise mostly animal-derived products, e.g. liver, meat, egg (yolk), milk and milk products, whereas vegan diets are basically vitamin B12-free (10).

Vitamin B12 is special in as far as its absorption depends on the availability of several secretory proteins, the most important being the so-called intrinsic factor (IF). IF is produced by the parietal cells of the fundic mucosa in man and is secreted simultaneously with HCl. In the small intestine, vitamin B12 (extrinsic factor) binds to the alkali-stable gastric glycoprotein IF. The molecules form a complex that resists intestinal proteolysis. In the ileum, the IF-vitamin B12-complex attaches to specific mucosal receptors of the microvilli as soon as the chymus reaches a neutral pH. Then either cobalamin alone or the complex as a whole enters the mucosal cell.

Mechanisms of Action

Vitamin B12 appears in two coenzymatic forms, namely methylcobalamin (cytosol) and 5'-deoxyadenosylcobalamin (mitochondria). Vitamin B12-dependent enzymes are (11):

1. Methylmalonyl-CoA mutase: 5'-deoxyadenosylcobalamin is part of dimethyl-benzimidazolecobamide coenzyme, a constituent of methylmalonyl-CoA mutase. This mutase catalyses the isomerisation of methylmalonyl-CoA to succinyl-CoA (anaplerotic reaction of the citric acid cycle).
2. Leucine 2,3-amino-mutase

V

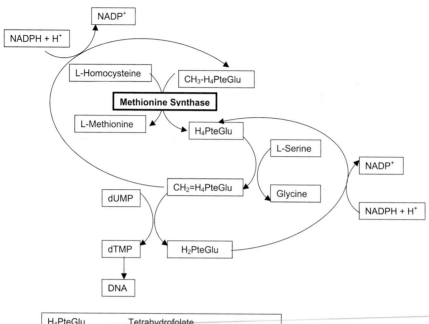

H₄PteGlu	Tetrahydrofolate
H₂PteGlu	Dihydrofolate
CH₃-H₄PteGlu	5-methyltetrahydrofolate
CH₂=H₄PteGlu	5,10-methylenetetrahydofolate
dUMP	desoxy uridine monophosphate
dTMP	desoxy thymidine monophosphate

Fig. 6 Selected reactions in which folic acid coenzymes are involved.

3. N5-Methyltetrahydrofolate homocysteine methyltransferase (= methionine synthesase). This reaction is essential to restore tetrahydrofolate from N5-methyltetrahydrofolate (Fig. 6).

Clinical Use (incl. side effects)

Vitamin B12 deficiency develops when the availability of intrinsic factor is reduced (atrophic gastritis, gastric mucosal defects, after gastrectomy), in persons with malabsorption syndromes, especially when the terminal ileum is involved, in breastfed infants whose mothers have lived on a vegan diet for years, in persons with congenital abnormalities in cobalamin metabolism and in persons having intestinal parasites, especially fish tapeworms (*Diphyllobothrium latum*). The characteristic symptoms of vitamin B12 deficiency include macrocytic hyperchromic ▶ anemia (common symptom in both vitamin B12 and folic acid deficiency) and ▶ funicular myelitis (neurological disorder, characteristic of vitamin B12 deficiency) (12).

Cyano- and hydroxocobalamin – both can be converted to the physiologically relevant coenzymes methyl- and 5′-deoxyadenosylcobalamin in the liver – are used for therapeutical applications. When pernicious anemia caused by chronic atrophic gastritis has been diagnosed it is treated as follows: During the first 7 days of treatment, 1000 µg of hydroxocobalamin/d are administered parenterally, usually intramuscularly. Then, the same dose is given once weekly for 4 to 6 weeks. The aim is to alleviate the deficiency symptoms and at the same time to replenish the stores. Afterwards, 1000 µg hydroxocobalamin should be given parenterally every 2 months lifelong to avoid relapse (12).

When funicular myelitis occurs in advanced stages of vitamin B12 deficiency, patients are given 250 µg vitamin B12/d during the first 2 weeks of treatment to alleviate the symptoms and to replenish the stores. If the deficiency has been caused by disturbed vitamin B12 absorption, lifelong monthly injections of 100 µg vitamin B12 are indicated (13).

Whether supplementation of vitamin B12 is useful in the therapy of a number of neurological disorders is still subject to discussion and further investigations.

Biotin

Synonyms

The chemical structure of biotin (hexahydro-2-oxo-1H-thieno [3,4-d] imidazol-4-valeric acid) is shown in Fig. 7. Of the 8 stereoisomers, only d-(+)-biotin occurs naturally and is biologically active.

Definition

Biotin can be synthesised by the human colon flora. The question to which extent this production contributes to covering the host-organism's requirements is, however, subject to discussion. In most foods of animal origin as well as in cereals, biotin prevails in the protein (= enzyme)-bound form as ε-N-biotinyl-L-lysine (= biocytin). Brewer's yeast, liver, soya beans and peanuts number among the biotin rich foods (14).

Mechanisms of Action

Biotin is involved in carboxylation and decarboxylation reactions. It is covalently bound to its enzyme. In the carboxylase reaction, CO_2 is first attached to biotin at the ureido nitrogen opposite the side chain in an ATP-dependent reaction. The activated CO_2 is then transferred from carboxybiotin to the substrate. The four enzymes of the

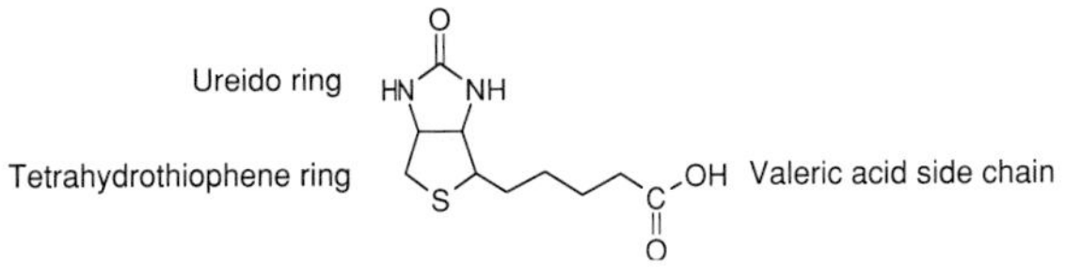

Fig. 7 Structure of biotin.

intermediary metabolism requiring biotin as a prosthetic group are pyruvate carboxylase (pyruvate → oxaloacetate), propionyl-CoA-carboxylase (propionyl-CoA → methylmalonyl-CoA), 3-methylcrotonyl-CoA-carboxylase (metabolism of leucine) and actyl-CoA-carboxylase (acetyl-CoA → malonyl-CoA) (15).

Clinical Use (incl. side effects)

Alimentary biotin deficiency is rare. It may, however, occur in patients on long-term parenteral nutrition lacking biotin or in persons who frequently consume raw egg white. Raw egg white contains a biotin-binding glycoprotein, called avidin, which renders biotin biologically unavailable. Pharmacological doses of the vitamin (1–10 mg/d) are then used to treat deficiency symptoms. There are no reports of toxicity for daily oral doses up to 200 mg and daily intravenous doses of up to 20 mg (15).

Folic acid

Synonyms

Folic acid or folate (Fig. 8) is the collective name for more than 100 derivatives of pteroyl-mono-L-glutamate. In plant and animal tissue, folic acid mostly occurs as pteroyloligo-L-glutamate ($PteGlu_n$), with up to 8 glutamyl residues.

Definition

Folic acid is sensitive to photo- as well as oxidative degradation and as an acid only slightly soluble in water, but in the salt form well soluble. 5,6,7,8-tetrahydro-folic acid ($H_4PteGlu$) is derived from folic acid by two consecutive reductions using $NADPH_2$. $H_4PteGlu$ and its derivatives are the biologically active vitamers. Reduced folates ($H_2PteGlu$ or $H_4PteGlu$) are less stable than folic acid itself. Folate losses during food preparation are high, especially when foods are excessively heated or soaked in water. Bioavailability of natural folate from foods averages 50%, while folic acid from supplements or fortified foods is absorbed to more than 90%.

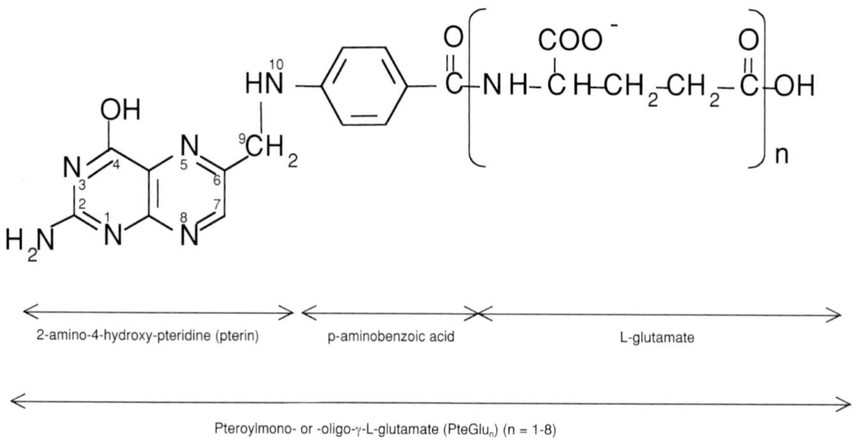

2-amino-4-hydroxy-pteridine (pterin)   p-aminobenzoic acid   L-glutamate

Pteroylmono- or -oligo-γ-L-glutamate (PteGlu$_n$) (n = 1-8)

Fig. 8 Structure of folic acid.

Spinach, salad, cereal germ and bran as well as pulses are good sources of folic acid. Liver and yeast contain high amounts of this vitamin, too, but are not consumed frequently enough to be relevant for the coverage of daily requirements (16,17).

Mechanisms of Action

Tetrahydrofolic acid (H$_4$PteGlu) accepts and transfers activated one-carbon units in the form of 5-methyl-, 10-formyl-, 5-formyl-, 5,10-methenyl-, 5,10-methylene-, and 5-formiminotetrahydrofolate (Fig. 9). These activated metabolites are involved in the methylation of homocysteine to methionine, the conversion of glycine to serine, in histidine metabolism as well as in choline, purine and pyrimidene biosynthesis.

5-methyl-tetrahydro folic acid is furthermore, together with vitamin B12 and B6, required to regenerate homocysteine (Fig. 6). Homocysteine results when methionine is used as a substrate for methyl group transfer. During the last few years, homocysteine has been acknowledged as an independent risk factor in atherosclerosis etiology. Folic acid supplementation can help reduce elevated homocysteine plasma levels and is therefore supposed to reduce the risk of atherosclerosis as well (17).

Clinical Use (incl. side effects)

Folic acid deficiency is common even in industrial countries. High-risk groups to develop folic acid deficiency are pregnant and breastfeeding women, people who regularly take anticonvulsant drugs, oral contraceptives or tuberculostatics, patients suffering from malabsorption and chronic alcoholics. As folic acid is involved in cell proliferation, deficiency symptoms first become evident in tissues and cells with high proliferation rates, such as erythrocytes and epithelia.

It is recommended that women of childbearing age take 400 µg/d synthetic folic acid as a supplement in order to reduce the risk of neural tube defects of the embryo when they later become pregnant (periconceptional folic acid supplementation) (17). When supplementing folic acid, it should be considered that this vitamin can mask the simultaneous presence of vitamin B12 deficiency. The typical symptom of vitamin B12 deficiency, megaloblastic anemia, will be reduced by high doses of folic acid, yet the nervous system will – in the long run – be irreversibly damaged (= funicular myelitis) when vitamin B12 is not provided as well.

Overall, supplementation with folic acid is considered safe as the vitamin has a low acute and chronic toxicity.

Niacin

Synonyms

Niacin (Fig. 10) is a collective name for all vitamers having the biological activity associated with

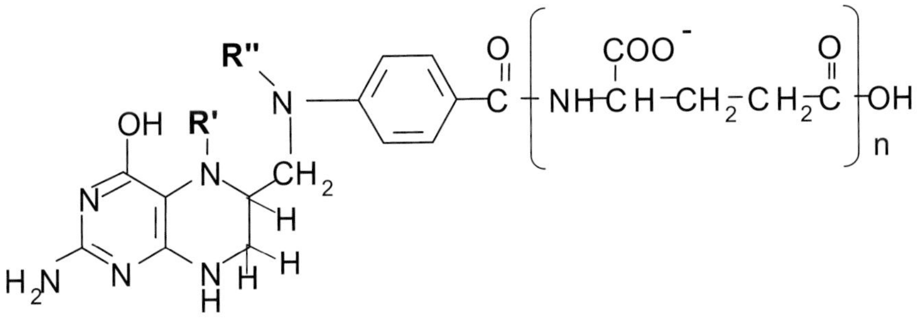

Coenzyme	R'	R''
Tetrahydro folic acid	-H	-H
5-methyl-tetrahydro folic acid	-CH₃	-H
5,10-methylene-tetrahydro folic acid	-CH₂-	
5,10-methenyl-tetrahydro folic acid	-CH=	
5-formyl-tetrahydro folic acid	-HCO	-H
10-formyl-tetrahydro folic acid	-H	-HCO
5-formimino-tetrahydro folic acid	-HCNH	-H

Fig. 9 Coenzyme forms of folic acid.

nicotinamide (= pyridine-3-carboxamide), including nicotinic acid (= pyridine-3-carboxylic acid) and a variety of pyridine nucleotide structures.

Definition

Nicotinamide and nicotinic acid are both white crystalline substances. Their aqueous solution has a maximal UV absorbance at 263 nm. Both vitamers have the same biological activity as they can be converted into each other. Fig. 11 shows the structure of the coenzyme forms NAD⁺ and NADP⁺.

Fig. 10 Structure of nicotinic acid and nicotinamide.

Most foods of animal origin contain nicotinamide in the coenzyme form (high bioavialability). Liver and meat are particularly rich in highly bioavailable niacin. Most of the niacin in plants, however, occurs as nicotinic acid in overall lower concentrations and with a lower bioavailability. The major portion of niacin in cereals is found in the outer layer and its bioavailability is as low as 30% because it is bound to protein (niacytin). If the diet contains a surplus of L-tryptophan (Trp), e.g. more than is necessary for protein synthesis, the liver can synthesise NAD from Trp. Niacin requirements are therefore declared as niacin equivalents (1 NE = 1 mg niacin = 60 mg Trp).

Mechanisms of Action

NAD⁺ and NADP⁺ are coenzymes of dehydrogenases. NADH/NADPH are intermediate carriers of both hydrogen and electrons. Most NAD-dependent enzymes are located in the mitochondria and deliver H₂ to the respiratory chain whereas NADP-dependent enzymes take part in cytosolic syntheses (reductive biosyntheses).

NAD⁺ possesses some non-redox functions as well. The glycosidic linkage between nicotinamide and ribose is a high-energy bond. The energy provided by breaking this bond allows the addition of ADP-ribose to a variety of nucleophilic acceptors.

Researchers found that NAD serves as a substrate in poly(ADP-ribose) synthesis, a reaction important for DNA repair processes. In addition, it takes part in mono(ADP-ribosyl)ation reactions that are involved in endogenous regulation of many aspects of signal transduction and membrane trafficking in eukaryotic cells.

V

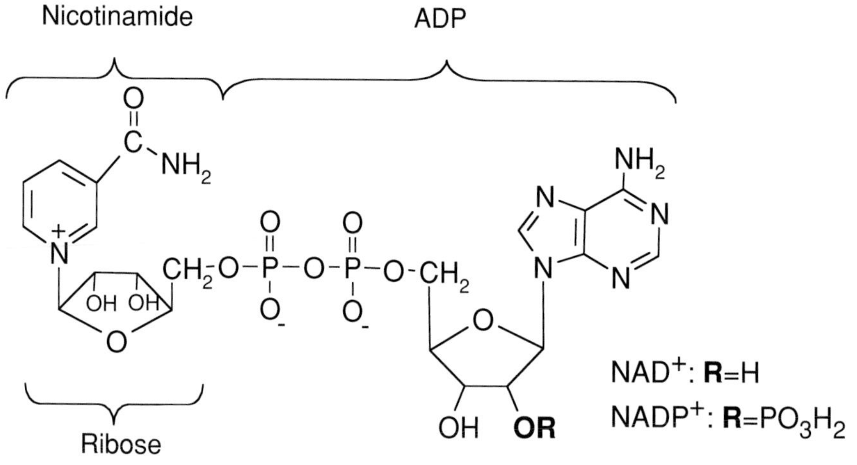

Fig. 11 Structure of the coenzymes NAD$^+$ (= nicotinamide-adenine dinucleotid) and NADP$^+$ (= nicotinamide-adenine dinucleotid phosphate).

NAD$^+$: **R**=H
NADP$^+$: **R**=PO$_3$H$_2$

NADP can be converted to nicotinic acid adenine dinucleotide phosphate (NAADP), which has distinct functions in the regulation of intracellular calcium stores. The studies of these new roles of NAD(P) in metabolism are in their early stages, but they might soon help to better understand and explain the symptoms of niacin deficiency (▸ pellagra) (18).

Clinical Use (incl. side effects)

Nicotinic acid is used in the treatment of hyperlipidemia. It causes various changes in lipid and lipoprotein metabolism when administered in high doses (up to 5 g/d):

The maximum changes achieved in a study were –20% total serum cholesterol, –40% serum triglycerides and +15% HDL-cholesterol (19). However, there are considerable short- and long-term side effects. The treatment should therefore be monitored by a doctor.

Nicotinamide potentiates the cytotoxic effects of chemotherapy and radiation treatment against tumor cells. This effect is probably attributable to increased blood flow and oxygenation of the tumor tissue. Furthermore, insulin-dependent diabetes mellitus might be prevented by the administration of high doses of nicotinamide (about 3 g/d) according to recent studies. The mechanisms have yet so far not been fully elucidated and potential side effects not completely explored (18).

Pantothenic acid

Synonyms

Fig. 12 shows the structure of pantothenic acid ((R)-(+)-N-(2,4-dihydroxy-3,3-dimethyl-1-oxobutyl-β-alanine). Only D(+)-pantothenic acid occurs naturally and is biologically active. The alcohol (R)-pantothenol (= (D)-panthenol) shows biological activity as well.

Definition

Pantothenic acid is an unstable, highly hygroscopic viscous water and alcohol soluble oil of light yellow colour. The vitamin is stable to heat and light. In pharmaceutical preparations, Na$^+$- or

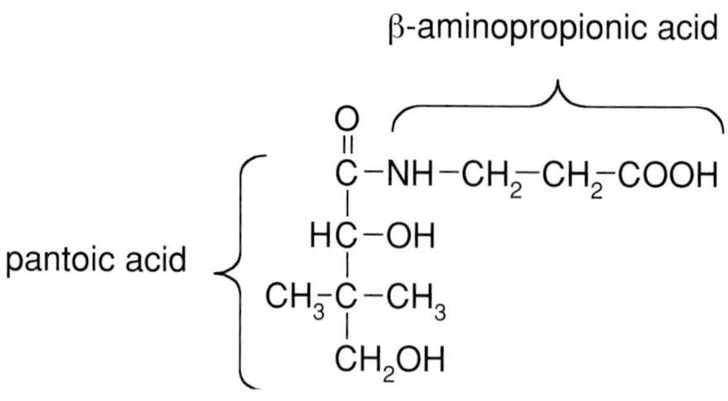

Fig. 12 Structure of pantothenic acid.

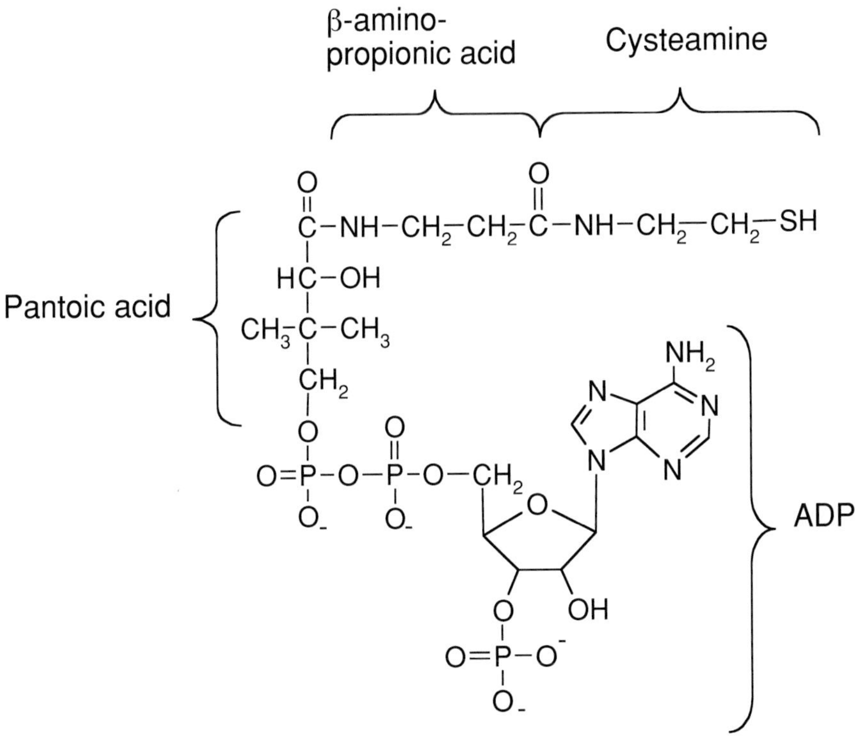

Fig. 13 Structure of coenzyme A.

Ca^{2+}-salts of the alcohol panthenol are more commonly used because it has an overall higher stability. Pantothenic acid occurs in most food stuffs. Liver, kidney and brain contain particularly high concentrations of pantothenic acid, yet numerous small contributions from other dietary sources, e.g. fruits, vegetables, milk and milk products, cereals or pulses, are more important for the coverage of daily requirements (20,21).

Mechanisms of Action

Pantothenic acid is an essential component of coenzyme A (CoA) (Fig. 13) and, as pantetheine, of fatty acid synthesase. The HS-group of cysteamine is in both cases the active site for the binding of acyl- or acetyl-residues. There is also a pantothenate-depending step in the synthesis of leucine, arginine and methionine.

The main role of CoA is acyl- and acetyl-group transfer and condensation. CoA plays a vital role in the metabolism of carbohydrates, fatty acids and nitrogen compounds. In addition to the role in energy generation and molecular syntheses, pantothenic acid participates in regulating numerous proteins by donating acetyl-and fatty acyl-modifying groups, which alter the location and/or activity of the acylated protein (21).

Clinical Use (incl. side effects)

Panthenol is frequently used in ointments and solutions for the treatment of burns, anal fissures and inflammation of the conjunctiva. The vitamin has to be substituted in patients on total parenteral nutrition and in those who regularly undergo dialysis. Hypervitaminosis has not been observed for doses up to 5 g/d (22). Furthermore, the administration of pantothenic acid leads to improved surgical wound healing due to its antiinflammatory properties.

Vitamin C

Synonyms

Vitamin C or L-ascorbic acid (Fig. 14) is chemically defined as 2-oxo-L-theo-hexono-4-lactone-

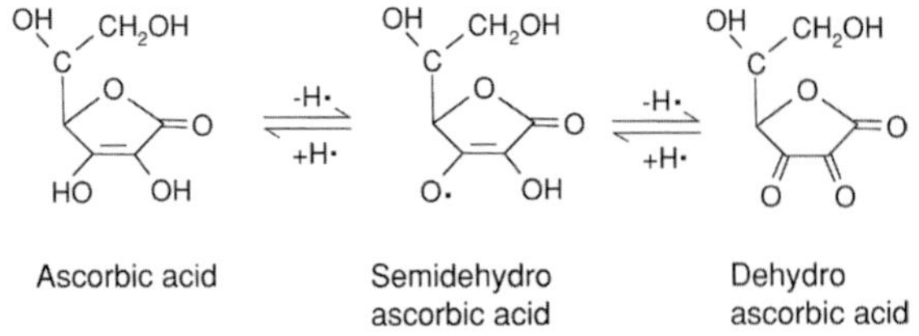

Fig. 14 Structure of ascorbic acid, semidehydro ascorbic acid and dehydro asorbic acid.

2,3-enediol. Ascorbic acid can be reversibly oxidised to semidehydro-L-ascorbic acid and further to dehydro ascorbic acid.

Definition

Ascorbic acid is photosensitive and unstable in aqueous solution at room temperature. During storage of foods, vitamin C is inactivated by oxygen. This process is accelerated by heat and the presence of catalysts. Ascorbic acid concentration in human organs is highest in adrenal and pituitary glands, eye lens, liver, spleen and brain. Potatoes, citrus fruits, blackcurrant, sea backthorn, acerola, hips and paprika peppers are among the most valuable vitamin C sources (23).

Mechanisms of Action

Ascorbic acid scavenges reactive oxygen and nitrogen species. The resulting ascorbate radical converts quickly to ascorbic acid and dehydroascorbic acid, but does usually not react with other surrounding molecules. This is why ascorbic acid is such an important physiological antioxidant. Dehydroascorbic acid is enzymatically reduced to ascorbic acid in biological systems. This recycling helps to maintain the ascorbic acid stores in the tissue at a high level. In addition to its antioxidant function, ascorbic acid plays a role as a cofactor of mono- and dioxygenases in norepinephrine synthesis, hormone activation, collagen biosynthesis, carnitine biosynthesis, and tyrosine metabolism (24). Furthermore, ascorbic acid improves intestinal absorption of inorganic iron by reducing Fe^{3+} to Fe^{2+} (only the latter has a high affinity to the mucosal iron receptor). In the stomach, ascorbic acid inhibits the formation of nitrosamines and thus might be important in protecting the stomach from ulcers and cancer. Finally, ascorbic acid competitively inhibits the glycosylation of proteins, a process that could be important for the long-term prognosis of diabetes (23).

Vitamin C status is supposed to play a role in immune function and to influence the progression of some chronic degenerative diseases like atherosclerosis, cancer, cataracts and osteoporosis. The role of vitamin C in immune function, especially during common cold and upper respiratory tract infection, is the subject of lively debate. The exact mechanisms of action have not yet been fully elucidated, but the results of several trials point to a reduced duration and intensity of infections in subjects consuming high amounts of vitamin C (200–1000 mg/d). However, the incidence of common cold was not influenced significantly (24).

Ascorbic acid is able to regenerate vitamin E from tocopheryl radicals. This reaction might be important in the context of atherosclerosis prevention. The role of vitamin C in cancer prevention is still unclear. Its importance in the etiology of various types of cancer has not yet been proven. The observed high vitamin C intake levels in groups with low cancer rates might simply have been a marker for high fruit and vegetable intake (23).

Clinical Use (incl. side effects)

Presently, the full clinical picture of vitamin C-deficiency, called scurvy, is rarely seen. The typical symptoms include mucosal and subcutaneous bleedings, follicular hyperkeratosis and gingivitis. Current issues regarding this vitamin include the question where the optimal dose lies to gain optimum health benefits. A daily intake of 75 mg for adults is considered sufficient to prevent vitamin C deficiency symptoms. The RDA for adults was recently increased by 25–50%, from 60 mg to 75 mg for females and 90 mg for males, acknowledging the fact that increased doses might help prevent chronic diseases. The results of numerous studies suggest that optimum health benefits are achieved (i.e. maintenance of maximum plasma and tissue stores) at even higher daily intakes of about 100–200 mg/d (24).

Vitamin C is not toxic and a hypervitaminosis has not yet been described in the literature. The statement that high vitamin C intake increases the risk of kidney stones could not be maintained.

Vitamin C requirements are increased during pregnancy and lactation, in patients undergoing hemodialysis and in smokers. Seniors often have suboptimal intakes.

On the basis of available results, persons suffering from common cold might benefit from taking 1–2 g/d of vitamin C. However, the usefulness of taking high amounts of vitamin C to prevent common cold has yet to be proven (23).

So far, it is not possible to give any recommendations concerning the vitamin C intake required for the prevention of osteoporosis, cataracts, cancer or cardiovascular disease.

References

1. Bitsch R (2002) Vitamin B1 (Thiamin). In: Biesalski HK, Köhrle J, Schümann K (eds) Vitamine, Spurenelemente und Mineralstoffe – Prävention und Therapie mit Mikronährstoffen. Georg Thieme Verlag Stuttgart, p 85–94
2. Tanphaichitr V (2001) Thiamine. In: Rucker RB, Suttie JW, McCormick DB, Machlin LJ (eds) Handbook of vitamins (third edition, revised and expanded). Marcel Dekker, Inc. New York, Basel, p 275–316
3. Bitsch R (1997). Vitamin B1 (Thiamin). In: Biesalski HK, Schrezenmeir J, Weber P, Weiß H (eds). Vitamine – Physiologie, Pathophysiologie, Therapie. Georg Thieme Verlag Stuttgart, p 67–74
4. Bitsch R (2002) Vitamin B2 (Riboflavin). In: Biesalski HK, Köhrle J, Schümann K (eds) Vitamine, Spurenelemente und Mineralstoffe – Prävention und Therapie mit Mikronährstoffen. Georg Thieme Verlag Stuttgart, p 95–103
5. Rivlin RS, Pinto JT (2001) Riboflavin (Vitamin B2) In: Rucker RB, Suttie JW, McCormick DB, Machlin LJ (eds) Handbook of vitamins (third edition, revised and expanded). Marcel Dekker, Inc. New York, Basel, p 255–273
6. Bitsch R (1997). Vitamin B2 (Riboflavin). In: Biesalski HK, Schrezenmeir J, Weber P, Weiß H (eds). Vitamine – Physiologie, Pathophysiologie, Therapie. Georg Thieme Verlag Stuttgart, p 75–84
7. Frank J (2002) Vitamin B6. In: Biesalski HK, Köhrle J, Schümann K (eds) Vitamine, Spurenelemente und Mineralstoffe – Prävention und Therapie mit Mikronährstoffen. Georg Thieme Verlag Stuttgart, p 70–74
8. Leklem JE (2001) Vitamin B6. In: Rucker RB, Suttie JW, McCormick DB, Machlin LJ (eds) Handbook of vitamins (third edition, revised and expanded). Marcel Dekker, Inc. New York, Basel, p 339–396
9. Zempleni J (1997) Vitamin B6. In: Biesalski HK, Schrezenmeir J, Weber P, Weiß H (eds). Vitamine – Physiologie, Pathophysiologie, Therapie. Georg Thieme Verlag Stuttgart, p 85–95
10. Frank J (2002) Vitamin B12. In: Biesalski HK, Köhrle J, Schümann K (eds) Vitamine, Spurenelemente und Mineralstoffe – Prävention und Therapie mit Mikronährstoffen. Georg Thieme Verlag Stuttgart, p 75–79
11. Beck WS (2001) Cobalamin (Vitamin B12). In: Rucker RB, Suttie JW, McCormick DB, Machlin LJ (eds) Handbook of vitamins (third edition, revised and expanded). Marcel Dekker, Inc. New York, Basel, p 463–512
12. Kurrle E (1997) Mangel an Vitamin B12 und an Folsäure: megaloblastäre Anämien. In: Biesalski HK, Schrezenmeir J, Weber P, Weiß H (eds). Vitamine – Physiologie, Pathophysiologie, Therapie. Georg Thieme Verlag Stuttgart, p 257–263
13. Nix WA (1997) Vitamin-B12-Mangel: funikuläre Myelose. In: Biesalski HK, Schrezenmeir J, Weber P, Weiß H (eds). Vitamine – Physiologie, Pathophysiologie, Therapie. Georg Thieme Verlag Stuttgart, p 263–265
14. Krause KH (2002) Biotin. In: Biesalski HK, Köhrle J, Schümann K (eds) Vitamine, Spurenelemente und Mineralstoffe – Prävention und Therapie mit Mikronährstoffen. Georg Thieme Verlag Stuttgart, p 104–110
15. Mock DM (2001) Biotin. In: Rucker RB, Suttie JW, McCormick DB, Machlin LJ (eds) Handbook of vitamins (third edition, revised and expanded). Marcel Dekker, Inc. New York, Basel, p 397–426
16. Brody T, Shane B (2001) Folic acid. In: Rucker RB, Suttie JW, McCormick DB, Machlin LJ (eds) Handbook of vitamins (third edition, revised and expanded). Marcel Dekker, Inc. New York, Basel, p 427–462
17. Frank J (2002) Folsäure. In: Biesalski HK, Köhrle J, Schümann K (eds) Vitamine, Spurenelemente und Mineralstoffe – Prävention und Therapie mit Mikronährstoffen. Georg Thieme Verlag Stuttgart, p 80–85

18. Kirkland JB, Rawling JM (2001) Niacin. In: Rucker RB, Suttie JW, McCormick DB, Machlin LJ (eds) Handbook of vitamins (third edition, revised and expanded). Marcel Dekker, Inc. New York, Basel, p 213–254

19. Wolfram G (1997) Dyslipoproteinämien. In: Biesalski HK, Schrezenmeir J, Weber P, Weiß H (eds). Vitamine – Physiologie, Pathophysiologie, Therapie. Georg Thieme Verlag Stuttgart, p 375–380

20. Biesalski HK, Hanck A (2002) Pantothensäure. In: Biesalski HK, Köhrle J, Schümann K (eds) Vitamine, Spurenelemente und Mineralstoffe – Prävention und Therapie mit Mikronährstoffen. Georg Thieme Verlag Stuttgart, p 111–116

21. Plesofsky NS (2001) Pantothenic Acid. In: Rucker RB, Suttie JW, McCormick DB, Machlin LJ (eds) Handbook of vitamins (third edition, revised and expanded). Marcel Dekker, Inc. New York, Basel, p 317–337

22. Biesalski HK, Hanck (1997) Pantothensäure. In: Biesalski HK, Schrezenmeir J, Weber P, Weiß H (eds). Vitamine – Physiologie, Pathophysiologie, Therapie. Georg Thieme Verlag Stuttgart, p 126–131

23. Weber P (2002) Vitamin C. In: Biesalski HK, Köhrle J, Schümann K (eds) Vitamine, Spurenelemente und Mineralstoffe – Prävention und Therapie mit Mikronährstoffen. Georg Thieme Verlag Stuttgart, p 57–69

24. Johnston CS, Steinberg FM, Rucker RB (2001) Ascorbic acid. In: Rucker RB, Suttie JW, McCormick DB, Machlin LJ (eds) Handbook of vitamins (third edition, revised and expanded). Marcel Dekker, Inc. New York, Basel, p 529–554

25. Bässler KH (1997) Niacin. In: Biesalski HK, Schrezenmeir J, Weber P, Weiß H (eds). Vitamine – Physiologie, Pathophysiologie, Therapie. Georg Thieme Verlag Stuttgart, p 122–125

26. Bässler KH, Biesalski HK (2002) Niacin. In: Biesalski HK, Köhrle J, Schümann K (eds) Vitamine, Spurenelemente und Mineralstoffe – Prävention und Therapie mit Mikronährstoffen. Georg Thieme Verlag Stuttgart, p 117–123

27. Hanck A, Weber P (1997) Vitamin C. In: Biesalski HK, Schrezenmeir J, Weber P, Weiß H (eds). Vitamine – Physiologie, Pathophysiologie, Therapie. Georg Thieme Verlag Stuttgart, p 132–140

28. Krause KH (1997) Biotin. In: Biesalski HK, Schrezenmeir J, Weber P, Weiß H (eds). Vitamine – Physiologie, Pathophysiologie, Therapie. Georg Thieme Verlag Stuttgart, p 117–125

29. Pietrzik K, Prinz-Langenohl R (1997) Folsäure. In: Biesalski HK, Schrezenmeir J, Weber P, Weiß H (eds). Vitamine – Physiologie, Pathophysiologie, Therapie. Georg Thieme Verlag Stuttgart, p 104–116

VLDL

▶ Very Low Density Lipoprotein

VMAT

VMAT is short for Vesicular Monoamine Transporter.

▶ Vesicular Transporters

Voltage-dependent Ca^{2+} Channels

FRANZ HOFMANN
Technische Universität München,
München, Germany
Pharma@ipt.med.tu-muenchen.de

Synonyms

High voltage-activated (HVA) calcium channels; low voltage–activated (LVA) calcium channels.

Definition

Voltage-dependent calcium channels are a family of multi-subunit complexes of 5 proteins, which respond to membrane depolarisation with channel opening allowing the influx of calcium into a cell. Voltage-dependent calcium channels are subdivided into three subfamilies: the HVA DHP-sensitive L-type calcium channels, the HVA DHP-insensitive calcium channels and the LVA T-type calcium channels (1,2).

Basic Characteristics

Voltage-dependent calcium channels regulate the intracellular calcium concentration and thereby contribute to calcium signalling in numerous cell types. These channels are widely distributed in the animal kingdom and are an essential part of many excitable and non-excitable mammalian cell signalling pathways. Electrophysiological studies characterized different calcium currents identified as L-, N-, P-, Q-, R-, and T-type current (1,2). The opening of these channels is primarily triggered by depolarisation of the membrane potential, but is also modulated by a wide variety of hormones, protein kinases, protein phosphatases, toxins and drugs. Site-directed mutagenesis has identified sites on these channels that interact specifically with other proteins, inhibitors and ions.

High voltege-activated (HVA) calcium channels are biochemically heterooligomeric complexes of five proteins encoded by four gene families (Fig. 1): The α_1 subunits of approximately 190–250 kD contain the voltage-sensor, the selectivity filter, the ion-conducting pore, the binding sites for most calcium channel blockers, and the interaction sites for G protein subunits and other proteins. Seven α_1 genes have been identified (Fig. 1). Four genes (Ca$_V$1.x) encode the L-type dihydropyridine sensitive channels. Three genes (Ca$_V$2.x) encode the dihydropyridine-sensitive, neuronal N-, P-, Q-, R-current. These α_1 subunits are associated with four auxiliary proteins (Fig. 2). The $\alpha_2\delta$ subunits, which are disulfide-linked dimers, are transcribed from four different genes and are clipped posttranslational into the extracellular located α_2- and the transmembrane δ-protein. The intracellular located β subunit and the transmembrane γ subunit are encoded by 4 and up to 8 distinct genes, respectively. With the exception of the skeletal muscle calcium channel, a heterooligomer containing the Ca$_V$1.1 (α_{1S}), β1, $\alpha_2\delta$-1 and γ1 subunit, the exact composition of individual channels is not known. The identity of these complexes is further complicated by the existence of several splice variants for most genes that confer significant effects on the electrophysiological and/or pharmacological properties of the channels.

The exact subunit composition of the low-voltage activated (LVA) channels is unknown (3). Three α_1 subunits, Ca$_V$3.x, have been identified that induce large T-type current after expression in Xenopus oocytes and in HEK cells in the absence of additional subunits. The T-type current is affected by the $\alpha_2\delta$ subunit suggesting a minimal subunit composition of $\alpha_1/\alpha_2\delta$.

Properties of the α_1 Subunits

Each α_1 subunit contains four repeats that are composed of six transmembrane helices and a pore region between helix S5 and S6. The selectivity filter of the channels is located in the pore region and calcium selectivity of the HVA channels is created by four glutamates (E) in each pore, whereas the LVA channels have glutamates in the pore of repeat I and II and aspartates (D) in that of repeat III and IV. Conformational changes of the protein allow the channel to occupy one of three states: the closed, open or inactivated state. The change in membrane potential is sensed by the S4 helices of each repeat, which contain a number positive charged amino acids. Movement of these helices induces opening of the channel pore. HVA channels are activated approximately at a membrane potential of –30 mV with a maximal activation around 0 mV, whereas the LVA channels activate at potentials around –60 mV and have a maximal inward current around –10 mV. The LVA channels activate and inactivate faster than the HVA channels. Inactivation of all channels is voltage-dependent and accelerated if the membrane is depolarised for prolonged time. ▶ Voltage-dependent inactivation may be mediated by sequences present in repeat I and II. Some of the HVA channels, especially the Ca$_V$1.2 channel, show calcium-dependent inactivation. Calcium flowing through the channel binds on the internal side to calmodulin, a calcium binding protein tethered to the carboxy terminal tail of the α_1 protein by an isoleucine/glutamine (IQ)-motive. The calcium-calmodulin complex induces a conformational change in the α_1 protein that leads to inactivation of the channel. LVA channels do not have this type of inactivation.

V

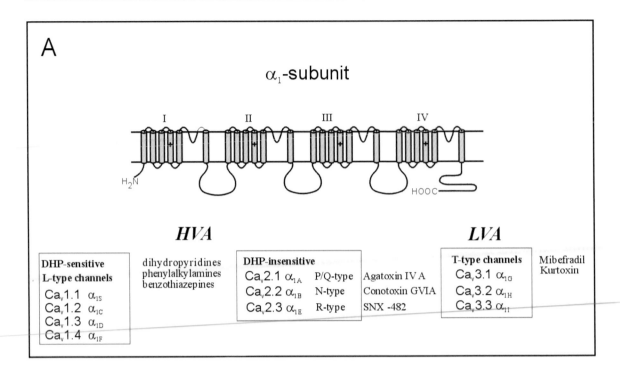

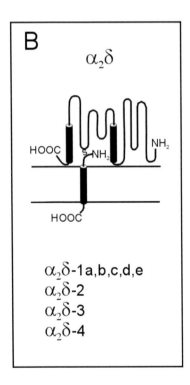

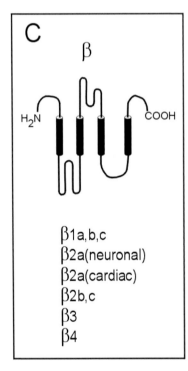

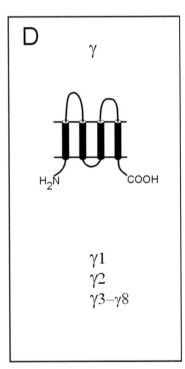

Fig. 1 Structure, identity and blockers of calcium channel subunits.

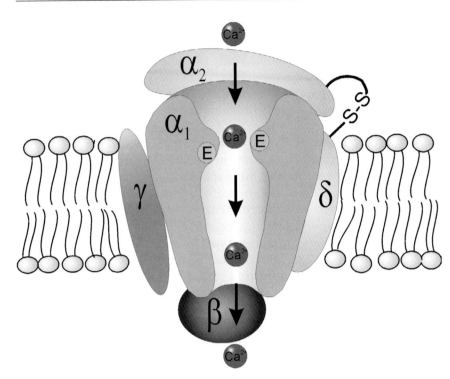

Fig. 2 Subunit composition of a HVA calcium channel. The selectivity filter of the channel is created by four glutamates (E).

The intracellular loop between repeat II and III couples and signals to intracellular ▶ effectors. The II-III loop of the Ca$_v$1.1 protein couples directly with the ryanodine receptor 1 located at the sarcoplasmatic reticulum in the skeletal muscle triad. In contrast, the cardiac Ca$_v$1.2 channel is in close proximity but not in direct contact with the cardiac ryanodine receptor 2. This cardiac ryanodine receptor channel is activated by calcium flowing through the open Ca$_v$1.2 channel. The II-III loops of the neuronal presynaptic localised Ca$_v$2.1 and Ca$_v$2.2 channels interact directly with the SNARE complex of the neurotransmitter-containing vesicles and facilitates together with the inflowing calcium fusion of the vesicle and plasma membrane resulting in opening of the vesicle. Similar interactions occur probably between the Ca$_v$1.2 II-III loop and insulin-containing vesicles of the pancreatic islets.

Neurotransmitter receptors inhibit the neuronal Ca$_v$2.x channels by activation of G-proteins. The β/γ subunit of the ▶ G-proteins binds to a QxxER sequence that is located at the I-II loop. Binding of the β/γ subunits confers the "reluctant phenotype" to these channels. This phenotype includes a reduced channel activation and current

at normal depolarised membrane potentials. The I-II loop interacts also with the calcium channel β subunit with high affinity allowing transport of the α$_1$ protein from the Golgi to the membrane surface and a shift in the voltage-dependence of channel opening and closing.

Channel Blockers

Distinct blockers have been identified for the various HVA calcium channels, which are listed in Fig. 1. ▶ Dihydropyridines, ▶ phenylalkylamines and ▶ benzothiazepines block all Ca$_v$1.x L-type calcium channels. These compounds are used mainly to lower the blood pressure in hypertensive patients. In therapeutic concentrations, they block mainly the smooth muscle Ca$_v$1.2 channel. The dihydropyridines bind with high affinity to the inactivated state of the L-type channels. Binding requires amino acids on the IIIS5, IIIS6 and IVS6 helices. Mutation of Thr1061 in IIIS5 to tyrosine abolishes the high affinity interaction of dihydropyridines with the Ca$_v$1.2 channel protein. The difference in the sensitivity between the cardiac and the smooth muscle L-type calcium channel is in part caused by the use of alternative exons (No. 8) coding for the IS6 helix (4). The phenylalkylamine

V

and benzothiazepine binding sites contain amino acids present in the IIIS6 and IVS6 helices and the glutamates in the pore region of repeat III and IV. The latter two groups include compounds that block neuronal $Ca_V2.x$ channels at similar concentrations as the $Ca_V1.x$ channels.

The LVA α_1 subunits are blocked by moderate to low (10 µM) concentrations of nickel and bind the channel blocker mibefradil and kurotoxin. Both compounds are not specific LVA channel blockers because they also block $Ca_V1.x$ and $Ca_V2.x$ channels at about 10 fold higher concentrations. Interestingly, the endogenous cannabinoid anandamide binds to LVA channels and stabilizes the inactivated state. This effect decreases T-type calcium current and neuronal firing activities.

The $\alpha_2\delta$ subunit 1 and 2 bind gabapentin with high affinity. This interaction may be causally related to its antiepileptic and neuropathic pain alleviating property.

Localization of Channels

The $Ca_V1.1$ channel is present in skeletal muscle at the triad. The $Ca_V1.2$ channel is widely distributed and represents the major L-type calcium channel in most tissues. In contrast, the $Ca_V1.4$ channel has been detected only in the retina, so far. The $Ca_V1.3$ (α_{1D}) channel is mainly found in neuro-endocrine cells and the inner ear. The $Ca_V2.1$, $Ca_V2.2$ and $Ca_V2.3$ are mainly localized presynaptically. The $Ca_V2.1$ and $Ca_V2.2$ channels interact with the vesicular release machinery and regulate the release of neurotransmitters.

The LVA channels are expressed in a wide variety of tissues. In the cardiac sinus node and the thalamus, activation of LVA channels seems to be necessary to generate action potentials upon depolarising the membrane.

Mutation and Deletion

Deletion of the $Ca_V1.1$ and $Ca_V1.2$ gene is not compatible with viable mouse pups (5). The $Ca_V1.2$ channel is absolutely required for the contraction of the developing mouse heart after embryonal day 14. Mutation of the human $Ca_V1.1$ gene is associated with hypokalemic periodic paralysis. Deletion of the $Ca_V1.3$ gene leads to viable pups that are deaf and have cardiac arrhythmia at rest. Mutation of the human $Ca_V1.4$ gene is associated with X-linked congenital stationary night blindness.

Mutation in the neuronal $Ca_V2.1$ channel is associated with familial hemiplegic migraine and episodic ataxia (▶ Episodic Ataxia/Myokymia) in humans. Deletion of the $Ca_V2.1$, $Ca_V2.2$ and $Ca_V2.3$ gene is compatible with life accompanied by a variety of central and peripheral defects.

Deletion of the $Ca_V3.1$ channel in thalamocortical relay neurons prevents ▶ absence epilepsy. A block of the neuronal LVA-channels alleviates certain forms of epilepsy.

Deletion of the β1 subunit is lethal, whereas deletion or mutation of the $\alpha_2\delta$-2, β3, β4, γ1 and γ2 genes is associated either with no or various neuronal phenotypes.

More recent analysis of tissue specific gene deletions showed that the $Ca_V1.2$ channel is involved in a wide variety of functions including hippocampal learning, insulin secretion, intestine and bladder motility. Further analysis will be required to unravel the functional significance of voltage-dependent calcium channels for specific cellular functions.

Drugs

Numerous dihydropyridine calcium channel blockers have been introduced to treat hypertension and stable angina pectoris. Nifedipine, Nitrendipine, Nisoldipine, Nilvadipine, Nicardipine, Amlodipine, Felodipine, Isradipine block preferentially the vascular, smooth muscle $Ca_V1.2$ calcium channel at therapeutic doses. Nimodipine, which has a short half-life, has been used to alleviate cerebral vasospasms after subarachnoidal bleeding. The phenylalkylamines Verapamil and Gallopamil and the benzothiazepine Diltiazem have been used as antihypertensive drugs and to treat supraventricular tachyarrhythmia. Mibefradial, a preferential T-type channel blocker has been used for a short period as an antihypertensive drug. It has been removed from the market due to intolerable interactions with other drugs.

Gabapentin is prescribed in certain epileptic diseases such as absence epilepsy and in neuropathic pain, although its therapeutic target is unknown.

References

1. Hofmann F, Lacinova L, Klugbauer N (1999) Voltage-dependent calcium channels: from structure to function. Rev Physiol Biochem Pharmacol 139: 33–87

2. Catterall WA (2000) Structure and regulation of voltage-gated Ca2+ channels. Annu Rev Cell Dev Biol 16: 521–555

3. Lacinova L, Klugbauer N, Hofmann F (2000) Low voltage activated calcium channels: from genes to function. Gen Physiol Biophys 19:121–136

4. Welling A, Ludwig A, Zimmer S, Klugbauer N, Flockerzi V, Hofmann F (1997) Alternatively spliced IS6 segments of the α 1C gene determine the tissue-specific dihydropyridine sensitivity of cardiac and vascular smooth muscle L-type Ca2+ channels. Circ Res 81:526–532

5. Muth JN, Varadi G, Schwartz A (2001) Use of transgenic mice to study voltage-dependent Ca2+ channels. Trends Pharmacol Sci 22:526–532

Voltage-dependent Inactivation

Voltage-dependent inactivation is channel inactivation at depolarised membrane potentials.

▶ Voltage-dependent Ca^{2+} Channels

Voltage-dependent Na$^+$ Channels

KEIJI IMOTO
National Institute for Physiological Sciences and School of Life Science, The Graduate University for Advanced Studies, Okazaki, Japan
keiji@nips.ac.jp

Synonyms

Voltage-gated sodium channel, Na$^+$ channel

Definition

Voltage-dependent sodium channels are a family of membrane proteins that mediate rapid Na$^+$ influx in response to membrane depolarization to generate action potentials in excitable cells.

▶ Table appendix: Membrane Transport Proteins
▶ Antiarrhythmic Drugs
▶ Epithelial Na$^+$ Channel
▶ Local Anaesthetics

Basic Characteristics

Voltage clamp and patch clamp studies revealed the essential properties of the sodium channels; kinetics of channel ▶ gating and selective ion permeation. Sodium channels are closed at negative resting membrane potentials. Membrane depolarization evokes very rapid activation of the channel, followed by inactivation within several milliseconds. The sodium channels recover quickly from fast inactivation when the membrane is repolarized. When the membrane is depolarized for a longer period (from hundreds of milliseconds to seconds), the sodium channels undergo slow inactivation. There are probably multiple types of slow inactivation. Recovery from slow inactivation requires a longer time of repolarization.

The sodium channels are very selective for Na$^+$ over K$^+$, allowing Na$^+$ influx down the electrochemical gradient to generate positive membrane potentials. The sodium channels are also permeable to Li$^+$ and NH$_4^+$. The narrowest portion of the channel pore is estimated to be rectangular (3.1 ×5.2 Å).

In addition to the ionic current, membrane depolarization evokes the gating current even in the absence of permeant ions. This tiny current represents the movements of charged parts of the sodium channel proteins. Comparison of the voltage-dependence of ionic currents and gating currents together with other lines of evidence, suggests that the sodium channels undergo multiple conformational transitions between the resting and open states. Conformational changes are essential for state-dependent effects of various drugs acting on the sodium channels.

The primary role of the sodium channels is to generate action potentials in excitable cells. In the

V

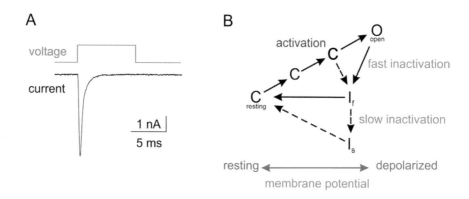

Fig. 1 A. Typical sodium current recorded from a CHO cell heterologously expressing sodium channels using the whole-cell mode of patch-clamp. Depolarization from the holding membrane potential (the upper trace showing the command potential) evokes an inward current (downward) of rapid activation and inactivation. **B. A state diagram showing conformational changes of the sodium channel.**

case of neurons, the sodium channel density is high at axon hillocks or axon initial segment where action potentials start to propagate. The sodium channels are also present in dendrites. The sodium channels are actively involved in ▶ back propagation of action potentials into dendrites. Subtle differences in the properties of sodium channels influence the dendritic processes of synaptic integration in complex ways.

Molecular Structure

Mammalian voltage-dependent sodium channels are composed of the main pore forming α subunit and smaller auxiliary β subunits. The rat brain sodium channel contains the 260 kD α subunit, the 36 kD β1 subunit and the 33 kD β2 subunit. The subunit stoichiometry is α:β1:β2 at 1:1:1.

The α subunit is the main component of the sodium channels, consisting of ~2,000 amino acid residues. Amino acid sequence analysis reveals four repeated units of homology (repeat I–repeat IV), each containing six hydrophobic, putative transmembrane segments. The N- and C-termini and the linking regions between the repeats are assumed to reside in the cytoplasmic side. The fourth hydrophobic segment, S4, of each repeat has a well conserved motif of positively charged residues appearing every third residue. This motif is found in other voltage-dependent channels and contributes to sensing voltage changes (▶ Voltage Sensor). S4 moves outward in response to depo-

larization and becomes accessible from the extracellular side. Among sodium channel subtypes, the linker regions between repeats are less homologous than the transmembrane regions, except for the linker connecting repeats III and IV.

The conserved linker between repeats III and IV is critical for fast inactivation. Cleavage of the III–IV linkage causes a strong reduction in the rate of inactivation. A cluster of three hydrophobic residues (IFM) in the linker is an essential component, probably serving as a hydrophobic latch to stabilize the inactivated state. Other parts of the α subunit are also involved in fast inactivation. Conformational changes in the P region contribute to the slow inactivation process

The region between S5 and S6 of each repeat is commonly called "P region" (P for "pore") and is important for forming the narrow part of the ion conducting pathway and the selectivity filter. Mutagenesis studies identified the most critical amino acid residues, D, E, K and A for repeats I–IV, respectively. Interestingly, alteration of K to E in repeat III, and A to E in repeat IV dramatically change the ion selectivity properties to resemble those of calcium channels, suggesting that these amino acid residues participate in forming the selectivity filter. This observation also suggests a close evolutionary relationship between the voltage-dependent sodium and calcium channels, although a prokaryotic voltage-gated sodium channel has been reported recently that is encoded

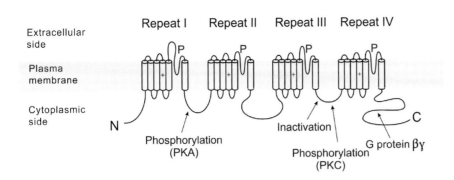

Fig. 2 A schematic model of the sodium channel α subunit. "P" the P region, "+" S4 voltage sensor.

by a single domain. The "P region" also forms the binding site for ▶ tetrodotoxin (TTX) and ▶ saxitoxin (STX), which block the channel pore from the outer side. The difference in tetrodotoxin sensitivity among the sodium channels is caused by a single amino acid difference in the "P region" of repeat I; the sensitive channels have aromatic amino acids (phenylalanine or tyrosine), while the resistant channels have cysteine or serine residues at the position. The S6 segments contribute to forming the inner pore of the channel.

Molecular cloning has detected multiple α subunit genes, more than expected from electrophysiological and pharmacological measurements. A new standard nomenclature has been proposed (Na$_V$1.1–Na$_V$1.9). The primary transcript from a sodium channel gene undergoes a developmentally regulated complex pattern of alternative splicing, generating further heterogeneity.

The sodium channels are practically classified into two major classes based on the sensitivity to tetrodotoxin. The brain types (Na$_V$1.1, Na$_V$1.2, Na$_V$1.3, Na$_V$1.6), the skeletal muscle type (Na$_V$1.4) and a peripheral nerve type (Na$_V$1.7) are sensitive to TTX, whereas the cardiac type (Na$_V$1.5) and peripheral nerve types (Na$_V$1.8, Na$_V$1.9) are TTX-resistant. The sodium channels show relatively similar properties, showing rapid activation and inactivation.

The β subunits (β1–β3) are membrane proteins with a single transmembrane domain and an extracellular immunoglobulin-like motif, and perform the regulatory roles of sodium channels. The β1 subunit accelerates the activation and inactivation kinetics. The β2 subunit is covalently linked to the α subunit, and is necessary for the efficient assembly of the channel. The more recently identified β3 subunit is homologous to β1, but differs in

its distribution within the brain and in a weaker accelerating property.

The three-dimensional strucutre of the sodium channel (from electric eel) was determined at 19 Å resolution using cryo-electron microscopy and single-particle image analysis. The sodium channel has a bell-shaped outer surface of 135 Å in height, 100 Å in side length at the square bottom, and 65 Å in diameter of the spherical top. An interesting finding is that there are several inner cavities connected to outer orifices.

Functions and Associated Disorders of Sodium Channel Subtypes

CNS neurons express at least four types of sodium channels, Na$_V$1.1, Na$_V$1.2, Na$_V$1.3, and Na$_V$1.6. Na$_V$1.1 is found in the somatodendritic membrane, whereas Na$_V$1.2 is predominantly found on axons and at or near axon terminals. A sequence of 9 amino acid residues has been identified in the cytoplasmic C-terminus of Na$_V$1.2, which mediates axonal compartmentalization. Na$_V$1.2 is likely to be involved in action potential initiation at the initial segment. Knockout of Na$_V$1.2 is lethal. Na$_V$1.3 is expressed predominantly in embryonic and early postnatal stages. Na$_V$1.6 is localized at nodes of Ranvier and dendrites.

In cerebellar Purkinje cells, a TTX-sensitive inward current is elicited when the membrane is partially repolarized after strong depolarization. This current is named "resurgent current" and is considered to contribute to repetitive firing of Purkinje neurons. Because the null and mis-sense mutation of Na$_V$1.6 (*med* and *med^{jo}* mice) disrupts spontaneous and repetitive firing, Na$_V$1.6 is suggested to underlie the resurgent current, although the resurgent current is so far observed only in Purkinje cells despite of a wide distribu-

V

Tab. 1 Mammalian sodium channel α subunits.

Type	Conventional names	Gene symbol (human)	Primary tissues
Na$_V$1.1	Brain type I	SCN1A	CNS, PNS
Na$_V$1.2	Brain type II, type IIA	SCN2A	CNS
Na$_V$1.3	Brain type III	SCN3A	CNS, PNS
Na$_V$1.4	μ1, SkM1, SCN4A	SCN4A	Skeletal muscle
Na$_V$1.5	heart 1, SkM2, hH1, SCN5A	SCN5A	heart
Na$_V$1.6	NaCh6, Scna8, PN4, CerIII	SCN8A	CNS, PNS
Na$_V$1.7	hNE-Na, Na$_s$, PN1, Scn9a	SCN9A	PNS
Na$_V$1.8	SNS, PN3, NaNG, Scn10a	SCN10A	PNS
Na$_V$1.9	NaN, SNS2	SCN11A	PNS
Na$_X$	Na$_V$2.1, Na$_V$2.3, NaG, SCL-11	SCN7A	CNS, PNS, heart, uterus

Note that the numbering of the new system is not the same as for the gene symbols.
Closely related sodium channel-like proteins have been identified and named Na$_X$. Functional properties of these proteins are not known, except for the NaG protein, which functions as a sodium sensor of body fluid.

tion of Na$_V$1.6. The *med* mutant mice show defective synaptic transmission in the neuromuscular junction and degeneration of cerebellar Purkinje cells.

Generalized epilepsy with febrile seizures plus (GEFS+) is an autosomal dominantly-inherited syndrome, which is distinct from febrile seizures, displaying seizures persisting beyond 6 years of age and generalized epilepsies. GEFS+ is associated with mutations in the genes encoding the sodium channel β1 subunit (GEFS+ type 1), the Na$_V$1.1 α subunit (GEFS+ type 2), and the Na$_V$1.2 α subunit. GEFS+ also results from GABA$_A$ receptor dysfunction.

In peripheral nervous system Na$_V$1.7, Na$_V$1.8, and Na$_V$1.9 are expressed in addition to the CNS sodium channel subtypes. Whereas large diameter neurons in dorsal root ganglia (DRG) generate TTX-sensitive currents (presumably mediated by Na$_V$1.6 and Na$_V$1.7), small cells also generate TTX-resistant currents (presumably mediated by Na$_V$1.8, possibly by Na$_V$1.9). Since small diameter neurons in DRG are the parent cell bodies of nociceptive nerve fibers (C-fibers and small myelinated Aδ fibers), the TTX-resistant Na$_V$1.8 channel is supposed to play a major role in pain pathways. When peripheral nerves are damaged, expression of Na$_V$1.8 and Na$_V$1.9 are downregulated, whereas Na$_V$1.3 is upregulated. The β3 subunit is also upregulated in injured nerves. This deranged sodium channel expression may cause aberrant ectopic activity in sensory neurons, generating ▶ neuropathic pains.

Mutations of the NaV1.4 channel gene cause various types of muscle diseases, including hyperkalemic periodic paralysis, paramyotonia congenita, ▶ myotonia fluctuans, acetazolamide-sensitivie myotonia. Mutations disrupt inactivation and cause both myotonia (enhanced excitability) and attacks of paralysis (inexcitability resulting from depolarization).

In the ▶ Long QT Syndrome (LQTS), the repolarization phase of the cardiac muscle is delayed, rendering the heart vulnerable to an "arrhythmia" known as torsade de pointes. LQTS is associated with five genes encoding ion channels. LQTS type 3 (LQT3) results from mutations of Na$_V$1.5, which cause a persistent sodium current. In contrast, sodium channel mutations associated with Brugada syndrome reduce the expression level of cardiac sodium channels.

Channel Modulation

Protein kinase A attenuates sodium current amplitude by phosphorylating serines located in the I–II linker. There is a consensus protein kinase C phosphorylation site in the III–IV linker. Activation of protein kinase C decreases peak sodium current and slows its inactivation. Sodium channels interact with G proteins. Coexpression of G protein $\beta\gamma$ subunits greatly enhances sodium currents, slows inactivation and shifts the steady state inactivation curve to the depolarizing direction. The C-terminal region of the sodium channel contains the G$\beta\gamma$-binding motif Q-X-X-E-R, suggesting that the sodium channel is directly modulated by G$\beta\gamma$ subunits. The sodium channel has the IQ-motif sequence of non-Ca^{2+}-dependent calmodulin binding in the C-terminal region. This motif is conserved in various types of sodium channels, but its physiological function remains to be elucidated.

Drugs

The sodium channels are targets of various chemicals and drugs. TTX and saxitoxin block the channel pore from the outside. Lidocaine and other local anesthetics act on the S6 transmembrane segment of repeat IV (IVS6) and delay the recovery from the inactivated state. Batrachotoxin, aconitine and grayanotoxin interact with IS6 to shift voltage-dependent activation and to slow inactivation. Scorpion toxins slow inactivation (α-toxins) and shift the voltage dependence of activation to more negative potentials (β-toxins). The peptide toxin μ-conotoxin GIIIB is a specific blocker for Na$_V$1.4, but no other pharmacological tools are available to specifically discriminate the sodium channel subtypes.

References

1. Hille B (2001) Ion channels of excitable membranes, 3rd ed. Sinauer Associates, Sunderland, MA
2. Catterall WA (2000) From ionic currents to molecular mechanisms: the structure and function of voltage-gated sodium channels. Neuron 26:13–25
3. Goldin AL (2001) Resurgence of sodium channel research. Ann Rev Physiol 63:871–894

Voltage-gated Ion Channels

▶ Voltage-dependent Ca^{2+} Channels
▶ Cl$^-$ Channels
▶ Voltage-dependent Na$^+$ Channels
▶ Voltage-gated K$^+$ Channels

Voltage-gated K⁺ Channels

OLAF PONGS
Institut für Neurale Signalverarbeitung,
Zentrum für Molekulare Neurobiologie
Hamburg, Hamburg, Germany
pointuri@uke.uni-hamburg.de

Synonyms

▶ Kv-channels

Definition

Voltage-gated potassium (Kv) channels are membrane-inserted protein complexes, which form potassium-selective pores that are gated by changes in the potential across the membrane. The potassium current flow through the open channel is determined by the electrochemical gradient as defined by the Nernst equation. In general, Kv channels are localized to the plasma membrane.

▶ Antiarrhythmic Drugs
▶ ATP-dependent K$^+$ Channel
▶ Inward Rectifier K$^+$ Channels
▶ K$^+$ Channels

Basic Characteristics

Functional Characteristics

Kv channels may be important determinants of cellular activities correlated with changes in membrane potential. Examples range from neural signal transduction, action potential wave forms, action potential propagation, action potential frequency, pacemaking and secretion to the regulation of cell volume and cell proliferation. In addi-

V

tion to changes in voltage, Kv-channel activities may be regulated by various physical and/or chemical stimuli. They include Na$^+$, Ca^{2+}, Mg^{2+}, ATP, O$_2$, pH, pressure, redox potential, phosphorylation/dephosphorylation, G protein binding, interaction with cytoskeletal proteins and more [1]. Once Kv channels have been activated, they permit a rapid passage of K$^+$ through the open pore along the electrochemical gradient as defined by the Nernst-equation. Many activated Kv-channels tend to inactivate [2,3]. The kinetics of inactivation may occur in time ranges of ms to tens of seconds. The inactivation mechanism of ▸ Shaker-channels, which inactivate rapidly, has been thoroughly investigated. The mechanism uses an amino-terminal inactivating domain. This domain is able to bind to the open pore of *Shaker*-channels. Thereby, the pore becomes both occluded and locked in an open state. Upon repolarisation, inactivated Kv-channels recover from inactivation. Inactivated Kv-channels are refractory to activation. In most circumstances, intracellular K$^+$ concentrations are higher than the extracellular ones, and the membrane potential is positive to the Nernst potential. Therefore, the direction of K$^+$ current flow through Kv-channels is mostly outward. But there are important exceptions, where either the membrane potential at which the Kv-channel opens is negative to the Nernst potential or the extracellular K$^+$-concentration is not very different from the intracellular one. For example, inactivated Kv-channels like ▸ HERG-channels (see above) may recover from inactivation at very negative membrane potentials. During recovery they pass through an open state permitting an inward flow of K$^+$-current. Depending on the particular conditions, hyperpolarizing Kv-channel activity may attenuate cellular excitability, e.g. the firing of action potentials, or they may balance depolarizing activities, e.g. clamp the membrane potential to a certain value to allow a steady inward flow of calcium ions. Frequently, depolarizing Kv-channel activity shifts the membrane potential into a hyperpolarizing direction.

Kv-channels are closed in the resting state. Upon depolarization of the cellular membrane potential closed Kv channels undergo a series of voltage-dependent activating steps until they reach an activated state from which they can open and close in a voltage-independent manner.

The open Kv-channel conducts potassium selectively. The flow of potassium ions is governed by the electrochemical gradient. Thus, the usual direction of potassium currents is from the cytoplasm to the extracellular space. A particularly interesting example of Kv-channel inactivation is represented by HERG-channels. HERG-channels have faster inactivation than activation kinetics, and they very rapidly recover from inactivation at negative membrane potentials. This behaviour may result in a situation where most of the current carried by HERG-channels occurs during their recovery from inactivation at negative potentials, i.e. represents an inward, rather than outward current.

Structural Characteristics of Kv-Channels

Kv-channels are frequently heteromultimeric protein assemblies of pore-forming membrane-integrated α-subunits and of auxiliary subunits [2,3]. The first Kv-channel subunits were cloned from *Drosophila*. This work initiated the subsequent identification and cloning of many more Kv-channel genes constituting a superfamily of related proteins. The design of the proteins is structurally and functionally highly conserved. Kv-channel α-subunits have cytoplasmic amino- and carboxy-termini, which frame a membrane-spanning core domain. The core domain consists of six hydrophobic membrane-spanning segments S1 to S6. Segments S5 and S6 are linked by the so-called P-loop. This P-loop enters and exits the plasma membrane from the extracellular face. Fig. 1A shows a cartoon of the most likely membrane topology of Kv-channel α-subunits. Four subunits are necessary to form a functional channel. Homo- as well as heterotetrameric assembly of Kv-channels is possible (Fig. 1B). Kv-channels can be expressed *in vitro* in heterologous expression systems (Fig. 1C). The relative ease to *in vitro* mutagenise Kv-channel cDNAs and to express Kv-channel cDNAs heterologously in the *Xenopus* oocyte or tissue culture expression systems has produced a detailed understanding of many basic features concerning Kv-channel activity. The results showed that the voltage-sensing apparatus of Kv-channels is mainly formed by amino-acids residing in segments S2 to S4. Most notably is the occurrence of a repeat sequence $(R/KXX)_{n=3-5}$ in segment S4 lining up several positive charges in

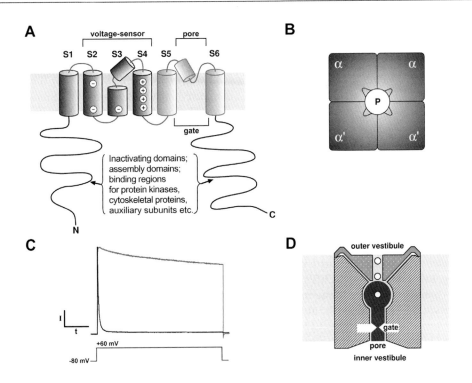

Fig. 1 Basic features of voltage-gated potassium channels. A. Schematic drawing of the membrane topology of Kvα-subunits. Transmembrane segments are numbered S1 to S6. The linker regions between segments S3/S4 and S5/S6 contain small α-helical regions marked as cylinders. Negative charges (-) in segments S2 and S3 and positive charges (+) in segment S4 contribute to the voltage-sensor of Kv-channels. Pore-forming residues are located within the S5/S6 linker region and segment S6. The gate which opens and closes Kv channels is not exactly known. Amino-acid residues of the S4/S5 linker region, segment S5 and segment S6 are directly and/or indirectly involved in the gating machinery. Brackets give examples for additional functions and properties associated with sequences and domains of the cytoplasmic amino- and/or carboxy-termini. **B. Assembly of four Kvα-subunits is needed to form functional Kv-channels with a central pore P. α and α′ indicate that assembly of homo- and hetero-multimers is possible. C. Typical examples of potassium outward currents (I) mediated by Kv-channels upon jumping from a holding potential of –80 mV to a test potential of +60 mV.** Black trace. rapidly-inactivating outward current; gray trace. non inactivating delayed-rectifyer type current. Time-scale (t) is in ms. Upon repolarisation from a depolarising test potential to a hyperpolarising holding potential an inward current or tail current can be observed that reflects the closure of open channels. **D. Schematic diagram of pore structure.** Shown is a hypothetical sagittal section through the pore. The pore has an outer vestibule, a selectivity filter (dotted gray) in the upper third of the membrane, an aqueous cavity, a gate (black), and an inner water filled vestibule. Potassium ions are drawn approximately to scale as white circles.

the membrane electric field. The charges apparently move in the electric field when the Kv channels become activated giving rise to a gating current across the membrane. Gating currents are observed during the voltage-dependent activation of Kv-channels.

Amino-acid residues residing in the S5-P-S6 region are engaged in forming the pore, most notably a highly-conserved P-loop sequence TVGY/FGD/N, which has been dubbed the K-channel signature sequence. This sequence forms part of the selectivity filter of the Kv-channel pore. It has been possible to crystallize a bacterial K-channel (KcsA). The crystals provide a high-resolution picture of the pore of a K-channel with its surrounding transmembrane helices [4]. A crystal structure of a Kv-channel is not available yet. However, the preservation of K-channel pore

V

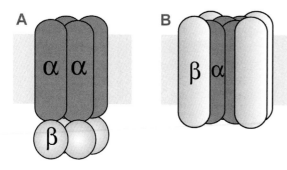

Fig. 2 Schematic drawing of voltage-gated potassium channels as heteromultimeric assemblies of pore-forming Kvα-subunits and auxiliary subunits. A. Assembly of *Shaker*-type Kv-channels with cytoplasmic subunits, e.g. Kvβ-subunits and KChIPs; B. Assembly of Kv-channels with membrane-integrated auxiliary subunits, e.g. MinK and MirPs. Membrane is shaded gray.

structures during evolution makes it likely that Kv-channels have pore structures with a selectively filter for potassium that is similar to the one of KcsA-channels.

According to the KcsA crystal structure data, hallmarks of the pore structure are an outer-vestibule with a relatively flat surface. Beneath lies a narrow selectivity filter in the upper-third of the membrane. This is followed by a central aqueous cavity narrowing into the internal mouth of the pore (Fig. 1D). Kv-channels, during voltage-dependent activation and opening, undergo marked conformational changes. In the resting state it is assumed that the pore is closed by a "gate" and that upon activation the gate opens. Amino-acid residues in the carboxy-terminal half of the S6 region seem to play a pivotal role for the structure and function of the Kv-channel gate. Other Kv channel domains may also contribute to channel gating, likely by indirect and/or allosteric mechanisms.

In addition to the membrane-inserted core domain of Kv channels, their cytoplasmic domains have many roles important for Kv-channel function [5]. Many of these functions are related to subunits assembly, channel trafficking to and from the plasma membrane, and interactions with cytoskeletal components (Fig. 1A). A tetrameriza-tion (T) domain for subunit assembly has been well-defined in *Shaker*-channels, where it is localized in the amino-terminus. Other Kv-channels (e.g. eag, HERG, ▸ KvLQT1) may have comparable domains within the cytoplasmic carboxy-terminus. ER retention and retrieval signals have been found in the cytoplasmic amino- or carboxy-termini. Also, cytoplasmic Kv-channel domains may contain recognition sequences for a variety of serin/threonine and/or tyrosine kinases. Finally, motifs have been characterized that interact with a variety of cytoskeletal components. E.g., the conserved carboxy-terminal amino-acid motif TDV is recognized by MAGUK(PSD)-proteins of the post- and presynaptic densities.

Auxiliary Subunits

Kvα-subunits may co-assemble with auxiliary subunits (see Table 1). Auxiliary subunits, e.g. Kvβ-subunits, may bind to cytoplasmic regions of the Kvα-subunits extending the reach of the membrane-integrated core channel into the cytoplasm (Fig. 2A). A particular interesting group is the KChIP-family. KChIP stands for K-channel inter-acting protein. The proteins are small Ca^{2+}-binding proteins being related to the superfamily of neuronal calcium sensors. They are tightly associated with somato-dendritic rapidly-inactivating Kv-channels (Kv4.1, Kv4.2, Kv4.3). Alternatively, the auxiliary subunits may be membrane integrated proteins like Kvα-subunits (Fig. 2B). Examples are members of the KCNE-family of auxiliary subunits that may assemble with a great variety of Kv-channels including ▸ KCNQ-channels, HERG-channels and *Shaker*-related Kv-channels.

Tab. 1 Auxiliary subunits and their reported interactions with Kvα-subunits.

Auxiliary Subunit	Kvα-subunits
Kvβ1, Kvβ2, Kvβ3	Kv1-family, *Shaker*
MIRP2	Kv3.4
KChIPs (KChIP1,2,3,4)	Kv4.1, Kv4.2, Kv4.3
KCNE1-KCNE4	KCNQ1-KCNQ5 HERG, Kv3.4, Kv4.3
sloβ1-sloβ4	BK(slo)α-subunits

Voltage-gated K$^+$ Channels

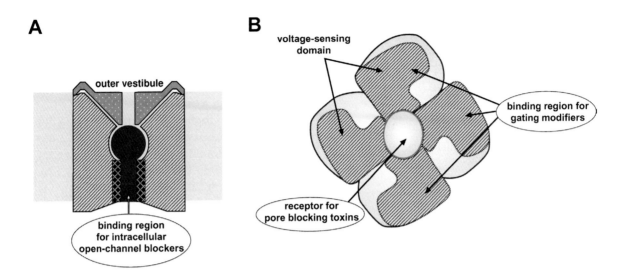

Fig. 3 Schematic drawing of Kv-channel binding sites for toxins and drugs. A. Side view of a cut-open Kv-channel. Intracellular open-channel blockers may bind to the inner vestibule of Kv-channels (hatched) formed by segment S6. **B. View of a Kv-channel from the top.** Pore-blocking toxins bind to receptor sites formed by the Kv-channel pore and the outer vestibule. Gating-modifiers have binding sites outside of the pore (striped) and interfere with the voltage-sensing machinery.

Functional activities of auxiliary subunits may include chaperone-activities during assembly, e.g. Kvβ-subunits have been shown to exert a chaperone-function for the assembly of *Shaker* α-subunits, or the recognition of ER-retention signals as discussed for KChIPs. Notably, auxiliary subunits may modulate the biophysical and pharmacological properties of Kv-channels. Certain Kvβ (Kvβ1.1 and Kvβ3.1) confer a rapid-inactivation behaviour to otherwise non-inactivating Kv-channels. Association of KCNE1 with KvLQT1 leads to a significant slowing of Kv-channel activation, a depolarizing shift in the voltage-dependence of activation and a change in drug sensitivity, e.g. for mefenamide. On the other hand association of KCNE3 with KvLQT1 leads to channels that are no longer activated by voltage, but behave like potassium-selective pores in the membrane.

Drugs

A great number of toxins in the animal kingdom, ranging from snakes to scorpions, insects, spiders and sea anemones have been identified that block various Kv-channels with nano- to picomolar affinities. Two kinds of block may be discerned in general. The toxin may bind to the outer vestibule of the Kv-channel pore and thereby occlude the pore (Fig. 3A). In this case, the binding of one toxin per channel may suffice to block channel activity. Alternatively, the toxin may interfere with the voltage-sensing machinery and modify Kv-channel gating. The voltage-sensing machinery is located in the periphery of the pore. As each subunit appears to have its own voltage-sensing apparatus, gating-modifying toxins may have four binding sites per Kv-channel (Fig. 3A). Characteristically, gating-modifying toxins induce a positive shift in the current-voltage relationship of Kv-channels and accelerate channel-deactivation (closing of the open channel).

Many non-peptidergic compounds are known to block Kv-channels. Where the mechanism of block is known, it is related to pore occlusion. Most frequently, non-peptidergic drugs block the pore by interacting with amino-acid residues located in the carboxy-terminal part of segment S6 (Fig. 3B). This part is particularly hydrophobic in the pore of HERG-channels. Apparently, it distinguishes HERG-channels from other Kv-chan-

Tab. 2 Kv-channel genes correlated with heritable diseases.

Gene	Trivial Name	Kv-channel Type	Disease
KCNA 1	Kv1.1	Shaker-channel	EA
KCNH 2	HERG	IKR-channel	LQT
KCNE 1	MinK	Auxiliary subunit	LQT
KCNE 2	MirP1	Auxiliary subunit	LQT
KCNE 4	MirP2	Auxiliary subunit	Myopathy
KCNQ 1	KvLQT1	Delayed rectifier	LQT/JLN
KCNQ 2	-	M-channel	BFNC
KCNQ 3	-	M-channel	BFNC
KCNQ 4	-	M-channel	DFNB2

EA – episodic ataxia; LQT – long QT syndrome; JLN – Jervyll-Lange-Nielson syndrome; BFNC – benign familial epilepsy; DFNB2 – deafness syndrome.

nels and renders HERG-channels exceptionally sensitive to block by many pharmaceuticals. Since HERG-channels make an important contribution to cardiac action potential repolarization, HERG-channel block may be frequently responsible for cardiac side-effects of drugs. Tetraethylammonium, 4-aminopyridine, and quinidine are unspecific drugs blocking Kv-channels by binding to the inner entrance of the pore. TEA may also bind to the outer entrance of Kv-channel pores.

Mutations in Human Kv-genes Associated with Hereditary Channelopathies

Mutations in human Kv-channel genes have been detected that are associated with hereditary diseases ranging from heart arrythmia (long QT-syndrome) and deafness to epilepsy and ataxia (see Table 2). Typically, many Kv-channel-related channelopathies are correlated with a mutant phenotype that is episodic in nature and appears as a dominant hereditary trait.

References

1. Hille B (2001) Ionic Channels of Excitable membranes, 3rd edn., Sinauer Associates, Sunderland, MA, USA.
2. Jan LY and JanYN (1997) Cloned Potassium Channels from Eukaryotes and Prokariotes. Annu. Rev. Neurosci 20:91–123
3. Pongs O (1999) Voltage-gated potassium channels: from hyperexcitability to excitement. FEBS Letters 452:31–35
4. Zhou Y, Morais-Cabral JH, Kaufman A and MacKinnon R (2001) Chemistry of ion coordination and hydration revealed by a K+ channel-Fab complex at 2.0 Å resolution. Nature 414:43–48
5. 5.Yi BA, Minor Jr. DL, Lin Y-F, Jan YN and Jan LY (2001) Controlling potassium channel activities: Interplay between the membrane and intracellular factors. PNAS 98:11016–11023

Voltage Sensor

The voltage sensor is the part of a channel protein responsible for detection of the membrane potential. A voltage sensor of the voltage-dependent Na^+ channel was predicted by Hodgkin and Huxley in 1952. Positively charged amino acid residues in S4 of each repeat play an essential role as the voltage sensor.

▶ Voltage-dependent Na^+ Channels

Vomiting

The act of vomiting is a complex process accompanied by several events apart from activation of the motor nerves and various voluntary muscles involved in the increase of intragastric pressure and evacuation of the stomach contents. Vomiting is preceded by a deep inspiration, closure of the glottis and raising of the soft palate to prevent vomitus entering the trachea and nasopharynx, respectively. There is also increased heart rate, pallor, salivation, sweating and lacrimation.

▶ Emesis
▶ Serotonin (vomiting)

von Willebrand Factor

The von Willebrand factor (vWf) is a heterogeneous multimeric plasma glycoprotein produced by megakaryocytes and endothelial cells which is found in platelets, plasma and the subendothe-

lium. Subendothelial vWf facilitates platelet adhesion, especially under high shear stress, by binding to glycoprotein GPIb-V-IX, a complex of four leucine-rich repeat proteins on platelets.

▶ Antiplatelet Drugs

V-type ATPase

▶ Table appendix: Membrane Transport Proteins

vWf

von Willebrand factor

VZV

▶ Varizella Zoster Virus

V

Water Channel

▶ Table appendix: Membrane Transport Proteins

Watson-Crick Base Pairing

The rules of base pairing (or nucleotide pairing) are:
A with T: the purine adenine (A) always pairs with the pyrimidine thymine (T) .
C with G: the pyrimidine cytosine (C) always pairs with the purine guanine (G).

This is consistent with there not being enough space (20 Å) for two purines to fit within the helix and too much space for two pyrimidines to get close enough to each other to form hydrogen bonds between them. These relationships are often called the rules of Watson-Crick base pairing.

▶ Antisense Oligonucleotides

Wernicke's Syndrome / Encephalopathy

Wernicke's syndrome is a serious consequence of alcoholism and thiamine (vitamin B_1) deficiency. Certain characteristic signs of this disease, notably ophthalmoplegia, nystagmus, and ataxia, respond rapidly to the administration of thiamine but to no other vitamin. Wernicke's syndrome may be accompanied by an acute global confusional state that may also respond to thiamine. Left untreated, Wernicke's syndrome frequently leads to a chronic disorder in which learning and memory are strongly impaired. This so-called Korsakoff's psychosis is characterized by confabulation, and is less likely to be reversible once established.

▶ Drug Addiction/Dependence
▶ Ethanol
▶ Vitamin B1

Wheal

The classical skin response to local release of histamine that results from contact with an allergen, irritant or following an insect bite. A central wheal develops as a direct result of local inflammation and the oedema follows the increased capillary permeability caused by histamine acting on H_1-receptors on vascular endothelial cells.

▶ Histaminergic System

Withdrawal

The abrupt cessation of a repeatedly or continuously administered opioid agonist, or the administration of an antagonist typically results in the withdrawal syndrome. Signs and symptoms include sweating, tachycardia, hypertension, diarrhea, hyperventilation and hyperreflexia.

▶ Drug Addiction / Dependence

X

Xanthine

▶ Anti-gout Drugs

Xanthine Oxidase

Xanthine oxidase (XOD) is the key enzyme in purine catabolism. XOD catalyses the conversion of hypoxanthine to xanthine and of xanthine to uric acid, respectively. The uricostatic drug allopurinol and its major metabolite alloxanthine (oxypurinol) inhibit xanthine oxidase.

▶ Anti-gout Drugs

Xenobiotic

Xenobiotics are chemicals not naturally belonging to or originating from a particular organism or an ecosystem (from Greek *xenos:*foreign). Environmental pollutants like agricultural pesticides, food constitutents, especially those produced by charbroiling, many drugs and cosmetics are typical xenobiotics. The drug-metabolizing system of vertebrates provides a chemical protection aimed at detoxifying xenobiotics.

▶ P450 Mono-oxygenase System

Y

YAC

A yeast artificial chromosome (YAC) is a vector that allows the propagation of large exogenous DNA fragments, up to several megabases, in yeast.

▶ Transgenic Animal Models

Z

Zero-order Kinetic

Zero-order kinetics describe the time course of disappearance of drugs from the plasma, which do not follow an exponential pattern, but are initially linear (i.e. the drug is removed at a constant rate that is independent of its concentration in the plasma). This rare time course of elimination is most often caused by saturation of the elimination processes (e.g. a metabolizing enzyme), which occurs even at low drug concentrations. Ethanol or phenytoin are examples of drugs, which are eliminated in a time-dependent manner which follows a zero-order kinetic.

▶ Pharmacokinetics

ZES

▶ Zollinger-Ellison Syndrome

Zinc Finger

Zinc fingers are structural motifs which were first recognized in DNA-binding domains of various proteins but which are now known to occur also in proteins that do not bind to DNA. In the classical C_2H_2 zinc finger domain, three secondary structures, an α-helix and two β-strands with an antiparallel orientation, form a finger-like bundle, which is held together by a zinc ion. Zinc ions are bound by 2 cysteine and 2 histidine residues, which are localized in the β-strands and the α-helix. The C_2H_2 zinc finger domain, which can insert its α-helix into the major groove of DNA, is one of the most common DNA-binding motifs in eukaryotic transcription factors. A second type of zinc finger structure, designated the C_4 zinc finger, is found in ▶ nuclear receptors. While C_2H_2 zinc finger proteins generally contains 3 or more repeating zinc finger motifs and bind as monomers to DNA, nuclear receptors contain only 2 C_4 zinc finger units and bind to DNA as homodimers or heterodimers. The C_4 zinc finger motif is structurally quiet as distinct from the C_2H_2 zinc finger domain.

Zollinger-Ellison Syndrome

Zollinger-Ellison syndrome (ZES) is characterized by the development of a tumor (gastrinoma) or tumors that secrete excessive levels of gastrin, a hormone that stimulates production of acid by the stomach. In most cases, the tumor or tumors arise within the pancreas and/or the upper region of the small intestine (duodenum).

▶ Proton Pump Inhibitors

Zona Glomerulosa

The adrenal cortex is functionally divided into three zones, the zonae glomerulosa, fasciculata and reticularis. Only the outermost zone, the zona glomerulosa, synthesizes ▶ aldosterone. The other zones are responsible for the generation of gluco-corticoids and androgens.

▶ Epithelial Na$^+$Channel (ENaC)
▶ Gluco-/Mineralcorticoid Receptors

Zymogen

Zymogen is a precursor protein that is converted to an active protease when one or more of its peptide bonds are cleaved, zymogens involved in coagulation include factors II (prothrombin), VII, IX, X, and XI.

▶ Anticoagulants
▶ Coagulation/Thrombosis

Appendix

Tables of Proteins
List of Drugs

Tables Index

Receptor Proteins

Receptor proteins are specialized structures that are able to recognize mostly diffusable molecules with a very high specificity and that are able to reversibly bind them with a high affinity. Ligand binding to the receptor initiates a signal transduction process which propagates the message of the ligand. There are many different types of receptors that differ especially in their mode of signal propagation. Most receptors are cell-surface receptors and respond to ligands that usually cannot enter the cell. Lipophilic molecules (e.g. steroids), however, are able to enter the cell and can act on intracellular receptors.

The group of **cell-surface receptors** can be subdivided into those with an intrinsic effector function (enzymes, ion channels) and others without intrinsic effector function. The first group consists of *receptor operated ion channels* or receptors with intrinsic enzymatic activity. In both cases the intrinsic effector function is regulated by ligand binding. Receptors linked to an intrinsic enzymatic activity are *receptor tyrosine kinases, receptor serine/threonine kinases* or *receptor guanylyl cyclases.*

Receptors without intrinsic effector function interact with proteins that are either effectors themselves or that can regulate effectors. The largest group of such receptors are the *G-protein coupled receptors (GPCRs). Via* heterotrimeric G-proteins they are able to regulate the activity of a variety of effector proteins (enzymes, ion channels). Other receptors such as the *cytokine receptors* interact with and activate cytosolic protein kinases (Jak-family) upon ligand binding. A third group of receptors (*TNF-receptor superfamily, IL-1/Toll-like receptors*) recruit adaptor proteins (e.g. TRADD, MyD88) following ligand-dependent activation which then serve as a platform for the formation of an effector complex consisting of various other proteins.

The majority of **intracellular receptors** are so-called "*nuclear receptors*". They are transcription factors that reside in the cytoplasm or nucleus and upon ligand binding translocate to the nucleus to become transcriptionally active.

Ligand-gated ion channels

Ligand-operated ion channels generate electrical signals in response to specific chemical neurotransmitters and are specialized in mediating the fast chemical synaptic transmission. Depending on their ion selectivity, ligand-gated ion channels are either excitatory (glutamate-, P2X-, nicotinic, $5-HT_3$-receptors) or inhibitory ($GABA_A$-, glycine-receptors). Ligand-gated ion channels can be grouped in three distinct families based on the architecture of the channel. Most known ligand-operated ion channels consist of five subunits. This pentamer contains different subunits two of which bind the ligand. Each subunit has four transmembrane domains. Heteropentameric channels are formed by $GABA_A$-, glycine- nicotinic acetylcholine and, $5-HT_3$-receptors. In contrast, the cation-selective ionotropic glutamate receptors have four subunits. Each subunit is able to bind glutamate. P2X purinoceptors subunits, finally, have only two transmembrane segments. P2X receptors are made up of three or four subunits. (▶ Nicotinic Receptor, ▶ Ionotropic Glutamate Receptor, ▶ GABAergic System, ▶ Glycine Receptor).

Cation channels

Receptor-subunit	Ion selectivity	Endogenous Ligand
Ionotropic glutamate receptors		
NMDA receptors (tetrameric)		
NR1	$Na^+/K^+/(Ca^{2+})$	Glutamate, Glycine
NR2A	$Na^+/K^+/(Ca^{2+})$	Glutamate, Glycine
NR2B	$Na^+/K^+/(Ca^{2+})$	Glutamate, Glycine
NR2C	$Na^+/K^+/(Ca^{2+})$	Glutamate, Glycine
NR2D	$Na^+/K^+/(Ca^{2+})$	Glutamate, Glycine
NR3	$Na^+/K^+/(Ca^{2+})$	Glutamate, Glycine
AMPA receptors (tetrameric)		
GluR1 (GluR-A)	Na^+/K^+	Glutamate
GluR2 (GluR-B)	Na^+/K^+	Glutamate
GluR3 (GluR-C)	Na^+/K^+	Glutamate
GluR4 (GluR-D)	Na^+/K^+	Glutamate

Cation channels (Continued)

Receptor-subunit	Ion selectivity	Endogenous Ligand
Kainate receptors (tetrameric)		
GluR5	Na^+/K^+	Glutamate
GluR6	Na^+/K^+	Glutamate
GluR7	Na^+/K^+	Glutamate
KA1	Na^+/K^+	Glutamate
KA2	Na^+/K^+	Glutamate
Purinoceptors (P2X) (trimeric)		
$P2X_1$	$Na^+/K^+/(Ca^{2+})$	ATP
$P2X_2$	$Na^+/K^+/(Ca^{2+})$	ATP
$P2X_3$	$Na^+/K^+/(Ca^{2+})$	ATP
$P2X_4$	$Na^+/K^+/(Ca^{2+})$	ATP
$P2X_5$	$Na^+/K^+/(Ca^{2+})$	ATP
$P2X_6$	$Na^+/K^+/(Ca^{2+})$	ATP
$P2X_7$	$Na^+/K^+/(Ca^{2+})$	ATP
Nicotinic acetylcholine receptors (nAChR) (pentameric)		
Ligand-binding		
α1	Na^+/K^+	Acetylcholine
α2	Na^+/K^+	Acetylcholine
α3	Na^+/K^+	Acetylcholine
α4	Na^+/K^+	Acetylcholine
α6	Na^+/K^+	Acetylcholine
α7	Na^+/K^+	Acetylcholine
α8	Na^+/K^+	Acetylcholine
α9	Na^+/K^+	Acetylcholine
α10	Na^+/K^+	Acetylcholine
Non-ligand-binding		
β1	Na^+/K^+	
β2	Na^+/K^+	
β3	Na^+/K^+	
β4	Na^+/K^+	
γ	Na^+/K^+	
δ	Na^+/K^+	
ε	Na^+/K^+	
Ionotropic serotonin receptors (5-HT$_3$) (pentameric)		
5-HT$_{3A}$	Na^+/K^+	Serotonin
5-HT$_{3B}$	Na^+/K^+	Serotonin

Anion channels

Receptor-subunit	Ion selectivity	Endogenous Ligand
GABA$_A$ receptors (pentameric)		
Ligand-binding		
α1	Cl^-	γ-Aminobutyric acid, (Benzodiazepines)
α2	Cl^-	γ-Aminobutyric acid, (Benzodiazepines)
α3	Cl^-	γ-Aminobutyric acid, (Benzodiazepines)
α4	Cl^-	γ-Aminobutyric acid
α5	Cl^-	γ-Aminobutyric acid, (Benzodiazepines)
α6	Cl^-	γ-Aminobutyric acid

Anion channels (Continued)

Receptor-subunit	Ion selectivity	Endogenous Ligand
Non-ligand-binding		
β1	Cl⁻	
β2	Cl⁻	
β3	Cl⁻	
γ1	Cl⁻	
γ2	Cl⁻	
γ3	Cl⁻	
δ	Cl⁻	
ε	Cl⁻	
θ	Cl⁻	
ρ1	Cl⁻	
ρ2	Cl⁻	
ρ3	Cl⁻	

Glycine receptors (GlyR) (pentameric)

Ligand-binding		
α1	Cl⁻	Glycine
α2	Cl⁻	Glycine
α3	Cl⁻	Glycine
α4	Cl⁻	Glycine
Non-ligand-binding		
β	Cl⁻	

Receptors with intrinsic enzyme function

Receptor tyrosine kinases (RTKs)

Receptor tyrosine kinases (RTKs) are a group of transmembrane receptors with an intrinsic tyrosine kinase activity. RTKs possess an extracellular ligand binding domain and an intracellular conserved tyrosine kinase domain. Almost 60 genes encoding RTKs have been identified in the mammalian genome (Robinson et al., 2000, Oncogene 19, 5548-5557). With the exception of members of the insulin-receptor family that form $\alpha_2\beta_2$ heterodimers, all known RTKs are monomers which dimerize upon ligand binding resulting in autophosphorylation of their cytoplasmic domains. Tyrosine autophosphorylation of RTKs induces recruitment and activation of various signaling molecules *via* the interaction of SH2 (src homology 2) or PTB (phosphotyrosine binding) domains with tyrosine autophosphorylation sites at the cytoplasmic region. Some RTK ligands (e.g. FGFs) require accessory molecules for receptor activation. While some RTKs homodimerize, heterodimerization is a common feature among different RTK subfamilies. (▶ Growth Factors, ▶ Neurotrophic Factors, ▶ Insulin Receptor).

Receptor tyrosine kinases (RTKs)

Receptor	Endogenous ligand(s)
ErbB receptor family	
ErbB1 (EGFR)	Epidermal growth factor (EGF), Heparin-binding (HB)-EGF, Transforming growth factor α (TGFα), Amphiregulin (AR), Betacellulin (BTC), Epiregulin (EPR)
ErbB2 (Neu, HER2)	dimerization partner for ErbB1,3,4 , no ligand so far found
ErbB3 (HER3)	Neuregulin-1 (Heregulin), Neuregulin-2
ErbB4 (HER4)	Neuregulin-1, -2, -3, -4; BTC, HB-EGF, EPR
Insulin-receptor family	
InsR	Insulin
IGF-1R	Insulin-like growth factor-1 (IGF-1), IGF-2
InsRR (IRR)	?
Platelet-derived growth factor-receptor family	
PDGFR-α / PDGFR-α	PDGF-CC, PDGF-AA, PDGF-AB, PDGF-BB
PDGFR-β / PDGFR-β	PDGF-BB, PDGF-DD
PDGFR-α / PDGFR-β	PDGF-AA, PDGF-AB
CSF-1R	Colony stimulating factor (CSF)
Kit/SCFR	Stem cell factor (SCF, Steel factor)
Flk2/Flt3	Flt3 Ligand
Vascular endothelial growth factor (VEGF) receptor family	
VEGF-R1 (Flt-1)	Placenta growth factor (PlGF), VEGF-A, VEGF-B
VEGF-R2 (Flk-1)	VEGF-A, VEGF-C, VEGF-D
VEGF-R3 (Flt-4)	VEGF-C, VEGF-D
Fibroblast growth factor (FGF) receptor family	
FGF-R-1	FGF-1, -2, -3, -4, -5, -6, -10
FGF-R-2	FGF-1, -2, -3, -4, -5, -6, -7, -8, -9, -10
FGF-R-3	FGF-1, -2, -4, -8, -9
FGF-R-4	FGF-1, -2, -4, -6, -8, -9
KLG/CCK receptor family	
CCK4/PTK7	?
Nerve growth factor (NGF) receptor family	
TrkA	Nerve growth factor (NGF)
TrkB	Brain derived neurotrophic factor (BDNF), Neurotrophin 4 (NT4), Neurotrophin 5, (NT5)
TrkC	Neurotrophin 3 (NT3)

Receptor tyrosine kinases (RTKs)   (Continued)

Receptor	Endogenous ligand(s)
Hepatocyte growth factor (HGF) receptor family	
Met	HGF (Scatter factor)
Ron/Skt	Macrophage-stimulating protein (MSP)
Eph family receptors	
EphA1	Ephrin-A1
EphA2	Ephrin-A1, -A3, -A4, -A5
EphA3	Ephrin-A1, -A2, -A3, -A5
EphA4	Ephrin-A1, -A2, -A3, -A5, -B2, -B3
EphA5	Ephrin-A1, -A2, -A3, -A4, -A5
EphA6	Ephrin-A1, -A2, -A3, -A4, -A5
EphA7	Ephrin-A1, -A2, -A3
EphA8	Ephrin-A2, -A3, -A5
EphB1	Ephrin-A3, -B1, -B2
EphB2	Ephrin-B1, -B2, -B3
EphB3	Ephrin-B1, -B2, -B3
EphB4	Ephrin-B1, -B2
EphB5	
EphB6	
Axl	
Axl	Growth arrest-specific protein 6 (Gas6)
Mer	Gas6
Tyro3 (Sky, Rse)	Gas6, Protein S
Tie	
Tie-1	?
Tie-2 (Tek)	Angiopoietin-1, -4 (Agonists); Angiopoietin-2, -3 (Antagonists)
Ryk	
Ryk	?
Dicoid domain receptor (DDR) family	
DDR1	Collagen
DDR2	Collagen
Ret	
Ret	Glial cell derived neurotrophic factor (GDNF; + GFRα1), Neuturin (+GFRα2), Artemin (+GFRα3), Persephin (+GFRα4)
Ros	
Ros	?
Leukocyte tyrosine kinase (Ltk) family	
Ltk	?
Alk	Pleiotrophin
Ror	
Ror1	?
Ror2	?
MuSK	
MuSK	Agrin
LMR	
AATYK	?
AATYK2	?
AATYK3	?
Others	
RTK106	?

Receptor serine/threonine kinases

Receptor serine/threonine kinases function as hetero-oligomeric complexes and consist of type II and type I serine/threonine kinase receptors. Ligand binding induces oligomerization. Type II-receptors primarily bind the ligand and phosphorylate type I-receptors (also termed "activin receptor-like kinases" (ALK)) which then specifically phosphorylate receptor regulated Smad-proteins (R-Smads). In response, R-Smads dimerize with Co-Smads in the cytosol. The R-Smad/Co-Smad complex translocates to the nucleus where it binds to regulatory sequences in combination with specific transcription factors.

Type II receptor	Ligand(s)	Type I receptor	R-Smads	Co-Smads
TβR-II	TGFβ-1/2/3	TβR-I (ALK-5)	Smad 2/3	Smad 4
ActR-II A		ALK-1		
ActR-II A	Activins	ActR-I B (ALK-4)	Smad 2/3	Smad 4
ActR-II B	Activins, Nodals	ActR-I B (ALK-4)	Smad 2/3	Smad 4
BMPR-II	BMP-6/7	ActR-I A (ALK-2)	Smad 1/5	
BMPR-II	BMP-2/4/7	BMPR-I A (ALK-3)	Smad 1/5/8	Smad 4
BMPR-II	GDF-5, BMP-2/4/7	BMPR-I B (ALK-6)	Smad 1/5/8	Smad 4
AHMR-II	MIS/AMH (Anti-Müller hormone)	BMPR-I B (ALK-6)	Smad 1	Smad 4

Receptor-linked guanylyl cyclases

Receptor-linked guanylyl cyclases belong to the group of receptor-linked enzymes. The receptor-linked (membrane-bound) guanylyl cyclases have one transmembrane region and function as homodimers. They share a conserved intracellular catalytic domain but differ in their extracellular ligand-binding domains (▶ Guanylyl Cyclases).

Receptor	Endogenous ligand(s)
GC-A	Atrial natriuretic peptide (ANP), B-type natriuretic peptide (BNP)
GC-B	C-type natriuretic peptide (CNP)
GC-C	Guanylin, Uroguanylin, (*E. coli* heat-stable enterotoxin)
GC-D	?
GC-E	?
GC-F	?
GC-G	?

G-protein coupled receptors (GPCRs)

Receptors

G-protein coupled receptors (GPCRs) represent the largest family of transmembrane receptors. The majority of GPCRs in mammalian organisms (depending on species up to more than 1000) belong to the group of olfactory, pheromone and taste receptors which respond to exogenous stimuli. Currently, more than 300 cDNAs encoding distinct mammalian GPCRs which are supposed to bind endogenous ligands like hormones, neurotransmitters or paracrine factors can be found in public databases (http://www.gpcr.org/ and http://www.expasy.org/cgi-bin/lists?7tmrlist.txt). For about 200 of these GPCRs endogenous ligands have been identified (see list below). GPCRs without an identified endogenous ligand are called "orphan" GPCRs. Their number is currently not well defined and may be in the range of 100-300. Based on structural similarity to rhodopsin (type A), calcitonin/secretin receptors (type B) and metabotropic glutamate receptors (type C), GPCRs can be grouped into three major classes (▶ G-protein Coupled Receptors). The cellular and physiological effects induced by activation of GPCRs are determined by the specific coupling of the receptor to subgroups of heterotrimeric G-proteins (G_s, $G_{i/o}$, $G_{q/11}$, $G_{12/13}$). A comprehensive list of drugs that act specifically on GPCRs

can be found under http://pdsp.cwru.edu/PDSP.asp as well as in the *TIPS Nomenclature Supplement* published by *Trends in Pharmacological Sciences*. (▶ G-protein Coupled Receptors, ▶ α-adrenergic System, ▶ β-adrenergic System, ▶ Cannabinoid Receptor, ▶ Chemokine Receptor, ▶ Dopamine System, ▶ Endothelins, ▶ Galanin Receptors, ▶ Histaminergic System, ▶ Kinins, ▶ Leukotrienes, ▶ Lysophospholipids, ▶ Metabotropic Glutamate Receptors, ▶ Muscarinic Receptors, ▶ Neuropeptide Y, ▶ Opioid System, ▶ Prostanoids, ▶ Protease-activated Receptors, ▶ Purinergic System, ▶ Serotoninergic System, ▶ Somatostatin, ▶ Transmembrane Signalling, ▶ Vasopressin/Oxytocin.)

Class A (Rhodopsin-like)

Receptor	Endogenous ligand(s)	Coupling
(Rhod)opsins		
Rhodopsin	11-cis-retinal	G_{t-r}
Blue-sensitive opsin	11-cis-retinal	G_{t-c}
Green-sensitive opsin	11-cis-retinal	G_{t-c}
Red-sensitive opsin	11-cis-retinal	G_{t-c}
Melanopsin	11-cis-retinal	?
Amines		
Adrenoceptors		
α_{1A}	Adrenaline = Noradrenaline	$G_{q/11}$
α_{1B}	Adrenaline = Noradrenaline	$G_{q/11}$
α_{1D}	Adrenaline = Noradrenaline	$G_{q/11}$
α_{2A}	Adrenaline > Noradrenaline	$G_{i/o}$
α_{2B}	Adrenaline > Noradrenaline	$G_{i/o}$
α_{2C}	Adrenaline > Noradrenaline	$G_{i/o}$
β_1	Noradrenaline > Adrenaline	G_s
β_2	Adrenaline > Noradrenaline	G_s
β_3	Adrenaline = Noradrenaline	G_s
Histamine receptors		
H_1	Histamine	$G_{q/11}$
H_2	Histamine	G_s
H_3	Histamine	$G_{i/o}$
H_4	Histamine	$G_{i/o}$
Dopamine receptors		
D_1	Dopamine	G_s
D_2	Dopamine	$G_{i/o}$
D_3	Dopamine	$G_{i/o}$
D_4	Dopamine	$G_{i/o}$
D_5	Dopamine	G_s
Acetylcholine receptors		
M_1	Acetylcholine	$G_{q/11}$
M_2	Acetylcholine	$G_{i/o}$
M_3	Acetylcholine	$G_{q/11}$
M_4	Acetylcholine	$G_{i/o}$
M_5	Acetylcholine	$G_{q/11}$

Class A (Rhodopsin-like) (Continued)

Receptor	Endogenous ligand(s)	Coupling
Serotonin receptors		
5-HT$_{1A}$	Serotonin	$G_{i/o}$
5-HT$_{1B}$	Serotonin	$G_{i/o}$
5-HT$_{1D}$	Serotonin	$G_{i/o}$
5-HT$_{1E}$	Serotonin	$G_{i/o}$
5-HT$_{1F}$	Serotonin	$G_{i/o}$
5-HT$_{2A}$	Serotonin	$G_{q/11}$
5-HT$_{2B}$	Serotonin	$G_{q/11}$
5-HT$_{2C}$	Serotonin	$G_{q/11}$
5-HT$_4$	Serotonin	G_s
5-HT$_{5A}$	Serotonin	$G_{i/o}$, G_s
5-HT$_{5B}$	Serotonin	?
5-HT$_6$	Serotonin	G_s
5-HT$_7$	Serotonin	G_s
Melatonin receptors		
MT$_1$	Melatonin	$G_{i/o}$
MT$_2$	Melatonin	$G_{i/o}$
MT$_3$	Melatonin, N-acetyl serotonin	
Trace amines		
TA1	Tyramine, β-Phenylethylamine	G_s
TA2	Tryptamine, β-Phenylethylamine	G_s
Nucleotide-like		
Adenosine receptors (P1)		
A$_1$	Adenosine	$G_{i/o}$
A$_{2A}$	Adenosine	G_s
A$_{2B}$	Adenosine	G_s
A$_3$	Adenosine	$G_{i/o}$
Purinoceptors (P2)		
P2Y$_1$	ADP > ATP	$G_{q/11}$
P2Y$_2$	UTP/ATP	$G_{q/11}$
P2Y$_4$	UTP > ATP	$G_{q/11}$
P2Y$_6$	UDP	$G_{q/11}$
P2Y$_{11}$	ATP	$G_{q/11}$, G_s
P2Y$_{12}$	ADP	$G_{i/o}$
P2Y$_{13}$	ADP	$G_{i/o}$
P2Y$_{14}$	UDP-glucose	$G_{i/o}$
Peptide receptors		
Opioid receptors		
δ	β-Endorphin, Met/Leu-enkephalin	$G_{i/o}$
κ	Dynorphin A	$G_{i/o}$
μ	β-Endorphin > Dynorphin A > Met/Leu-enkephalin	$G_{i/o}$
ORL1	Nociceptin/Orphanin FQ	$G_{i/o}$
Somatostatin receptors		
SST$_1$	Somatostatin-14 = Somatostatin-28	$G_{i/o}$
SST$_2$	Somatostatin-14 = Somatostatin-28	$G_{i/o}$
SST$_3$	Somatostatin-14 = Somatostatin-28	$G_{i/o}$
SST$_4$	Somatostatin-14 = Somatostatin-28	$G_{i/o}$
SST$_5$	Somatostatin-28 > Somatostatin-14	$G_{i/o}$
Melanin-concentrating hormone receptors		
MCH1	Melanin-concentrating hormone	$G_{i/o}$?
MCH2	Melanin-concentrating hormone	$G_{q/11}$

Class A (Rhodopsin-like)   (Continued)

Receptor	Endogenous ligand(s)	Coupling
Neuropeptide Y receptors		
Y_1	Neuropeptide Y (NPY) > Peptide YY (PYY)	$G_{i/o}$
Y_2	NPY > PYY	$G_{i/o}$
Y_4	Pancreatic Polypeptide (PP) > NPY = PYY	$G_{i/o}$
Y_5	NPY > PYY > PP	$G_{i/o}$
Y_6	NPY = PYY > PP	$G_{i/o}$
Bradykinin receptors		
B_1	Bradykinin	$G_{q/11}$
B_2	Bradykinin	$G_{q/11}$
Angiotensin receptors		
AT_1	Angiotensin II > Angiotensin III	$G_{q/11}$, $G_{12/13}$, $G_{i/o}$
AT_2	Angiotensin II = Angiotensin III	?
Vasopressin/Oxytocin receptors		
V_{1a}	Vasopressin > Oxytocin	$G_{q/11}$
V_{1b}	Vasopressin > Oxytocin	$G_{q/11}$
V_2	Vasopressin > Oxytocin	G_s
OT	Oxytocin > Vasopressin	$G_{q/11}$, $G_{i/o}$
Endothelin receptors		
ET_A	Endothelin-1 = Endothelin-2	$G_{q/11}$, $G_{12/13}$, G_s
ET_B	Endothelin-1 = Endothelin-2 = Endothelin-3	$G_{q/11}$, $G_{i/o}$
Orexin/Hypocretin receptors		
OX1	OrexinA/B	G_s, $G_{q/11}$
OX2	OrexinA/B	G_s, $G_{q/11}$
Neuropeptide FF receptor		
NPFF1	RFamide-related peptide 1 & 3, NPFF	$G_{i/o}$
NPFF2	Neuropeptide FF & AF (NPFF & NPAF)	$G_{i/o}$
Galanin receptors		
GAL1	Galanin > Galanin-like peptide	$G_{i/o}$
GAL2	Galanin-like peptide > Galanin	$G_{q/11}$, $G_{i/o}$, $G_{12/13}$
GAL3	Galanin	$G_{i/o}$
Protease-activated receptors		
PAR-1	Thrombin, Trypsin, Factor Xa, APC	$G_{q/11}$, $G_{12/13}$, $G_{i/o}$
PAR-2	Trypsin, Factor Xa, TF/Factor VIIa	$G_{q/11}$
PAR-3	Thrombin, Trypsin	$G_{q/11}$
PAR-4	Thrombin, Trypsin	$G_{q/11}$, $G_{12/13}$, $G_{i/o}$
Bombesin receptors		
BB1	Neuromedin B > Bombesin	$G_{q/11}$
BB2	Gastrin-releasing peptide > Bombesin	$G_{q/11}$
BB3		$G_{q/11}$
Tachykinin receptors		
NK_1	Substance P	$G_{q/11}$
NK_2	Neurokinin A (Substance K)	$G_{q/11}$
NK_3	Neurokinin B, Neuromedin K	$G_{q/11}$
Melanocortin receptors		
MC_1	α-Melanocortin (α-MSH) > β-MSH	G_s
MC_2	Adrenocorticotrophin (ACTH)	G_s
MC_3	γ-MSH = β-MSH	G_s
MC_4	β-MSH > α-MSH = ACTH	G_s
MC_5	α-MSH > β-MSH	G_s

Class A (Rhodopsin-like) (Continued)

Receptor	Endogenous ligand(s)	Coupling
Neurotensin receptors		
NTS1	Neurotensin	$G_{q/11}$
NTS2	Neurotensin	$G_{q/11}$
Cholecystokinine receptors		
CCK_1	Cholecyctokinin (CCK-8)	$G_{q/11}$, G_s
CCK_2	CCK-8, Gastrin	$G_{q/11}$
Thyrotropin-releasing hormone		
TRH-1	Thyrotropin-releasing hormone (TRH)	$G_{q/11}$
TRH-2	Thyrotropin-releasing hormone (TRH)	$G_{q/11}$
Others		
PrRP (GPR10)	Prolactin-releasing peptide	$G_{q/11}$
GRP7	Neuropeptide W-23, W-30, Neuropeptide B	$G_{i/o}$
GPR8	Neuropeptide W-23, W-30	$G_{i/o}$
GPR54	Metastin, Kisspeptins	$G_{q/11}$
UT-II (GPR14)	Urotensin II	$G_{q/11}$
APJ	Apelin	$G_{i/o}$
NMU1 (FM-3)	Neuromedin U	$G_{q/11}$
NMU2 (FM-4)	Neuromedin U	$G_{q/11}$
GHS-R	Ghrelin	$G_{q/11}$
GPR38	Motilin	$G_{q/11}$
PK-R1	Prokineticin-1, -2	$G_{q/11}$
PK-R2	Prokineticin-1, -2	$G_{q/11}$
Chemokine receptors		
CC chemokine receptors		
CCR1	CCL3, CCL5, CCL7, CCL8, CCL13, CCL14, CCL15, CCL23	$G_{i/o}$
CCR2	CCL2, CCL7, CCL8, CCL13	$G_{i/o}$
CCR3	CCL5, CCL7, CCL8, CCL11,CCL13, CCL14, CCL15, CCL24, CCL26	$G_{i/o}$
CCR4	CCL17, CCL22	$G_{i/o}$
CCR5	CCL3, CCL4, CCL5, CCL8, CCL11, CCL13, CCL14	$G_{i/o}$
CCR6	CCL20	$G_{i/o}$
CCR7	CCL19, CCL21	$G_{i/o}$
CCR8	CCL1, CCL16	$G_{i/o}$
CCR9	CCL25	$G_{i/o}$
CCR10	CCL27, CCL28	$G_{i/o}$
CXC chemokine receptors		
CXCR1	CXCL5, CXCL6, CXCL8	$G_{i/o}$
CXCR2	CXCL1, CXCL2, CXCL3, CXCL5, CXCL7, CXCL8	$G_{i/o}$
CXCR3	CXCL9, CXCL10, CXCL11	$G_{i/o}$
CXCR4	CXCL12	$G_{i/o}$
CXCR5	CXCL13	$G_{i/o}$
CXCR6	CXCL16	$G_{i/o}$
CX_3C chemokine receptors		
CX_3CR1	XCL1, XCL2	$G_{i/o}$
XCR1	CX3L1	$G_{i/o}$
(Glyco)protein hormone receptors		
FSH	Follicle-stimulating hormone (FSH)	G_s
LSH	Luteinizing hormone (LH), Choriogonadotropin	G_s,G_i

Class A (Rhodopsin-like)   (Continued)

Receptor	Endogenous ligand(s)	Coupling
TSH	Thyrotropin (TSH)	G_s, $G_{q/11}$, G_i, $G_{12/13}$
GnRH	Gonadotropin-releasing hormone	$G_{q/11}$
Relaxin receptors		
LGR7	Relaxin	G_s
LGR8	Relaxin, Relaxin-like factor	G_s
Cannabinoid receptors		
CB_1	Anandamide, 2-Arachidonoyl glycerol	$G_{i/o}$
CB_2	Anandamide, 2-Arachidonoyl glycerol	$G_{i/o}$
Prostanoid receptors		
FP	Prostaglandin $F_{2\alpha}$ (PGF)	$G_{q/11}$
TP	Thromboxane A_2 (TXA_2)	$G_{q/11}$, $G_{12/13}$
DP	Prostaglandin D_2(PGD_2)	G_s
IP	Prostacyclin (PGI_2)	G_s
EP_1	Prostaglandin E_2(PGE_2)	$G_{q/11}$
EP_2	Prostaglandin E_2(PGE_2)	G_s
EP_3	Prostaglandin E_2(PGE_2)	G_s, $G_{q/11}$, G_i
EP_4	Prostaglandin E_2(PGE_2)	G_s
CRTH2	PGD_2	$G_{i/o}$
Leukotriene receptors		
BLT	Leukotrinene B_4 (LTB_4)	$G_{i/o}$
CysLT1	$LTC_4 = LTD_4$	$G_{q/11}$
CysLT2	$LTC_4 > LTD_4$	$G_{q/11}$
Platelet-activating factor receptor		
PAF	Platelet-activating factor (PAF)	$G_{q/11}$
Chemotactic substances		
C3a	C3a	$G_{i/o}$
C5a	C5a	$G_{i/o}$
FPR	Formyl-Met-Leu-Phe (fMLP)	$G_{i/o}$
FPRL1 (ALXR)	LXA_4	$G_{i/o}$
FPRL2		
Free fatty acids		
GPR40	Free fatty acids (C_{12}-C_{20})	$G_{q/11}$
GPR41	Fatty acids (C_2-C_5)	$G_{i/0}$
GPR43	Fatty acids (C_2-C_5)	$G_{i/0}$, $G_{q/11}$
Lysophospholipid receptors		
$S1P_1$ (Edg1)	Spingosine-1-phosphate (S1P)	G_i
$S1P_2$ (Edg5)	S1P	G_i, $G_{q/11}$, $G_{12/13}$
$S1P_3$ (Edg3)	S1P	G_i, $G_{q/11}$, $G_{12/13}$
$S1P_4$ (Edg6)	S1P, Spingosylphosphorylcholine (SPC)	G_i
$S1P_5$ (Edg8)	S1P, SPC	G_i
LPA_1 (Edg2)	Lysophosphatidic acid (LPA)	G_i, $G_{q/11}$, $G_{12/13}$
LPA_2 (Edg4)	LPA	G_i, $G_{q/11}$, $G_{12/13}$
LPA_3 (Edg7)	LPA	G_i, $G_{q/11}$
SPC_1 (OGR1)	SPC	G_i
SPC_2 (GPR4)	SPC, Lysophosphatidylcholine (LPC)	G_i
LPC_1 (G2A)	LPC	$G_{q/11}$, $G_{12/13}$
PSY_1 (TDAG8)	Psychosine	

Class B (Calcitonin/Secretin-like)

Receptor	Endogenous ligand(s)	Coupling
Secretin	Secretin	G_s
GHRH	Growth hormone releasing hormone	G_s
GIP	Gastric inhibitory peptide	G_s
PTH/PTHrP	Parathyroid hormone (related peptide)	G_s, $G_{q/11}$
Calcitonin/CGRP-receptors		
CT	Calcitonin	G_s, $G_{q/11}$
AMY_1 (CT+RAMP1)	Amylin	G_s
AMY_2 (CT+RAMP2)	Amylin	G_s
AMY_3 (CT+RAMP3)	Amylin	G_s
$CGRP_1$ (CL+RAMP1)	Calcitonin gene-related peptide (CGRP)	G_s, $G_{q/11}$
AM_1 (CL+RAMP2)	Adrenomedullin	G_s
AM_2 (CL+RAMP3)	Adrenomedullin	G_s
Corticitropin-releasing factor		
CRF_1	Corticitropin-releasing factor (CRF), Urocortin	G_s
CRF_2	CRF, Urocortin, Urocortin II	G_s
Glucagon/Glucagon-like peptide receptors		
Glucagon	Glucagon	G_s
GLP1	Glucagon-like peptide	G_s
GLP2	Glucagon-like peptide	G_s
VIP/PACAP receptors		
$VPAC_1$	Vasoactive intestinal peptide (VIP), Pituitary adenylyl cyclase activating peptide (PACAP)	G_s
$VPAC_2$	VIP, PACAP	G_s
PAC_1	PACAP	G_s

Class C (Metabotropic glutamate-like)

Receptor	Endogenous ligand(s)	Coupling
CaSR	Ca^{2+}	$G_{q/11}$, $G_{i/o}$
Metabotropic GABA receptors		
$GABA_{B1}$ (binding)	γ-Aminobutyric acid	
$GABA_{B2}$ (signalling)	γ-Aminobutyric acid	$G_{i/o}$
Metabotropic glutamate receptors		
mGluR1	Glutamate	$G_{q/11}$
mGluR2	Glutamate	$G_{i/o}$
mGluR3	Glutamate	$G_{i/o}$
mGluR4	Glutamate	$G_{i/o}$
mGluR5	Glutamate	$G_{q/11}$
mGluR6	Glutamate	$G_{i/o}$
mGluR7	Glutamate	$G_{i/o}$
mGluR8	Glutamate	$G_{i/o}$

Heterotrimeric G-proteins

Heterotrimeric G-proteins couple seven transmembrane receptors (▶ G-protein Coupled Receptors; GPCR) to various effectors such as enzymes and ion channels. G-protein regulated effectors produce intracellular signals which result in specific cellular responses. G-protein functions are highly diverse and the cellular response to the activation of a GPCR depends on the pattern of G-protein subtypes activated through the receptor. The diversity of G-proteins is due to their composition of different α-, β-and γ-subunits, each of which is a product of a different gene. The α-subunit possesses structural and functional homologies to other members of the guanine nucleotide binding protein superfamily.

The β- and γ-subunits of heterotrimeric G-proteins form an non-dissociable complex and represent a functional unit. The functional properties of a heterotrimeric G-protein are primarily defined by the identity of its α-subunit. Both, the α-subunit and the β/γ-complex can regulate effectors such as inward rectifier K^+-channels (GIRKs), voltage-dependent Ca^{2+}-channels (VDCC), adenylyl cyclases (AC) or phospholipase C β-isoforms (PLC-β); (▶ Transmembrane Signalling, ▶ Adenylyl Cyclases, ▶ G-protein Coupled Receptors, ▶ K^+ Channels, ▶ Voltage-dependent Ca^{2+} Channels, ▶ Phospholipases).

Name	Gene symbol	Expression	Effectors
α-subunits			
$G\alpha_s$ class			
$G\alpha_s$	GNAS	ubiquitous	Adenylyl cyclase (AC) ↑
$G\alpha_{olf}$	GNAL	olfact. epithelium, brain	AC ↑
$G\alpha_{i/o}$ class			
$G\alpha_{i1}$	GNAI1	widely distributed	AC↓, GIRK1-4 (Kir3.1-3.4) ↑ (via G$\beta\gamma$)
$G\alpha_{i2}$	GNAI2	ubiquitous	AC↓, GIRK1-4 (Kir3.1-3.4) ↑ (via G$\beta\gamma$)
$G\alpha_{i3}$	GNAI3	widely distributed	AC↓, GIRK1-4 (Kir3.1-3.4) ↑ (via G$\beta\gamma$)
$G\alpha_o$	GNAO	neuronal, neuroendocrine	N-, P/Q-, R-type VDCC (Ca$_v$2.1-2.3) ↓, GIRK ↑ (via G$\beta\gamma$)
$G\alpha_z$	GNAZ	neuronal, platelets	AC ↓, ?
$G\alpha_{gust}$	GNAG	taste cells, brush cells	?
$G\alpha_{t-r}$	GNAT1	retinal rods, taste cells	cGMP PDE ↑
$G\alpha_{t-c}$	GNAT2	retinal cones	cGMP PDE ↑
$G\alpha_{q/11}$ class			
$G\alpha_q$	GNAQ	ubiquitous	PLC-β ↑
$G\alpha_{11}$	GNA11	almost ubiquitous	PLC-β ↑
$G\alpha_{14}$	GNA14	kidney, lung, spleen	PLC-β ↑
$G\alpha_{15/16}$	GNA15	hematopoietic cells	PLC-β ↑
$G\alpha_{12/13}$ class			
$G\alpha_{12}$	GNA12	ubiquitous	Rho GEF
$G\alpha_{13}$	GNA13	ubiquitous	Rho GEF
β-subunits			
β_1	GNB1	widely, retinal rods	
β_2	GNB2	widely distributed	
β_3	GNB3	widely, retinal cones	adenylyl cyclase type I ↓
β_4	(GNB4)	widely distributed	adenylyl cyclase types II, IV ↑
β_5	GNB5	mainly brain	
			phospholipase C-β (β3>β2>β1) ↑
γ-subunits			
γ_1, γ_{rod}	GNGT1	Retinal rods, brain,	GIRK1-4 (Kir3.1-3.4) ↑
γ_{14}, γ_{cone}, γ_8	GNGT2	Retinal cones, brain	phospholipase A$_2$ ↑
γ_2, γ_6	GNG2	widely	
γ_3	GNG3	Brain, blood	receptor kinases (GRK 2 and 3) ↑
γ_4	GNG4	Brain and other tissues	phosphoinositide 3 kinase β, γ ↑
γ_5	GNG5	widely	
γ_7	GNG7	widely	N-,P/Q-,R-type VDCC (Ca$_v$2.1-2.3) ↓
γ_{10}	GNG10	widely	
γ_{11}	GNG11	widely	
γ_{12}	GNG12		
γ_{13}	GNG13	Taste buds	

RGS proteins

Regulators of G-protein signaling (RGS) proteins play an important role in GPCR signal transduction. RGS proteins contain a conserved RGS box that is often accompanied by other signaling regulatory elements. RGS proteins acceler- ate the deactivation of G-proteins resulting in the reduction of GPCR signaling. Some RGS proteins also have an effector function and transmit signals. ▶ Transmembrane Signalling, ▶ G-protein Coupled Receptors.

RGS proteins

Name	G-protein interaction	Expression
A- or RZ-subfamily		
RGS19 (GAIP)	G_i, G_q	ubiquitous, low in brain
RGS17 (RGS-Z2)	G_i ($G_z\alpha$)	
RGS20 (RGS-Z1)	G_i ($G_z\alpha$)	brain
B- or R4-subfamily		
RGS4	G_i, G_q	brain, heart
RGS1	G_i, G_q	B-lymphocytes, lung
RGS2 (GOS8)	$G_q \gg G_i$	ubiquitous
RGS3	G_i, G_q	ubiquitous
RGS5	G_i, G_q	ubiquitous
RGS8	G_i	brain
RGS13	ND	lung
RGS16	G_i, G_q	retina, pituitary, liver, ubiquitous?
RGS18	G_i, G_q	
C- or R7-subfamily		
RGS9	G_i	retina, neurons
RGS6	G_i ($G_o\alpha$)	brain
RGS7	$G_i(G_o\alpha > G_i\alpha_2 > G_i\alpha_1)$	brain, B-cells
RGS11	G_i ($G_o\alpha$)	brain
D- or R12-subfamily		
RGS12	G_i	lung, brain, spleen, testis
RGS10	G_i	brain
RGS14	G_i	brain, spleen, lung
E- or RA-subfamily		
Axin	ND	ubiquitous, greatest in thymus, testis
Axil	ND	lung, thymus
F- or GEF-subfamily		
p115-RhoGEF	G_{13}	ubiquitous, leukocytes
PDZ-RhoGEF	$G_{12/13}$	ubiquitous, low in liver, lung, colon
LARG	$G_{12/13}$	
H- or SNX-subfamily		
SNX13 (RGS-PX1)	G_s	
SNX14	ND	
SNX25	ND	
D-AKAP2		
D-AKAP2	ND	ubiquitous, greatest in testis

Cytokine receptors (Jak/STAT-coupled)

The group of cytokine receptors directly coupled to the Jak/STAT pathway is subdivided in class I-cytokine receptors (also known as "hematopoietin receptors") and class II-cytokine receptors (also known as the "interferon receptor family"). The class I receptors fall into four subgroups which are functioning as homodimers or heterooligomers. The heterooligomeric group consists of the ligand binding receptor that heterooligomerizes with a second subunit required for signaling (gp130, βc-subunit/gp140, γc-subunit). Binding of the ligand results in homodimerization or heterooligomerization of receptor components, followed by the activation of cytosolic tyrosine protein kinases of the Jak-family (Jak1, Jak2, Tyk2) and the subsequent phosphorylation of the receptor as well as of transcription factors (STAT1-6). The class II cytokine receptor subfamily consists of at least two subunits, which are not associated in the absence of ligand. Ligand binding results in dimerization or oligomerization, and *via* the activation of a preassociated tyrosine kinase of the Jak-family to the activation of the Jak/STAT-pathway. (▶ Interferons, ▶ Cytokines, ▶ Jak/STAT Pathway, ▶ Hematopoietic Growth Factors).

Cytokine receptors (Jak/STAT-coupled)

Receptor	Endogenous ligand(s)	Tyrosine kinase	Transcription factor
Homodimeric receptors			
EPO-R	Erythropoietin	Jak2	STAT5
GH-R	Growth hormone	Jak2	STAT1/3/5
PRL-R	Prolactin	Jak2	STAT5
Mpl	Thrombopoietin	**Jak2**	STAT1/3/5
Receptor-heterooligomers (gp130)			
IL-6-R	Interleukin-6 (IL-6)	Jak1/2,Tyk2	STAT1/3
IL-11-R	Interleukin-11(IL-11)	Jak2	STAT1/3
IL-12-R	Interleukin-12 (IL-12)	Jak2,Tyk2	STAT4
LIF-R	Leukemia inhibitory factor (LIF), Cardiotrophin-1	Jak1/2	STAT1/3
CNTFR-R	Ciliary neurotrophic factor (CNTFR)	Jak1/2,Tyk2	STAT1/3
OSM-R	Oncostatin M	Jak1/2	STAT1/3
G-CSF-R	Granulocyte-colony stimulating factor (G-CSF)	Jak2	STAT3
Ob-R	Leptin	**Jak2**	STAT3
Receptor-heterodimers (βc-subunit)			
GM-CSF-R	GM-CSF	Jak2	STAT5
IL-3-R	Interleukin-3 (IL-3)	Jak2	STAT5
IL-5-R	Interleukin-5 (IL-5)	Jak2	STAT5
Receptor-heterodimers (γc-subunit)			
IL-2-R	Interleukin-2 (IL-2)	Jak1/3	STAT3/5
IL-4-R	Interleukin-4 (IL-4)	Jak1/3	STAT6
IL-7-R	Interleukin-7 (IL-7)	Jak1/3	STAT5
IL-9-R	Interleukin-9 (IL-9)	Jak1/3	STAT1/3/5
IL-13-R	Interleukin-13 (IL-13)	Jak1/3	STAT6
IL-15-R	Interleukin-15 (IL-15)	Jak1/3	STAT3/5
Interferon/IL-10-like receptors (class II)			
INFα-R1/2	INF α/β	Jak1/Tyk2	STAT1/2/3/5
INFγ-R1/2	INF γ	Jak1/Jak2	STAT1/5
IL-10-R1/2	Interleukin-10 (IL-10)	Jak1/Tyk2	STAT1/3
IL-20-R1/2	Interleukin-19/20/24 (IL-19/20/24)	Jak1/ ?	STAT3
IL-22-R/IL-20-R2	Interleukin-20/24 (IL-20/24)		STAT3
IL-22-R/IL-10-R2	Interleukin-22 (IL-22), IL-TIF	Jak1/Tyk2	STAT3

TNF receptor superfamily

The TNF receptor superfamily currently comprises about 25 receptors which share some structural features (Locksley et al., 2001, Cell 104, 487-501; Baud and Karin, 2001, Trends Cell Biol. 11, 372-377; http://www.gene.UCL.ac.uk/usres/hester/tnfinfo.html). The signaling mechanism of this receptor family has recently been elucidated by exemplary studies on the TNF and the Fas receptor. Binding of the inherently trimeric ligand TNFα or FasL induces receptor trimerization and recruitment of several signaling proteins to the cytoplasmic domains of the receptors. TNF receptors recruit the TNFR1-associated death domain protein (TRADD) that serves as a platform to recruit several other mediators including receptor-interacting protein 1 (RIP1), Fas-associated death domain protein (FADD) and TNF-receptor-associated factor 2 (TRAF2). TNFR2-activation results in the recruitment of TRAF1 and TRAF2. TRAF2 plays a central role in the induction of downstream events such as activation of IκB-kinase (IKK) and MAP-kinases. Fas activation does not result in the recruitment of TRAF2 but recruits FADD and subsequently leads to the activation of caspase 8. ▶ Apoptosis, ▶ MAP Kinase Cascade.

TNF receptor superfamily

Receptor	Ligand	Interacting proteins
NGFR	Nerve growth factor (NGF)	TRAF 2, 4, 6
Troy	?	TRAF 1, 2, 3, 5
EDAR	Ectodysplasin-A1 (EDA-A1)	TRAF 1, 3
XEDAR	Ectodysplasin-A2 (EDA-A2)	TRAF 3, 6
CD40	CD40Ligand (CD40L/CD154)	TRAF 2, 3, 5, 6
DcR3	LIGHT, Fas Ligand (FasL)	-
FAS (CD 95)	Fas Ligand (FasL)	FADD
OX40 (CD 134)	OX40Ligand (OX40L)	TRAF 1. 2, 3, 5
AITR	AITRLigand (AITRL)	TRAF 1, 2, 3
CD30	CD30L (CD153)	TRAF 1. 2, 3, 5
HveA	LIGHT, Lymphotoxin α (LTα)	TRAF 1. 2, 3, 5
4-1BB (CDw 137)	4-1BBL (CDw137L)	TRAF 1, 2
TNFR2 (TNF-R75 / CD120b)	Tumour necrosis factor α (TNFα), LTα	TRAF 2
DR3	TWEAK?	FADD
CD27	CD27L (CD 70)	TRAF 2
TNFR1 (TNF-R55 / CD120a)	TNFα, LTα	TRADD, FADD
LTβR	LIGHT, LTα, Lymphotoxin β (LTβ)	TRAF 3, 5
RANK	RANKL	TRAF 1, 2, 3, 5, 6
TACI	APRIL, BLYS	TRAF 2, 5, 6
BCMA	APRIL, BLYS	TRAF 1, 2, 3
DR6	RANKL, "TNF receptor-related, apoptosis-inducing ligand" (TRAIL)	TRADD
OPG	RANKL, TRAIL?	-
DR4	TRAIL	FADD
DR5	TRAIL	FADD
DcR1	TRAIL	-
DcR2	TRAIL	-

IL-1 / toll-like receptors

The interleukin-1 / toll-like receptor superfamily is involved in the rapid defense response to infection and injury. Currently, 10 human Toll-like receptors have been identified, TLRs 1 to 10. They share structural homologies and are involved in innate immunity by recognizing microbial particles. Their intracellular domains show homology with that of the IL-1 receptor subfamily (TIR-domain). Activation of downstream signaling events *via* IL-1/toll-like receptors involves receptor association with the MyD88 protein. MyD88 acts as an adaptor and recruites various proteins including IRAK-1, IRAK-2 and TRAF-6, eventually resulting in the activation of NF-κB and MAP kinases (Kaisho and Akira, 2002, Biochim. Biophys. Acta 1589,1-13; Vasselon and Detmers, 2002, Infect. Immul. 70, 1033-1041; Sims et al., 2002, Curr. Opin. Immunol., 14, 117-122). ▶ MAP Kinase Cascade, ▶ Toll-like Receptors.

IL-1 / toll-like receptors

Receptor	Ligand
toll-like receptors	
TLR1	Lipoprotein
TLR2	Lipoproteins, Peptidoglycan, Lipopeptides, Zymosan, Lipoarabinomannan, Bacterial lipopolysaccharide (LPS),
TLR3	Viral dsRNA
TLR4	Bacterial lipopolysaccharide (LPS)
TLR5	Flagellin
TLR6	?
TLR7	?
TLR8	?
TLR9	Unmethylated CpG DNA
TLR10	?
IL-1 / IL-18 receptor subfamily	
IL-1RI / IL-RacP	Interleukin-1α, Interleukin-1β
IL-1RII / IL-RacP	Interleukin-1β
IL-18R / IL-18RacP	Interleukin-18
T1 / ST2	
IL-1Rrp2	IL-1F9 ?
APL	
TIGIRR (APL-2)	
SIGIRR	

Nuclear receptors

Nuclear receptors bind to DNA as either homodimers or heterodimers. They function as ligand-activated gene expression regulatory proteins. In the inactive state they reside in the nucleus or in the cytoplasm, usually associated with an inhibitory protein. Ligand binding to the receptor results in its activation, translocation to the nucleus, binding to specific receptor binding elements on the DNA and activation of target gene transcription. Nuclear receptors are activated by a variety of small hydrophobic molecules, including hormones and intracellular metabolites. For a variety of nuclear receptors, the so called "orphan nuclear receptors", the physiological ligands are not known. (▶ Gluco-/Mineralocorticoid Receptor, ▶ Sex Steroid Receptor, ▶ Selective Sex Steroid Receptor Modulators).

Nuclear receptors

Receptor	Gene name	Ligand
Homodimers		
ERα	NR3A1	Estradiol
ERβ	NR3A2	Estradiol
PR	NR3C3	Progestins
AR	NR3C4	Androgens
MR	NR3C2	Mineralocorticoids
GR	NR3C1	Glucocorticoids
RXR (α, β, γ)-Heterodimers		
RXRα	NR2B1	
RXRβ	NR2B2	
RXRγ	NR2B3	
RARα	NR1B1	Retinoic acids
RARβ	NR1B2	Retinoic acids
RARγ	NR1B3	Retinoic acids
TRα	NR1A1	Thyroid hormone (T_3)
TRβ	NR1A2	Thyroid hormone (T_3)
VDR	NR1I1	1,25 $(OH)_2$ Vitamin D_3
FXR	NR1H4	Bile acids
LXRα	NR1H2	Oxysterols
LXRβ	NR1H3	Oxysterols
CAR	NR1I3/4	Xenobiotics, Phenobarbital, Androstane metabolites
SXR / PXR	NR1I2	Xenobiotics, Steroids, Rifampicin, Hyperforin
PPARα	NR1C1	Fatty acids, Fibrates
PPARβ	NR1C2	Fatty acids, Carboprostacyclin
PPARγ	NR1C3	Fatty acids, Eicosanoids, Thiazolidinediones
Orphan receptor		
SF-1, FTZ-F1	NR5A1	
LRH-1, FTZ-F1β	NR5A2	
DAX-1	NR0B1	
SHP	NR0B2	
TLL, TLX	NR2E1	
PNR, RNR	NR2E3	
NGFI-Bα	NR4A1	
NGFI-Bβ	NR4A2	
NGFI-Bγ	NR4A3	
RORα	NR1F1	Stearic acid
RORβ	NR1F2	
RORγ	NR1F3	
ERRα	NR3B1	Diethylstilbestrol, 4-Hydroxytamoxifen
ERRβ	NR3B2	

Nuclear receptors (Continued)

Receptor	Gene name	Ligand
ERRγ	NR3B3	
Rev-erbα	NR1D1	
Rev-erbβ	NR1D2	
GCNF	NR6A4	
TR 2	NR2C1	
TR 4	NR2C2	
HNF-4α	NR2A1	Palmitic acid
HNF-4γ	NR2A3	
COUP-TFα	NR2F1	
COUP-TFβ	NR2F2	
COUP-TFγ	NR2F6	

Membrane transport proteins

Membrane transport proteins are integral transmembrane proteins and transport substances with a high degree of specificity. Due to differences in their mechanism of action, the rate of transport differs considerably between different types of transport proteins.

Channel proteins transport water or specific ions down their concentration gradients or electric potential gradients. In the open state they form passages across the membrane through which either multiple water molecules or ions can move simultaneously. The transport rate of channel proteins is very high (10^7-10^8 ions/sec.).

In contrast to channel proteins, **solute carriers (transporters)** transport only one or a few substrate molecules at a time. In order to transport a substrate molecule across the plasma membrane, the transporter has to undergo a conformational change. Their transport rate is much lower than that of ion channels being in the range of 10^2-10^4 molecules/ sec. Solute carriers can transport specific molecules down a concentration gradient (uniporters). Other carriers func-

tion as coupled carriers, in which the transfer of one solute strictly depends on the transport of a second one. Coupled transport involves the simultaneous transfer of two or more solutes either in the same direction (cotransporter/symporter) or in the opposite directions (antiporter/exchanger). Coupled solute transporters usually couple the movement of one type of ion or molecule up its concentration gradient to the movement of a different ion or molecule down its concentration gradient. In this case an energetically unfavorable reaction is coupled to an energetically favorable reaction.

The third major group of membrane transport proteins is able to move ions or small molecules across the membrane against a chemical concentration gradient or electric potential by using the energy of ATP hydrolysis. They are called "**transport ATPases**", "**ATP-powered pumps**" or simply "pumps". ATP-powered pumps have a relatively low transport rate (10^0-10^3 molecules/sec.).

Channel proteins

Sodium channels

Sodium channels can be divided in voltage-dependent channels and non-voltage-dependent channels. **Voltage-dependent Na$^+$-channels** are mainly found in excitable cells where they become activated by membrane depolarization and are involved in the generation of action potentials. They consist of a pore-forming α-subunit, which is structurally related to the pore forming α-subunit of voltage-gated Ca^{2+}-channels. In addition, the voltage-dependent Na$^+$-channels contain auxillary β subunits (▶ Voltage-dependent Na$^+$ Channels). Non-voltage-dependent Na$^+$-channels belong to the family of **degenerin/epithelial Na$^+$-channel family**. Epi-

thelial sodium channels (ENaC) mediate Na$^+$-transport in epithelia and are essential for sodium homeostasis. Acid sensing channels (ASIC) are proton-gated cation channels with a preference for Na$^+$ ions, which are present both in the central and peripheral nervous system. Epithelial Na$^+$-channels are heteromultimeric channels, whose pore may be formed by three ENaC subunits. However, other models for their subunit arrangement have been proposed [Kellenberger and Schild, Physiol. Rev. 82, 735-767 (2002)]. (▶ Epithelial Na$^+$ Channels).

Sodium channels

Gene symbol	Name	Aliases	Expression
Voltage-dependent Na$^+$-channels			
Pore forming α-subunits			
SCN1A	Na$_v$1.1	rat I, HBSCI, GPBI, SCN1A	CNS, PNS
SCN2A	Na$_v$1.2	rat II, HBSCII, HBA	CNS
SCN3A	Na$_v$1.3	rat III	CNS
SCN4A	Na$_v$1.4	SkM1, μ1	skeletal muscle
SCN5A	Na$_v$1.5	SkM2, H1	uninnerv. skeletal muscle, heart
SCN8A	Na$_v$1.6	NaCh6, PN4, Scn8a, CerIII	CNS, PNS
SCN9A	Na$_v$1.7	NaS, hNE-Na, PN1	PNS, Schwann cells
SCN10A	Na$_v$1.8	SNS, PN3, NaNG	DRG
SCN11A	Na$_v$1.9	NaN, SNS2, PN5, NaT, SCN12A	PNS

Sodium channels (Continued)

Gene symbol	Name	Aliases	Expression
β-subunits			
SCN1B	β1	GEFSP1	
SCN2B	β2		
SCN4B	-		
Degenerin / epithelial Na⁺ channel family			
Epithelial Na⁺-channels			
SCNN1A	ENaCα		epithelial cells
SCNN1B	ENaCβ		epithelial cells
SCNN1D	ENaCδ		epithelial cells
SCNN1G	ENaCγ	PHA1	epithelial cells
Acid-sensing channels			
ACCN1	ASIC1	BNC1, BNaC1, MDEG	CNS, PNS
ACCN2	ASIC2	BNaC2	CNS, PNS
ACCN3	ASIC3	TNaC1, DRASIC	CNS, PNS

Potassium channels

Potassium channels are a diverse family of membrane proteins which selectively conduct K^+ ions across the cell membrane along its electrochemical gradient. More than 80 genes that encode subunits of potassium channels have been identified, including non-pore forming auxiliary subunits. The general feature of potassium channels are the α subunits forming the conducting pore. In some cases, additional auxiliary subunits are required for proper function and/or regulation of the tetrameric K^+ channel. Based on their primary amino acid sequence, potassium channels can be grouped into three major families. The voltage-gated K^+ channels are composed of four subunits, each containing six transmembrane segments and a conducting pore between segment five and segment six with a voltage sensor (positive charge of amino acid residues) located at S4 (e.g. KCNA-KCNH, KCNM-KCNT). The inward rectifier K^+ channels (Kir; KCNJ) consist of four subunits, each containing two transmembrane segments with a P-loop between the transmembrane segments. Finally, the KCNK subgroup of potassium channel subunits has four putative transmembrane with two pore forming domains. (▶ ATP-dependent K^+ Channels; ▶ Inward Rectifier K^+ Channels; ▶ K^+ Channels; ▶ Voltage-gated K^+ Channels).

Potassium channels

Gene symbol	Name	Aliases	Expression
KCNA (Shaker)			
KCNA1	Kv1.1	AEMK, HUK1, MBK1	neurons, heart, retina pancreas
KCNA2	Kv1.2	HK4	brain, heart, pancreas
KCNA3	Kv1.3	MK3, HLK3, HPCN3	lymphocyte, brain, lung
KCNA4	Kv1.4	HK1, HPCN2	brain, heart, pancreas
KCNA5	Kv1.5	HK2, HPCN1	brain, heart, lung, skeletal muscle
KCNA6	Kv1.6	HBK2	brain
KCNA7	Kv1.7	HAK6	heart, pancreas, skeletal muscle
KCNA10	Kv1.8		aorta, brain, kidney

Potassium channels (Continued)

Gene symbol	Name	Aliases	Expression
Auxillary subunits			
KCNAB1	Kvβ1	KCNA1B, Kvb1.3	
KCNAB2	Kvβ2	KCNA2B, Kvb2.1, 2.2	
KCNAB3	Kvβ3	KCNAB3	
KCNB (Shab)			
KCNB1	Kv2.1	DRK1	brain, heart, kidney, retina, skeletal muscle
KCNB2	Kv2.2		brain, heart, kidney, retina, skeletal muscle
KCNC (Shaw)			
KCNC1	Kv3.1		brain, muscles, lymphocytes
KCNC2	Kv3.2		brain
KCNC3	Kv3.3		brain, liver
KCNC4	Kv3.4	HKSHIIIC	brain, skeletal muscle
KCND (Shal)			
KCND1	Kv4.1		brain, heart, liver, kidney, lung, placenta, pancreas
KCND2	Kv4.2	KIAA1044, RK5	brain
KCND3	Kv4.3		brain, heart
KCNE (auxillary subunits for KCNQ1-5, KCNH2, KCNC4, KCND3)			
KCNE1		minK/Isk	
KCNE1L		AMMECR2	
KCNE2		MiRP1	
KCNE3		MiRP2	
KCNE4		MiRP3	
KCNF			
KCNF1	Kv5.1	IK8, kH1	brain
KCNG			
KCNG1	Kv6.1	K13, kH2	brain
KCNG2	Kv6.2	KCNF2	heart
KCNG3	Kv6.3		
KCNH (Ether-a-go-go)			
KCNH1	Kv10.1	meag, reag	brain
KCNH2	Kv11.1	LQT2, HERG	brain, heart
KCNH3	Kv12.2	BEC1	
KCNH4	Kv12.3	BEC2	
KCNH5	Kv10.2	Eag2,	
KCNH6	Kv11.2	HERG2	brain
KCNH7	Kv11.3	HERG3	brain
KCNH8	Kv12.1		
KCNJ (inward rectifyer)			
KCNJ1	Kir1.1	ROMK1	kidney, pancreas
KCNJ2	Kir2.1	IRK1	heart, brain, smooth muscle, skeletal muscle, lung, placenta, kidney
KCNJ3	Kir3.1	GIRK1	cerebellum
KCNJ4	Kir2.3	HIR, HRK1, HIRK2	heart, brain, skeletal muscle
KCNJ5	Kir3.4	CIR, GIRK4	heart, pancreas

Potassium channels (Continued)

Gene symbol	Name	Aliases	Expression
KCNJ6	Kir3.2	BIR1, GIRK2	cerebellum, pancreatic islets
KCNJ8	Kir6.1		various
KCNJ9	Kir3.3		
KCNJ10	Kir4.1, Kir1.2		glia
KCNJ11	Kir6.2	BIR, IKATP	various
KCNJ12	Kir2.2		ventricle
KCNJ13	Kir7.1, Kir1.4		glia, kidney, cerebellum, hippocampus, thyroid gland
KCNJ14	Kir2.4		brain, retina
KCNJ15	Kir4.2, Kir1.3		kidney, lung, brain
KCNJ16	Kir5.1		brain, periphery
KCNJN1	Kir2.2v		
KCNK (Two-pore K$^+$ channels)			
KCNK1		DPK, TWIK1	brain, kidney, heart
KCNK2		TREK-1	brain, lung
KCNK3		TASK	brain, heart, pancreas, placenta
KCNK4		TRAAK	brain, spinal cord, retina
KCNK5		TASK2	kidney
KCNK6		TOSS, TWIK2, KCNK8	eyes, lung, stomach, embryo
KCNK7			
KCNK9		TASK-3	
KCNK10		TREK2	
KCNK12		THIK2	
KCNK13		THIK-1	
KCNK15		TASK5, KCNK11, 14	
KCNK16		TALK1	
KCNK17		TALK2, TASK4	
KCNM			
α-subunit			
KCNMA1	Kca1.1	SLO	brain, smooth muscle
β-subunit			
KCNMB2		slo-β	
KCNMB3			
KCNMB3L			
KCNMB4			
KCNN (Ca^{2+}-activated)			
KCNN1	Kca2.1	hSK1	brain, heart
KCNN2	Kca2.2	hSK2	brain, adrenal gland, Jurkat T cells
KCNN3	Kca2.3	hSK3	brain, heart, liver
KCNN4	Kca3.1	hSK4, hKCa4, hIKCa1	lymphocytes, intestine, smooth muscle, prostate, red blood cells, neurons, placenta, thyroid gland

Potassium channels (Continued)

Gene symbol	Name	Aliases	Expression
KCNQ (slow delayed rectifyer)			
KCNQ1	Kv7.1	KVLQT1, LQT1	heart, kidney, lung, placenta, colon, cochlea
KCNQ2	Kv7.2	KvEBN1	brain, Neuron
KCNQ3	Kv7.3	KvEBN2	brain, Neuron
KCNQ4	Kv7.4		outer hair cells, inner ear, central auditory pathway
KCNQ5	Kv7.5		brain, skeletal muscle
KCNS			
KCNS1	Kv9.1		brain
KCNS2	Kv9.2		brain
KCNS3	Kv9.3		brain, lung, artery
KCNT			
KCNT1	Kca4.1		
KCNT2	Kca4.2	Slack, Slo2	
KCNU			
KCNU1	Kca5.1		
KCNV			
KCNV1	Kv8.1	KCNB3, Kv2.3	brain

Voltage-dependent Ca^{2+}-channels

Voltage-dependent Ca^{2+}-channels are a family of multi-subunit complexes, consisting of 5 proteins, which allow the influx of Ca^{2+} into a cell in response to membrane depolarization. The 5 subunits of these channels are encoded by 4 different gene families. The α_1 subunit is the pore-forming unit which contains the voltage-sensor, the selectivity filter and the interaction sites for regulatory proteins. The electrophysiological properties of voltage-dependent Ca^{2+}-channels are mainly determined by the identity of their α_1 subunit (▶ Voltage-dependent Ca^{2+}-channels).

Voltage-dependent Ca^{2+}-channels

Gene symbol	Name	Aliases	Expression
L-type channel(α_1-subunit)			
CACNA1S	Ca$_v$1.1	α_{1S}, α_{1Skm}, CaCh1	skeletal muscle
CACNA1C	Ca$_v$1.2a	$\alpha_{1C\text{-a}}$, rbC, CaCh2	heart
	Ca$_v$1.2b	$\alpha_{1C\text{-b}}$	smooth muscle
	Ca$_v$1.3c	$\alpha_{1C\text{-c}}$	brain, pituitary, adrenal
CACNA1D	Ca$_v$1.3	α_{1D}, rbD, CaCh3	brain, pancreas, kidney, ovary, cochlea
CACNA1F	Ca$_v$1.4	α_{1F}	retina
P/Q-type channel (α_1-subunit)			
CACNA1A	Ca$_v$2.1a	α_{1A}, rbA, CaCh4, BI1	brain, cochlea, pituitary
	Ca$_v$21b	BI2	brain, cochlea, pituitary
N-type channel (α_1-subunit)			
CACNA1B	Ca$_v$2.2a	$\alpha_{1B\text{-1}}$, rbB, CaCh5, BIII	brain, nervous system
	Ca$_v$2.2b	$\alpha_{1B\text{-2}}$	brain, nervous system

Voltage-dependent Ca^{2+}-channels (Continued)

Gene symbol	Name	Aliases	Expression
R-type channel (α_1-subunit)			
CACNA1E	Ca$_v$2.3a	α_{1E}, rbB, CaCh6, BII	brain, cochlea, pituitary, retina, heart
	Ca$_v$2.3b	BII2	brain, cochlea, retina
T-type channel(α_1-subunit) BII			
CACNA1G	Ca$_v$3.1	α_{1G}	brain, nervous system
CACNA1H	Ca$_v$3.2	α_{1H}	brain, heart, kidney, liver
CACNA1I	Ca$_v$3.3	α_{1I}	brain
$\alpha_2\delta$-subunit			
CACNA2D1	$\alpha_2\delta1$		ubiquitously
CACNA2D2	$\alpha_2\delta2$		heart
CACNA2D3	$\alpha_2\delta3$		brain
β-subunit			
CACNB1	$\beta1$		skeletal muscle, brain, spleen
CACNB2	$\beta2$		heart, aorta, lung, brain
CACNB3	$\beta3$		brain, smooth muscle
CACNB4	$\beta4$		brain
γ-subunit			
CACNG1	$\gamma1$		skeletal muscle
CACNG2	$\gamma2$		brain
CACNG3	$\gamma3$		brain
CACNG4	$\gamma4$		
CACNG5	$\gamma5$		
CACNG6	$\gamma6$		
CACNG7	$\gamma7$		
CACNG8	$\gamma8$		

Chloride channels

Several classes of chloride channels have been found: they include **ligand-gated chloride channels** (GABA$_A$- and glycine-receptors; ▶ Ligand-gated ion channels), the cystic fibrosis transmembrane conductance regulator (CFTR; ▶ ABC transporters), and the **CLC family of chloride channels**. CLIC proteins and CaCC proteins are proposed chloride channels. However, their function as chloride channels has not yet been proven. The CLC chloride channels form a large family of which many are gated in a voltage-dependent manner. Nine different CLC genes have been found in mammals. CLC channels are present in the plasma membrane as well as in intracellular organelles. They function as dimers, with each monomer having its own pore. Some CLC channels have accessory β-subunits (▶ Cl$^-$ channels).

Chloride channels

Gene Symbol	Name	Alias	Expression
CLCN1	ClC-1		skeletal muscle
CLCN2	ClC-2		broad
CLCN3	ClC-3		brain, kidney, liver etc.

Chloride channels (Continued)

Gene Symbol	Name	Alias	Expression
CLCN4	ClC-4		brain, muscle etc.
CLCN5	ClC-5	DENTS, XLRH	kidney, intestine, liver etc.
CLCN6	ClC-6		broad
CLCN7	ClC-7		broad
CLCNKA	ClC-Ka		kidney, inner ear
CLCNKB	ClC-Kb		kidney, inner ear

Cation channels

TRP channels. The TRP superfamily comprises a variety of non-voltage-gated cation channels that are distinguished by their selectivity and mode of action. They all are similar to the first member of the family, the *Drosphila* TRP ("transient receptor potential"). TRP cation channels are subdivided in three families, the TRPC, TRPV and TRPM. The TRP-canonical (TRPC) subfamily, is most highly related to *Drosphila* TRP and at least some of the members of the TRPC subfamily play a role as Ca^{2+} store-operated channels.

The TRPV subfamily comprises TRP channels that are related to the vanilloid receptor1 (VR1). Members of this family can be regulated by heat, osmolarity and other stimuli. The third subfamily, TRPM, is related to the first member of this family, melastatin, and is structurally characterized by its increased length compared to the other subfamilies. For details of the nomenclature and recent review: Molecular Cell, 9, 229-231 (2002); Cell 108, 595-598 (2002).

TRP channels

Name	Alias	Expression
TRPC Subfamily		
TRPC1	TRP1	ubiquitous
TRPC2	TRP2	VNO, testis (pseudogene in human)
TRPC3	TRP3	Brain
TRPC4	TRP4	Brain, endothel, adrenal gland, retina, testis
TRPC5	TRP5	Brain
TRPC6	TRP6	Smooth muscle, lung, brain
TRPC7	TRP7	Eye, heart, lung
TRPV Subfamily		
TRPV1	VR1, OTRPC1	Trigeminal & dorsal root ganglia (DRG)
TRPV2	VRL-1, OTRPC2	DRG, spinal cord, brain, spleen, intestine
TRPV3		Keratinocytes
TRPV4	OTRPC4, VR-OAC, TRP12, VRL-2	Kidney, lung, spleen, testis, endothelium, liver, heart
TRPV5	ECaC1, CaT2	Kidney, duodenum, jejunum, placenta, pancreas
TRPV6	CaT1, EcaC2, CaT-L	Small intestine, pancreas, placenta, prostate cancer
TRPM Subfamily		
TRPM1	Melastatin	Eye, melanocytes
TRPM2	TRPC7, LTRPC2	Brain
TRPM3	KIAA1616, LTRPC3	?
TRPM4	TRPM4, LTRPC4	Prostate, colon, heart, kidney
TRPM5	MTR1, LTRPC5	Small intestine, liver, lung, taste buds
TRPM6	Chak2	Kidney, intestine
TRPM7	TRP-PLIK, Chak1, LTRPC7	ubiquitous
TRPM8	TRP-p8	Sensory ganglia, prostatic tumour

Cyclic nucleotide-regulated cation channels. The activation of cyclic nucleotide-gated cation channels is regulated or modulated by cyclic AMP or cyclic GMP. While the **cyclic nucleotide-gated (CNG) channels** obligatorily require the binding of cyclic nucleotides in order to activate, **hyperpolarization-** **activated cyclic nucleotide-gated (HCN) channels** are primarily activated by membrane hyperpolarization and are modulated in their activity by cyclic nucleotides (▶ Cyclic nucleotide-regulated cation channels).

Cyclic nucleotide-regulated cation channels

Gene Symbol	Previous name	Alias	Expression
Cyclic nucleotide-gated (CNG) channels			
α-subunits			
CNGA1	CNCG1	RCNC1, CNG1	rods, brain
CNGA2	CNCA1	CNG2, OCNC1	olfactory epithelium, brain
CNGA3	CNCG3, ACHM2	CCNC1, CNG3	cones, brain
CNGA4	CNCA2, CNGB2	OCNC2, CNG5	olfactory epithelium, brain
β-subunits			
CNGB1	CNCG2, CNCG3L	RCNC2, GARP, GAR1	rods, olfactory epithelium
CNGB3			retina (cones)
Hyperpolarization-activated cyclic nucleotide-gated (HCN) channels			
HCN1	BCNG1	BCNG-1, HAC-2	heart, brain (hippocampus)
HCN2	BCNG2	BCNG-2, HAC-1	brain, heart
HCN3			brain
HCN4			heart (SA node), brain (thalamus)

Calcium Release Channels. The Ca^{2+} release channels are abundant in some regions of the sarcoplasmic or endoplasmic reticulum. **Ryanodine receptors** (which bind the plant alkaloid ryanodine) consist of homotetramers that can be opened by Ca^{2+} (Ca^{2+}-induced Ca^{2+} release occurs in heart muscle). In skeletal muscle, the ryanodine Ca^{2+} release channel is gated by a conformational change of a voltage sensor, the α_{1S} subunit of voltage-dependent calcium chan- nels. **Inositol-1,4,5-triphosphate receptors** have a general structure similar to ryanodine receptors. They mediate the release of intracellularly stored Ca^{2+} in response to the production of Inositol-1,4,5-triphosphate (IP_3). Calcium release channels have a low selectivity for individual cations, but at physiological conditions mainly allow the passage of Ca^{2+} ions (▶ Ryanodine receptor).

Calcium Release Channels

Gene symbol	Name	Alias	Expression
Ryanodine receptor			
RYR1	RyR1	Type I, MHS1	skeletal muscle (high levels)
RYR2	RyR2	Type II	cardiac muscle, brain
RYR3	RyR3	Type III	ubiquitous (low levels)
Inositol-1,4,5-triphosphate receptors			
ITPR1	IP_3 receptor 1	Type I IP_3 receptor	CNS, ubiquitous
ITPR2	IP_3 receptor 2	Type II IP_3 receptor	widely
ITPR3	IP_3 receptor 3	Type III IP_3 receptor	Kidney, brain, gastrointest. tract, pancreas

Water channels

The aquaporins (AQPs) are a family of small integral membrane proteins related to the major intrinsic protein (MIP, or AQP0) of the lens. Whereas most AQPs function as water-selective channels, a subgroup, AQP3, AQP7, AQP9, and AQP 10, is also permeable for neutral solutes such as glycerol and urea. The membrane topology of AQPs is characterized by intracellular N- and C-termini and two tandem repeats, each formed from three transmembrane helices. Two highly conserved loops (intracellular loop B and extracellular loop E, each containing a signature motif asn-pro-ala) fold into the bilayer and form the water pore. AQPs increase the water permeability of biological membranes, thereby allowing rapid transcellular movements of water. AQPs are constitutively active. Most AQPs are inhibited by mercury. Mercury sensitivity is conferred by a cysteine residue in the extracellular pore-forming loop E. An exception is AQP4, which lacks a corresponding cysteine residue. Other chemical modulators of AQP activity are not known.

The prototypical AQP is AQP1. AQP1 forms tetramers with each subunit containing its own water pore. Determination of its atomic structure revealed insight into the permeation of water molecules through the pore. With the exception of AQP2, the biological function of most AQPs is not well understood. AQP2, highly expressed in epithelial (principal) cells of the renal collecting duct, is regulated by vasopressin (syn.: antidiuretic hormone). Vasopressin-induced insertion of AQP2 in the apical membrane of principal cells greatly facilitates the reabsorption of water from the collecting duct. Mutations in the AQP2 gene are the cause of autosomal forms of nephrogenic diabetes insipidus, a disease characterized by a major loss of water through the kidney (▶ Vasopressin/Oxytocin).

Water channels

Gene Symbol	Name	Alias	Expression
AQP1	Aquaporin 1	CHIP28, HGNC:2177	erythrocytes, kidney, lung
AQP2	Aquaporin 2	WCH-CD, Aquaporin-CD	kidney (collecting duct), inner ear
AQP3	Aquaporin 3		kidney, lungs, eye, urinary bladder, skin, gastrointestinal tract
AQP4	Aquaporin 4	MIWC	kidney, brain, retina, inner ear, skeletal muscle
AQP5	Aquaporin 5		salivary glands, lacrimal glands, sweat glands, eye, lung
AQP6	Aquaporin 6	AQP2L	kidney
AQP7	Aquaporin 7	AQP7L, AQPap, AQP9	testis, adipose tissue
AQP8	Aquaporin8		pancreas , colon
AQP9	Aquaporin9		leukocytes, liver, lung, spleen
AQP10	Aquaporin10		small intestine

Solute Carriers (Transporters)

Solute carriers comprise a huge family of membrane transport proteins, which specifically bind a variety of ions and molecules. The solute carrier then undergoes a conformational change, which results in the transport of the ion or molecule across the membrane. Solute carriers are not directly coupled to an energy consuming process. If two or more ions/molecules are transported in a coupled fashion in one direction, the solute carrier is called **cotransporter (symporter)**. If ions/molecules are transported in opposite directions, the solute carrier is called **antiporter (exchanger)**. The tight coupling between the transport of two solutes allows these carriers to use the energy that is stored in the electrochemical gradient of one solute, typically an ion, to transport the other solute. This way the free energy which is released during the movement of an inorganic ion down its electrochemical gradient is used as a driving force to pump other solutes uphill, against their electrochemical gradient. This principle is called "secondary active transport" in contrast to "primary active transport" carried out by transport ATPases (see below). The latter is carried out by transporters, which generate the required energy directly. The third type of solute carrier transports certain molecules just down a concentration gradient (**uniporter**). (▶ Glucose transporters; ▶ Neurotransmitter transporters; ▶ Organic cation transporters; ▶ Vesicular transporters).

Solute Carriers (Transporters)

Gene	Name/Aliases	Function
Na+/dicarboxylate cotransporters (excitatory amino acid transporters)		
SLC1A1	EAAC1, EAAT3	neuronal/epithelial high affinity glutamate transporter
SLC1A2	GLT-1, EAAT2	glial high affinity glutamate transporter
SLC1A3	GLAST, EAAT1	glial high affinity glutamate transporter
SLC1A4	SATT, ASCT1	glutamate/neutral amino acid transporter
SLC1A5	AAAT, ASCT2	neutral amino acid transporter
SLC1A6	EAAT4	high affinity aspartate/glutamate transporter
SLC1A7	EAAT5	glutamate transporter
Facilitated glucose transporters (Uniporter)		
SLC2A1	GLUT1, GLUT	facilitated glucose transporter
SLC2A2	GLUT2	facilitated glucose transporter
SLC2A3	GLUT3	facilitated glucose transporter
SLC2A4	GLUT4	facilitated glucose transporter
SLC2A5	GLUT5	facilitated glucose/fructose transporter
SLC2A6	GLUT9, GLUT6	facilitated glucose transporter
SLC2A7		facilitated glucose transporter
SLC2A8	GLUTX1, GLUT8	facilitated glucose transporter
SLC2A9	Glut9, GLUTX	facilitated glucose transporter
SLC2A10	GLUT10	facilitated glucose transporter
SLC2A11	GLUT11,GLUT10	facilitated glucose transporter
SLC2A12	GLUT12, GLUT8	facilitated glucose transporter
SLC2A13	HMIT	H^+/myo-inositol cotransporter
SLC2A4RG	GEF	SLC2A4 regulator
Heavy chains of heteromeric amino acid transporters (SLC7)		
SLC3A1	rBAT, CSNU1	Heavy chain of SLC7A5,6,7,8,10,11
SLC3A2	4F2hc, CD98	Heavy chain of SLC7A9
Anion antiporters, Na$^+$/bicarbonate cotransporters		
SLC4A1	AE1, RTA1A	Cl^-/HCO_3^- antiporter
SLC4A2	AE2, HKB3	Cl^-/HCO_3^- antiporter
SLC4A3	AE3, SLC2C	Cl^-/HCO_3^- antiporter
SLC4A4	NBC1, NBC2	Na^+/HCO_3^- cotransporter
SLC4A5	NBC4	Na^+/HCO_3^- cotransporter
SLC4A7	NBC3, SBC2	Na^+/HCO_3^- cotransporter
SLC4A8	NBC3	Na^+-dependent anion exchanger

Solute Carriers (Transporters) (Continued)

Gene	Name/Aliases	Function
SLC4A9	AE4	Na$^+$/bicarbonate cotransporter ?
SLC4A10		Na$^+$-dependent anion exchanger
SLC4A11	BTR1	Na$^+$/bicarbonate transporter-like
SLC4A1AP	kanadaptin	kidney anion exchanger adaptor protein

Na$^+$-coupled ions/sugars/nutrient transporters

Gene	Name/Aliases	Function
SLC5A1	SGLT1	Na$^+$/glucose cotransporter
SLC5A2	SGLT2	Na$^+$/glucose cotransporter
SLC5A3	SMIT	Na$^+$/myo-inositol cotransporters
SLC5A4	SAAT1, SGLT3	low affinity Na$^+$/glucose cotransporter
SLC5A5	NIS	Na$^+$/iodine cotransporter
SLC5A6	SMVT	Na$^+$/vitamin cotransporter
SLC5A7	hCHT, CHT1	Na$^+$/choline cotransporter

Na$^+$/Cl$^-$-dependent neurotransmitter transporters (NTS)

Gene	Name/Aliases	Function
SLC6A1	GAT1	Na$^+$,Cl$^-$/GABA cotransporter
SLC6A2	NET1, NAT1	Na$^+$,Cl$^-$/noradrenalin cotransporter
SLC6A3	DAT1	Na$^+$,Cl$^-$/dopamine cotransporter
SLC6A4	SERT	Na$^+$,Cl$^-$/serotonin cotransporter
SLC6A5	GLYT2	Na$^+$,Cl$^-$/glycin cotransporter
SLC6A6	TAUT	Na$^+$,Cl$^-$/taurine cotransporter
SLC6A7	PROT	Na$^+$,Cl$^-$/L-proline cotransporter
SLC6A8	CRTR, CT1	Na$^+$,Cl$^-$/creatine cotransporter
SLC6A9		Na$^+$,Cl$^-$/glycine cotransporter
SLC6A10	CT-2	Na$^+$,Cl$^-$/creatine cotransporter
SLC6A11	GAT3	Na$^+$,Cl$^-$/GABA cotransporter
SLC6A12	BGT-1	Na$^+$,Cl$^-$/betaine, GABA cotransporter
SLC6A13	GAT2	Na$^+$,Cl$^-$/GABA cotransporter
SLC6A14		Neurotransmitter transporter
SLC6A15	hv7-3	Neurotransmitter transporter
SLC6A16		Neurotransmitter transporter

Amino acid – polyamine – choline (APC) transporters

Cationic amino acid transporters

Gene	Name/Aliases	Function
SLC7A1	CAT-1, REC1L	cationic AA transporter, y$^+$ system
SLC7A2	CAT-2	cationic AA transporter, y$^+$ system
SLC7A3	CAT-3, ATRC3	cationic AA transporter, y$^+$ system
SLC7A4	CAT-4	cationic AA transporter, y$^+$ system

Heteromeric amino acid transporters

Gene	Name/Aliases	Function
SLC7A5	LAT1, E16	heterom. AA transp., L system; + SLC3A2
SLC7A6	y+LAT-2, LAT3	heterom. AA transp., y$^+$L system; + SLC3A2
SLC7A7	y+LAT-1	heterom. AA transp., y$^+$L system; + SLC3A2
SLC7A8	LAT2, LPI-PC1	heterom. AA transp., y$^+$ system; + SLC3A2
SLC7A9		heterom. AA transp., b$^{0,+}$ system; + SLC3A1
SLC7A10	asc-1	heterom. AA transp., asc system; + SLC3A2
SLC7A11	xCT	heterom. AA transp., x$_c$ system; + SLC3A2

Na$^+$/Ca^{2+} antiporter

Gene	Name/Aliases	Function
SLC8A1	NCX1	Na$^+$/Ca^{2+} antiporter
SLC8A2	NCX2	Na$^+$/Ca^{2+} antiporter
SLC8A3	NCX3	Na$^+$/Ca^{2+} antiporter

Na$^+$/H$^+$ antiporter

Gene	Name/Aliases	Function
SLC9A1	NHE1, APNH	Na$^+$/H$^+$ antiporter
SLC9A2	NHE2	Na$^+$/H$^+$ antiporter
SLC9A3	NHE3	Na$^+$/H$^+$ antiporter
SLC9A4	NHE4	Na$^+$/H$^+$ antiporter

Solute Carriers (Transporters) (Continued)

Gene	Name/Aliases	Function
SLC9A5	NHE5	Na^+/H^+ antiporter
SLC9A6	NHE6	Na^+/H^+ antiporter
SLC9A7	NHE7	Na^+/H^+ antiporter
SLC9A3R1	NHERF, EBP50	Na^+/H^+ antiporter, isoform 3 regulatory factor 1
SLC9A3R2	SIP-1, NHERF-2,	Na^+/H^+ antiporter, isoform 3 regulatory factor 2

Na^+/bile acid cotransporter

SLC10A1	NTCP	Na^+/bile acid cotransporter
SLC10A2	ASBT, ISBT	Na^+/bile acid cotransporter

H^+-coupled divalent metal ion transporters

SLC11A1	LSH, NRAMP	H^+-coupled divalent metal ion transporters
SLC11A2	DCT1, DMT1	H^+-coupled divalent metal ion transporters
SLC11A3	MTP1	H^+-coupled divalent metal ion transporters

Cation/Cl^- cotransporters

SLC12A1	NKCC2	$Na^+/K^+/Cl^-$ cotransporter
SLC12A2	NKCC1	$Na^+/K^+/Cl^-$ cotransporter
SLC12A3	NCC	Na^+/Cl^- cotransporter
SLC12A4	KCC1	K^+/Cl^- cotransporter
SLC12A5		K^+/Cl^- cotransporter
SLC12A6	KCC3	K^+/Cl^- cotransporter
SLC12A7	KCC4	K^+/Cl^- cotransporter
SLC12A8		K^+/Cl^- cotransporter

Na^+-dependent dicarboxylate/sulfate transporters

SLC13A1	NaSi-1	Na^+/SO_4^{2-} cotransporters
SLC13A2	NaDC-1	Na^+/dicarboxylate cotransporter
SLC13A3	NADC3, SDCT2	Na^+/ dicarboxylate cotransporter
SLC13A4	SUT-1	Na^+/SO_4^{2-} cotransporters

Urea transporters (Uniporter)

SLC14A1	JK	urea transporter
SLC14A2	HUT2, UT2	urea transporter

H^+/peptide transporters

SLC15A1	PEPT1	H^+/peptide cotransporter
SLC15A2	PEPT2	H^+/peptide cotransporter

H^+/monocarboxylic acid (lactate/pyruvate etc.) cotransporters

SLC16A1	MCT1	H^+/monocarboxylic acid cotransporter
SLC16A2	XPCT, MCT8	H^+/monocarboxylic acid cotransporter
SLC16A3	MCT4	H^+/monocarboxylic acid cotransporter
SLC16A4	MCT5	H^+/monocarboxylic acid cotransporter
SLC16A5	MCT6	H^+/monocarboxylic acid cotransporter
SLC16A6	MCT7	H^+/monocarboxylic acid cotransporter
SLC16A7	MCT2	H^+/monocarboxylic acid cotransporter
SLC16A8	MCT3	H^+/monocarboxylic acid cotransporter
SLC16A10	TAT1	aromatic amino acid transporter

Anion/cation cotransporters

SLC17A1	NPT1, NAPI-1	Na^+/PO_4^{2-} cotransporters
SLC17A2	NPT3	Na^+/PO_4^{2-} cotransporters
SLC17A3	NPT4	Na^+/PO_4^{2-} cotransporters
SLC17A4		Na^+/PO_4^{2-} cotransporters
SLC17A5	AST	anion/sugar transporter
SLC17A6	DNPI, VGLUT2	vesicular glutamate transporter
SLC17A7	BNPI, VGLUT1	vesicular glutamate transporter

Vesicular monoamine/acetylcholine transporters

Solute Carriers (Transporters) (Continued)

Gene	Name/Aliases	Function
SLC18A1	VMAT1, VAT1	$2H^+$/vesicular monoamine antiorter
SLC18A2	VMAT2	$2H^+$/vesicular monoamine antiporter
SLC18A3	VAchT	$2H^+$/vesicular acetylcholine antiporter
Folate/Thiamine transporter		
SLC19A1	FOLT	folate transporter
SLC19A2	THTR1	thiamine transporter
SLC19A3	THTR2	thiamine transporter
Na^+/PO_4^{2-}-cotransporters		
SLC20A1	PiT-1, Glvr-1	Na^+/PO_4^{2-} cotransporter
SLC20A2	PiT-2, Glvr-2	Na^+/PO_4^{2-} cotransporter
Organic anion transporter		
SLC21A1		organic anion transporter
SLC21A2	PGT	organic anion transporter
SLC21A3	OATP	organic anion transporter
SLC21A4	OAT-K1, OAT-K2	organic anion transporter
SLC21A5	Oatp2	organic anion transporter
SLC21A6	OATP-C, LST-1	organic anion transporter
SLC21A7	Oatp3	organic anion transporter
SLC21A8	OATP8	organic anion transporter
SLC21A9	OATP-B	organic anion transporter
SLC21A10	lst-1, Oatp4	organic anion transporter
SLC21A11	OATP-D	organic anion transporter
SLC21A12	OATP-E	organic anion transporter
SLC21A13	Oatp5	organic anion transporter
SLC21A14	OATP-F	organic anion transporter
Organic cation/anion transporter		
SLC22A1	OCT1	organic cation transporter
SLC22A2	OCT2	organic cation transporter
SLC22A3	OCT3, EMT	extraneuronal monoamine transporter
SLC22A4	OCTN1	organic cation transporter
SLC22A5	OCTN2, SCD	organic cation transporter
SLC22A6	OAT1, PAHT	organic anion / dicarboxylate antiporter
SLC22A7	OAT2, NLT	organic anion transporter
SLC22A8	OAT3	organic anion transporter
SLC22A9	OAT4	organic anion/cation transporter
SLC22A10	OAT5	organic anion/cation transporter
SLC22A11	OAT4	organic anion/cation transporter
SLC22A12	OAT4L URAT1	organic anion/cation transporter
SLC22A1L	BWR1A, TSSC5	organic cation transporter
SLC22A1LS	BWR1B	organic cation transporter
Na^+/ascorbic acid cotransporters		
SLC23A1	YSPL2, SVCT2	Na^+/ascorbic acid cotransporter
SLC23A2	YSPL3, SVCT1	Na^+/ascorbic acid cotransporter
Na^+/Ca^{2+}, K^+ antiporter		
SLC24A1	NCKX1	Na^+/Ca^{2+}, K^+ antiporter
SLC24A2	NCKX2	Na^+/Ca^{2+}, K^+ antiporter
SLC24A3	NCKX3	Na^+/Ca^{2+}, K^+ antiporter
SLC24A4	NCKX4	Na^+/Ca^{2+}, K^+ antiporter
Mitochondrial transporter		
SLC25A1	CTP	citrate transporter
SLC25A3	PHC	phosphate carrier
SLC25A4	T1, ANT1, PEO2	adenine nucleotide translocator

Solute Carriers (Transporters) (Continued)

Gene	Name/Aliases	Function
SLC25A5	T2, ANT2	adenine nucleotide translocator
SLC25A6	ANT3	adenine nucleotide translocator
SLC25A10	DIC	dicarboxylate transporter
SLC25A11	OGC	oxoglutarate carrier
SLC25A12	Aralar	mitochondrial carrier, Aralar
SLC25A13	CTLN2	citrin
SLC25A14	BMCP1	mitochondrial carrier, brain
SLC25A15	ORNT1, HHH	ornithine transporter
SLC25A16	GDA, HGT.1,ML7	mitochondrial carrier; Graves disease autoantigen
SLC25A17	PMP34	mitochondrial carrier
SLC25A18		mitochondrial carrier
SLC25A19	DNC, MUP1	mitochondrial deoxynucleotide carrier
SLC25A20	CACT	carnitine/acylcarnitine translocase
SLC25A21	ODC1	mitochondrial oxodicarboxylate carrier
SLC25A15P		mitochondrial carrier; ornithine transporter
SLC25A20P	CACTP	carnitine/acylcarnitine translocase
SLC25A5L		adenine nucleotide translocator

Anion transporters, anion antiporters

Gene	Name/Aliases	Function
SLC26A1	SAT-1, EDM4	SO_4^{2-}/anion antiporter
SLC26A2	DTD	SO_4^{2-} transporter
SLC26A3	DRA, CLD	Cl^-/HCO_3^- antiporter
SLC26A4	DFNB4, PDS	anion transporter
SLC26A6		
SLC26A7	SUT2	Cl^-, SO_4^{2-}, oxalate transporter
SLC26A8	TAT1	Cl^-, SO_4^{2-}, oxalate transporter
SLC26A9		Cl^-, SO_4^{2-}, oxalate transporter
SLC26A10		
SLC26A11		

Fatty acid transporters

Gene	Name/Aliases	Function
SLC27A1	FATP1	fatty acid transporter
SLC27A2	FATP2	fatty acid transporter
SLC27A3	FATP3	fatty acid transporter
SLC27A4	FATP4	fatty acid transporter
SLC27A5	FATP5	fatty acid transporter
SLC27A6	FATP6	fatty acid transporter

Na^+/nucleoside cotransporters (concentrative)

Gene	Name/Aliases	Function
SLC28A1	CNT1	Na^+/nucleoside cotransporter (pyrim. + adenosine)
SLC28A2	CNT2, SPNT1	Na^+/nucleoside cotransporter (purin + uridin)
SLC28A3	CNT3	Na^+/nucleoside cotransporter

Nucleoside transporter (equilibrative)

Gene	Name/Aliases	Function
SLC29A1	ENT1	nucleoside uniporter (purins, pyrimidines)
SLC29A2	ENT2, DER12	nucleoside uniporter (purins, pyrimidines)

Zinc transporter

Gene	Name/Aliases	Function
SLC30A1	ZnT1	zinc transporter
SLC30A2	ZnT2	zinc transporter
SLC30A3	ZnT3	zinc transporter
SLC30A4	ZnT4	zinc transporter

Copper transporter

Gene	Name/Aliases	Function
SLC31A1	COPT1, CTR1	copper transporter
SLC31A2	COPT2, CTR2	copper transporter

Solute Carriers (Transporters) (Continued)

Gene	Name/Aliases	Function
Vesicular H$^+$/GABA,glycin antiporter		
SLC32A1	VGAT	vesicular H$^+$/GABA, glycin antiporter
Na$^+$/PO$_4^{2-}$ cotransporter		
SLC34A1	NPT2, NAPI-3	Na$^+$/PO$_4^{2-}$ cotransporter
SLC34A2	NAPI-3B	Na$^+$/PO$_4^{2-}$ cotransporter
Nucleotide sugar transporters		
SLC35A1	CMPST, hCST	CMP-sialic acid transporter
SLC35A2	UGAT, UGT	UDP-galactose transporter
SLC35A3		UDP-N-acetylglucosamine transporter
Glycerol-3-phosphate transporter		
SLC37A1		glycerol-3-phosphate transporter
Na$^+$/neutral amino acid cotransporter		
SLC38A1	ATA1, NAT2, SAT1	Na$^+$/neutral amino acid cotransporter
SLC38A2	SAT2, ATA2	Na$^+$/neutral amino acid cotransporter
SLC38A3	G17, SN1	Na$^+$/neutral amino acid cotransporter
SLC38A4	PAAT, NAT3, ATA3	Na$^+$/neutral amino acid cotransporter
SLC38A5	SN2, JM24	Na$^+$/neutral amino acid cotransporter
Zinc transporter		
SLC39A1	ZIP1	zinc transporter
SLC39A2	ZIP2	zinc transporter
SLC39A3	ZIP3	zinc transporter
SLC39A4	ZIP4	zinc transporter

Transport ATPases (ATP-powered pumps)

Transport ATPases are primarily active transporters that use the energy of ATP hydrolysis to move ions or small molecules across the membrane against a chemical concentration gradient or electrical potential. There are two major groups of active transport ATPases. Those which actively transport ions (P-ATPases, V-ATPases, F-ATPases) and those of the superfamily of ATP-binding cassette (ABC) transporters, which couple the hydrolysis of ATP with the transport of a huge variety of small molecules as well as ions. Many **P-class ion pumps (P-ATPases)** are tetramers, composed of two α and two β subunits. The α subunit contains an ATP-binding site. During the transport process, at least one of the α subunits is phosphorylated (P) and the transported ions are thought to move through the phosphorylated subunit. The smaller β subunit may have regulatory functions. **F-class and V-class ion pumps (F-ATPases and V-ATPases)** have much more complicated structures than P-class pumps. They contain at least three kinds of transmembrane proteins and five kinds of extrinsic polypeptides that form the cytosolic domain. V-class pumps are mainly found in lysosomes and other acidic vesicles, whereas F-class pumps are found in mitochondria. Both transport protons (H^+) in a process that does not involve a phosphoprotein intermediate. While V-class pumps use the energy derived from ATP hydrolysis to pump protons into vesicles, F-class pumps power the synthesis of ATP from ADP and P_i by moving protons from the exoplasmic to the cytosolic of the membrane down the proton electrochemical gradient. F-class pumps are important in ATP synthesis in mitochondria. The class of **ATP-binding cassette (ABC) transporters** is much larger and more diverse than the ion pumps. Each ABC transporter is specific for a single substrate or a group of related substances including ions and many small molecules. ABC transporters share a common organization of four "core" domains: two transmembrane domains, forming the passageway used by transported molecules, and two cytosolic ATP-binding domains. These four "core" domains can either be present on four separate proteins or the "core" domains are fused into one or two multidomain proteins. In all ATP-powered pumps, the hydrolysis of ATP is tightly coupled to the transport process. (▶ Multidrug transporter).

P-type ATPases

Gene	Name/Aliases	Function
ATP1A1	NaKα1	Na^+/K^+ transporting ATPase, α1 polypeptide
ATP1A2	NaKα2	Na^+/K^+ transporting ATPase, α2 (+) polypeptide
ATP1A3	NaKα3	Na^+/K^+ transporting ATPase, α3 polypeptide
ATP1A4	NaKα4	Na^+/K^+ transporting ATPase, α4 polypeptide
ATP1B1		Na^+/K^+ transporting ATPase, β1 polypeptide
ATP1B2		Na^+/K^+ transporting ATPase, β2 polypeptide
ATP1B3		Na^+/K^+ transporting ATPase, β3 polypeptide
ATP1B4		Na^+/K^+ transporting ATPase, β4 polypeptide
ATP1BL1		Na^+/K^+ transporting ATPase, β polypeptide-like 1
ATP2A1	SERCA1	Ca^{2+} transporting ATPase, cardiac muscle, fast twitch 1
ATP2A2	SERCA2	Ca^{2+} transporting ATPase, cardiac muscle, slow twitch 2
ATP2A3	SERCA3	Ca^{2+} transporting ATPase, ubiquitous
ATP2B1	PMCA1	Ca^{2+} transporting ATPase, plasma membrane 1
ATP2B2	PMCA2	Ca^{2+} transporting ATPase, plasma membrane 2
ATP2B3	PMCA3	Ca^{2+} transporting ATPase, plasma membrane 3
ATP2B4	PMCA4	Ca^{2+} transporting ATPase, plasma membrane 4
ATP2C1	PMR1	Ca^{2+} transporting ATPase, type 2C, member 1
ATP3		Mg^{2+} transporting ATPase
ATP4A	ATP6A	H^+/K^+ exchanging ATPase, α polypeptide
ATP4B	ATP6B	H^+/K^+ exchanging ATPase, β polypeptide
ATP7A	MNK	Cu^{2+} transporting ATPase, α polypeptide (Menkes syndrome)
ATP7B	WND	Cu^{2+} transporting ATPase, β polypeptide (Wilson disease)
ATP8A1	ATPIA, APLT	ATPase, aminophospholipid transporter, Class I, 8A/1

P-type ATPases (Continued)

Gene	Name/Aliases	Function
ATP8A2	ATPIB, ML-1	ATPase, aminophospholipid transporter-like, Class I, 8A/2
ATP8B1	ATPIC, PFIC	ATPase, Class I, type 8B, member 1
ATP8B2	ATPID	ATPase, Class I, type 8B, member 2
ATP8B3	ATPIK	ATPase, Class I, type 8B, member 3
ATP8B4	ATPIM	ATPase, Class I, type 8B, member 4
ATP8B5	ATPIN	ATPase, Class I, type 8B, member 5
ATP9A	ATPIIA	ATPase, Class II, type 9A
ATP9B	ATPIIB	ATPase, Class II, type 9B
ATP10A	ATPVA	ATPase, Class V, type 10A
ATP10B	ATPVB	ATPase, Class V, type 10B
ATP10C	ATPVC	ATPase, Class V, type 10C
ATP10D	ATPVD	ATPase, Class V, type 10D
ATP11A	ATPIH, ATPIS	ATPase, Class VI, type 11A
ATP11B	ATPIF, ATPIR	ATPase, Class VI, type 11B
ATP11C	ATPIG, ATPIQ	ATPase, Class VI, type 11C
ATP12A	ATP1AL1	H^+/K^+ transporting ATPase, nongastric, α polypeptide

V-type ATPases

Gene	Name/Aliases	Function
ATP6IP1	ORF, XAP-3	H^+ transporting ATPase, lysosomal interacting protein 1
ATP6IP2	APT6M8-9	H^+ transporting ATPase, lysosomal interacting protein 2
ATP6V0A1	a1, vph1	H^+ transporting ATPase, lysosomal V0 subunit a isoform 1
ATP6V0A2	TJ6, ATP6a2	H^+ transporting ATPase, lysosomal V0 subunit a isoform 2
ATP6V0A4	VPP2	H^+ transporting ATPase, lysosomal V0 subunit a isoform 4
ATP6V0B	VMA16	H^+ transporting ATPase, lysosomal 21kD, V0 subunit c"
ATP6V0C	VATL, Vma3	H^+ transporting ATPase, lysosomal 16kD, V0 subunit c
ATP6V0D1	VATX	H^+ transporting ATPase, lysosomal 38kD, V0 subunit d 1
ATP6V0D2		H^+ transporting ATPase, lysosomal 38kD, V0 subunit d 2
ATP6V0E	Vma21p	H^+ transporting ATPase, lysosomal 9kD V0 subunit e
ATP6V1A1	Vma1	H^+ transporting ATPase, lysosomal 70kD, V1 subunit A 1
ATP6V1B1	VATB, Vma2	H^+ transporting ATPase, lysosomal 56/58kD, V1 subunit B1
ATP6V1B2	VATB, Vma2	H^+ transporting ATPase, lysosomal 56/58kD, V1 subunit B2
ATP6V1C1	VATC, Vma5	H^+ transporting ATPase, lysosomal 42kD, V1 subunit C1
ATP6V1C2		H^+ transporting ATPase, lysosomal 42kD, V1 subunit C2
ATP6V1D	VATD, VMA8	H^+ transporting ATPase, lysosomal 34kD, V1 subunit D
ATP6V1E1	P31, Vma4	H^+ transporting ATPase, lysosomal 31kD, V1 subunit E1
ATP6V1E2	MGC9341	H^+ transporting ATPase, lysosomal 31kD, V1 subunit E-like 2
ATP6V1El1		H^+ transporting ATPase, lysosomal 31kD, V1 subunit E-like 1
ATP6V1F	VATF, Vma7	H^+ transporting ATPase, lysosomal 14kD, V1 subunit F
ATP6V1G1	Vma10	H^+ transporting ATPase, lysosomal 13kD, V1 subunit G1
ATP6V1G2	Vma10	H^+ transporting ATPase, lysosomal 13kD, V1 subunit G2
ATP6V1G3	Vma10	H^+ transporting ATPase, lysosomal 13kD, V1 subunit G3
ATP6V1H	SFD, VMA13	H^+ transporting ATPase, lysosomal 50/57kD V1 subunit H

F-type ATPases

Gene	Name/Aliases	Function
ATP5A1	hATP1	H^+ transp. ATP synthase, mitochondr. F1 complex, α 1 (cardiac)
ATP5A2		H^+ transp. ATP synthase, mitochondr. F1 complex, α 2, (non-cardiac)
ATP5AL1		H^+ transp. ATP synthase, mitochondr. F1 complex, α1 cardiac-like 1
ATP5AL2		H^+ transp. ATP synth., mitochondr. F1 complex, α 2, non-cardiac-like 2
ATP5B	ATPSB	H^+ transp. ATP synthase, mitochondr. F1 complex, β polypeptide
ATP5BL1	ATPSBL1	H^+ transp. ATP synthase, mitochondr. F1 complex, β polypeptide -like 1
ATP5BL2	ATPSBL2	H^+ transp. ATP synthase, mitochondr. F1 complex, β polypeptide -like 2
ATP5C1	ATP5CL1	H^+ transp. ATP synthase, mitochondr. F1 complex, γ polypeptide 1
ATP5C2	ATP5CL2	H^+ transp. ATP synthase, mitochondr. F1 complex, γ polypeptide 2
ATP5D		H^+ transp. ATP synthase, mitochondr. F1 complex, δ subunit
ATP5E		H^+ transp. ATP synthase, mitochondr. F1 complex, ε subunit
ATP5F1		H^+ transp. ATP synthase, mitochondr. F0 complex, subunit b, isoform 1
ATP5G1	ATP5G	H^+ transp. ATP synthase, mitochondr. F0 complex, subunit c, isoform 1
ATP5G2		H^+ transp. ATP synthase, mitochondr. F0 complex, subunit c, isoform 2
ATP5G3		H^+ transp. ATP synthase, mitochondr. F0 complex, subunit c, isoform 3
ATP5H	ATPQ, ATP5JD	H^+ transp. ATP synthase, mitochondr. F0 complex, subunit d
ATP5I		H^+ transp. ATP synthase, mitochondr. F0 complex, subunit e
ATP5J		H^+ transp. ATP synthase, mitochondr. F0 complex, subunit F6
ATP5J2	F1Fo-ATPase	H^+ transp. ATP synthase, mitochondr. F0 complex, subunit f, isoform 2
ATP5L	ATP5JG	H^+ transp. ATP synthase, mitochondr. F0 complex, subunit g
ATP5O	OSCP, ATPO	H^+ transp. ATP synthase, mitochondr. F1 complex, O subunit

ABC-Transporter

Gene	Name/Aliases	Function
ABCA1	ABC1	cholesterol efflux onto HDL
ABCA2	ABC2	drug resistance
ABCA3	ABCC	
ABCA4	ABCR	rod photoreceptor retinoid transport
ABCA5		
ABCA6		
ABCA7		
ABCA8		
ABCA9		
ABCA10		
ABCA12		
ABCA13		
ABCB1	PYG1, MDR	multidrug resistance
ABCB2	TAP1	peptide transport
ABCB3	TAP2	peptide transport
ABCB4	PGY3	Phosphatidylcholine (PC) transport
ABCB5		
ABCB6	MTABC3	iron transport

ABC-Transporter (Continued)

Gene	Name/Aliases	Function
ABCB7	ABC7	Fe/S cluster transport
ABCB8	MTABC1	
ABCB9		
ABCB10	MTABC2	
ABCB11	SPGP	bile salt transport
ABCC1	MRP1	drug resistance, LTC_4 transport
ABCC2	MRP2	organic anion efflux
ABCC3	MRP3	drug resistance, organic anion transport
ABCC4	MRP4	nucleoside transport, cyclic nucleotide transport
ABCC5	MRP5	nucleoside transport, cyclic nucleotide transport
ABCC6	MRP6	
ABCC7	CFTR	chloride ion channel
ABCC8	SUR	sulfonylurea receptor
ABCC9	SUR2	
ABCC10	MRP7	
ABCC11		
ABCC12		
ABCD1	ALD	very long chain fatty acid transport regulation
ABCD2	ALDL1	
ABCD3	PXMP1	
ABCD4	PMP69	
ABCE1	OABP	oligoadenylate binding protein
ABCF1	ABC50	
ABCF2		
ABCF3		
ABCG1	White	cholesterol transport?
ABCG2	ABCP	toxin efflux, drug resistance
ABCG4	White2	
ABCG5	White3	sterol transport
ABCG8		sterol transport

Adhesion molecules

Adhesion molecules are transmembrane proteins. Through their extracellular part they mediate the interaction of one cell with another or with extracellular components such as the extracellular matrix. On the basis of structural and functional similarities, most adhesion molecules can be grouped into families such as cadherins, integrins, selectins, the immunoglobulin superfamily or the syndecans. While some adhesion molecules are passive in their adhesive function, the adhesiveness of other adhesive molecules can be regulated. Some adhesive proteins are very similar to receptors; they not only bind other molecules with high selectivity and affinity, but they are also able to transduce the binding into an intracellular signal.

Cadherins

Cadherins are characterized by the presence of four to seven cadherin repeats of about 110 amino acids that are present in the extracellular part of the protein. Cadherins mediate Ca^{2+}-dependent homophilic adhesion. The specificity of this homophilic interaction is generated by sequence differences at the adhesive face of the N-terminal cadherin domain. Cadherins have to dimerize in order to bind cadherins in a Ca^{2+}-dependent manner on different cells. Cadherins are divided into two subfamilies, the classic cadherins and the protocadherins. Classic cadherins are subdivided into four subfamilies, the type I classic cadherins, the type II classic cadherins, the desmosomal cadherins and the so-called "other classic cadherins". The protocadherins represent a recently discovered subfamily and contain more than five extracellular cadherin domains. The protocadherin subfamily consists of far more than 50 protocadherins and is less well studied, but may also mediate Ca^{2+}-dependent homophilic adhesion.

▶ Cadherins

Classic Cadherins

Classic Cadherins	Symbol	Distribution
type I		
E-Cadherin	CDH1	Non-neural epithelial cells during development
N-Cadherin	CDH2	Adult neural tissue, cardiac and skeletal muscle, lens, endothelial cells in the embryo
P-Cadherin	CDH3	Placenta, epidermis and mammary gland
R-Cadherin	CDH4	Developing epithelia in the kidney, lung, thymus, early optic nerve glia
type II		
VE-Cadherin	CDH5	Endothelium, intercellular junctions
K-Cadherin	CDH6	Kidney, brain, cerebellum
Cadherin-7	CDH7	
Cadherin-8	CDH8	Brainstem, cerebellum, thymocytes
T1-Cadherin	CDH9	
T2-Cadherin	CDH10	
OB-Cadherin	CDH11	Bone
Br-Cadherin	CDH12	Central nervous system
Cadherin-14	CDH14	Central nervous system
M-Cadherin	CDH15	Myoblasts, regenerating skeletal muscle myoblasts
Ey-Cadherin	CDH18	
Cadherin-19	CDH19	
Cadherin-20	CDH20	
other		
H-Cadherin	CDH13	Heart and breast epithelium, vascular smooth muscle cells
Ksp-Cadherin	CDH16	Kidney
LI-Cadherin	CDH17	Liver and intestine
desmosomal		
Desmocollin 1	DSC1	Epidermis
Desmocollin 2	DSC2	Epithelia, lymph nodes, heart
Desmocollin 3	DSC3	Keratinocytes
Desmoglein 1	DSG1	Keratinizing epodermis
Desmoglein 2	DSG2	Simple and stratified epithelia
Desmoglein 3	DSG3	Epidermis, tongue, tonsil, oesophagus

Protocadherins

Protocadherins	Symbol	Alias
protocadherin 1 (cadherin-like 1)	PCDH1	PC42
BH-protocadherin (brain-heart)	PCDH7	BH-PCDH
protocadherin 8	PCDH8	PAPC, ARCADLIN
protocadherin 9	PCDH9	
protocadherin 10	PCDH10	OL-PCDH, KIAA1400
protocadherin 11	PCDH11	
protocadherin 12	PCDH12	LOC51294, VE-Cadherin-2
protocadherin 14	PCDH14	
protocadherin 15	PCDH15	
protocadherin 16	PCDH16	FIB1
protocadherin 17	PCDH17	PCDH68, PCH68
protocadherin 18	PCDH18	KIAA1562, PCDH68-like
protocadherin 19	PCDH19	
protocadherin 20	PCDH20	PCDH13
protocadherin α locus	PCDHA@	CNRS1
protocadherin β locus	PCDHB@	PCDH3
protocadherin γ locus	PCDHG@	PCDH2, PCDH4
protocadherin α 1	PCDHA1	
protocadherin α 2	PCDHA2	
protocadherin α 3	PCDHA3	
protocadherin α 4	PCDHA4	Crnr1, Cnr1
protocadherin α 5	PCDHA5	Crnr6, Cnr6, CNRS6
protocadherin α 6	PCDHA6	Crnr2, Cnr2, CNRS2
protocadherin α 7	PCDHA7	Crnr4, Cnr4, CNRS4
protocadherin α 8	PCDHA8	
protocadherin α 9	PCDHA9	
protocadherin α 10	PCDHA10	Crnr8, Cnr8, CNRS8
protocadherin α 11	PCDHA11	Crnr7, Cnr7, CNRS7
protocadherin α 12	PCDHA12	
protocadherin α 13	PCDHA13	Crnr5, Cnr5, CNRS5
protocadherin α subfamily C1	PCDHAC1	
protocadherin α subfamily C2	PCDHAC2	
protocadherin α constant	PCDHACT	PCDHAC
protocadherin β 1	PCDHB1	
protocadherin β 2	PCDHB2	
protocadherin β 3	PCDHB3	
protocadherin β 4	PCDHB4	
protocadherin β 5	PCDHB5	
protocadherin β 6	PCDHB6	
protocadherin β 7	PCDHB7	
protocadherin β 8	PCDHB8	
protocadherin β 9	PCDHB9	
protocadherin β 10	PCDHB10	
protocadherin β 11	PCDHB11	
protocadherin β 12	PCDHB12	

Protocadherins (Continued)

Protocadherins	Symbol	Alias
protocadherin β 13	PCDHB13	
protocadherin β 14	PCDHB14	
protocadherin β 15	PCDHB15	
protocadherin γ subfamily A, 1	PCDHGA1	
protocadherin γ subfamily A, 2	PCDHGA2	
protocadherin γ subfamily A, 3	PCDHGA3	
protocadherin γ subfamily A, 4	PCDHGA4	
protocadherin γ subfamily A, 5	PCDHGA5	
protocadherin γ subfamily A, 6	PCDHGA6	
protocadherin γ subfamily A, 7	PCDHGA7	
protocadherin γ subfamily A, 8	PCDHGA8	
protocadherin γ subfamily A, 9	PCDHGA9	
protocadherin γ subfamily A, 10	PCDHGA10	
protocadherin γ subfamily A, 11	PCDHGA11	
protocadherin γ subfamily A,12	PCDHGA12	KIAA0588
protocadherin γ subfamily B, 1	PCDHGB1	
protocadherin γ subfamily B, 2	PCDHGB2	
protocadherin γ subfamily B, 3	PCDHGB3	
protocadherin γ subfamily B, 4	PCDHGB4	
protocadherin γ subfamily B, 5	PCDHGB5	
protocadherin γ subfamily B, 6	PCDHGB6	
protocadherin γ subfamily B, 7	PCDHGB7	
protocadherin γ subfamily C, 3	PCDHGC3	PCDH2, PC-43
protocadherin γ subfamily C, 4	PCDHGC4	
protocadherin γ subfamily C, 5	PCDHGC5	
protocadherin γ constant	PCDHGCT	PCDHGC

Integrins

Integrins consist of an α and β subunit that form a dimer. They mediate the interaction of cells with the extracellular matrix or with proteins on other cells. Both, the α and the β subunit take part in ligand binding. Integrin function is modulated by signals from within the cell. Signals are delivered *via* other receptor systems ("inside-out signalling") and are mediated through complex cytoskeletal interactions with the cytoplasmic tails of the integrin subunits. Binding of a ligand to an integrin can result in an intracellular signal ("outside-in signalling").

▶ Integrins

Integrins

Integrin	Ligand	Distribution
$\alpha_1\beta_1$	Collagen, Laminin	Widespread, embryogenesis, smooth muscle cells and liver, haemopoietic cells
$\alpha_2\beta_1$	Echovirus 1, Fibronectin, Collagen types I-IV, Laminin	Stimulated T cells, fibroblasts, endothelium, peripheral nerves, platelets
$\alpha_3\beta_1$	Epiligrin, Fibronectin, Invasin, Thrombospondin	Monocytes, B and T cells, kidney, thyroid, most non-lymphoid adherent cell lines
$\alpha_4\beta_1$	Fibronectin, Invasin, VCAM-1, Thrombospondin	Leukocytes, haemopoietic precursors, muscle
$\alpha_4\beta_7$	Fibronectin, MAdCAM-1, VCAM-1	Mucosal lymphocytes, NK cells, eosinophils
$\alpha_5\beta_1$	Fibronectin, Fibrinogen, Invasin, Denatured collagen	Widespread in embryonic and adult tissues
$\alpha_6\beta_1$	Invasin, Laminin, Sperm fertilin	Epithelia, haemopoietic tissues
$\alpha_6\beta_4$	Laminin	Stratified epithelia, Schwann cells and some endothelia
$\alpha_7\beta_1$	Laminin types 1,2,4	Expression during myogenesis, developing nervous system
$\alpha_8\beta_1$	Cytotactin/tenascin-C, Fibronectin, Osteopontin	Smooth muscle, kidney
$\alpha_9\beta_1$	Cytotactin/tenascin-C	Epithelia, muscle, liver
$\alpha_{10}\beta_1$	Collagen type II	Chondrocytes, skeletal muscle, heart
$\alpha_E\beta_7$	E-cadherin	Intraepithelial lymphocytes, subpopulation of T cells in the lamina propria
$\alpha_L\beta_2$	ICAM-1, ICAM-2,3,4,5	Lymphocytes, monocyte lineage cells and other leucocytes, during T cell activation
$\alpha_M\beta_2$	*Candida albicans*, Factor X, Fibrinogen, Complement fragment iC3b, ICAM-1, Neutrophil inhibitory factor	Neutrophils, monocytes, eosinophils and basophils, NK cells
$\alpha_D\beta_2$	ICAM-3, VCAM-1	Peripheral leucocytes, tissue macrophages
$\alpha_x\beta_2$	Fibrinogen, Complement fragment iC3b	Tissue macrophages and monocytes
$\alpha_v\beta_1$	Fibronectin, Vitronectin	
$\alpha_v\beta_3$	Adenovirus penton base protein, Bone sialoprotein, Denatured collagen, Cytotactin/tenascin-C, Disintegrins, Fibronectin, Fibrinogen, HIV Tat protein, Laminin, Matrix metalloproteinase-2, Osteopontin, Prothrombin, Thrombospondin, Vitronectin, von Willebrand factor	Endothelium, smooth muscle, some activated macrophages and T cells, platelets
$\alpha_v\beta_5$	Adenovirus penton base protein, Bone sialoprotein, Fibronectin, HIV Tat protein, Vitronectin	More widely than $\alpha_v\beta_3$, regulated in angiogenesis
$\alpha_v\beta_6$	Cytotactin/tenascin-C, Fibronectin	Epithelial cells
$\alpha_v\beta_8$	Fibronectin	Placenta, kidney, brain, ovary, uterus, synapses, glia
$\alpha_{IIb}\beta_3$	Fibrinogen, Plasminogen, Prothrombin, Collagens, *Borrelia burgdorferi*, Denatured collagen, Decorsin, Disintegrins, Fibronectin, Thrombospondin, Vitronectin, von Willebrand factor	Platelets, megacaryocytes

Selectins

The three known selectins are structurally and functionally related. They are transmembrane proteins with an N-terminal C-type actin domain, followed by an EGF repeat and a variable number of complement control protein (CCP) domains. Selectins bind carbohydrates that are present on various glycoproteins.

Selectins

Selectin	Ligands	Distribution
E-Selectin	ESL-1, PSGL-1, leukocyte L-selectin	Activated endothelial cells
L-Selectin	CD34, GlyCAM-1, MAdCAM-1, PSGL-1	Leucocytes
P-Selectin	PSGL-1, CD24	Megakaryocytes, activated platelets, activated endothelial cells

Syndecans

Syndecans are transmembrane proteins which are modified by the addition of heparan sulphate glycosaminoglycan (GAG) chains and other sugars. Syndecans bind a wide variety of different ligands *via* their heparan sulphate chains. Binding specificities may vary depending on the cell-type specific modifications of the heparan sulphate chains.

Syndecans

Syndecan	Ligands	Distribution
Syndecan-1	Growth factors, extracellular matrix components (fibronectin, laminin, collagens), other adhesion receptors (L-selectin, NCAM, CD31) and enzymes	Epithelial cells, vascular smooth muscle cells, endothelium, neural cells, pre-B cells, immature B cells and plasma cells
Syndecan-2	Growth factors, extracellular matrix components (fibronectin, laminin, collagens), other adhesion receptors (L-selectin, NCAM, CD31) and enzymes	Fibroblasts during development, primary human monocytes, in response to differentiation/activation
Syndecan-3	Growth factors, extracellular matrix components (fibronectin, laminin, collagens), other receptors (L-selectin, NCAM, CD31) and enzymes	Neuronal cells, during development
Syndecan-4	Include growth factors, extracellular matrix components (fibronectin, laminin, collagens), other receptors (L-selectin, NCAM, CD31) and enzymes	Many epithelial and fibroblastic cells, localized to focal adhesion

Immunoglobulin superfamily

The immunoglobulin superfamily represents a very large group of transmembrane proteins. They are characterized by the presence of one or more extracellular immunoglobulin domains of approximately 100 amino acids each. This structural motif is very widely used in transmembrane proteins. It is estimated that up to 1/3 of all transmembrane proteins belong to this superfamily. However, not all of them function as adhesion molecules. Examples of immunoglobulin superfamily proteins that do function as adhesion molecules are listed below.

Immunoglobulin superfamily

Member	Ligand	Distribution
ALCAM	CD6, homophilic adhesion, NgCAM	Neurons, epithelial cells, fibroblasts, activated T cells, activated monocytes
CD22	Sialoglycoconjugate NeuAcα2-6Galβ1-4GlcNAc present on *N*-linked carbohydrates	Mature peripheral B cells

Immunoglobulin superfamily (Continued)

Member	Ligand	Distribution
CD31 (PECAM-1)	Homophilic adhesion, integrin $\alpha_v\beta_3$, glycosaminoglycans	Endothelial cells, platelets, monocytes, granulocytes and other leucocytes
CD33	Sialoglycoconjugate NeuAcα2-3Galβ1-3(4)GlcNAc and NeuAcα2-3Galβ1-3GlcNAc on glycoproteins	Myelomonocytic precursors
CD96	Not known	Up-regulated following T cells activation, expressed by most T cell lines
CD147	Interstitial collagenase (MMP-1)	Widely expressed in embryonic and adult tissues
CEACAM family	Mediates homophilic cell-cell adhesion, E-selectin	Granulocytes, epithelial cells
Contactin-1	CASPR	Adult brain
ICAM-1	Integrins $\alpha_L\beta_2$, $\alpha_M\beta_2$ and $\alpha_X\beta_2$, rhinoviruses, *Plasmodium falciparum*-infected erythrocytes	Wide range of both haematopoietic and non-haematopoietic cells
ICAM-2	Integrins $\alpha_L\beta_2$ and $\alpha_M\beta_2$	Subpopulation of lymphocytes, monocytes, splenic sinusoids, dendritic cells, platelets, stromal cells and at high levels on vascular endothelium
ICAM-3	Integrins $\alpha_L\beta_2$ and $\alpha_D\beta_2$, DC-SIGN	Leucocytes, epidermal Langerhans cells
ICAM-4	Integrins $\alpha_L\beta_2$, $\alpha_M\beta_2$ and $\alpha_X\beta_2$	Erythrocytes, subsets of both B and T cells
ICAM-5	Integrins $\alpha_L\beta_2$	Brain
JAM	Presumed to be homotypic	Endothelial and epithelial cells, mesothelial cells, megacaryocytes
L1	Homophilic binding, integrins $\alpha_V\beta_3$ and $\alpha_5\beta_1$	Adult and embryonic nervous system, 10-20% of peripheral blood lymphocytes
MAdCAM-1	Integrin $\alpha_4\beta_7$, L-selectin	High endothelial venules of Peyer's patches and mesenteric lymph nodes, vascular endothelium
MAG	Sialoglycoconjugate NeuAcα2-3Galβ1-3GlcNAc on *N*- and *O*- linked oligosaccharides and gangliosides, CD22, CD33, collagens I-VI	Oligodendrocytes, Schwann cells
MUC18	None identified	Endothelial, smooth muscle, trophoblast, subpopulation of activated T cells
NCAM	Homophilic binding, chondroitin sulphate proteoglycans	Adult neural tissue and muscle, NK cells
P(0)	Homophilic interaction,	Schwann cells
Sialoadhesin	Sialoglycoconjugate NeuAcα2-3Galβ1-3(4)GlcNAc and NeuAcα2-3Galβ1-3GlcNAc on glycoproteins and glycolipids	Subsets of macrophages in bone marrow and secondary lymphoid organs
TAG-1	L1 family members	Neural tissue
VCAM-1	Integrins $\alpha_4\beta_1$ and $\alpha_4\beta_7$, integrin $\alpha_D\beta_2$	Activated endothelial cells, tissue macrophages, dendritic cells, bone marrow fibroblasts, myoblasts

Protein Kinases

Protein kinases catalyse the transfer of the terminal (γ) phosphoryl group of ATP to a hydroxyl residue on an amino acid side-chain. Phosphorylation of proteins by protein kinases represents the most prevalent reversible modification which regulates the activities of many enzymes, ion channels and other proteins. Reversible protein phosphorylation is involved in basically all cellular processes including signal transduction, metabolism, transcription, cell cycle progression, cell movement, apoptosis or cell differentiation. There are two principal classes of protein kinases: Those that transfer phosphoryl groups to specific serine and threonine residues (**Serine/Threonine Kinases**) on those that transfer them to specific tyrosine residues (**Tyrosine Kinases**). Protein phosphorylation occurs inside of cells where the substrate ATP is present in abundance. The effects of protein kinases are reversed by protein phosphatases which remove phosphoryl groups from proteins by catalysing the hydrolysis of the phosphate bond.

Protein kinases represent one of the largest families of genes in eukaryotes. The protein kinase complement of the human genome has recenty been catalogued [Manning et al., Science 298, 1912 (2002)]. The following list of protein kinases is based on the classification used by Manning et al. for the description of the human "kinome".

▶ JAK-STAT-pathway
▶ MAP Kinase Cascades
▶ Neurotrophic Factors
▶ Transmembrane Siganlling
▶ Tyrosine Kinases

Serine/Threonine Kinases

AGC Group (containing PK<u>A</u>, PK<u>G</u> and PK<u>C</u> families)

AGC Group (containing PK<u>A</u>, PK<u>G</u> and PK<u>C</u> families)

Family	Subfamily	Name
PKA (Protein kinase A)		PKA-Cα
		PKA-Cβ
		PKA-Cγ
		PRKX
		PRKY
AKT/ PKB (Protein kinase B)		AKT1 (PKB α)
		AKT2 (PKB β)
		AKT3 (PKB γ)
PKC (Protein kinase C)	α	PKCα
	α	PKCβ
	α	PKCγ
	δ	PKCδ
	δ	PKCθ
	η	PKCη
	η	PKCε
	ι	PKCι
	ι	PKCζ
PKG (cGMP-dependent protein kinase)		PKG1 (cGK-I)
		PKG2 (cGK-II)
PKN (Protein kinase N)		PKN1
		PKN2
		PKN3
DMPK (Dystrophia myotonica protein kinase)	GEK (Genghis Khan)	DMPK1
	GEK	DMPK2

AGC Group (containing PK<u>A</u>, PK<u>G</u> and PK<u>C</u> families) (Continued)

Family	Subfamily	Name
	GEK	MRCKβ (myotonic dystrophy kinase-related Cdc42-binding kinase)
	GEK	MRCKα
	ROCK (Rho-kinase)	ROCK2
	ROCK	ROCK1
	ROCK	CRIK (Citron)
GRK (G-protein coupled receptor kinase)	βARK (β-adrenoceptor kinase)	βARK1 (GRK2) βARK2 (GRK3)
	GRK	RHOK (Rhodopsin kinase; GRK1)
	GRK	GRK4
	GRK	GRK5
	GRK	GRK6
	GRK	GRK7
MAST (Microtubuli-associated serine/threonine Kinase)		MAST3
		MAST2
		MAST1
		MASTL
		MAST4
PDK1 (Phosphoinositide-dependent kinase 1)		PDK1
NDR		NDR1
		LATS1
		LATS2
		NDR2
RSK (ribosomal protein S6 kinase)	MSK (mitogen and stress-activated kinase)	MSK1 MSK2
	p70	p70S6K
	p70	p70S6Kb
	RSK	RSK1
	RSK	RSK2
	RSK	RSK3
	RSK	RSK4
		SgK494
RSKL		RSKL2
		RSKL1
SGK (serum/glucocorticoid regulated kinases)		SGK
		SGK2
		SGK3
YANK		YANK1
		YANK2
		YANK3

CAMK Group (Calcium-calmodulin dependent protein kinase)

CAMK Group (Calcium-calmodulin dependent protein kinase)

Family	Subfamily	Name
CaMK I		CaMK Iγ
		CaMK Iα
		CaMK IV
		CaMK Iδ
		CaMK Iβ
CaMK II		CaMK IIα
		CaMK IIβ
		CaMK IIγ
		CaMK IIδ
CaMKL	AMPK (AMP-activated kinase)	AMPKα1
	AMPK (AMP-activated kinase)	AMPKα2
	BRSK	BRSK2
	BRSK	BRSK1
	CHK1	CHK1
	HUNK	HUNK
	LKB	LKB1
	MARK	MARK3
	MARK	MARK2
	MARK	MARK1
	MARK	MARK4
	MELK	MELK
	NIM1	NIM1
	NuaK	NuaK1
	NuaK	NuaK2
	PASK	PASK
	QIK	QSK
	QIK	QIK
	QIK	SIK
	SNRK	SNRK
CaMK-Unique		VACAMKL
		STK33
		SgK495
CASK (Ca^{2+}/calmodulin-dependent serine protein kinase)		CASK
DAPK (death associated protein kinase)		DAPK1
		DAPK2
		DRAK1
		DRAK2
		DAPK3
DCAMKL (double cortin and Ca^{2+}/calmodulin-dependent protein kinase-like)		DCAMKL1
		DCAMKL3
		DCAMKL2
MAPKAPK (MAP kinase-activated protein kinase)	MAPKAPK	MAPKAPK2
	MAPKAPK	MAPKAPK3
	MAPKAPK	MAPKAPK5
	MINK	MNK1
	MINK	MNK2
MLCK (myosin light chain kinase)		smMLCK
		Titin

CAMK Group (Calcium-calmodulin dependent protein kinase)   (Continued)

Family	Subfamily	Name
		caMLCK
		skMLCK
		sgMLCK
PhK (phosphorylase kinase)		PhKγ1
		PhKγ2
Pim (proviral integration site)		Pim3
		Pim1
		Pim2
PDK		PDK1
		PDK2
		PDK3
Psk (putative protein-serine kinase)		PskH1
		PskH2
RAD53		CHK2 (checkpoint kinase 2)
Trbl		Trb1
		Trb2
Trio		Trio
		Trad
		SPEG
		Obscn
TSSK (testis specific serine/ threonine kinase)		TSSK3
		TSSK2
		SSTK
		TSSK4
		TSSK1

CK1 Group (Casein kinase 1)

CK1 Group (Casein kinase 1)

Family	Name
CK1 (casein kinase 1)	CK1α
	CK1δ
	CK1ε
	CK1γ2
	CK1γ3
	CK1α2
	CK1γ1
TTBK (tau tubulin kinase)	TTBK2
	TTBK1
Vrk (vaccinia related kinase)	Vrk1
	Vrk2
	Vrk3

CMGC Group (Containing Cdk, MAPK, GSK3, Clk families)

CMGC Group (Containing Cdk, MAPK, GSK3, Clk families)

Family	Subfamily	Name
Cdk (cyclin-dependent kinase)	Cdc2	Cdc2
	Cdc2	Cdk2
	Cdc2	Cdk3
	Cdk10	Cdk10
	Cdk4	Cdk4
	Cdk4	Cdk6
	Cdk5	Cdk5
	Cdk7	Cdk7
	Cdk8	Cdk8
	Cdk8	Cdk11
	Cdk9	Cdk9
	Crk7	Ched
	Crk7	Crk7
	PITSLRE	PITSLRE
	TAIRE	PCTAIRE1
	TAIRE	PCTAIRE2
	TAIRE	PCTAIRE3
	TAIRE	PFTAIRE1
	TAIRE	PFTAIRE2
		CCRK
Cdkl (cyclin-dependent kinase-like)		Cdkl2
		Cdkl1
		Cdkl5
		Cdkl4
		Cdkl3
Clk (cdc2/CDC28-like kinase)		Clk1
		Clk2
		Clk3
		Clk4

CMGC Group (Containing Cdk, MAPK, GSK3, Clk families) (Continued)

Family	Subfamily	Name
Dyrk (dual-specificity tyrosine-(Y)-phosphorylation regulated kinase)	Dyrk1	Dyrk1A
	Dyrk1	Dyrk1B
	Dyrk2	Dyrk2
	Dyrk2	Dyrk3
	Dyrk2	Dyrk4
	HIPK (Homeodomain-interacting protein kinase) HIPK2	HIPK1
	HIPK	HIPK3
	HIPK	HIPK4
	PRP4	PRP4
GSK (Glycogen synthase kinase 3)		GSK3α
		GSK3β
MAPK (Mitogen activated protein kinase)	Erk	Erk1
	Erk	Erk2
	Erk	Erk3
	Erk	Erk4
	Erk	Erk5
	Erk7	Erk7
	Jnk	Jnk1
	Jnk	Jnk2
	Jnk	Jnk3
	nmo	NLK
	p38	p38α
	p38	p38β
	p38	p38γ
	p38	p38δ
RCK (related to the cdc2 kinase)		Mak
		ICK
		MOK
SRPK (serine/arginine-rich protein specific kinase)		SRPK1
		SRPK2
		MSSK1

RGC Group (Receptor Guanylyl Cyclases; ▶ Guanylyl Cyclases)

RGC Group (Receptor Guanylyl Cyclases)

Family	Name
RGC (Receptor guanylyl cyclases)	GC-A (ANPa)
	GC-B (ANPb)
	GC-D (CYGD)
	GC-F (CYGF)
	GC-C (HSER)

STE Group (Homologues of yeast sterile-7, -11, -20 kinases; ▶ MAP Kinase Cascades)

STE Group (Homologues of yeast sterile-7, -11, -20 kinases)

Family	Subfamily	Name
STE11 (sterile 11)		MAP3K1 (Mekk1)
		MAP3K2 (Mekk2)
		MAP3K3 (Mekk3)
		MAP3K4 (Mekk4)
		MAP3K5 (Mekk5)
		MAP3K6 (Ask2)
		MAP3K7
		MAP3K8 (Tpl2)
STE20 (sterile 20)	FRAY	OSR1
	FRAY	STLK3
	KHS (kinase homologous to SPS1/STE20)	GCK (MAP4K2)
	KHS	HPK1 (MAP4K1)
	KHS	KHS1 (MAP4K5)
	KHS	KHS2
	MSN	ZC1/HGK (MAP4K4)
	MSN	ZC2/TNIK (Traf2)
	MSN	ZC3/MINK (Misshapen)
	MSN	ZC4/NRK (Nesk)
	MST	MST1 (Stk4; Krs-2)
	MST	MST2 (Stk3; Krs-1)
	NinaC	MYO3B
	NinaC	MYO3A
	PAKA (p21-activated kinase)	PAK1
	PAK2	
	PAK2	PAK3
	PAKB	PAK6
	PAKB	PAK4
	PAKB	PAK5
	SLK	SLK
	SLK	LOK (Stk10)
	STLK	STLK5
	STLK	STLK6
	TAO (Thousand-and-one amino acid kinase)	TAO2
		TAO3
		TAO1
	YSK	MST3 (Stk24)
	YSK	YSK1 (Sok1; Stk25)
	YSK	MST4 (Mask)
STE7 (sterile 7)		MAP2K1 (Mek1)
		MAP2K2 (Mek2)
		MAP2K5 (Mek5)
		MAP2K6 (Mek6)
		MAP2K7 (Mek7)
		MAP2K3 (Mek3)
		MAP2K4 (Mek4)
STE-Unique		COT
		NIK (MAP3K14)

TKL Group (Tyrosine kinase-like families)

TKL Group (Tyrosine kinase-like families)

Family	Subfamily	Name
IRAK (interleukin-1 receptor-associated kinase)		IRAK1
		IRAK2
		IRAK3
		IRAK4
LISK (LIMK/TESK)	LIMK	Limk2
	LIMK	Limk1
	TESK (Testis-specific protein kinase)	Tesk1
		Tesk2
LRRK		LRRK2
		LRRK1
Mlk (mixed lineage kinase)	HH498	HH498
	ILK	ILK (Integrin linked kinase)
	LZK	DLK (MAP3K12)
	LZK	LZK (MAP3K13)
	Mlk	Mlk1 (MAP3K9)
	Mlk	Mlk2 (MAP3K10)
	Mlk	Mlk3 (MAP3K11)
	Mlk	ZAK (Mltk)
	Mlk	Mlk4
	TAK1	TAK1 (TGF-β activated-kinase 1)
Raf		A-Raf
		B-Raf
		KSR1 (Kinase suppressor of ras-1)
		Raf1 (C-Raf)
		KSR2
RIPK (receptor-interacting protein kinase)		RIPK1
		RIPK2
		RIPK3
		ANKRD3
		SgK288
STKR (receptor serine/threonine kinases ▶ Receptors)	Type I	ALK-1
	Type I	ActR-I A (ALK-2)
	Type I	BMPR-I A (ALK-3)
	Type I	ActR-I B (ALK-4)
	Type I	TGFβR-I (ALK-5)
	Type I	BMPR-I B (ALK-6)
	Type I	ALK-7
	Type II	ActR-II A
	Type II	ActR-II B
	Type II	MISR-II
	Type II	BMPR-II
	Type II	TGFβR-II
TKL	Unique	MLKL

Atypical Group

Atypical Group

Family	Subfamily	Name
A6		A6
		A6r
ABC1	ABC1-A	ADCK4
	ABC1-A	ADCK3
	ABC1-B	ADCK1
	ABC1-B	ADCK5
	ABC1-C	ADCK2
Alpha	ChaK	ChaK1
	ChaK	ChaK2
	eEF2K	eEF2K
	eEF2K	AlphaK2
		AlphaK3
		AlphaK1
BCR (breakpoint cluster region)		BCR
BRD		BRD2
		BRD3
		BRD4
		BRDT
FAST		FASTK
G11		G11
H11		H11
PDHK (pyruvate dehydrogenase kinase)		BCKDK
		PDHK1
		PDHK2
		PDHK3
		PDHK4
PIKK	ATM	ATM
	ATR	ATR
	DNAPK	DNAPK
	FRAP	FRAP
	SMG1	SMG1
	TRRAP	TRRAP
RIO	RIO1	RIOK1
	RIO2	RIOK2
	RIO3	RIOK3
TAF1		TAF1
		TAF1L
TIF1		TIF1α
		TIF1β
		TIF1γ

Other Groups

Other Groups

Family	Subfamily	Name
AUR		AurC
		AurB
		AurAC
BUB (budding uninhibited by benzimidazoles 1 homolog)		BUBR1
		BUB
Bud32		PRPK
CAMKK (Ca^{2+}/calmodulin-dependent protein kinase kinase)	Meta	CaMKK2
	Meta	CaMKK1
Cdc7		Cdc7
CK2 (Casein kinase 2)		CK2α1
		CK2α2
Haspin (Germ cell-specific gene 2)		Haspin
IKK (IκB kinase)		IKKα
		IKKβ
		IKKε
		TBK1
Ire (Inositol-requiring)		Ire1 (Ern1)
		Ire2 (Ern2)
Mos (Moloney sarcoma oncogene)		Mos
Nak (Numb-associated kinase)		Gak
		Aak1
		MPSK1
		BIKE
Nek (NimA-related expressed kinase)		Nek1
		Nek2
		Nek3
		Nek4
		Nek6
		Nek7
		Nek9
		Nek8
		Nek5
		Nek11
		Nek10
NKF1		SgK069
		SgK110
		SBK
NKF2		PINK1
NKF3		SgK223
		SgK269
NKF4		CLIK1L
		CLIC1
NKF5		SgK307
		SgK424
NRBP		NRBP1
		NRBP2
Other-Unique		SgK493
		SgK496

Other Groups (Continued)

Family	Subfamily	Name
		SgK071
		SgK196
		SgK396
		KIS
		RNAseL
PEK	GCN2	GCN2
	PEK	PEK
		PKR
		HRI
Plk (Polo-like kinase)		Plk1
		Plk3
		Plk4
		Plk2
SCY1		SCYL1
		SCYL3
		SCYL2
Slob		Slob
TBCK		TBCK
Tlk (Tousled-like kinase)		Tlk1
		Tlk2
TOPK		PBK
Ttk (Embryonal carcinoma kinase)		Ttk
Ulk (Unc-51-like kinase)		Fused
		Ulk1
		Ulk2
		Ulk3
		Ulk4
VPS15		PIK3R4
Wee (Wee 1 homolog)		MYT1
		Wee1
		Wee1B
Wnk (With-no-lys kinase)		Wnk2
		Wnk1
		Wnk4
		Wnk3

Tyrosine Kinases

RTK Group (Receptor tyrosine kinases; ▶ Table appendix: Receptor Proteins)

RTK Group (Receptor tyrosine kinases)

Family	Name
EGFR (epidermal growth factor receptor; ErbB)	EGFR/ErbB1
	HER2/ErbB2
	HER3/ErbB3
	HER4/ErbB4
InsR (insulin receptor)	IGF1R
	INSR
	IRR
PDGFR (platelet derived growth factor)	FMS
	Flt3/Flk2
	Kit/SCFR
	PDGFRα
	PDGFRβ
VEGFR (vascular endothelial growth factor)	VEGF-R1; Flt1
	VEGF-R3; Flt4
	VEGF-R2; Flk1; KDR
FGFR (fibroblast growth factor)	FGFR1
	FGFR2
	FGFR3
	FGFR4
KLG/CCK (kinase-like gene)	CCK4/PTK7
NGF (nerve growth factor; Trk)	TrkA
	TrkB
	TrkC
HGF (hepatocyte growth factor; Met)	Met
	Ron/Skt
Eph (kinase detected in erythropoietin-producing hepatoma)	EphA1
	EphA2
	EphA3
	EphA4
	EphA5
	EphA8
	EphB1
	EphB2
	EphB3
	EphB4
	EphB6
	EphA7
	EphA10
	EphA6
Axl (anexelekto)	Axl
	Mer
	Tyro3
Tie (tyrosine kinase with Ig and EGF homology)	Tie2 (tek)
	Tie1
Ryk	Ryk
DDR (discoid domain receptor)	DDR1

RTK Group (<u>R</u>eceptor <u>t</u>yrosine <u>k</u>inases)   (Continued)

Family	Name
	DDR2
Ret	Ret
Sev (sevenless)	Ros
Alk (anaplastic lymphoma kinase)	Alk
	Ltk (Leukocyte tyrosine kinase)
Ror	Ror1
	Ror2
Musk	Musk
LMR	LMR1 (AATYK)
	LMR2 (AATYK2)
	LMR3 (AATYK3)
TK-Unique	SuRTK106

NRTK Group (<u>N</u>on-<u>r</u>eceptor <u>t</u>yrosine <u>k</u>inases; ▶ Tyrosine Kinases)

NRTK Group (<u>N</u>on-<u>r</u>eceptor <u>t</u>yrosine <u>k</u>inases)

Family	Name
Abl (abelson murine leukemia oncogene)	Abl
	Arg (Abl-related gene)
Ack (activated Cdc42-associated kinase)	Ack (Tnk2)
	Tnk1 (Tyrosine kinase, non-receptor 1)
Csk (C-terminal Src kinase)	Csk
	Ctk (Csk-type protein tyrosine kinase)
Fak (Focal adhesion kinase)	Fak
	Pyk2
Fer (Fps/Fes-related tyrosine kinase)	Fer (TYK3)
	Fes (Feline sarcoma oncogene)
JAKA	Jak1 (Janus kinase-1)
	Jak2 (Janus kinase-2)
	Jak3 (Janus kinase-3)
	Tyk2 (Transducer of interferon α/β signals)
Src (rous sarcoma virus oncogene)	Blk (B lymphocyte kinase)
	Brk (Breast tumor kinase; PTK6)
	Fgr (Gardner-Rasheed sarcoma virus oncogene)
	Fyn (Related to Fgr and Yes)
	Hck (Hemopoietic cell kinase; Bmk)
	Lck (Lymphocyte protein tyrosine kinase)
	Lyn (JTK8)
	Src
	Yes (Yamaguchi 73 sarcoma virus oncogene)
	Frk (Fyn-related kinase; Gtk; Lyk; Rak)
	Srm
Syk (spleen tyrosine kinase)	Syk (p72Syk)
	Zap70 (ζ-chain associated protein kinase)
Tec (tyrosine kinase expressed in hepatocellular carcinoma)	Btk (Bruton's tyrosine kinase)
	Itk (IL-2 inducible T-cell kinase ; Tsk)
	Tec
	Txx
	Bmx (Bone marrow kinase, X-linked; Etk)

List of Drugs

Drug	Group/Class	Link
Abacavir	Reverse transcriptase inhibitor	▶ Antiviral Agents
Abciximab	GPIIb/IIIa-inhibitor	▶ Anti-platelet Drugs
Acarbose	α-glucosidase inhibitor	▶ Oral Antidiabetic Drugs ▶ Diabetes mellitus
Acebutolol	β-adrenergic antagonist (blocker)	▶ β-adrenergic System
Acetaminophen	Analgetic/antipyretic drug	▶ Analgesics
Acetazolamide	Carbonic anhydrase inhibitor	▶ Diuretics
Acetylsalicylic Acid	Analgetic/Antipyretic/ Antiinflammatory drug	▶ Analgesics ▶ Cycloxygenase ▶ Non-steroidal Anti-inflammatory Drugs
Aciclovir / Acyclovir	Antiviral drug	▶ Antiviral drugs
Acitretin	Retinoid	▶ Retinoids
Adenosine	Nucleoside	▶ Purinergic System ▶ Antiarrhythmic Drugs
Adrenaline (Epinephrin)	Adrenoceptor agonist	▶ β-adrenergic Sstem ▶ α-adrenergic System
Ajmalin	Antiarrhythmic drug	▶ Antiarrhyrthmic Drugs
Albuterol	β-adrenergic agonist	▶ β-adrenergic System
Alendronate	Biphosphonate	▶ Bone Metabolism
Alfentanil	Opioid, analgesic	▶ Opioid System ▶ Analgesics
Alfuzosin	α-adrenergic antagonist	▶ α-adrenergic System
Allopurinol	Anti-gout drug	▶ Anti-gout Drugs
Alprazolam	Benzodiazepine	▶ Benzodiazepines
Alteplase (t-PA)	Fibrinolytic	▶ Fibrinolytics
Amantadine	Anti-parkinson drug	▶ Anti-parkinson Drugs ▶ Antiviral Drugs
Amikacin	Aminoglycoside (antibacterial drug)	▶ Aminoglycosides
Amiloride	Potassium-sparing diuretic	▶ Diuretics ▶ Epithelial Sodium Channels
Amiodarone	Antiarrhythmic drug	▶ Antiarrhyrthmic Drugs
Amitriptyline	Non-selective monoamine reuptake inhibitor (NSMRI)	▶ Antidepressants ▶ Neurotransmitter Transporter
Amlodipine	Dihydropyridine	▶ Calcium Channel Blockers ▶ Voltage-dependent Calcium Channels
Amoxicillin	β-lactam antibiotic	▶ β-lactam Antibiotics
Amphetamine	Indirect sympathomimetic	▶ Psychostimmulants
Amphotericin B	Polyene	▶ Antifungal Drugs
Ampicillin	β-lactam antibiotic	▶ β-lactam Antibiotics
Amprenavir	Viral protease inhibitor	▶ Antiviral Drugs ▶ Viral Proteases
Amrinone	PDE-inhibitor	▶ Phosphodiesterases
Anakinra	Recombinant IL-1-receptor antagonist	▶ Cytokines

Drug	Group/Class	Link
Anastrozole	Aromatase inhibitior	▶ Aromatase
Apomorphine	Dopamine receptor agonist, emetic	▶ Emesis
Aprepitant	NK1 receptor antagonist	▶ Emesis
Atenolol	β-adrenergic antagonist (β-blocker)	▶ β-adrenergic System
Atipamezole	α-adrenergic antagonist	▶ α-adrenergic System
Atorvastatin	HMG-CoA-reductase inhibitor (statin)	▶ HMG-CoA-Reductase Ihibitors (Statin)
Atovaquone	Antimalarial agent	▶ Antiprotozoal Drugs
Atracurium	Neuromuscular blocking drug	▶ Nicotinic Receptors
Atropine	Muscarinic antagonist (parasympatholytic)	▶ Muscarinic Receptors
Auranofin	Antirheumatoid drugs	▶ Gold Compounds
Azathioprine	Immunosuppressant	▶ Immunosuppressants
	Antineoplastic drugs	▶ Antineoplastic Drugs
Azithromycin	Macrolide (antibacterial drugs)	▶ Ribosomal Protein Synthesis Inhibitors
Aztreonam	β-lactam antibiotic	▶ β-lactam Antibiotics
Baclofen	Muscle relaxant	▶ GABAergic System
Basiliximab	Anti-IL-2-receptor antibody	▶ Immune System
		▶ Cytokines
Beclomethason-diproprionat	Glucocorticoid	▶ Glucocorticoids
Benazepril	ACE inhibitor	▶ ACE Inhibitors
		▶ Renin-angiotensin-aldosterone System
Benperidole	Butyrophenone	▶ Antipsychotic Drugs
Benserazid	Dopa decarboxylase inhibitor	▶ Anti-parkinson Drugs
Benzbromarone	Uricosuric agent	▶ Anti-gout Drugs
Betamethason	Glucocorticoid	▶ Glucocorticoids
Betaxolol	β-adrenergic antagonist (β-blocker)	▶ β-adrenergic System
Bethanechol	Muscarinic receptor agonist (parasympathomimetic)	▶ Muscarinic Receptors
Bezafibrate	Fibrate	▶ Fibrates
Bicuculline	GABA$_A$-receptor antagonist	▶ GABAergic System
Biperiden	Anticholinergic agent	▶ Antiparkinson Drugs
		▶ Muscarinic Receptors
Bisoprolol	β-adrenergic antagonist (β-blocker)	▶ β-adrenergic System
Bleomycin	Antineoplastic agent	▶ Antineoplastic Agents
Bosentan	Endothelin receptor antagonist	▶ Endothelins
Botulinum toxin	Toxin	▶ Bacterial Toxins
Botezomib	Proteasome inhibitor	▶ Ubiquitin / Proteasome System
Bromocriptine	Dopamine receptor agonist	▶ Dopamine System
Budesonide	Glucocorticoid	▶ Glucocorticoids
Bumetanide	Loop diuretic	▶ Diuretics
Bupivacaine	Local anaesthetic	▶ Local Anaesthetics
		▶ Votage-Dependent Sodium Channels
Buprenorphine	Opioid, analgesic	▶ Opioid System
		▶ Analgesics

Drug	Group/Class	Link
Bupropion	Antidepressant	▶ Antidepressants
Buspirone	Serotonin receptor agonist	▶ Serotoninergic System
Buserelin	GnRH receptor antagonist	▶ GnRH
Busulphan	Alkylating agent	▶ AntineOplastic Agents
Butorphanol	Opioid, analgesic	▶ Opioid System, Analgesics
Butylscopolamin	Muscarinic receptor antagonist (parasympatholytic)	▶ Muscarinic Receptors
Caffeine	PDE inhibitor / adenosine receptor antagonist	▶ Phosphodiesterases
Calcitonin	Hormone	▶ Bone Metabolism
Calcitriol	Vitamin D metabolite	▶ Bone Metabolism
Candesartan	Angiotensin receptor Antagonist	▶ Renin-angiotensin-aldosterone System
Capecitabine	Antimetabolite	▶ Antineoplastic Agents
Capsaicin	TRP channel activator	▶ Nociceptive System
Captopril	ACE inhibitor	▶ ACE Inhibitors ▶ Renin-angiotensin-aldosterone System
Carbachol	Muscarinic receptor agonist (parasympatholytic)	▶ Muscarinic receptors
Carbamazepine	Antiepileptic drug	▶ Antiepileptic Drugs
Carbidopa	Antiparkinson drug	▶ Anti-parkinson Drugs
Carbimazole	Antithyroid drug	▶ Antithyroid Drugs
Carboplatin	Antineoplastic agent	▶ Antineoplastic Agents
Carmustin	Alkylating agent	▶ Antineoplastic Agents
Carvedilol	β-adrenergic antagonist (β-blocker)	▶ β-adrenergic System
Cefachlor	Cephalosporin	▶ β-lactam Antibiotics
Cefadroxil	Cephalosporin	▶ β-lactam Antibiotics
Cefazolin	Cephalosporin	▶ β-lactam Antibiotics
Cefepime	Cephalosporin	▶ β-lactam Antibiotics
Cefixime	Cephalosporin	▶ β-lactam Antibiotics
Cefotaxime	Cephalosporin	▶ β-lactam Antibiotics
Cefotetan	Cephalosporin	▶ β-lactam Antibiotics
Ceftazidime	Cephalosporin	▶ β-lactam Antibiotics
Ceftriaxone	Cephalosporin	▶ β-lactam Antibiotics
Cefuroxime	Cephalosporin	▶ β-lactam Antibiotics
Celecoxib	Antiinflammatory agent	▶ Cyclooxygenases ▶ Non-steroidal Anti-inflammatory Drugs
Cephalexin	Cephalosporin	▶ β-lactam Antibiotics
Cetirizine	Histamin receptor antagonist	▶ Histaminergic System, Allergy
Chlorambucil	Alkylating agent	▶ Anti-neoplastic Agents
Chloroquine	Antimalaria drug	▶ Antiprotozoal Drugs
Chlorpheniramine	Histamin receptor antagonist	▶ Histaminergic System
Chlorpromazine	Phenothiazine	▶ Antipsychotic Drugs
Chlorprothixene	Thioxanthene	▶ Antipsychotic Drugs
Chlorthalidone	Thiazide	▶ Diuretics

Drug	Group/Class	Link
Cholestyramine	Anion exchange resin	▶ Lipid-lowering Drugs
Ciclopirox	Hydroxypyridone	▶ Antifungal Drugs
Cidofovir	Antiviral drug	▶ Antiviral Drugs
Cilastatin	β-lactamase inhibitor	▶ β-lactam Antibiotics
Cilostazol	PDE-inhibitor	▶ Phosphodiesterases
Cimetidine	Histamin receptor antagonist	▶ Histaminergic System
Ciprofloxacin	Quinolone	▶ Quinolones
Cisapride	Serotonin receptor agonist	▶ Serotoninergic System
Cisplatin	Antineoplastic agent	▶ Antineoplastic Agents
Citalopram	Selectiv serotonine reuptake inhibitor (SSRI)	▶ Antidepressants ▶ Neurotransmitter Transporters
Clarithromycin	Macrolide (antibacterial drugs)	▶ Ribosomal Protein Synthesis Inhibitors
Clavulanate	β-lactamase inhibitor	▶ β-lactam Antibiotics
Clemastine	Histamin receptor antagonist	▶ Histaminergic System
Clenbuterol	β-adrenergic agonist	▶ β-adrenergic System
Clindamycin	Antibacterial agent	▶ Ribosomal Protein Synthesis Inhibitors
Clofibrate	Fibrate	▶ Fibrates
Clomiphene	Oestrogen receptor antagonist	▶ Sex Steroid Receptors
Clomipramine	Non-selective monoamine reuptake inhibitor (NSMRI)	▶ Antidepressants ▶ Neurotransmitter Transporters
Clonazepam	Benzodiazepine	▶ Benzodiazepines
Clonidine	α-adrenergic agonist	▶ α-adrenergic System
Clopidogrel	Thienopyridine	▶ Anti-platelet Drugs
Clorazepate	Benzodiazepine	▶ Benzodiazepines
Clotrimazole	Antifungal drugs	▶ Antifungal Drugs
Clozapine	Atypical neuroleptic	▶ Antipsychotic Drugs ▶ Neurotransmitter Transporters
Cocaine	Psychostimulant	▶ Psychostimulants ▶ Drug Addiction Dependence
Codeine	Opioid	▶ Opioid Systems
Colchicine	Antigout drug	▶ Anti-gout Drugs ▶ Cytoskeleton
Colestipol	Anion exchange resin	▶ Lipid-lowering Drugs
Cortisone-Acetat	Glucocorticoid	▶ Glucocorticoids
Cromoglycate (cromoglycin)	Cromone	▶ Allergy
Cyclophosphamide	Alkylating agent	▶ Antineoplastic Agents
Cyclosporine	Immunosuppressive agent	▶ Immunosuppressive Agents
Cyproterone	Androgen receptor antagonist	▶ Sex Steroid Receptors
Cytarabine	Antimetabolite	▶ Antineoplastic Agents
Daclizumab	Anti-IL-2-receptor antibody	▶ Immune system ▶ Cytokines
Danaparoid	Glycosaminoglycans	▶ Anticoagulants
Dapsone	Antibacterial drug	▶ Antibacterial Drugs/Antiprozotoal Drugs
Daunorubicin	Anthracycline	▶ Antineoplastic Agents

Drug	Group/Class	Link
Delavirdine	Reverse transcriptase inhibitor	▶ Antiviral Agents
Desirudin	Hirudin-analogue	▶ Anticoagulants
Desmopressin	Vasopressin receptor agonist	▶ Vasopressin/Oxytocin
Dexamethasone	Glucocorticoid	▶ Glucocorticoids
Diamorphin (heroin)	Opioid	▶ Opioid System ▶ Drug Addiction/Dependence
Diazepam	Benzodiazepine	▶ Benzodiazepines
Diazoxide	Vasorelaxant	▶ ATP-dependent Potassium Channels
Diclofenac	Analgetic/ Antipyretic/ Antiinflammatory drug	▶ Analgesics ▶ Cycloxygenase ▶ Non-steroidal Antiinflammatory Drugs
Dicloxacillin	β-lactam antibiotic	▶ β-lactam Antibiotics
Didanosine	Reverse transcriptase inhibitor	▶ Antiviral Drugs
Digitoxin	Cardiac glycoside	▶ Cardiac Glycosides
Digoxin	Cardiac glycoside	▶ Cardiac Glycosides
Diltiazem	Benzothiazepine	▶ Calcium Channel Blockers ▶ Voltage-dependent Calcium Channels
Dimenhydrinate	Histamin receptor antagonist	▶ Histaminergic System
Diphenhydramine	Histamin receptor antagonist	▶ Histaminergic System
Disopyramide	Antiarrhythmic drugs	▶ Antiarryrthmic Drugs
Dizocilpine	NMDA-receptor antagonist blocker	▶ Glutamate Receptors
Dobutamine	β adrenergic receptor agonist	▶ β Adrenergic System
Docetaxel	Taxane	▶ Antineoplastic Agents ▶ Cytoskeleton
Dofetilide	Antiarrhythmic drug	▶ Antiarrhythmic Drugs ▶ Potassium Channels
Dolasetron	Antiemetic drug, serotonin receptor antagonist	▶ Emesis ▶ Serotoninergic System
Donepezil	Acetylcholinesterase inhibitor	▶ Acetylcholinesterase
Doxazosin	α-adrenergic antagonist	▶ α-adrenergic System
Doxepin	Non-selective monoamine reuptake inhibitor (NSMRI)	▶ Antidepressants ▶ Neurotransmitter Transporters
Doxorubicin	Anthracycline	▶ Antineoplastic Agents
Doxycycline	Tetracycline	▶ Ribosomal Protein Synthesis Inhibitors
Dronabinol	Cannabinoid receptor agonist	▶ Cannabinoid Receptors
Edrophonium	Acetylcholinesterase	▶ Acetylcholinesterase Inhibitor
Efavirenz	Reverse transcriptase inhibitor	▶ Antiviral Agents
Eflornithine	Antitrypanosomal drug	▶ Antiprotozoal Drugs
Enalapril	ACE inhibitor	▶ ACE Inhibitors ▶ Renin-angiotensin-aldosterone System
Enalaprilat	ACE inhibitor	▶ ACE Inhibitors ▶ Renin-angiotensin-aldosterone System
Enflurane	General anaesthetics	▶ General Anaesthetics
Enfuvirtide	HIV fusion inhibitor	▶ Antiviral Agents
Enoxaparin	Low-molecular-weight heparin	▶ Anticoagulants

Drug	Group/Class	Link
Entacapone	COMT-inhibitor	▶ Anti-parkinson drugs ▶ Catechol-O-methyltransferase
Ephedrine		
Epinephrine (adrenalin)	Adrenoceptor agonist	▶ β-adrenergic System ▶ α-adrenergic system
Epirubicin	Anthracycline	▶ Antineoplastic Agents
Eplerenone	Aldosterone receptor antagonist	▶ Antihypertensive Agents / Blood Pressure Control
Epoetin α	Haematopoietic growth factor	▶ Haematopoietic Growth Factors
Eprosartan	Angiotensin receptor antagonist	▶ Renin-angiotensin-aldosterone System
Eptifibatide	GPIIb/IIIa inhibitor	▶ Antiplatelet Drugs
Ergometrine	Ergot alkaloid	▶ Ergot Alkaloids
Ergotamine	Ergot alkaloid	▶ Ergot Alkaloids
Erythromycin	Macrolide (antibacterial drug)	▶ Ribosomal Protein Synthesis Inhibitors
Esmolol	β-adrenergic antagonist (β-blocker)	▶ β-adrenergic System
Estradiol	Oestrogen receptor agonist	▶ Sex Steroid Receptors
Etanercept	Soluble TNF receptor construct	▶ Immune System
Ethacrynic acid	Loop diuretic	▶ Diuretics
Ethambutol	Antituberculotic agent	▶ Antituberculotic Drugs
Ethinylesteradiol	Oestrogen receptor agonist	▶ Sex Steroid Receptors
Ethosuximide	Antiepileptic drugs	▶ Antiepileptic Drugs
Etodolac	Analgetic/ Antipyretic/ Antiinflammatory drug	▶ Analgesics ▶ Cycloxygenase ▶ Non-steroidal Antiinflammatory
Etoposide	Antineoplastic agent	▶ Antineoplastic Agents
Etretinate	Retinoid	▶ Retinoids
Exemestane	Aromatase inhibitor	▶ Aromatase
Ezetimib	Cholestorol absorbtion inhibitor	▶ Lipid Lowering Drugs
Famotidine	Histamin receptor antagonist	▶ Histaminergic System
Felbamate	Antiepileptic drugs	▶ Antiepileptic Drugs
Felodipine	Dihydropyridine	▶ Calcium Channel Blockers ▶ Voltage-dependent Calcium Channels
Fenoterol	β-adrenergic agonist	▶ β-adrenergic System
Fentanyl	Opioid, analgesic	▶ Opioid system ▶ Analgesics
Fexofenadine	Histamin receptor antagonist	▶ Histaminergic System ▶ Allergy
Filgrastim	Haematopoietic growth factor	▶ Haematopoietic Growth Factors
Finasteride	Antiandrogen	▶ Sex Steroid Receptors
Flecainide	Antiarrhythmic drug	▶ Antiarrhythmic Drugs
Fluconazole	Azole	▶ Antifungal Drugs
Fludarabine	Antimetabolite	▶ Antineoplastic Agents
Fludrocortisone	Glucocorticoid	▶ Glucocorticoids ▶ Gluco/Mineralocorticoid Receptors
Flumazenil	Benzodiazepine	▶ Benzodiazepines

Drug	Group/Class	Link
Flunisolid-acetonid	Glucocorticoid	▶ Glucocorticoids
Flunitrazepam	Benzodiazepine	▶ Benzodiazepines
5-Fluorouracil	Antimetabolite	▶ Antineoplastic Agents
Fluoxetine	Selective serotonine reuptake inhibitor (SSRI)	▶ Antidepressants ▶ Neurotransmitter Transporters
Fluphenazine	Phenothiazine	▶ Antipsychotic Drugs
Flupenthixol	Thioxanthene	▶ Antipsychotic Drugs
Fluspirilen	Antipsychotic drug	▶ Antipsychotic Drugs
Fluticasone	Glucocorticoid	▶ Glucocorticoids
Flurbiprofen	Analgetic/ Antipyretic/ Antiinflammatory drug	▶ Analgesics ▶ NSAID ▶ Cycloxygenase
Flutamide	Androgen receptor antagonist	▶ Sex Steroid Receptors
Fluvastatin	HMG-CoA-reductase inhibitor (statin)	▶ HMG-CoA-reductase Inhibitors (Statin)
Fluvoxamine	Selective serotonine reuptake inhibitor (SSRI)	▶ Antidepressants ▶ Neurotransmitter Transporters
Fondaparinux	Synthetic pentasaccharide	▶ Anticoagulants
Formoterol	β-adrenergic agonist	▶ β-adrenergic System
Formestane	Aromatase inhibitor	▶ Aromatase
Fulvestrant	Estrogene receptor antagonist	▶ Sex Steroid Receptors
Furosemide	Loop diuretic	▶ Diuretics
Gabapentin	Antiepileptic drug	▶ Antiepileptic Drugs
Gallamine	Neuromuscular blocking drug	▶ Nicotinic Receptors
Gallopamil	Phenylalkylamine	▶ Calcium Cannel Blockers ▶ Voltage-Dependent Calcium Channels
Ganciclovir	Antiviral drug	▶ Antiviral Drugs
Gatifloxacin	Quinolone	▶ Quinolones
Gefitinib	Receptor tyrosine kinase inhibitor	▶ Growth Factor1
Gemcitabine	Antimetabolite	▶ Antineoplastic Agents
Gemfibrozil	Fibrate	▶ Fibrates
Gentamicin	Aminoglycoside (antibacterial drug)	▶ Ribosomal Protein Synthesis Inhibitor
Glibenclamide	Sulphonylurea	▶ ATP-dependent Potassium Channels ▶ Oral Antidiabetic Drugs
Glimepiride	Sulphonylurea	▶ ATP-dependent Potassium Channels ▶ Oral Antidiabetic Drugs
Glipizide	Sulphonylurea	▶ ATP-dependent Potassium Channels ▶ Oral Antidiabetic Drugs
Glyburide	Sulphonylurea	▶ ATP-dependent Potassium Channels ▶ Oral Antidiabetic Drugs
Glyceryltrinitrate	Organic nitrate	▶ Guanylyl Cyclases
Granisetron	Antiemetic drug, serotonin receptor antagonist	▶ Emesis ▶ Serotoninergic System
Griseofulvin	Antifungal drug	▶ Antifungal Drugs
Haloperidol	Butyrophenone	▶ Antipsychotic Drugs
Halothane	General Anaesthetics	▶ General Anaesthetics

Drug	Group/Class	Link
Heparin	Anticoagulant	▶ Anticoagulants
Human Insulin	Antidiabetic drug	▶ Insulin Receptors ▶ Diabetes mellitus
Hydralazine	Vasodilator	▶ Antihypertensive Agents
Hydrochlorthiazide	Thiazide	▶ Diutetics
Hydroxychloroquine	Antimalaria drug	▶ Antiprotozoal Drugs
Hydroxyurea	Antineoplastic agent	▶ Antineoplastic Agents
Ibritumomab	Anti-CD20 antibody	▶ Antineoplastic Agents
Ibuprofen	Analgetic/ Antipyretic/ Antiinflammatory drug	▶ Analgesics ▶ Cycloxygenase ▶ NSAID
Idarubicin	Anthracycline	▶ Antineoplastic Agents
Ifosfamide	Alkylating agent	▶ Antineoplastic Agents
IL-2	Cytokine	▶ Cytokines
Imatinib (STI 571)	Tyrosine kinase inhibitor	▶ Tyrosine Kinases
Imipenem	β-lactam antibiotic	▶ β-Lactam Antibiotics
Imipramine	Non-selective monoamine reuptake inhibitor (NSMRI)	▶ Antidepressants ▶ Neurotransmitter Transporters
Indinavir	Protease inhibitor	▶ Antiviral Drugs ▶ Viral Proteases
Indomethacin	Analgetic/ Antipyretic/ Antiinflammatory drug	▶ Analgesics ▶ Cycloxygenase ▶ Non-steroidal Anti-inflammatory Drugs
Infliximab	Anti-TNFα antibody	▶ Humanised Monoclonal Antibodies ▶ Immune Defense
Insulin	Antidiabetic drug	▶ Insulin Receptors ▶ Diabetes mellitus
Insulin Aspart	Insulin analogue	▶ Insulin Receptors ▶ Diabetes mellitus
Insulin Glargine	Insulin analogue	▶ Insulin Receptors ▶ Diabetes mellitus
Insulin Lispro	Insulin analogue	▶ Insulin Receptors ▶ Diabetes mellitus
Interferon α	Immunomodulator	▶ Interferons ▶ Cytokines
Interferon β	Immunomodulator	▶ Interferons ▶ Cytokines
Interferon γ	Immunomodulator	▶ Interferons ▶ Cytokines
Ipratropium	Muscarinic receptor antagonist (parasympatholytic)	▶ Muscarinic Receptors
Irbesartan	Angiotensin receptor antagonist	▶ Renin-angiotensin-aldosterone System
Irinotecan	Topoisomerase-I-inhibitor	▶ Antineoplastic Agents
Isoflurane	General anaesthetics	▶ General Anaesthetics
Isoniazid	Antituberculotic agent	▶ Antituberculotic Agents

Drug	Group/Class	Link
Isoprenaline	Adrenoceptor agonist	▶ β-adrenergic System ▶ α-adrenergic System
Isoproterenol	Adrenoceptor agonist	▶ β-adrenergic System ▶ α-adrenergic System
Isosorbide-dinitrate	Organic nitrate	▶ Guanylyl Cyclases
Isosorbidmononitrate	Organic nitrate	▶ Guanylyl Cyclases
Isradipine	Dihydropyridine	▶ Calcium Channel Blockers ▶ Voltage-dependent Calcium Channels
Itraconazole	Azole	▶ Antifungal Drugs
Ivermectin	Antiparasitic agent	▶ Antiparasitic Agents
Ketamine	NMDA receptor antagonist, channel blocker	▶ General Anaesthetics ▶ NMDA-receptor ▶ Psychomimetic Drugs
Ketoconazole	Azole	▶ Antifungal Drugs
Ketoprofen	Analgetic/ Antipyretic/ Antiinflammatory drug	▶ Analgesics ▶ Cycloxygenase ▶ NSAID
Ketorolac	Analgetic/ Antipyretic/ Antiinflammatory drug	▶ Analgesics ▶ Cycloxygenase
Lactulose	Laxative	▶ Laxatives
Lamivudine	Reverse transcriptase inhibitor	▶ Antiviral Agents
Lamotrigine	Antiepileptic drug	▶ Antiepileptic Drugs
Lansoprazole	Proton pump inhibitor	▶ Proton Pump Inhibitors
L-dopa	Antiparkinson drug	▶ Anti-parkinson Drugs
Lenograstim	Haematopoietic growth factor	▶ Haematopoietic Growth Factor
Lepirudin	Hirudin-analogue	▶ Anticoagulants
Letrozole	Aromatase inhibitior	▶ Aromatase
Levetiracetam	Antiepileptic drug	▶ Antiepileptic Drugs
Levodopa	Antiparkinson drug	▶ Anti-parkinson Drugs
Levofloxacin	Quinolone	▶ Quinolones
Levomepromazine	Phenothiazine	▶ Antipsychotic Drugs
Levomethadon	Opioid	▶ Opioid System
Lidocaine	Local anaesthetic, Antiarrhythmic drug	▶ Local Anaesthetics ▶ Antiarrhythmic Drugs ▶ Voltage-dependent Sodium Channels
Lisinopril	ACE inhibitor	▶ ACE Inhibitors ▶ Renin-angiotensin-aldosterone System
Lisuride	Dopamine receptor agonist	▶ Dopamine System
Lithium	Mood stabilizer	▶ Mood Stabilizer
Loperamide	Opioid	▶ Opioid System
Lopinavir	Viral protease inhibitor	▶ Antiviral Drugs ▶ Viral Proteases
Loratadine	Histamin receptor antagonist	▶ Histaminergic System, Allergy
Lorazepam	Benzodiazepine	▶ Benzodiazepines
Losartan	Angiotensin receptor antagonist	▶ Renin-angiotensin-aldosterone System

Drug	Group/Class	Link
Lovastatin	HMG-CoA-reductase inhibitor (Statin)	▶ HMG-CoA-reductase Inhibitors (Statin)
Lysergic Acid Diethylamide	Serotonin receptor agonist	▶ Psychomimetic Drugs
Mebendazole	Anthelmintic drug	▶ Anti-malaria Drugs ▶ Antiprotozoal Drugs
Medroxyprogesterone	Progesterone receptor agonist	▶ Sex Steroid Receptors
Mefloquine	Anti-malaria drug	▶ Antiprotozoal Drugs
Melarsoprol	Antiprotozoal drug	▶ Antiprotozoal Drugs
Meloxicam	Analgetic/ Antipyretic/ Antiinflammatory drug	▶ Analgesics ▶ Cycloxygenase ▶ NSAID
Melperone	Butyrophenone	▶ Antipsychotic Drugs
Melphalan	Alkylating agent	▶ Antineoplastic Agents
Meperidine	Opioid, Analgesic	▶ Opioid System, Analgesics
Mercaptopurine	Antimetabolite	▶ Antineoplastic Agents
Meropenem	β-lactam antibiotic	▶ β-lactam Antibiotics
Mescaline	Psychotomimetic drug	▶ Psychotomimetic Drugs
Metamizol	Analgetic/ Antipyretic drug	▶ Analgesics
Metformin	Biguanide	▶ Oral Antidiabetic Drugs ▶ Diabetes mellitus
Methadone	Opioid	▶ Opioid System
Methotrexate	Antimetabolite	▶ Antineoplastic Agents
Methylphenidate	Indirect sympathomimetic	▶ Psychostimulants
Methylprednisolone	Glucocorticoid	▶ Glucocorticoids
Methysergide	Serotonin receptor antagonist	▶ Serotoninergic System
Metixene	Muscarinic receptor antagonist	▶ Antiparkinson Drugs ▶ Muscarinic Receptors
Metoclopramide	Serotonin receptor antagonist	▶ Serotoninergic System
Metoprolol	β-adrenergic antagonist (β-blocker)	▶ β-adrenergic System
Metronidazole	Antibacterial agent, Antiprozotoal agent	▶ Antiprozotoal Drugs
Mexiletine	Antiarrhythmic drugs	▶ Antiarrhyrthmic Drugs
Mianserin	Antidepressant	▶ Antidepressants
Midazolam	Benzodiazepine	▶ Benzodiazepines
Mifepristone (RU 486)	Progesterone receptor antagonist	▶ Sex steroid Receptors
Miglitol	α-glucosidase inhibitor	▶ Oral Antidiabetic Drugs
Milrinone	PDE-inhibitor	▶ Phosphodiesterases
Minocycline	Tetracycline	▶ Ribosomal Protein Synthesis Inhibitor
Mirtazapine	Antidepressants	▶ Antidepressants
Misoprostol	Prostaglandin derivative	▶ Prostanoids
Mivacurium	Neuromuscular blocking drug	▶ Nicotinic Receptors
Moclobemide	MAO$_A$-inhibitor	▶ Antidepressants
Molsidomine	NO-donator	▶ Guanylyl Cyclases
Montelukast	Leukotriene receptor antagonist	▶ Leukotrienes
Morphine	Opiate, Analgesics	▶ Opioid System ▶ Analgsics

Drug	Group/Class	Link
Moxifloxacin	Quinolone	▶ Quinolones
Moxonidine	α-adrenergic agonist	▶ α-adrenergic System
Muromonab	Anti-T-cell receptor antibody	▶ Cytokines
Mycophenolate	Immunosuppressant	▶ Immunosuppressants
Mycophenolate-mofetil	Immunosuppressant	▶ Immunosuppressants
Na-aurothiomalate	Antirheumatoid drugs	▶ Gold Compounds
Nabumetone	Analgetic/ Antipyretic/ Antiinflammatory drug	▶ Analgesics ▶ Cycloxygenase ▶ NSAID
Naftifine	Allylamine	▶ Antifungal Drugs
Nalbuphine	Opioid, Analgesic	▶ Opioid System ▶ Analgesics
Nalmefene	Opioid receptor antagonist	▶ Opioid System
Naloxone	Opioid receptor antagonist	▶ Opioid System
Nandrolon-decanoate	Anabolic	▶ Sex Steroid Receptors
Naproxen	Analgetic/ Antipyretic/ Antiinflammatory drug	▶ Analgesics ▶ Cycloxygenase ▶ NSAID
Naratriptan	Serotonin receptor agonist	▶ Serotoninergic System
Nateglinide	Meglitinide	▶ Oral Antidiabetic Drugs
Nedocromil	Cromone	▶ Allergy
Nelfinavir	Viral protease inhibitor	▶ Antiviral Drugs ▶ Viral Proteases
Neomycin	Aminoglycoside (Antibacterial drug)	▶ Ribosomal Protein Synthesis Inhibitor
Neostigmine	Acetylcholinesterase inhibitor	▶ Acetylcholinesterase
Nevirapine	Reverse transcriptase inhibitor	▶ Antiviral Agents
Nicardipine	Dihydropyridine	▶ Calcium Channel Blockers ▶ Voltage-dependent Calcium Channels
Nicotine	Nicotinic receptor agonist	▶ Nicotinic Receptors
Nicotinic Acid	Lipid lowering drug, Vitamine	▶ Lipid Lowering Drugs
Nifedipine	Dihydropyridine	▶ Calcium Channel Blockers ▶ Voltage-dependent Clcium Channels
Nitrenpidine	Dihydropyridine	▶ Calcium Channel Blockers ▶ Voltage-dependent Calcium Channels
Nitrofurantoin	Antimicrobial agent	▶ Antimicrobial Drugs
Nitroglycerin	Organic nitrate	▶ Guanylyl Cyclases
Nitroprussidnatrium	NO-donator	▶ Guanylyl Cyclyses
Noradrenalin	Adrenoceptor agonist	▶ β-adrenergic System ▶ α-adrenergic System
Norethisteron-Acetat	Oestrogen receptor agonist	▶ Sex Steroid Receptors
Nortriptyline	Non-selective monoamine reuptake inhibitor (NSMRI)	▶ Antidepressants ▶ Neurotransmitter Transporters
Nystatin	Antifungal agent	▶ Antifungal Agents
Octreotide	Somatostatin receptor agonist	▶ Somatostatin
Ofloxacin	Quinolone	▶ Quinolones

Drug	Group/Class	Link
Olanzapine	Atypical neuroleptic	▶ Antipsychotic Drugs
Omeprazole	Proton pump inhibitor	▶ Proton Pump Inhibitors
Ondansetron	Antiemetic drug, Serotonin receptor antagonist	▶ Emesis ▶ Serotoninergic System
Orlistat	Lipase inhibitor	▶ Anti-obesity Drugs
Oseltamivir	Neuraminidase inhibitor	▶ Antiviral Drugs
Oxacilin	β-lactam antibiotic	▶ β-lactam Antibiotics
Oxacepam	Benzodiazepine	▶ Benzodiazepines
Oxcarbazepine	Antiepileptic drug	▶ Antiepileptic Drugs
Oxybutynin	Muscarinic receptor antagonist	▶ Muscarinic Receptors
Oximetazoline	α-adrenergic agonist	▶ α-adrenergic System
Oxytocin	Hormone	
Paclitaxel	Taxane	▶ Antineoplastic Agents ▶ Cytoskeleton
Pancuronium	Neuromuscular blocking drug	▶ Nicotinic Receptors
Pantoprazol	Proton pump inhibitor	▶ Proton Pump Inhibitors
Paracetamol (acetaminophen)	Analgetic-/ Antipyretic drug	▶ Analgesics
Parathion	Acetylcholinesterase inhibitor	▶ Acetylcholinesterase
Paroxetine	Selectiv serotonine reuptake inhibitor (SSRI)	▶ Antidepressants ▶ Neurotransmitter Transporters
Penicillin	β-lactam antibiotic	▶ β-lactam Antibiotics
Pergolid	Dopamine receptor agonist	▶ Dopamine System
Perphenazine	Phenothiazine	▶ Antipsychotic Drugs
Pentazocine	Opioid, Analgesic	▶ Opioid system ▶ Analgesics
Pentostatin	Antimetabolite	▶ Antineoplastic Agents
Phencyclidine	NMDA receptor antagonist, Channel blocker	▶ General Anaesthetics ▶ NMDA-receptor ▶ Psychomimetic Drugs
Pethidine	Opioid / analgesic	▶ Opioid System ▶ Analgesics
Phenobarbital	Barbiturate	▶ Antiepileptic Drugs
Phenprocoumon	Coumarinderivative	▶ Anticoagulants ▶ Vitamin K
Phenylephrine	α-adrenergic agonist	▶ α-adrenergic System
Phenytoin	Antiepileptic drug	▶ Antiepileptic Drugs
Physostigmine	Acetylcholinesterase inhibitor	▶ Acetylcholinesterase
Pilocarpine	Muscarinic agonist (Parasympathomimetic)	▶ Muscarinic Receptors
Pimozide	Neuroleptic	▶ Antipsychotic Drugs
Pindolol	β-adrenergic antagonist (β-blocker)	▶ β-adrenergic System
Pioglitazone	Thiazolidinedione	▶ Oral Antidiabetic Drugs ▶ Diabetes mellitus
Pipamperon	Butyrophenone	▶ Antipsychotic Drugs

Drug	Group/Class	Link
Piretanide	Loop diuretic	▶ Diuretics
Piroxicam	Analgetic- /Antipyretic- / Antiinflammatory drug	▶ Analgesics ▶ Cycloxygenase ▶ NSAID
Pizotifen	Serotonin receptor antagonist	▶ Serotoninergic System
Pramipexole	Dopamine receptor agonist	▶ Dopamine System ▶ Antiparkinson Drugs
Pravastatin	HMG-CoA-reductase inhibitor (statin)	▶ HMG-CoA-Reductase Inhibitors (statin)
Praziquantel	Anthelmintic agent	▶ Anthelmintic Agents
Prazosin	α-adrenergic antagonist	▶ α-adrenergic System
Prednisolone	Glucocorticoid	▶ Glucocorticoids
Prednisone	Glucocorticoid	▶ Glucocorticoids
Prilocaine	Local anaesthetic	▶ Local Anaesthetics ▶ Voltage-dependent Sodium Channels
Primaquine	Anti-malaria drug	▶ Antiprotozoal Drugs
Probenecid	Uricosuric agent	▶ Anti-gout Drugs
Procainamide	Local anaesthetic	▶ Local Anaesthetics
Proguanil	Anti-malaria drug	▶ Antiprotozoal Drugs
Promazine	Phenothiazine	▶ Antipsychotic Drugs
Promethazine	Histamin receptor antagonist	▶ Histaminergic System
Propofol	Anaesthetic	▶ General Anaesthetics ▶ GABAergic System
Propranolol	β-adrenergic antagonist (β-blocker)	▶ β-adrenergic System
Pyridostigmine	Acetylcholinesterase inhibitor	▶ Acetylcholinesterase
Pyrimethamin	Antiprozotoal drug	▶ Antiprozotoal Drugs
Quetiapine	Atypical neuroleptic	▶ Antipsychotic Drugs
Quinidine	Antiarrhythmic drugs	▶ Antiarrhyrthmic Drugs
Quinine	Anti-malaria drug	▶ Antiprotozoal Drugs
Rabeprazole	Proton pump inhibitor	▶ Proton Pump Inhibitors
Raloxifene	Selective oestrogen receptor modulator (SERM)	▶ Selective Oestrogen Receptor Modulators (SERM)
Ramipril	ACE inhibitor	▶ ACE Inhibitors ▶ Renin-angiotensin-aldosterone System
Ranitidine	Histamin receptor antagonist	▶ Histaminergic System
Rapacuronium	Neuromuscular blocking drug	▶ Nicotinic Receptors
Reboxetine	Selective noradrenaline reuptake inhibitor (SNRI)	▶ Antidepressants
Remifentanil	Opioid, Analgesic	▶ Opioid System ▶ Analgesics
Repaglinide	Meglitinide	▶ ATP-dependent Potassium Channels ▶ Oral Antidiabetic Drugs
Reteplase	Fibrinolytic	▶ Fibrinolytics
Ribavirin	Antiviral agent	▶ Antiviral Drugs
Rifabutin	Antituberculotic agent	▶ Antituberculotic Drugs
Rifampin	Antituberculotic agent	▶ Antituberculotic Drugs

Drug	Group/Class	Link
Risperidone	Atypical neuroleptic	▶ Antipsychotic Drugs
Ritonavir	Viral protease inhibitor	▶ Antiviral Drugs ▶ Viral Proteases
Rituximab	Anti-CD20 antibody	▶ Antineoplastic Agents
Rivastgmine	Acetylcholinesterase inhibitor	▶ Acetylcholinesterase
Rizatriptan	Serotonin receptor agonist	▶ Serotoninergic System
Rofecoxib	Anti-inflammatory agent	▶ Cyclooxygenases ▶ Non-steroidal Anti-inflammatory Drugs
Rolipram	PDE-inhibitor	▶ Phosphodiesterases
Ropinirole	Dopamine receptor agonist	▶ Dopamine System
Rosiglitazone	Thiazolidinedione	▶ Oral Antidiabetic Drugs ▶ Diabetes mellitus
Roxithromycin	Macrolide (Antibacterial drugs)	▶ Ribosomal Protein Synthesis Inhibitors
Salbutamol	β-adrenergic agonist	▶ β-adrenergic System
Salmeterol	β-adrenergic agonist	▶ β-adrenergic System
Saquinavir	Viral protease inhibitor	▶ Antiviral Drugs ▶ Viral Proteases
Sargramostim	Haematopoietic growth factor	▶ Haematopoietic Growth Factors
Scopolamine	Muscarinic receptor antagonist (Parasympatholytic)	▶ Muscarinic Receptors
Selegiline	MAO_B-inhibitor	▶ Antiparkinson Drugs
Sertindol	Atypical neuroleptic	▶ Antipsychotic Drugs
Sertraline	Selective serotonine reuptake inhibitor (SSRI)	▶ Antidepressants ▶ Neurotransmitter Transporters
Sibutramine	Reuptake inhibitor	▶ Antidepressants ▶ Appetite Control ▶ Anti Obesity Drugs
Sildenafil	PDE-inhibitor	▶ Phosphodiesterases
Simvastatin	HMG-CoA-reductase inhibitor (statin)	▶ HMG-CoA-reductase Inhibitors (Statin)
Sirolimus (rapamycin)	Immunosuppressant	▶ Immunosuppressive Agents
Spironolactone	Aldosterone receptor antagonist	▶ Gluco-/Mineralocorticoid Receptors ▶ Renin-angiotensin-aldosterone System
Sotalol	Antiarrhythmic drug, β adrenergic receptor antagonist	▶ Antiarrhythmic Drugs ▶ β adrenergic receptor antagonists
Stavudine	Reverse transcriptase inhibitor	▶ Antiviral Agents
Streptokinase	Fibrinolytic	▶ Fibrinolytics
Streptomycin	Aminoglycoside (Antibacterial drug)	▶ Ribosomal Protein Synthesis Inhibitor
Strophantine	Cardiac glycoside	▶ Cardiac Glycosides
Strychnine	Glycine receptor antagonist	▶ Glycine Receptors
Sufentanil	Opioid, Analgesic	▶ Opioid System ▶ Analgesics
Sulfamethoxazole	Sulfonamide	▶ Sufonamides
Sulfasalazine	Anti-inflammatory drug	▶ Non-steroidal Anti-inflammatory Drugs
Sulfipyrazone	Uricosuric agent	▶ Anti-gout Drugs
Sulfisoxazole	Sulfonamide	▶ Sulfonamides

Drug	Group/Class	Link
Sulindac	Analgetic/ Antipyretic/ Antiinflammatory drug	▶ Analgesics ▶ Cycloxygenase ▶ NSAID
Sulpirid	Atypical neuroleptic	▶ Antipsychotic Drugs
Sumatriptan	Serotonin receptor agonist	▶ Serotoninergic System ▶ Analgesics
Suxamethonium	Nicotine receptor agonist	▶ Nicotinic Receptors
Tacrine	Acetylcholinesterase inhibitor	▶ Acetylcholinesterase
Tacrolimus (FK 506)	Immunosuppressant	▶ Immunosuppressive Agents
Tamoxifen	Selective estrogen receptor modulator (SERM)	▶ Selective Estrogen Receptor Modulators (SERM)
Tamsulosin	α-adrenergic antagonist	▶ α-adrenergic System
Tegaserod	Serotonin receptor antagonist	▶ Serotoninergic System
Terazosin	α-adrenergic antagonist	▶ α-adrenergic System
Terbinafin	Allylamine	▶ Antifungal Drugs
Terbutaline	β-adrenergic agonist	▶ β-adrenergic System
Teriparatide	Hormone	▶ Bone Metabolism
Testosteron-propionat	Androgen receptor agonist	▶ Sex Steroid Receptors
Tetracaine	Local anaesthetic	▶ Local Anaesthetics ▶ Votage-dependent Sodium Channels
Tetracycline	Tetracycline	▶ Ribosomal Protein Synthesis Inhibitors
Theophylline	PDE inhibitor, Adenosine receptor antagonist	▶ Phosphodiesterases
Thiamazol	Antithyroid drug	▶ Antithyroid Drugs
Thiethylperazine	Phenothiazine	▶ Antipsychotic Drugs
Thioguanine	Antimetabolite	▶ Antineoplastic Agents
Thiopental	Barbiturate	▶ General Anaesthetics
Thioridazine	Phenothiazine	▶ Antipsychotic Drugs
Thiotepa	Alkylating agent	▶ Antineoplastic Agents
Tiagabine	Antiepileptic drug	▶ Antiepileptic Drugs
Ticlopidine	Thienopyridine	▶ Antiplatelet Drugs
Tilidin	Opioid, Analgesic	▶ Opioid System ▶ Analgesics
Tirofiban	GPIIb/IIIa inhibitor	▶ Antiplatelet Drugs
Tobramycin	Aminoglycoside (Antibacterial drug)	▶ Ribosomal Protein Synthesis Inhibitors
Tocainide	Antiarrhythmic drugs	▶ Antiarrhyrthmic Drugs
Tolbutamide	Sulphonylurea	▶ ATP-dependent Potassium Channels ▶ Oral Antidiabetic Drugs
Tolcapone	COMT-inhibitor	▶ Antiparkinson Drugs ▶ Catechol-O-methyltransferase
Tolterodine	Muscarinic receptor antagonist	▶ Muscarinic Receptors
Topiramate	Antiepileptic drug	▶ Antiepileptic Drugs
Topotecan	Topoisomerase-I-inhibitor	▶ Antineoplastic Agents
Torasemide	Loop diuretic	▶ Diuretics

Drug	Group/Class	Link
Toremifene	Selective estrogen receptor modulator (SERM)	▶ Selective Estrogen Receptor Modulators (SERM)
Tramadol	Opioid, Analgesic	▶ Opioid System ▶ Analgesics
Trandolapril	ACE inhibitor	▶ ACE Inhibitors ▶ Renin-angiotensin-aldosterone System
Trastuzumab	Receptor tyrosine kinase blocking antibody	▶ Growth Factors
Trazodone	Antidepressant	▶ Antidepressants
Triamterene	Potassium-sparing diuretic	▶ Diuretics ▶ Epithelial Sodium Channels
Triazolam	Benzodiazepine	▶ Benzodiazepines
Trimethoprim	Antibacterial agent	▶ Antibacterial Agents
Trimipramin	Non-selective monoamine reuptake inhibitor (NSMRI)	▶ Antidepressants ▶ Neurotransmitter Transporters
Tropicamide	Muscarinic antagonist (Parasympatholytic)	▶ Muscarinic Receptors
Tropisetron	Antiemetic drug, Serotonin receptor antagonist	▶ Emesis ▶ Serotoninergic System
Tubocurarin	Neuromuscular blocking agent	▶ Nicotinic Receptors
Urapidil	α-adrenergic antagonist	▶ α-adrenergic System
Urokinase	Fibrinolytic	▶ Fibrinolytics
Valacyclovir	Antiviral drug	▶ Antiviral Drugs
Valproic Acid	Antiepileptic drug	▶ Antiepileptic Drugs
Valsartan	Angiotensin receptor antagonist	▶ Renin-angiotensin-aldosterone System
Vancomycin	Antibacterial agent	▶ Antibacterial Agents
Venronium	Neuromuscular blocking agent	▶ Nicotinic Receptors
Venlafaxine	Selective noradrenaline, Serotonine reuptake inhibitor (SSRNI)	▶ Antidepressants ▶ Neurotransmitter Transporters
Verapamil	Phenylalkylamine	▶ Calcium Channel Blockers ▶ Voltage-Dependent Calcium Channels
Vigabatrin	Antiepileptic drug	▶ Antiepileptic Drugs
Vinblastine	Vinca alkaloid	▶ Antineoplastic Agents ▶ Cytoskeleton
Vincristine	Vinca alkaloid	▶ Antineoplastic Agents ▶ Cytoskeleton
Vindesine	Vinca alkaloid	▶ Antineoplastic Agents ▶ Cytoskeleton
Warfarin	Coumarinderivative	▶ Anticoagulants ▶ Vitamin K
Xipamide	Thiazide	▶ Diuretics
Xylometazoline	α-adrenergic antagonist	▶ α-adrenergic System
Yohimbine	α-adrenergic antagonist	▶ α-adrenergic System
Zafirlukast	Leukotriene receptor antagonist	▶ Leukotrienes
Zalcitabine	Reverse transcriptase inhibitor	▶ Antiviral Agents
Zaleplon	Sedative	▶ GABAergic System

Drug	Group/Class	Link
Zanamivir	Neuraminidase inhibitor	▶ Antiviral Drugs
Zaprinast	PDE-inhibitor	▶ Phosphodiesterases
Zidovudine	Reverse transcriptase inhibitor	▶ Antiviral Agents
Zileuton	5-Lipoxygenase inhibitor	▶ Leukotrienes
Zolmitriptan	Serotonin receptor agonist	▶ Serotoninergic System
Zolpidem	Sedative	▶ GABAergic System
Zopiclone	Sedative	▶ GABAergic System

List of Entries

Essays are shown in blue

ABC Proteins
ABC Transporters
Aβ Amyloid
ABPs
Absence Epilepsy
Absorption
Abstinence Syndrome
Abused Drugs
ACE Inhibitors
Acetylcholine
Acetylcholinesterase
Acetyltransferase
ACPD
ACTH
Actin
Actin Binding Proteins
Action Potential
Activated Partial Thromboplastin Time
Activation-induced Cell Death
Active Site
Active Transport
Activins
Acute Phase Reactants
Acyl-CoA
Adaptive Immunity
Adaptor Proteins
Addiction
Additive Interaction
Aδ-fibres
Adenosine
Adenosine Receptors
Adenoviruses
Adenylyl Cyclases
ADH
ADHD
Adhesion Molecules
AdoMet
Adrenal Gland
Adrenaline
Adrenergic or Noradrenergic Synapses, Receptors and
    Drugs
Adrenoceptor
Adrenocorticotropic Hormone
Adrenomedullin
Adverse/Unwanted Reactions
Affective Disorders
Affinity
Agonist
Agouti-related Protein
AgRP
Ah Receptor
AIDS
Airway Hyperresponsiveness
Airway Surface Liquid
AKAP

Akt
Alcohol
Alcohol Dehydrogenase
Aldehyde Dehydrogenase
Aldosterone
AlF4⁻
Alkaloid
Alkylating Agents
Allele
Allergen
Allergy
Allodynia
Alloimmunity
Allosteric Modulators
Allylamine
α1-acid Glycoprotein
a-Adrenergic System
α-2 Antiplasmin
α-Glucosidase
5α-Reductase
α and β tubulin
ALS
Alternative Splicing
Alzheimer's Disease
Ames test
Amiloride-sensitive Na⁺ Channel
Aminoglycosides
AMP, cyclic
AMPA Receptors
AMP-activated Protein Kinase
Amphetamine
AMPK
Amyloid Precursor Protein
Amyotrophic Lateral Sclerosis
Anabolic Steroids
Anaesthesia
Anaesthetics, general
Anaesthetics, local
Analeptics
Analgesia
Analgesics
Anandamide
Anaphylactic Shock
Androgen Receptor
Androgens
Anemia, macrocytic hyperchromic
Angel Dust
Angina Pectoris
Angioblast
Angiogenesis and Vascular Morphogenesis
Angiogenic Switch
Angiopoietins
Angiotensin
Angiotensin Converting Enzyme
Angiotensin Receptors

11β-Hydroxysteroid Dehydrogenase Type II
β-Lactam Antibiotics
β-Lactamases
BH4
BH Domain
Bicuculline
BID
Biguanides
Bimodal Distribution
Bioavailability
Biogenic Amines
Bioinformatics
Biopterin
Biotin
BiP
Bipolar Disorder
Bisphosphonates
Bisubstrate Analogs
BK$_{Ca\ channel}$
Blastocyst
Blood-brain Barrier
Blood: Gas Partition Coefficient of Anaesthetics
Blood Pressure Control
B Lymphocyte
BMPs
Body Mass Index
Bombesin-like Peptides
Bone Formation
Bone Metabolism
Bone Morphogenetic Proteins
Bone Remodelling
Bone Resorption
Botulinum Toxin
Botulism
Bradykinesia
Bradykinin
Brain Derived Neurotrophic Factor
Brain Natriuretic Peptide
Breast Cancer
Bronchial Asthma
Bronchodilators
Btk
Butyrophenones
Butyrylcholinesterase

C2 Domain
C-fibres
Ca^{2+}-ATPase
Ca^{2+} Channels
Ca^{2+} Channel Blockers
Ca^{2+}-induced Ca^{2+} Release
Ca^{2+} Release Channel
Ca^{2+} Spark
Ca^{2+} Transient
Cadherins
Cadherins/Catenins
cAK
Calcineurin
Calcitonin
Calcitonin Gene Related Peptide
Calmodulin
cADP-ribose

cAMP
cAMP- and cGMP-dependent Protein Kinases
cAMP-binding Guanine Nucleotide Exchange Factors
cAMP-GEFs
Campothecins
Cancer, molecular mechanisms of therapy
Cannabinoid Receptor
Cannabinoids
Cannabis
Capsaicin
Capsid
CAR
Carbon Monoxide
Carbonic Anhydrase
Carcinogens
Carcinogenesis
Cardiac Glycosides
CART
Caspase
Catabolism
Catecholamines
Catechol-O-Methyltransferase and its Inhibitors
Cathepsins
Causalgia
Caveolae
CCK
CD26
cdk
Cell Adhesion Molecule
Cell-cycle Arrest
Cell-cycle Checkpoints
Cell-cycle Control
Cellular Immmunity
Central Diabetes Insipidus
Centrosome
Cephalosporins
CFTR
CG
cGK
cGMP
cGMP Kinase
cGMP-regulated Phosphodiesterases
CGRP
Channelopathies
Channels, ion
Chaperone Protein
Chemical Library
Chemical Neurotransmission
Chemokine Receptors
Chemokines
Chemoreceptor Trigger Zone
Chemotaxis
Chemotherapy
Cholecystokinin
Cholegraphic Contrast Agents
Cholera Toxin
Cholesterol
Cholinergic Transmission
Cholinesterase
Chorionic Gonadotropin
Chromosomal Translocations
Chromosomes

Dermatomycoses
Dermatophytes
Descending Inhibitory Pathway
Desensitization
Desmoplakin
DHOD
DHPR
Diabesity
Diabetes Insipidus
Diabetes Mellitus
Diacylglycerol
Dicer
DICR
Differential Display
Dihydrofolate Reductase
Dihydropyridine Receptor
Dihydropyridines
Dimer, Trimer, Oligomer
Dioxins
Dipeptidylpeptidase IV
Discharge
Dissociation Constant
Dissociative Anesthetic
Distribution of Drugs
Diuretics
DNA Fragmentation
DNA Methylation
DNA Replication
DNA Response Elements
Domain
Dopa Decarboxylase
Dopamine
Dopamine-β-hydroxylase
Dopamine System
Dose-response Curves
Double Stranded (ds) RNA
Drug Addiction/Dependence
Drug Discovery
Drug Interactions
Drug Metabolism
Drug Reinforcement
Drug-Receptor Interaction
DSI
DTH
Dyskinesias
Dyslipidemia
Dysrhythmias

EC_{50}
ECaC
EC Coupling
ECE
Ecogenetics
Ecstasy
ED_{50}
Edg Receptors
EEG
Effector
Efficacy
EGF
Eicosanoids
Elastase-like Proteinases

Electrochemical Driving Force
Electrospray Ionization Mass Spectrometry
Elimination Half-life
Elimination of Drugs
Emesis
ENaC
Endocannabinoid System
Endogenous Opioid Peptides
Endoplasmic Reticulum
Endorphins
Endothelial Cells
Endothelin Converting Enzyme
Endothelins
Endotoxin
Enkephalin
Entamoeba Histolytica
Envelope
Enzyme
Eosinophil
Eotaxin
Eph Receptor Tyrosine Kinase
Ephrin-B
Ephrins
Epidermal Growth Factor
Epidermal Growth Factor Receptor Family
Epidural (Space)
Epigenetic
Epilepsy
Epinephrine
Episodic Ataxia/Myokymia
Episome
Epithelial Ca^{2+} Channel 1
Epithelial Na^+ Channel
EPS
EPSP
ER
ERT
ERGIC
ER/Golgi Intermediate Compartment
ErbB Receptor Family
Erectile Dysfunction
Ergot Alkaloids
Erythropoietin
ESI-MS
EST
Estrogen Receptor
Estrogen Replacement Therapy (ERT)
Estrogens
Ethanol
Euglycaemia
Eukaryotic Expression Cassette
Excitability
Excitation-contraction Coupling
Excitatory Amino Acids
Excitotoxicity
Exocytosis
Exon
Exportins
Extrapyramidal Side Effects

F-actin
Fab Fragments

Factor IIa
FAD
Familial Persistent Hyperinsulinemic Hypoglycemia of
    Infancy
Farnesyl Transferase Inhibitors
FasL
Favism
Fever
Fibrates
Fibrin
Fibrinogen
Fibrinolysis
Fibrinolytics
Fibroblast Growth Factors
First-order Kinetics
First-pass (presystemic) Metabolism
Flare
Flavin Adenine Dinucleotide
Flavin Mononucleotide
Flp/FRT
Fluorides
Fluoroquinolones
FMN
Folate
Folic Acid
Follicle-stimulating Hormone
Follitrophin
Force Fields / Molecular Mechanics
Forskolin
Frontal Cortex
FSH
F-type ATPase
Functional Genomics
Functional Proteomics
Fungi
Fungicidal Effect
Fungistasis/Fungistatic
Funicular Myelitis
Furin
Furin-like Protease
Fyn
FYVE Domain

GABA
GABA$_A$ Receptor
GABA$_B$ Receptors
GABAergic System
G-actin
Gaddum, method of
Galanin
Galanin Receptors
GALP
γ-Aminobutyric Acid
γ-Glutamyl-transpeptidase
GAPs
Gastric Emptying Rate
Gastric H, K-ATPase
Gastrin
Gastrin Releasing Peptide
Gastroesophageal Reflux Disease
Gating
G-CSF

GDIs
GEFs
Gene Activity Profile
Gene-environment Interaction
Gene Expression
Gene Expression Analysis
Gene Gun
Gene Products
Gene Promoter
Gene Therapy
General Anaesthetics
Genetic Polymorphism
Genetic Vaccination
Genome
Genomics
Genotype
Gephyrin
GERD
GH
Ghrelin
Giardia Lamblia
GIRK
Gitelman's Syndrome
Glial Cells
Glomerular Filtration Rate
Glucagon
Glucagon-like Peptide-1
Gluco-/Mineralocorticoid Receptors
Glucocorticoids
Glucocorticoids, inhalable
Glucocorticosteroids
Gluconeogenesis
Glucose Transport Facilitators
Glucose Transporters
GLUT
Glutamate
Glutamate Receptors
Glycine
Glycine Receptors
Glycogen Synthase Kinase 3
Glycopeptide Antibiotics
Glycoprotein IIb/IIIa Receptor Antagonists
Glycoproteins
Glycosaminoglycan
Glycosides, cardiac
Glycosylphosphatidylinositol Anchor
Glycylcyclines
GM-CSF
GMP, cyclic
GnRH
Gold Compounds
Golgi Apparatus
Gonadorelin
Gonadotropin-releasing Factor/Hormone (GnRH)
Gonadotropins
Gout
GPIIb/IIIa Receptor Antagonists
GPCR
GPI Anchor
G-protein-coupled Receptors
G-protein-coupled Receptor Kinases
G-proteins

Integrase
INR
Integrins
Integrin, $\alpha IIb\beta 3$
Integrin, $\alpha 4\beta 1$
Integrin, $\alpha 4\beta 7$
Integrin, $\alpha v\beta 5$
Integrin, $\alpha v\beta 3$
Interactions
Interferons
Interleukin-1
Interleukin-2
Intermediate Filaments
Internalization
International Normalized Ratio (INR)
Intracellular Transport
Intrathecal Space
Intrinsic Efficacy
Intron
Inverse Agonist
Inward Rectification
Inward Rectifier K^+ Channels
Inwardly Rectifying K^+ Channel Family
Iodide
Iodine
Ion Channels
Ionic Contrast Media
Ionotropic (channel-linked) Receptors
Ionotropic Glutamate Receptors
IPC
IPSP
IRAG
Irreversible Antagonists
Irritable Bowel Syndrome
Ischemic Preconditioning
Islet Amyolid Peptide
Isoform
Isoprenoid
Ito

JAK-STAT Pathway

K^+ Channels
K^+ Channel Openers
K^+ Homeostasis
K^+-sparing Diuretics
Kainate Receptor
Kallidin
Kallikrein
K_{ATP} Channels
KCNQ-channels
KCOs
K_D
KDEL Receptor
KELL Blood Group Antigen
K_i Values
Kinase
Kinase Domain
Kinetochore
Kinins
Kir Channels
K_{NDP} Channel
Knockout Mice

k_{off}
Korsakoff Psychosis
$Kv\beta$-subunits
Kv-channels
KvLQT1-channels
Kynurenine Pathway

L-Arginine
Lasofoxifene
Lateral Hypothalamic Area
Laxatives
LD_{50}
L-dihydroxyphenylalanine
LDL-receptors
L-DOPA / Levodopa
Lead
Leptin
Lethal Dose
Leucin Zipper
Leukemia
Leukopoiesis
Leukotriene Receptor Antagonists
Leukotrienes
Levodopa
Lewy Bodies
Liddle's Syndrome
Ligand
Ligand-gated Ion Channels
Limbic System
Lipid Modifications
Lipid Phosphate Phosphohydrolases
Lipid Rafts
Lipid-lowering Drugs
Lipopolysaccharide
Lipoprotein
5-lipoxygenase
Lipoxygenases
Lithocholic Acid
L-NAME
Local Anaesthetics
Locus Ceruleus
Long-QT Syndromes
Long-term Depression
Long-term Potentiation
Loop Diuretics
Low-density-lipoprotein (LDL)-cholesterol
Low-dose Oral Contraceptives
LPS
LTD
3',5',3,5-L-tetraiodothyronine
LTP
3',5,3-L-triiodothyronine
L-type Ca^{2+} Channel
Luteinizing Hormone
Lymphangiogenesis
Lymphocytes
Lysophosphatidic Acid
Lysophospholipids

Macrolides
Macrophage
Macula Densa
Major Histocompatibility Complex

Parasympatholytics
Parasympathomimetics
Parathyroid Hormone
Paraventricular Nucleus
Parkin
Parkinson's Disease
PAS Domain
Patch-clamp Method
PCI
PDE
PDGF
PDK1
PDZ Domain
Pellagra
Pemphigus Blistering Disease
Penicillin
Penicillin-binding Protein
Pentasaccharide
Peptide Mass Fingerprinting
Peptide YY
Peptidoglycans
Peptidyl Transferase Center
Percutaneous Coronary Intervention
Periaqueductal Grey
Pericytes
Peripheral Nerve
Peripheral Neuropathy
Peroxisome Proliferator Activated Receptor
Peroxisome Proliferator Chemicals
Pertussis Toxin
PEST Sequences
PGI$_2$
P-glycoprotein
PH Domain
PHHI
Phage
Phagocyte/Phagocytosis
Pharmacodynamics
Pharmacogenetics
Pharmacogenomics
Pharmacokinetics
Pharmocodynamic Tolerance
Pharmocokinetic Tolerance
Phenothiazines
Phenotype
Phenylalkylamines
Phorbol Esters
Phosphatases
Phosphatidic Acid
Phosphatidylinositol 3-kinase
Phosphatidylinositol 4,5-bisphosphate
Phosphatidylinositol Phophate
Phosphatodylinositol
Phosphodiesterases
Phospholipases
Phospholipid
Phospholipid Kinases
Phospholipid Phosphatases
Phosphorylation
Phosphotyrosine-binding (PTB) Domain
Photoaging
Phototransduction

Phthalate Esters
Physical Dependence
PIAS
Picornaviruses
Picrotoxin
PI3-Kinase
PIP
PI Response
Pituitary Adenylyl Cyclase- activating Polypeptide
PKA
PKB/Akt
PKC
PKD2
Placenta Growth Factor
Plasmid
Plasmin
Platelet-activating Factor
Platelet-derived Growth Factor
Platelets
Pleckstrin Homology Domain
Plexins
PMF
Polyamines
Polyenes
Polyethylene Glycol
Polymorphism
POMC
Poor Metabolizer
Population Pharmacokinetics
Positron Emission Tomography
Post-translational Modification
Potentiation
PP
PPAR
PPCs
PR
Pregnane X Receptor
Preintegration Complex
Prenylation
Prepro-opiomelanocortin
Presynaptic Receptors
Primary Aldosteronism
Primary Hemostasis
Prodrug
Progesterone
Progesterone Receptor
Progestins
Programmed Cell Death
Prolactin
Promoter
Proopiomelanocortin
Prostacyclin
Prostaglandins
Prostanoids
Protamine Sulfate
Protease-activated Receptors
Proteases
Proteasome
Protein Folding
Protein Kinase
Protein Kinase A